DATE DUE

YAO & ARTUSIO'S

ANESTHESIOLOGY

PROBLEM-ORIENTED PATIENT MANAGEMENT

Sixth Edition

YAO & ARTUSIO'S

ANESTHESIOLOGY

PROBLEM-ORIENTED PATIENT MANAGEMENT

Sixth Edition

Editor-in-Chief

FUN-SUN F. YAO, MD

Professor, Department of Anesthesiology,
Weill Medical College of Cornell University;
Attending Anesthesiologist,
New York Presbyterian Hospital,
New York

Associate Editors

VINOD MALHOTRA, MD

Professor,
Department of Anesthesiology,
Weill Medical College of Cornell University;
Vice-Chair for Clinical Affairs,
Clinical Director of Operating Rooms,
Department of Anesthesiology,
New York Presbyterian Hospital,
New York

MANUEL L. FONTES, MD

Associate Professor of Anesthesiology
and Critical Care,
Weill Medical College of Cornell University;
Co-Director of Cardiothoracic Intensive Care
Unit,
Associate Attending Anesthesiologist,
Department of Anesthesiology,
New York Presbyterian Hospital,
New York

WITH 77 CONTRIBUTORS

Lippincott Williams & Wilkins
a Wolters Kluwer business

Philadelphia · Baltimore · New York · London
Buenos Aires · Hong Kong · Sydney · Tokyo

Acquisitions Editor: Brian Brown
Managing Editor: Nicole Dernoski
Project Manager: Bridgett Dougherty
Manufacturing Manager: Kathleen Brown
Marketing Manager: Angela Panetta
Director of Creative Services: Doug Smock
Compositor: Laserwords Private Limited, Chennai, India

Library of Congress Cataloging-in-Publication Data
Yao & Artusio's anesthesiology : problem-oriented patient management / editor-in-chief
Fun-Sun F. Yao ; [editors], Manuel L. Fontes, Vinod Malhotra.—6th ed.
   p. ; cm.
   Includes bibliographical references and index.
   ISBN-13: 978-0-7817-6510-7
   ISBN-10: 0-7817-6510-2
   1. Anesthesia—Case studies. 2. Anesthesia—Examinations, questions, etc. 3.
Anesthesiology—Examinations, questions, etc. I. Yao, Fun-Sun F., 1942- II. Fontes,
Manuel L. III. Malhotra, Vinod. IV. Title: Anesthesiology. V. Title: Yao and Artusio's
anesthesiology.
   [DNLM: 1. Anesthesia—Examination Questions. WO 218.2 Y25 2008]
   RD82.45.A54 2008
   617.9′6—dc22

                                                     2007022037

Care has been taken to confirm the accuracy of the information presented and to describe generally accepted practices. However, the authors, editors, and publisher are not responsible for errors or omissions or for any consequences from application of the information in this book and make no warranty, expressed or implied, with respect to the currency, completeness, or accuracy of the contents of the publication. Application of this information in a particular situation remains the professional responsibility of the practitioner.

The authors, editors, and publisher have exerted every effort to ensure that drug selection and dosage set forth in this text are in accordance with current recommendations and practice at the time of publication. However, in view of ongoing research, changes in government regulations, and the constant flow of information relating to drug therapy and drug reactions, the reader is urged to check the package insert for each drug for any change in indications and dosage and for added warnings and precautions. This is particularly important when the recommended agent is a new or infrequently employed drug.

Some drugs and medical devices presented in this publication have Food and Drug Administration (FDA) clearance for limited use in restricted research settings. It is the responsibility of the health care provider to ascertain the FDA status of each drug or device planned for use in their clinical practice.

To purchase additional copies of this book, call our customer service department at (800) 638-3030 or fax orders to (301) 223-2320. International customers should call (301) 223-2300.

Visit Lippincott Williams & Wilkins on the Internet: at LWW.com. Lippincott Williams & Wilkins customer service representatives are available from 8:30 am to 6 pm, EST.

10 9 8 7 6

This book is dedicated
to
Joseph F. Artusio Jr., MD
who
has taught us
not only
to be good anesthesiologists
but also
to become better persons.

CONTENTS

Contributors List   xiii
Preface   xix
Acknowledgments   xxi

SECTION I
The Respiratory System
1

CHAPTER 1   Asthma and Chronic Obstructive Pulmonary Disease   1
                  Fun-Sun F. Yao

CHAPTER 2   Bronchoscopy, Mediastinoscopy, and Thoracotomy   29
                  Alessia Pedoto • Paul M. Heerdt • Fun-Sun F. Yao

CHAPTER 3   Aspiration Pneumonitis and Acute Respiratory Failure   48
                  Manuel L. Fontes • Jeffrey S. Berger • Fun-Sun F. Yao

CHAPTER 4   Lung Transplantation   87
                  Paul M. Heerdt • Charles W. Hogue, Jr.

CHAPTER 5   Tracheoesophageal Fistula   105
                  Jacques H. Scharoun

CHAPTER 6   Congenital Diaphragmatic Hernia   115
                  Fun-Sun F. Yao • David Stein • John J. Savarese

SECTION II
The Cardiovascular System
131

CHAPTER 7   Ischemic Heart Disease and Coronary Artery Bypass Grafting   131
                  Fun-Sun F. Yao • Nikolaos Skubas • Manuel L. Fontes

CHAPTER 8   Valvular Heart Disease   198
                  Gregg S. Hartman • Stephen J. Thomas

CHAPTER 9   Pacemakers and Implantable Cardioverter-Defibrillators   229
                  Alan Cheng • Fun-Sun F. Yao

CHAPTER 10   Thoracoabdominal Aortic Aneurysms   252
Manu Sethi • Charles D. Collard • Manuel L. Fontes

CHAPTER 11   Abdominal Aortic Aneurysm Repair   271
Lori A. Rubin

CHAPTER 12   Hypertension   296
Manuel L. Fontes • Fun-Sun F. Yao

CHAPTER 13   Cardiac Tamponade   322
Manuel L. Fontes • Nikolaos Skubas • James Osorio

CHAPTER 14   Heart Transplantation and Subsequent Noncardiac Surgery   355
Davy C.H. Cheng • Jeff T. Granton

CHAPTER 15   Ischemic Heart Disease and Noncardiac Surgery   372
Marbelia Gonzalez • J. Patricio Escandon • Paul G. Barash

CHAPTER 16   Tetralogy of Fallot   403
James A. DiNardo

CHAPTER 17   Transposition of the Great Arteries   426
James A. DiNardo

CHAPTER 18   Patent Ductus Arteriosus and Prematurity   451
Rajesh Bhat • Isobel Russell • Fun-Sun F. Yao

SECTION III
The Gastrointestinal System
471

CHAPTER 19   Intestinal Obstruction   471
Joseph Tjan

CHAPTER 20   Liver Transplantation   486
Wilton C. Levine • Robert A. Peterfreund • Rae M. Allain

CHAPTER 21   Pyloric Stenosis   514
Vinod Malhotra • Aarti Sharma

SECTION IV
The Nervous System
527

CHAPTER 22   Brain Tumor and Craniotomy   527
Kane O. Pryor • Hugh C. Hemmings, Jr.

CHAPTER 23   Carotid Endarterectomy   548
Maria Bustillo • Cynthia A. Lien

CHAPTER 24   Awake Craniotomy for Deep Brain Stimulation   577
Elizabeth A.M. Frost • J. Lance LaFleur

CHAPTER 25   Management of Head Injury   597
Eugene S. Fu • Jonathan Jagid • Leo T. Harris

CHAPTER 26   Cerebral Aneurysm   617
Patricia Fogarty Mack

SECTION V
Pain Management and Neuraxial Blocks
641

CHAPTER 27   Brachial Plexus Block   641
Joseph Tjan • Vinod Malhotra

CHAPTER 28   Nerve Blocks of the Lower Extremity   655
Jeffrey Y.F. Ngeow • Philip S.L. Chan • David Y. Wang

CHAPTER 29   Complex Regional Pain Syndromes   669
Sudhir A. Diwan • Edward S. Rubin • Vinod Malhotra

CHAPTER 30   Cancer Pain   682
Sudhir A. Diwan • Shakil Ahmed

CHAPTER 31   Low Back Pain and Sciatica   699
David Y. Wang • Jeffrey Y. F. Ngeow

CHAPTER 32   Perioperative Pain Management   720
Narinder Rawal • Vinod Malhotra

CHAPTER 33   Acupuncture   746
Yuan-Chi Lin

SECTION VI
The Endocrine System
753

CHAPTER 34   Thyrotoxicosis   753
Dana L. Gurvitch

CHAPTER 35   Pheochromocytomas   767
                  Gregory E. Kerr • Manuel L. Fontes

CHAPTER 36   Diabetes Mellitus   782
                  Klaus Kjaer • Vinod Malhotra

SECTION VII
The Genitourinary System
797

CHAPTER 37   Transurethral Resection of the Prostate   797
                  Fun-Sun F. Yao • Vinod Malhotra • Vijayendra Sudheendra

CHAPTER 38   Kidney Transplant   822
                  Fun-Sun F. Yao • Panchali Dhar

CHAPTER 39   Laparoscopic Surgery   848
                  Judith Weingram

SECTION VIII
The Reproductive System
881

CHAPTER 40   Peripartum Hemorrhage   881
                  Klaus Kjaer • Eric Cappiello

CHAPTER 41   Hypertensive Disorders of Pregnancy   904
                  Sharon Abramovitz • Barbara Leighton

CHAPTER 42   Transverse Lie, Fetal Distress, and Mitral Stenosis   925
                  Jill Fong

CHAPTER 43   Appendectomy for a Pregnant Patient   948
                  Farida Gadalla

SECTION IX
The Hematologic System
963

CHAPTER 44   Hemophilia and Coagulation Disorders   963
                  Jonathan Leff • Linda Shore-Lesserson • Robert E. Kelly

CHAPTER 45   Sickle Cell Disease   980
                   Chris R. Edmonds • Vinod Malhotra

SECTION X
Eye, Ear, Nose, and Throat
993

CHAPTER 46   Airway Trauma   993
                   Richard P. Dutton

CHAPTER 47   Open-Eye Injury   1007
                   Theresa T. Kudlak

CHAPTER 48   Laser Treatment for Laryngeal Lesions   1025
                   Marcus Gutzler • Matthew C. Gomillion

CHAPTER 49   Airway Obstruction in Childhood: Stridor and Croup Syndromes   1038
                   Miles Dinner

CHAPTER 50   Cleft Palate   1049
                   Aarti Sharma

CHAPTER 51   Congenital Heart Disease with a Cervical Mass in Infancy   1061
                   Miles Dinner

SECTION XI
Miscellaneous
1075

CHAPTER 52   Myasthenia Gravis   1075
                   Cephas P. Swamidoss • Cynthia A. Lien

CHAPTER 53   Malignant Hyperthermia   1091
                   Henry Rosenberg • Vinod Malhotra • Dana Lynn Gurvitch

CHAPTER 54   Prolonged Postoperative Apnea   1105
                   Peter Savard • Matthew R. Belmont

CHAPTER 55   Burns   1113
                   Michael Tjeuw

CHAPTER 56   Trauma   1134
                   Ralph L. Slepian • Jaideep K. Malhotra

CHAPTER 57   Scoliosis   1155
Victor M. Zayas

CHAPTER 58   Hypoxia and Equipment Failure   1179
James B. Eisenkraft • Andrew B. Leibowitz

CHAPTER 59   Electroconvulsive Therapy   1201
Patricia Fogarty Mack

CHAPTER 60   Ambulatory Surgery   1209
Kathryn E. McGoldrick • Matthew C. Gomillion

CHAPTER 61   Magnetic Resonance Imaging   1231
Matthew C. Gomillion • Jung Hee Han

CHAPTER 62   Morbid Obesity and Obstructive Sleep Apnea   1249
Jon D. Samuels • Fun-Sun F. Yao

Index   **1285**

CONTRIBUTORS LIST

Sharon Abramovitz, MD
Associate Attending Physician, Department of
Anesthesiology, New York Presbyterian
Hospital, New York

**Shakil Ahmed, MD, MB, BS, FRCS (RCS
Glasgow)**
Assistant Professor of Anesthesiology,
Department of Anesthesiology, Weill Medical
College of Cornell University;
Attending Anesthesiologist, Department of
Anesthesiology, New York Presbyterian
Hospital, New York

Rae M. Allain, MD
Instructor in Anesthesia, Department of
Anesthesia and Critical Care, Harvard
University;
Assistant in Anesthesia, Department of
Anesthesia and Critical Care, Massachusetts
General Hospital, Boston, Massachusetts

Paul Barash, MD
Professor, Department of Anesthesiology, Yale
University School of Medicine;
Attending Anesthesiologist, Yale-New Haven
Hospital, New Haven, Connecticut.

Matthew R. Belmont, MD
Associate Professor of Anesthesiology,
Department of Anesthesiology, Weill Medical
College of Cornell University;
Associate Attending Anesthesiologist,
Department of Anesthesiology, New York
Presbyterian Hospital, New York

Jeffery S. Berger, MD
Assistant Professor of Anesthesiology, New York
University Medical School;
Attending Anesthesiologist, New York University
Hospital, New York

Rajesh Bhat, MB, BS
Assistant Professor, Department of
Anesthesiology, University of California, San
Francisco, School of Medicine;
Attending Anesthesiologist, Moffit Hospital, San
Francisco, California

Eric Cappiello, MD
Instructor in Aneasthesia, Harvard Medical
School, Brighan and Women's Hospital,
Boston, Massachusetts

Alan Cheng, MD
Assistant Professor of Medicine, Department of
Medicine, Division of Cardiovascular Diseases,
Johns Hopkins School of Medicine;
Cardiac Electrophysiologist, Department of
Medicine, Division of Cardiovascular Diseases,
Johns Hopkins Hospital, Baltimore,
Maryland

Philip S.L. Chan, MD
Fellow of Pain Medicine, Weill Medical College
of Cornell University;
New York Presbyterian Hospital, New York

Davy C. H Cheng, MD, MSc, FRCPC
Professor and Chair, Department(s) of
Anesthesia and Preoperative Medicine, The
University of Western Ontario;
Department(s) of Anesthesia and Preoperative
Medicine, London Health Sciences Center,
London

Charles D. Collard, MD
Division of Cardiovascular Anesthesia, Texas
Heart Institute;
Associate Professor, Division of Cardiovascular
Anesthesia, Baylor College of Medicine at the
Texas Heart Institute, St. Luke's Episcopal
Hospital, Houston, Texas

Panchali Dhar, MD
Assistant Professor of Clinical Anesthesiology,
    Weill Medical College of Cornell University;
Assistant Attending Anesthesiologist, New York
    Presbyterian Hospital, New York

James A. DiNardo, MD
Associate Professor of Anaesthesia, Department
    of Anesthesia, Children's Hospital Boston,
    Harvard Medical School;
Senior Associate in Cardiac Anesthesia, Cardiac
    Anesthesia Fellowship Director, Children's
    Hospital Boston, Boston, Massachusetts

Miles Dinner, MD
Professor of Clinical Anesthesiology, Cornell
    University Medical College, New York
    Presbyterian Hospital, New York

Sudhir Diwan, MD, MS
Director, Division of Pain Medicine, New York
    Presbyterian Hospital;
Associate Professor of Clinical Anesthesiology,
    Department of Anesthesiology, Weill Medical
    College of Cornell University, New York

Richard P. Dutton, MD, MBA
Associate Professor, Department of
    Anesthesiology, University of Maryland School
    of Medicine;
Director of Trauma Anesthesiology, R Adams
    Cowley Shock Trauma Center, University of
    Maryland Medical System, Baltimore

Chris Edmonds, MD
Clinical Assistant Professor of Anesthesiology,
    Weill Medical College of Cornell University;
Assistant Attending Anesthesiologist, Hospital
    for Special Surgery, New York

James B. Eisenkraft, MD
Professor, Department of Anesthesiology, Mount
    Sinai School of Medicine of New York
    University;
Attending Anesthesiologist, Department of
    Anesthesiology, The Mount Sinai Medical
    Center, New York

Jill Fong, MD
Associate Professor of Clinical Anesthesiology,
    Department of Anesthesiology, Weill Medical
    College of Cornell University, New York

Patricio Escandon, MD
Associate Professor, Department of
    Anesthesiology, Yale University;
Staff Anesthesiologist, Department of
    Anesthesia, Yale-New Haven Hospital,
    New Haven, Connecticut

Manuel L. Fontes, MD
Associate Professor of Anesthesiology and
    Critical Care, Department of Anesthesiology,
    Weill Medical College of Cornell University;
Co-Director Cardiothoracic Intensive Care Unit,
    Department of Anesthesiology, New York
    Presbyterian Hospital, New York

Elizabeth A.M. Frost, MD
Professor, Dept of Anesthesiology, Mount Sinai
    Medical Center;
Attending professor, Dept of Anesthesiology,
    Mount Sinai Medical Center, New York

Eugene S. Fu, MD
Associate Professor, Department of
    Anesthesiology, University of Miami;
Chief of Neuroanesthesia, Department of
    Anesthesiology, Jackson Memorial Hospital,
    Miami, Florida

Farida Gadalla, MD
Professor of Clinical Anesthesiology,
    Department of Anesthesiology, Weill Cornell
    Medical College, New York Presbyterian
    Hospital, New York

Matthew C. Gomillion, MD
Associate Professor of Clinical Anesthesiology,
    Weill Medical College of Cornell University,
    New York

Marbelia Gonzalez, MD
Staff Anesthesiologist, Department of
    Anesthesia, Hartford Hospital,
    Hartford, Connecticut

Jeff T. Granton, MD, FRCPC
Assistant Professor, Anesthesia and
    Perioperative Medicine, University of Western
    Ontario;
Cardiac Anesthesiologist and Intensivist,
    Anesthesia and Perioperative Medicine,
    London Health Sciences Centre, London,
    Ontario, Canada

Dana L. Gurvitch, MD
Assistant Professor, Department of Anesthesia,
Weill Medical College of Cornell University;
Department of Anesthesia, New York
Presbyterian Hospital, New York

Marcus Gutzler, MD
Instructor in Anesthesiology, Department of
Anesthesiology, Weill Medical College of
Cornell University;
Assistant Attending Anesthesiologist,
Department of Anesthesiology, New York
Presbyterian Hospital, New York

Jung Hee Han, MD
Clinical Instructor, Department of
Anesthesiology, Weill Medical College of
Cornell University;
Assistant Attending, Department of
Anesthesiology, New York Presbyterian
Hospital, New York

Leo T. Harris, MPH
Physician Assistant, Department of
Neurosurgery, University of Miami;
Physician Assistant, Department of
Neurosurgery, Jackson Memorial Hospital,
Miami, Florida

Gregg S. Hartman, MD
Professor, Department of Anesthesiology,
Dartmouth-Hitchcock Medical Center,
Lebanon

Paul M. Heerdt, MD, PhD
Professor, Department of Anesthesiology and
Pharmacology, Weill Medical College of
Cornell University, New York

Hugh C. Hemmings Jr., MD, PhD
Professor and Vice Chair of Research,
Department of Anesthesiology and
Pharmacology, Weill Medical College of
Cornell University,
New York

Charles W. Hogue, Jr., MD
Associate Professor of Anesthesiology, Johns
Hopkins School of Medicine;
Attending Anesthesiologist, Johns Hopkins
Hospital, Baltimore,
Maryland

Jagid Jonathan R., MD
Assistant Professor of Neurological Surgery,
Department of Neurosurgery,
University of Miami;
Assistant Professor of Neurological Surgery,
Department of Neurosurgery, Jackson
Memorial Hospital, Miami, Florida

Robert E. Kelly, MD
Professor Clinical Anesthesiology, Department
of Anesthesiology, Weill Medical College of
Cornell University;
Attending Anesthesiologist, Department
Anesthesiology, New York Presbyterian
Hospital, New York

Gregory E. Kerr, MD
Associate Professor of Anesthesiology, Weill
Medical College of Cornell University;
Associate Attending Anesthesiologist, Director,
Cardiac Anesthesia, New York Presbyterian
Hospital, New York

Klaus Kjaer-Pedersen, MD
Assistant Professor of Anesthesiology,
Department of Anesthesiology, Weill Medical
College of Cornell University;
Attending Anesthesiologist, Department of
Anesthesiology, New York Presbyterian
Hospital, New York

Theresa T. Kudlak, MD
Attending Anesthesiologist, Maine Medical
Center, Portland, Maine Clinical Associate
Professor, University of Vermont College of
Medicine, Burlington, Vermont

J. Lance LaFleur, MD, MBA
Department of Anesthesiology, University of
Texas Medical School at Houston,
Houston, Texas

Jonathan Leff, MD
Assistant Professor of Anesthesiology, Mount
Sinai Medical College, Montefoire Medical
Center, Bronx, New York

Wilton C. Levine, MD
Instructor of Anesthesiology, Harvard Medical
School;
Massachusetts General Hospital, Department of
Anesthesia and Critical Care,
Boston, Massachusetts

Andrew B. Leibowitz, MD
Associate Professor, Department of
    Anesthesiology and Surgery, Mount Sinai
    School of Medicine of New York University;
Executive Vice Chair, Department of
    Anesthesiology, Mount Sinai Hospital,
    New York

Barbara Leighton, MD
Professor of Anesthesiology, Professor of
    Obstetrics and Gynecology, Washington
    University School of Medicine in St. Louis;
Attending Anesthesiologist, Chief, Division of
    Obstetric Anesthesia, Barnes Jewish Hospital,
    St. Louis, Missouri

Cynthia A. Lien, MD
Professor of Anesthesiology, Department of
    Anesthesiology, Weill Medical College of
    Cornell University

Yuan-Chi Lin, MD, MPH
Associate Professor of Anaesthesia and
    Pediatrics, Department of Anaesthesia,
    Harvard Medical School;
Director, Medical Acupuncture Service,
    Department of Anesthesiology, Perioperative
    and Pain Medicine, Children's Hospital
    Boston, Boston, Massachusetts

Jaideep K. Malhotra, MD
Assistant Professor of Clinic Anesthesiology,
    Weill Medical College of Cornell University;
Assistant Attending Anesthesiologist, New York
    Presbyterian Hospital, New York

Vinod Malhotra, MD
Professor, Department of Anesthesiology, Weill
    Medical College of Cornell University;
Vice-Chair for Clinical Affairs, Clinical Director
    of Operating Rooms, Department of
    Anesthesiology, New York Presbyterian
    Hospital, New York

Kathryn E. McGoldrick, MD
Professor and Chair, Department of
    Anesthesiology, New York Medical
    College;
Director, Department of Anesthesiology,
    Westchester Medical Center, Valhalla,
    New York

Jeffrey Y. Ngeow, MBBS
Clinical Associate Professor, Department of
    Anesthesiology, Weill Medical College of
    Cornell University;
Attending Anesthesiologist, Department of
    Anesthesiology, Hospital for Special Surgery,
    New York

James Albert Osorio, MD
Assistant Professor, Anesthesiology and Critical
    Care, Department of Anesthesiology, Weill
    Medical College of Cornell University;
Assistant Attending Anesthesiologist,
    Anesthesiology and Critical Care, Department
    of Anesthesiology, New York Presbyterian
    Hospital, New York

Alessia C. Pedoto, MD
Assistant Member, Level I, Memorial
    Sloane-Kettering Cancer Center;
Assistant Attending Anesthesiologist,
    Anesthesiology and Critical Care Medicine,
    Memorial Hospital for Cancer and Allied
    Diseases, New York

Robert A. Peterfreund, MD, PhD
Associate Professor of Anesthesia, Department
    of Anesthesia, Harvard Medical School;
Anesthetist, Department of Anesthesia and
    Critical Care, Massachusetts General Hospital,
    Boston, Massachusetts

Kane O. Pryor, MD
Assistant Professor, Department of
    Anesthesiology, Weill Medical College of
    Cornell University;
Assistant Attending Anesthesiologist,
    Department of Anesthesiology, New York
    Presbyterian Hospital, New York

Narinder Rawal, MD, PhD
Professor, Dept of Anesthesiology and Intensive
    Care, Örebro University Hospital,
    Grev Rosengatan, Sweden

Henry Rosenberg, MD
Professor, Department of Anesthesiology, Mount
    Sinai School of Medicine, New York;
Director, Department of Medical Education and
    Clinical Research, Saint Barnabas Medical
    Center, Livingston, New Jersey

Lori A. Rubin, MD
Assistant Professor of Anesthesiology, New York
  Presbyterian Hospital, Weill Medical College
  of Cornell University,
  New York

Isobel Russell, MD, PhD, FACC
Professor, Department of Anesthesia, University
  of California, San Francisco;
Chief of Cardiac Anesthesia, University of
  California, San Francisco Medical Center,
  San Francisco, California

Jon D. Samuels, MD
Assistant Professor, Department of
  Anesthesiology, Weill Medical College of
  Cornell University;
Attending Anesthesiologist, Department of
  Anesthesiology, New York Presbyterian
  Hospital, New York

John J. Savarese, MD
Professor and Chair, Department of
  Anesthesiology, Weill Medical College of
  Cornell University;
Anesthesiologist-in-Chief, New York
  Presbyterian Hospital,
  New York

Jacques H. Scharoun, MD
Assistant Professor, Department of
  Anesthesiology, Weill Medical College of
  Cornell University;
Attending Professor, Department of
  Anesthesiology, New York Presbyterian
  Hospital, New York

Manu Sethi, MD
Division of Cardiovascular Anesthesia, Texas
  Heart Institute;
Assistant Professor, Division of Cardiovascular
  Anesthesia, Baylor College of Medicine at the
  Texas Heart Institute, St. Luke's Episcopal
  Hospital, Houston, Texas

Aarti Sharma, MD
Assistant Professor, Department of Anesthesia,
  Weill Medical College of Cornell University;
Assistant Attending, Department of Anesthesia,
  New York Presbyterian Hospital,
  New York

Linda Shore-Lesserson, MD
Associate Professor of Anesthesiology, Mount
  Sinai Medical College;
Chief, Division of Cardiothoracic Anesthesiology,
  Montefoire Medical Center, Bronx, New York

Vijayendra Sudheendra, MD
Clinical Assistant Professor, Department of
  Surgery and Anesthesiology, Brown University
  School of Medicine, Providence,
  Rhode Island;
Director of Cardiothoracic Anesthesia, Miriam
  Hospital, Providence, Rhode Island;
Medical Director, Southern New England
  Surgicenter, Attleboro, Massachusetts

Nikolaos Skubas, MD
Assistant Professor, Department of
  Anesthesiology, Weill Medical College of
  Cornell University;
Director, Perioperative Echocardiography,
  Department of Anesthesiology, New York
  Hospital, New York

Ralph L. Slepian, MD
Associate Professor of Clinical Anesthesiology,
  Weill Medical College of Cornell University;
Associate Attending Anesthesiologist, New York
  Presbyterian Hospital, New York

David G. Stein, MD
Assistant Professor of Anesthesiology,
  Department of Anesthesiology, Weill Medical
  College of Cornell University;
Attending Anesthesiologist, Department of
  Anesthesiology, New York Presbyterian
  Hospital, New York

Cephas P. Swamidoss, MD, MS, MPH
Associate Professor of Clinical Anesthesia,
  Department of Anesthesiology, Weill Medical
  College of Cornell University;
Associate Attending Anesthesiologist,
  Department of Anesthesiology, New York
  Presbyterian Hospital, New York

Stephen J. Thomas, MD
Topkins Van Poznak Professor, Department of
  Anesthesiology, Weill Medical College of
  Cornell University;
Vice Chair, Department of Anesthesiology,
  New York Presbyterian Hospital, New York

Joseph Tjan, MD
Assistant Professor, Department of
    Anesthesiology, Weill Medical College of
    Cornell University, New York

Michael Tjeuw, MD
Senior Consultant, Department of Anesthesia,
    Westmead Hospital, University of Sydney,
    Sydney, NSW, Australia;
Honorary Professor of Anesthesiology, Burn
    center, South West hospital, The Third
    Military Medical University,
    Chongqing, China

David Wang, MD
Clinical Assistant Professor, Department of
    Anesthesiology, Weill Medical College of
    Cornell University;
Attending Physician, Department of
    Anesthesiology, Hospital for Special Surgery,
    New York

Judith Weingram, MD
Assistant Professor, Department of
    Anesthesiology, Weill Medical College of
    Cornell University;
Attending Anesthesiologist, Department of
    Anesthesiology, New York Presbyterian
    Hospital, New York

Fun-Sun F. Yao, MD
Professor, Department of Anesthesiology, Weill
    Medical College of Cornell University;
Attending Anesthesiologist, New York
    Presbyterian Hospital, New York

Victor M. Zayas, MD
Clinical Assistant Professor of Anesthesiology
    and Pediatrics, Department of Anesthesiology
    and Pediatrics, Weill Medical College of
    Cornell University;
Director, Pediatric Anesthesiology, Department
    of Anesthesiology, Hospital for Special
    Surgery, New York

PREFACE

Important advances in surgical procedures and clinical practice of anesthesiology have prompted the production of a new edition of this text. The book has been published in four languages: English, German, Japanese, and Chinese. The remarkable popularity of the first five editions in the anesthesiology community both in the United States and abroad, encouraged us to update and expand its subject matter. The sixth edition is written to further improve anesthesia management for sophisticated surgery.

As with our previous editions, *Yao & Artusio's Anesthesiology: Problem-Oriented Patient Management* was written to present a group of important clinical entities covering the most critical anesthetic problems. It is intended to provide logical and scientific fundamentals for individualized patient management.

In this sixth edition, *Yao & Artusio's Anesthesiology* is organized by organ systems into eleven sections consisting of 62 chapters. Each chapter begins with a brief case presentation, followed by essential problems of each disease covering four areas: (a) medical disease and differential diagnosis, (b) preoperative evaluation and preparation, (c) intraoperative management, and (d) postoperative anesthetic management. The book is designed to stress anesthetic problems and to give the anesthesiologist the opportunity to organize his or her own ideas of patient care. A reasonable answer, with updated references, follows each question.

To maintain the fresh quality of the textbook, approximately one third of the sixth edition consists of new chapters or contributions by new authors. We have added 3 new chapters: acupuncture, perioperative pain management and electroconvulsive therapy.

The text originally reflected the clinical experience of the Department of Anesthesiology at Weill Medical College of Cornell University, The New York Presbyterian Hospital. In this edition, experts from other prestigious institutions have contributed their invaluable opinions to make this book more universally acceptable. The material in the book is prepared for the education of the resident and the practicing anesthesiologist; It also serves as a review source for the continuing education of the anesthesiologist. The question-and-answer format, combined with current references, enhances its educational value.

ACKNOWLEDGMENTS

I wish to express my personal gratitude to the individual contributors. I am grateful to the associate editors: Vinod Malhotra, MD and Manuel L. Fontes, MD. This book would not have been possible without their hard work and dedication. I would also like to thank Marlene Augustine for her help with typing. In addition, I am especially indebted to John J. Savarese, MD for his constructive advice and support. Above all, my deepest appreciation goes to my family, Tong-Yi, Ning-Yen, Jean-Kuan and especially to my dear compassionate wife Baw-Chyr Peggy Yao. Her understanding, patience, and encouragement made this book possible.

Editor-in-Chief
Fun-Sun F. Yao, MD

The Respiratory System

CHAPTER 1

Asthma and Chronic Obstructive Pulmonary Disease

FUN-SUN F. YAO

A 55-YEAR-OLD MAN

with cholelithiasis was scheduled for cholecystectomy. He had a long history of asthma and developed dyspnea with only moderate exertion. He slept on two pillows. There was no peripheral edema. Arterial blood gases showed the following: pH 7.36; P_{CO_2}, 60 mm Hg; P_{O_2}, 70 mm Hg; CO_2 content, 36 mEq per L.

A. Medical Disease and Differential Diagnosis

1. What differential diagnosis is compatible with these symptoms?
2. What is the prevalence of asthma?
3. What is the etiology of asthma?
4. Discuss the pathogenesis of asthma.
5. What are the predisposing factors of asthmatic attacks?
6. What is the universal finding in arterial blood gases during asthmatic attacks: hypoxemia or CO_2 retention?
7. What changes are seen in spirometry, lung volumes, and lung capacities during an asthmatic attack?

B. Preoperative Evaluation and Preparation

1. What preoperative workup would you order?
2. How would you distinguish obstructive lung disease from restrictive lung disease by spirometry?

3. Define normal lung volumes and lung capacities and their normal values in the average adult male.

4. What are flow–volume loops? Draw flow–volume loops in a healthy subject, in a patient with chronic obstructive pulmonary disease (COPD), and in a patient with restrictive lung disease.

5. Define closing capacity (CC) and closing volume (CV). What is the normal value of CV?

6. What are the effects of age and posture on functional residual capacity (FRC) and CC?

7. What are the effects of anesthesia on FRC and CC?

8. Why is the FRC important in oxygenation?

9. Are there methods to measure FRC and CV?

10. Give the equations for shunt (Qs/Qt) and dead space/tidal volume (VD/VT). What are their normal values?

11. Interpret the following arterial blood gases: pH, 7.36; P_{CO_2}, 60 mm Hg; P_{O_2}, 70 mm Hg; CO_2 content, 36 mEq per L.

12. What are the common physiologic causes of hypoxemia?

13. Would you order any special preoperative preparations for asthmatic patients with COPD?

14. How long would you postpone elective surgery if the patient had a recent upper respiratory infection (URI)?

15. What medicines would you expect the patient to have taken in the past or be taking at the present time?

16. Would you order preoperative steroid preparation? Why?

17. What is the onset of action of intravenous steroid therapy in asthma?

18. What are the effects of cimetidine on asthmatic patients?

19. How would you premedicate the patient? Why?

C. **Intraoperative Management**

1. What are the disadvantages of administering atropine to the asthmatic patient?

2. If the patient had a severe asthmatic attack in the operating room before the induction of anesthesia, would you put the patient to sleep or postpone the surgery?

3. The patient did not have an asthmatic attack in the operating room. How would you induce anesthesia? Would you use a laryngeal mask airway (LMA) instead of an endotracheal tube?

4. Why would you use methohexital instead of thiopental?

5. Would you use propofol, etomidate, or ketamine for induction?

6. Would you use lidocaine for intubation?

7. If this is emergency surgery and rapid sequence induction is indicated, how would you induce anesthesia in this patient?

8. What is your choice of agents for maintenance of anesthesia? Why?

9. What are the mechanisms of halothane that produce bronchodilation?

10. Why would you choose an inhalational instead of an intravenous technique?

11. Is regional anesthesia better than general anesthesia in this situation?

12. Which muscle relaxants would you use? Why?

13. In the middle of surgery, the patient developed a severe wheezing attack. How do you manage it?

14. How would you give β_2-agonists? What problems may arise when isoproterenol is given during halothane anesthesia? What is its mechanism of action on asthma?

15. Would you administer aminophylline? How does aminophylline relieve bronchospasm? What is the mechanism of action? What are the therapeutic blood levels of aminophylline? What are the toxic effects of aminophylline?

16. If the patient does not respond to the aforementioned treatment and becomes cyanotic, what would you do?

17. What are the differential diagnoses of intraoperative bronchospasm?

18. The asthmatic attack was finally relieved and the surgery was completed. The patient was found to be hypoventilating. What are the common causes of hypoventilation? Would you like to reverse the muscle relaxant?

D. Postoperative Management

1. Would you extubate the asthmatic patient while he or she was deeply anesthetized?

2. When the patient cannot be extubated early in the recovery room, how would you keep the endotracheal tube in place without causing bronchoconstriction?

3. In asthmatic patients, are narcotics contraindicated for postoperative pain control?

4. The patient was breathing well and was extubated. How much oxygen would you give to this asthmatic patient with COPD in the recovery room?

A. Medical Disease and Differential Diagnosis

A.1. What differential diagnosis is compatible with these symptoms?

The differential diagnosis of wheezing and dyspnea includes bronchial asthma, acute left ventricular failure (cardiac asthma), upper airway obstruction by tumor or laryngeal edema, endobronchial disease such as foreign body aspiration, neoplasms, bronchial stenosis, carcinoid tumors, recurrent pulmonary emboli, chronic bronchitis, eosinophilic pneumonias, chemical pneumonias, and occasionally polyarteritis. To differentiate asthma from other diseases with wheezing and dyspnea is usually not difficult. The triad of dyspnea, coughing, and wheezing, in addition to a history of periodic attacks, is quite characteristic. A personal or family history of allergic diseases is valuable contributory evidence. A patient with long-standing asthma may develop chronic obstructive lung disease and suffer from exertional dyspnea and orthopnea. Cardiac asthma is a misnomer and refers to acute left ventricular failure. Although the primary lesion is cardiac, the disease manifests itself in the lungs. The symptoms and signs may mimic bronchial asthma, but the findings of moist basilar rales, gallop rhythms, blood-tinged sputum, peripheral edema, and a history of heart disease allow the appropriate diagnosis to be reached.

Gould BE. *Pathophysiology for the health professions*, 3rd ed. Philadelphia: Saunders Elsevier, 2006:393–398.

Kasper DL, Braunwald E, Fauci AS, et al. eds. *Harrison's principles of internal medicine*, 16th ed. New York: McGraw-Hill, 2005:1508–1516.

A.2. What is the prevalence of asthma?

Approximately 4% to 5% of adults and 7% to 10% of children in the United States and Australia have asthma. It occurs at all ages but is predominant in early life. Approximately half the number of the patients develop asthma before age 10 and another one third of them before age 40. In childhood, there is a 2:1 male/female preponderance, which equalizes by age 30.

Kasper DL, Braunwald E, Fauci AS, et al. eds. *Harrison's principles of internal medicine*, 16th ed. New York: McGraw-Hill, 2005:1508–1516.

Stoelting RK, Dierdorf SF. *Anesthesia and co-existing disease*, 4th ed. New York: Churchill Livingstone, 2002:194.

A.3. What is the etiology of asthma?

Asthma is a heterogeneous disease, the etiology of which is difficult to define. The common denominator that underlies the asthmatic diathesis is a nonspecific hyperirritability of the tracheobronchial tree. Clinically, asthma is classified into two groups: allergic (extrinsic) and idiosyncratic (intrinsic). Allergic asthma is usually associated with a personal or a family history of allergic diseases, positive skin reactions to extracts of airborne antigens, and increased levels of immunoglobulin E (IgE) in the serum. Immunologic mechanisms appear to be causally related to 25% to 35% of all cases and contributory in another one third of them. Idiosyncratic asthma cannot be classified on the basis of immunologic mechanisms, and it is probably due to abnormality of the parasympathetic nervous system. Bronchospasm is provoked when certain agents stimulate tracheobronchial receptors. Intraoperative bronchospasm is probably usually cholinergically mediated. Afferent receptors in the bronchial mucosa can be an initiating event although such an event is not always identifiable. Efferent parasympathetic fibers travel to bronchial smooth muscle and can then result in bronchoconstriction by stimulation of the M3 cholinergic receptors on bronchial smooth muscle. Following release of acetylcholine (Ach) at the M3 receptor, the Ach will stimulate the M2 muscarinic receptor, which is an inhibitory receptor that limits further release of Ach. Alterations of M2 receptor function may contribute to bronchospasm.

Brusse WW, Lemanske RF. Asthma. *N Engl J Med* 2001;344:350–362.

Kasper DL, Braunwald E, Fauci AS, et al. eds. *Harrison's principles of internal medicine*, 16th ed. New York: McGraw-Hill, 2005:1508–1516.

A.4. Discuss the pathogenesis of asthma.

Asthma is a chronic disease characterized by chronic airway inflammation, reversible expiratory airflow obstruction resulting from narrowing of the airways in response to various stimuli, and airway hyperreactivity. The common denominator underlying the asthmatic diathesis is a nonspecific hyperirritability of the tracheobronchial tree. The basic mechanism of the persistent subacute airway hyperirritability remains unknown. The most popular hypothesis is that of subacute airway inflammation. Even when asthmatics are in remission, bronchial biopsy reveals infiltration by inflammatory cells and epithelial shedding from the mucosa. After exposure to an initiating stimulus, mast cells, eosinophils, lymphocytes, epithelial cells, and macrophages can be activated to release various mediators that lead to contraction of airway smooth muscle (bronchospasm), vascular congestion, increased capillary permeability (edema of bronchial mucosa), and thick tenacious secretions, thereby evoking an intense inflammatory reaction (Fig. 1.1). The net result is a reduction in airway diameter, an increase in airway resistance, decreased forced expiratory volumes and flow rates, hyperinflation of the lungs and thorax, increased work of breathing, alterations in respiratory tract muscle function, mismatched ventilation/perfusion, and altered blood gases.

Brusse WW, Lemanske RF. Asthma. *N Engl J Med* 2001;344:350–362.

Djukanvic R, Roche WR, Wilson JW, et al. State of the art: mucosal inflammation in asthma. *Am Rev Respir Dis* 1990;142:434–457.

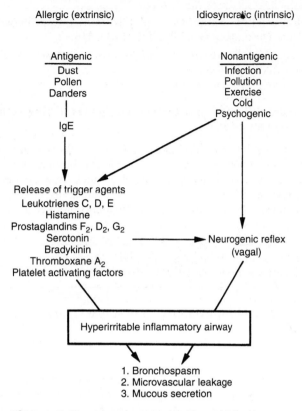

Figure 1.1 The pathogenesis of bronchial asthma.
IgE, immunoglobulin E.

Kasper DL, Braunwald E, Fauci AS, et al. eds. *Harrison's principles of internal medicine,*
16th ed. New York: McGraw-Hill, 2005:1515–1516.

A.5. What are the predisposing factors of asthmatic attacks?

- *Allergens.* Airborne allergens are the most common.
- *Pharmacologic stimuli.* The drugs most commonly associated with the induction of acute asthmatic attacks are aspirin, coloring agents such as tartrazine, β-adrenergic antagonists, and sulfiting agents. Aspirin and other nonsteroidal anti-inflammatory drugs (NSAIDs) such as indomethacin, mefenamic acid, ibuprofen, fenoprofen, flufenamic acid, naproxen, and phenylbutazone make the asthma worse because of inhibition of prostaglandin G/H synthase 1 (cyclooxygenase type 1).
- *Environment and air pollution.* Some types of asthma, such as Tokyo-Yokohama or New Orleans asthma, tend to occur in individuals who live in heavy industrial or dense urban areas.
- *Occupational factors.* Various compounds used in industry can cause asthma in susceptible individuals. Various names have been applied to this condition, such as meat wrapper's asthma, baker's asthma, and woodworker's asthma.
- *Infections.* Respiratory tract infections are among the most common stimuli that evoke acute asthmatic attacks.
- *Exercise.* Asthma can be induced or made worse by physical exertion.
- Emotional stress is also a factor.

Kasper DL, Braunwald E, Fauci AS, et al. eds. *Harrison's principles of internal medicine*, 16th ed. New York: McGraw-Hill, 2005:1515–1516.

Stoelting RK, Dierdorf SF. *Anesthesia and co-existing disease*, 4th ed. New York: Churchill Livingstone, 2002:196–198.

A.6. What is the universal finding in arterial blood gases during asthmatic attacks: Hypoxemia or CO_2 retention?

Hypoxemia is a universal finding during asthmatic attacks. However, frank ventilatory failure with CO_2 retention is relatively uncommon because CO_2 has a diffusion capacity that is 20 times higher than that of oxygen. During acute asthmatic attacks, most patients try to overcome airway obstruction and hypoxia by hyperventilation. This results in hypocarbia and respiratory alkalosis. CO_2 retention is a late finding and indicates severe and prolonged airway obstruction, as in status asthmaticus.

Kasper DL, Braunwald E, Fauci AS, et al. eds. *Harrison's principles of internal medicine*, 16th ed. New York: McGraw-Hill, 2005:1515–1516.

A.7. What changes are seen in spirometry, lung volumes, and lung capacities during an asthmatic attack?

The forced vital capacity (FVC) is usually normal but may be decreased during a severe attack. The forced expiratory volume at 1 second (FEV_1) is sharply reduced, usually to less than 50% of the FVC, typically less than 40% of that predicted. The maximum midexpiratory flow rate (MMEFR) and maximum breathing capacity (MBC) are sharply reduced as well. Residual volume (RV) is markedly increased, frequently approaching 400% of normal, and expiratory reserve volume (ERV) is moderately decreased. Therefore, FRC and total lung capacity (TLC) are increased. FRC frequently doubles.

Gold MI, Han YH, Helrich M. Pulmonary mechanics and blood gas tensions during anesthesia in asthmatics. *Anesthesiology* 1966;27:216.

Kasper DL, Braunwald E, Fauci AS, et al. eds. *Harrison's principles of internal medicine*, 16th ed. New York: McGraw-Hill, 2005:1515–1516.

Kingston HGG, Hirshman CA. Perioperative management of the patient with asthma. *Anesth Analg* 1984;63:844.

B. Preoperative Evaluation and Preparation

B.1. What preoperative workup would you order?

The goal of preoperative evaluation is to formulate an anesthesia plan that prevents or blunts obstruction to expiratory airflow. In addition to routine tests such as complete blood cell count; serum electrolytes; urinalysis; electrocardiogram; and coagulation screening; special attention should be paid to cardiopulmonary function; chest x-ray film; pulmonary function test results, including response to bronchodilator; and baseline arterial blood gases. A history of allergy and symptoms and signs of cardiac or respiratory failure must be checked carefully.

Stoelting RK, Dierdorf SF. *Anesthesia and co-existing disease*, 4th ed. New York: Churchill Livingstone, 2002:200.

B.2. How would you distinguish obstructive lung disease from restrictive lung disease by spirometry?

Table 1.1 summarizes the distinctions between the two types of lung diseases. In restrictive lung disease (e.g., pulmonary fibrosis and ankylosing spondylitis), the FVC is low because of limited expansion of the lungs or chest wall. However, the FEV_1 is often not reduced proportionately, because airway resistance is normal. Therefore, the FEV_1/FVC percentage is normal or high.

In obstructive lung disease (e.g., emphysema), the FEV_1/FVC is grossly reduced because the airway resistance is high. MBC and MMEFR are reduced early in small airway obstruction. MMEFR is also called $FEF_{25\%-75\%}$ (forced expiratory flow). MMEFR is obtained by dividing the volume between 75% and 25% of the vital capacity (VC) by the corresponding elapsed time. Unlike FEV_1, MMEFR is independent of patient effort.

Normally, FEV_1 is more than 80% of FVC and VC should be more than 80% of predicted value. The predicted values depend on body size, age, and sex. The TLC is increased in obstructive lung disease and decreased in restrictive lung disease. However, TLC cannot be obtained by routine screening spirometry. Normal MBC is more than 125 L per minute and normal MMEFR is more than 300 L per minute.

Barash PG, Cullen BF, Stoelting RK, eds. *Clinical anesthesia*, 5th ed. Philadelphia: Lippincott Williams & Wilkins, 2006:807.

Crapo RO. Pulmonary function testing. *N Engl J Med* 1994;331:25–30.

Kasper DL, Braunwald E, Fauci AS, et al. eds. *Harrison's principles of internal medicine*, 16th ed. New York: McGraw-Hill, 2005:1499–1500.

B.3. Define normal lung volumes and lung capacities and their normal values in the average adult male.

There are four basic "volumes" and four derived "capacities" that are combinations of these volumes (Fig. 1.2).

Tidal volume (VT) is the volume of air inhaled or exhaled during normal breathing. Normal VT is 500 mL or approximately 6 to 8 mL per kg.

Inspiratory reserve volume (IRV) is the maximum volume of gas that can be inhaled after a normal inspiration while at rest. Normal IRV is 2,000 to 3,000 mL.

Table 1.1 Differences between Obstructive and Restrictive Lung Diseases.

	OBSTRUCTIVE	RESTRICTIVE
Vital capacity	N or ↓	↓
Total lung capacity	N or ↑	↓
Residual volume	↑	↓
FEV_1/FVC	↓	N or ↑
Maximum midexpiratory flow rate	↓	N
Maximum breathing capacity	↓	N

N, normal; ↓, decreased; ↑, increased; FEV_1, forced expiratory volume in 1 second; FVC, forced vital capacity.

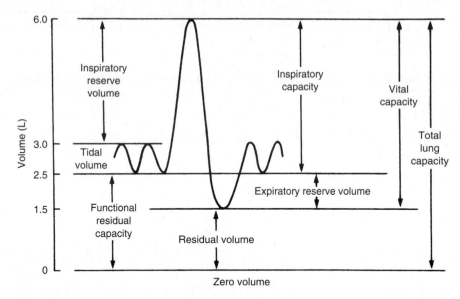

Figure 1.2 Lung volumes and lung capacities.

Expiratory reserve volume (ERV) is the maximum volume of gas that can be exhaled after a normal expiration. Normal ERV is 1,000 mL.

Residual volume (RV) is the volume of gas remaining in the lungs after a forced exhalation. Normal RV is 1,500 mL.

Vital capacity (VC) is the maximum amount of gas that can be exhaled after a maximum inhalation. VC is the sum of V_T, ERV, and IRV. Normal VC is approximately 60 mL per kg.

Inspiratory capacity (IC) is the maximum amount of gas that can be inhaled from the resting expiratory position after a normal exhalation. It is the sum of V_T and IRV. Normal IC is 3,500 mL.

Functional residual capacity (FRC) is the remaining lung volume at the end of a normal quiet expiration. It is the sum of RV and ERV. Normal FRC is 2,500 mL.

Total lung capacity (TLC) is the lung volume at the end of a maximum inspiration. It is the sum of VC and RV. Normal TLC is 5,000 to 6,000 mL.

Barash PG, Cullen BF, Stoelting RK, eds. *Clinical anesthesia*, 5th ed. Philadelphia: Lippincott Williams & Wilkins, 2006:804–805

Lumb AB. *Nunn's applied respiratory physiology*, 6th ed. Philadelphia: Elsevier Butterworth-Heinemann, 2005:33–35.

B.4. What are flow–volume loops? Draw flow–volume loops in a healthy subject, in a patient with COPD, and in a patient with restrictive lung disease.

Flow–volume loops provide a graphic analysis of flow at various lung volumes. Both flow and volume are plotted simultaneously on an X–Y recorder as subjects inspire fully to TLC and then perform an FVC maneuver. This is immediately followed by maximum inhalation as fast as possible back to TLC (Fig. 1.3). The entire inspiratory portion of the loop and the expiratory curve near TLC are highly effort dependent, and the expiratory flow at 75% to 25% of VC is effort independent. The normal expiratory flow/inspiratory flow ratio at 50% of VC (mid-VC flow ratio) is approximately 1.0. This ratio is particularly useful in identifying the presence of upper airway obstruction. In patients with restrictive lung disease such as pulmonary fibrosis and scoliosis,

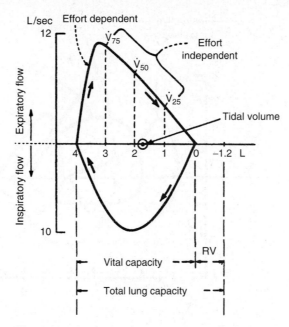

Figure 1.3 Flow–volume loop in a healthy subject. $\dot{V}_{75}$, $\dot{V}_{50}$, and $\dot{V}_{25}$ represent flow at 75%, 50%, and 25% of vital capacity, respectively. RV, residual volume. (From Goudsouzian N, Karamanian A. *Physiology for the anesthesiologist*, 2nd ed. Norwalk, CT: Appleton-Century-Crofts, 1984, with permission.)

a reduction is seen in FVC, with a relatively normal FEV_1. The TLC is markedly reduced, and $FEF_{25\%-75\%}$ and mid-VC flow ratio are usually normal (Fig. 1.4). In patients with obstructive lung disease, peak expiratory flow rate, $FEF_{25\%-75\%}$, and mid-VC flow ratio are reduced, but TLC is increased secondary to the increase in RV, as shown in Fig. 1.4.

A variable obstruction is defined as a lesion with influence that varies with the phase of respiration. In variable extrathoracic obstructions such as vocal cord paralysis or tracheal stenosis, during forced inspiration the respiratory flow is reduced because the negative transmural pressure inside the airway tends to collapse the airway. During expiration, the expiratory flow is reduced far less and may be normal because the positive pressure inside the airway tends to decrease the obstruction (Fig. 1.4). On the contrary, in variable intrathoracic obstruction, the expiratory flow is markedly reduced because the high positive intrapleural pressures during forced expiration decrease airway diameter, and the inspiratory flow is far less reduced because the negative intrapleural pressure tends to increase the diameter of the airway. (Also see Fig. 34.1 in Chapter 34.)

Barash PG, Cullen BF, Stoelting RK, eds. *Clinical anesthesia*, 5th ed. Philadelphia: Lippincott Williams & Wilkins, 2006:806.

Goudsouzian N, Karamanian A. *Physiology for the anesthesiologist*, 3rd ed. Norwalk, CT: Appleton-Century-Crofts, 1984:212–213.

Miller RD, ed. *Miller's anesthesia*, 6th ed. Philadelphia: Elsevier Churchill Livingstone, 2005:1008–1009.

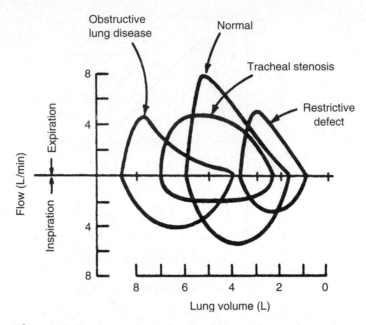

Figure 1.4 Flow–volume loops relative to lung volumes in a healthy subject, a patient with chronic obstructive pulmonary disease (COPD), a patient with fixed obstruction (tracheal stenosis), and a patient with pulmonary fibrosis (restrictive defect). Note the concave expiratory form in the patient with COPD and the flat inspiratory curve in the patient with a fixed obstruction. (From Goudsouzian N, Karamanian A. *Physiology for the anesthesiologist,* 2nd ed. Norwalk, CT: Appleton-Century-Crofts, 1984, with permission.)

B.5. Define closing capacity (CC) and closing volume (CV). What is the normal value of CV?

CC is the lung volume at which the small airways in the dependent parts of the lung begin to close. CC is the sum of CV and residual volume (RV). CV is the gas volume expelled during phase IV of the single-breath nitrogen test; it denotes the lung volume from the beginning of airway closure to the end of maximum expiration. Therefore, CV = CC–RV (Fig. 1.5).

In healthy young people, CV is approximately 10% of the VC, or 400 to 500 mL. CV and CC increase with age. CV is increased in patients with small airway disease and in chronic *smokers*.

Buist AS. The single-breath nitrogen test. *N Engl J Med* 1975;293:438.

Closing volume [Editorial]. *Lancet* 1972;2:908.

Lumb AB. *Nunn's applied respiratory physiology*, 6th ed. Philadelphia: Elsevier Butterworth-Heinemann, 2005:44.

B.6. What are the effects of age and posture on FRC and CC?

FRC is either independent of age in adults or increases very slightly with age, increasing by around 16 mL per year. CC, however, increases with age. Normally, CC becomes equal to FRC at the age of 66 in the upright position and at the age of 44 in the supine position.

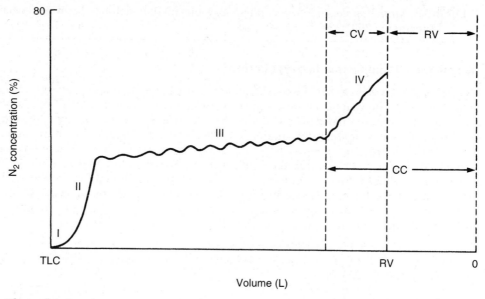

Figure 1.5 Closing volume measurement by single-breath nitrogen test. CC, closing capacity; CV, closing volume; RV, residual volume; TLC, total lung capacity.

FRC increases by approximately 30% by changing from the supine position to the upright position. CC, on the other hand, is independent of body position. It is important to remember that the effects of age on CC and posture on FRC determine whether airway closure exists.

Lumb AB. *Nunn's applied respiratory physiology*, 6th ed. Philadelphia: Elsevier Butterworth-Heinemann, 2005:34, 44.

Rehder K, Marsh HM, Rodarte JR, et al. Airway closure. *Anesthesiology* 1977;47:40.

B.7. What are the effects of anesthesia on FRC and closing capacity (CC)?

During anesthesia, FRC is reduced by approximately 20% with spontaneous breathing and by approximately 16% with artificial ventilation. This is due to changes in the chest wall shape and diaphragm position. After induction of general anesthesia, a reduction occurs in the cross-sectional area of the rib cage corresponding to a decrease in lung volume of approximately 200 mL. Recent studies have consistently shown a cephalad movement of the dependent regions of the diaphragm, with little or no movement of the nondependent regions. However, the change in FRC that can be ascribed to changes in diaphragm is on average less than 30 mL.

CC was previously reported to be unchanged during anesthesia, but later studies concluded that CC reduced in parallel to FRC during anesthesia.

Bergman NA, Tien YK. Contribution of the closure of pulmonary units to impaired oxygenation during anesthesia. *Anesthesiology* 1983;59:395.

Gilmour I, Burnham M, Craig DB. Closing capacity measurements during general anesthesia. *Anesthesiology* 1976;45:477.

Juno P, Marsh HM, Knopp TJ, et al. Closing capacity in awake and anesthetized-paralyzed man. *J Appl Physiol* 1978;44:238.

Lumb AB. *Nunn's applied respiratory physiology*, 6th ed. Philadelphia: Elsevier Butterworth-Heinemann, 2005:304.

B.8. Why is the FRC important in oxygenation?

First, when FRC is decreased to below CC, airways close in the dependent parts of the lung during certain periods of normal tidal ventilation. Airway closure results in shunting of pulmonary blood flow through the unventilated alveoli. Therefore, Qs/Qt is increased and arterial oxygenation is decreased. Second, pulmonary circulation and alveolar gas exchange are continuous during both inspiratory and expiratory phases of respiration. Irrespective of whether there is airway closure or not, blood oxygenation during the expiratory phase is mainly dependent on the remaining lung volume, which is FRC. Therefore, when the FRC is high, blood oxygenation is better and there is more time for oxygenation before hypoxemia occurs during apnea. FRC is decreased in the supine position during general anesthesia and in patients with acute respiratory distress syndrome. Positive end-expiratory pressure (PEEP) increases FRC and decreases airway closure.

Lumb AB. *Nunn's applied respiratory physiology*, 6th ed. Philadelphia: Elsevier Butterworth-Heinemann, 2005:34, 44.

B.9. Are there methods to measure FRC and closing volume?

FRC may be measured by helium dilution, nitrogen washout, and body plethysmography. CV may be determined by two techniques, the single-breath nitrogen test (residual gas technique) and the bolus technique with an inert tracer gas such as helium, xenon, or argon.

Buist AS. The single-breath nitrogen test. *N Engl J Med* 1975;293:438.

Lumb AB. *Nunn's applied respiratory physiology*, 6th ed. Philadelphia: Elsevier Butterworth-Heinemann, 2005:36–37, 52–53.

B.10. Give the equations for shunt (QS/QT) and dead space/tidal volume (VD/VT). What are their normal values?

$$\text{Qs/Qt} = \frac{\text{Cco}_2 - \text{Cao}_2}{\text{Cco}_2 - \text{C}\overline{\text{v}}\text{o}_2} \qquad \text{Vd/Vt} = \frac{\text{Paco}_2 - \text{P}\overline{\text{E}}\text{co}_2}{\text{Paco}_2}$$

Normal Qs/Qt is 4% to 5% and Vd/Vt is approximately 0.3.

Barash PG, Cullen BF, Stoelting RK, eds. *Clinical anesthesia*, 5th ed. Philadelphia: Lippincott Williams & Wilkins, 2006:803–804.

Lumb AB. *Nunn's applied respiratory physiology*, 6th ed. Philadelphia: Elsevier Butterworth-Heinemann, 2005:33–35.

B.11. Interpret the following arterial blood gases: pH, 7.36; PCO$_2$, 60 mm Hg; PO$_2$, 70 mm Hg; CO$_2$ content, 36 mEq per L.

The fraction of inspired oxygen (Fio$_2$) is essential to evaluate Pao$_2$. We assume the blood is taken while the patient is breathing room air. The blood gases show mild hypoxemia and respiratory acidosis, compensated by metabolic alkalosis. The blood gases are compatible with COPD.

B.12. What are the common physiologic causes of hypoxemia?

From the shunt equation, arterial oxygen content is related to the change in pulmonary capillary oxygen content, venous oxygen content, and venous admixture. It is easier to classify hypoxemia into the following three categories.

Decreased Pulmonary Capillary Oxygen Tension

- Hypoventilation
- Low F_{IO_2}
- Ventilation/perfusion abnormalities from pulmonary parenchymal change
- Diffusion abnormality (rare)

Increased Shunting, Either Intrapulmonary or Cardiac
Reduced Venous Oxygen Content

- Congestive heart failure—low cardiac output
- Increased metabolism—fever, hyperthyroidism, shivering
- Decreased arterial oxygen content—anemia

Braunwald E, Fauci AS, Kasper DL, et al. eds. *Harrison's principles of internal medicine*, 16th ed. New York: McGraw-Hill, 2005:1503–1504.

Malley WJ. *Clinical blood gases, assessment and intervention*, 2nd ed. St. Louis: Elsevier Saunders, 2005:236–239.

Shapiro BA, Peruzzi WT, Templin R. *Clinical application of blood gases*, 5th ed. Chicago: Year Book Medical Publishers, 1994:47–52.

B.13. Would you order any special preoperative preparations for asthmatic patients with COPD?

Yes. The preoperative preparation should include the following:

- Eradication of acute and chronic infection with appropriate antibiotics
- Relief of bronchial spasm with a bronchodilator
- Chest physiotherapy to improve sputum clearance and bronchial drainage
- Reversal of uncompensated or borderline cor pulmonale with diuretics, digitalis, improved oxygenation, and correction of acidemia by more efficient ventilation
- Correction of dehydration and electrolyte imbalance
- Familiarization with respiratory therapy equipment likely to be used in the postoperative period
- Cessation of smoking, if possible for 2 months, to improve mucociliary clearance and to decrease sputum production
- Abstinence from smoking for 2 days (at least 12 hours), to reduce carboxyhemoglobin levels, resulting in improvement of blood oxygen content and increasing the release of oxygen in hemoglobin
- Continuation of prophylactic cromolyn inhalation up to the time of surgery to prevent the degranulation of mast cells and the subsequent release of chemical mediators responsible for bronchoconstriction
- Initiation of a tapered steroid therapy in the week before surgery for patients with ongoing wheezing and scheduled elective surgery

Barash PG, Cullen BF, Stoelting RK, eds. *Clinical anesthesia*, 5th ed. Philadelphia: Lippincott Williams & Wilkins, 2006:484.

Bishop MJ. Bronchospasm, avoiding an anesthetic disaster. In: Barash PG, ed. *ASA refresher courses in anesthesiology*. Park Ridge, IL: American Society of Anesthesiologists, 1991: 15–27.

Miller RD, ed. *Miller's anesthesia*, 6th ed. Philadelphia: Elsevier Churchill Livingstone, 2005:1858–1859.

B.14. How long would you postpone elective surgery if the patient had a recent URI?

Respiratory tract infections are the most common stimuli that evoke acute exacerbations of asthma. The airway responsiveness of even healthy subjects to nonspecific stimuli is transiently increased after a viral infection. Increased airway responsiveness can last from 2 to 8 weeks after the infection in both healthy subjects and asthmatics. Recently Cohen and Cameron reported that if a child had a URI and had endotracheal anesthesia, the risk of a respiratory complication increased 11-fold. In addition, Tait and Knight found that laryngospasm and bronchospasm were significantly increased even in healthy children 2 weeks after a URI. Therefore, it has been recommended to wait for 2 to 3 weeks after clinical recovery from a URI in asthmatics even if clinical symptoms are not present.

Bishop MJ. Bronchospasm, avoiding an anesthetic disaster. In: Barash PG, ed. *ASA refresher courses in anesthesiology*. American Society of Anesthesiologists, 1991:15–27.

Cohen MM, Cameron CB. Should you cancel the operation when a child has an upper respiratory infection? *Anesth Analg* 1991;72:282–288.

Tait AR, Knight PR. Intraoperative respiratory complications in patients with upper respiratory tract infections. *Can J Anaesth* 1987;34:300–303.

B.15. What medicines would you expect the patient to have taken in the past or to be taking at the present time?

The asthmatic patient might take bronchodilators such as methylxanthines and sympathomimetics. Special attention is required if the patient has taken systemic glucocorticoids. Recently, aerosol therapy has become quite popular because it provides optimal local therapeutic effects and minimizes the systemic side effects. Various relatively selective β_2-agonists (albuterol, fenoterol, terbutaline, and bitolterol), anticholinergic bronchodilators (ipratropium bromide and methylatropine nitrate), mast cell stabilizer (cromolyn), leukotriene receptor antagonists such as zafirlukast (Accolate) and montelukast (Singulair) and various steroids are now available as aerosols and are frequently able to control most cases of chronic asthma.

Brusse WW, Lemanske RF. Asthma. *N Engl J Med* 2001;344:350–362.

Gould BE. *Pathophysiology for the health professions*, 3rd ed. Philadelphia: Saunders Elsevier, 2006:393–398.

Kasper DL, Braunwald E, Fauci AS, et al. eds. *Harrison's principles of internal medicine*, 16th ed. New York: McGraw-Hill, 2005:1508–1516.

Stoelting RK, Dierdorf SF. *Anesthesia and co-existing disease*, 4th ed. New York: Churchill Livingstone, 2002:198–199.

B.16. Would you order preoperative steroid preparation? Why?

It is recommended that preoperative glucocorticoid replacement therapy be given to all patients with known or suspected adrenal insufficiency. Patients who have been treated with high-dose glucocorticoids within the previous year should also be assumed to have an unknown element of adrenocortical suppression that should be treated with full replacement therapy. The human adrenal glands normally secrete approximately 30 mg of hydrocortisone (cortisol) per day under baseline conditions; however, under stress up to 200 to 500 mg a day may be secreted. It is reasonable to replace 300 mg of hydrocortisone per day during perioperative periods. The night before surgery, 100 mg of hydrocortisone acetate may be given intramuscularly. In addition, a 100-mg dose of hydrocortisone phosphate is given intravenously before induction and during surgery. Postoperatively, hydrocortisone phosphate, 100 mg intravenously, is given every 8 hours for 48 hours and then the steroid therapy is tapered. The biologic half-life of hydrocortisone is 8 to 12 hours. If the patient had less than 1 week of systemic steroid therapy more than 6 months previously and there are no signs of adrenal insufficiency, routine steroid preparation is not advised. However, intravenous steroid preparations should be available in the operating room in case intractable hypotension from adrenal insufficiency occurs during surgery.

The increasing emphasis on reactive airways as an inflammatory disease has led to greater appreciation of the importance of steroids in controlling the incidence of attacks and in aborting acute attacks. It has been recommended that systemic steroid preparation be used preoperatively in patients with moderate to severe asthma and a history of a need for steroids in the past. One day of high-dose steroids should not significantly affect wound healing. In the face of ongoing wheezing and scheduled elective surgery, a steroid course in the week or weeks before surgery may be useful. The concern that steroids will increase the rate of wound-healing problems or infection are not well founded. A recent study of asthmatics treated with steroids preoperatively found no increase in the incidence of wound infections or wound-healing problems.

Barash PG, Cullen BF, Stoelting RK, eds. *Clinical anesthesia*, 5th ed. Philadelphia: Lippincott Williams & Wilkins, 2006:484.

Bishop MJ. Editorial views: preoperative corticosteroids for reactive airway. *Anesthesiology* 2004;100:1047–1048.

Bishop MJ. Bronchospasm: successful management. In: *ASA annual meeting refresher course lectures*, Park Ridge, IL: American Society of Anesthesiologists, 2005:408.

Kabalin CS, Yarnold PR, Grammer LC. Low complication rate of corticosteroid-treated asthmatics undergoing surgical procedures. *Arch Intern Med* 1995;155:1379–1384.

Sheffer AL. Expert panel on the management of asthma. *J Allergy Clin Immunol* 1991;88: 425–534.

Silvanus M-T, Groeben H, Peters J. Corticosteroids and inhaled salbutamol in patients with reversible airway obstruction markedly decrease the incidence of bronchospasm after tracheal intubation. *Anesthesiology* 2004;100:1052–1057.

B.17. What is the onset of action of intravenous steroid therapy in asthma?

The bronchial effects of intravenous steroids are not immediate and may not be seen for 6 to 12 hours after the initial administration. When severe bronchospasm does not resolve despite intense optimal bronchodilator therapy, intravenous corticosteroid administration is indicated. A loading dose of hydrocortisone, 4 mg per kg, is given to achieve plasma cortisol levels above 100 μg per dL, followed by 3 mg per kg every 6 hours. Alternatively, methylprednisolone, 60 to 125 mg, may be given every 6 hours.

Kasper DL, Braunwald E, Fauci AS, et al. eds. *Harrison's principles of internal medicine*, 16th ed. New York: McGraw-Hill, 2005:1508–1516.

Parker SD, Brown RH, Darowski MJ, et al. Time related decrease in airway reactivity by corticosteroids [Abstract]. *Anesthesiology* 1989;71:A1077.

Stoelting RK, Dierdorf SF. *Anesthesia and co-existing disease*, 4th ed. New York: Churchill Livingstone, 2002:194.

B.18. What are the effects of cimetidine on asthmatic patients?

Cimetidine is an H_2-receptor antagonist. Nathan et al. found that histamine mediates bronchoconstriction through the H_1-receptor (blocked by chlorpheniramine), and bronchodilation is mediated by H_2-receptor agonists (blocked by cimetidine). H_2-receptors are thought to be responsible for inhibitory feedback control of mediator release. Cimetidine may potentiate histamine H_1-receptor bronchoconstrictions. It should be avoided in asthmatic patients. Cimetidine also slows clearing of theophylline by inhibiting microsomal metabolism. Therefore, theophylline dosage should be decreased to avoid toxicity.

Nathan R, Segall N, Schocket A. A comparison of the actions of H_1 and H_2 antihistamines on histamine-induced bronchoconstriction and cutaneous wheal response in asthmatic patients. *J Allergy Clin Immunol* 1981;67:171.

Stoelting RK, Dierdorf SF. *Anesthesia and co-existing disease*, 4th ed. New York: Churchill Livingstone, 2002:201.

B.19. How would you premedicate the patient? Why?

No good controlled studies have been performed on premedication used in asthmatic patients. The asthmatic patient may be premedicated with atropine and diphenhydramine alone or in combination with droperidol. Atropine is an anticholinergic drug. It decreases airway resistance, and diminishes secretion-initiated airway reactivity. Diphenhydramine is an H_1-receptor–blocking drug. It inhibits histamine-mediated bronchoconstriction and possesses a sedative effect. The sedative effect of diphenhydramine may prevent bronchospasm induced by psychologic stress. Hydroxyzine hydrochloride (Vistaril) is a frequently used alternative because of its sedative, antihistaminic, and bronchodilating effects.

Inhaled or systemic steroids may be given to patients with moderate to severe asthma to decrease the incidence of asthmatic attacks.

Inhaled β_2-agonists, cromolyn, or steroids should be continued up to the time of surgery.

Bishop MJ. Bronchospasm, avoiding an anesthetic disaster. In: Barash PG, ed. *ASA refresher courses in anesthesiology*. Park Ridge, IL: American Society of Anesthesiologists, 1991:15–27.

Stoelting RK, Dierdorf SF. *Anesthesia And co-existing disease*, 4th ed. New York: Churchill Livingstone, 2002:200–201.

C. Intraoperative Management

C.1. What are the disadvantages of administering atropine to the asthmatic patient?

Some physicians consider atropine relatively contraindicated because it causes drying of secretions, further plugging, and perhaps the initiation of a severe attack of asthma. This assumption has proved more theoretic than real in the reasonably well-managed asthmatic patient. However, atropine blocks the formation of cyclic guanosine monophosphate (GMP) and therefore has a bronchodilation effect. Inhaled atropine improves FEV_1 in 85% of patients with COPD.

Barash PG, Cullen BF, Stoelting RK, eds. *Clinical anesthesia*, 5th ed. Philadelphia: Lippincott Williams & Wilkins, 2006:819.

Barrett JP. Editorial views: clinical epilog on bronchomotor tone. *Anesthesiology* 1975;42: 1–3.

C.2. If the patient had a severe asthmatic attack in the operating room before the induction of anesthesia, would you put the patient to sleep or postpone the surgery?

First of all, medical treatment should be given to relieve the asthmatic attack. Elective surgery should be postponed and the patient should be reevaluated carefully and better prepared preoperatively. In case of emergency surgery such as acute appendicitis, the surgery can be performed after the asthmatic attack is terminated with medical treatment. During surgery, the medical treatment should be continued.

C.3. The patient did not have an asthmatic attack in the operating room. How would you induce anesthesia? Would you use an LMA instead of an endotracheal tube?

The principles of anesthetic management for the asthmatic patient are threefold: to block airway reflexes before laryngoscopy and intubation, to relax airway smooth muscle, and to prevent release of biochemical mediators. Before induction of anesthesia, I would like to ask the patient to take two to three puffs of albuterol from a metered-dose inhaler (MDI). Methohexital is used for induction. Then oxygen and a potent inhalation agent, such as halothane, sevoflurane, or isoflurane, are administered by mask to achieve adequate depth of anesthesia before endotracheal intubation after injection of succinylcholine or other muscle relaxants. Topical endotracheal spray of 80 to 120 mg of lidocaine through a laryngotracheal anesthesia (LTA) kit may be used before intubation to suppress the cough reflex induced by intubation, but the introduction of lidocaine itself may cause the cough reflex when the depth of anesthesia is light.

As a supraglottic airway, the LMA seems to be suitable for asthmatic patients. The LMA provides a unique opportunity for the clinician to control the airway without having to introduce a foreign body into the trachea. Therefore, it may be an ideal airway tool in the asthmatic patient who is not at risk of reflux and aspiration. However, the patient is undergoing cholecystectomy, which may need manipulating and packing of stomach and bowels; the patient is at risk of regurgitation and aspiration. Meanwhile, the patient may need a nasogastric tube for decompression of gastrointestinal tract. The classic LMA device (except LMA-ProSeal) is not compatible with the use of a nasogastric tube intraoperatively. I would not choose a classic LMA instead of an endotracheal tube for this procedure. However, the introduction of the LMA-ProSeal with a gastric drain tube and larger cuff reduces both the risk of gastric inflation and the risk of aspiration of refluxed gastric contents. The LMA-ProSeal has been successfully used for laparoscopic cholecystectomy in obese patients.

Barash PG, Cullen BF, Stoelting RK, eds. *Clinical anesthesia*, 5th ed. Philadelphia: Lippincott Williams & Wilkins, 2006:605–607.

Malthy JR, Beriault MT, Watson NC, et al. The LMA ProSeal is an effective alternative to tracheal intubation in laparoscopic cholecystectomy. *Can J Anaesth* 2002;49:857.

C.4. Why would you use methohexital instead of thiopental?

Hirshman et al., using human skin mast cell preparations, demonstrated histamine release by thiopental and thiamylal, but not by methohexital and pentobarbital. Thiopental and thiamylal are thiobarbiturates, and methohexital and pentobarbital are oxybarbiturates. This suggests that the sulfur atom is important in barbiturate-induced histamine release. Moreover, they further found that thiobarbiturates, but not oxybarbiturates, constricted guinea pig tracheas and that this constriction was mediated by thromboxane. Therefore, methohexital may be preferred as the induction agent in patients showing extreme sensitivity to histamine (asthmatics) or increased histamine releasability (atopics). However, thiopental itself does not cause bronchospasm. Because it provides only a light plane of anesthesia, airway instrumentation under thiopental anesthesia alone may trigger bronchospasm. Therefore, clinically, both barbiturates have been used successfully in the asthmatic patient, provided that an adequate depth of anesthesia is achieved before stimulating the airway.

Bishop MJ. Bronchospasm: successful management. In: *ASA annual meeting refresher course lectures*. Park Ridge, IL: American Society of Anesthesiologists, 2005:408.

Curry C, Lenox WC, Spannhake EW, et al. Contractile responses of guinea pig trachea to oxybarbiturates and thiobarbiturates. *Anesthesiology* 1991;75:679–683.

Lorenz W, Doenicke A. Editorial views: anaphylactoid reactions and histamine release by barbiturate induction agents: clinical relevance and pathomechanisms. *Anesthesiology* 1985;63:351.

Hirshman CA, Edelstein RA, Ebertz JM, et al. Thiobarbiturate-induced histamine release. *Anesthesiology* 1985;63:353.

C.5. Would you use propofol, etomidate, or ketamine for induction?

Propofol may be the induction agent of choice for the patient with reactive airways who was hemodynamically stable. A recent report found that induction of asthmatics with 2.5 mg per kg of propofol per kg of body weight resulted in a significantly lower incidence of wheezing after tracheal intubation when compared with induction with 5 mg per kg of thiopental or thiamylal or with 1.75 mg per kg of methohexital per kg of body weight. The incidence of wheezing was 0%, 45%, and 26% in patients who received propofol, a thiobarbiturate, and oxybarbiturate, respectively. Another study found that in unselected patients, propofol resulted in a significantly lower respiratory resistance after tracheal intubation than induction with thiopental or etomidate.

Etomidate does not depress myocardial function. Therefore, it provides hemodynamic stability in critically ill patients. Although it was advertised as an ideal agent for asthmatic patients, little evidence supports the claim except that etomidate does not release histamine. A recent study suggests that neither etomidate nor thiopental prevents wheezing after intubation, as opposed to the marked protection afforded by propofol.

Ketamine produces bronchodilation both through neural mechanisms and through release of catecholamines. In an actively wheezing patient, ketamine is the induction agent of choice, particularly when hemodynamics are unstable.

Bishop MJ. Bronchospasm: successful management. In: *ASA annual meeting refresher course lectures*. Park Ridge, IL: American Society of Anesthesiologists, 2005:408.

Eames WO, Rooke GA, Wu RS, et al. Comparison of the effects of etomidate, propofol, and thiopental on respiratory resistance following tracheal intubation. *Anesthesiology* 1996;84:1307–1311.

Pizov R, Brown RH, Weis YS, et al. Wheezing during induction of general anesthesia in patients with and without asthma. A randomized, blind trial. *Anesthesiology* 1995;82: 1111–1116.

Stoelting RK, Dierdorf SF. *Anesthesia and co-existing disease*, 4th ed. New York: Churchill Livingstone, 2002:194.

C.6. Would you use lidocaine for intubation?

Intravenous lidocaine, 1 mg per kg, may be given 1 to 2 minutes before intubation to prevent reflex-induced bronchospasm. Topical endotracheal spray of lidocaine must be used cautiously because it may provoke reflex bronchoconstriction if adequate depth of anesthesia has not been achieved. Lidocaine infusion, 1 to 2 mg per kg per hour, may be used in cardiac or elderly patients with COPD whose airways need more anesthesia than their cardiovascular system can tolerate.

Hirshman CA. Anesthesia and bronchospastic disease. In: Barash PG, ed. *ASA refresher courses in anesthesiology*. Chicago: American Society of Anesthesiologists, 1985:81–95.

McAlpine LG, Thomson NC. Lidocaine-induced bronchoconstriction in asthmatic patients. Relation to histamine airway responsiveness and effect of preservative. *Chest* 1989; 96:1012–1015.

C.7. If this is emergency surgery and rapid sequence induction is indicated, how would you induce anesthesia in this patient?

All the precautions to prevent aspiration of gastric contents and asthmatic attack must be considered simultaneously. Rapid sequence induction and tracheal intubation using propofol, thiopental or methohexital, and succinylcholine are necessary to prevent aspiration, but light anesthesia may precipitate severe bronchospasm.

Ketamine, 2 mg per kg, may be the induction agent of choice in noncardiac asthmatic patients, because ketamine increases catecholamine release with resultant bronchodilation.

In asthmatic patients who have ischemic heart disease, we give a moderate dose of fentanyl, 5 μg per kg, 2 to 3 minutes before the administration of propofol, 1.5 mg per kg, or methohexital, 1.5 mg per kg, to suppress airway reflexes and prevent tachycardia and hypertension caused by intubation.

Intravenous lidocaine, 1 to 2 mg per kg, given immediately before the administration of ketamine or fentanyl, and succinylcholine, are useful adjunct drugs to prevent reflex bronchospasm, particularly in an emergency situation when deep anesthesia cannot be achieved before intubation.

A full stomach should be emptied by a functioning nasogastric tube. The patient should be denitrogenated with 100% oxygen by mask. Cisatracurium or vecuronium, 1 mg, should be given 3 minutes before administration of succinylcholine.

If the patient has a wheezing attack before anesthesia, inhalation of sympathomimetics such as albuterol may be used as the first-line therapy for acute asthmatic attacks.

Bishop MJ. Bronchospasm, avoiding an anesthetic disaster. In: Barash PG, ed. *ASA refresher courses in anesthesiology*. Park Ridge, IL: American Society of Anesthesiologists, 1991: 15–27.

Kingston HGG, Hirshman CA. Perioperative management of the patient with asthma. *Anesth Analg* 1984;63:844.

Martin DE, Rosenberg H, Aukburg SJ, et al. Low-dose fentanyl blunts circulatory responses to tracheal intubation. *Anesth Analg* 1982;61:680.

C.8. What is your choice of agents for maintenance of anesthesia? Why?

We use inhalation agents such as sevoflurane, halothane, and isoflurane with nitrous oxide and oxygen. Sevoflurane, enflurane, and isoflurane are preferable to halothane, because halothane sensitizes the myocardium to arrhythmic effects of circulating catecholamines more than sevoflurane, enflurane, and isoflurane. However, some authorities prefer halothane and sevoflurane to isoflurane and desflurane because the latter anesthetics have a pungent odor that may cause airway irritation and trigger bronchospasm. At lower doses (<1.0 minimum alveolar concentration [MAC]), the inhaled anesthetics inhibit chemically induced tracheal contractions in the order: halothane > enflurane ≥ isoflurane > sevoflurane. However, more recent clinical observations in humans indicate that sevoflurane at 1.1 MAC may be the most effective agent, particularly in the presence of airway instrumentation. In addition, sevoflurane may have a more rapid onset of bronchodilation than isoflurane or halothane.

Barash PG, Cullen BF, Stoelting RK, eds. *Clinical anesthesia*, 5th ed. Philadelphia: Lippincott Williams & Wilkins, 2006:408.

Rock GA, Choi JH, Bishop MJ. The effect of isoflurane, halothane, sevoflurane and thiopental nitrous oxide on respiratory system resistance after tracheal intubation. *Anesthesiology* 1997;86:1294–1299.

Stoelting RK, Dierdorf SF. *Anesthesia and co-existing disease*, 4th ed. New York: Churchill Livingstone, 2002:202.

C.9. What are the mechanisms of halothane that produce bronchodilation?

The major component of bronchodilation elicited by halothane is mediated through β-adrenergic receptor stimulation, which is decreased by β-blocking agents. The β-agonistic effect works through two intracellular mechanisms. The first mechanism is direct relaxation of bronchial musculature mediated by an increase in intracellular cyclic 3′,5′-adenosine monophosphate (cAMP). Increased cAMP may bind free calcium within bronchial myoplasm and thereby promote relaxation by a negative feedback mechanism. The second mechanism may arise from the first inasmuch as elevated levels of cAMP seem to impede antigen-/antibody-mediated enzyme production and release of histamine from leukocytes. However, a study by Hirshman et al. suggests that the mechanism of action involves the depression of airway reflexes and direct effects on airway smooth muscle. Halothane may also have protective effects by acting on bronchial epithelium through a nonadrenergic, noncholinergic mechanism, possibly involving the nitric oxide pathway.

Barash PG, Cullen BF, Stoelting RK, eds. *Clinical anesthesia*, 5th ed. Philadelphia: Lippincott Williams & Wilkins, 2006:408.

Hirshman CA, Edelstein G, Peetz S, et al. Mechanism of action of inhalational anesthesia on airways. *Anesthesiology* 1982;56:107.

Linderman KS, Baker SG, Hirshman CA. Interaction between halothane and the nonadrenergic, noncholinergic inhibitory system in porcine trachealis muscle. *Anesthesiology* 1994;81:641.

C.10. Why would you choose an inhalational instead of an intravenous technique?

First, inhalation agents such as sevoflurane, halothane, enflurane, and isoflurane have dose-related direct bronchodilator effects. Ketamine has an indirect bronchodilator effect, which is not dose related and not predictable. Large doses of morphine produce bronchoconstriction because morphine increases central vagal tone and releases histamine. Droperidol has an α-blocking effect that may relieve bronchospasm induced by α stimulation. Meperidine was shown to have a spasmolytic effect in asthmatic patients, but not in experimental dogs. Fentanyl does not have a significant effect on bronchial tone. Second, cholinesterase inhibitors can induce bronchospasm. Inhalation agents potentiate muscle relaxants; therefore, lower doses of relaxants are needed for surgery. The use of cholinesterase inhibitors to reverse the effect of muscle relaxants may be avoided or decreased.

Barash PG, Cullen BF, Stoelting RK, eds. *Clinical anesthesia*, 5th ed. Philadelphia: Lippincott Williams & Wilkins, 2006:408.

Kingston HGG, Hirshman CA. Perioperative management of the patient with asthma. *Anesth Analg* 1984;63:844.

C.11. Is regional anesthesia better than general anesthesia in this situation?

This issue is controversial. The use of regional anesthesia avoids the possibility of bronchospasm that may be induced by endotracheal tube stimulation. However, if high levels of sensory and motor block are required, they may produce severe anxiety and actually incite bronchospasm. Another concern is the associated blockade of sympathetic input to the lungs. Some case reports have speculated about a resultant increase in airway resistance. Respiratory complications were reported to be quite common (83%) in patients undergoing intraperitoneal surgery who had relatively high spinal anesthesia (T6-4). Low spinal, epidural, and caudal anesthesia for surgery of the perineum, lower extremities, and pelvic extraperitoneal organs resulted in fewer respiratory complications than did general anesthesia. A study of patients with asthma demonstrated no differences between those anesthetized with high epidurals (T2-4) and those undergoing general anesthesia with ketamine and isoflurane.

Endotracheal general anesthesia is advantageous because it provides a controlled airway to deliver the desirable oxygen concentration, but the endotracheal tube may also induce bronchospasm during light anesthesia.

Bishop MJ. Bronchospasm: successful management. In: *ASA annual meeting refresher course lectures*. Park Ridge, IL: American Society of Anesthesiologists, 2005:408.

Gold MI, Helrich M. A study of the complications related to anesthesia in asthmatic patients. *Anesth Analg* 1963;42:283–293.

Ramanathan J, Osborne B, Sibai B. Epidural anesthesia in asthmatic patients. *Anesth Analg* 1990;70:S317–S318.

C.12. Which muscle relaxants would you use? Why?

Muscle relaxants that cause histamine release should be avoided (Table 1.2). Pancuronium, rocuronium, cisatracurium, and vecuronium are the preferred relaxants because the histamine released is insignificant. Vecuronium, rocuronium, and cisatracurium may be better choices of relaxant because of their intermediate action durations, allowing early recovery without reversal

Table 1.2 Histamine Release from Nondepolarizing Muscle Relaxants.

MUSCLE RELAXANT	HISTAMINE RELEASE[a]
Benzylisoquinolinium compounds	
D-Tubocurarine	0.6
Metocurine	2.0
Doxacurium	>4.0
Mivacurium	3.0
Atracurium	2.5
Cisatracurium	None
Steroidal compounds	
Pancuronium	None
Vecuronium	None
Pipecuronium	None
Rocuronium	None
Others	
Alcuronium	None
Gallamine	None

[a]Defined as the number of multiples of the ED_{95} for neuromuscular blockade required to produce histamine release.

with an anticholinesterase, which may precipitate bronchospasm. D-Tubocurarine can cause bronchospasm by histamine release. Metocurine and succinylcholine also cause histamine release, but to a lesser extent. Gallamine has minimal histamine release but has been reported to cause bronchospasm in patients. Atracurium, mivacurium, and doxacurium in high doses increase histamine release. Therefore, they are not the relaxants of choice.

Basta SJ. Modulation of histamine release by neuromuscular blocking drugs. *Curr Opin Anesth* 1992;5:572.

Caldwell JE, Lau M, Fisher DM. Atracurium versus vecuronium in asthmatic patients. A blinded, randomized comparison of adverse events. *Anesthesiology* 1995;83:985–991.

Mehr EH, Hirshman CA, Lindeman KS. Mechanism of action of atracurium on airways. *Anesthesiology* 1992;76:448–454.

Miller RD, ed. *Miller's anesthesia*, 6th ed. Philadelphia: Elsevier Churchill Livingstone, 2005:511–512.

C.13. In the middle of surgery, the patient developed a severe wheezing attack. How do you manage it?

First, deepen the level of anesthesia and increase FIO_2. Remember that the patient is under anesthesia and surgery. Therefore, medical intervention, such as β-agonist administration, is not the first choice of treatment. The most common cause of asthmatic attack during surgery is inadequate anesthesia. The asthmatic patient has an extremely sensitive tracheobronchial tree. When the level of anesthesia is too light, he may develop bucking, straining, or coughing as a result of the foreign body (endotracheal tube) in his trachea and go on to develop bronchospasm. First the blood pressure is taken to ensure it is normal or high, and then anesthesia is deepened by increasing the concentration of inhalation agents, such as sevoflurane, halothane, enflurane, or isoflurane, which are direct bronchodilators as well. An incremental dose of ketamine may be a quick way of maintaining blood pressure, rapidly deepening anesthesia, achieving bronchodilation, and avoiding the problem of delivering an inhaled anesthetic to a patient with poor ventilation. At the same time, oxygenation can be improved by increasing the oxygen concentration and decreasing the nitrous oxide. The patient should be continuously ventilated with a volume-cycled ventilator.

Second, relieve mechanical stimulation. Pass a catheter through the endotracheal tube to suction secretions and to determine whether there is any obstruction or kinking of the tube. The cuff of the endotracheal tube can be deflated, the tube moved back 1 to 2 cm, and the cuff reinflated. Occasionally, the endotracheal tube slips down and stimulates the carina of the trachea, causing severe bronchospasm during light anesthesia. Surgical stimulation, such as traction on the mesentery, intestine, or stomach, should be stopped temporarily, because it causes vagal reflex and can cause bronchospasm.

Third, medical intervention is necessary if the previously mentioned treatment cannot break the bronchospasm or the anesthesia cannot be increased because of hypotension. The cornerstone of the treatment of the intraoperative bronchospasm is inhalation of β_2-agonists such as albuterol, which induce further bronchodilation even in the presence of adequate inhalational anesthesia. β_2-Agonists produce more rapid and effective bronchodilation than intravenous aminophylline. When severe bronchospasm is not resolving despite intense optimal bronchodilation therapy, intravenous corticosteroid is indicated (see sections B.16 and B.17).

Fourth, bring in an intensive care unit (ICU) ventilator. Anesthesia ventilators are not designed for patients with high airway resistance. It is impossible to deliver adequate alveolar ventilation because the anesthesia circuit has too much compressible volume (tubing compliance) and the anesthesia ventilator does not have enough driving power. An ICU ventilator can generate inspiratory pressures as high as 120 cm H_2O. With low tubing compliance, little ventilation is wasted into the circuit. High inspiratory flow rate allows for shorter inspiratory time with adequate time for expiration and lower auto-PEEP. The major disadvantage of an ICU ventilator is its inability to use inhalational anesthetics. However, the Siemens 900D anesthesia machine incorporates an ICU-type ventilator with vaporizers and oxygen mixers. It may be ideal for this situation.

Bishop MJ. Bronchospasm: successful management. In: *ASA annual meeting refresher course lectures*. Park Ridge, IL: American Society of Anesthesiologists, 2002:411.

Brusse WW, Lemanske RF. Asthma. *N Engl J Med* 2001;344:350–362.

Tobias JD, Hirshman CA. Attenuation of histamine-induced airway constriction by albuterol during halothane anesthesia. *Anesthesiology* 1990;72:105–110.

C.14. How would you give β_2-agonists? What problems may arise when isoproterenol is given during halothane anesthesia? What is its mechanism of action on asthma?

In the past it was fashionable to treat episodes of severe asthma with intravenous sympathomimetics such as isoproterenol. This approach no longer appears justifiable. Isoproterenol infusions can induce ventricular arrhythmias during halothane anesthesia. In addition, isoproterenol infusion can clearly cause myocardial damage, and even the β_2-selective agents such as terbutaline and albuterol when given intravenously offer no advantages over the inhaled route.

β_2-Agonists such as albuterol, terbutaline, fenoterol, and pirbuterol may be administered through MDI adapters or small-volume jet nebulizers to the anesthetic circuit. Because MDI adapters are not very efficient in the intubated patient, more than two puffs are needed to break acute bronchospasms.

Adrenergic stimulants produce bronchodilation through action on β-adrenergic receptors. β-Agonists increase intracellular cAMP by activating adenyl cyclase, which produces cAMP from adenosine triphosphate (ATP). Increased cAMP promotes bronchial relaxation and inhibits the release of mediators from mast cells (Fig. 1.6).

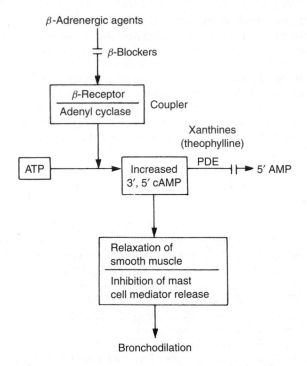

Figure 1.6 Cyclic adenosine monophosphate (cAMP) pathways involved in bronchodilator action. 3', 5' cAMP, cyclic 3',5'-adenosine monophosphate; AMP, adenosine monophosphate; ATP, adenosine triphosphate; PDE, phosphodiesterase. (From Hirshman C. Airway reactivity in humans: anesthetic implications. *Anesthesiology* 1983;58:170, with permission.)

Barnes PJ. A new approach to the treatment of asthma. *N Engl J Med* 1989;321:1517–1527.

Kasper DL, Braunwald E, Fauci AS, et al. eds. *Harrison's principles of internal medicine*, 16th ed. New York: McGraw-Hill, 2005:1508–1516.

Stoelting RK, Dierdorf SF. *Anesthesia and co-existing disease*, 4th ed. New York: Churchill Livingstone, 2002:199.

C.15. Would you administer aminophylline? How does aminophylline relieve bronchospasm? What is the mechanism of action? What are the therapeutic blood levels of aminophylline? What are the toxic effects of aminophylline?

Currently, aminophylline is rarely used for acute bronchospasm because of its narrow therapeutic–toxic window and its relatively weak bronchodilating effect. In addition, aminophylline does not add to the bronchodilating efficacy of inhaled halothane.

The usual intravenous loading dose is 6.0 mg per kg given slowly, followed by a continuous infusion of 1.0 mg per kg per hour for smokers, 0.5 mg per kg per hour for nonsmokers, and 0.3 mg per kg per hour for severely ill patients, such as those with congestive heart failure, pneumonia, and liver disease. Maintenance doses must also be reduced to 0.3 mg per kg per hour for patients taking cimetidine, which interferes with hepatic microsomal enzymes.

It was formerly thought that aminophylline increases intracellular cAMP through inhibition of the enzyme phosphodiesterase (PDE), which inactivates cAMP (Fig. 1.6). However, the available evidence does not support this concept. The therapeutic plasma levels of aminophylline range from 5 to 15 μg per mL. The common side effects of aminophylline include nervousness, nausea, vomiting, anorexia, and headache; cardiac arrhythmias and seizures occur with high plasma levels.

Hirshman CA. Airway reactivity in humans: anesthetic implications. *Anesthesiology* 1983;58:170.

Kasper DL, Braunwald E, Fauci AS, et al. eds. *Harrison's principles of internal medicine*, 16th ed. New York: McGraw-Hill, 2005:1508–1516.

Tobias JD, Kubos KL, Hirshman CA. Aminophylline does not attenuate histamine-induced airway constriction during halothane anesthesia. *Anesthesiology* 1989;71:723–729.

C.16. If the patient does not respond to the aforementioned treatment and becomes cyanotic, what would you do?

The values of arterial blood gases should be determined immediately. In a severe, prolonged asthmatic attack, there will be combined respiratory and metabolic acidosis resulting from CO_2 retention and lactic acidosis from tissue hypoxia. $NaHCO_3$ should be given to correct the acidosis, because aminophylline and β-agonists are not effective in severe acidosis. At the same time, bronchodilator therapy should be continued or increased. Consultation with senior staff or a physician in pulmonary medicine may be necessary.

Kampschulte S, March J, Safar P. Simplified physiologic management of status asthmaticus in children. *Crit Care Med* 1973;1:69–74.

C.17. What are the differential diagnoses of intraoperative bronchospasm?

The causes of wheezing and increased airway pressure include the following:

- Kinked endotracheal tube
- Solidified secretions or blood
- Pulmonary edema
- Tension pneumothorax
- Aspiration pneumonitis
- Pulmonary embolism
- Endobronchial intubation
- Persistent coughing and straining
- Negative pressure expiration

Stoelting RK, Dierdorf SF. *Anesthesia and co-existing disease*, 4th ed. New York: Churchill Livingstone, 2002:203.

C.18. The asthmatic attack was finally relieved and the surgery was completed. The patient was found to be hypoventilating. What are the common causes of hypoventilation? Would you like to reverse the muscle relaxant?

The following are common causes of apnea or hypoventilation at the end of surgery:

- Respiratory center depression by inhalational anesthetics, narcotics, or hyperventilation (low Pa_{CO_2})
- Peripheral blockade by muscle relaxants

Because the patient is a severe asthmatic, it is better to avoid the use of an anticholinesterase, such as neostigmine, to reverse a nondepolarizing relaxant. Neostigmine may trigger bronchospasm by a cholinergic mechanism. Although atropine given simultaneously with neostigmine may prevent bronchospasm, the action duration of neostigmine is longer than that of atropine. If reversal is required, it appears prudent to administer larger than customary doses of glycopyrrolate (>0.5 mg) or atropine (>1.0 mg) to minimize the possibility of bronchospasm. It is advisable to use inhalation agents to potentiate relaxants and to use smaller amounts of intermediate-acting relaxants for surgery. If spontaneous respiration is not adequate, artificial ventilation should be continued.

Gal TJ. Reactive airway disease: anesthetic perspectives. In: *International anesthesia research society review course lectures*. Cleveland, OH: International Anesthesia Research Society, 2002:45–53.

Hazizai A, Hatija A. Bronchospasm caused by neostigmine. *Eur J Anaesthesiol* 2006;23: 85–86.

D. Postoperative Management

D.1. Would you extubate the asthmatic patient while he or she was deeply anesthetized?

To avoid bronchospasm triggered by coughing and bucking caused by laryngeal and pharyngeal reflexes during emergence and extubation, patients may be extubated at surgical (deep) levels of anesthesia. However, the risks of aspiration, airway obstruction, and hypoventilation should be weighed against the benefits. With a history of severe COPD, chronic hypoxemia, and CO_2 retention, the patient was not a good candidate for extubation while deeply anesthetized. A systematic approach for emergence and extubation is illustrated in Fig. 1.7. However, the guidelines do not include all possible patient-surgical-anesthetic conditions. Certainly the practitioner's clinical judgment is of utmost importance in the decision about whether to extubate the patient.

Lien CA, Koff H, Malhotra V, et al. Emergence and extubation: a systemic approach. *Anesth Analg* 1997;85:1177.

Miller KH, Harkin CP, Bailey PL. Postoperative tracheal extubation. *Anesth Analg* 1995; 80:148–172.

D.2. When the patient cannot be extubated early in the recovery room, how would you keep the endotracheal tube in place without causing bronchoconstriction?

Loading doses of lidocaine or aminophylline, followed by continuous infusion, as described in the sections C.6 and C.15, may be administered intravenously to prevent bronchoconstriction induced by stimulation of the endotracheal tube. β_2-Agonists such as albuterol may be administered

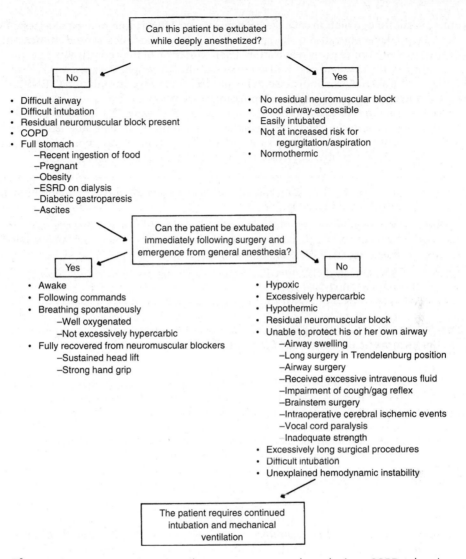

Figure 1.7 A systemic approach to emergence and extubation. COPD, chronic obstructive pulmonary disease; ESRD, end-stage renal disease.

through MDI adapter to prevent bronchospasm. Alternatively, an LMA may be used to replace the endotracheal tube for control of ventilation and to avoid tracheal stimulation.

Barash PG, Cullen BF, Stoelting RK, eds. *Clinical anesthesia*, 5th ed. Philadelphia: Lippincott Williams & Wilkins, 2006:604–605.

D.3. In asthmatic patients, are narcotics contraindicated for postoperative pain control?

Narcotics should be used very carefully because prolonged respiratory depression may further compromise the airway. Morphine is avoided because of possible histamine release and increased central vagal tone, which may cause bronchospasm. Meperidine may be a better choice for postoperative analgesia because of its spasmolytic action. Narcotics should be titrated carefully to control pain and not depress respiration. Poor pain control may compromise respiration because of splinting of the thoracic cage and decreased ability to cough. Paravertebral or intercostal nerve blocks, epidural analgesia, or transcutaneous electrical nerve stimulation (TENS) may be used to control postoperative pain without depressing respiration.

NSAIDs precipitate acute bronchospasm in an estimated 8% to 20% of adult asthmatics. NSAIDs block the cyclooxygenase-mediated conversion of arachidonic acid to prostaglandins, thereby shunting arachidonic acid toward the formation of bronchoconstrictor leukotrienes. Therefore, it may be prudent to avoid NSAIDs for postoperative pain control.

Barash PG, Cullen BF, Stoelting RK, eds. *Clinical anesthesia*, 5th ed. Philadelphia: Lippincott Williams & Wilkins, 2006:358–361.

Marsh HM. Anesthesia for patients with chronic pulmonary disease. In: Hershey SG, ed. *ASA refresher courses in anesthesiology*. Park Ridge, IL: American Society of Anesthesiologists, 1984:133.

Stoelting RK, Dierdorf SF. *Anesthesia and co-existing disease*, 4th ed. New York: Churchill Livingstone, 2002:197, 201.

D.4. The patient was breathing well and was extubated. How much oxygen would you give to this asthmatic patient with COPD in the recovery room?

Forty percent oxygen by mask is usually used postoperatively in the recovery room. However, for a small proportion of patients with COPD, the hypoxic drive might be taken away by increased FIO_2. Moreover, oxygen therapy may abolish hypoxic pulmonary vasoconstriction in poorly ventilated areas, increasing blood flow to these areas and so decreasing blood flow to other lung regions with normal or high ventilation/perfusion ratios. These regions will then contribute to alveolar dead space and thereby cause an increase in $Paco_2$. It is important to monitor the patient's respiration, oxygenation, and $Paco_2$ very carefully during oxygen therapy. Venturi masks with FIO_2 of 0.24 to 0.4 may be used for patients with COPD. Nevertheless, adequate oxygen concentration must be used in the presence of hypoxemia. Hypoventilation can be assisted or controlled by artificial ventilation.

Lumb AB. *Nunn's applied respiratory physiology*, 6th ed. Philadelphia: Elsevier Butterworth-Heinemann, 2005:191, 381.

CHAPTER 2

Bronchoscopy, Mediastinoscopy, and Thoracotomy

ALESSIA PEDOTO • PAUL M. HEERDT • FUN-SUN F. YAO

A 60-YEAR-OLD MAN

has suffered from cough, intermittent hemoptysis, and weight loss for 2 months. He has been smoking one pack of cigarettes per day for 40 years. A chest x-ray 1 month ago revealed a right middle lobe infiltrate that was treated with antibiotics, without improvement. Subsequent evaluation revealed a carcinoma. He is now scheduled for fiberoptic bronchoscopy (FOB), mediastinoscopy, and possible thoracotomy for lobectomy or pneumonectomy.

A. Medical Disease and Differential Diagnosis

1. How are lung carcinomas diagnosed, and what is your prediction for the most likely type of malignancy?
2. What are the less common manifestations of bronchogenic carcinoma?
3. The patient has a long history of cigarette smoking. What is the significance of this finding?

B. Preoperative Evaluation and Preparation

1. How would you evaluate the patient preoperatively?
2. What are the pulmonary function guidelines that indicate increased risk of morbidity and mortality?

C. Intraoperative Management

1. How would you premedicate, monitor, and anesthetize this patient?
2. How many types of bronchoscopes are available and what are the intraoperative considerations of each?
3. What are the indications for mediastinoscopy? Are there potential complications?
4. The decision was made to proceed with thoracotomy and right middle lobectomy. How would you alter your management?
5. What are the indications for one-lung ventilation (OLV) and how can it be accomplished?

6. What are the contraindications to the use of double-lumen endotracheal tubes (ETTs)?

7. Would you use a right- or left-sided double-lumen tube (DLT)?

8. How do you know that the tube is in correct position?

9. How many types of bronchial blockers are available? What are the advantages and disadvantages of bronchial blockers?

10. How will systemic oxygenation be monitored during OLV? What is the mechanism of oxymetry?

11. The patient was placed in the lateral decubitus position for thoracotomy. Describe the effects of lateral positioning on pulmonary blood flow and respiration.

12. What is hypoxic pulmonary vasoconstriction (HPV)?

13. What are the effects of anesthetic agents on HPV and what are their clinical implications?

14. Discuss pulmonary blood flow distribution, shunt flow, and PaO_2 ($FIO_2 = 1.0$) during OLV.

15. How could you improve oxygenation during OLV?

16. Right middle lobectomy was performed. Would you extubate the trachea at the end of the procedure?

D. Postoperative Management

1. What are the immediate life-threatening complications that follow lobectomy or pneumonectomy?

2. Why is it important to control postoperative pain? How would you achieve this?

A. Medical Disease and Differential Diagnosis

A.1. How are lung carcinomas diagnosed, and what is your prediction for the most likely type of malignancy?

Symptoms of nonproductive cough and hemoptysis, along with unresolved lung infiltrate, usually suggest carcinoma. The diagnosis and extent of the disease are confirmed with sputum cytology, bronchoscopy and brush biopsy, biopsy of palpable lymph nodes in the neck or axilla, needle aspiration biopsy, mediastinoscopy, and possibly exploratory thoracotomy. Prior to thoracotomy, an extensive work up is aimed to diagnose metastases that would contraindicate surgery.

Cancers of the lung comprise 16% of all malignancies and account for approximately 30% of cancer deaths worldwide. *Bronchogenic carcinomas* comprise the vast majority of lung cancers presenting for surgical resection and can be classified into four major types: small cell, large cell, squamous cell, and adenocarcinoma. For surgical purposes, small cell tumors are kept distinct and the others grouped into a "non–small cell" category. In general, non–small cell carcinomas are amenable to surgical resection whereas small cell tumors tend to be nonresectable and are treated medically. Further subclassification of tumors involves the TNM system where T represents tumor site, size, and local extent; N represents presence and location of regional lymph node involvement; and M represents presence of distal metastases beyond the ipsilateral hemithorax. The TNM classification is used in the staging of bronchogenic carcinomas and helps predict response to therapy. In general, small cell carcinomas that spread beyond the bounds of possible resection by the time of presentation are primarily managed with chemotherapy, with or without radiation. The 5-year survival after chemotherapy and radiation is approximately 3% to 8%. In contrast, non–small cell cancers found to be localized at the time of presentation should be considered for resection. The 5-year survival after primary resection is dependent on tumor staging, but can be as high as 85% for small tumors without regional lymph node involvement or metastases (stage I). Approximately 45% of patients present with circumscribed extrapulmonary extension and/or lymphatic spread to the ipsilateral mediastinal or subcarinal lymph nodes (stage IIIA) and exhibit a 5-year postresection survival of less than 20%.

Kasper DL, Braunwald E, Fauci AS, et al. eds. *Harrison's principles of internal medicine*, 16th ed. New York: McGraw-Hill, 2005:506–515.

Shibutani HC. Pulmonary resection. In: Youngberg JA, Lake CL, Wilson RS, eds. *Cardiac, vascular and thoracic anesthesia*. New York: Churchill Livingstone, 2000:639–659.

A.2. What are the less common manifestations of bronchogenic carcinoma?

Other manifestations of lung tumors are primarily related to mass effects or altered metabolism. In addition to bronchial obstruction (evident in this patient), mass effects include invasion into the chest wall, compression of great vessels (e.g., superior vena cava syndrome), tracheobronchial displacement, paresis of the recurrent laryngeal or phrenic nerves, and Pancoast's syndrome (pain and upper extremity weakness secondary to invasion of the brachial plexus, first and second thoracic and eighth cervical nerve roots). Recognized metabolic manifestations of lung tumors include symptoms that resemble those of myasthenia gravis, peripheral neuritis involving both motor and sensory components, Cushing's syndrome, carcinoid syndrome, hypercalcemia and hypophosphatemia (from ectopic secretion of parathyroid hormone [PTH]/PTH-related peptide by epidermoid cancer), hypokalemia (from ectopic secretion of adrenocorticotropic hormone [ACTH] by small cell cancer), and hyponatremia (from inappropriate secretion of antidiuretic hormone or possibly atrial natriuretic factor by small cell cancer).

Kasper DL, Braunwald E, Fauci AS, et al. eds. *Harrison's principles of internal medicine*, 16th ed. New York: McGraw-Hill, 2005:508–509.

Slinger PD, Johnston MR. Preoperative assessment for pulmonary resection. *J Cardiothorac Vasc Anesth* 2000; 14:202–211.

Wirtz PW, Wintzen AR, Verschuuren JJ. Lambert-Eaton myasthenic syndrome has a more progressive course in patients with lung cancer. *Muscle Nerve* 2005; 32(2):226–229.

A.3. The patient has a long history of cigarette smoking. What is the significance of this finding?

Cigarette smoking promotes the development of chronic obstructive pulmonary disease (COPD), which includes chronic bronchitis and emphysema. Evidence of chronic changes can be found in preoperative pulmonary function testing. Pulmonary hypertension and cor pulmonale are also more common in this patient population. Patients who continue to smoke until surgery are at greater risk for postoperative pulmonary complications such as atelectasis and hypoxemia. Although carboxyhemoglobin concentrations decline substantially within 12 hours of smoking cessation, it remains unclear as to how long smoking must be discontinued to see a significant reduction of post-thoracotomy complications. In cardiac surgery patients, smoking must be discontinued for 2 months before an impact upon postoperative pulmonary function, mainly related to improved mucociliary function.

Licker MJ, Widikker I, Robert J, et al. Operative mortality and respiratory complications after lung resection for cancer: impact of chronic obstructive pulmonary disease and time trends. *Ann Thorac Surg* 2006;81(5):1830–1837.

Slinger PD, Johnston MR. Preoperative assessment for pulmonary resection. *J Cardiothorac Vasc Anesth* 2000;14:202–211.

Tisi GM. Preoperative evaluation of pulmonary function: validity, indications, and benefits. *Am Rev Respir Dis* 1979;119:293.

B. Preoperative Evaluation and Preparation

B.1. How would you evaluate the patient preoperatively?

Preoperative evaluation should include a complete history, physical examination, and laboratory tests (e.g., complete blood count, SMA7, coagulation as well as electrocardiogram and chest x-ray). A history of smoking, cough, sputum production, orthopnea, and dyspnea are hallmarks of cardiopulmonary disease and should be further investigated. Abnormal exercise tolerance (such as inability to climb at least three flights of stairs) can be helpful in anticipating the patient's response to the stress of anesthesia and surgery. Most patients are admitted to the hospital on the day of surgery. A brief review of symptoms, physical limitations, interval changes, and airway anatomy should be performed at this time.

In addition to routine electrocardiogram and blood analysis, patients should have preoperative pulmonary function testing to help define the relative risks for the magnitude of planned resection. Respiratory function can be assessed using the following parameters:

- *Respiratory mechanics.* Forced vital capacity (FVC), forced expiratory volume in the first second (FEV_1), maximum voluntary ventilation (MVV), and the residual volume (RV)/total lung capacity (TLC) ratio
- *Cardiopulmonary reserve.* Maximal oxygen uptake (Vo_2max), stair climbing, 6-minute walk
- *Lung parenchymal function.* Diffusing capacity (DLCO) and arterial Pao_2 and $Paco_2$

Datta D, Lahiri B. Preoperative evaluation of patients undergoing lung resection surgery. *Chest* 2003; 123:2096–2103.

Slinger PD, Johnston MR. Preoperative assessment for pulmonary resection. *J Cardiothorac Vasc Anesth* 2000; 14:202–211.

B.2. What are the pulmonary function guidelines that indicate increased risk of morbidity and mortality?

The reported mortality from lung resection is between 2% and 4%, mainly due to pneumonia, respiratory failure, bronchopleural fistula, empyema, and pulmonary embolism. Respiratory insufficiency occurs in approximately 5% of patients following lung resection, which is associated with a 50% mortality rate. Advanced age and a relatively high incidence of concomitant nonpulmonary disease seem to contribute to this outcome. An increased risk of postoperative complications can be predicted by the following parameters:

Spirometry

- FVC less than 50% of predicted value
- FEV_1 less than 50% of FVC or 2 L
- MVV less than 50% of predicted value or 50 L per minute
- Diffusion capacity less than 50% of predicted value
- RV/TLC greater than 50%

Table 2.1   Minimal Pulmonary Function Test Criteria for Various-Sized Pulmonary Resections.

TEST	UNIT	NORMAL	PNEUMONECTOMY	LOBECTOMY	BIOPSY OR SEGMENTAL
MBC	Liters/minute (L/min)	>100	>50	>40	>25
MBC	Percentage (%) predicted	100	>50	>40	>25
FEV_1	Liters (L)	>4	>2.1–1.7	>1.2–1.0	>0.6–0.9
FEV_1	Percentage (%)	>80% FVC	>50% FVC	>40% FVC	>40% FVC
$FEV_{25\%-75\%}$	Liters (L)	>2	>1.6	>0.6–1.6	>0.6

FEV_1, forced expiratory volume in the first second; $FEV_{25\%-75\%}$, forced expiratory volume from 25% to 75% of forced vital capacity; MBC, maximum breathing capacity.

Arterial Blood Gases

- $PaCO_2$ greater than 45 mm Hg
- PaO_2 less than 50 mm Hg

In addition, the location of the tumor, the extent of the proposed resection and the presence of preoperative induction chemotherapy seem to be associated with further risks (Table 2.1). Better preoperative evaluation and care has contributed to improved outcome, especially in patients with severe emphysematous disease undergoing lung volume reduction surgery (i.e. $FEV_1 < 1$/min). The development of minimally invasive techniques for pulmonary resection-including pneumonectomy - has helped lessen perioperative morbidity and mortality. Therefore, the evaluation of risk factors for pulmonary resection has changed with time. Pulmonary function tests are valid indices of physiologic performance, but the actual predictive use of a range of values for a single parameter is poorly defined. Emphasis has now been directed toward the integration of various aspect of preoperative evaluation (e.g. respirometry, ventilation-perfusion scanning, and the extent of planned resection) to estimate postoperative function. With this technique, the utility of FEV_1 as a predictor of pulmonary complications is substantially improved. Patients shown to have a predicted postoperative FEV_1 less than 40% of the predicted value are now considered to be at increased risk for the more sophisticated regimen of thrombosis prophylaxis of postoperative complications. Even so, continuing refinements of intraoperative and postoperative management, the use of goal-specific analgesia techniques, and more sophisticated thrombosis prevention regimens have probably attenuated the incidence of complications in the high-risk group.

Hartigan PM, Pedoto A. Anesthetic considerations for lung volume reduction surgery and lung transplantation. *Thorac Surg Clin* 2005;15(1):143–157.

Matsubara Y, Takeda S, Mashimo T. Risk stratification for lung cancer surgery: impact of induction therapy and extended resection. *Chest* 2005;128(5):3519–3525.

Miller RD, ed. *Miller's anesthesia*, 5th ed. New York: Churchill Livingstone, 2005:1853.

Slinger PD, Johnston MR. Preoperative evaluation of the thoracic surgery patient. In: Kaplan JA, Slinger PD, eds. *Thoracic anesthesia*, 3rd ed. Philadelphia: Churchill Livingstone, 2003:1–23.

Tisi GM. Preoperative evaluation of pulmonary function: validity, indications, and benefits. *Am Rev Respir Dis* 1979;119:293.

Triantafillou AN. Anesthetic management for bilateral volume reduction surgery. *Semin Thorac Cardiovasc Surg* 1996;8(1):94–98.

C. Intraoperative Management

C.1. How would you premedicate, monitor, and anesthetize this patient?

Current practice at most institutions dictates that patients arrive at the hospital the day of surgery, thereby rendering largely obsolete the traditional oral or parenteral premedication before transport to the operating suite. Bronchoscopy and mediastinoscopy are generally ambulatory procedures, necessitating relatively rapid hospital discharge. Because bronchoscopy followed by mediastinoscopy and thoracotomy in this patient is only a possibility, intravenous midazolam immediately upon entry into the operating room is sufficient for anxiolysis and subsequent amnesia. In addition, a small intravenous dose (0.2 mg) of glycopyrrolate can be useful as an antisialagogue, particularly in patients who smoke. However, the potential of tachycardia should be considered, especially in patients with coronary artery disease (CAD) or atrial fibrillation.

During mediastinoscopy, intermittent compression or occlusion of the innominate artery can occur. The blood pressure cuff should, therefore, be placed on the left arm and the pulse oximeter on the right hand. In case of innominate artery compression, a dampening of the pulse oximetry trace will be evident while blood pressure measurements remain accurate. Finally, along with the electrocardiogram (ECG), temperature should be monitored and a warming blanket applied; despite the potential for a short procedure, elderly patients, in particular, can become hypothermic. Induction, maintenance of anesthesia, and muscle relaxation can be achieved with relatively short-acting agents. Propofol is usually used for induction followed by rocuronium, vecuronium, or cisatracurium to facilitate tracheal intubation through a single-lumen ETT. Anesthesia is maintained with a potent inhalational agent in oxygen/air, if oxygen saturation tolerates it, and 3 to 4 μg per kg of fentanyl often provides sufficient analgesia for the procedure. In addition, a local anesthetic can be infiltrated in the wound. Many clinicians choose to avoid nitrous oxide because of the potential for the mediastinoscope to enter the pleural space and create a pneumothorax.

Ehrenwerth J, Brull SJ. Anesthesia for thoracic diagnostic procedures. In: Kaplan JA, Slinger PD, eds. *Thoracic anesthesia*, 3rd ed. Philadelphia: Churchill Livingstone, 2003: 174–195.

Molins L, Fibla JJ, Perez J, et al. Outpatient thoracic surgical programme in 300 patients: clinical results and economic impact. *Eur J Cardiothorac Surg* 2006;29(3):271–275.

Wilson RS. Anesthesia for bronchoscopy and mediastinoscopy. In: Youngberg JA, Lake CL, Wilson RS, eds. *Cardiac, vascular and thoracic anesthesia*. New York: Churchill Livingstone, 2000:660–669.

C.2. How many types of bronchoscopes are available and what are the intraoperative considerations of each one?

There are three types of bronchoscopes currently in use: flexible fiberoptic, rigid ventilating, and rigid venturi.

The flexible *FOB* can be used in sedated patients either under local anesthesia (allowing examination of vocal cords movements), or under general anesthesia with laryngeal mask airway

(LMA) or endotracheal intubation. For awake sedated examination, local anesthesia of the upper airway can be accomplished by gargling 4% viscous lidocaine. Lower airway anesthesia can be produced with 4% lidocaine administered through an atomizer with a long nozzle or a nebulizer mask. Bilateral superior laryngeal nerve blocks and/or transtracheal block can be added. Intravenous sedation is supplemented with 0.5-mg increments of midazolam and/or 10 μg of remifentanyl boluses, until the patient is calm and cooperative but not obtunded. If the oropharynx is adequately anesthetized, an LMA can be inserted without discomfort and used to assist ventilation and provide higher F_{IO_2} concentrations.

In contrast, rigid bronchoscopy usually necessitates general anesthesia and muscle relaxation to avoid coughing or moving, which could cause tracheal trauma. The *rigid ventilating bronchoscope* has a side-arm adapter that can be attached to the anesthesia machine. A variable air leak usually exists around the bronchoscope, so high flow rates of inspired gases and/or packing of the oropharynx are needed. Volatile anesthetics can leak and contaminate the operating room, therefore total IV anesthesia is a valid alternative.

The *rigid Venturi-effect bronchoscope* relies on an intermittent (10 to 12 times/minute) high-pressure oxygen jet to entrain air and insufflate the lungs. The jet is delivered through a reducing valve into a 16- or 18-gauge needle inside and parallel to the lumen. Major disadvantages of this bronchoscope are lack of control of the inspired oxygen concentration and inability to administer inhaled anesthetics. Accordingly, anesthesia must be maintained by intravenous techniques.

Bronchoscopic procedures can be relatively short, therefore continuous succinylcholine infusion still remains an option. If not contraindicated, mivacurium is also a valid alternative for muscle relaxation. When followed by another procedure (such as the mediastinoscopy scheduled for this patient), an intermediate duration nondepolarizing muscle relaxant is often desirable.

Ehrenwerth J, Brull SJ. Anesthesia for thoracic diagnostic procedures. In: Kaplan JA, Slinger PD, eds. *Thoracic anesthesia*, 3rd ed. Philadelphia: Churchill Livingstone, 2003: 174–195.

Wilson RS. Anesthesia for bronchoscopy and mediastinoscopy. In: Youngberg JA, Lake CL, Wilson RS, eds. *Cardiac, vascular and thoracic anesthesia*. New York: Churchill Livingstone, 2000:660–669.

C.3. What are the indications for mediastinoscopy? Are there potential complications?

Mediastinoscopy is usually performed to establish diagnosis of specific lesions within the mediastinum or as a staging procedure for malignancy to determine mediastinal lymph node spread. If lymph nodes are positive for malignancy on frozen section, the patient is probably not a candidate for surgery and the planned lung resection is aborted.

Conventional cervical mediastinoscopy involves a small incision at the sternal notch for introduction of the scope and sampling of lymph nodes within the mediastinum. The pleural space is generally not entered intentionally and therefore, a chest tube is not indicated. However, occult pneumothorax can occur. Examination of the intrapleural space can be performed either with a mediastinoscope inserted through an extension of a cervical incision or through a small anterior thoracotomy. In this case, the chest may be evacuated through a catheter after closure or after a chest tube is inserted. Complications during mediastinoscopy are relatively rare (1% to 2%) and generally result from nerve injury (recurrent laryngeal or phrenic) or trauma to adjacent structures (pleura, trachea, esophagus, superior vena cava, azygous vein innominate artery, pulmonary artery, and aorta). Should a major vascular structure be perforated, blood loss can be rapid and profound, necessitating emergent sternotomy. Because packing or vascular clamps may be applied to the superior vena cava, clinicians should always have a plan for establishing venous access in the lower extremity.

Ehrenwerth J, Brull SJ. Anesthesia for thoracic diagnostic procedures. In: Kaplan JA, Slinger PD, eds. *Thoracic anesthesia*, 3rd ed. Philadelphia: Churchill Livingstone, 2003: 174–195.

Wilson RS. Anesthesia for bronchoscopy and mediastinoscopy. In: Youngberg JA, Lake CL, Wilson RS, eds. *Cardiac, vascular and thoracic anesthesia*. New York: Churchill Livingstone, 2000:660–669.

C.4. The decision was made to proceed with thoracotomy and right middle lobectomy. How would you alter your management?

Although not uniformly regarded as necessary for lung resection, an arterial catheter will be placed in the left (dependent) radial artery and the single-lumen ETT replaced with a left-sided double-lumen tube. Although right middle lobectomy is not an absolute indication for lung isolation, this has become common practice because of improved surgical exposure. Nonetheless, OLV is associated with certain disadvantages and complications. The most notable is the large and variable alveolar-to-arterial oxygen tension difference (P_{AO_2}–Pa_{O_2}) that occurs as a result of continued perfusion to the nondependent, nonventilated lung. The incidence of severe hypoxemia and hypercarbia, however, is relatively small and primarily results from incorrect positioning of the DLT. Other complications include traumatic laryngitis and tracheobronchial rupture.

Brodsky JB, Fitzmaurice B. Modern anesthetic techniques for thoracic operations. *World J Surg* 2001; 25(2):162–166.

Campos JA. Lung separation techniques. In: Kaplan JA, Slinger PD, eds. *Thoracic anesthesia*, 3rd ed. Philadelphia: Churchill Livingstone, 2003:159–173.

Shibutani HC. Pulmonary resection. In: Youngberg JA, Lake CL, Wilson RS, eds. *Cardiac, vascular and thoracic anesthesia*. New York: Churchill Livingstone, 2000:639–659.

C.5. What are the indications for OLV and how can it be accomplished?

Absolute Indications

- Isolation from spillage or contamination
  - Infection—bronchiectasis and lung abscess
  - Massive hemorrhage
- To control the distribution of ventilation
  - Bronchopleural fistula
  - Bronchopleural cutaneous fistula
  - Giant unilateral lung cyst or bulla
  - Tracheobronchial tree disruption/trauma
  - Surgical procedures on major conducting airway
  - Life-threatening hypoxemia due to unilateral lung disease
  - Unilateral bronchopulmonary lavage (pulmonary alveolar proteinosis)
- To facilitate surgical exposure
  - Video and robotic-assisted thoracoscopic surgery (VATS)

Relative Indications

- Facilitation of surgical exposure—high priority
  - Thoracic aortic aneurysm
  - Pneumonectomy
  - Upper lobectomy
  - Mediastinal exposure
  - Pulmonary resection through median sternotomy
- Facilitation of surgical exposure—low priority
  - Esophageal resection
  - Middle and lower lobectomies and segmental resection
  - Procedures on the thoracic spine
- Post–cardiopulmonary bypass status after removal of totally occluding chronic unilateral pulmonary emboli
- Severe hypoxemia due to unilateral lung disease

Several techniques can be used to provide OLV: conventional ETTs passed endobronchially, special single-lumen ETTs with incorporated bronchial blocking catheters (Univent endotracheal tube), bronchial blocking catheters passed outside or inside the ETT, and double-lumen endobronchial tubes. Currently, the use of DLTs remains the most common method for achieving lung isolation. Although DLTs of variant design and material have been used clinically (e.g., Robertshaw, Carlens, and White), the models most commonly used now are disposable and are made of polyvinylchloride (PVC). Such a tube was chosen for this procedure. Double-lumen ETTs are available in five sizes: 28, 35, 37, 39, and 41 French catheter gauge (size in French equals 3.14 times external diameter in millimeters or 4 times the internal diameter plus 2). Choosing the size of a DLT is an important step in decreasing the likelihood of airway trauma or malposition. Although there is a general rule that average-sized men usually accommodate a No. 39 ETT and average-sized women a No. 37 ETT, there is apparently no clear correlation between age, height, weight, and DLT size. A variety of techniques have been described on the basis of measurements of airway size derived from radiographic or computed tomographic (CT) imaging, but these have been questioned across gender and ethnic lines. Ultimately, a properly sized DLT should pass atraumatically through the glottis, advance easily into the trachea and bronchus, and exhibit any air leak when the bronchial cuff is deflated.

Campos JA. Lung separation techniques. In: Kaplan JA, Slinger PD, eds. *Thoracic anesthesia*, 3rd ed. Philadelphia: Churchill Livingstone, 2003:159–173.

Miller RD, ed. *Miller's anesthesia*, 5th ed. New York: Churchill Livingstone, 2005:1873–1875.

Slinger PD. Lung isolation. In: Youngberg JA, Lake CL, Wilson RS, eds. *Cardiac, vascular and thoracic anesthesia*. New York: Churchill Livingstone, 2000:660–669.

C.6. What are the contraindications to the use of double-lumen ETTs?

Placement of a double-lumen ETT should be carefully considered in the following situations:

- Patients whose upper airway anatomy may preclude safe insertion of the tube (recessed jaw, prominent teeth, bull neck, anterior larynx)
- Patients with lesions present somewhere along the pathway of the tube that could be traumatized such as airway stricture or endoluminal tumors
- Small patients for whom a 35 French tube is too large to fit comfortably through the larynx and a 28 French tube is considered too small

- Critically ill patients who have a single-lumen tube already in place and who cannot tolerate cessation of mechanical ventilation and positive end-expiratory pressure (PEEP) ventilation for a short period of time

Under these circumstances, OLV can be achieved through an endobronchial blocker or endobronchial tube placed into a mainstem bronchus.

Brodsky JB, Fitzmaurice B. Modern anesthetic techniques for thoracic operations. *World J Surg* 2001; 25(2)**:**162–166.

Campos JA. Lung separation techniques. In: Kaplan JA, Slinger PD, eds. *Thoracic anesthesia*, 3rd ed. Philadelphia: Churchill Livingstone, 2003:159–173.

Miller RD, ed. *Miller's anesthesia*, 5th ed. New York: Churchill Livingstone, 2005:1883.

Slinger PD. Lung isolation. In: Youngberg JA, Lake CL, Wilson RS, eds. *Cardiac, vascular and thoracic anesthesia*. New York: Churchill Livingstone, 2000:660–669.

C.7. Would you use a right- or left-sided DLT?

A left-sided DLT is preferable for most procedures because the origin of the right upper lobe (RUL) approximately 0.5 to 1.0 cm below the carina complicates placement of a right-sided tube. The left mainstem bronchus is much longer than the right one (approximately 50–55 mm vs. 15–20 mm), thereby providing a greater margin for error in positioning. A right-sided DLT is indicated in case of large exophytic lesions within the left mainstem bronchial, tight left mainstem bronchus stenosis, distortion of the left mainstem bronchus by an adjacent tumor or a thoracoabdominal aneurysm, and tracheobronchial disruption. Relative indications are left pneumonectomy or lung transplantation because the surgical field is not encumbered by a "foreign body" that could be included into the staple line. At the end of the procedure, the stump or bronchial anastomosis can be protected from positive pressure ventilation. Right DLTs are contraindicated in case of anomalous takeoff of the right upper bronchus above tracheal carina.

Brodsky JB, Fitzmaurice B. Modern anesthetic techniques for thoracic operations. *World J Surg* 2001;25(2):162–166.

Campos JA. Lung separation techniques. In: Kaplan JA, Slinger PD, eds. *Thoracic anesthesia*, 3rd ed. Philadelphia: Churchill Livingstone, 2003:159–173.

Slinger PD. Lung isolation. In: Youngberg JA, Lake CL, Wilson RS, eds. *Cardiac, vascular and thoracic anesthesia*. New York: Churchill Livingstone, 2000:660–669.

C.8. How do you know that the tube is in the correct position?

The DLT position may be confirmed by listening to breath sounds of each lung while clamping each lumen of the DLT. However, in emphysematous patients breath sounds may be decreased, making auscultation difficult and unreliable; therefore, FOB is often helpful before placing the patient in lateral decubitus position. During bronchoscopy, the tracheal cartilaginous rings are anterior and the tracheal membrane is posterior. Therefore, the right and left sides can be discerned by the relation of the mainstem bronchi to the anterior cartilaginous ring and the posterior membrane (Fig. 2.1A). In addition, looking for the RUL takeoff (which usually arises from the lateral aspect of right mainstem bronchus just below the tracheal carina) is a useful landmark when the airway anatomy has been obscured by bleeding, edema, or radiation-induced changes, or it has been distorted by extrinsic compression. Left DLT position and depth are confirmed by inserting the FOB in the tracheal lumen. The entire right mainstem bronchus

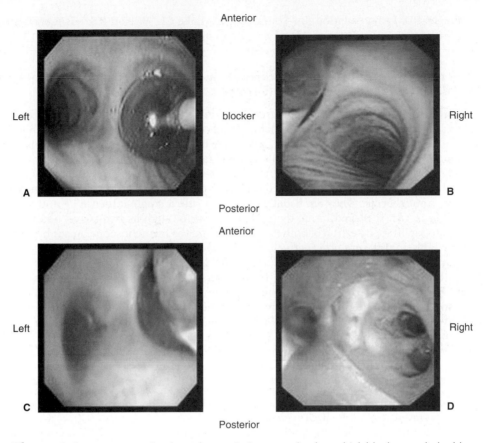

Figure 2.1 Representative bronchoscopic images of a bronchial blocker and double-lumen endotracheal tube placement. **A:** Depicts normal tracheal anatomy with cartilaginous rings anteriorly and membranous trachea posteriorly; this helps define left versus right sides. A bronchial blocking catheter is seen in the right main bronchus. **B:** Depicts placement of a left-sided double-lumen tube; upper portion of endobronchial cuff is evident as is the orifice of the right upper lobe just below the tracheal carina. **C:** Depicts placement of a right-sided double-lumen tube; the upper portion of the endobronchial cuff is evident. **D:** Depicts the orifice of the right upper lobe visualized through the port on the lateral aspect of a right-sided double-lumen tube.

should be visible and the tracheal lumen orifice should be 1 to 2 cm above the tracheal carina. When properly positioned, the upper surface of the blue endobronchial cuff is visualized just below the tracheal carina in the left mainstem bronchus (Fig. 2.1B). If a right DLT is used, correct positioning is confirmed both by visualization of the bronchial cuff in the right main bronchus (Fig. 2.1C) and by visualization of the RUL orifice through a port on the lateral surface of the DLT (Fig. 2.1D). For both left and right tubes, the bronchoscope should also be inserted in the bronchial lumen to evaluate the distance between the tip of the tube and distal bifurcation of the bronchus. Position should be reconfirmed after the patient is laterally positioned.

Campos JA. Lung separation techniques. In: Kaplan JA, Slinger PD, eds. *Thoracic anesthesia*, 3rd ed. Philadelphia: Churchill Livingstone, 2003:159–173.

Slinger PD. Lung isolation. In: Youngberg JA, Lake CL, Wilson RS, eds. *Cardiac, vascular and thoracic anesthesia*. New York: Churchill Livingstone, 2000:660–669.

C.9. How many types of bronchial blockers are available? What are the advantages and disadvantages of bronchial blockers?

The bronchial blockers most often used for adults are the Fogarty occlusion catheter or the Arndt catheter (wire-guided endobronchial blocker). Fogarty catheters come with either a 12- or a 20-mL high pressure, low volume balloon in both latex and nonlatex models. They have a metallic stylet that can be bent into shape to facilitate endobronchial placement. In case of dislodgment, the stylet can be reinserted and the blocker repositioned. Fogarty catheters have no communicating central channel, therefore continuous positive airway pressure (CPAP) or suction cannot occur. They are usually placed outside a single-lumen ETT and positioned with FOB (Fig. 2.1A). If placed inside the ETT, a connector such as two swivel adaptors in series is needed to facilitate insertion of both the catheter and the bronchoscope. Arndt bronchial blockers are available in different sizes with elliptical or spherical cuffs (low pressure, high volume), and are particularly advantageous to isolate the RUL. They are usually inserted through the ETT via a three-way connector (catheter, bronchoscopy, ventilation circuit) and are made with a guide suture loop at the tip that can be placed around a bronchoscope to facilitate positioning. This suture loop is then removed, leaving an inner lumen that allows for suctioning, CPAP, or jet ventilation. Other devices made for endobronchial placement of a blocking cuff through a catheter within the ETT include the Univent tube (a blocker built inside an ETT) and the Cohen endobronchial blocker that is similar to the Arndt catheter but includes a device for mechanically moving the catheter tip. In addition, the use of gauze tampons, a Magill balloon-tipped luminal blocker, and Foley catheters have been reported.

Advantages. Bronchial blockers are relatively simple and can be used in children and adults who are too small for DLTs. Also, they can
  * facilitate OLV in patients with a difficult airway or where a DLT is contraindicated;
  * be placed through an existing single-lumen ETT in emergent situations;
  * eliminate the need to change ETTs for postoperative mechanical ventilation.

Disadvantages. In comparison to DLTs, bronchial blockers present
  * inability to suction efficiently or intermittently ventilate the lung distal to the blocker without deflating the balloon;
  * the need for bronchoscopic positioning;
  * difficulty in maintaining position in the right mainstem/isolating the RUL efficiently if the takeoff is close to carina
  * obstruction of the trachea if the bronchial blocker dislodges proximally or bilateral lung ventilation if the cuff is not inflated properly;
  * potential risk of being stapled in the bronchial stump if not retracted at an appropriate time.

Arndt GA, DeLessio ST, Kranner PW, et al. One-lung ventilation when intubation is difficult—presentation of a new endobronchial blocker. *Acta Anaesthesiol Scand* 1999; 43(3):356–358.

Campos JH. An update on bronchial blockers during lung separation techniques in adults. *Anesth Analg* 2003;97:1266–1274.

Ginsberg RJ. New technique for one-lung anesthesia using an endobronchial blocker. *J Thorac Cardiovasc Surg* 1981;82(4):542–546.

Miller RD. *Miller's anesthesia*, 5th ed. New York: Churchill Livingstone, 2005:1853.

Slinger PD. Lung isolation. In: Youngberg JA, Lake CL, Wilson RS, eds. *Cardiac, vascular and thoracic anesthesia*. New York: Churchill Livingstone, 2000:660–669.

C.10. How will systemic oxygenation be monitored during OLV? What is the mechanism of oxymetry?

Pulse oximetry has become the hallmark for monitoring arterial oxygenation during lung resection, decreasing the need for repeated measurements of arterial blood gases. This technique uses spectrophotoelectric oximetric principles to determine oxygen saturation. Pulse oximeters are multiple wavelength plethysmographs. The amplitude of the pulse is a function of arterial distension, hemoglobin oxygen saturation of arterial blood inflow, and light wavelength. Hemoglobin saturation in the arterial blood is the result of the ratio between the pulse amplitude of red (660 nm = deoxyhemoglobin) and infrared light (940 nm = oxyhemoglobin). Because pulsatile waveform is a characteristic of arterial blood flow, there is no interference from surrounding venous blood, skin, connective tissue, or bone. Arterial pulsations cause changes in light absorption, which are used to calculate oxygen saturation. Adequate finger pulsation is generally lost with hypothermia of a few degrees, hypotension (mean blood pressure <50 mm Hg), and infusion of vasoconstrictive drugs. Dyshemoglobinemias (such as carboxyhemoglobin, methemoglobin, and sulfhemoglobin) and intravenous dye injection can also affect the oximeter accuracy.

Other methods include transcutaneous oxygen tension ($PtcO_2$) and arterial oxygen tension using an indwelling electrode. $PtcO_2$ requires special site preparation, airtight probe mantling, and a potentially harmful local source of heat to induce arterialization. Moreover, $PtcO_2$ fails to perfectly reflect true arterial oxygenation. An indwelling arterial oxygen electrode is inserted into the arterial line and may increase the incidence of thromboembolism.

Brodsky JB, Fitzmaurice B. Modern anesthetic techniques for thoracic operations. *World J Surg* 2001;25(2):162–166.

Tremper KK, Barker SJ. Pulse oximetry. *Anesthesiology* 1989;70:98–108.

C.11. The patient was placed in the lateral decubitus position for thoracotomy. Describe the effects of lateral positioning on pulmonary blood flow and respiration.

In both upright and supine positions, the right lung receives approximately 55% of the total blood flow, whereas the left lung receives the remaining 45%. Gravity causes a vertical gradient in the distribution of blood flow in the lateral decubitus. Therefore, blood flow to the dependent lung is significantly greater than that to the nondependent lung. When the right lung is nondependent, it receives 45% of the total blood flow, whereas 55% perfuses the dependent left lung. When the left lung is nondependent, it receives 35% of the total blood flow, whereas the dependent right lung receives 65%. Therefore, the average blood flow of the nondependent lung is approximately 40% of the total blood flow, whereas the dependent lung is perfused with the remaining 60%.

Respiratory effects

Lateral decubitus position causes mechanical interference with chest wall movement, decreasing lung expansion. The dependent chest wall is constricted by the operating room table, and lateral movements are limited by the bolsters or bean-bags used to hold the patient in position. In addition, the increase in intra-abdominal pressure that occurs with general anesthesia, decreases diaphragmatic movements. Mismatching of ventilation and perfusion in the lateral position is the result of (a) gravity, with redistribution of blood flow toward the dependent lung, and (b) compression of the dependent lung by the mediastinum and abdominal contents. In awake, spontaneously breathing subjects the lower (dependent) diaphragm is still able to contract more efficiently, maintaining ventilation to the dependent lung and matching increased perfusion. In contrast, when the patient is anesthetized, with or without paralysis, most ventilation is preferentially switched to the upper lung, because of an increase in compliance in these areas. The preferential ventilation of the upper lung, coupled with greater perfusion of the lower lung, results in an increased degree of ventilation–perfusion mismatch.

Rehder K, Hatch DJ, Sessler AD, et al. The function of each lung of anesthetized and paralyzed man during mechanical ventilation. *Anesthesiology* 1972;37:16.

Shibutani HC. Pulmonary resection. In: Youngberg JA, Lake CL, Wilson RS, eds. *Cardiac, vascular and thoracic anesthesia*. New York: Churchill Livingstone, 2000:639–659.

Walff KE, Aulin I. The regional lung function in the lateral decubitus position during anesthesia and operations. *Acta Anesthesiol Scand* 1972;16:195–205.

C.12. What is HPV?

HPV is an autoregulatory mechanism to prevent ventilation–perfusion mismatch and improve arterial oxygenation. HPV involves a redox-based O_2 sensor within pulmonary artery smooth muscle cells and is triggered by decreased PaO_2 within the lung from low FIO_2, hypoventilation, or atelectasis. The selective increase of vascular resistance in the hypoxic parenchyma diverts blood away to the better-ventilated normoxic lung, decreasing the amount of shunt flow.

Brimioulle S, LeJeune P, Naeije R. Effects of hypoxic pulmonary vasoconstriction on pulmonary gas exchange. *Appl Physiol* 1996; 81(**4**):1535–1543.

Nagendran J, Stewart K, Hoskinson M, et al. An anesthesiologist's guide to hypoxic pulmonary vasoconstriction: implications for managing single-lung anesthesia and atelectasis. *Curr Opin Anaesthesiol* 2006;19(1):34–43.

C.13. What are the effects of anesthetic agents on HPV and what are their clinical implications?

Several clinical studies have failed to demonstrate a decrease in HPV during one-lung ventilation and total intravenous anesthesia (TIVA). Intravenous anesthetics, such as thiopental, ketamine, morphine, and fentanyl, have no direct effect on HPV. In contrast, inhalational anesthetics have been shown to inhibit HPV in a dose-related manner but usually at concentrations much higher than those used clinically. Other nonanesthetic drugs such as β-agonists and antagonists, calcium channel blockers, nitrovasodilators and theophylline may influence the effects of inhalation anesthetics on shunting and arterial oxygenation during OLV.

- The effect of increased shunt on PaO_2 depends on the absolute level of the initial shunt and the inspired oxygen concentration. In practice, almost 100% oxygen is used during OLV. Even when shunt is increased, PaO_2 usually remains well above 100 mm Hg, and oxygen saturation and oxygen content hardly change.
- The direct inhibition of HPV due to inhaled anesthetics can be antagonized by their secondary effects, such as a decrease in cardiac output, mixed venous oxygen tension and pulmonary pressure. All these can intensify HPV in the nondependent lung. Furthermore, the presence of chronic, irreversible disease in the vessels of the nondependent lung may impair HPV response.

- The presence of disease in the dependent lung will decrease the ability of accepting redistribution of blood flow, thereby decreasing the HPV effect of the nondependent lung.
- Surgical interference with blood flow to the nondependent lung also decreases the anesthetic effect on HPV.

Boldt J, Müller M, Uphus D, et al. Cardiorespiratory changes in patients undergoing pulmonary resection using different anesthetic management techniques. *J Cardiothorac Vasc Anesth* 1996;10:854–859.

Nagendran J, Stewart K, Hoskinson M, et al. An anesthesiologist's guide to hypoxic pulmonary vasoconstriction: implications for managing single-lung anesthesia and atelectasis. *Curr Opin Anaesthesiol* 2006;19(1):34–43.

Reid CW, Slinger PD, Lewis S. A comparison of the effects of propofol-alfentanil versus isoflurane anesthesia on arterial oxygenation during one-lung ventilation. *J Cardiothorac Vasc Anesth* 1996;10:860–863.

C.14. Discuss pulmonary blood flow distribution, shunt flow, and PaO_2 ($FIO_2 = 1.0$) during OLV.

When the nondependent lung is collapsed, HPV will increase pulmonary vascular resistance and decrease lung blood flow in this area. If no complicating factors exist, HPV should decrease blood flow to that lung by approximately 50%. Consequently, the nondependent lung should be able to reduce its blood flow from 40% to 20% of the total, and the nondependent/dependent lung blood flow ratio during OLV should be 20%/80%.

In atelactasis, all the blood flow to the nonventilated lung is shunt flow. Therefore, OLV creates an obligatory right-to-left transpulmonary shunt that was not present during two-lung ventilation. If no shunt existed during two-lung ventilation (ignoring the normal 1% to 3% shunt flow due to the bronchial, pleural, and thebesian circulation), an ideal total shunt flow of 20% would be expected during OLV. PaO_2 with fractional inspired O_2 concentration (FIO_2) equal to 1 should be approximately 280 mm Hg if hemodynamic and metabolic states are normal. Clinically, PaO_2 ($FIO_2 = 1$) ranges from 150 to 250 mm Hg.

Marshall BE, Marshall C. Continuity of response to hypoxic pulmonary vasoconstriction. *J Appl Physiol* 1980;59:189–196.

Shibutani HC. Pulmonary resection. In: Youngberg JA, Lake CL, Wilson RS, eds. *Cardiac, vascular and thoracic anesthesia*. New York: Churchill Livingstone, 2000:639–659.

C.15. How could you improve oxygenation during OLV?

The following interventions can be used to improve oxygenation:

- Use 100% oxygen.
- Check the position of the DLT with an FOB.
- Ventilate manually to determine whether higher or lower tidal volumes/inspiratory pressures are beneficial.
- Set minute ventilation to maintain $PaCO_2$ at 40 mm Hg (hypocapnia may inhibit HPV in the nondependent lung; hyperventilation may increase airway pressure and promote blood flow to the nonventilated lung).
- Insufflate oxygen to the nonventilated lung—a flow of approximately 3 L per minute allowed to circulate freely will often increase arterial oxygen saturation by 3% to 4%.

- Apply PEEP of 5 cm H_2O to the dependent lung—it may be beneficial if larger tidal volumes delivered manually improved arterial saturation (i.e., recruitable alveoli). Alternatively, if tidal volumes are too large, adding PEEP may overdistend alveoli that are already open and compress blood vessels, diverting blood to the nonventilated lung and worsening the shunt.
- Partially re-expand the nonventilated lung and then cease ventilation but keep the lumen to the nonventilated side closed. This could interfere with surgical exposure.
- Use differential lung CPAP/PEEP. Use CPAP to the nonventilated lung alone or in combination with PEEP to the ventilated lung in the effort of matching shunt with ventilation (rarely necessary):
  - Add CPAP of 5 cm H_2O to the nondependent lung during the deflation phase of a large tidal volume breath to overcome critical opening pressure in the atelectatic lung. Disadvantage of this maneuver is that although the lung is not ventilated, it may remain distended.
  - Apply PEEP of 5 cm H_2O to the dependent lung.
  - Increase the nondependent lung CPAP to 10 cm H_2O whereas the dependent lung is maintained at PEEP of 5 cm H_2O.
  - Increase dependent lung PEEP to 10 cm H_2O to match the nondependent lung CPAP. The differential lung CPAP/PEEP search discussed in the preceding text is conducted in this way to find the optimal (best) end-expiratory pressure for each lung and minimum Q_S/Q_T for the patient as a whole.
- Use two-lung ventilation intermittently.
- Clamp the pulmonary artery of the nondependent lung temporarily (rarely necessary).

Benumof JL. *Anesthesia for thoracic surgery*, 2nd ed. Philadelphia: WB Saunders, 1995: 408–428.

Brodsky JB, Fitzmaurice B. Modern anesthetic techniques for thoracic operations. *World J Surg* 2001;25(2):162–166.

Miller RD, ed. *Miller's anesthesia*, 5th ed. New York: Churchill Livingstone, 2005:1894–1899.

Shibutani HC. Pulmonary resection. In: Youngberg JA, Lake CL, Wilson RS, eds. *Cardiac, vascular and thoracic anesthesia*. New York: Churchill Livingstone, 2000:639–659.

C.16. Right middle lobectomy was performed. Would you extubate the trachea at the end of the procedure?

After routine lung resection, the trachea can be extubated as long as the patient meets all criteria and has adequate analgesia. If the patient cannot maintain adequate oxygenation and ventilation, postoperative mechanical support is indicated. Under most circumstances, when patients require postoperative ventilatory support, it is advantageous to change the DLT to a single-lumen ETT. Since spontaneous ventilation avoids the potential hazards of positive pressure on the suture lines of the new bronchial stump or parenchymal air leaks, the combination of modest CPAP and pressure support ventilation is usually preferable to controlled intermittent mandatory ventilation.

D. Postoperative Management

D.1. What are the immediate life-threatening complications that follow lobectomy or pneumonectomy?

Serious complications after lobectomy include lobar collapse, massive hemorrhage caused by loosening of a ligature from a pulmonary vessel, bronchopleural fistula from disruption of a bronchial stump, and pulmonary torsion due to increased mobility of a lobe.

Pneumonectomy can be complicated by herniation of the heart (in case of intrapericardial approach), acute right heart failure, right-to-left shunting across a patent foramen ovale due to increased pulmonary vascular resistance and right ventricular pressure, nerve injuries (phrenic, vagus, or recurrent laryngeal) during radical hilar dissection or excision of mediastinal tumors, and acute respiratory insufficiency.

Higgins TL. Postthoracotomy complications. In: Kaplan JA, Slinger PD, eds. *Thoracic anesthesia*, 3rd ed. Philadelphia: Churchill Livingstone, 2003:159–173.

Reed CE. Physiologic consequences of pneumonectomy. Consequences on the pulmonary function. *Chest Surg Clin N Am* 1999;9(2):449–457.

D.2. Why is it important to control postoperative pain? How would you achieve this?

Postoperative pain control is important not only for patient comfort but also to minimize pulmonary complications, allowing the patient to breathe deeply, cough effectively, and ambulate. Systemic administration of opiates is often used alone or in combination with other modalities to control postoperative pain. Morphine in 2-mg increments can be titrated during emergence from anesthesia to achieve adequate pain relief, avoiding respiratory depression. This can be followed postoperatively by patient-controlled analgesia (PCA), often in combination with nonsteroidal anti-inflammatory drugs (NSAIDs). However, when used as a single modality, systemic opioids require plasma concentrations that are usually associated with sedation and potential respiratory depression. Even when used with PCA, pain control is often suboptimal, because of fluctuations in the drug plasma concentration. NSAIDs such as ketorolac, diclofenac, ketoprofen, and indomethacin are usually used as adjuvants to parenteral opiates, particularly for the treatment of shoulder pain associated with chest tube placement. The main short-term concerns for NSAIDs are the potential for exacerbating renal insufficiency and inducing platelet dysfunction. Alternative methods for pain control include epidural local anesthetic with or without opiate, intrathecal opiates, intercostal or paravertebral nerve block, cryoanalgesia, interpleural regional analgesia, and transcutaneous electrical nerve stimulation (TENS).

Epidural and intrathecal analgesia

Thoracic or lumbar epidural analgesia may be achieved by a single injection or a continuous infusion of local anesthetic, alone or in combination with an opiate. In order to reduce the volume required to produce an effect and lessen the chance of hypotension and motor weakness, the catheter should be placed as close as possible to the dermatomes to be covered. A low concentration of local anesthetic such as 0.1% or 0.05% bupivacaine combined with an opiate (e.g., fentanyl 10 μg/mL or sufentanil 0.1 μg/mL) produces synergistic effects that help reduce the sympathetic blockade that may occur with more concentrated local anesthetic alone. In addition, the presence of local anesthetics seems to increase the affinity of the narcotic for the opioid receptors. The use of thoracic epidural analgesia with local anesthetic plus opiate has been shown to improve postoperative pulmonary function. Potential complications of the thoracic epidural technique include inadvertent dural puncture, trauma to the spinal cord, and intravascular injection of local anesthetics with resultant cardiovascular and central nervous system toxicity.

Intrathecal injection of opiates has been successfully used preoperatively or intraoperatively to provide postoperative pain relief for 18 to 24 hours. However, in comparison to epidural injection, intrathecal opiate (in particular morphine) is associated with an increased incidence of late respiratory depression (4% to 7% as compared with <1% for epidural administration). The advantages of neuraxial opiates as compared with systemic opiates include selective blockade of spinal pain with minimal sympathetic blockade and no loss of motor function, and greater predictability of pain relief. Epidural analgesia and opiates in combination with local anesthetics block the presynaptic and postsynaptic neuron cells of the substantia gelatinosa of the spinal cord by passive diffusion across the dura into the cerebrospinal fluid. The lipophilic narcotics, such as fentanyl, methadone, and meperidine, in doses of 0.1 mg, 5 mg, and 30 mg to 100 mg, respectively, have a relatively short onset of action of less than 12 minutes. They provide significant pain relief in 20 to 30 minutes and have a duration of action of 6 to 7 hours. In contrast, a lipophobic narcotic, such as morphine, in a 5-mg dose, has a relatively slow onset of action of 15 to 30 minutes, provides maximal pain relief in 40 to 60 minutes, and has a duration of action of more than 12 hours. The most serious complications of epidural narcotics are early and late respiratory depression. The other side effects include urinary retention, pruritus, and nausea and vomiting. The narcotic antagonist, naloxone, can reverse all the earlier side effects but will reverse the analgesic effect as well, and therefore must be used cautiously.

Intercostal or paravertebral nerve block

Intercostal nerve blocks with long-acting local anesthetics can be used to control pain after thoracoscopy or thoracotomy and can be done by the surgeon intraoperatively. The blocks to the intercostal nerves are placed at the level of the incision and two or three interspaces above and below this level. Catheters that can be injected postoperatively when pain occurs may be placed in the appropriate intercostal grooves at the time of thoracotomy closure. Paravertebral blocks in combination with parenteral opiates and NSAIDs are an alternative to thoracic epidural analgesia. However, the failure rate for this technique is relatively high (6% to 10%). Pneumothorax (especially if bilateral blocks are attempted), hypotension, local anesthetic toxicity due to the high vascularization of the area, and inadvertent total spinal block are the potential risks.

Cryoanalgesia

Long-lasting (3 to 4 weeks up to 6 months) intercostal nerve block can be obtained by cryoablation. Two 30-second freeze cycles ($-60°C$), separated by a 5-second thaw period, are applied to each of the nerves selected. Although cryoanalgesia was initially shown to effectively relieve pain and improve postoperative pulmonary function, a more detailed study has revealed a significant incidence of paresthesia and postthoracotomy pain syndrome.

Interpleural regional analgesia

This technique involves percutaneous introduction of a catheter into the thoracic cage between the parietal and visceral pleura for injection of local anesthetic. Analgesia is thought to occur as a result of (a) diffusion of local anesthetic through the parietal pleura and the innermost intercostal muscle to the intercostal nerves (where the block occurs), (b) block of the intrathoracic sympathetic chain, and (c) direct action of local anesthetic on nerve endings within the pleura. However, efficacy is not uniform because of the loss of anesthetic through thoracotomy drainage, the presence of extravasated blood and tissue fluid in the pleural space diluting the local anesthetic, and possible sequestration and channeling of local anesthetic by the decreased movements of the operated lung. Moreover, in the sitting position, the local anesthetic pools in the costophrenic angle, limiting the quality of analgesia. The use of multiple or fenestrated catheters may achieve more even distribution of local anesthetic over the pleura and improve the quality of analgesia.

Transcutaneous electrical nerve stimulation

The advantages of TENS include low cost, ease of application, and lack of undesirable side effects. However, TENS has a weak analgesic effect. It is generally reserved for adjunctive use with narcotics to relieve postthoracotomy pain if mild to moderate. It is ineffective if the pain is severe.

Ali J, Yaffe CS, Serrette C. The effect of transcutaneous electric nerve stimulation in treatment of postoperative pain. *Surgery* 1981;89:507–512.

Brodsky JB, Fitzmaurice B. Modern anesthetic techniques for thoracic operations. *World J Surg* 2001;25(2):162–166.

Cousins MJ, Mather LE, Wilson PR. Intrathecal and epidural administration of opioid analgesic. *Anesthesiology* 1984;61:276.

Ferrante FM, Chan VWS, Arthur R, et al. Interpleural analgesia after thoracotomy. *Anesth Analg* 1991;72:105–109.

Kaplan JA, Slinger PD. *Thoracic anesthesia*, 3rd ed. New York: Churchill Livingstone, 2003: 445–456.

Kavanagh BP, Katz J, Sandler AN. Pain control after thoracic surgery. A review of current techniques. *Anesthesiology* 1994;81:737–759.

Maiwand MO, Makey AR, Rees A. Cryoanalgesia after thoracotomy: improvement of technique and review of 600 cases. *J Thorac Cardiovasc Surg* 1986;92:291.

Miller RD, ed. *Miller's anesthesia*, 5th ed. New York: Churchill Livingstone, 2005:1906–1909.

CHAPTER 3

Aspiration Pneumonitis and Acute Respiratory Failure

MANUEL L. FONTES • JEFFREY S. BERGER • FUN-SUN F. YAO

A 20-YEAR-OLD FULL-TERM PREGNANT WOMAN

was rushed to the operating room for emergency cesarean section because of fetal distress. During emergence from general anesthesia, the patient vomited and aspirated.

A. Management of Aspiration

1. Delineate the risk factors for aspiration pneumonitis.
2. What is Mendelson syndrome?
3. What is the critical pH value and volume of aspirate to cause Mendelson syndrome?
4. How does aspiration pneumonitis differ from aspiration pneumonia?
5. You suspect the patient has aspirated; what is your initial management strategy?
6. Would you give prophylactic antibiotics?
7. Would you give steroid therapy?
8. Would you irrigate the bronchial tree with bicarbonate or saline solution?
9. How would you prevent aspiration during emergency surgery?

B. Acute Lung Injury

The patient was extubated in the recovery room. Chest x-ray films showed questionable mottled density in the posterior segments of the right upper lobe. Six hours after being transferred to the floor, she was found to be dyspneic and cyanotic. On auscultation of the chest, significant wheezing was noted and the most recent analysis of arterial blood gases showed the following: pH 7.26; $PaCO_2$, 55 mm Hg; PaO_2, 55 mm Hg; and HCO_3^-, 20 mEq per L on room air.

1. Define acute lung injury (ALI) and acute respiratory distress syndrome (ARDS).
2. What are the common causes of ARDS?
3. Describe the pathogenesis of ALI.
4. What are the radiographic findings in ARDS?
5. Describe protective-ventilation strategy in ALI and ARDS.
6. Define pulmonary compliance.

C. Mechanical Ventilation

The patient did not improve after receiving 50% oxygen through face mask. A second arterial blood gas analysis showed the following: pH, 7.25; $PaCO_2$, 50 mm Hg; PaO_2, 55 mm Hg; and CO_2 content, 22 mEq per L. The respiratory rate was 40 breaths per minute.

1. Interpret the blood gases.
2. What is your clinical plan?
3. What are the criteria for mechanical ventilation?
4. Describe the basic modes of mechanical ventilation. Discuss the advantages and disadvantages of pressure-controlled and volume-controlled modes.
5. What control mode would you select for this patient?
6. What initial ventilator settings will you prescribe for this patient (tidal volume, respiratory frequency, inspiratory oxygen fraction, etc.)?
7. Describe the potential hemodynamic effects of positive pressure ventilation (PPV).
8. What are the adverse effects of mechanical ventilation?

D. Therapeutic Approaches for Ventilatory Support

After intubation and mechanical ventilation, the oxygenation did not improve. On FIO_2, 0.7, the arterial blood gas analysis showed the following: pH, 7.30; $Paco_2$, 40 mm Hg; Pao_2, 57 mm Hg; and CO_2 content, 18 mEq per L.

1. What factors determine oxygen delivery?
2. How will you treat the hypoxemia?
3. What are the major factors governing oxygen toxicity?
4. What is the mechanism of oxygen toxicity?
5. What are your criteria to start positive end-expiratory pressure (PEEP)?
6. How does PEEP improve arterial oxygenation?
7. How would you determine the best PEEP and the optimal PEEP?
8. What are the cardiopulmonary effects of PEEP?
9. What is pressure-support ventilation (PSV)? Discuss its advantages.
10. What is inverse-ratio ventilation (IRV)?
11. Describe the rationale for prone-position ventilation and its effect on oxygenation.
12. How is liquid ventilation accomplished?
13. What are the indications and contraindications for extracorporeal membrane oxygenation? How many ways can it be used? What are its results?
14. What is high-frequency positive pressure ventilation (HFPPV)? What are its characteristics?
15. What are the frequencies used in high-frequency ventilation (HFV)? How are they classified?
16. What are the indications and precautions for HFV?
17. What is nitric oxide (NO)? What is the role of inhaled NO in the treatment of ARDS?

E. Weaning from Ventilatory Support

The patient's condition improved after respiratory support with 12 cm H_2O PEEP. Arterial blood gas analysis showed the following: pH, 7.45; $Paco_2$, 35 mm Hg; Pao_2, 150 mm Hg; and FIO_2, 0.75.

1. What would you do now?
2. The patient continued to improve. When would you consider weaning the patient from the respirator? Discuss the criteria for weaning.
3. Describe weaning by synchronized intermittent mandatory ventilation (IMV), pressure support, continuous positive airway pressure (CPAP), and T-piece.

A. Management of Aspiration

A.1. Delineate the risk factors for aspiration pneumonitis.

Aspiration pneumonitis arises most often from aspiration of gastric content that is both acidic and voluminous. It can also occur from aspiration of oropharyngeal content. Several patient characteristics lead to the development of aspiration. These include:

- Neurologic dysphagia
- Disruption of gastroesophageal junction
- Anatomic abnormalities of the upper aerodigestive tract
- General anesthesia
- Pharmacologic agents that alter consciousness (e.g., sedatives, antipsychotics, antidepressants, narcotics). Extremes of age (elderly, neonates)

The risk of aspiration pneumonitis is approximately 10% in patients presenting to the hospital after a drug overdose. This condition used to be very common in general anesthesia and accounted for most obstetric morbidity and mortality. The most recent report suggests an incidence of 1 in 3,000 patients receiving general anesthetics; however, the mortality remains very high and accounts for 10% to 30% of all deaths related to anesthesia. The elderly, particularly the nursing home population, is at increased risk of aspiration secondary to both an increased incidence of pharyngeal dysmotility and gastroesophageal reflux. Aspiration pneumonia and pneumonitis are the most common causes of death in patients with dysphagia caused by neurologic disorders, a condition that affects approximately 300,000 to 600,000 people yearly in the United States.

Irwin RS. Aspiration. In: Irwin RS, Cerra FB, Rippe JM, eds. *Irwin and Rippe's intensive care medicine*, 4th ed. Vol. 1. Philadelphia: Lippincott-Raven Publishers, 1999:685–692.

Janssens JP. Pneumonia in the elderly (geriatric) population. *Curr Opin Pulm Med* 2005;11(3):226–230.

Jaovisidha K, Csuka ME, Almagro UA, et al. Severe gastrointestinal involvement in systemic sclerosis: report of five cases and review of the literature. *Semin Arthritis Rheum* 2005; 34(4):689–702.

Marik P. Aspiration pneumonitis and aspiration pneumonia. *N Engl J Med* 2001;344:665–671.

Ng A, Smith G. Gastroesophageal reflux and aspiration of gastric contents in anesthetic practice. *Anesth Analg* 2001;93:494–513.

A.2. What is Mendelson syndrome?

Mendelson first described acute chemical aspiration pneumonitis in 1946. The triphasic sequence beginning with immediate respiratory distress, bronchospasm, cyanosis, tachycardia, and dyspnea, following with partial recovery, and concluding with a final phase of gradual respiratory recovery is characteristic of Mendelson syndrome. No signs of mediastinal shift are seen, but chest x-ray films usually show irregular mottled densities. This syndrome is due to the irritation of bronchioles by gastric hydrochloric acid, producing bronchiolar spasm, a peribronchiolar exudates, and congestion.

James CF, Modell JH, Gibbs CP, et al. Pulmonary aspiration—effects of volume and pH in the rat. *Anesth Analg* 1984;63:665–668.

Knight PR, Rutter T, Tait AR, et al. Pathogenesis of gastric particulate lung injury: a comparison and interaction with acidic pneumonitis. *Anesth Analg* 1993;77:754–760.

Mendelson CC. The aspiration of stomach contents into the lungs during obstetric anesthesia. *Am J Obstet Gynecol* 1946;52:191–205.

Schwartz DJ, Wynne JW, Gibbs CP, et al. The pulmonary consequences of aspiration of gastric contents at pH values greater than 2.5. *Am Rev Respir Dis* 1980;121:119–126.

Teabeault JR. Aspiration of gastric contents: experimental study. *Am J Pathol* 1952;28:51–67.

A.3. What is the critical pH value and volume of aspirate to cause Mendelson syndrome?

The critical pH value is 2.5. At a pH value higher than 2.5, the response is similar to that of distilled water. Maximal pulmonary damage is achieved at an aspirate pH value of 1.5. A patient is thought to be at risk when there is more than 25 mL (0.4 mL/kg) of gastric contents and the pH value of the gastric contents is less than 2.5.

Hong JY, Oh JI. Effects of preoperative anxiety on gastric fluid acidity and volume. *J Korean Med Sci* 2005;20(2):232–235.

Pisegna JR, Martindale RG. Acid suppression in the perioperative period. *J Clin Gastroenterol* 2005;39(1):10–16.

Teabeault JR. Aspiration of gastric contents: experimental study. *Am J Pathol* 1952;28:51–67.

A.4. How does aspiration pneumonitis differ from aspiration pneumonia?

Aspiration pneumonitis is generally attributed to a chemical injury of the lungs from aspiration of gastric content. The more acidic the pH value and the more voluminous the gastric content, the more severe the chemical burn. Food particles, independent of the acidity, can also cause a chemical injury. Aspiration pneumonitis consists of two phases: the first stage peaks within the first few hours after the aspiration and is mostly related to the caustic effect of the low pH value of the aspirate on the cells lining the alveolar-capillary interface; the second phase generally peaks at approximately 6 hours and is characterized both by infiltration of neutrophils into the alveoli and the lung interstitium and by an inflammatory process identical to that observed in other types of acute lung injury.

Aspiration pneumonia, on the other hand, differs from aspiration pneumonitis on the basis of microbiology. The latter is sterile, and the former contains bacterial agents. As such, the incidence of aspiration pneumonia in the population at risk (see section A.1) is much greater because a small amount of either oropharyngeal or gastric content that is colonized with bacteria is sufficient to cause injury, particularly in the elderly and the immunocompromised host. In the community, both *Haemophilus influenzae* and *Streptococcus pneumoniae* first colonize the oropharynx and access the tracheobronchial tree and alveoli after aspiration to cause community-acquired pneumonia. The term *aspiration pneumonia* is used specifically to describe radiographic evidence of infiltrate in a patient who is at risk of oropharyngeal aspiration. More than 50% of adults aspirate some amount of oropharyngeal secretion during sleep; however, very little sequelae arise from this for several reasons: first, the burden of virulent bacteria in "normal" pharyngeal secretions is low; second, the host is able to clear the aspirate through ciliary transport and cough reflexes; and third, the status of the immune system is noncompromised.

Cassiere HA, Niederman MS. Aspiration pneumonia, lipoid pneumonia, and lung abscess. In: Baum GL, Crapo JD, Celli BR, et al, eds. *Textbook of pulmonary diseases*, 6th ed. Vol. 1. Philadelphia: Lippincott-Raven Publishers, 1998:645–655.

Irwin RS. Aspiration. In: Irwin RS, Cerra FB, Rippe JM, eds. *Irwin and Rippe's intensive care medicine*, 4th ed. Vol. 1. Philadelphia: Lippincott-Raven Publishers, 1999:685–692.

Marik P. Aspiration pneumonitis and aspiration pneumonia. *N Engl J Med* 2001;344:665–671.

Mylotte JM, Goodnough S, Gould M. Pneumonia versus aspiration pneumonitis in nursing home residents: prospective application of a clinical algorithm. *J Am Geriatr Soc* 2005; 53(5):755–761.

A.5. You suspect the patient has aspirated. What is your initial management strategy?

Rapidly tilt the operating table to a 30-degree head-down position to have the larynx at a higher level than the pharynx and to allow gastric content to drain to the outside. While an assistant maintains cricoid pressure, suction the mouth and pharynx as rapidly as possible. Next, endotracheal intubation should be performed (if the patient had been extubated) with immediate inflation of the endotracheal cuff to prevent further aspiration. Quickly suction through the endotracheal tube before administering 100% oxygen by PPV. This is to prevent pushing aspirated material beyond your reach. Suction should be brief to avoid cardiac arrest from hypoxia. Give 100% oxygen before and after suctioning.

An orogastric tube should be inserted to empty the stomach. The pH value of the gastric content should be determined.

Tracheobronchial aspirate is collected for culture and sensitivity tests. Auscultation of the chest will determine whether diminished breathing sounds, wheezing, rales, and rhonchi are present. If bronchospasm is noted, β_2-agonists such as albuterol or terbutaline may be administered through metered-dose inhaler adapters to the anesthetic circuit.

The earliest and most reliable sign of aspiration is hypoxemia, which follows aspiration of even the mildest and most benign aspirate. Therefore, analysis of arterial blood gases should be performed to determine the severity of hypoxemia. Early application of PEEP is recommended to improve pulmonary function.

Abouleish E, Grenvik A. Vomiting, regurgitation, and aspiration in obstetrics. *Pa Med* 1974; 77:45–58.

Barash PG, Cullen BF, Stoelting RK, eds. *Clinical anesthesia*, 5th ed. Philadelphia: Lippincott Williams & Wilkins, 2006:1393–1395.

d'Escrivan T, Guery B. Prevention and treatment of aspiration pneumonia in intensive care units. *Treat Respir Med* 2005;4(5):317–324.

Stoelting RK, Dierdorf SP. *Anesthesia and co-existing disease*, 4th ed. New York: Churchill Livingstone, 2002:580–581.

A.6. Would you give prophylactic antibiotics?

The initial aspirate, excluding feculent aspirate, is usually sterile and remains so for the first 24 hours. Thereafter, the aspiration pneumonitis can become aspiration pneumonia either from contamination of the initial aspirate or secondarily from aspiration of a colonized oropharyngeal secretion in a host that now has tracheobronchial and alveolar damage. Colonization cultures may demonstrate gram-positive or gram-negative superinfection or both, usually with *Escherichia, Klebsiella, Staphylococcus, Pseudomonas,* and *Bacteroides* or with anaerobes. Prophylactic antibiotic has *not* been shown to improve mortality or reduce secondary infection rates. Cultures must be taken as soon as possible after aspiration and thereafter as clinically indicated. The antibiotic therapy is given according to the sensitivity test result. Prophylactic use of broad-spectrum antibiotics may lead to drug-resistant bacterial and fungal superinfection. However, if intestinal obstruction is a possibility, antimicrobial therapy for the possibility of anaerobic and gram-negative infection may be warranted. Although data supporting the use of prophylactic antibiotics are lacking, it is not unusual for clinicians to prescribe such therapy in settings in which the host is considered immunocompromised (e.g., elderly and critically ill patients). If one or several antibiotics have been administered, prompt withdrawal should occur with laboratory or clinical evidence of no infection. In contrast, the use of antibiotics in aspiration pneumonia is unequivocally indicated (e.g., third-generation cephalosporins, fluoroquinolones, or piperacillin).

Allewelt M, Schuler P, Bolcskei PL, et al. Study Group on Aspiration Pneumonia. Ampicillin + sulbactam vs clindamycin +/− cephalosporin for the treatment of aspiration pneumonia and primary lung abscess. *Clin Microbiol Infect* 2004;10(2):163–170.

Barash PG, Cullen BF, Stoelting RK, eds. *Clinical anesthesia*, 5th ed. Philadelphia: Lippincott Williams & Wilkins, 2006:1393–1395.

Genne D, Sommer R, Kaiser L, et al. Analysis of factors that contribute to treatment failure in patients with community-acquired pneumonia. *Eur J Clin Microbiol Infect Dis* 2006;25(3):159–166.

Rebuck JA, Rasmussen JR, Olsen KM. Clinical aspiration-related practice patterns in the intensive care unit: a physician survey. *Crit Care Med* 2001;29(12):2239–2244.

A.7. Would you give steroid therapy?

The value of systemic corticosteroids is controversial. The rationale for immediate use of corticosteroids is to reduce inflammation and stabilize lysosomal membranes. In addition, they have been shown to prevent pulmonary cellular damage by protecting type II alveolar pneumocytes and to attenuate agglutination of leukocytes and platelets.

In experimental studies, the effectiveness of corticosteroid therapy appeared to be related to the pH value of aspirates. When the pH value of the aspirate was in the narrow range of 1.5 to 2.5, corticosteroid therapy was beneficial in treating acid-aspiration pneumonitis. Dexamethasone, given 0.08 mg per kg every 6 hours, decreased pulmonary water content significantly starting at 24 hours, with return to the normal range by 72 hours. When the pH value of the aspirate was less than 1.5, the pulmonary parenchymal damage was maximal. Therefore, the steroid therapy was not effective. When the pH value of the aspirate was higher than 2.5, the response was similar to that of water.

Wolfe, Bone, and Ruth found that pneumonia caused by gram-negative bacteria was more frequent after aspiration in patients treated with corticosteroids than in those who were not. Similarly, studies in animals have failed to demonstrate a beneficial effect of corticosteroids on pulmonary function, lung injury, alveolar-capillary permeability, or outcome after acid aspiration. Furthermore, because of the failure of two multicenter, randomized, controlled trials to demonstrate a benefit of high-dose corticosteroids in patients with ARDS, the administration of corticosteroids cannot be recommended.

Barash PG, Cullen BF, Stoelting RK, eds. *Clinical anesthesia*, 5th ed. Philadelphia: Lippincott Williams & Wilkins, 2006:1395.

Bernard GR, Luce JM, Sprung CL, et al. High-dose corticosteroids in patients with the adult respiratory distress syndrome. *N Engl J Med* 1987;317:1565–1570.

Downs JB, Chapman RL Jr, Modell JH, et al. An evaluation of steroid therapy in aspiration pneumonitis. *Anesthesiology* 1974;40:129–135.

Dudley WR, Marshall BE. Steroid treatment for acid-aspiration pneumonitis. *Anesthesiology* 1974;40:136–141.

Lee M, Sukumaran M, Berger HW, et al. Influence of corticosteroid treatment on pulmonary function after recovery from aspiration of gastric contents. *Mt Sinai J Med* 1980;47:341–346.

Lowrey LD, Anderson M, Calhoun J, et al. Failure of corticosteroid therapy for experimental acid aspiration. *J Surg Res* 1982;32:168–172.

Miller RD, ed. *Anesthesia*, 5th ed. New York: Churchill Livingstone, 2000:2222.

Sukumaran M, Granada MJ, Berger HW, et al. Evaluation of corticosteroid treatment in aspiration of gastric contents: a controlled clinical trial. *Mt Sinai J Med* 1980;47:335–340.

Wolfe JE, Bone RC, Ruth WE. Effects of corticosteroids in the treatment of patients with gastric aspiration. *Am J Med* 1997;63:719–722.

Wynne JW, DeMarco FJ, Hood CI. Physiological effects of corticosteroids in foodstuff aspiration. *Arch Surg* 1981;116:46–49.

A.8. Would you irrigate the bronchial tree with bicarbonate or saline solution?

No. In acid-aspiration pneumonitis, Bannister, Sattilaro, and Otis demonstrated that pulmonary lesions were aggravated by irrigation with sodium bicarbonate, normal saline, and sodium hydroxide. This was explained on the basis that (a) the large volume of fluid served to push the hydrochloric acid deeper into the lungs; (b) mixing of the acid and treatment solution was impossible because of the minute size of the interface; (c) hydrochloric acid probably causes damage within a very short time; (d) if equal volumes of hydrochloric acid (e.g., with a pH value of 1.6) and sodium chloride are mixed, the pH value increases only to 1.8; and (e) neutralization of hydrochloric acid with sodium bicarbonate produces heat, and a thermal burn of the bronchial mucosa may occur.

Bronchial irrigation is indicated only in the obstructive type of aspiration. Five to ten milliliters of normal saline is instilled into the tracheobronchial tree, followed immediately by suction. Bronchial irrigation is preceded and followed by oxygenation. The sequence is repeated until the aspirate fluid is clear.

Bannister WK, Sattilaro AJ, Otis RD. Therapeutic aspects of aspiration pneumonitis in experimental animals. *Anesthesiology* 1961;22:440–443.

Barash PG, Cullen BF, Stoelting RK, eds. *Clinical anesthesia*, 5th ed. Philadelphia: Lippincott Williams & Wilkins, 2006:1395.

A.9. How would you prevent aspiration during emergency surgery?

An ounce of prevention is worth a pound of cure. The following principles of preoperative preparation are of extreme importance:

- Application of gastric decompression by a wide-bore orogastric tube
- Use of regional anesthesia whenever possible
- Preoperative administration of a clear antacid, such as 30 mL of 0.3-M. sodium citrate
- Premedication with anticholinergic agents, such as atropine or glycopyrrolate
- Administration of metoclopramide to stimulate gastric emptying and to increase lower esophageal sphincter tone
- Preoperative administration of an H_2-receptor antagonist or proton inhibitors (pantoprazole sodium) to decrease further secretion of additional acid
- Extubation only when the patient is fully awake

Barash PG, Cullen BF, Stoelting RK, eds. *Clinical anesthesia*, 5th ed. Philadelphia: Lippincott Williams & Wilkins, 2006:1055–1056, 1234, 1395.

DiSario JA. Future considerations in aspiration pneumonia in the critically ill patient: what is not known, areas for future research, and experimental methods. *JPEN J Parenter Enteral Nutr* 2002;26(6 Suppl):S75–S78; discussion S79.

Miller RD, ed. *Miller's anesthesia*, 6th ed. New York: Churchill Livingstone, 2005:2599–2601.

Pisegna JR, Martindale RG. Acid suppression in the perioperative period. *J Clin Gastroenterol* 2005;39(1):10–16.

Smith G, Ng A. Gastric reflux and pulmonary aspiration in anaesthesia. *Minerva Anestesiol* 2003;69(5):402–406.

B. Acute Lung Injury

The patient was extubated in the recovery room. Chest x-ray films showed questionable mottled density in the posterior segments of the right upper lobe. Six hours after being transferred to the floor, she was found to be dyspneic and cyanotic. On auscultation of the chest, significant wheezing was noted and the results of the most recent analysis of arterial blood gases showed the following: pH, 7.26; $PaCO_2$, 55 mm Hg; PaO_2, 55 mm Hg; and HCO_3, 20 mEq per L on room air.

B.1. Define ALI and ARDS.

ARDS is the most severe form of ALI. To standardize definitions, a consensus panel of experts developed a set of criteria characterizing ARDS and ALI. The criteria include onset that is acute, bilateral infiltrates on chest radiography, hypoxemia, and no evidence of cardiogenic failure (i.e., pulmonary artery occlusion pressure, <18 mm Hg). Additionally, this group defined hypoxemia in ALI as a PaO_2/FIO_2 ratio of less than 300 mm Hg and selected a threshold ratio of PaO_2/FIO_2 of less than 200 mm Hg for ARDS, reflecting the more severe nature of the disease.

Bernard GR, Artigas A, Brigham KL, et al. The American-European Consensus Conference of ARDS: definitions, mechanisms, relevant outcomes, and clinical trial coordination. *Am J Respir Crit Care Med* 1994;149:818–824.

Murray JF, Matthay MA, Luce JM, et al. An expanded definition of the adult respiratory distress syndrome. *Am Rev Respir Dis* 1988;138:720–723.

Putensen C, Wrigge H. Ventilator-associated inflammation in acute lung injury. *Intensive Care Med* 2000;26:1515–1522.

Tobin MJ. Advances in mechanical ventilation. *N Engl J Med* 2001;344:1986–1996.

B.2. What are the common causes of ARDS?

ARDS can occur as a result of pulmonary injury arising primarily from the lung pathology or secondarily from extrapulmonary processes. These include multiple trauma, massive blood transfusion, septic shock, fat or air embolism, disseminated intravascular coagulation, aspiration pneumonitis, fluid overload, burns, smoke or gas inhalation, and viral and mycobacterial pneumonia. The following conditions are also associated with ARDS: acute renal failure, oxygen toxicity, drug overdose, radiation, immunosuppression, neurogenic pulmonary edema, acute vasculitis, pancreatitis, cardioversion, cardiopulmonary bypass, and Goodpasture syndrome.

Barash PG, Cullen BF, Stoelting RK, eds. *Clinical anesthesia*, 5th ed. Philadelphia: Lippincott Williams & Wilkins, 2006:1485–1486.

Stoelting RK, Dierdorf SP. *Anesthesia and co-existing disease*, 4th ed. New York: Churchill Livingstone, 2002:225.

Tobin MJ. Advances in mechanical ventilation. *N Engl J Med* 2001;344:1986–1996.

B.3. Describe the pathogenesis of acute lung injury.

The histopathology reveals areas of hyaline membrane, alveolar hemorrhage, increased endothelial and epithelial permeability, and neutrophilic infiltration. Increased permeability allows passage of protein-rich plasma both in the alveolar and in the interstitial spaces, resulting in poor lung compliance and ineffective gas exchange. As the injury process progresses, dependent lung regions beneath the diseased and edematous lung become collapsed, worsening oxygenation. Additionally, alveolar surfactant content diminishes, and its space becomes filled with fibrin and other cellular materials. Ultimately, a fibroproliferative phase is entered whereby further destruction of the lungs occurs with varying degrees of collagen deposition and pulmonary fibrosis.

Complement activation may also play a major role in the pathogenesis of ARDS. Activation of the complement cascade through the alternative pathway by endotoxin or lipopolysaccharides results in the production of C5a complement. C5a complement causes microvascular occlusion and pulmonary granulocyte aggregation and embolization. The resultant damage to the endothelium leads to capillary leakage and pulmonary interstitial edema, ultimately producing terminal airway and alveolar edema and collapse. However, studies have shown limitations of the complement-neutrophil theory. Complement activation does not necessarily correlate with the development or severity of ARDS. ARDS can develop in patients with neutropenia, and pulmonary sequestration of neutrophils may not produce lung injury. As a result, the complement-neutrophil theory of ARDS has been expanded to include central roles for additional humoral mediators (such as endotoxin, tumor necrosis factor, interleukins, and thromboxane) and cellular mediators (e.g., the macrophage-monocyte system). The lung in patients with ARDS is now viewed as one of the organs involved in the multiorgan system dysfunction that occurs as a result of the systemic inflammatory response syndrome. Increased mediator levels are found in bronchoalveolar lavage fluid from patients with ARDS.

Barash PG, Cullen BF, Stoelting RK, eds. *Clinical anesthesia*, 5th ed. Philadelphia: Lippincott Williams & Wilkins, 2006:1485–1486.

Parsons PE. Mediators and mechanism of acute lung injury. *Clin Chest Med* 2000;21:467–476.

Raghavendran K, Davidson BA, Mullan BA, et al. Acid and particulate-induced aspiration lung injury in mice: importance of MCP-1. *Am J Physiol* 2005;289(1):L134–L143.

van Westerloo DJ, Knapp S, van't Veer C, et al. Aspiration pneumonitis primes the host for an exaggerated inflammatory response during pneumonia. *Crit Care Med* 2005;33(8):1770–1778.

B.4. What are the radiographic findings in ARDS?

The chest radiograph typically shows bilateral, fluffy involvement that initially led clinicians to think the pathology was homogenous. Now, however, pulmonary imaging techniques have provided convincing evidence that the injury is segmental. Although the vascular permeability is widespread and homogenous in all lung regions, both total and extravascular lung water is greatest in the dependent lung region. The computed tomography (CT) scans of patients with ARDS are several folds more dense than those of healthy individuals and in severe cases can involve up to 80% of lung fields. Based on the findings of Gattinoni et al., the lungs in patients with ARDS may be divided in thirds, wherein one third represents a completely consolidated, nonventilated region; one third is healthy with normal ventilation/perfusion matching; and one third is a region that is hyperdistended with bullae formation. Contrary to previous belief, the compliance of the lung in patients with ARDS is normal for one third of the lung parenchyma and "stiff" for the rest. The healthy portion is frequently referred to as *baby lung* and is subject to injury because of injudicious assignment of tidal volume. By selecting tidal volume on the basis of body weight (≥ 10 mL/kg), clinicians have overlooked the important fact that only a small fraction of the total lung in patients with ARDS participates in gas exchange. Therefore, a disproportionate share of the tidal volume will travel to the better compliant baby lung, subjecting it to overdistention and injury. Proponents of using lower tidal volume in ALI and in ARDS stress that utilizing a larger tidal volume in such settings is as inappropriate as ventilating an infant's lung with a tidal volume equivalent to that of an adult.

Gattinoni L, Bombino M, Lissoni A, et al. Lung structure and function in different stages of severe adult respiratory distress syndrome. *JAMA* 1994;271:1772–1779.

Gattinoni L, Pesenti A, Bombino M, et al. Relationships between lung computed tomographic density, gas exchange, and PEEP in acute respiratory failure. *Anesthesiology* 1988;69:824–832.

Puybasset L, Cluzel P, Chao N, et al. A computed tomography scan assessment of regional lung volume in acute lung injury. *Am J Respir Crit Care Med* 1998;158:1644–1655.

Rossi UG, Owens CM. The radiology of chronic lung disease in children. *Arch Dis Child* 2005;90(6):601–607.

B.5. Describe protective-ventilation strategy in acute lung injury (ALI) and ARDS.

Many investigators have demonstrated a direct association between mechanical ventilation and lung injury that is independent of barotrauma and functionally and histoanatomically identical to injury observed in ARDS. ALI can occur at both low and high lung volumes (Fig. 3.1). At the lower end (below functional residual capacity [FRC]), cyclical opening and closure of alveolar units during tidal breathing may lead to lung injury from generated sheer forces. The regions most subject to this type of injury are at the interface between lung units that are edematous and nonfunctional with regions that are recruitable and mildly affected by the ARDS process. At the other extreme of lung volume, high airway pressure can cause segmental alveolar overdistention.

During the 1990s, use of a protective-ventilation strategy in patients with ALI or ARDS was shown to improve survival rates. Hickling, Henderson, and Jackson were the first to report a 60% reduction in the expected mortality for patients with ARDS. In a subsequent prospective randomized trial of patients with ARDS treated by a protective lung strategy versus a conventional approach, Amato et al. also demonstrated significant survival improvement in the experimental group. The basic principles of the lung protection strategy include: maintenance of lower inspiratory driving pressures (<20 cm H_2O above PEEP); use of lower tidal volumes (6 mL/kg); acceptance of permissive hypercapnia over higher airway pressures; providing liberal sedation to improve patient-ventilator synchronization; and circumvention of alveolar collapse through judicious use of PEEP. PEEP maintains the end-expiratory pressure above the lower inflexion point on the static pressure–volume curve of the respiratory system (Fig. 3.1). This contrasts to management by the conventional approach employing a tidal volume of 12 mL per kg; selection of lowest PEEP to achieve adequate oxygenation; and keeping the arterial carbon dioxide levels

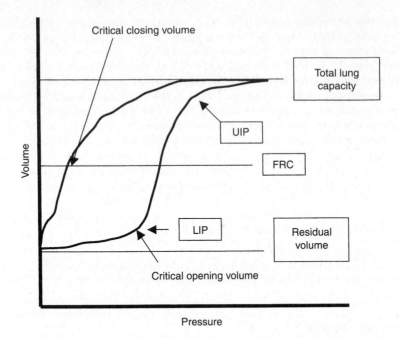

Figure 3.1 Static pressure–volume curve depicting low inflexion point and high inflexion point. On the basis of the concept of a protective-ventilation strategy in acute lung injury (ALI) and acute respiratory distress syndrome (ARDS), there are two critical regions in which pulmonary compliance is very poor. The first region is slightly above the residual volume and denotes a critical opening volume whereby recruitable alveoli have the propensity to collapse during tidal breathing. Cyclic opening and closing of these alveolar units has been implicated as a cause of ventilator-induced lung injury. On a static pressure-volume curve, the determination of this lower inflexion point (LIP) allows the clinician to set the positive end-expiratory pressure (PEEP) to 2 cm H_2O above this critical opening volume to prevent alveolar collapse and promote recruitment. The compliance of the lung markedly improves beyond this point until it reaches higher lung volumes, labeled upper inflexion point (UIP). The ideal tidal volume can be extracted from this exercise as the volume contained between the LIP and the UIP. Similarly, ideal compliance can be derived from the slope of this steep portion (region between LIP and UIP). FRC, functional residual capacity.

between 35 and 38 mm Hg. Fifty-three patients were enrolled in Amato's study (29 were assigned to a protective strategy and 24 were assigned to conventional management). After 28 days, the mortality in the protective-ventilation group was significantly reduced (38% vs. 71%). Further, the rates of weaning from mechanical ventilation were 66% and 29% for the protective-ventilation group and conventional group, respectively.

Following the work of Amato et al., a multicenter study sponsored by the National Institutes of Health (NIH), the Acute Respiratory Distress Syndrome Network, which included 861 patients, reported the same results. Briefly, 432 patients were ventilated with 6 mL per kg of tidal volume, and 429 patients received 12 mL per kg of tidal volume. The mean airway pressures were 25 ± 6 and 33 ± 8 cm H_2O. The trial was stopped prematurely after an interim analysis revealed an overall mortality reduction of 22% in the protective-ventilation group (31% vs. 39%, $p = 0.01$). This trial measured plasma level of interleukin-6 at days 0 through 3 and found it to be markedly reduced in the lower tidal volume group, suggesting fewer systemic inflammatory processes associated with the protective approach.

Acute Respiratory Distress Syndrome Network. Ventilation with lower tidal volumes as compared with traditional tidal volumes for acute lung injury and the acute respiratory distress syndrome. *N Engl J Med* 2000;342:1301–1308.

Amato MB, Barbas CS, Medeiros DM, et al. Beneficial effects of the "open lung approach" with low distending pressures in acute respiratory distress syndrome: a prospective randomized study on mechanical ventilation. *Am J Respir Crit Care Med* 1995;152: 1835–1846.

Amato MBP, Barbas CSV, Medeiros DM, et al. Effect of a protective-ventilation strategy on mortality in the acute respiratory distress syndrome. *N Engl J Med* 1998;338:347–354.

Fontes ML. Progress in mechanical ventilation. *Curr Opin Anesthesiol* 2002;15:45–51.

Hickling KG, Henderson SJ, Jackson R. Low mortality associated with low volume pressure limited ventilation with permissive hypercapnia in severe adult respiratory distress syndrome. *Intensive Care Med* 1990;16:372–377.

Stewart TE, Meade MO, Cook DJ, et al. Evaluation of a ventilation strategy to prevent barotrauma in patients at high risk for acute respiratory distress syndrome. *N Engl J Med* 1998;338:355–361.

B.6. Define pulmonary compliance.

Lung compliance is defined as the change in lung volume per unit change in trasmural pressure gradient, (i.e. between the alveolus and pleural space). Compliance is measured by adding a known amount of volume to a system and recording the pressure change. The ratio between this volume change and the respective pressure change defines compliance. The reciprocal of this relationship is called *elastance*. The lungs are said to be compliant or noncompliance depending on the pressure change that occurs after a given volume (tidal volume) is delivered. The overall lung compliance is rarely measured during clinical practice; rather, inspiratory pressures (peak airway and plateau pressures) are used to infer the status of overall compliance (lungs and thoracic). In actuality, assessing lung compliance is very difficult because different regions of the lungs exhibit different states of compliance, reflecting the heterogeneity of alveolar compliance. For example, in the upright position, the upper lung fields have the poorest compliance relative to the middle and lower lung segments. Evolutionarily speaking, blood flow is directed to lung regions that have the best compliance (i.e., the dependent regions). As described in the previous section, pulmonary compliance changes as the lung volume is increased from residual volume to total lung volume. At the extremes of volume, compliance becomes reduced. Therefore, the ideal compliance occurs at a lung volume between FRC and the resultant lung volume contributed by a normal tidal volume (7 mL/kg).

Pulmonary compliance changes with aging. Compliance is worse at the extremes of age. In addition, several disease states can compromise pulmonary compliance such as ALI, ARDS, congestive heart failure, barotraumas, neuromuscular disease, obesity, and pregnancy.

Gropper MA, Wiener-Kronish JP. Acute lung injury and acute respiratory distress syndrome. In: Murray MJ, Coursin DB, Pearl RG, et al, eds. *Critical care medicine: perioperative management*. Philadelphia: Lippincott-Raven Publishers, 1997.

Lumb AB. *Nunn's applied respiratory physiology*, 6th ed. Philadelphia: Elsevier Butterworth-Heinemann, 2005:25–33.

C. Mechanical Ventilation

The patient did not improve after receiving 50% oxygen through a face mask. A second arterial blood gas analysis showed the following: pH value, 7.25; $Paco_2$, 50 mm Hg; Pao_2, 55 mm Hg; and CO_2 content, 22 mEq per L. The respiratory rate was 40 breaths per minute.

C.1. Interpret the blood gases.

The patient is demonstrating significant signs of respiratory failure. She is hypoxemic, hypercarbic, and dyspneic, and has an acid-base disturbance marked by a combined respiratory and metabolic acidosis. A 10 mm Hg rise in $Paco_2$ should have reduced the pH value by 0.08 (pH = 7.32). Therefore, a component of metabolic acidosis is present, lowering the pH value to 7.25.

C.2. What is your clinical plan?

Several approaches can be used for the initial management of this patient. A noninvasive approach using PPV by nasal or face bilevel positive airway pressure (BiPAP) is a temporary measure. BiPAP is typically reserved for patients who are experiencing mild to moderate respiratory failure and who are not at increased risk of aspiration. Given this patient's presentation, the severity of respiratory failure will likely not improve rapidly. In fact, the clinical picture suggests that the patient has suffered ALI resulting in transpulmonary shunting and ineffective ventilation. The safest approach is to electively intubate the trachea and provide mechanical ventilation. Once successfully intubated, sedation can be given to allow for better patient-ventilator synchronization and comfort. If the pulmonary compliance is poor, as is commonly the case in the setting of ALI and ARDS, "deep" sedation may be required as well as muscle relaxation to facilitate gas exchange and to reduce barotrauma.

C.3. What are the criteria for mechanical ventilation?

The physiologic criteria for mechanical ventilation are as follows:

Mechanics

- Respiratory rate of more than 35 breaths per minute
- Vital capacity of less than 15 mL per kg
- Rapid shallow breathing index (respiratory rate/tidal volume) more than 200 breaths per minute per L

Oxygenation

- Pao_2 less than 70 mm Hg on mask oxygen
- PAo_2–Pao_2 more than 350 mm Hg on 100% FIo_2 or Qs/Qt more than 20%

Ventilation

- $Paco_2$ more than 55 mm Hg, except in patients with chronic hypercarbia
- VD/VT more than 0.60

The trend of values and clinical state is important. The numerical guidelines should not be followed to the exclusion of clinical judgment. Also, frequently, the blood gas analysis results reflect what the patient's status had been at the time the sample was obtained. Depending on the time interval required to perform the analysis and to receive the result, there can be significant exacerbation or resolution in both oxygenation and ventilation, emphasizing the role of clinical judgment.

Pontoppidan H, Geffin B, Lowenstein E. Acute respiratory failure in the adult. *N Engl J Med* 1972;287:743–751.

Stoelting RK, Dierdorf SP. *Anesthesia and co-existing disease*, 4th ed. New York: Churchill Livingstone, 2002:224.

C.4. Describe the basic modes of mechanical ventilation. Discuss the advantages and disadvantages of pressure-controlled and volume-controlled modes?

Fundamentally, the various modes of mechanical ventilation, both new and old, share the following variables: trigger, control, limit, cycle, and baseline.

Trigger mode

The trigger is the first and most important component of the inspiratory phase, marking the end of exhalation. Examples of triggering mechanisms include time, flow, and pressure. In the nonparalyzed and nonanesthetized state, the patient triggers a mechanical or assisted breath by generating negative transpulmonary pressure that is sensed by the ventilator as a pressure change in the airway (the ventilator circuit including the endotracheal tube). The threshold for triggering a breath (i.e., the set sensitivity) can be altered depending on the clinical setting; however, the greatest challenge in mechanical ventilation is determining the level at which sensitivity pressure should be set (usually at 1 to 2 cm H_2O). If the threshold is set too low, the ventilator will be triggered by any process that causes the airway pressure to surpass the set threshold. These include patient motion, external compression, gastric suctioning, and air leaks in the circuit or in the chest tubes. Conversely, if the threshold is set too high, the work of breathing increases; that is, to trigger every breath, the patient must make a significant effort to overcome the threshold limit for inspiratory flow to occur. At high levels of ventilatory assistance, as much as one third of the patient's inspiratory efforts may be insufficient to trigger the ventilator. In a 2001 review, Tobin explained that "breaths that do not reach the threshold for triggering the ventilator have higher tidal volumes and shorter expiratory times than do breaths that do trigger the ventilator." In the setting of acute respiratory failure, the inspiratory effort exhausted by the patient is approximately four to six times the normal value. This level of respiratory work frequently causes breath stacking, generating intrinsic PEEP, which in turn imposes a tremendous burden on inspiratory muscle and if sustained can result in muscle fatigue and cardiopulmonary collapse.

Control mode

The delivered breath can be either pressure regulated (pressure control) or volume targeted (volume control). In the pressure-controlled mode, the amount of volume delivered is inversely related to the resistance encountered. When the resistive forces are low (i.e., normal compliance), the tidal volume for a given pressure will be relatively larger than if compliance were poor. For adults, the recommended upper limit of pressure control is 35 cm H_2O. Higher pressures may directly cause ALI or delay healing of the already injured lung. When the resistive forces are high, the resultant tidal volume may be inadequate for ventilation or oxygenation, even at high levels of inspiratory pressures. Typically, these patients have ARDS, and lower levels of arterial oxygen tension (PaO_2) are tolerated along with higher levels of arterial carbon dioxide tension (permissive hypercapnia).

Volume-controlled mode is the most common control mode used to ventilate patients mechanically. Examples include assist-control ventilation and synchronous intermittent mandatory ventilation (SIMV). The ventilator will attempt to deliver a preset volume regardless of the pressure generated. For patients with poorly compliant lungs, volume-controlled mode may promote barotrauma and acute lung injury (ALI).

Limit mode

The limit is an essential feature in mechanical ventilation. Its variables include volume, pressure, and flow. The upper and lower limits of these variables should be preselected for each patient and adjusted in a manner consistent with the goals of the protective lung strategy employed.

Cycle mode

As discussed in the previous section, cycling has several variables: time, flow, and pressure. As such, the inspiratory phase and the expiratory phase becomes controlled. The challenge faced is in synchronizing the machine's cycling of inspiration and exhalation with the patient's "neural" respiratory cycle. Although pressure, flow, and time can be used to affect cycling, the manipulation of one or all three variables, both intrabreath and interbreath, to coincide precisely with the demands of the patient is virtually impossible (Fig. 3.2).

Baseline mode

The baseline variable is the function that is controlled during exhalation and generally indicates the level of PEEP.

Fontes ML. Progress in mechanical ventilation. *Curr Opin Anesthesiol* 2002;15:45–51.

Hess D, Branson R. Ventilators and weaning modes. *Respir Care Clin N Am* 2000;6:407–435.

Tobin MJ. Advances in mechanical ventilation. *N Engl J Med* 2001;344:1986–1996.

C.5. What control mode would you select for this patient?

For adult patients, volume-controlled mode is most often chosen for ventilatory management. Examples include assist-control ventilation, SIMV, and PSV. A targeted tidal volume is selected (7 to 12 mL/kg), and the ventilator will attempt to deliver this volume regardless of the pressure generated. If the resistance to ventilation is great, the pressure change can be excessive, resulting in barotrauma and ALI. Occasionally, the pressure increase is acute, reflecting some reversible condition, such as mucous plugging, bronchospasm, and patient anxiety. These conditions can be treated appropriately without having to switch to a different ventilatory mode. Alternatively, patients with ALI may have very poor compliance for which volume-controlled mode may be ineffective or prohibitive.

Some alternative modes of mechanical ventilation combine pressure control that is volume compensated or vice versa. Examples include pressure-regulated volume-controlled (PRVC) ventilation, proportional assist ventilation, adaptive support ventilation, and many other combinations of volume control, volume support, pressure support, and pressure control. These alternative modes attempt to improve patient comfort and synchronization with the ventilator. Older modes were overly simplistic, and incorrect assumptions were made regarding the role of ventilatory assistance. The concept was to make the ventilator the "boss" and allow it to drive the respiratory cycles. The important insight gained from today's clinical research is that the ventilator should be a "helper" aimed at assisting the patient in a manner determined by the patient.

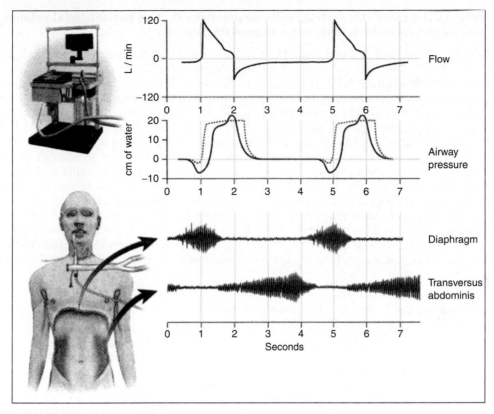

Figure 3.2 Activation of expiratory muscle during a mechanical inspiratory cycle. The airway flow, pressure, and electromyogram recording of two mechanically assisted respiratory cycles are illustrated. The start of inspiration is reflected by diaphragmatic activity that begins before the commencement of the inspiratory flow or airway pressure. The diaphragm stops contracting, marking the end of inspiratory effort. The expiratory muscle activity begins with contraction of the transversus abdominis muscle **(lower panel)**; however, the ventilator continued to deliver inspiratory flow while the patient was attempting to exhale. This illustrates a common problem with all ventilation modes that cannot fully adapt and synchronize with the patient's neuronal timing of inspiration and expiration. In the case mentioned earlier, the ventilator's inspiratory time exceeded the patient's inspiratory cycle, resulting in dyssynchrony and in some instances high airway pressure, predisposing to barotrauma. (From Tobin MJ. Advances in medical ventilation. *N Engl J Med* 2001;344:1986–1996, with permission.)

Brochard L. Pressure support ventilation. In: Tobin MJ, ed. *Principles and practice of mechanical ventilation*. New York: McGraw-Hill, 1994:239–257.

Esteban A, Anzueto A, Alia I, et al. How is mechanical ventilation employed in the intensive care unit? An international utilization review. *Am J Respir Crit Care Med* 2000;161: 1450–1458.

Sassoon CSH. Intermittent mandatory ventilation. In: Tobin JM, ed. *Principles and practice of mechanical ventilation*. New York: McGraw-Hill, 1994:221–237.

Tobin MJ. Mechanical ventilation. *N Engl J Med* 1994;330:1056–1061.

C.6. What initial ventilator settings will you prescribe for this patient (tidal volume, respiratory frequency, inspiratory oxygen fraction, etc.)?

Initially, an attempt will be made to ventilate the patient with a volume-controlled mode. The tidal volume will be set at 5 to 8 mL/kg, respiratory frequency at 10 breaths per minute, F_{IO_2} of 70%, PEEP of 10 cm H_2O. The limits for alarming will be standard. After this initial setting, an arterial blood gas analysis should be performed to determine the adequacy of ventilation and oxygenation. Should lung compliance be poor, large tidal volumes must be avoided, which will predispose the lungs to barotrauma. The patient should be adequately sedated, and both the patient and the ventilator should be examined to rule out correctable causes of elevated inspiratory pressures. Alternatively, a pressure-controlled mode can be selected to ensure the driving pressure (plateau or mean airway pressure) does not exceed 35 cm H_2O. The PEEP level should be adjusted to improve oxygenation. A Pa_{O_2} level of more than 60 mm Hg is acceptable, and the level of Pa_{CO_2} can rise in excess of 60 or 70 mm Hg (permissive hypercapnia). Treating the ensuing acidemia, particularly, respiratory acidemia is no longer recommended, unless the pH value becomes less than 7.20. The use of sodium bicarbonate is reserved for profound acidemia. Once administered, this agent is chemically converted to byproducts that include H_2O and CO_2. The latter can diffuse easily through the cell membrane to make the intercellular milieu more acidotic.

Cuhaci B, Lee J, Ahmed Z. Sodium bicarbonate and intracellular acidosis: myth or reality? *Crit Care Med* 2001;29(5):1088–2090.

Levraut J, Giunti C, Ciebiera JP, et al. Initial effect of sodium bicarbonate on intracellular pH depends on the extracellular nonbicarbonate buffering capacity. *Crit Care Med* 2001;29(5):1033–1039.

C.7. Describe the potential hemodynamic effects of positive pressure ventilation (PPV).

During spontaneous inspiration, air is delivered to the lungs by generating a pressure gradient between pleural (negative pressure) and atmospheric pressures (1 atmospheric pressure). During exhalation, the reverse process occurs and air is expelled as pleural pressure increases (never positive) and the rib cage recoils returning lung volume to FRC. The hemodynamic consequence of physiologic breathing is minor but is associated with alterations in systemic blood pressure. For example, during inspiration, blood flow to the right ventricle is promoted and blood flow to the left side of the heart is diminished. This results in a decrease in stroke volume and systemic systolic pressure (approximately 5 to 10 mm Hg). In contrast, during positive pressure inspiration, the ventilator applies positive pressure to overcome alveolar pressure. Overall, transthoracic pressure increases, impeding or diminishing venous return to the heart. Both the right and the left ventricular output can decrease depending on the thoracic compliance, intravascular volume status, and biventricular function; that is, PPV will cause a decrease in cardiac output and blood pressure when the overall lung compliance is poor, the intravascular volume is inadequate, and/or ventricular function is compromised.

The hemodynamic consequences of both spontaneous pressure ventilation and PPV may be profound and may have opposite effects on cardiovascular stability in different patient populations. Therefore, no firm rules apply about the specific response that will be seen in all patients and under all conditions. Some generalities, however, are probably reasonable. In patients with markedly increased work of breathing, hypervolemia, or impaired left ventricular pump function, the institution of mechanical ventilatory support can be life saving because of its ability to support the cardiovascular system, independent of any beneficial effects that mechanical ventilation may have on gas exchange. In patients with decreased pulmonary elastic recoil, increased pulmonary vascular resistance, hypovolemic, or airflow obstruction, the institution of mechanical ventilatory support may induce cardiovascular instability, which if not corrected can lead to total cardiovascular collapse.

The initiation of intermittent positive pressure ventilation (IPPV) is associated with a decrease in cardiac output and in arterial blood pressure in patients without significant lung consolidation. Cardiac output and stroke volume decrease as the peak airway pressure increases. There is also a decrease in cardiac output with increasing inspiratory/expiratory ratios. IPPV increases intrathoracic pressure, resulting in decreased venous return and cardiac output. Patients with healthy lungs behave differently from patients with significant cardiopulmonary disease. When pulmonary compliance decreases, the transmission of airway pressure to intrathoracic pressure decreases. Patients with more rigid lungs can tolerate higher airway pressures.

IPPV decreases transmural pulmonary artery pressure as well. There is no change in pulmonary vascular resistance. The systemic vascular resistance increases slightly when IPPV is begun. The decrease in cardiac output during IPPV is rarely of any clinical significance because it is compensated by an increase in peripheral vascular resistance in nonanesthetized patients. When patients are hypovolemic, the decrease in blood pressure can be significant.

Pinsky MP. Cardiovascular effects of ventilatory support and withdrawal. *Anesth Analg* 1995;79:567–576.

Shapiro BA, Kacmarek RM, Cane RD, et al. eds. *Clinical application of respiratory care*. St. Louis: Mosby-Year Book, 1991:285–286.

C.8. What are the adverse effects of mechanical ventilation?

Physiologic Complications

- Decreased cardiac output resulting from increased intrathoracic pressure
- Respiratory alkalosis from hyperventilation
- Increased venous admixture (Q_S/Q_T) from prolonged low tidal volume ventilation

Pulmonary Complications

- Infection
- Acute lung injury
- Barotrauma/pneumothorax, mediastinal, interstitial, and subcutaneous emphysema in 10% to 15% of adults
- Oxygen toxicity if the inspired oxygen concentration is more than 60%
- Atelectasis caused by immobilization and ineffective humidification

Complications from Endotracheal Intubation

- Endobronchial intubation, kinking or obstruction, leaking cuffs
- Nasal damage from nasal intubation, nose bleeding, fractured turbinates, septal perforation, partial loss of alae nasi, nasal synechiae
- Laryngeal damage and edema, vocal cord paresis and granulomas, laryngotracheal membranes, subglottic fibrotic stenosis
- Tracheal damage and tracheal erosion, tracheoesophageal fistula, tracheomalacia, tracheal stenosis
- Complications from mechanical device malfunction

Dreyfuss D, Saumon G. Ventilator-induced lung injury: lessons from experimental studies. *Am J Respir Crit Care Med* 1998;157:294–323.

Pierson DJ. Barotrauma and bronchopleural fistula. In: Tobin MJ, ed. *Principles and practice of mechanical ventilation*. New York: McGraw-Hill, 1994:813–836.

Pinsky MP. Cardiovascular effects of ventilatory support and withdrawal. *Anesth Analg* 1995; 79:567–576.

Puybasset L, Cluzel P, Chao N, et al. A computed tomography scan assessment of regional lung volume in acute lung injury. *Am J Respir Crit Care Med* 1998;158:1644–1655.

Stoelting RK, Dierdorf SP. *Anesthesia and co-existing disease*, 4th ed. New York: Churchill Livingstone, 2002:221–222.

D. Therapeutic Approaches for Ventilatory Support

After intubation and mechanical ventilation, the oxygenation did not improve. On FIO_2 0.7, the arterial blood gas analysis showed the following: pH, 7.30; $PaCO_2$, 40 mm Hg; PaO_2, 57 mm Hg; and CO_2 content, 18 mEq per L.

D.1. What factors determine oxygen delivery?

Oxygen delivery is dependent on blood flow (cardiac output) and the content of oxygen carried in blood (hemoglobin and dissolved oxygen). The actual amount is reflected by the following formula:

$$\text{oxygen delivery} = CO[(Hgb \times 1.39)SaO_2 + PaO_2 \times 0.003],$$

where *CO* is cardiac output; *Hgb*, hemoglobin content in blood; SaO_2, percent arterial oxygen saturation; and PaO_2, partial pressure of oxygen dissolved in blood.

Based on this formula, oxygenation can be improved by several modalities. First, it is important to determine where the physiologic derangement lies. If the cardiac output is inadequate, the appropriate therapy should be to improve the elements of cardiac output (rate and rhythm, preload, contractility, and afterload); next, should the hemoglobin content be too low, the patient should undergo a transfusion with red blood cells; last, oxygen delivery to the lungs and uptake should be maximized. The latter can be accomplished by increasing the inspired oxygen concentration, increasing the level of PEEP, and by other maneuvers that will improve ventilation/perfusion matching and decrease intrapulmonary shunting (e.g., chest physiotherapy, prone position, bronchodilators, and diuresis).

Ginosa Y, Pizov R, Sprung C. Arterial and pulmonary artery catheters. In: Parrillo J, Bone R, eds. *Critical care medicine, principles of diagnosis and management*. St Louis: Mosby-Year Book, 1995:27–49.

D.2. How will you treat the hypoxemia?

The arterial blood gas analyses suggest that the patient is hypoxemic but is adequately ventilated and has a component of metabolic acidosis. As discussed previously, it is *not* appropriate to correct this level of metabolic acidosis with sodium bicarbonate or to attempt to hyperventilate the patient and induce respiratory alkalosis. The underlying problem producing the hypoxemia is lung injury from the aspiration pneumonitis, whose effect has led to significant intrapulmonary shunting. The FIO_2 is set at 0.7. The most appropriate maneuver is to increase the PEEP level, ensure good patient-ventilator synchronization (i.e., the patient is not fighting the ventilator), and avoid excessive tidal volumes or inspiratory driving pressures. Other ventilatory modalities that can be applied include IRV, pressure-controlled ventilation, prone position, use of NO, jet ventilation, and partial liquid ventilation (PLV).

D.3. What are the major factors governing oxygen toxicity?

Oxygen toxicity is governed by the duration of exposure, the partial pressure of oxygen, and the susceptibility of the individual to pulmonary oxygen injury. The degree of toxicity is related to the partial pressure, but not to the percentage of oxygen inspired, as demonstrated during U.S. space flights, where astronauts tolerate 100% oxygen for 2 to 4 weeks at a tension of 250 mm Hg. Systemic oxygen toxicity is related to arterial oxygen tension, whereas pulmonary oxygen toxicity depends on alveolar oxygen tension. Retrolental fibroplasia (retinopathy of prematurity) in the premature neonate has been reported after exposure to PaO_2 at more than 80 to 150 mm Hg for a few hours. Pulmonary toxicity can develop after prolonged exposure to oxygen at concentrations between 0.5 and 1.0 atmospheres. It must be emphasized that the adult patient can generally tolerate 1 atmosphere of oxygen partial pressure for at least 24 hours. Moreover, there is no evidence that clinically relevant pulmonary oxygen toxicity occurs in humans at inspired partial pressures less than 0.5 atmosphere. Lastly, no patients should ever experience life-threatening levels of hypoxemia to avoid possible oxygen toxicity.

Deneke SM, Fanburg BL. Normobaric oxygen toxicity of the lung. *N Engl J Med* 1980; 303:76–86.

Frank L, Massaro D. Oxygen toxicity. *Am J Med* 1980;69:117.

Lumb AB. *Nunn's applied respiratory physiology*, 6th ed. Philadelphia: Elsevier Butterworth-Heinemann, 2005:348–358.

D.4. What is the mechanism of oxygen toxicity?

The so-called free-radical theory of oxygen toxicity proposed in the early 1960s has garnered a great deal of recent experimental support and is now accepted as the most probable molecular-level explanation for oxygen toxicity. Various highly reactive and potentially cytotoxic free-radical products of oxygen are generated metabolically in the cell. These short-lived O_2 metabolites, including superoxide anion (O_2^-), hydroxyl radical ($OH^·$), hydrogen peroxide (H_2O_2), and singlet oxygen (O), have been shown to be capable of effects such as inactivation of sulfhydryl enzymes, interaction with and disruption of DNA, and peroxidation of unsaturated membrane lipids with resultant loss of membrane integrity. The cell is also equipped with an array of antioxidant defenses, including the enzymes superoxide dismutase (SOD), catalase, glutathione peroxidase, vitamin E, and ascorbate. Under hyperoxia, the intracellular generation and influx of free radicals is believed to increase markedly and may overwhelm the detoxifying capacity of the normal complement of antioxidant defenses, with resultant cytotoxicity.

The pathology of oxygen toxicity is nonspecific and consists of atelectasis, edema, alveolar hemorrhage, inflammation, fibrin deposition, and thickening and hyalinization of alveolar membranes. There are exudative and proliferative phases. Capillary endothelium is damaged early and plasma leaks into interstitial and alveolar spaces. Pulmonary surfactant may be altered. Type I alveolar lining cells are injured early, and bronchiolar and tracheal ciliated cells can be damaged by 80% to 100% oxygen. Resolution of exudative changes, hyperplasia of alveolar type II cells, fibroplastic proliferation, and interstitial fibrosis occur with recovery or with the development of tolerance to oxygen. Total resolution is possible if the initial hyperoxia is not overwhelming.

Deneke SM, Fanburg BL. Normobaric oxygen toxicity of the lung. *N Engl J Med* 1980; 303:76–86.

Frank L, Massaro D. The lung and oxygen toxicity. *Arch Intern Med* 1979;139:347–350.

Freeman BA, Crapo JD. Free radicals and tissue injury. *Lab Invest* 1982;47:412.

Lumb AB. *Nunn's applied respiratory physiology*, 6th ed. Philadelphia: Elsevier Butterworth-Heinemann, 2005:348–358.

D.5. What is your criteria to start PEEP?

The role of PEEP in mechanical ventilation is evolving. Previously, it was reserved for patients who had significant pulmonary pathology and hypoxemia. Either in apparently healthy lungs or in disease lungs, there can be significant heterogeneity in alveolar compliance and ventilation. Therefore, at normal levels of PEEP (physiologic), while in the supine position, alveolar components can collapse during tidal breathing, particularly, when there exist underlying comorbid states (e.g., ALI, ARDS, chronic obstructive pulmonary disease [COPD], congestive heart failure, obesity, and general anesthesia). To prevent cyclical closure of alveolar units and to ensure that the lung volume is maintained at or slightly above FRC, PEEP should be instituted accordingly. One should not wait for physiologic or laboratory evidence of inadequate gas exchange to initiate PEEP. Five to 10 cm H_2O is often sufficient and is not associated with hemodynamic disturbances. In the setting of ALI and ARDS, application of PEEP is essential for achieving adequate oxygenation.

Acute Respiratory Distress Syndrome Network. Ventilation with lower tidal volumes as compared with traditional tidal volumes for acute lung injury and the acute respiratory distress syndrome. *N Engl J Med* 2000;342:1301–1308.

Amato MB, Barbas CS, Medeiros DM, et al. Beneficial effects of the "open lung approach" with low distending pressures in acute respiratory distress syndrome: a prospective randomized study on mechanical ventilation. *Am J Respir Crit Care Med* 1995;152:1835–1846.

Amato MBP, Barbas CSV, Medeiros DM, et al. Effect of a protective-ventilation strategy on mortality in the acute respiratory distress syndrome. *N Engl J Med* 1998;338:347–354.

Gattinoni L, Pesenti A, Bombino M, et al. Relationships between lung computed tomographic density, gas exchange, and PEEP in acute respiratory failure. *Anesthesiology* 1988;69:824–832.

D.6. How does PEEP improve arterial oxygenation?

The mechanism is related to an increase in the FRC and redistribution of extravascular lung water. The FRC expands linearly with increases in the end-expiratory pressure, usually at a rate of 400 mL or more for each 5 cm H_2O of end-expiratory pressure; however, recruitment of alveolar units is both variable and unpredictable in patients with ARDS. This increase in FRC represents alveoli that remain open and available for gas exchange during all phases of the respiratory cycle. The increase in FRC improves the relationship between FRC and closing capacity and therefore decreases intrapulmonary shunt or venous admixture.

PEEP therapy changes the distribution of interstitial lung water but does not directly decrease lung water. PEEP facilitates the movement of water from the less compliant interstitial spaces (between the alveolar epithelium and capillary endothelium, where gas exchange occurs) to the more compliant interstitial spaces (toward the peribronchial and hilar areas). This redistribution of interstitial lung water improves oxygen diffusion across the alveolar-capillary membrane, resulting in increased arterial oxygenation. Approximately 25% of patients with ARDS are unresponsive to increases in PEEP as measured by an increase in PaO_2.

Abbound N, Rehder K, Rodarte JR, et al. Lung volume and closing capacity with continuous positive airway pressure. *Anesthesiology* 1975;42:138–142.

Acute Respiratory Distress Syndrome Network. Ventilation with lower tidal volumes as compared with traditional tidal volumes for acute lung injury and the acute respiratory distress syndrome. *N Engl J Med* 2000;342:1301–1308.

Miller WC, Rice DL, Unger KM, et al. Effect of PEEP on lung water content in experimental noncardiogenic pulmonary edema. *Crit Care Med* 1981;9:7.

Pare PD, Warriner B, Baile M, et al. Redistribution of pulmonary extravascular water with positive and expiratory pressure in canine pulmonary edema. *Am Rev Respir Dis* 1983;127:590.

D.7. How would you determine the best PEEP and the optimal PEEP?

Suter, Fairley, and Isenberg described best conventional PEEP in 1975. The best PEEP is defined as the level of PEEP with the highest oxygen transport, which is the product of cardiac output and oxygen content. This PEEP correlates with the highest total respiratory compliance, the highest mixed venous oxygen tension, and the lowest Vd/Vt (Fig. 3.3). Arterial oxygen tension and intrapulmonary shunt are not good indicators of the best conventional PEEP. They continue to improve even after this level has been reached. Oxygen transport decreases after the best PEEP is reached, because the cardiac output decreases.

Civetta, Barnes, and Smith described optimal high PEEP in 1975. It is defined as the level of PEEP with the lowest intrapulmonary shunt and without compromising cardiac output. The PEEP used in this report is so-called high or super PEEP, more than 25 cm H_2O, whereas the PEEP in the article by Suter, Fairley, and Isenberg is conventional PEEP, ranging from 5 to 20 cm H_2O. However, the concept of best or optimal PEEP has evolved over the years. More recently, the endpoint for PEEP application is the lowest level of PEEP that provides an adequate PaO_2 at an FIO_2 of less than 0.5. Increasing PEEP beyond this level to obtain optimum values for various other endpoints, such as the production of maximum oxygen transport, maximum static pulmonary compliance, shunt less than 15% to 20%, minimal arterial end-tidal CO_2 gradient, decreased mixed venous oxygen tension, and minimum FIO_2 will not be clinically helpful and may be harmful.

Albert RK. Least PEEP: primum non nocere. *Chest* 1985;87:2–3.

Benumof JL. *Anesthesia for thoracic surgery*, 2nd ed. Philadelphia: WB Saunders, 1995:725.

Carrol GC, Tuman KJ, Braverman B, et al. Minimal positive end-expiratory pressure (PEEP) may be best PEEP. *Chest* 1988;93:1020–1025.

Civetta JM, Barnes TA, Smith LO. Optimal PEEP and intermittent mandatory ventilation in the treatment of acute respiratory failure. *Respir Care* 1975;20:551–557.

Pelosi P. DVD: vertical gradient of regional lung inflation in adult respiratory distress syndrome. *Am J Respir Crit Care Med* 1994;149:8.

Suter PM, Fairley HB, Isenberg MD. Optimum end-expiratory airway pressure in patients with acute pulmonary failure. *N Engl J Med* 1975;292:284–288.

D.8. What are the cardiovascular effects of PEEP?

The cardiovascular effects of PEEP depend on the severity of respiratory failure, the level of PEEP, the intravascular volume, the contractility of the heart, and the pulmonary vasculature.

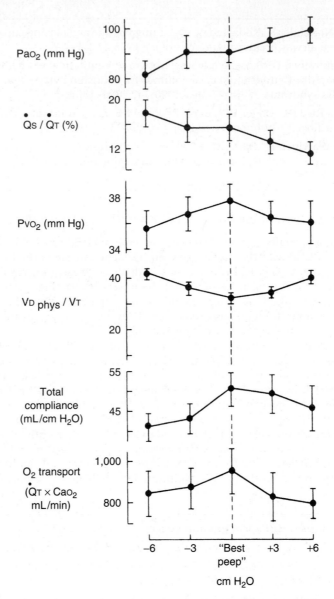

Pao$_2$ (mm Hg)

$\overset{\bullet}{Q}$s / $\overset{\bullet}{Q}$t (%)

Pvo$_2$ (mm Hg)

Vd phys / Vt

Total compliance (mL/cm H$_2$O)

O$_2$ transport ($\overset{\bullet}{Q}$t × Cao$_2$ mL/min)

−6   −3   "Best peep"   +3   +6

cm H$_2$O

Figure 3.3 Best positive end-expiratory pressure. (From Suter PM, Fairley HB, Isenberg MD. Optimal end-expiratory airway pressure in patients with acute pulmonary failure. *N Engl J Med* 1975;292:284−288, with permission.)

In healthy subjects without respiratory failure, **PEEP** decreases cardiac output mainly because of increased intrathoracic pressure resulting in decreased venous return. **PEEP** also causes pulmonary parenchymal overdistention, which makes the lung come in close contact with the left ventricle, changing compliance and interfering with ventricular function. In addition, **PEEP** increases pulmonary pressure and resistance, resulting in right ventricular dilation, which causes an intraventricular septum shift toward the left ventricle. The leftward septal shift decreases left ventricular diastolic filling, resulting in decreased stroke volume and cardiac output. Also, unilateral pulmonary hyperinflation may cause neural reflex, resulting in a decreased cardiac output and heart rate. Moreover, humoral depression of myocardial contractility may also be a factor. The aforementioned deleterious effect of PEEP is more apparent in individuals with limited cardiovascular reserve. Although PEEP is applied only at the end of expiration, in actuality, the alveolar and transpulmonary pressures are highest during inspiration (driving pressures exceeding 20 to 30 cm H_2O in some patients) and are associated with the greatest negative hemodynamic effects.

In persons with respiratory failure, PEEP, up to optimum levels, usually increases or does not change cardiac output because of an increase in oxygenation with resultant improvement of cardiac performance. Cardiac output decreases when PEEP exceeds the individual's optimum PEEP. Hypotension during PEEP therapy may be exacerbated by hypovolemia.

In patients with underlying left ventricular failure and filling pressure more than 18 mm Hg, PEEP may increase cardiac output by increasing coronary arterial oxygen content, augmenting systolic function, or reducing venous return. The decreased venous return may produce a shift in the Starling curve to filling pressures associated with better myocardial function.

Pinsky MP. Cardiovascular effects of ventilatory support and withdrawal. *Anesth Analg* 1995;79:567–576.

Robotham JL, Lixfeld W, Holland L, et al. The effects of positive end-expiratory pressure on right and left ventricular performance. *Am Rev Respir Dis* 1980;121:677–683.

D.9. What is pressure support ventilation (PSV)? Discuss its advantages.

PSV is pressure-limited, flow-controlled PPV during which each spontaneous inspiratory effort is assisted by mechanically maintaining a predetermined inspiratory pressure plateau throughout inspiration. Whereas PSV is most often flow cycled, both pressure and time can be secondary cycling mechanisms. That is, pressure support can cycle to the exhalation phase when flow decelerates to a ventilator-determined level or to a pressure-determined level and/or when the inspiratory time has reached a predetermined level. PSV can be used for patients who are breathing completely spontaneously or who are being supported with IMV, and it can be used for patients receiving CPAP (Fig. 3.4).

PSV, which is an adjunct form of ventilatory support, is controlled with a microprocessor incorporated into the mechanical ventilator's circuit. When the patient makes the initial inspiratory effort, a very sensitive pressure transducer detects the slight negative pressure change and application of a constant support pressure is begun. Pressure is applied continuously throughout inspiration at the value selected by the operator.

The advantages of PSV are as follows:

- Achieving larger tidal volumes with lower airway pressures
- Decreasing work of breathing
- Improving spontaneous breathing patterns, including decreased respiratory rate, longer expiratory phase, and better synchrony with mechanical ventilation
- Promoting weaning from mechanical ventilation because of decreased respiratory muscle fatigue

Although theoretic advantages and safety of the mode in appropriately monitored patients support its use, few clinical studies have documented the efficacy of PSV.

Barash PG, Cullen BF, Stoelting RK, eds. *Clinical anesthesia*, 4th ed. Philadelphia: Lippincott Williams & Wilkins, 2001:1470.

Berger KI, Barry Sorkin I, Norman RG, et al. Mechanism of relief of tachypnea during pressure support ventilation. *Chest* 1996;109:1320–1327.

Braun NMT, Faulkner J, Hughes RL, et al. When should respiratory muscles be rested? *Chest* 1986;84:76–84.

Hess D, Branson R. Ventilators and weaning modes. *Respir Care Clin N Am* 2000;6:407–435.

MacIntyre NR. Respiratory function during pressure support ventilation. *Chest* 1986;89: 677–683.

D.10. What is inverse-ratio ventilation (IRV)?

During the normal respiratory cycle, the duration of inspiration is one half to one third shorter than the duration of exhalation. In IRV, the inspiratory cycle time is increased to two or more times greater than expiratory cycle time. This mode of ventilation can be applied during pressure-controlled ventilation (pressure controlled, time cycled) or in volume-controlled ventilation (by decreasing the inspiratory flow rate and applying a decelerating waveform). The intended benefits of IRV in ARDS are several: (a) lower peak airway pressures are generated; (b) improved gas exchange as a result of allowing greater time for exchange and mixing to take place; (c) sustained elevation of airway pressure and maintenance of higher mean airway pressure can both prevent alveolar collapse and improve alveolar recruitment; and (d) reduction in dead space with improvement in carbon dioxide elimination. By shortening the exhalation cycle, several problems can arise. First, the propensity for gas trapping increases, resulting in an increase in intrinsic PEEP. With the development of intrinsic PEEP, the work of breathing becomes excessive, along with patient-ventilator dyssynchrony. Consequently, most patients require heavy sedation and paralysis while on IRV mode. The proposed improvement in gas exchange and possibly in alveolar recruitment may come solely from the effects of intrinsic PEEP. In fact, Zavala et al. investigated the effect of gas exchange during four ventilator settings: (a) volume-controlled mechanical ventilation (VC-MV) without PEEP; (b) VC-MV with PEEP; (c) volume-controlled IRV (VC-IRV); and (d) pressure-controlled IRV (PC-IRV). In each mode of ventilation, the level of PEEP (8 cm H_2O) was assigned equally, whereas the tidal volume, respiratory rate, and inspired oxygen fraction

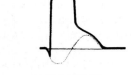

[IN][LIM][CYC]
Pressure Pressure Flow

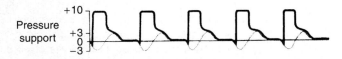

Pressure support
+10
+3
0
−3

Figure 3.4 Airway pressure tracings of pressure-support ventilation (*solid line*) and spontaneous ventilation (*dotted line*). CYC, cycle; IN, initiation; LIM, limit;. (From Shapiro BA, Kacmarek RM, Cane RD, et al. *Clinical application of respiratory care,* 4th ed. St. Louis; Mosby-Year Book, 1991:317, with permission.)

were maintained unchanged from baseline values. The following observations were made: (a) The peak airway pressure was lower during IRV than VC-MV PEEP; however, the plateau pressure was similar for all three modes (VC-MV PEEP, VC-IRV, and PC-IRV); (b) the mean airway pressure was higher in the IRV group, particularly, in the PC-IRV; (c) the arterial PaO_2 improved with the addition of PEEP in VC-MV and VC-IRV but not in PC-IRV; and (d) the level of $PaCO_2$ significantly decreased and the pH increased in IRV mode as compared with the controlled mechanical ventilation modes. These findings suggest that in IRV mode, whether in pressure-controlled or volume-controlled mode, there is no short-term benefit in gas exchange relative to controlled mechanical ventilation when the same level of PEEP is applied. Whereas the peak airway pressures were lower in the IRV than in the VC-MV PEEP mode, the lack of differences in plateau pressure between these ventilator modalities can be explained by the resistive pressure decrease (differences in peak airway pressure and plateau pressure) that is predominantly determined by the endotracheal tube. At present, no prospective randomized trial has been conducted to assess the beneficial effect of IRV compared with conventional ventilation on outcome in ARDS; consequently, opposing opinions exist regarding the application of IRV in the management of ALI and ARDS.

Barash PG, Cullen BF, Stoelting RK, eds. *Clinical anesthesia*, 4th ed. Philadelphia: Lippincott Williams & Wilkins, 2001:1471.

Fontes ML. Progress in mechanical ventilation. *Curr Opin Anesthesiol* 2002;15:45–51.

McIntyre RC Jr, Pulido EJ, Bensard DD, et al. Thirty years of clinical trials in acute respiratory distress syndrome. *Crit Care Med* 2000;28(9):3314–3331.

Smith RP, Fletcher R. Pressure-controlled inverse ratio ventilation after cardiac surgery. *Eur J Anaesthesiol* 2001;18(6):401–406.

Zavala E, Ferrer M, Polese G, et al. E ratio ventilation on pulmonary gas exchange in acute respiratory distress syndrome. *Anesthesiology* 1998;88:35–42.

D.11. Describe the rationale for prone-position ventilation and its effect on oxygenation.

The concept of improving oxygenation and gas exchange in patients with ARDS was proposed more than 20 years ago. The mechanisms for improvement in oxygenation in the prone position are unclear, and whether such physiologic benefit alters outcome is equally unknown. For gas exchange to improve, several respiratory processes must occur: (a) better matching of ventilation and perfusion in those lung regions affected by either too little perfusion but normal ventilation or normal perfusion but inadequate ventilation; (b) improvement in pulmonary diffusion capacity of oxygen and carbon dioxide (i.e., reduced interstitial edema and inflammation); (c) improvement in mobilization and delivery of these gases from the tissues to the lungs (better cardiac output and end-organ function); and (d) reduction in ventilator-induced lung injury in the prone position as compared with supine. In ARDS, the whole lung is affected by endothelial and epithelial hyperpermeability with resulting edema. In the supine position, dependent lung regions are subjected to a relatively greater regional pleural pressure gradient secondary to the forces of gravity acting on the ribcage, the diaphragm, the abdomen, the heart, and the mediastinal structures. Such increases in transpulmonary pressures overstretch normal alveoli, cause epithelial and endothelial disruption, and induce a state of pulmonary edema. Studies of animal models of ALI have shown that while in the supine position, high levels of PEEP are required to maintain the injured and surfactant-depleted alveoli open. Failure to do this promotes ventilator-related lung injury. Additionally, perfusion of these dependent regions may be reduced from regional compression by the weight of the edematous upper lung units and from the effects of hypoxic pulmonary vasoconstriction. In contrast, positioning the patient prone allows for a more uniform gravitational gradient for alveolar ventilation and redistribution of alveolar ventilation to dorsal lung regions. Several other processes may account for the observed improvement in physiologic parameters in the prone position:

- The airway orientation is such that it tends to promote drainage of airway liquids toward the airway opening while in prone position and toward the dorsal regions when lying supine
- Redistribution of perfusion along a gravitational gradient to less injured lung regions
- Increased FRC
- Change in regional diaphragm motion

Pelosi et al. measured the change in thoracoabdominal compliance in the supine versus the prone position and compared this to changes in oxygenation. They found a direct correlation between improvement in compliance in the prone position and improvement in oxygenation that was most likely attributed to positioning the more rigid ribcage and vertebrae in the superior position while splinting the mobile anterior chest by the mattress. This maneuver favored redistribution of ventilation to the dorsal lung segments and alveolar recruitment.

Clinical improvement in oxygenation is reported in up to 90% of patients after transition from the supine to the prone position. Jolliet et al. studied the effects of 12 hours of prone positioning in 19 patients with ARDS who were heavily sedated and paralyzed. Patients were defined as responders if an increase in PaO_2 of greater than or equal to 10 mm Hg or in PaO_2/FiO_2 ratio of greater than or equal to 20 was observed in the prone position. Fifty-seven percent of the subjects in this study responded to prone placement. At the end of 12 hours, the patients were repositioned supine and had repeated measurements of respiratory parameters. Interestingly, the measures of oxygenation did not change after the first 30 minutes of resuming supine ventilation as compared with the previous prone position. In fact, oxygenation was improved from the baseline value. Jolliet et al. also reported that repeated trials of supine-to-prone and prone-to-supine maneuvers revealed a positive response in 71% of the initial responders versus a 25% positive response in the former nonresponders. Unfortunately, the study could not identify patient characteristics that predicted positive response, magnitude of positive or negative response, or the effect of positive response on survival and outcome. Others have also reported similar findings. Voggenreiter compared the effects of intermittent prone ventilation in 22 patients (11 of whom had severe and moderate posttraumatic lung injury and 11 had ARDS). Statistically significant improvements in respiratory parameters were observed in the prone position relative to the supine position for the following variables: (a) oxygenation; (b) $PAO_2 - PaO_2$ and Qs/QT; (c) total static lung compliance; and (d) reduction in pulmonary densities.

Although the advantages of the prone position have been shown in many case reports and in animal studies of ALI, the definitive study (large, randomized, and prospective) has not been done. The risks of proning patients also need to be tested prospectively. Several of the known risks include accidental extubation, inadvertent removal of intravenous lines and central venous catheters, and pressure injury of soft tissues.

Albert RK, Hubmayr RD. The prone position eliminates compression of the lungs by the heart. *Am J Respir Crit Care Med* 2000;161:1660–1665.

Fontes ML. Progress in mechanical ventilation. *Curr Opin Anesthesiol* 2002;15:45–51.

Gattinoni L, Bombino M, Lissoni A, et al. Lung structure and function in different stages of severe adult respiratory distress syndrome. *JAMA* 1994;271:1772–1779.

Gattinoni L, Pelosi P, Vitale G, et al. Body position changes redistribute lung computed-tomographic density in patients with acute respiratory failure. *Anesthesiology* 1991;74:15–23.

Jolliet P, Bulpa P, Chevrolet JC, et al. Effects of the prone position on gas exchange and hemodynamics in severe acute respiratory distress syndrome. *Crit Care Med* 1998;26:1977–1985.

Mure M, Domino KB, Lindahl SG, et al. Regional ventilation-perfusion distribution is more uniform in the prone position. *J Appl Physiol* 2000;88:1076–1083.

Mutoh T, Guest RJ, Lamm WJ, et al. Prone position alters the effect of volume overload on regional pleural pressures and improves hypoxemia in pigs *in vivo*. *Am Rev Respir Dis* 1992;146:300–306.

Pelosi P, Tubiolo D, Mascheroni D, et al. Effects of the prone position on respiratory mechanics and gas exchange during acute lung injury. *Am J Respir Crit Care Med* 1998;157:387–393.

Voggenreiter G, Neudeck F, Aufmkok M, et al. Intermittent prone positioning in the treatment of severe and moderate posttraumatic lung injury. *Crit Care Med* 1999;27:2375–2382.

D.12. How is liquid ventilation accomplished?

Kylstra, who demonstrated that salt solutions could be saturated with oxygen at high pressures, first introduced the concept of fluid breathing in the 1960s. In 1966, Leland Clark uncovered that both oxygen and carbon dioxide were soluble in fluorocarbon liquids. The earlier methods of liquid ventilation with fluorocarbons met limited success as a result of impurities and chemical compositions of the fluorocarbons that caused ALI. Advances in perfluorocarbon (PFC) technology, however, have led to the development of improved generations of oxygen carriers that incorporated nontoxic carriers. The PFC compounds are inert organic chemicals produced by replacement of fluorine for hydrogen in specific sites within the carbon chain. These agents do not undergo metabolism in the body and are eliminated through the pulmonary, gastrointestinal and renal systems.

The proposed mechanisms for both improvement in oxygenation and hastening of recovery from ALI include a high solubility coefficient for oxygen and carbon dioxide relative to hemoglobin and a density that is twice that of water. As such, replacement of the FRC by PFC eliminates the alveolar membrane-air-liquid interface, reduces surface tension in the surfactant-depleted lung, and physically maintains the alveoli open. Because of its high density, it tends to gravitate toward the more dependent lung region that is most affected by lung edema and ALI. This effect stabilizes alveolar units in these regions and aids in alveolar recruitment. The use of partial liquid ventilation (PLV) with PFC may alter regional blood flow by diverting blood from dependent to nondependent lung regions, thereby improving ventilation/perfusion matching (i.e., fluid **PEEP**). An additional benefit of PLV is the displacement of alveolar proteinaceous edema, inflammatory cells, debris, and other mediators from the alveolar spaces that are less dense.

Several clinical trials investigating the effect of PFC for PLV have shown a dose-dependent improvement in oxygenation. Leach et al. studied the efficacy of PLV using perflubron—an eight carbon PFC—in 13 premature infants with severe ARDS in whom conventional therapy using various modalities, including surfactant replacement, had failed. An amount of PFC equaling the infant's FRC was infused endotracheally while standard mechanical ventilation was maintained. Within 1 hour after installation of PFC, the PaO_2 increased by 138% and the dynamic compliance improved by 61%. Whereas the duration of PLV was 24 to 72 hours and no direct complications occurred during the trial, the overall mortality rate was 50%. In 2001, Schuster et al. investigated whether or not the distribution of PFC in PLV is inhomogeneous, resulting in either inadequate improvement or deterioration in oxygenation, particularly during the first 24 hours after initiation of PLV. Inhomogeneity in distribution may arise from regional obstruction of airway components by (a) cellular debris, edema, and inflammatory factors; (b) local destruction of lung parenchyma; and (c) regional uptake of the PFC by blood. In this study, the chest radiograph of 16 patients who had received PLV for 48 hours were reviewed. The best predictor of inhomogeneous filling was the initial dose of PFC (10 mL/kg as compared with 20 mL/kg). Although other investigators have shown a dose-dependent improvement in oxygenation, several others have confirmed the findings of Schuster et al.

PLV has been combined with several ventilatory approaches to maximize oxygen delivery. Suh et al. showed, in an animal model of ALI, that PLV has a dose-dependent increase in PaO_2 with PEEP or proning as compared with volume-controlled mechanical ventilation mode. Additionally, lung histology revealed significantly less hyaline membrane formation in the PLV group, suggesting that this modality of ventilation allows the lungs to heal after an acute injury process. Relative to lungs from conventionally ventilated animals, similar histologic findings have been described whereby the use of PLV resulted in less alveolar hemorrhage, decreased lung fluid accumulation, and diminished neutrophilic infiltration. This antiinflammatory benefit may be attributed to the mechanical lavage of alveolar debris by the PFC and by a direct effect on alveolar macrophages. Despite these proven benefits, the use of PFC for PLV remains investigative for management of ARDS and ALI. Additional larger randomized clinical trials addressing the efficacy and safety of PLV need to be performed before any definitive recommendation can be made.

Leach CL, Greenspan JS, Rubenstein SD, et al. Partial liquid ventilation with perflubron in premature infants with severe respiratory distress syndrome. *N Engl J Med* 1996; 335:761–767.

Lewis DA, Colton D, Johnson K, et al. Prevention of ventilator-induced lung injury with partial liquid ventilation. *J Pediatr Surg* 2001;36(9):1333–1336.

Ricard JD, Lemaire F. Liquid ventilation. *Curr Opin Crit Care* 2001;7(1):8–14.

Schuster DP, Lange NR, Tutuncu A, et al. Study group: clinical correlation with changing radiographic appearance during partial liquid ventilation. *Chest* 2001;119(5):1503–1509.

Suh GY, Chung MP, Park SJ, et al. Partial liquid ventilation shows dose-dependent increase in oxygenation with PEEP and decreases lung injury associated with mechanical ventilation. *J Crit Care* 2000;15:103–112.

Valls-I-Soler A, Alvarez FJ, Gastiasoro E. Liquid ventilation: from experimental use to clinical application. *Biol Neonate* 2001;80(Suppl 1):29–33.

D.13. What are the indications and contraindications for extracorporeal membrane oxygenation? How many ways can it be used? What are its results?

Extracorporeal membrane oxygenation (ECMO) should be used for patients in severe acute respiratory failure with reversible lung disease, who are dying of severe hypoxemia despite maximal conventional ventilatory care (e.g., tracheal intubation, mechanical ventilation with 10 to 15 cm H_2O PEEP, diuresis, chest physical therapy, antibiotics, normothermia or mild hypothermia, sedation, paralysis, and increased oxygen concentration). Indications for ECMO by the NIH are as follows: PaO_2 less than 50 mm Hg for more than 2 hours with FIO_2 of 1.0 and conventional PEEP; and a PaO_2 less than 50 mm Hg for more than 12 hours with FIO_2 of more than 0.6 and conventional PEEP. Active bleeding is the only absolute contraindication to use of the artificial lung. The three routes for ECMO are as follows: venovenous perfusion from the inferior vena cava by way of the femoral vein to the oxygenator and then to the superior vena cava; venoarterial perfusion from the femoral vein to the oxygenator and then to the femoral artery; and venovenous arterial perfusion from the femoral vein to the oxygenator and then to both the internal jugular vein and the femoral artery.

A collaborative study on ECMO has been completed under the auspices of the National Heart, Lung, and Blood Institute of the NIH. The results of this controlled study are as follows:

- Compared with the control group of conventional respiratory therapy, ECMO did not improve mortality (90%), and the predominant cause of death was still progressive respiratory failure.

- ECMO did not affect the progress of disease (or lung pathology in those patients who died) any differently from conventional respiratory therapy.
- Although ECMO is an effective means of short-term life support, its clinical application for the treatment of ARDS is not appropriate or economically justified.

However, data analyzed from a national registry series of 715 neonatal ECMO patients (1980 to 1987) demonstrated an overall survival of 81%, which in earlier series had been the overall mortality rate with conventional therapy. As neonatal ECMO has evolved, entry criteria have been used, and experience with ECMO technology has been shown to improve survival. ECMO is now a proven support modality for neonatal respiratory failure that is due to several causes, such as meconium aspiration syndrome, persistent pulmonary hypertension of the newborn, congenital diaphragmatic hernia, and infant respiratory distress syndrome.

Kirshbom PM, Bridges ND, Myung RJ, et al. Use of extracorporeal membrane oxygenation in pediatric thoracic organ transplantation. *J Thorac Cardiovasc Surg* 2002; 123(1):130–136.

Mamprin F, Pesenti A, Fumagalli R. Extracorporeal circulation for acute respiratory failure. *Intensive Care Med* 2001;27(5):934–936.

National Heart, Lung, and Blood Institute. *Extracorporeal support for respiratory insufficiency. A collaborative study.* Bethesda, MD: US Department of Health, Education and Welfare, 1979.

Schumacher RE, Baumgart S. Extracorporeal membrane oxygenation 2001. The odyssey continues. *Clin Perinatol* 2001;28(3):629–653.

Taghavi S, Ankersmit HJ, Wieselthaler G, et al. Extracorporeal membrane oxygenation for graft failure after heart transplantation: recent Vienna experience. *J Thorac Cardiovasc Surg* 2001;122(4):819–820.

D.14. What is high frequency positive pressure ventilation (HFPPV)? What are its characteristics?

HFV was originally used as a technique to provide adequate oxygenation and alveolar ventilation for rigid bronchoscopy and laryngeal surgery. Since that time, the literature is replete with clinical applications of HFV. The major characteristics of the ventilatory pattern of volume-controlled HFPPV are as follows:

- A ventilatory frequency of approximately 60 to 100 per min and an inspiration/expiration ratio of less than 0.3
- Smaller tidal volumes and therefore lower maximum and mean airway and transpulmonary pressures, yet a higher FRC than in conventional PPV
- Positive intratracheal and negative intrapleural pressures throughout the ventilatory cycle
- Less circulatory interference than in IPPV and/or continuous positive pressure ventilation (CPPV)
- Reflex suppression of spontaneous respiratory rhythmicity during normoventilation
- Decelerating inspiratory flow without an end-inspiratory plateau
- More efficient pulmonary gas distribution than in IPPV and/or CPPV

Barash PG, Cullen BF, Stoelting RK, eds. *Clinical anesthesia*, 4th ed. Philadelphia: Lippincott Williams & Wilkins, 2001:1471.

Sjostrand U. High frequency positive-pressure ventilation (HFPPV): a review. *Crit Care Med* 1980;8:345–364.

D.15. What are the frequencies used in HFV? How are they classified?

HFV is a generic term encompassing any form of mechanical ventilation operating at a frequency at least four times higher than the natural breathing frequency of the subject being ventilated. Smith categorized HFV into three groups:

- HFPPV, 60 to 110 per minute
- High-frequency jet ventilation (HFJV), 110 to 400 per minute
- High-frequency oscillatory ventilation (HFOV), 400 to 2,400 per minute

Froese summarized HFV into five groups as shown in Fig. 3.5.

Sjostrand, in Sweden, first introduced HFPPV. It was administered with a very low compliant ventilator with high gas flow rates. This produces a flow profile with rapid upstroke to a high peak flow rate, followed by a passive expiration. Because it is a closed circuit, there was no entrainment of additional gas during inspiration.

HFJV delivers a small tidal volume at a high flow rate by means of a narrow orifice at an adjustable drive pressure, rate, and inspiratory time or I/E ratio. Gas is regulated by a solenoid

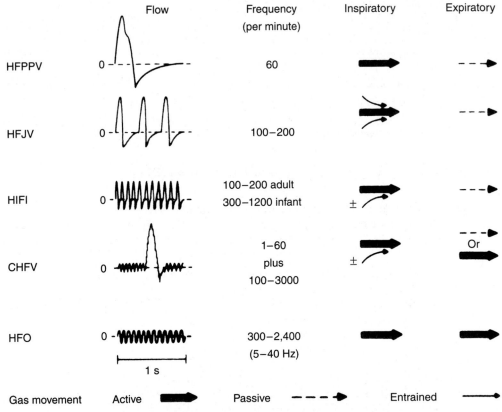

Figure 3.5 Summary of features of several commonly encountered high-frequency modalities. See text for details. CHFV, combined high-frequency ventilation; HFJV, high-frequency jet ventilation; HFOV, high-frequency oscillatory ventilation; HFPPV, high-frequency positive pressure ventilation; HIFI, high fidelity. (From Froese AB. High-frequency ventilation; uses and abuses. *ASA refresher courses in anesthesiology.* Park Ridge, IL: American Society of Anesthesiologists, 1986:127–138, with permission.)

or fluidic mechanism. Because jet flow is delivered to a small-lumen tube, entrainment occurs due to subambient pressure created at the distal end of a cannula. Exhalation occurs around the tube or through another lumen and is passive. Frequencies are commonly 100 to 200 per minute, occasionally up to 400 per minute.

High-frequency flow interrupters (HFFI) are closely related to jet ventilators. Gas from a high-pressure source is "chopped" into pulses by a rotating ball valve and directed into the lung. The frequencies are usually 100 to 200 per minute in adults and 300 to 1,200 per minute in infants.

CHFV means combined high-frequency ventilation. Combined approaches usually superimpose some form of HFV onto backup conventional mechanical ventilation. The reported combinations vary considerably, with the slow component ranging from 1 to 60 per minute, and the fast component being delivered at 100 to 3,000 per minute.

HFOV is delivered by an oscillator-type ventilator consisting of a rotary-driven piston to produce to-and-fro movement of gas within the airway. Unlike all the other modalities, during HFOV the ventilator actively drives both inspiratory and expiratory flows.

Barash PG, Cullen BF, Stoelting RK, eds. *Clinical anesthesia*, 4th ed. Philadelphia: Lippincott Williams & Wilkins, 2001:1172–1173.

Butler WJ, Bohn DJ, Bryan AC, et al. Ventilation by high frequency oscillation in humans. *Anesth Analg* 1980;59:577–584.

Carlon GC, Kahn RC, Howland WS, et al. Clinical experience with high frequency jet ventilation. *Crit Care Med* 1981;9:1–6.

El-Baz N, Faber LP, Doolas A. Combined high frequency ventilation for management of terminal respiratory failure: a new technique. *Anesth Analg* 1983;62:39–49.

Froese AB. High frequency ventilation: uses and abuses. In: Barash PG, ed. *ASA refresher courses in anesthesiology*. Park Ridge, IL: American Society of Anesthesiologists, 1986: 127–138.

Smith RB. Ventilation at high respiratory frequencies. *Anaesthesia* 1983;37:1011.

D.16. What are the indications and precautions for high frequency ventilation (HFV)?

The indications for HFV include the following:

- Respiratory failure with bronchopleural fistula, tracheoesophageal or bronchoesophageal fistula, barotrauma, pulmonary fibrosis, and pulmonary hemorrhage, because of low airway pressure with HFV.
- Anesthesia for special procedures, such as bronchoscopy, laryngoscopy, tracheal reconstruction over a T-tube, and laser resection of a bronchial lesion, because HFV uses a small cannula for ventilation, leaving adequate room for surgeons to operate.
- Anesthesia for open thoracic surgery because of a moderately expanded lung and minimal respiratory movement with HFV.
- Improving oxygenation in adult and infant respiratory distress syndrome when hypoxemia persists in spite of maximal conventional ventilatory support.
- Enhancement of CO_2 elimination when conventional mechanical ventilation has been unable to support adequate CO_2 elimination despite multiple adjustments of ventilator settings in situations such as persistent fetal circulation in the neonate. HFV could prove advantageous in achieving a respiratory alkalosis by hyperventilation at low peak and mean airway pressures.

The precautions with HFV include the following:

- HFV must never be used in a situation in which expiratory outflow of gas from the lung is impeded. Under such circumstances, lethal barotrauma can occur.

- HFV should never be used with inadequate humidification, because serious tracheal injury may occur.
- HFV system pressure should be accurately and appropriately sampled and monitored in order to drive an automatic shutoff mechanism so gas entry into the lungs can be terminated immediately if an overpressure situation occurs.
- HFV should never be used without adequate training.

Borg U, Eriksson I, Sjostrand U. High frequency positive pressure ventilation (HFPPV): a review based upon its use during bronchoscopy and for laryngoscopy and microlaryngeal surgery under general anesthesia. *Anesth Analg* 1980;59:594–603.

Carlon GC, Howland WS, Ray C, et al. High frequency jet ventilation. A prospective randomized evaluation. *Chest* 1983;84:551–559.

Carlon GC, Kahn RC, Howland WS, et al. Clinical experience with high frequency jet ventilation. *Crit Care Med* 1981;9:1–6.

Cartotto R, Cooper AB, Esmond JR, et al. Early clinical experience with high-frequency oscillatory ventilation for ARDS in adult burn patients. *J Burn Care Rehabil* 2001;22(5): 325–333.

Dalton HJ. Lung volume measurement during high-frequency ventilation: a new role for an old technique? *Crit Care Med* 2001;29(12):2394–2395.

El-Baz N, Holinger L, El-Ganzouri A, et al. High frequency positive-pressure ventilation for tracheal reconstruction supported by tracheal T-tube. *Anesth Analg* 1982;61:796–800.

Froese AB. High frequency ventilation: uses and abuses. In: Barash PG, ed. *ASA refresher courses in anesthesiology*. Park Ridge, IL: American Society of Anesthesiologists, 1986: 127–138.

Fujino Y, Kacmarek RM, Hess DR. Nitric oxide delivery during high-frequency oscillatory ventilation. *Respir Care* 2000;45(9):1097–1104.

Imai Y, Nakagawa S, Ito Y, et al. Comparison of lung protection strategies using conventional and high-frequency oscillatory ventilation. *J Appl Physiol* 2001;91(4):1836–1844.

Keszler M, Durand DJ. Neonatal high-frequency ventilation. Past, present, and future. *Clin Perinatol* 2001;28(3):579–607.

Varkul MD, Stewart TE, Lapinsky SE, et al. Successful use of combined high-frequency oscillatory ventilation, inhaled nitric oxide, and prone positioning in the acute respiratory distress syndrome. *Anesthesiology* 2001;95(3):797–799.

Whitwam JG, Chakrabarti MK, Cody M, et al. Intermittent high frequency ventilation. Clinical evaluation of a new mode of ventilation. *Anaesthesiol Scand* 1990;34(6): 447–451.

D.17. What is nitric oxide (NO)? What is the role of inhaled NO in the treatment of ARDS?

In 1987, endothelium-derived relaxing factor was identified as NO. NO produced by the endothelium diffuses into vascular smooth muscle where NO activates soluble guanylate cyclase. The subsequent increase in intracellular cyclic guanosine monophosphate (cGMP) causes smooth muscle vasodilation. Endothelium-independent nitrovasodilators such as nitroglycerin and nitroprusside also act through guanylate cyclase activation to directly release NO.

Inhaled NO is a selective pulmonary vasodilator. NO is not effective during systemic administration because it is rapidly inactivated by hemoglobin. Therefore, inhaled NO may diffuse from the alveoli to pulmonary vascular smooth muscle and produce pulmonary vasodilation without systemic vasodilation because any NO that diffuses into blood will be inactivated by hemoglobin. Inhaled NO has been shown to be effective in treating primary pulmonary hypertension, as well as decreasing pulmonary hypertension and improving oxygenation after mitral valve replacement and in the newborn with persistent pulmonary hypertension.

Pulmonary hypertension and hypoxemia universally occur in ARDS. Pulmonary hypertension in ARDS may be due to active vasoconstriction from local alveolar hypoxic pulmonary vasoconstriction and other vasoconstrictor mediators. Hypoxemia in ARDS is due to ventilation/perfusion mismatch, intrapulmonary shunting, or anatomic shunting. Intravenous pulmonary vasodilator therapy with agents such as nitroglycerin, nitroprusside, prostaglandin E, prostacyclin, adenosine, and nifedipine produces small reduction in pulmonary artery pressure but large reduction in systemic blood pressure and arterial oxygenation. The adverse effect on oxygenation is primarily due to reversal of hypoxic pulmonary vasoconstriction. On the contrary, inhaled NO may decrease pulmonary hypertension and improve oxygenation in patients with ARDS because inhaled NO may be distributed according to ventilation so the associated vasodilation increases blood flow to well-ventilated alveoli.

Rossaint et al. published the first major report of the use of inhaled NO in patients with ARDS. They found that inhaled NO (5 to 20 parts per million [ppm]) effectively decreased pulmonary hypertension and improved oxygenation. In a subsequent study, they showed that inhaled concentrations of only 60 to 250 parts per billion could increase PaO_2 by 30%. These concentrations had little or no effect on pulmonary artery pressure. The other major study by Bigatello et al. demonstrated that inhaled NO produced dose-related decreases in pulmonary artery pressure with 50% of the maximal effect occurring at 5 ppm. Inhaled NO also increased oxygenation, but dose-response effects could not be demonstrated.

Inhaled NO has been effective on ARDS in combination with other therapies. The combination of inhaled NO (5 to 10 ppm) and almitrine bismesylate, a potentiator of hypoxic pulmonary vasoconstrictor, had additive effects on improving oxygenation in ARDS and simultaneously decreased pulmonary hypertension. Dcering et al. studied intravenous phenylephrine, 50 to 200 μg per minute, titrated to a 20% increase in mean arterial pressure; inhaled NO, 40 ppm; and the combination of phenylephrine and NO. They found that phenylephrine alone can improve PaO_2 in patients with ARDS. In phenylephrine-responsive patients, phenylephrine augments the improvement in PaO_2 seen with inhaled NO. These results may reflect selective enhancement of hypoxic pulmonary vasoconstriction by phenylephrine, which complements selective vasodilation by inhaled NO

However, an important unsolved issue is the potential pulmonary toxicity of inhaled NO. Toxicity may be due to NO itself, or to its reactive metabolite, NO_2. NO can combine with superoxide anion to produce peroxynitrite anion, which is a powerful oxidizing agent. The effects of NO and NO_2 on repair versus fibrosis in injured lung and on pulmonary host defenses are unknown. Therefore, the effects of inhaled NO on outcome in patients with ARDS are not predictable.

Overall, the data on NO therapy in the setting of ARDS demonstrate that it can improve oxygenation in some patients, but this is limited over time and it does *not* improve survival. Currently, NO is not recommended for use in the setting of ARDS.

Bigatello LM, Hurford WE, Kacmarek RM, et al. Prolonged inhalation of low concentrations of nitric oxide in patients with severe adult respiratory distress syndrome. Effect on pulmonary hemodynamics and oxygenation. *Anesthesiology* 1994;80:761–770.

Dcering EB, Hanson CW III, Reily DJ, et al. Improvement in oxygenation by phenylephrine and nitric oxide in patients with adult respiratory distress syndrome. *Anesthesiology* 1997;87:18–25.

Ferguson ND, Granton JT. Inhaled nitric oxide for hypoxemic respiratory failure: passing bad gas? *Can Med Assoc J* 2000;162(1):85–86.

Finer NN, Sun JW, Rich W, et al. Randomized, prospective study of low-dose versus high-dose inhaled nitric oxide in the neonate with hypoxic respiratory failure. *Pediatrics* 2001;108(4):949–955.

Gerlach H, Pappert D, Lewandowski K, et al. Long-term inhalation with evaluated low doses of nitric oxide for selective improvement of oxygenation in patients with adult respiratory distress syndrome. *Intensive Care Med* 1993;19:443–449.

Hurfold WE. Inhaled nitric oxide—current concepts. In: *ASA annual meeting refresher course lectures*, Park Ridge, IL, American Society of Anesthesiologists, 2001;431.

Matthews BD, Noviski N. Management of oxygenation in pediatric acute hypoxemic respiratory failure. *Pediatr Pulmonol* 2001;32(6):459–470.

Mercier JC. Franco-Belgium Neonatal Study Group on Inhaled NO. Uncertainties about the use of inhaled nitric oxide in preterm infants. *Acta Paediatr Suppl* 2001;90(436): 15–18.

Rossaint R, Falke KJ, Lopez F, et al. Inhaled nitric oxide for the adult respiratory disease syndrome. *N Engl J Med* 1993;328:399–405.

Weinacker AB, Vaszar LT. Acute respiratory distress syndrome: physiology and new management strategies. *Annu Rev Med* 2001;52:221–237.

Zwissler B, Welte M, Habler O, et al. Effects of inhaled prostacyclin as compared with inhaled nitric oxide in a canine model of pulmonary microembolism and oleic acid edema. *J Cardiothorac Vasc Anesth* 1995;9:634–640.

E. Weaning from Ventilatory Support

The patient's condition improved after respiratory support with 20 cm H_2O PEEP. Arterial blood gases showed pH, 7.45; $Paco_2$, 35 mm Hg; Pao_2, 150 mm Hg; Fio_2 0.75.

E.1. What would you do now?

The arterial blood gas analysis suggests that the oxygenation has improved markedly; nevertheless, there continues to be significant intrapulmonary shunting and the level of PEEP remains high. Before making any drastic changes, it is important to examine the patient thoroughly to determine that in fact the lung injury is resolving and that there is no evidence of infection, systemic inflammatory involvement, and metabolic derangements. The most appropriate ventilatory change is to lower the Fio_2 to less than 0.5 or 0.6. This should be well tolerated. Next, the PEEP should be lowered gradually. The suggested criteria to lower PEEP level are a stable, nonseptic patient; Pao_2/Fio_2 more than 200 mm Hg; effective compliance, more than 25 mL per cm H_2O; Pao_2- Pao_2, less than 200 mm Hg at Fio_2 0.5. PEEP should not be decreased by more than 5 cm H_2O during a trial. At least 6 hours should elapse before undertaking a further attempt at lowering the PEEP level.

Esteban A, Alia I, Tobin MJ, et al. Effect of spontaneous breathing trial duration on outcome of attempts to discontinue mechanical ventilation. *Am J Respir Crit Care Med* 1999;159:512–518.

Luterman A, Hororvitz JH, Carrico CJ, et al. Withdrawal from PEEP. *Surgery* 1978;39: 328–332.

Tobin MJ. 1999 Donald F Egan scientific lecture: weaning from mechanical ventilation: what have we learned? *Respir Care* 2000;45:417–431.

E.2. The patient continued to improve. When would you consider weaning the patient from the respirator? Discuss the criteria for weaning.

The criteria for discontinuance of mechanical ventilation are essentially the converse of the criteria for the institution of mechanical support and are as follows:

- Clear consciousness with adequate gag and cough reflex
- Cardiovascular stability
- Stable metabolic state without hypothermia, hyperpyrexia, metabolic acidosis, or alkalosis
- Adequate pulmonary function

Mechanics

- A vital capacity of more than 10 mL per kg or more than twice the normal tidal volume
- Rapid shallow breathing index (respiratory frequency/tidal volume) of less than 100 breaths per minute per L
- A maximum inspiratory force of at least -20 to -30 cm H_2O

Oxygenation

- Pa_{O_2} more than 80 mm Hg with F_{IO_2} at 0.4
- $PA_{O_2} - Pa_{O_2}$ less than 300 mm Hg with F_{IO_2} at 1.0
- Qs/Q_T less than 15%

Ventilation

- Pa_{CO_2} less than 45 mm Hg
- V_D/V_T less than 0.6

Lumb AB. *Nunn's applied respiratory physiology*, 6th ed. Philadelphia: Elsevier Butterworth-Heinemann, 2005:430–431.

E.3. Describe weaning by synchronized IMV, pressure support, CPAP, and T-piece.

Mechanical ventilatory assistance is often an obligatory step during management of critically ill patients; however, complete withdrawal from this support represents a significant clinical problem in approximately 25% of intubated patients. Frequently employed weaning techniques have included PSV, T-piece, CPAP, and SIMV. Several studies have compared these various weaning approaches, but the results have been conflicting. Brochard et al. compared weaning by PSV, T-piece, and SIMV and found weaning by PSV to be superior to weaning by T-piece and by SIMV. In contrast, in a large multicenter trial of nonsurgical patients with diverse medical problems, Esteban et al. demonstrated that the duration of weaning by T-piece once a day was significantly less than weaning by PSV, which in turn was less than weaning by SIMV. Recently, Kollef et al. showed that a protocol-guided weaning by nurses and respiratory therapists was safe and led to extubation more rapidly than physician-directed weaning. Therefore, in addition to differences in study design, weaning modalities, and weaning techniques, there are selection and physician biases that interfere with the process of weaning. Although employment of protocol-driven weaning may control for physician bias, it is also data driven, time consuming, and costly.

Conventional T-piece technique

When the patient meets the criteria for weaning, a T-piece adapter and heated nebulizer are connected to the patient's endotracheal tube. The patient should be in a semisitting or sitting position. The inspired oxygen concentration is set at a level 5% to 10% higher than what the patient was receiving during mechanical ventilation. The vital signs and cardiac rhythm are monitored carefully every 5 to 10 minutes. Arterial blood gases are determined 15 minutes after weaning is begun and then every hour. The patient who tolerates the T-piece very well is extubated after 2 to 4 hours. Oxygen is then administered through a face mask with a heated nebulizer, at the same inspired oxygen concentration as during the T-piece trial.

The high success associated with T-piece weaning is related primarily to the fact that the clinician biases are removed from the process. In other words, the patient becomes the sole controller of his or her weaning and readiness for extubation. No guessing is involved. One is either ready or not for weaning, and the best way to determine this is to apply no support. The weaning process is very difficult because the patient's need varies on a breath-by-breath basis, such that the clinician is incapable of predicting such changes. The common error is to be too conservative, thereby prolonging the weaning process.

Synchronized intermittent mandatory ventilation technique

Weaning is accomplished by a gradual decrease in the SIMV rate that the ventilator delivers, allowing the patient slowly to take over spontaneous ventilation. This system allows the patient to breathe spontaneously between the preset mechanical ventilation. This system ensures intermittent hyperinflation of the lung.

Weaning by SIMV is the least effective approach in terms of weaning time. It promotes dependence on the ventilator and can be "confusing" to the respiratory center. The delivery of the mechanical breath must coincide with the central inspiratory time. The same rule applies during exhalation. Prolonging the mechanical breath will overlap with the neural start of exhalation; that is, although the neural input is telling the patient to exhale, the ventilator continues to inflate the lungs. This is frequently seen in patients with COPD whose airway flow changes more slowly and the expiratory muscle becomes active during ventilator-induced inflation. A mismatch can also occur if the patient's inspiratory drive occurs before exhalation is complete, leading to "breath stacking."

Another important aspect of synchronization during PPV is the flow rate that changes on an intrabreath and an interbreath basis. Frequently, patients will show signs of "air hunger" and tachypnea if the inspiratory flow rate is inadequate. In most ventilators, the flow rate is set at 60 L per minute. Too much flow is also problematic. Occasionally, the flow rate is increased to lower the inspiratory time while increasing the exhalation time. Unfortunately, the patient may respond adversely by becoming tachypneic, resulting in shortened expiratory times, which then potentiates dynamic hyperinflation (intrinsic PEEP). Several studies have shown a flow-related inspiratory termination reflex. Activating such reflexes can result in curtailing the neural inspiration producing shallow inspiratory efforts. Overall, the consequences of poor synchronization include increase in work of breathing, anxiety, patient discomfort, ineffective ventilation, and increased morbidity and mortality.

Pressure-support weaning

Pressure-support weaning can be combined with IMV and with CPAP weaning. Its proposed advantages include reducing the work of breathing, improving synchronization between the patient and the ventilator, reducing inspiratory pressures, and facilitating weaning. While on IMV, once the patient has been weaned to a minimum rate (i.e., IMV of 4 to 6 breaths per minute), the level of pressure support is gradually reduced (2 to 3 cm H_2O at a time). In some cases, this level of change is performed only once a day, whereas in other cases, the changes may be made several times a day. When the pressure-support level is at a minimum (<8 cm H_2O), weaning parameters are obtained in preparation for complete withdrawal from the mechanical ventilation. Attention to the pressure–volume and flow waveforms, which are available in most mechanical ventilators, can facilitate the weaning process and help determine other important aspects of respiratory mechanics (Fig. 3.6).

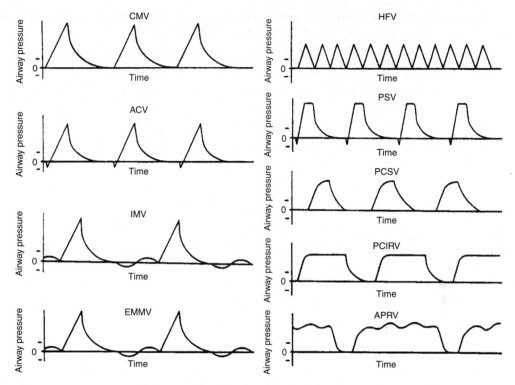

Figure 3.6 Airway pressure waveforms. ACV, assist/control ventilation; APRV, airway pressure-release ventilation; CMV, controlled mechanical ventilation; EMMV, extended mandatory minute ventilation; HFV, high-frequency ventilation; IMV, intermittent mandatory ventilation; PC–IRV, pressure-controlled inverse-ratio ventilation; PCV, pressure-controlled ventilation; PSV, pressure-support ventilation. (From Barash PG, Cullen BF, Stoelting RK, eds. *Clinical anesthesia,* 4th ed. Philadelphia: Lippincott Williams & Wilkins, 2001:1470, with permission.)

As with IMV, the inherent problem with pressure-support weaning is the clinical biases that exist. Once again, the technology and the knowledge that allow for minute-to-minute assessment and adjustment of the dynamic environment of the patient's physiology needs are lacking. Consequently, we make predictions about the level of support the patient needs and await clinical and laboratory signs of problems or success.

Overall, difficulties with weaning can be ascribed in part to the heterogeneity of underlying pulmonary diseases and to inconsistencies in clinical practice. Data-driven approaches to weaning are often nonpredictive of outcome and may fail to provide clinicians with signs of impending respiratory muscle fatigue. The patient's respiratory demand can vary considerably, requiring appropriate and timely ventilatory adjustments. A potential solution to this labor-intensive and costly task is to employ a computer-driven automated weaning process.

Benumof JL. *Anesthesia for thoracic surgery*, 2nd ed. Philadelphia: WB Saunders, 1995:738–740.

Brochard L, Rauss A, Benito S, et al. Comparison of three methods of gradual withdrawing from ventilatory support during weaning from mechanical ventilation. *Am J Respir Crit Care Med* 1994;150:896–903.

Esteban A, Frutos F, Tobin MJ, et al. A comparison of four methods of weaning patients from mechanical ventilation. *N Engl J Med* 1995;332:345–350.

Kollef MH, Shapiro SD, Silver P, et al. A randomized, controlled trial of protocol-directed versus physician-directed weaning from mechanical ventilation. *Crit Care Med* 1997;25:567–574.

CHAPTER 4

Lung Transplantation

PAUL M. HEERDT • CHARLES W. HOGUE, JR.

A 52-YEAR-OLD MAN

with progressively worsening dyspnea on exertion, limitation of daily activity despite supplemental oxygen, and radiographic and spirometric evidence of severe obstructive pulmonary disease was scheduled for single-lung transplantation. History was remarkable for a one pack per day for 30 years smoking history (although none for 10 years) and mild hypertension.

A. Medical Disease and Differential Diagnosis
1. What were the expected manifestations of severe obstructive pulmonary disease in this patient, and why was he a transplant candidate?
2. What other end-stage lung diseases can also be treated with transplantation?
3. How many lung transplantations have been performed?
4. What are the selection criteria for recipients?
5. How is the decision made to transplant one or both lungs, and does this influence preoperative management?
6. How does a single-lung transplantation differ technically from a double-lung transplantation?

B. Preoperative Evaluation and Preparation
1. What preoperative evaluation is desirable?
2. How would you premedicate this patient?
3. What vascular access is required?
4. Is preoperative epidural catheter placement advantageous?

C. Intraoperative Management
1. What special equipment is necessary?
2. How would you monitor this patient?
3. How would you induce anesthesia in this patient?
4. How would you ventilate this patient? What kind of endotracheal tube would you use?
5. How does the physiology of single-lung ventilation influence the procedure?
6. Should volatile anesthetics be avoided during single-lung ventilation?
7. At what specific points in the procedure are problems anticipated?
8. What problems are associated with the lateral position?
9. How does single-lung ventilation affect cardiopulmonary function? What are the problems of single-lung ventilation in this patient? How would you treat them?
10. How would you deal with problems related to clamping of the pulmonary artery (PA)?

11. What hemodynamic alterations would you expect during graft implantation and reperfusion? How would you correct them?

12. When is cardiopulmonary bypass (CPB) necessary for lung transplantation?

13. Should fluid administration be restricted, and are blood products commonly required?

14. Would you extubate the patient upon conclusion of the procedure?

D. Postoperative Management

1. What are the major complications after lung transplantation?

2. How is postoperative ventilation managed, and for how long is it required?

3. What special precautions should be taken when a lung transplant recipient requires general anesthesia for subsequent nonpulmonary surgery?

4. What are the long-term outcomes of lung transplantation?

5. Are there surgical alternatives to lung transplantation?

A. Medical Disease and Differential Diagnosis

A.1. What were the expected manifestations of severe obstructive pulmonary disease in this patient, and why was he a transplant candidate?

This patient suffered from increased airway resistance, reduced expiratory flow rates, and high residual lung volumes. When expiratory airway obstruction and lung hyperinflation become so severe that the chest cannot physically expand to accommodate a normal tidal volume, restrictive physiology becomes superimposed on obstructive disease. This condition is usually refractory to medical management and substantially limits daily activity. This patient's age and lack of other major systemic illness allowed him to be considered a transplant candidate.

Chronic obstructive pulmonary disease (COPD) (often secondary to smoking), emphysema secondary to α_1-antitrypsin deficiency, and cystic fibrosis are the most common obstructive disorders in adults undergoing lung transplantation. At one time, concerns about mediastinal displacement and profound ventilation/perfusion mismatch secondary to hyperinflation of the remaining native lung prevented surgeons from attempting single-lung transplantation for emphysema. However, clinical experience has demonstrated that many emphysemic patients can be successfully treated by single-lung transplantation. Because of the severe shortage of organs for transplant, single-lung procedures have been advocated as a means to increase the number of recipients. However, increasing experience suggests that bilateral lung transplantation for COPD is associated with improved functional outcomes and perhaps improved long-term survival compared with single-lung transplantation. Nonetheless, although transplantation may improve the quality of life for patients with severe COPD, recent data question whether either single or bilateral lung transplant has significant survival benefit.

Stavem K, Bjortuft O, Borgan O, et al. Lung transplantation in patients with chronic obstructive pulmonary disease in a national cohort is without obvious survival benefit. *J Heart Lung Transplant* 2006;25(1):75–84.

Sundaresan RS, Shiraishi Y, Trulock EP, et al. Single or bilateral lung transplantation for emphysema? *J Thorac Cardiovasc Surg* 1996;112:1485.

A.2. What other end-stage lung diseases can also be treated with transplantation?

The first successful (i.e., the patient left the hospital) single-lung transplantations were performed in 1983 for idiopathic pulmonary fibrosis. Since that time, the procedure has been applied

Table 4.1 Lung Transplants Categorized by Disease.

END-STAGE LUNG DISEASE	SINGLE-LUNG TRANSPLANT (% OF TOTAL)	BILATERAL/DOUBLE-LUNG TRANSPLANT (% OF TOTAL)
Cystic fibrosis	3	33
Retransplant	3	2
Primary pulmonary hypertension	4	9
α_1-Antitrypsin deficiency	11	10
Miscellaneous	11	18
Idiopathic pulmonary fibrosis	21	8
Emphysema	47	20

to patients suffering from various end-stage pulmonary diseases (Table 4.1). In general, the underlying disease processes produce lung dysfunction that can be broadly characterized as obstructive, restrictive, infectious (e.g., cystic fibrosis and bronchiectasis), or vascular. As of 2005, most single-lung transplantations have been performed for obstructive lung disease, followed by idiopathic pulmonary fibrosis. The most common indications for bilateral lung transplantation are cystic fibrosis and obstructive lung disease.

Reflecting a loss of lung parenchymal elasticity and compliance, end-stage restrictive disease is characterized by profoundly reduced lung volumes and diffusing capacity but relative preservation of ventilatory flow rates. Comparison of flow–volume loops representing obstructive and restrictive diseases is shown in Fig. 4.1. The underlying disease process also tends to obliterate

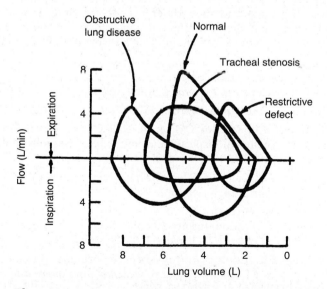

Figure 4.1 Representative tracings of flow–volume loops from a healthy subject, a patient with parenchymal obstructive disease, a patient with tracheal stenosis, and a patient with restrictive disease from parenchymal fibrosis. (From Goudsouzian N, Karamanian A. *Physiology for the anesthesiologist,* 2nd ed. Norwalk: Appleton-Century-Crofts, 1984:213, with permission.)

pulmonary microvasculature, thereby chronically increasing vascular resistance, producing pulmonary hypertension, and predisposing to cor pulmonale. Most patients with restrictive disease are good candidates for a single-lung transplantation because the stiff, vasoconstricted native lung will receive relatively little ventilation and perfusion and can therefore usually be left without compromising the transplanted lung.

Infectious lung disease such as cystic fibrosis is the most frequent indication for lung transplantation in patients younger than 18 years. Characterized by chronic infection and the production of copious purulent secretions, patients with cystic fibrosis primarily exhibit functional abnormalities that are obstructive with increased airway reactivity. Under most circumstances, residual volumes and functional residual capacity are increased and bronchodilators have little effect on expiratory flow rates. Because of potential infectious cross-contamination of the transplanted lung, chronic infectious disease represents a contraindication to single-lung transplantation. However, single-lung transplantation with contralateral pneumonectomy has been performed and suggested as an alternative solution.

Pulmonary vascular disease with severe pulmonary hypertension and right ventricular dysfunction has also emerged as an indication for transplantation. Pathologically, severe PA hypertension can result from idiopathic proximal vascular processes such as persistent pulmonary hypertension (PPH) or secondary to chronically increased pulmonary blood flow (e.g., left-to-right intracardiac shunt, leading to Eisenmenger's syndrome) or pulmonary venous hypertension. Pulmonary hypertension may precipitate chronic hypoxemia if it is associated with an intracardiac defect that allows for development of a right-to-left shunt. Because a native lung can usually be left intact without compromising a transplanted lung (which will receive most of blood flow), some patients with pulmonary vascular disease may be reasonable candidates for single-lung transplantation, with concurrent repair of any cardiac anomalies. Early reports indicated poorer functional recovery and higher mortality after single versus bilateral lung transplantation for PPH. Subsequent studies, however, have failed to show differences in outcome. In addition, improved medical therapy for PPH, particularly with continuous long-term intravenous prostacyclin infusions, has affected the numbers of patients undergoing lung transplantation for this disease at some centers.

Gammie JS, Keenan RJ, Pham SM, et al. Single- versus double-lung transplantation for pulmonary hypertension. *J Thorac Cardiovasc Surg* 1998;115:397–402.

Hinson KFW. Diffuse pulmonary fibrosis. *Hum Pathol* 1970;1:825–847.

Pasque MK, Kaiser LR, Dresler CM, et al. Single lung transplantation for pulmonary hypertension. Technical aspects and immediate hemodynamic results. *J Thorac Cardiovasc Surg* 1992;130(3):475–482.

Shennib H, Massard G, Gauthier R, et al. Single lung transplantation for cystic fibrosis: is it an option? *J Heart Lung Transplant* 1993;12(2):288–293.

Trulock EP, Edwards LB, Taylor DO, et al. Registry of the International Society for Heart and Lung Transplantation: twenty-second official adult lung and heart-lung transplant report–2005. *J Heart Lung Transplant* 2005;24(8):956–967.

Voelkel NF, Weir EK. Etiologic mechanisms in primary pulmonary hypertension. In: Weir EK, Reeves JT, eds. *Pulmonary vascular physiology and pathophysiology*. New York: Marcel Dekker Inc, 1989:513–539.

A.3. How many lung transplantations have been performed?

Although the first human lung allograft was performed in 1963, transplantation of one or both lungs did not emerge as a viable therapeutic option for patients with end-stage lung disease until the 1980s. The ultimate emergence of this procedure can be largely attributed to advances in the prevention and treatment of airway complications, infections, and rejection. Since initiation of an international registry for lung transplantation in the mid-1980s, the number of procedures reported yearly rose sharply, until beginning to slow in 1993. To date, the highest yearly total was 1,767 in 2002. Despite this volume, the number of patients awaiting lung transplantation continues to exceed the limited donor supply. As of the 2005 international registry, 19,197 lung transplantations had been reported.

Hardy JD, Webb WR, Dalton ML, et al. Lung homotransplantation in man. *JAMA* 1963;186: 1065–1074.

Trulock EP, Edwards LB, Taylor DO, et al. Registry of the International Society for Heart and Lung Transplantation: twenty-second official adult lung and heart-lung transplant report–2005. *J Heart Lung Transplant* 2005;24(8):956–967.

Trulock EP. Lung transplantation. *Am J Respir Crit Care Med* 1997;155:789–818.

A.4. What are the selection criteria for recipients?

In general, patients with severe end-stage lung disease are considered candidates for transplantation when their life expectancy is less than 2 to 3 years, they have minimal disease of other organ systems, and they are mentally and psychologically capable of following strict regimens for rehabilitation and immunosuppressive therapy. Specific criteria, including age, are dependent on the type of lung disease and whether the planned procedure is single or bilateral lung transplantation. Recent data reveal that the age of lung transplant recipients is increasing with approximately 20% now 60 years of age and above. In contrast to criteria formulated when lung transplantation was in its infancy, concomitant steroid therapy, previous intrathoracic surgery, mechanical ventilation, and right ventricular failure are no longer considered absolute contraindications.

Bigham M, Dickstein ML, Hogue CW Jr. Cardiac and lung transplantation. In: Estafanous FG, Barash PG, Reves JG, eds. *Cardiac anesthesia*. Philadelphia: Lippincott Williams & Wilkins, 2001:636.

Myles PS. Pulmonary transplantation. In: Kaplan JA, Slinger PD, eds. *Thoracic anesthesia*. Philadelphia: Elsevier Science, 2003:295–314.

Trulock EP, Edwards LB, Taylor DO, et al. Registry of the International Society for Heart and Lung Transplantation: twenty-second official adult lung and heart-lung transplant report–2005. *J Heart Lung Transplant* 2005;24(8):956–967.

A.5. How is the decision made to transplant one or both lungs, and does this influence preoperative management?

Single-lung transplantation is often preferred because of the extreme shortage of donor organs. The only absolute contraindication to single-lung transplantation is infectious lung disease (e.g., cystic fibrosis and bronchiectasis), with which leaving the native lung could endanger long-term viability of the transplanted lung. As noted earlier, severe emphysema was once thought of as a contraindication to single-lung transplantation because of the probability of mediastinal shift and marked ventilation mismatch between the highly dispensable native lung and the graft. This is only rarely of clinical significance, and it is now accepted that single-lung transplantation can be successfully performed in patients with obstructive disease. Although single-lung transplantation is technically easier and advocated for more difficult recipients, such as those with prior thoracic surgery or coexisting illnesses, functional improvements are often better with bilateral lung transplantation. In addition, the status of the donor lungs further influences the decision of whether to perform a single or bilateral procedure. Finally, transplantation of two lobes from two living related donors for patients with inflammatory disease who are unlikely to survive the wait for a cadaver donor is gaining acceptance. From a practical standpoint, the decision to perform a single-lung or a bilateral lung transplant has little impact on preoperative management because both procedures necessitate the same level of preparation.

Date H, Tanimoto Y, Goto K, et al. A new treatment strategy for advanced idiopathic interstitial pneumonia: living-donor lobar lung transplantation. *Chest* 2005;128(3):1364–1370.

Myles PS. Pulmonary transplantation. In: Kaplan JA, Slinger PD, eds. *Thoracic anesthesia*. Philadelphia: Elsevier Science, 2003:295–314.

Sundaresan RS, Shiraishi Y, Trulock EP, et al. Single or bilateral lung transplantation for emphysema? *J Thorac Cardiovasc Surg* 1996;112:1485.

A.6. How does a single-lung transplantation differ technically from a double-lung transplantation?

It is extremely important that anesthesiologists be broadly familiar with the surgical methods, because manipulation of the heart and lungs at specific points during the transplantation can produce marked cardiopulmonary disturbances. Ideally, the anesthesiologist will anticipate these changes and adapt the anesthetic management accordingly. Description of the detailed technical aspects of lung transplantation are readily available.

Single-lung transplantation is usually performed in the lateral decubitus position through a thoracotomy incision, often with the upper leg and pelvis angled to allow groin exposure for potential femoral cannulation and CPB. In contrast, bilateral sequential lung transplantation is usually performed with the patient supine through a "clamshell" incision (bilateral anterior thoracotomies with or without transverse sternotomy). For both single-lung and bilateral lung transplantation, intermittent single-lung ventilation is required during dissection of the native lung to be removed and implantation of the graft. Once stable single-lung ventilation is established, dissection of the lung to be transplanted is initiated with isolation of the PA. To assess the cardiopulmonary response to diverting the entire cardiac output through one lung, progressive temporary occlusion of the vessel is first performed manually; if well tolerated, the vessel is then clamped and stapled. After ligation of the PA, the pneumonectomy is completed. Implantation of the graft begins with anastomosis of the airway. In the past, the bronchial anastomosis was wrapped with an omental pedicle, mobilized through a small abdominal incision in an effort to improve blood supply to the airway and promote healing. However, the use of a "telescoping" bronchial anastomosis has now largely obviated the need for omental wrapping. The PA branch is then attached to the graft, followed by anastomosis of a cuff of the left atrium containing the pulmonary veins. The implanted lung is then partially inflated, the left atrial cuff and pulmonary veins de-aired, and circulation to the organ restored. Patients presenting for single-lung transplantation with chronic persistent pulmonary hypertension (PPH) of primary or secondary etiology often exhibit severe functional compromise of the right ventricle. To avoid additional right ventricular stress, many institutions choose to institute partial normothermic CPB during single-lung transplantation for PPH or in patients with severe pulmonary hypertension and right ventricular dysfunction secondary to restrictive or obstructive disease. Cannulation is typically through the femoral artery and the right atrium unless simultaneous correction of an intracardiac defect is planned. In such patients, conventional aortic and single- or double-stage atrial cannulation are performed. Implantation of the lung is otherwise performed in the same manner as described earlier.

Double-lung transplantation was first described by the Toronto Lung Transplant Group in the mid-1980s as en bloc implantation of both lungs simultaneously. The procedure is performed through a median sternotomy using hypothermic CPB, cardioplegic cardiac arrest, and single tracheal (or double bronchial) anastomosis of the trachea and main PA. Although the procedure initially produced encouraging results, considerable limitations related to technical complexity, morbidity, mortality, and application to many patients with end-stage lung disease soon became apparent. Not surprisingly, use of the procedure declined sharply and has now been largely replaced by the bilateral sequential implantation technique, which does not uniformly require hypothermic CPB. Introduced in 1990, bilateral sequential (or bilateral single) lung transplantation has become the surgical procedure of choice when replacement of both lungs is necessary. As noted earlier, in contrast to single-lung transplantation, bilateral sequential lung transplantation procedures are performed in the supine position. In general, the procedure can be regarded as having two phases. First, the most severely compromised lung (as determined by preoperative ventilation/perfusion lung scanning) is removed during ventilation of the "good" contralateral lung. Implantation is achieved through a bronchial anastomosis as with a single-lung transplantation. The second lung is then removed and transplanted during ventilation of the new lung alone.

Kaiser LR, Cooper JD. Adult lung transplantation. In: Flye MW, ed. *Atlas of organ transplantation*. Philadelphia: WB Saunders, 1995:296–312.

Pasque MK, Cooper JD, Kaiser LK, et al. An improved technique for bilateral single lung transplantation; rationale and clinical experience. *Ann Thorac Surg* 1990;49:785–789.

B. Preoperative Evaluation and Preparation

B.1. What preoperative evaluation is desirable?

At most centers, an extensive physical examination, psychologic evaluation, and numerous tests of cardiopulmonary function are performed before acceptance into the transplant program. This facilitates the preanesthetic evaluation that ideally is performed when the patient is first accepted into the transplant program. Familiarity with pulmonary function tests, ventilation/perfusion lung scan results, heart catheterization, echocardiographic data (including evidence of intracardiac shunts), exercise tolerance, oxygen use, and dependence on continuous pulmonary vasodilator infusion (i.e., prostacyclin) are beneficial for formulating an anesthetic plan. Although many of these parameters are regularly reassessed, the interval between evaluation and transplantation necessitates that a careful history and physical examination be performed before the procedure, focusing on signs of pulmonary hypertension and cardiac dysfunction.

Bigham M, Dickstein ML, Hogue CW Jr. Cardiac and lung transplantation. In: Estafanous FG, Barash PG, Reves JG, eds. *Cardiac anesthesia*. Philadelphia: Lippincott Williams & Wilkins, 2001:636.

Myles PS. Pulmonary transplantation. In: Kaplan JA, Slinger PD, eds. *Thoracic anesthesia*. Philadelphia: Elsevier Science, 2003:295–314.

B.2. How would you premedicate this patient?

As with all critically ill patients, considerations regarding preoperative sedation are governed primarily by the functional limitations imposed by the underlying disease. Consideration must also be given to the possibility that the donor lungs will be deemed unacceptable at final inspection, and therefore, the procedure canceled and the patient discharged from the hospital. When indicated, parenteral sedation is usually chosen because of insufficient time to effectively administer oral anxiolytics. Midazolam alone or with diphenhydramine (potentially protecting the lung against drug-induced histamine release) is often sufficient. Clinically, most patients with end-stage restrictive, obstructive, or infectious lung disease are tachypneic while breathing room air and cannot be aggressively sedated. In contrast, patients with persistent pulmonary hypertension and no intracardiac defect often appear reasonably normal and will benefit from sedation because of the potential for stress-related increases in pulmonary vascular resistance. Alternatively, patients with pulmonary hypertension and significant right-to-left intracardiac shunting (i.e., Eisenmenger physiology) are often cyanotic despite oxygen supplementation and may not tolerate sedation well. In addition, consideration needs be given to immunosuppression protocols, and in appropriate patients supplemental bronchodilator therapy.

Hartigan PM, Pedoto A. Anesthetic considerations for lung volume reduction surgery and lung transplantation. *Thorac Surg Clin* 2005;15(1):143–157.

Myles PS. Pulmonary transplantation. In: Kaplan JA, Slinger PD, eds. *Thoracic anesthesia*. Philadelphia: Elsevier Science, 2003:295–314.

B.3. What vascular access is required?

Typically, a large-bore intravenous catheter and central venous access for PA catheter placement are secured before surgery. In many centers, additional central venous cannulation is performed with a multiple-lumen catheter to provide intraoperative and postoperative venous access. For patients with chronic infectious lung disease or a history of previous intrathoracic procedures, a second large-bore intravenous catheter is often started because of the potential for brisk blood loss during dissection of pulmonary adhesions. Meticulous removal of air from venous infusion lines should be performed, particularly in patents with known or suspected right-to-left shunts. At many institutions, cannulation of a femoral artery, instead of the radial artery, is performed under local anesthesia in the operating room, because radial arterial pressures may become damped during the procedure secondary to positioning of the arms.

Hartigan PM, Pedoto A. Anesthetic considerations for lung volume reduction surgery and lung transplantation. *Thorac Surg Clin* 2005;15(1):143–157.

Heerdt PM, Triantafillou AN. Anesthesia for lung transplantation. In: Flye MW, ed. *Atlas of organ transplantation*. Philadelphia: WB Saunders, 1995:313–318.

B.4. Is preoperative epidural catheter placement advantageous?

Pain control after lung transplantation can be critical in facilitating patient extubation and rehabilitation. Both lumbar and thoracic epidural catheters have been used for postoperative pain management. At many institutions, catheters are placed immediately before the procedure in most patients, despite the rare possibility of anticoagulation and CPB during the transplantation procedure. This practice is supported by data indicating no adverse sequelae to preoperatively placed epidural catheters, including patients who required emergent heparinization and CPB. Obvious exceptions to this approach are patients anticoagulated preoperatively or those in whom CPB is planned. Delaying placement of the epidural catheter until the postoperative period may actually increase the potential risk of complications, because both hemodilution and immunosuppression tend to promote a coagulopathy.

Hartigan PM, Pedoto A. Anesthetic considerations for lung volume reduction surgery and lung transplantation. *Thorac Surg Clin* 2005;15(1):143–157.

Myles PS. Pulmonary transplantation. In: Kaplan JA, Slinger PD, eds. *Thoracic anesthesia*. Philadelphia: Elsevier Science, 2003:295–314.

C. Intraoperative Management

C.1. What special equipment is necessary?

Items advantageous for lung transplantation procedures include an anesthesia machine with a ventilator capable of delivering a wide range of inspiratory/expiratory (I : E) ratios, differing ventilatory modes, and efficacy at higher airway pressures. Apparatus to deliver continuous positive airway pressure (CPAP) should be readily available, as should a fiberoptic bronchoscope to confirm double-lumen tube (DLT) positioning, to provide guided airway suctioning, and for inspecting anastomosis. Access to transesophageal echocardiography (TEE) is often beneficial and a CPB machine should always be immediately available for lung transplantation. Though not specifically approved for this indication, a nitric oxide (NO) delivery system is highly desirable during lung transplantation.

C.2. How would you monitor this patient?

Intraoperatively, hemodynamic, and respiratory changes are often acute and profound, so extensive monitoring is imperative. In addition to the electrocardiogram, arterial blood pressure, and peripheral arterial oxygen saturation, PA catheter placement is routine for lung transplantation at most institutions because of the profound changes in pulmonary and systemic hemodynamics that often occur. During single-lung transplantations, PA catheters often migrate to the operative side after the patient has been laterally positioned even when radiographically confirmed to be in the nonoperative lung. Therefore, the surgeon should be reminded to palpate the PA and withdraw the catheter if necessary before cross-clamping the vessel. PA catheters capable of measuring mixed venous oxygen saturation have become widely used. TEE is often employed during lung transplantation to evaluate right ventricular function, particularly during clamping of the PA, to assess for intracardiac shunts, and to evaluate vascular anastomosis.

Bigham M, Dickstein ML, Hogue CW Jr. Cardiac and lung transplantation. In: Estafanous FG, Barash PG, Reves JG, eds. *Cardiac anesthesia*. Philadelphia: Lippincott Williams & Wilkins, 2001:636.

Miyaji K, Matsubara H, Nakamura K, et al. Equivalence of flow velocities through bilateral pulmonary vein anastomoses in bilateral living-donor lobar lung transplantation. *J Heart Lung Transplant* 2005;24(7):860–864.

Myles PS. Pulmonary transplantation. In: Kaplan JA, Slinger PD, eds. *Thoracic anesthesia*. Philadelphia: Elsevier Science, 2003:295–314.

Schenk P, Globits S, Koller J, et al. Accuracy of echocardiographic right ventricular parameters in patients with different end-stage lung prior to lung transplantation. *J Heart Lung Transplant* 2000;19(2):145–154.

C.3. How would you induce anesthesia in this patient?

As with induction of anesthesia in any critically ill patent, multiple techniques have been safely used for patients undergoing lung transplantation. The only general rule is that induction be relatively gradual, because abrupt withdrawal of sympathetic tone in these patients with high sympathetic activity can result in marked cardiovascular compromise, particularly during the transition from spontaneous to mechanical ventilation. For this reason, injecting an epidural catheter with local anesthetic before induction of anesthesia can be problematic. Because effective alveolar ventilation and nitrogen washout are poor in the patient with severe obstructive lung disease and high residual volumes, prolonged (i.e., 15 to 20 minutes) preoxygenation is worthwhile, followed by a rapid-acting induction agent to shorten the excitement stage, expedite airway management, and prevent opiate-induced truncal rigidity. Thiopental, etomidate, propofol, and ketamine have all been used safely, but specific properties of each drug in the setting of the patient's underlying disease should be considered. Thiopental, for example, may not be desirable for patients with bronchospasm or pulmonary hypertension because of a propensity for histamine release. Alternatively, the sympathomimetic properties of ketamine may preclude use in the presence of pulmonary hypertension, whereas its bronchodilating effects may be beneficial in the setting of bronchospasm. After administration of the hypnotic, either fentanyl, 10 to 15 μg per kg, or sufentanil, 1 to 2 μg per kg, has been commonly used with either succinylcholine or a nondepolarizing muscle relaxant to complete induction. Benzodiazepines, scopolamine, and/or volatile anesthetic agents are frequently administered after induction to promote amnesia and in the case of volatile agents to promote bronchodilation.

Bigham M, Dickstein ML, Hogue CW Jr. Cardiac and lung transplantation. In: Estafanous FG, Barash PG, Reves JG, eds. *Cardiac anesthesia.* Philadelphia: Lippincott Williams & Wilkins, 2001:636.

Hartigan PM, Pedoto A. Anesthetic considerations for lung volume reduction surgery and lung transplantation. *Thorac Surg Clin* 2005;15(1):143–157.

C.4.   How would you ventilate this patient? What kind of endotracheal tube would you use?

After induction, the trachea is usually intubated with a left endobronchial double-lumen tube (DLT) for both single-lung and bilateral lung transplantation. Use of a single-lumen endotracheal tube with either an external or an internal bronchial blocking catheter has been described but does not appear to be clearly superior to the left endobronchial tube for most procedures. Furthermore, an endobronchial tube allows for differential lung ventilation if required postoperatively. One exception to this approach has been in patients with cystic fibrosis who exhibit thick tenacious secretions that are difficult to suction through the small-lumen suction catheters necessary for DLTs. In these patients, it is often helpful to first place a large single-lumen tube and perform extensive bronchoscopic-directed bronchial lavage and suctioning before placement of the DLT.

The transition from spontaneous to mechanical ventilation invariably produces hemodynamic alterations resulting from acute changes in intrathoracic pressure and chest wall compliance. With obstructive lung disease, mechanical ventilation magnifies airtrapping, leading to "pulmonary tamponade." Varying degrees of this phenomenon should be expected during anesthesia induction. The treatment consists of intermittent apnea with an open ventilator circuit, adjustment of the ventilatory pattern to an I : E ratio of 1 : 5 or less with moderate tidal volumes, and administration of bronchodilating drugs. Prompt restoration of blood pressure usually ensues. If hypotension persists, other causes of circulatory compromise must be excluded including pneumothorax. With restrictive disease, higher inflation pressures and positive end-expiratory pressure (PEEP) are often required. In both patients with obstructive and patients with restrictive disease, optimal balance of ventilation with hemodynamic stability often necessitates tolerating a degree of hypercapnia. In pulmonary hypertensive patients, mechanical ventilation usually produces less cardiovascular disturbance if caution is exercised not to increase pulmonary vascular resistance (e.g., from hypoxia, hypercarbia, or lung hyperinflation).

Because lung recipients have little pulmonary reserve, ventilation with 100% oxygen is commonly used intraoperatively. Although this approach is somewhat controversial, few data suggest acute oxygen toxicity to a transplanted lung. High PaO$_2$ may also directly promote pulmonary vasodilation and therefore be beneficial in reducing right ventricular afterload.

Hartigan PM, Pedoto A. Anesthetic considerations for lung volume reduction surgery and lung transplantation. *Thorac Surg Clin* 2005;15(1):143–157.

Triantafillou AN, Heerdt PM, Patterson GA. Lung transplantation. In: Youngberg JA, Lake CA, Roizen MF, et al. eds. *Cardiac, thoracic and vascular anesthesia*. New York: Churchill Livingstone, 2000:703.

Weir EK, Reeves JT, eds. *Pulmonary vascular physiology and pathophysiology*. New York: Marcel Dekker Inc, 1989:241–290.

C.5. How does the physiology of single-lung ventilation influence the procedure?

In laterally positioned patients, gravity helps redistribute blood away from the nonventilated lung during single-lung ventilation and lessen intrapulmonary shunt. In supine patients, this benefit is obviously lost and single-lung ventilation may not be well tolerated. In general, because of large residual lung volumes that will become filled with a high concentration of oxygen content during the initial stages of the procedure, lung recipients with severe obstructive lung disease may initially maintain oxygenation for the first 10 to 15 minutes of single-lung ventilation. However, rapid arterial desaturation may then occur once a substantial portion of the residual volume is absorbed. Alternatively, patients with restrictive lung disease and a low functional residual capacity may rapidly exhibit both hypoxia and hypercarbia. Multiple steps can be taken to improve oxygenation including insufflation of oxygen or CPAP to the nonventilated lung, bronchoscopic-guided suctioning of the ventilated lung, careful manipulation of the ventilatory pattern, and PEEP to the ventilated lung. Differential PEEP/CPAP should be done cautiously, however, because increased airway pressure in the ventilated lung can divert blood toward the nonventilated side. In some patients, intermittent ventilation of the operative lung may have to be performed before pneumonectomy. In general, oxygenation improves after the clamping of the PA supplying the nonventilated lung. For desaturation not responding to the usual maneuvers, tourniquets can be placed around the PA by the surgeon as a temporizing step until dissection permits proper stapling of this vessel.

Myles PS. Pulmonary transplantation. In: Kaplan JA, Slinger PD, eds. *Thoracic anesthesia*. Philadelphia: Elsevier Science, 2003:295–314.

Triantafillou AN, Heerdt PM, Patterson GA. Lung transplantation. In: Youngberg JA, Lake CA, Roizen MF, et al. eds. *Cardiac, thoracic and vascular anesthesia*. New York: Churchill Livingstone, 2000:703.

C.6. Should volatile anesthetics be avoided during single-lung ventilation?

Because of experimental evidence demonstrating inhibition of hypoxic pulmonary vasoconstriction (HPV) by the volatile anesthetic agents, some authors have suggested that these drugs be avoided in the anesthetic management of patients with end-stage lung disease requiring single-lung ventilation. However, true clinical significance of these experimental observations remains somewhat controversial. From a clinical standpoint, commonly used doses of isoflurane (e.g., end-tidal concentrations of ≤ 1.0) have not been empirically associated with worsening of intrapulmonary shunt and hypoxia. Therefore, isoflurane remains widely used in these patients and may actually benefit some lung recipients because of its bronchodilating properties. (See Chapter 2, section C.13.)

Benumof JL. Anesthesia for one-lung ventilation [Reply]. *Anesthesiology* 1988;69:631.

Bjertnaes J, Hauge A, Torgrinson T. The pulmonary vasoconstrictor response to hypoxia: the hypoxia sensitive site studied with a volatile inhibitor. *Acta Physiol Scand* 1980; 109:447–462.

Hartigan PM, Pedoto A. Anesthetic considerations for lung volume reduction surgery and lung transplantation. *Thorac Surg Clin* 2005;15(1):143–157.

Marshall BE. Anesthesia for one-lung ventilation [Letter]. *Anesthesiology* 1988;69:630–631.

Raffin L, Cherqui MM, Sperandio M, et al. Anesthesia for bilateral lung transplantation without cardiopulmonary bypass: initial experience and review of intraoperative problems. *J Cardiothorac Vasc Anesth* 1992;6(4):409–417.

C.7. At what specific points in the procedure are problems anticipated?

- Anesthesia induction
- Lateral positioning
- Single-lung ventilation
- Clamping of the PA
- Graft implantation
- Graft reperfusion

C.8. What problems are associated with the lateral position?

Single-lung transplantation is usually performed in the lateral decubitus position, often with the upper leg and pelvis angled to allow groin exposure for potential femoral cannulation and CPB. Not surprisingly, position-related changes in venous return, coupled with compression of the dependent lung by the mediastinum and diaphragm, may promote systemic hypotension and ventilation/perfusion mismatch. Furthermore, PA pressure usually tends to rise after lateral positioning, probably because of gravity-induced shifts in pulmonary blood flow distribution, vascular congestion, and increased vascular resistance.

Triantafillou AN, Heerdt PM, Patterson GA. Lung transplantation. In: Youngberg JA, Lake CA, Roizen MF, et al. eds. *Cardiac, thoracic and vascular anesthesia*. New York: Churchill Livingstone, 2000:703.

C.9. How does single-lung ventilation affect cardiopulmonary function? What are the problems of single-lung ventilation in this patient? How would you treat them?

Isolated ventilation of the dependent lung is often accompanied by a marked acute increase in peak inspiratory pressure and a subsequent gradual progressive rise in PA pressure. As noted earlier, because of the beneficial effect of gravity on redistributing blood away from the nondependent nonventilated lung, single-lung ventilation is often tolerated better from a respiratory standpoint by patients undergoing single-lung transplantation in the lateral position than those undergoing bilateral lung transplantation in the supine position. Close monitoring of right ventricular performance during conversion to single-lung ventilation is extremely important because of the increase in afterload produced by hypoxic vasoconstriction and redistribution of blood flow. Though unusual, if the right ventricle becomes hypokinetic and distended, and if the ejection fraction decreases, ventilation may have to be altered to minimize airway pressure.

Triantafillou AN, Pasque MK, Huddleston CB, et al. Predictors, frequency, and indications for cardiopulmonary bypass during lung transplantation in adults. *Ann Thorac Surg* 1994;57:1248–1251.

C.10. How would you deal with problems related to clamping of the PA?

To assess the cardiopulmonary response to diverting the entire cardiac output through one lung, progressive occlusion of the vessel is first performed manually (Fig. 4.2). Careful assessment of right ventricular function is performed with the TEE looking for evidence of right ventricular distension or hypokinesis. If well tolerated, the vessel is then clamped and stapled. If occlusion is poorly tolerated, the vessel is unclamped and a pulmonary vasodilator such as prostaglandin E_1 or NO and/or positive inotropic infusion begun. If severe respiratory or cardiovascular derangement persists after reclamping of the vessel despite pharmacologic intervention, heparin is administered and CPB instituted to avoid profound hypoxia or right ventricular failure. However, for most patients undergoing single-lung transplantation, hypoxemia during single-lung ventilation and after PA clamping is rarely a problem and right ventricular performance can be adequately maintained.

Triantafillou AN, Heerdt PM, Patterson GA. Lung transplantation. In: Youngberg JA, Lake CA, Roizen MF, et al. eds. *Cardiac, thoracic and vascular anesthesia.* New York: Churchill Livingstone, 2000:703.

C.11. What hemodynamic alterations would you expect during graft implantation and reperfusion? How would you correct them?

During the process of performing the vascular and bronchial anastomoses, major disturbances on cardiac filling and rhythm can be produced (Fig. 4.2). Though often transient, systemic hypotension and pulmonary hypertension can ensue. Transient hypotension may follow the introduction of the vasodilator-containing lung graft preservatives into the systemic circulation. Incomplete de-airing of the lung can lead to coronary air embolism, leading to transient myocardial ischemia. The latter is manifested by ST-segment elevation and regional wall

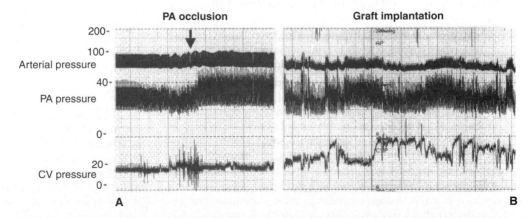

Figure 4.2 Tracings of femoral arterial blood pressure, along with pulmonary artery (PA) and central venous (CV) pressures, before and after occlusion of the left PA **(A)** and during implantation of a left lung graft **(B)**. (All pressures are in millimeters of mercury.)

motion abnormalities on TEE. This condition is typically responsive to intravenous nitroglycerin while maintaining perfusion pressures with phenylephrine. After reperfusion and subsequent ventilation of the new lung, PA pressures and arterial blood gases should be closely followed. PA pressure usually falls after reperfusion of the donor organ. If a substantial decrease is not observed, potential causes include anastomotic problems with the atrial cuff or the PA. When pulmonary anastomotic problems are suspected, the surgeon should palpate to assess whether the PA catheter is located proximal or distal to the anastomosis. If a proximal location is confirmed, direct measurement of PA pressures should be performed with a needle connected to pressure tubing handed off the operative field. Assessment of the PA and venous flow pattern by TEE can sometimes be of benefit in evaluating adequacy of the anastomoses. Early graft dysfunction can manifest shortly after reperfusion of the first lung and may be the result of various insults. Occurring in 15% to 35% of cases, early graft dysfunction ranges in severity from modest chest radiograph abnormalities to fulminant pulmonary edema with hypoxia and cardiovascular compromise. Immediate treatment includes adjustment of ventilation, addition of PEEP, and pulmonary vasodilators. Nitric oxide (NO) may be effective for improving oxygenation and reducing PA pressures, and some clinicians advocate "prophylactic" NO administration although benefit of this intervention has recently been questioned. Should graft dysfunction become evident after implantation of the first lung, but before completion of the second lung transplantation, consideration should be given to initiating CPB. When severe hypoxemia persists after lung transplantation despite maximal medical therapy including the use of inhaled NO, extracorporeal membrane oxygenation (ECMO) is indicated.

Date H, Triantafillou AN, Trulock EP, et al. Inhaled nitric oxide reduces human allograft dysfunction. *J Thorac Cardiovasc Surg* 1996;111:913–919.

Myles PS. Pulmonary transplantation. In: Kaplan JA, Slinger PD, eds. *Thoracic anesthesia*. Philadelphia: Elsevier Science, 2003:295–314.

Perrin G, Roch A, Michelet P, et al. Inhaled nitric oxide does not prevent pulmonary edema after lung transplantation measured by lung water content: a randomized clinical study. *Chest* 2006;129(4):1024–1030.

Trulock EP. Lung transplantation. *Am J Respir Crit Care Med* 1997;155:789.

C.12. When is CPB necessary for lung transplantation?

CPB may be used electively for patients with severe PA hypertension, in whom double-lumen endobronchial tubes cannot be placed, or when visualization of hilar structures is poor. However, in the absence of intraoperative complications, CPB is not desired because it can increase bleeding and blood product usage. It has also been suggested that CPB may aggravate postoperative lung dysfunction although this has not been evident in cases where lung transplant was performed in conjunction with cardiac surgery. Nonetheless, the use of CPB has been associated with longer duration of mechanical ventilation and hospitalization, although it is difficult to differentiate whether the latter results directly from CPB or is the result of a complicated procedure that resulted in the need for CPB. Indications for CPB include right ventricular dysfunction not responding to medical therapy, early graft dysfunction occurring during implantation of the second lung during bilateral procedures, and surgical misadventures. Unplanned CPB is reported to occur in 17% to 41% of lung transplantation procedures, but predicting which patients may require this intervention is extremely difficult. Some report that CPB is more likely to be necessary for restrictive lung diseases than obstructive diseases.

In an attempt to derive the benefits of CPB while reducing complications, some centers advocate the use of heparin-bound ECMO systems. This approach allows for pulmonary support both during and after the procedure with minimal systemic anticoagulation.

Aeba R, Griffith BP, Kormos RL, et al. Effect of cardiopulmonary bypass on early graft dysfunction in clinical lung transplantation. *J Thorac Cardiovasc Surg* 1994;57: 715–722.

de Hoyos A, Demajo W, Snell G, et al. Preoperative prediction for the use of cardiopulmonary bypass in lung transplantation. *J Thorac Cardiovasc Surg* 1993;106:787–795.

Lau CL, Hoganson DM, Meyers BF, et al. Use of an apical heart suction device for exposure in lung transplantation. *Ann Thorac Surg* 2006;81(4):1524–1525.

Parekh K, Meyers BF, Patterson GA, et al. Outcome of lung transplantation for patients requiring concomitant cardiac surgery. *J Thorac Cardiovasc Surg* 2005;130(3):859–863.

Triantafillou AN, Pasque MK, Huddleston CB, et al. Predictors, frequency and indications for cardiopulmonary bypass during lung transplantation in adults. *Ann Thorac Surg* 1994;57:1248–1251.

Wang Y, Kurichi JE, Blumenthal NP, et al. Multiple variables affecting blood usage in lung transplantation. *J Heart Lung Transplant* 2006;25(5):533–538.

C.13. Should fluid administration be restricted, and are blood products commonly required?

The amount of crystalloid that can be safely administered intraoperatively without adversely affecting the graft appears to be widely variable. Although efforts should be made to minimize fluid infusion intraoperatively, many patients undergoing lung transplantation require large amounts to maintain hemodynamic stability. Not uncommonly, central venous and pulmonary capillary wedge pressures of 3 to 5 mm Hg immediately after a transplantation are evident despite infusion of large amounts of crystalloid and colloid, as well as only moderate blood loss. Review of fluid management during 215 lung transplantations performed without CPB revealed that intraoperative crystalloid administration varied widely (4 to 32 mL/kg/hour), with a mean of 13 ± 6 mL/kg/hour. Using the PaO_2/FIO_2 ratio on arrival in the intensive care unit and time to extubation as indices of early graft function and initial outcome, this study showed no correlation between the amount of fluids administered and either of these indices.

Before the development of the bilateral lung transplantation procedure without CPB, patients with a history of surgery involving the lung or pleura or chronic infectious lung diseases were not deemed acceptable candidates for lung transplantation because of the anticipated excessive bleeding associated with dissecting a scarred lung after anticoagulation for CPB. Now, without the uniform requirement for heparinization, such patients are generally regarded as operative candidates. As with other surgical procedures in which hemorrhage is anticipated, continuous infusion of aprotinin has been proposed to reduce intraoperative bleeding in patients with cystic fibrosis or a history of previous intrathoracic surgery. Interestingly, aprotinin may also have beneficial effects on the function of the transplanted lung after reperfusion. Variables reported to increase the need for blood product usage include the use of CPB, double-lung procedures, and patients with cystic fibrosis. If blood products are to be administered, the anesthesiologist must know whether the patient has antibodies to cytomegalovirus (CMV) and must closely check blood products to confirm they coincide with the patient's status.

Bigham M, Dickstein ML, Hogue CW Jr. Cardiac and lung transplantation. In: Estafanous FG, Barash PG, Reves JG, eds. *Cardiac anesthesia*. Philadelphia: Lippincott Williams & Wilkins, 2001:636.

Kyriss T, Wurst H, Friedel G, et al. Reduced blood loss by aprotinin in thoracic surgical operations associated with high risk of bleeding. A placebo-controlled, randomized phase IV study. *Eur J Cardiothorac Surg* 2001;20(1):38–41.

Myles PS. Pulmonary transplantation. In: Kaplan JA, Slinger PD, eds. *Thoracic anesthesia*. Philadelphia: Elsevier Science, 2003:295–314.

Wang Y, Kuricni JE, Blumenthal NP, et al. Multiple variables affecting blood usage in lung transplantation. *J Heart Lung Transplant* 2006;25(5):533–538.

C.14. Would you extubate the patient upon conclusion of the procedure?

Because of the cardiopulmonary insult associated with the procedure, the large postoperative volume shifts, hypothermia, and the frequent need for postoperative bronchoscopy, the trachea of lung transplant recipients is not generally extubated immediately after the procedure. Accordingly, unless intraoperative events (e.g., hyperinflation of the remaining intact lung) suggest that postoperative differential lung ventilation will be required, or unless functional issues such as profound oropharyngeal edema or difficult intubation are present, the double-lumen endotracheal tube is exchanged for a single-lumen tube. In many patients, the endotracheal tube change can be facilitated by use of an exchange catheter. However, great care should be taken to not advance the catheter too far and damage the graft. It is often beneficial to perform fiberoptic bronchoscopy to examine bronchial anastomoses and aggressively suction secretions or blood after replacement of the DLT with a single-lumen endotracheal tube. As with many procedures, careful inspection of the upper airway for edema should be performed with a laryngoscope before removal of the double-lumen endobronchial tube for placement of the single-lumen endotracheal tube.

D. Postoperative Management

D.1. What are the major complications after lung transplantation?

Early graft dysfunction, episodes of rejection, infection, and airway complication are the major early complications of lung transplantation. Early graft dysfunction varies in severity from mild shunting and chest radiograph infiltrates to gross pulmonary edema. Management is with fluid restriction, diuretics, PEEP, NO, and ECMO for severe cases. Immunosuppression is usually initiated before surgery and the induction phase of therapy is continued for 5 to 10 days. The exact regimen varies between institutions but typically includes azathioprine, steroids, cyclosporine, and polyclonal antilymphocyte/antithymocyte globulins or interleukin-2 receptor antagonists. Acute rejection episodes are usually treated with intense steroid therapy and optimization of other immunosuppressant dosages. A challenge arises in differentiating acute rejection from infection as a source of shunting and chest radiograph infiltrates. Transbronchial biopsy is often necessary to make the distinction from histologic specimens. Bacterial pneumonia is the most frequent infection in the first 2 weeks. Though unusual in the first 2 weeks after transplantation, cytomegalovirus is the second most common source of infectious pneumonitis. This virus is treated with ganciclovir. Broad-spectrum antibiotics are given perioperatively, and the regimen is adjusted based on the results of donor and recipient cultures. Antibiotic therapy for patients with cystic fibrosis is challenging, and the drug chosen is dictated by the patient's cultures and prior history of the organisms colonizing his or her lungs. Prophylactic acyclovir appears to be effective in reducing infections caused by herpes simplex, and trimethoprim-sulfamethoxazole is given to prevent infections from *Pneumocystis carinii*.

Myles PS. Pulmonary transplantation. In: Kaplan JA, Slinger PD, eds. *Thoracic anesthesia*. Philadelphia: Elsevier Science, 2003:295–314.

Trulock EP, Edwards LB, Taylor DO, et al. Registry of the International Society for Heart and Lung Transplantation: twenty-second official adult lung and heart-lung transplant report–2005. *J Heart Lung Transplant* 2005;24(8):956–967.

D.2. How is postoperative ventilation managed, and for how long is it required?

After most procedures, the FIO_2 can be rapidly reduced and weaning from the ventilator can be initiated as soon as the patient is warm and stable. An exception to this approach is the patient who has undergone single-lung transplantation for pulmonary hypertension. Because of a propensity for episodes of cardiopulmonary instability during the first 24 to 48 hours postoperatively, it is usually advantageous to keep these patients sedated, paralyzed, and ventilated during this period.

Postoperatively, ventilation/perfusion mismatch and intrapulmonary shunt are often more pronounced after single-lung transplantation than bilateral lung transplantation. Not surprisingly, patients with restrictive disease usually display the best pulmonary function after single-lung transplantation, because the graft receives the majority of both ventilation and perfusion. Alternatively, after single-lung transplantation in emphysemic patients, the remaining native lung often receives a substantial portion of the tidal volume, whereas in pulmonary hypertensive patients, the native lung continues to be ventilated but receives very little blood flow. On rare occasions, differential ventilation of the transplanted and native lung is needed after single-lung transplantation for obstructive lung disease. In these situations, the double-lumen endobronchial tube is left in place and two ventilators are employed. The native lung is ventilated with low tidal volume (2 to 3 mL/kg) and rate, or even just connected to CPAP without intermittent mandatory ventilation. Nonetheless, the condition usually resolves rapidly with return of spontaneous ventilation. Postural changes in arterial oxygen saturation are often prominent in single-lung transplant recipients. In general, patients who received a single lung for pulmonary hypertension or emphysema display better postoperative pulmonary function with the "transplant side up," whereas the opposite may be true in certain patients with restrictive lung disease. The precise etiology of this response is unclear but probably reflects positional variation in ventilation/perfusion matching.

Bigham M, Dickstein ML, Hogue CW Jr. Cardiac and lung transplantation. In: Estafanous FG, Barash PG, Reves JG, eds. *Cardiac anesthesia*. Philadelphia: Lippincott Williams & Wilkins, 2001:636.

Triantafillou AN, Heerdt PM, Patterson GA. Lung transplantation. In: Youngberg JA, Lake CA, Roizen MF, et al. eds. *Cardiac, thoracic and vascular anesthesia*. New York: Churchill Livingstone, 2000.703.

D.3. What special precautions should be taken when a lung transplant recipient requires general anesthesia for subsequent nonpulmonary surgery?

In general, after lung transplantation, the patient can be treated like any other ill immunocompromised patient. Recipients have subsequently undergone various surgical procedures unrelated to their pulmonary disease after lung transplantation and have few anesthetic problems. Not surprisingly, differences in the compliance and expiratory flow rates of a native and transplanted lung after single-lung transplantation for emphysema can result in alterations in intraoperative capnography. This phenomenon has been described as producing a biphasic pattern of carbon dioxide exhalation, with the first peak reflecting exhalation from the transplanted lung and the second peak exhalation from the native lung. In addition, the transplanted lung is denervated so the cough reflex is present only in the proximal native airway and mucociliary function is impaired. In contrast, hypoxic pulmonary vasoconstriction is intact after lung transplantation and central respiratory control is unaffected. However, a blunted response to carbon dioxide may persist for patients with preoperative hypercapnia.

The major factor limiting long-term survival from lung transplantation is bronchiolitis obliterans. This progressive condition characterized by progressive narrowing of small airways must be considered in patients with prior lung transplantation presenting for surgery and anesthesia after the initial recovery phase. Other perioperative considerations for the patient with a prior lung transplant undergoing subsequent surgery are based on whether the patient was the recipient of one versus two lungs. In the former case, ventilation/perfusion of the remaining "diseased" native lung is influenced by the functional status of the transplanted lung. For patients with obstructive lung disease, overinflation of the native lung and resultant mediastinal shift with associated ventilation and hemodynamic consequences, although rare, must be considered when employing positive pressure ventilation.

Bigham M, Dickstein ML, Hogue CW Jr. Cardiac and lung transplantation. In: Estafanous FG, Barash PG, Reves JG, eds. *Cardiac anesthesia.* Philadelphia: Lippincott Williams & Wilkins, 2001:636.

Cerza RA. Cardiopulmonary bypass in a post-lung transplant patient. *J Cardiothorac Vasc Anesth* 1996;10:384–386.

Myles PS. Pulmonary transplantation. In: Kaplan JA, Slinger PD, eds. *Thoracic anesthesia.* Philadelphia: Elsevier Science, 2003:295–314.

Williams EL, Jellish WS, Modica PA, et al. Capnography in a patient after single lung transplantation. *Anesthesiology* 1991;74:621–622.

D.4. What are the long-term outcomes of lung transplantation?

Increased experience and improved techniques have made lung transplantation a realistic option for many patients. However, the procedure is not without substantial risk, and a favorable outcome is by no means ensured. Survival is better for patients with COPD compared with those with persistent pulmonary hypertension or idiopathic pulmonary fibrosis. However, there are data to suggest that lung transplant does not have significant survival benefit in patients with COPD. Since 1994, 1-, 3-, 5-, and 10-year survival rates after lung transplantation are 76%, 60%, 49%, and 24%, respectively. The major cause of early mortality is graft dysfunction and infection, and the major causes of late mortality are infection and rejection. Interestingly, there is a relatively high incidence of cancer in the lung transplantation population with over 11% of 5-year survivors developing lymphoma or other malignancy.

Trulock EP, Edwards LB, Taylor DO, et al. Registry of the International Society for Heart and Lung Transplantation: twenty-second official adult lung and heart-lung transplant report–2005. *J Heart Lung Transplant* 2005;24(8):956–967.

D.5. Are there surgical alternatives to lung transplantation?

Some patients with severe emphysema who are not deemed transplant candidates may benefit from lung volume reduction surgery (LVRS) or "reduction pneumoplasty." Performed either through a median sternotomy or through a bilateral thoracoscopy, the goal of LVRS is to remove up to 30% of the patient's most severely compromised lung tissue. Postoperatively, this allows the previously hyperexpanded chest and depressed diaphragm to resume a more normal shape, therefore improving chest wall mechanics and eventually pulmonary function. However, beneficial effects of the procedure are not immediately evident, usually requiring 1 to 2 months. Furthermore, whether the improvement in pulmonary function is sufficient to warrant the risk of the procedure remains controversial. Nonetheless, recent data indicate that for many patients, LVRS represents a viable alternative to transplantation.

Tutic M, Lardinois D, Imfeld S, et al. Lung-volume reduction surgery as an alternative or bridging procedure to lung transplantation. *Ann Thorac Surg* 2006;82(1):208–213.

CHAPTER 5

Tracheoesophageal Fistula

JACQUES H. SCHAROUN

A 12-HOUR-OLD FULL TERM INFANT

weighing 2.5 kg presents with choking and cyanosis during its first feed. Neonatal intensive care unit (NICU) staff is unable to pass a feeding tube into the stomach. The baby also has copious oral secretions. Before birth polyhydramnios was seen.

A. Pathophysiology and Differential Diagnosis

1. What is the diagnosis? What are the clinical features of this disease?
2. What is the pathophysiology of this disease?
3. How does this lesion occur during development?
4. How are different types of tracheoesophageal fistula (TEF) classified?
5. What other problems may this child have, and when should these be investigated?
6. What should the parents be told regarding perioperative risk?

B. Preoperative Evaluation and Preparation

1. What laboratory workup should be obtained before surgery?
2. What options are there if patient has severe lung disease?
3. Describe management in the NICU before surgery.
4. Should these patients be routinely intubated preoperatively for airway protection?

C. Intraoperative Management

1. What intravenous (IV) access and monitoring are appropriate before induction? After induction?
2. Discuss fluid and temperature management for this baby
3. What are the options regarding induction and intubation?
4. What is the role of fiberoptic bronchoscopy in this patient?
5. Discuss the surgical technique.
6. Discuss common intraoperative problems for this repair.

D. Postoperative Issues

1. When should the baby be extubated?
2. What pain control options are available?
3. What are early and late complications of TEF repair?

A. Pathophysiology and Differential Diagnosis

A.1. What is the diagnosis? What are the clinical features of this disease?

This patient has esophageal atresia with tracheoesophageal fistula. This occurs in 1 per 4,000 live births. The diagnosis is suspected prenatally by the presence of polyhydramnios caused by failure of the fetus to swallow amniotic fluid (secondary to esophageal atresia). After birth, the neonate will have copious drooling. Attempting to feed the baby will result in coughing and cyanosis. An orogastric tube (OGT) will coil up in the upper esophageal pouch rather than pass into the stomach.

Bissonnette B, Dalens B, eds. *Pediatric anesthesia: principles and practice*, 2nd ed. New York: McGraw-Hill, 2002:1016.

Brunicardi FC, Anderson DK, Billiar TR, et al. eds. *Schwartz's principles of surgery*, 8th ed. New York: McGraw-Hill, 2005:1482.

Motoyama EK, Davis PJ, eds. *Smith's anesthesia for infants and children*, 7th ed. Philadelphia: Mosby, Elsevier Science, 2006:550.

A.2. What is the pathophysiology of this disease?

In this abnormality the distal trachea is connected to the lower esophagus through a fistula. This causes three problems. First, inhaled air can bypass the lungs and distend the stomach, which will eventually impede ventilation and cause atelectasis. Second, acidic stomach contents are at continual risk of leaking back into and damaging lung tissue. Third, oral secretions tend to pool in the proximal esophageal pouch resulting in intermittent aspiration, coughing, and cyanosis.

Bissonnette B, Dalens B, eds. *Pediatric anesthesia: principles and practice*, 2nd ed. New York: McGraw-Hill, 2002:1016.

Brunicardi FC, Anderson DK, Billiar TR, et al. eds. *Schwartz's principles of surgery*, 8th ed. New York: McGraw-Hill, 2005:1482.

Hammer GB. Pediatric thoracic anesthesia. *Anesth Analg* 2001;92:1449–1464.

A.3. How does this lesion occur during development?

The median ventral diverticulum of the foregut differentiates into a separate esophagus and trachea by the end of the fifth week of gestation. New insights into the embryologic origin of TEF come from rat studies wherein fetal rats exposed to Adriamycin reliably produce TEF closely resembling the most common version seen in humans. In this model, the lung bud was found to trifurcate instead of normal bifurcation. Two branches become normal lung with pseudostratified columnar epithelium. The third branch grows caudally until it merges with the distal esophagus. Hence the fistula comes from respiratory tissue. Bolstering this conclusion is the finding that the fistula expresses thyroid transcription factor-1 (TTF-1), which is found only in respiratory tissue of the foregut. Human studies also corroborate this finding. Sonic Hedgehog (Shh) is a secreted signaling glycoprotein involved in directing differentiation of the foregut and lung. Defective Shh signaling is associated with VACTERL type anomalies (including TEF) in Shh-knockout mice studies. Tissue was surgically obtained from the esophageal pouch and fistula in neonates undergoing repair of TEF. This tissue was then stained to detect Shh. The proximal pouch, but not the fistula, stained positive for Shh. This suggests that the fistula is not an esophageal structure, despite superficial resemblance.

Brunicardi FC, Anderson DK, Billiar TR, et al. eds. *Schwartz's principles of surgery*, 8th ed. New York: McGraw-Hill, 2005:1481.

Crisera CA, Grau JB, Maldonado TS, et al. Defective epithelial-mesenchymal interactions dictate the organogenesis of Tracheoesophageal fistula. *Pediatr Surg Int* 2000;16:256–261.

Kim JH, Kim PCW, Hui C. The VACTERL association: lesions from the Sonic hedgehog pathway. *Clin Genet* 2001;59:306–315.

Motoyama EK, Davis PJ, eds. *Smith's anesthesia for infants and children*, 7th ed. Philadelphia: Mosby, Elsevier Science, 2006:550.

Spilde T, Bhatia A, Ostlie D, et al. A role for Sonic hedgehog signaling in the pathogenesis of human Tracheoesophageal fistula. *J Pediatr Surg* 2003;38(3):465–468.

A.4. How are different types of TEF classified?

There are five types of TEF according to the classic Gross classification Type A is pure esophageal atresia with no involvement of the respiratory tree. This occurs in 8% of cases. Gross Type B has esophageal atresia and a fistula connecting the proximal esophageal pouch to the trachea. This occurs in less than 1%. The most common is type C with esophageal atresia and fistula linking the distal esophagus to the trachea. This occurs in 75% to 80% of cases. Rarely, type D occurs with two fistula connecting both proximal and distal esophagus to the trachea (2%). Type E, known as an H-type fistula has no atresia. Instead, an intact esophagus has a linkage with trachea through a fistula, and it occurs in 4%.

Brunicardi FC, Anderson DK, Billiar TR, et al. eds. *Schwartz's principles of surgery*, 8th ed. New York: McGraw-Hill, 2005:1481.

Motoyama EK, Davis PJ, eds. *Smith's anesthesia for infants and children*, 7th ed. Philadelphia: Mosby, Elsevier Science, 2006:551.

A.5. What other problems may this child have, and when should these be investigated?

Unfortunately TEF often does not occur in isolation. Serious additional anomalies can occur in the spectrum known as *VACTERL* (formerly known as *VATER*)

V = vertebral anomalies
A = anal canal defect (anal atresia)
C = cardiac malformation (ventricular septal defect [VSD], atrial septal defect [ASD], Tetralogy of Fallot, right sided arch, patent ductus arteriosus [PDA])
TE = TEF
R = renal dysplasia
L = limb defect (radial aplasia)

A patient is considered to have VACTERL association with the presence of three or more of these lesions. Nearly one-third of TEF patients will have an additional VACTERL lesion and an additional one-fifth will have two VACTERL problems. Nearly half of children with TEF will have significant cardiac disease including ASD, bilateral superior vena cava (SVC), and VSD. Other possible gastrointestinal (GI) problems include malrotation of the midgut, and duodenal atresia. Renal problems can include malposition, hydronephrosis, and ureteral abnormalities.

Brunicardi FC, Anderson DK, Billiar TR, et al. eds. *Schwartz's principles of surgery*, 8th ed. New York: McGraw-Hill, 2005:1782.

Diaz LK, Akpek EA, Dinavahi R, et al. Tracheoesophageal fistula and associated congenital heart disease: implications for anesthetic management and survival. *Pediatr Anesth* 2005;15:862–869.

Krosnar S, Baxter A. Thoracoscopic repair of esophageal atresia with Tracheoesophageal fistula: anesthetic and intensive care management of a series of eight neonates. *Pediatr Anesth* 2005;15:541–546.

McMullen KP, Karnes PS, Moir CR, et al. Familial recurrence of tracheoesophageal fistula and associated malformations. *Am J Med Genet* 1996;63:525–528.

A.6. What should the parents be told regarding perioperative risk?

The survival of TEF babies has improved over the years because of improvements in intensive care unit (ICU) care, anesthesia, and surgical technique. Waterston developed the first classification of prognosis of TEF in 1962 as follows:

Group A: birth weight greater than 2.5 kg, healthy, survival 95%
Group B: birth weight 1.8 to 2.5 kg and healthy, or greater than 2.5 kg with moderate pneumonia, or other anomalies, survival 68%
Group C: birth weight less than 1.8 kg or greater than 1.8 kg with severe pneumonia or severe congenital anomaly, survival 6%

With improvements in neonatal care, the survival in groups A and B both approach 100%, so new classification systems have been developed to provide more useful information, as birth weight greater than 1.5 kg no longer independently predicts mortality. Of these perhaps the most useful is the Spitz classification, which is predicated on finding that cardiac disease is leading risk factor and/or cause of mortality in the TEF group.

Spitz group I: birth weight more than 1.5 kg, no major cardiac disease. Survival 97%
Spitz group II: birth weight less than 1.5 kg, or major cardiac disease. Survival 59%
Spitz group III: birth weight less than 1.5 kg and major cardiac disease. Survival 22%

This date was based on a review of 372 infants from 1980 to 1992. With ongoing improvement in care, A recent review of 188 cases from 1993 to 2004 found Spitz group I survival 99%, group II 82%, and group III 50%.

Choudhury SR, Ashcraft KW, Sharp RJ, et al. Survival of patients with esophageal atresia: influence of birth weight, cardiac anomaly, and late respiratory complications. *J Pediatr Surg* 1999;34:70–74.

Konkin DE, O'Hali WA, Webber EM, et al. Outcomes in esophageal atresia and Tracheoesophageal fistula. *J Pediatr Surg* 2003;38:1726–1729.

Lopez PJ, Keys C, Pierro A, et al. Oesophageal atresia: improved outcome in high-risk groups? *J Pediatr Surg* 2006;41:331–334.

Motoyama EK, Davis PJ, eds. *Smith's anesthesia for infants and children*, 7th ed. Philadelphia: Mosby, Elsevier Science, 2006:550.

B. Preoperative Evaluation and Preparation

B.1. What laboratory workup should be obtained before surgery?

Firstly, one must assess the presence and severity of pulmonary disease, especially looking for aspiration pneumonia, and respiratory distress associated with prematurity. Plain chest x-ray may show infiltrates. A radio-opaque orogastric tube (OGT) will be coiled in the proximal esophageal pouch, whereas an abdominal x-ray may show air in the bowels entering through the fistula. Because of the risk of aspiration, use of contrast dye to delineate the fistula should be used only when there is diagnostic uncertainty. Ideally, contrast would be given under fluoroscopy so that any aspiration can be immediately detected. This should only be done if the baby is stable enough to be transported to the fluoroscopy suite. Of note, an OGT that appears to enter the stomach may also reflect esophageal perforation caused by repeated traumatic insertion attempts.

Second, an echocardiogram is mandatory as major cardiac defects strongly influence survival and may impact on anesthetic management. In addition, one wants to look for presence of a right-sided aortic arch, because this may affect the positioning and surgical approach.

Spinal plain films should be done to exclude vertebral anomalies, especially if epidural pain management is being considered. Renal ultrasound should be done to rule out abnormalities, especially hydronephrosis. In addition, complete blood count (CBC), arterial blood gas, and electrolytes should be drawn, and at least 1 unit of packed red blood cells should be type and crossed.

Bissonnette B, Dalens B, eds. *Pediatric anesthesia: principles and practice*, 2nd ed. New York: McGraw-Hill, 2002:986, 1017.

Brunicardi FC, Anderson DK, Billiar TR, et al. eds. *Schwartz's principles of surgery*, 8th ed. New York: McGraw-Hill, 2005:1482.

Motoyama EK, Davis PJ, eds. *Smith's anesthesia for infants and children*, 7th ed. Philadelphia: Mosby, Elsevier Science, 2006:551.

B.2. What options are there if patient has severe lung disease?

In the past, most children with TEF were routinely given a gastrostomy (under local) followed by a staged repair. Beginning in the 80 s, this conservative management began to be questioned, and now primary repair is considered standard of care. However, there remains a subset of neonates with severe pneumonia or respiratory distress syndrome (RDS) who are considered a poor anesthetic and surgical risk (Waterston type C). If the child is intubated because of respiratory disease one technique to optimize ventilation while minimizing gastric distension (through the fistula) is to employ high frequency oscillator ventilation to minimize the peak inspiratory pressure.

If this is insufficient, a simple gastrostomy is placed to allow drainage of gastric fluid (to minimize further aspiration) and prevent or relieve gastric distension that can occur with positive pressure ventilation (PPV) in the setting of a type C TEF. This procedure can be performed under local and obviates the need for a thoracotomy. The problem with this approach is that by decompressing the stomach, gas from the trachea can now bypass the lungs and exit through the stomach. This is especially a concern if the baby's lungs are noncompliant from pneumonia or RDS. This can make it difficult or impossible to ventilate the baby adequately. Fortunately, this can be alleviated if the gastrostomy tube is placed underneath a water seal therefore allowing gas to escape when it exceeds a predetermined threshold.

More recently, Ratan SK et aldescribe another salvage technique which involves occluding the fistula retrograde through a gastrostomy: The child is given local anesthetic over the incision site and a styletted 10 French Foley catheter is advanced through a gastrostomy to a position just above the gastroesophageal junction using fluoroscopy. The balloon is then inflated and the catheter is either clamped or placed under water seal. In this way the baby could be ventilated with positive pressure while avoiding gastric distention or inadequate ventilation from gas bypassing lungs. This technique runs the risk of esophageal rupture and fatal pneumothorax if the catheter is not placed properly.

Brunicardi FC, Anderson DK, Billiar TR, et al. eds. *Schwartz's principles of surgery*, 8th ed. New York: McGraw-Hill, 2005:1483.

Oxford J, Cass DT, Glasson MJ. Advances in the treatment of oesophageal atresia over three decades: the 1970s and the 1990s. *Pediatr Surg Int* 2004;20:402–407.

Ratan SK, Rattan KN, Ratan J, et al. Temporary transgastric fistula occlusion as salvage procedure in neonates with esophageal atresia with wide distal fistula and moderate to severe pneumonia. *Pediatr Surg Int* 2005;21:527–531.

Shaul DB, Schwartz MZ, Marr CC, et al. Primary repair without routine gastrostomy is the treatment of choice for neonates with esophageal atresia and Tracheoesophageal fistula. *Arch Surg* 1989;124:1188–1190.

B.3. Describe management in the NICU before surgery.

After diagnosis of TEF is established and other coexisting anomalies investigated, the baby should be immediately made NPO (nothing by mouth). He should be kept in a warmed isolette with the head elevated at least 30 degrees to minimize reflux through the fistula. An nasogastric tube (NGT) should be placed in the proximal esophageal pouch and kept on intermittent suction to minimize aspiration of oral secretions. Antibiotics to treat aspiration pneumonia should be given when appropriate. Ampicillin and gentamicin should be given in those patients who have coexisting significant cardiac disease as prophylaxis. Ensure that blood is available from the blood bank. Because the patient will require a thoracotomy with lung retraction and intermittent compression of the trachea and great vessels, an arterial line is mandatory for the case. This should ideally be placed in the NICU. An umbilical artery line may be conveniently placed by a qualified neonatologist. Two additional IV lines should also be placed, as the patient will be NPO. Avoid placing lines in the right arm as this arm will most likely be elevated with limited access during right thoracotomy and access limited.

Bissonnette B, Dalens B, eds. *Pediatric anesthesia: principles and practice*, 2nd ed. New York: McGraw-Hill, 2002:986, 1017.

Brunicardi FC, Anderson DK, Billiar TR, et al. eds. *Schwartz's principles of surgery*, 8th ed. New York: McGraw-Hill, 2005:1483.

Hammer GB. Pediatric thoracic anesthesia. *Anesth Analg* 2001;92:1449–1464.

Motoyama EK, Davis PJ, eds. *Smith's anesthesia for infants and children*, 7th ed. Philadelphia: Mosby, Elsevier Science, 2006:551.

B.4. Should these patients be routinely intubated preoperatively for airway protection?

Unless mandated by severe pulmonary disease, the child is not intubated routinely preoperative to minimize the possibility of gastric distension from PPV through the fistula. It is noted that intubation does not protect the child from aspiration of gastric contents through the fistula.

Hammer GB. Pediatric thoracic anesthesia. *Anesth Analg* 2001;92:1449–1464.

C. Intraoperative Management

C.1. What IV access and monitoring are appropriate before induction? After induction?

At least one peripheral IV should be in place before induction. A second may be placed after patient is anesthetized. If the surgeon intends to give the child total parenteral nutrition (TPN) postoperatively, a central may be placed. Arterial line placement for blood gas and hemodynamic monitoring should be placed before incision if it has not already been inserted in the NICU. If a peripheral A-line is not feasible, an umbilical arterial line may be placed by someone experienced in this technique. ECG, oxygen saturation, end-tidal CO_2, and rectal temperature should be also be monitored. A precordial stethoscope should be placed over the left axilla to assess breath sounds in case of inadvertent movement of the endotracheal tube (ETT) during surgical retraction or positioning. A second precordial stethoscope placed over the stomach may be useful to assess if the fistula is being ventilated.

If a gastrostomy tube is present, the end may be placed underneath a water seal. The presence of bubbling indicates ventilation through the fistula, which will occur if the tip of the ETT is proximal to the opening of the fistula. A capnograph inserted into the gastrostomy tube will indicate the same thing.

Motoyama EK, Davis PJ, eds. *Smith's anesthesia for infants and children*, 7th ed. Philadelphia: Mosby, Elsevier Science, 2006:552.

C.2. Discuss fluid and temperature management for this baby.

As with all neonates undergoing surgery, meticulous attention to fluid management and temperature is essential. The child should be transported to the operating room (OR) (in head up position) in a warmed isolette, with a stocking cap on the head to minimize temperature shifts. The OR should be prewarmed to at least 85°F. Surgical irrigation and IV crystalloid should be warmed, as well as any blood products stored on ice. Using a forced-air convective warming system is strongly recommended. An appropriate size heat-moisture exchanger placed in the airway can be useful. Keep in mind that the neonate is more prone to develop hypothermia for a number of reasons including limited subcutaneous fat. One way the baby compensates is with brown fat nonshivering thermogenesis. When choosing anesthetic technique, keep in mind that volatile anesthetics including halothane and isoflurane can decrease thermogenesis by up to 70%.

Considering that the patient has been NPO since birth (and what ever was fed probably did not reach the stomach because of esophageal atresia, it is advisable to administer dextrose-containing solution at a controlled rate during the operation. D10/0.2 NS administered intravenously at maintenance rate using a controlled-infusion pump is an excellent way to avoid hypoglycemia. Insensible losses should be estimated at 3 to 4 mL/kg/hour and replaced with isotonic solution. Urine output (ideally 1 mL/kg/hour) may be difficult to assess accurately in a low–birth weight baby.

Bissonnette B, Dalens B, eds. *Pediatric anesthesia: principles and practice*, 2nd ed. New York: McGraw-Hill, 2002:1003, 1012.

Brunicardi FC, Anderson DK, Billiar TR, et al. eds. *Schwartz's principles of surgery*, 8th ed. New York: McGraw-Hill, 2005:1483.

Motoyama EK, Davis PJ, eds. *Smith's anesthesia for infants and children*, 7th ed. Philadelphia: Mosby, Elsevier Science, 2006:541.

C.3. What are the options regarding induction and intubation?

The goal is to intubate the baby to allow adequate gas exchange with the lowest possible inspiratory pressure needed to inflate the lungs, avoid atelectasis, and avoid distension of the abdomen. Positive pressure mask ventilation should be avoided. There are several options. First is to keep the child spontaneously ventilating until the fistula is ligated. This requires a deep inhalational technique with gentle assisting of each breath to minimize atelectasis. Intubation can performed either awake or after inhalation induction. In this way, the lowest inspiratory pressure is required, minimizing distension of the stomach. Awake intubation used to be common, but attention must be paid to the possibility of increased intracranial pressure or intraventricular hemorrhage in the premature infant, as well as the obvious discomfort to the child. Good intubating conditions can be achieved with deep volatile agent, but maintaining adequate ventilation and surgical conditions during a thoracotomy without relaxant may be challenging. Rapid sequence IV induction and intubation (to minimize face-mask ventilation) is another option provided attention is paid to minimizing inspiratory pressure.

As important as the intubation is the correct positioning of the ETT. The goal is to have the tip of the ETT distal to the fistula yet proximal to the carina. If the tube is deliberately placed deep (into the right mainstem) with the bevel facing forward, then slowly pulled back just until breath sounds occur on the left equal to the right, the tube is likely to be in good position. If the patient has a preexisting gastrostomy, the ETT should be pulled back almost until gas begins to bubble from the end of the gastric tube (which has been placed under water seal), then readvanced until the bubbling stops. If the tube is in good position, then the child can be paralyzed and normal positive pressure ventilation (PPV) maintained. The difficulty lies in maintaining good position of the ETT during surgical manipulation and turning the patient lateral.

Andropoulos DB, Rowe RW, Betts JM. Anaesthetic and surgical airway management during Tracheoesophageal fistula repair. *Pediatr Anaesth* 1998;8:313–319.

Bissonnette B, Dalens B, eds. *Pediatric anesthesia: principles and practice*, 2nd ed. New York: McGraw-Hill, 2002:1017.

Motoyama EK, Davis PJ, eds. *Smith's anesthesia for infants and children*, 7th ed. Philadelphia: Mosby, Elsevier Science, 2006:552.

C.4. What is the role of fiberoptic bronchoscopy in this patient?

Perioperative bronchoscopy before commencing TEF repair has become common for two reasons. First, the airway can be examined directly to help guide the surgical technique. Second, if deemed appropriate, the fistula can be occluded using a Fogarty occlusion catheter, thereby allowing unimpeded PPV without distending the abdomen. Kosloske AM et al. in 1988 reported a series of 42 neonates with TEF who underwent bronchoscopy before incision. They reported 31% had crucial findings impacting on the surgical technique, especially with regard to level of fistula (a cervical level fistula does not necessarily require thoracotomy). Identifying the level of the fistula can assist in correct positioning the ETT (11% may have it below the carina in one series). Reeves, Burt, and Smith report using a rigid bronchoscope to guide placement of a 2-French Fogarty arterial embolectomy catheter into the TEF and the balloon inflated. The bronchoscope was removed and the patient was then intubated using a 3.0 ETT. Andropoulos, Rowe and Betts describe 61 cases of TEF managed with rigid bronchoscopy. Three babies (those with large fistula) electively had their fistula occluded and all three experience immediate improvement in ventilation. If the fistula was small, it was deemed unlikely to cause ventilatory problems and was left unmodified. Another seven had a catheter placed in the fistula to help the surgeon identify it. This technique of isolating the trachea and esophagus before ligation may be useful in skilled hands. However, there is a real possibility that during positioning or surgical manipulation, the Fogarty balloon may slide back into the trachea. This could precipitate immediate complete airway obstruction if not promptly recognized and treated.

Andropoulos DB, Rowe RW, Betts JM. Anaesthetic and surgical airway management during Tracheoesophageal fistula repair. *Pediatr Anaesth* 1998;8:313–319.

Kosloske AM, Jewell PF, and Cartwright KC. Crucial bronchoscopic findings in esophageal atresia and Tracheoesophageal fistula. *J Pediatr Surg* 1988;23:466–70.

Motoyama EK, Davis PJ, eds. *Smith's anesthesia for infants and children*, 7th ed. Philadelphia: Mosby, Elsevier Science, 2006:552.

Reeves ST, Burt N, Smith CD. Is it time to reevaluate the airway management of Tracheoesophageal fistula? *Anesth Analg* 1995;81:866–869.

Veyckemans F, Hamoir M, Rombaux P, et al. Preoperative tracheoscopy in neonates with esophageal atresia (letter). *Anesth Analg* 2002;96:1827–1828.

C.5. Discuss the surgical technique.

First, the patient is positioned in the lateral position, usually left side down. If the patient has a right-sided aortic arch sometimes the surgeon may wish to position him with right side down. A retropleural approach is used which minimizes the danger from an anastomotic leak. The fistula is exposed and ligated (usually occurs within 45 minutes). The upper esophagus is mobilized, then the distal esophagus. The esophagus is joined together. Following this, a feeding tube is placed across the anastomosis to allow feeding (if the patient does not have a gastrostomy). The lung should be carefully reexpanded to eliminate atelectasis before closure.

Brunicardi FC, Anderson DK, Billiar TR, et al. eds. *Schwartz's principles of surgery*, 8th ed. New York: McGraw-Hill, 2005.

C.6. Discuss common intraoperative problems for this repair.

Interference with ventilation is the most common problem and can have many causes. Lung retraction with resulting atelectasis leads to frequent desaturation. It may be difficult if not impossible to maintain normocarbia. The P_{CO_2} may rise to 70–80 mm Hg despite all attempts to optimize ventilation. If the patient has a Fogarty catheter in the fistula, it may be displaced into the trachea causing total airway obstruction. Surgical manipulation of the soft trachea makes it vulnerable to kinking or displacement of ETT distal (into right mainstem) or proximally (above the fistula). Frequent compression of vital structures in the mediastinum can lead to profound hemodynamic compromise. Blood and secretions are a constant problem, which risk obstructing the tube. The ETT should be suctioned frequently, more so if blood is seen. (It does not require much blood to clog a 3.0 ETT.) The retracted lung may need to be intermittently reexpanded to avoid severe hypoxia. Severe gastric distension before ligation of the TEF may require emergent gastric needle decompression. It is crucial to maintain close communication with the surgeon. Avoid hypothermia.

Bissonnette B, Dalens B, eds. *Pediatric anesthesia: principles and practice*, 2nd ed. New York: McGraw-Hill, 2002:1017.

Motoyama EK, Davis PJ, eds. *Smith's anesthesia for infants and children*, 7th ed. Philadelphia: Mosby, Elsevier Science, 2006:552.

D. Postoperative Issues

D.1. When should the baby be extubated?

Although some surgeons prefer to have the baby extubated immediately in the OR to minimize tension on the suture line, this can be risky. Tracheomalacia can precipitate airway obstruction requiring immediate reintubation. Many of the children have lung disease from prematurity or aspiration pneumonia. After receiving narcotics for pain they may be prone to hypoventilation. If early extubation is planned an epidural technique might be helpful. However, if the child is to remain intubated, care should be made to limit inspiratory pressure to protect the repair from disruption.

Brunicardi FC, Anderson DK, Billiar TR, et al. eds. *Schwartz's principles of surgery*, 8th ed. New York: McGraw-Hill, 2005:1483.

Motoyama EK, Davis PJ, eds. *Smith's anesthesia for infants and children*, 7th ed. Philadelphia: Mosby, Elsevier Science, 2006:552.

D.2. What pain control options are available?

If the patient is going to remain intubated postoperative (most likely) then a narcotic technique is advisable. Fentanyl at 10 to 20 μg per kg with muscle relaxant will give hemodynamic stability and allow analgesia to be continued in the postoperative period. For experienced practitioners, epidural can also be placed. An epidural catheter threaded through the caudal space can be threaded up to the thoracic dermatomes. Check the placement of the catheter using fluoroscopy before using it. This technique should only be undertaken by someone highly experienced in regional anesthesia for children, with full awareness of the risks and ability to manage complications.

Bissonnette B, Dalens B, eds. *Pediatric anesthesia: principles and practice*, 2nd ed. New York: McGraw-Hill, 2002:549, 1017.

D.3. What are early and late complications of TEF repair?

Early anastomosis leakage occurs in up to 15%. This may require immediate exploration, or managed expectantly. Esophageal dysmotility, and gastroesophageal reflux disease (GERD) are common. Stricture of the esophageal anastomosis may require repeated dilatations. Tracheomalacia may be evident postoperative and vocal cord paresis has been reported.

Brunicardi FC, Anderson DK, Billiar TR, et al. eds. *Schwartz's principles of surgery*, 8th ed. New York: McGraw-Hill, 2005.

Diaz LK, Akpek EA, Dinavahi R, et al. Tracheoesophageal fistula and associated congenital heart disease: implications for anesthetic management and survival. *Pediatr Anesth* 2005;15:862–869.

Motoyama EK, Davis PJ, eds. *Smith's anesthesia for infants and children*, 7th ed. Philadelphia: Mosby, Elsevier Science, 2006:552.

CHAPTER 6

Congenital Diaphragmatic Hernia

Fun-Sun F. Yao • David Stein • John J. Savarese

A FULL-TERM MALE BABY

was born with respiratory distress and cyanosis. Physical examination showed barrel chest and scaphoid abdomen. The breath sounds were absent in the left side of the chest; the heart sounds were best heard in the right side of the chest. Labored respiration, nasal flaring, and sternal retraction were found. The baby weighed 2,800 g. Blood pressure was 60/30 mm Hg; heart rate, 160 beats per minute; respiration, 70 breaths per minute; temperature, 36°C (96.8°F). Arterial blood gas analysis on room air showed the following: pH, 7.20; PCO_2, 55 mm Hg; PO_2, 35 mm Hg; and CO_2 content, 19 mEq per L.

A. Medical Disease and Differential Diagnosis

1. What differential diagnoses are compatible with these signs and symptoms?
2. Describe the incidence and classification of congenital diaphragmatic hernia (CDH).
3. What are the causes of hypoxemia in patients with CDH?
4. How does the diaphragmatic hernia develop in the fetus? Why do varying degrees of pulmonary hypoplasia usually accompany CDH? How do they affect the prognosis?
5. How do you assess the severity of pulmonary hypoplasia?
6. Discuss persistent pulmonary hypertension (PPH) in the patient with CDH.
7. How do you make a diagnosis of right-to-left shunting through the ductus arteriosus or patent foramen ovale?
8. What other congenital anomalies are usually associated with CDH?

B. Preoperative Evaluation and Preparation

1. How would you interpret the following arterial blood gas analyses: pH, 7.20; PCO_2, 55 mm Hg; PO_2, 35 mm Hg; and CO_2 content, 19 mEq per L? How would you correct them?
2. What immediate treatment should be given to improve the newborn's respiratory status preoperatively?
3. Should CDH be repaired urgently once the diagnosis is made and confirmed?
4. How would you treat pulmonary hypertension and improve oxygenation?
5. What are the effects of nitric oxide (NO) on pulmonary and systemic circulation?

6. How is extracorporeal membrane oxygenation (ECMO) established?
7. What are the advantages of ECMO?
8. What are the indications and contraindications to ECMO?
9. When is the optimal time to repair CDH?
10. What other measures should you take to prepare the patient for surgery?
11. How would you premedicate this patient?

C. Intraoperative Management

1. What monitors would you use for this neonate during surgery?
2. How would you induce and maintain anesthesia?
3. Would you use nitrous oxide for anesthesia? Why?
4. Would you use 100% oxygen during anesthesia?
5. How would you ventilate the patient?
6. How would you maintain the neonate's body temperature?
7. The surgeon returned the intrathoracic stomach and intestine to the peritoneal cavity and the ipsilateral lung was found to be hypoplastic and collapsed. The resident anesthesiologist tried to expand the collapsed lung manually with positive airway pressure. Five minutes after the abdomen was closed, the blood pressure suddenly dropped from 70/40 to 30/20 mm Hg, the heart rate from 150 to 80 beats per minute, and the pulse oximeter from 95% down to 60% saturation. What would you do immediately?
8. Discuss fluid therapy in this patient.
9. At the conclusion of surgery, would you extubate the patient in the operating room?

D. Postoperative Management

1. What postoperative problems would you expect in this patient? What is the mortality rate in patients with CDH?
2. The neonate's blood gas analyses improved right after surgery. However, 3 hours later, severe hypoxemia recurred in spite of ventilatory support with high inspired oxygen concentration. What are the possible causes? How should this patient be treated?

A. Medical Disease and Differential Diagnosis

A.1. What differential diagnoses are compatible with these signs and symptoms?

Congenital cardiopulmonary anomalies should be considered whenever cyanosis and respiratory distress are present. A scaphoid abdomen is present due to the absence of abdominal contents. The presence of the barrel chest, bowel sounds in the chest, and the shift of heart sounds to the right definitely suggest the diagnosis of CDH. To confirm the diagnosis, a chest radiograph should be performed to demonstrate gas-filled loops of bowel and probably the spleen or liver in the chest. The lung on the side of the hernia is compressed into the hilum, and the mediastinum is shifted to the opposite side of the chest. If in doubt, radiopaque dye may be injected through a nasogastric tube to delineate the stomach and intestine in the chest.

Barash PG, Stoelting RK, eds. *Clinical anesthesia*, 5th ed. Philadelphia: Lippincott Williams & Wilkins, 2006:1194–1196.

Behrman RE, Kliegman RM, Jenson HB, et al. eds. *Nelson textbook of pediatrics*, 17th ed. Philadelphia: WB Saunders, 2004:1353–1355.

Gregory GA, ed. *Pediatric anesthesia*, 4th ed. New York: Churchill Livingstone, 2002: 435.

Motoyama EK, Davis PJ, eds. *Smith's anesthesia for infants and children*, 7th ed. Philadelphia: Mosby, Elsevier Science, 2006:545–550.

Stoelting RK, Dierdorf SF. *Anesthesia and co-existing disease*, 4th ed. New York: Churchill Livingstone, 2002:696–697.

A.2. Describe the incidence and classification of CDH.

The incidence of CDH is estimated to be 1 in 2,500 to 5,000 births. The male/female ratio is 2:1, and the left diaphragm is more frequently involved than the right (5:1).

The diaphragm is embryologically formed from the fusion of several components; therefore, a number of developmental defects may occur, resulting in herniation of abdominal contents into the chest. Embryologically, two fundamental types of defects may occur:

- Complete or partial absence of the diaphragm
- Failure of complete muscularization

Embryologic classification is not convenient clinically. A practical classification is used based on the anatomic location of the defects in the diaphragm:

- *Absent diaphragm.* Very rare
- *Diaphragmatic hernia.* (Fig. 6.1)
  - Posterolateral (Bochdalek): 80%
  - Anterior (Morgagni): 2%
  - Paraesophageal: 15% to 20%
- *Eventration.* Very rare

Barash PG, Stoelting RK, eds. *Clinical anesthesia*, 5th ed. Philadelphia: Lippincott Williams & Wilkins, 2006:1194–1196.

Behrman RE, Kliegman RM, Jenson HB, et al. eds. *Nelson textbook of pediatrics*, 17th ed. Philadelphia: WB Saunders, 2004:1353–1355.

Motoyama EK, Davis PJ, eds. *Smith's anesthesia for infants and children*, 7th ed. Philadelphia: Mosby, Elsevier Science, 2006:545–550.

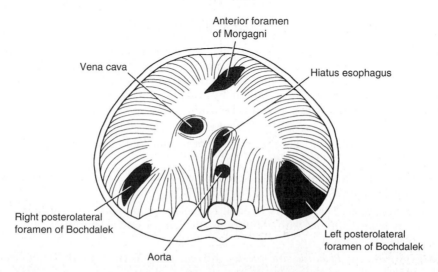

Figure 6.1 Potential sites of congenital diaphragmatic hernia.

A.3. What are the causes of hypoxemia in patients with CDH?

The causes of hypoxemia are as follows:

- Atelectasis resulting from compression of the developed lung by the herniated abdominal organs
- Pulmonary hypoplasia with a decrease in the number of alveoli and bronchial generations. The hypoplastic lung will have abnormal pulmonary vasculature resulting from a disruption of normal development of the lung tissue, secondary to the crowding of the herniated abdominal organs in the thorax.
- Persistent pulmonary hypertension, causing increased right-to-left shunting through a patent foramen ovale and ductus arteriosus

Behrman RE, Kliegman RM, Jenson HB, et al. eds. *Nelson textbook of pediatrics*, 17th ed. Philadelphia: WB Saunders, 2004:1353–1355.

Gregory GA, ed. *Pediatric anesthesia*, 4th ed. New York: Churchill Livingstone, 2002:435–436.

Motoyama EK, Davis PJ, eds. *Smith's anesthesia for infants and children*, 7th ed. Philadelphia: Mosby, Elsevier Science, 2006:545–550.

Stoelting RK, Dierdorf SF. *Anesthesia and co-existing disease*, 4th ed. New York: Churchill Livingstone, 2002:696–697.

A.4. How does the diaphragmatic hernia develop in the fetus? Why do varying degrees of pulmonary hypoplasia usually accompany CDH? How do they affect the prognosis?

Embryologic development of the diaphragm, gut, heart, and lungs takes place at about the same time, and abnormal development of one organ affects development of the others. Normally, the pleural and peritoneal cavities are separated by the diaphragm from the 8th to the 10th week of gestation. At about the same time, the gut physiologically herniates into the yolk stalk but then returns to the peritoneal cavity. The pleuroperitoneal canals progressively narrow and are finally closed by the 10th week. CDH may result either from the early return of the midgut to the peritoneal cavity or from delayed closure of the pleuroperitoneal canal.

The lung is also undergoing development at this time. Alveolar buds begin to differentiate by the 6th week; airways develop from the 10th to the 12th week. Bronchial branching continues until the 16th week of gestation. Alveolar multiplication continues until 8 years of age.

The degree of pulmonary hypoplasia is related to the timing of the herniation of abdominal organs into the pleural cavity. The earlier the herniation, the more severe the pulmonary hypoplasia. Hypoplasia of the left ventricle may also occur, resulting in cardiac insufficiency. The degree of pulmonary hypoplasia determines the prognosis of CDH. Severe bilateral hypoplasia predicts high mortality. With unilateral hypoplasia, the patient may survive with aggressive therapy. When pulmonary hypoplasia is insignificant, the prognosis is excellent.

Barash PG, Stoelting RK, eds. *Clinical anesthesia*, 5th ed. Philadelphia: Lippincott Williams & Wilkins, 2006:1194–1196.

Behrman RE, Kliegman RM, Jenson HB, eds. *Nelson textbook of pediatrics*, 17th ed. Philadelphia: WB Saunders, 2004:1353–1355.

Berdon WE, Baker DH, Amoury R, et al. The role of pulmonary hypoplasia in the prognosis of newborn infants with diaphragmatic hernia and eventration. *Am J Roentgenol* 1968;103:413–421.

Gregory GA, ed. *Pediatric anesthesia*, 4th ed. New York: Churchill Livingstone, 2002: 435.

Motoyama EK, Davis PJ, eds. *Smith's anesthesia for infants and children*, 7th ed. Philadelphia: Mosby, Elsevier Science, 2006:545–550.

A.5. How do you assess the severity of pulmonary hypoplasia?

The severity of pulmonary hypoplasia is assessed by the intrapulmonary shunt (Qs/Qt) or the alveolar–arterial difference in oxygen tension (PAO_2–PaO_2). A (PAO_2–PaO_2) of more than 500 mm Hg when breathing 100% oxygen is predictive of nonsurvival, and a (PAO_2–PaO_2) of less than 400 mm Hg is predictive of survival. A (PAO_2–PaO_2) between 400 and 500 mm Hg represents a zone of uncertain prognosis.

The severity of pulmonary hypoplasia may also be evaluated more aggressively by cardiac catheterization and pulmonary angiogram to define the size and branching pattern of the pulmonary arteries. Patients with severe pulmonary hypoplasia typically will have a fixed right-to-left shunting at the level of the patent ductus arteriosus or patent foramen ovale caused by pulmonary hypertension. Pulmonary angiography demonstrates a small diameter of affected pulmonary artery compared with the main pulmonary artery. The postductal PaO_2 never rises to more than 60 mm Hg in nonsurvivors.

Harrington J, Raphaely RC, Downes JJ, et al. Relationship of alveolar-arterial oxygen tension difference in diaphragmatic hernia of the newborn. *Anesthesiology* 1982;56: 473.

Vacanti JP, Crone RK, Murphy JD, et al. The pulmonary hemodynamic response to perioperative anesthesia in the treatment of high-risk infants with congenital diaphragmatic hernia. *J Pediatr Surg* 1984;19:672–679.

A.6. Discuss persistent pulmonary hypertension in the patient with CDH.

Pulmonary hypertension is one of the major causes of hypoxemia in CDH. There are several causes of pulmonary hypertension in these patients:

- Increased pulmonary vascular resistance and pressure result from a hypoplastic lung.
- The pulmonary vasculature is abnormal, with a decrease in volume and marked increase in muscular mass in the arterioles.
- Right-to-left shunting of oxygen depleted venous blood at the patent foremen ovale and the patent ductus arteriosus. This shunting results in varying degrees of hypoxemia, hypercarbia, and acidosis causing high pulmonary vascular resistance and pressure.

When pulmonary artery pressures are higher than systemic pressures, right-to-left shunting occurs across the ductus, resulting in higher PaO_2 in the upper extremities than in the lower extremities. When right ventricular failure (precipitated by pulmonary hypertension, progressive hypoxemia, and acidosis or by closure of the ductus) increases right atrial pressure to a level higher than the left atrial pressure, right-to-left atrial shunting ensues, producing further hypoxemia. Left ventricular failure from hypoxemia and acidosis induces systemic hypotension, resulting in increased ductal shunting and hypoxemia. A vicious cycle is established. Unless pulmonary artery pressure is decreased, progressive hypoxia and death may ensue.

Barash PG, Stoelting RK, eds. *Clinical anesthesia*, 5th ed. Philadelphia: Lippincott Williams & Wilkins, 2006:1194–1196.

Behrman RE, Kliegman RM, Jenson HB, et al. eds. *Nelson textbook of pediatrics*, 17th ed. Philadelphia: WB Saunders, 2004:1353–1355.

Gregory GA, ed. *Pediatric anesthesia*, 4th ed. New York: Churchill Livingstone, 2002:424–425, 435, 887.

Motoyama EK, Davis PJ, eds. *Smith's anesthesia for infants and children*, 7th ed. Philadelphia: Mosby, Elsevier Science, 2006:545–550.

A.7. How do you make a diagnosis of right-to-left shunting through the patent ductus arteriosus or patent foramen ovale?

If right-to-left shunting occurs through the patent ductus arteriosus, the preductal PaO_2 is at least 15 to 20 mm Hg higher than the postductal value. A right-to-left shunt of 20% is considered "normal" for a newborn infant. If shunting occurs through the patent foramen ovale, the preductal PaO_2 is below the value predicted for 20% shunt. When the degree of preductal shunting is severe, detection of ductal shunting is impossible. Echocardiography with color Doppler, cardiac catheterization, and pulmonary angiography will confirm the diagnosis.

Gregory GA, ed. *Pediatric anesthesia*, 4th ed. New York: Churchill Livingstone, 2002:1171–1173.

Nelson NM, Prod'Hom LS, Cherry RB, et al. Pulmonary function in the newborn infant: the alveolar-arterial oxygen gradient. *J Appl Physiol* 1963;18:534.

Stoelting RK, Dierdorf SF. *Anesthesia and co-existing disease*, 4th ed. New York: Churchill Livingstone, 2002:696–697.

A.8. What other congenital anomalies are usually associated with CDH?

The incidence of other congenital anomalies in newborns with CDH is as follows:

- *Cardiovascular system.* 13% to 23%; for example, atrial septal defect, ventricular septal defect, coarctation of aorta, and tetralogy of Fallot
- *Central nervous system.* 28%; for example, spina bifida, hydrocephalus, and acephalus
- *Gastrointestinal system.* 20%; for example, malrotation and atresia
- *Genitourinary system.* 15%; for example, hypospadias

David TJ, Illingworth CA. Diaphragmatic hernia in the southwest of England. *J Med Genet* 1976;13:253.

Gregory GA, ed. *Pediatric anesthesia*, 4th ed. New York: Churchill Livingstone, 2002:1171–1173.

B. Preoperative Evaluation and Preparation

B.1. How would you interpret the following arterial blood gas analyses: pH, 7.20; PCO_2, 55 mm Hg; PO_2, 35 mm Hg; and CO_2 content, 19 mEq per L? How would you correct them?

The blood gas analyses showed mixed respiratory and metabolic acidosis and severe hypoxemia. Severe hypoxemia is caused by the pulmonary pathologies and persistent pulmonary hypertension (PPH). Hypoxemia stimulates respiratory chemoreceptors and causes hyperventilation, resulting in respiratory alkalosis initially. However, if hypoxemia is not corrected, the patient will become exhausted and CO_2 retention ensues. Severe pulmonary hypoplasia may also cause CO_2 retention. Severe hypoxemia induces anaerobic metabolism, resulting in lactic acidosis.

Hypoxemia and respiratory acidosis should be treated with mechanical ventilation and oxygen therapy. Metabolic acidosis should be corrected by administration of sodium bicarbonate and improvement of circulation with fluid therapy.

Behrman RE, Kliegman RM, Jenson HB, et al. eds. *Nelson textbook of pediatrics*, 17th ed. Philadelphia: WB Saunders, 2004:1353–1355.

Gregory GA, ed. *Pediatric anesthesia*, 4th ed. New York: Churchill Livingstone, 2002:435–437.

Stoelting RK, Dierdorf SF. *Anesthesia and co-existing disease*, 4th ed. New York: Churchill Livingstone, 2002:696–697.

B.2. What immediate treatment should be given to improve the newborn's respiratory status preoperatively?

Immediate intervention should include decompression of the stomach with an orogastric or nasogastric tube and administration of supplemental oxygen by mask. Positive pressure ventilation by mask should be avoided to prevent distention of the intrathoracic stomach, which will further compress the lung and compromise respiration. If cyanosis and hypoxemia persist, awake intubation should be done to facilitate mechanical ventilation. Positive airway pressure during mechanical ventilation should not exceed 30 cm H_2O to reduce the risk of tension pneumothorax. Although pneumothorax can happen on either side, it occurs more frequently on the contralateral side of the hernia because the pressure needed to expand the hypoplastic lung is higher than that required to rupture the normal lung.

Behrman RE, Kliegman RM, Jenson HB, et al. eds. *Nelson textbook of pediatrics*, 17th ed. Philadelphia: WB Saunders, 2004:1353–1355.

Gregory GA, ed. *Pediatric anesthesia*, 4th ed. New York: Churchill Livingstone, 2002:435–437.

Stoelting RK, Dierdorf SF. *Anesthesia and co-existing disease*, 4th ed. New York: Churchill Livingstone, 2002:696–697.

B.3. Should CDH be repaired urgently once the diagnosis is made and confirmed?

In the past, CDH was considered a surgical emergency, in the belief that the herniated contents caused lung collapse and respiratory failure. However, recognition of the role of pulmonary hypertension, in addition to pulmonary hypoplasia and the effects of surgical repair on pulmonary function, has prompted critical reevaluation of that strategy. It is now clear that lung compression by the herniated viscera is a minor factor in the cardiopulmonary compromise compared with the pulmonary hypertension and hypoplasia. The consensus today is to delay surgery and concentrate on medical stabilization. The goal of preoperative therapy is to reverse the PPH that results in right-to-left shunting across the patent foramen ovale and the ductus arterious. Improvement in the infant's status is apparent by improved oxygenation and ventilation. Doppler echocardiography may be used to confirm the decreased pulmonary vascular resistance. The time it takes to stabilize the condition varies from 24 to 48 hours in infants with only mild pulmonary hypertension and hypoplasia up to 7 to 10 days in neonates with severe pulmonary hypertension and hypoplasia.

Barash PG, Stoelting RK, eds. *Clinical anesthesia*, 5th ed. Philadelphia: Lippincott Williams & Wilkins, 2006:1194–1196.

Behrman RE, Kliegman RM, Jenson HB, et al. eds. *Nelson textbook of pediatrics*, 17th ed. Philadelphia: WB Saunders, 2004:1353–1355.

Charlton AJ. The management of congenital diaphragmatic hernia without ECMO. *Paediatr Anaesth* 1993;3:201.

Gregory GA, ed. *Pediatric anesthesia*, 4th ed. New York: Churchill Livingstone, 2002:436–437.

Haugen SE, Linker D, Eik-Nes S, et al. Congenital diaphragmatic hernia: determination of the optimal time for operation by echocardiographic monitoring of the pulmonary arterial pressure. *J Pediatr Surg* 1991;26:560.

B.4. How would you treat persistent pulmonary hypertension (PPH) and improve oxygenation?

Pulmonary vascular resistance is greatly increased in the hypoplastic lung, and blood flow is minimal because of medial hyperplasia of pulmonary arterioles. When further aggravated by hypoxemia, acidosis, decreased FIO_2, or sudden changes in pulmonary blood volume, pulmonary vasoconstriction increases and fetal circulation persists. The treatment of pulmonary hypertension includes the following measures in sequence:

- Continue general anesthesia in the intensive care unit, using fentanyl 3 μg/kg/hour, and pancuronium 0.1 mg/kg/hour to blunt the autonomically mediated cardiovascular response (pulmonary vasoconstriction) to stimulation.
- Minimize endotracheal suctioning to avoid transient hypoxemia or decrease in FIO_2.
- Hyperventilate the neonate with low tidal volume and high respiratory rate (60 to 120 breaths/minute) to pH of 7.55 to 7.60. Respiratory alkalosis is the most consistently effective therapeutic modality to achieve pulmonary vasodilation.
- Moderately restrict fluid to 2 to 4 mL/kg/hour.
- Administer pharmacologic vasodilators if the aforementioned measures fail to control pulmonary hypertension. Morphine, prednisolone, chlorpromazine, phentolamine, acetylcholine, bradykinin, tolazoline, prostaglandin E_1, prostaglandin D_2, and inhaled NO have been tried with some success. Milrinone would be helpful if right ventricular failure is apparent.
- Ligate the patent ductus arteriosus to prevent shunting. This is theoretically possible but practically has been associated with sudden right ventricular failure.
- Support with ECMO if pharmacologic intervention fails. ECMO has been associated with a 50% to 65% survival rate.

Barash PG, Stoelting RK, eds. *Clinical anesthesia*, 5th ed. Philadelphia: Lippincott Williams & Wilkins, 2006:1194–1196.

Gregory GA, ed. *Pediatric anesthesia*, 4th ed. New York: Churchill Livingstone, 2002:436–437.

Vacanti JP, Crone RK, Murphy JD, et al. The pulmonary hemodynamic response to perioperative anesthesia in the treatment of high-risk infants with congenital diaphragmatic hernia. *J Pediatr Surg* 1984;19:672–679.

B.5. What are the effects of nitric oxide (NO) on pulmonary and systemic circulation?

When produced *in vivo*, NO is endothelium-derived relaxing factor (EDRF) producing smooth muscle relaxation and vasodilation. Inhaled NO is unique, as it is a selective pulmonary vasodilator and has no effect on systemic circulation because it is inactivated immediately on exposure to hemoglobin. Clinical studies are limited but have shown some improvement in oxygenation in neonates with persistent pulmonary hypertension (PPH) exposed to 20 to 80 parts per million (ppm) of NO. NO has been reported to be ineffective before ECMO therapy in those patients with both CDH and pulmonary hypoplasia. After ECMO followed by surgery, NO was effective in improving oxygenation. However, NO has not been shown to improve survival.

Behrman RE, Kliegman RM, Jenson HB, et al. eds. *Nelson textbook of pediatrics*, 17th ed. Philadelphia: WB Saunders, 2004:1353–1355.

Charlton AJ. The management of congenital diaphragmatic hernia without ECMO. *Paediatr Anaesth* 1993;3:201.

Gregory GA, ed. *Pediatric anesthesia*, 4th ed. New York: Churchill Livingstone, 2002:436–437.

Motoyama EK, Davis PJ, eds. *Smith's anesthesia for infants and children*, 7th ed. Philadelphia: Mosby, Elsevier Science, 2006:545–550.

Wheeler M. Practical anesthetic management of neonatal surgical emergencies. *ASA annual meeting refresher course lectures* Park Ridge, IL: American Society of Anesthesiologists, 2001:116.

B.6. How is ECMO established?

Venovenous or venoarterial bypass is used. Venovenous bypass is established with a double-lumen catheter through the internal jugular vein, with blood removed from and infused into the right atrium through separate ports. Venoarterial bypass is used preferentially by some centers because it provides the cardiac support that is often needed. The right atrium is cannulated through the internal jugular vein. Blood is allowed to passively flow by gravity into the ECMO circuit, where it is pumped with an occlusive blood pump into the membrane oxygenator. From the oxygenator, blood is returned through a catheter placed through the right common carotid artery into the ascending aorta.

Gregory GA, ed. *Pediatric anesthesia*, 4th ed. New York: Churchill Livingstone, 2002:436–437.

B.7. What are the advantages of ECMO?

The theoretical advantages are as follows:

- Diversion of as much as 80% of cardiac output from the right atrium into the extracorporeal circuit immediately reduces or eliminates right-to-left shunting through the foramen ovale or ductus arteriosus.
- Right ventricular work is decreased because of reduced pulmonary blood flow and pressure.
- Pulmonary vasoconstriction is reduced because hypoxemia and acidosis are corrected by ECMO. Improved systemic oxygenation and reduced ductal blood flow may lead to spontaneous closure of the ductus arteriosus.
- The hypoplastic lung is allowed to grow rapidly and alveolar size is increased.
- The incidence of bronchopulmonary dysplasia is reduced because FIO_2 and airway pressure are lowered by ECMO.

Gregory GA, ed. *Pediatric anesthesia*, 4th ed. New York: Churchill Livingstone, 2002: 437–438.

B.8. What are the indications and contraindications to ECMO?

Patients with severe hypoxemia, hypercarbia, and pulmonary hypertension who do not respond to maximal conventional respiratory and pharmacologic intervention are candidates for ECMO. However, due to the necessity for anticoagulation and the consumption and inactivation of platelets, ECMO is associated with serious complications of intracranial and pulmonary hemorrhage. The entry criteria include a gestational age of 34 weeks or greater, the presence of a reversible disease process, a minimal weight of 2,000 g, and a predicted mortality of greater than 80%. (Predicted mortality is commonly estimated by the oxygenation index [$F_{IO_2} \times$ mean airway pressure $\times 100/Pa_{O_2}$].) Values of oxygenation index in excess of 40 predict mortality greater than 80%.

The contraindications to ECMO include the following:

- Gestational age less than 34 weeks
- Weight less than 2,000 g
- Preexisting grade II or greater intracranial hemorrhage
- Congenital or neurologic abnormalities incompatible with good outcome
- More than 1 week of aggressive respiratory therapy
- Congenital heart disease

Dilley RE, Zwischenberger JB, Andrews AF, et al. Intracranial hemorrhage during extracorporeal membrane oxygenator in neonates. *Pediatrics* 1986;78:699.

Gregory GA, ed. *Pediatric anesthesia*, 4th ed. New York: Churchill Livingstone, 2002:438–439.

Redmond CR, Goldsmith JP, Sharp MJ, et al. Extracorporeal membrane oxygenation for neonates. *J La State Med Soc* 1986;138:40.

Stolar CJ, Snedecor SS, Bartlett RH. Extracorporeal membrane oxygenation and neonatal respiratory failure: experience from the extracorporeal life support organization. *J Pediatr Surg* 1991;26:563.

B.9. When is the optimal time to repair CDH?

The newborn should be maintained on ECMO until the pulmonary hypertension is reversed and improvement in lung function is evident. Doppler echocardiography may be used to confirm the reversal of PPH. This is usually seen within 7 to 10 days but in some infants is not apparent for up to 3 weeks. Newborns who do not demonstrate significant improvement over this time have pulmonary hypoplasia that will not benefit from further extracorporeal life support. Timing of repair of the CDH on ECMO is controversial. Some centers prefer early repair to allow a greater duration of postrepair ECMO, whereas many centers defer repair until the infant has demonstrated the ability to tolerate weaning from ECMO support.

Behrman RE, Kliegman RM, Jenson HB, et al. eds. *Nelson textbook of pediatrics*, 17th ed. Philadelphia: WB Saunders, 2004:1353–1355.

Gregory GA, ed. *Pediatric anesthesia*, 4th ed. New York: Churchill Livingstone, 1994:436–437.

Haugen SE, Linker D, Eik-Nes S, et al. Congenital diaphragmatic hernia: determination of the optimal time for operation by echocardiographic monitoring of the pulmonary arterial pressure. *J Pediatr Surg* 1991;26:560.

B.10. What other measures should you take to prepare the patient for surgery?

The patient should be examined carefully for the presence and severity of associated congenital anomalies as described in section A.8. Those patients with congenital heart disease in addition to CDH have significantly increased mortality.

Hypothermia should be prevented and corrected. Hypothermia can aggravate the hypoxemia and acidosis. Hypothermia can also lead to coagulopathy and arrhythmia. The neonate should be maintained in a neutral thermal environment of 36.5°C to 37.5°C (97.7°F to 99.5°F).

Laboratory studies should include arterial blood gases, complete blood cell count, electrolytes, blood sugar, blood type, and cross-match for blood products.

Venous access should be ready before surgery. Peripheral veins in the upper extremities are preferred because reduction of the hernia often increases abdominal pressure and partially obstructs the inferior vena cava, making lower extremity veins less reliable. Neck veins are avoided in case ECMO is required. Central venous access should be attempted through the umbilical or femoral vein.

B.11. How would you premedicate this patient?

No premedication should be given to the neonate with CDH. The newborn should not have any anxiety, and sedatives will further depress the already compromised cardiopulmonary function.

C. Intraoperative Management

C.1. What monitors would you use for this neonate during surgery?

Respiratory
- Precordial and esophageal stethoscope
- Two Pulse oximeters, for preductal and postductal oxygen saturation
- Capnometry
- Inspiratory pressure measurement
- Inspiratory oxygen concentration
- Intraoperative arterial blood gas analysis

Cardiovascular
- Five lead electrocardiogram
- Blood pressure cuff
- Precordial stethoscope
- Arterial line: right radial artery for preductal PaO_2
- Central venous pressure (CVP) line for evaluating volume status and right ventricular performance

Thermoregulatory
- Esophageal or rectal temperature probe

C.2. How would you induce and maintain anesthesia?

If the neonate has not been intubated, intubation should be performed with spontaneous ventilation. Positive pressure ventilation should be avoided before intubation to prevent gastric distention and further compromise of respiration. An awake intubation can be performed after preoxygenation. However, if the neonate is too vigorous for awake intubation, he can be intubated without a muscle relaxant after breathing sevoflurane and oxygen spontaneously.

The choice of maintenance anesthetics depends on the severity of cardiovascular dysfunction. Patients in shock and severe hypoxemia may tolerate only oxygen and a nondepolarizing relaxant such as rocuronium or vecuronium. If blood pressure is adequate and stable, inhalation agents and narcotics in addition to a muscle relaxant, may be titrated to maintain anesthesia. Narcotics and nondepolarizers may be continued postoperatively to control ventilation and minimize hormonal response to stress, which may increase pulmonary hypertension.

Barash PG, Stoelting RK, eds. *Clinical anesthesia*, 5th ed. Philadelphia: Lippincott Williams & Wilkins, 2006:1194–1196.

Dierdorf SF, Krichna G. Anesthetic management of neonatal surgical emergencies. *Anesth Analg* 1981;60:204–214.

Gregory GA, ed. *Pediatric anesthesia*, 4th ed. New York: Churchill Livingstone, 2002:437.

Motoyama EK, Davis PJ, eds. *Smith's anesthesia for infants and children*, 7th ed. Philadelphia: Mosby, Elsevier Science, 2006:545–550.

C.3. Would you use nitrous oxide for anesthesia? Why?

No. Nitrous oxide should not be used in patients with CDH before hernia reduction and abdominal closure. Because nitrous oxide has a higher diffusion capacity than nitrogen (35:1), the amount of nitrous oxide diffused from blood to the gut is much more than the amount of nitrogen diffused from the gut to the blood. Therefore, nitrous oxide may distend the intrathoracic gut and compress the functioning lung tissue, further compromising pulmonary function. Moreover, a distended gut may cause difficulty in abdominal closure and may increase abdominal pressure, compressing the inferior vena cava and resulting in hypotension.

Barash PG, Stoelting RK, eds. *Clinical anesthesia*, 5th ed. Philadelphia: Lippincott Williams & Wilkins, 2006:1194–1196.

Eger El II, Saidman LJ. Hazards of nitrous oxide anesthesia in bowel obstruction and pneumothorax. *Anesthesiology* 1975;26:61.

Fink R. Diffusion anoxia. *Anesthesiology* 1955;16:511–519.

Gregory GA, ed. *Pediatric anesthesia*, 4th ed. New York: Churchill Livingstone, 2002:437.

C.4. Would you use 100% oxygen during anesthesia?

Selection of the appropriate inspired concentration of oxygen depends on the severity of pulmonary dysfunction. Retrolental fibroplasia (retinopathy of prematurity) is a potential danger during neonatal anesthesia. Current guidelines suggest that infants are at risk of retrolental fibroplasia until 44 to 50 weeks of gestational age. However, hypoxia causes pulmonary vasoconstriction and pulmonary hypertension, which may increase right-to-left shunting of desaturated blood at preductal or ductal level. Serial arterial blood gases may be used to determine the optimal FIO_2. Air is added to oxygen if the PaO_2 on 100% oxygen is more than 90 to 100 mm Hg. The PaO_2 should be optimally kept at 80 to 100 mm Hg or the arterial oxygen saturation between 95% and 98%.

Dierdorf SF, Krishna G. Anesthetic management of neonatal surgical emergencies. *Anesth Analg* 1981;60:204–214.

Gregory GA, ed. *Pediatric anesthesia*, 4th ed. New York: Churchill Livingstone, 2002:436–437.

Motoyama EK, Davis PJ, eds. *Smith's anesthesia for infants and children*, 7th ed. Philadelphia: Mosby, Elsevier Science, 2006:545–550.

C.5. How would you ventilate the patient?

Ventilation is controlled either manually or by a respirator. Small tidal volumes should be used to keep the airway pressure below 30 cm H_2O to prevent contralateral pneumothorax. High respiratory rates (60 to 120 breaths/minute) should be adjusted to achieve hyperventilation to a $PaCO_2$ between 25 and 30 mm Hg to lower pulmonary vascular resistance and minimize right-to-left shunting through the patent ductus arteriosus.

Bray RJ. Congenital diaphragmatic hernia. *Anesthesia* 1979;34:567.

Gregory GA, ed. *Pediatric anesthesia*, 4th ed. New York: Churchill Livingstone, 2002:436–437.

C.6. How would you maintain the neonate's body temperature?

The neonate is particularly susceptible to heat loss because of a large surface to volume ratio, lack of insulating fat, and a naturally flaccid and open posture. Body temperature should be monitored carefully and maintained within the normal range. The following steps are used to maintain body temperature:

- Warm the operating room to 80.6°F (27°C).
- Use radiant warming lamps and a heating blanket.
- Use a Heat Moisture Exchanger on the ventilator circuit.
- Warm transfused blood and intravenous fluid to 37°C (99.5°F).

Dierdorf SF, Krishna G. Anesthetic management of neonatal surgical emergencies. *Anesth Analg* 1981;60:204–214.

Gregory GA, ed. *Pediatric anesthesia*, 4th ed. New York: Churchill Livingstone, 2002:430–437.

C.7. The surgeon returned the intrathoracic stomach and intestine to the peritoneal cavity and the ipsilateral lung was found to be hypoplastic and collapsed. The resident anesthesiologist tried to expand the collapsed lung manually with positive airway pressure. Five minutes after the abdomen was closed, the blood pressure suddenly dropped from 70/40 to 30/20 mm Hg, the heart rate from 150 to 80 beats per minute, and the pulse oximeter from 95% down to 60% saturation. What would you do immediately?

Any sudden deterioration in blood pressure, heart rate, oxygen saturation, or pulmonary compliance is suggestive of tension pneumothorax. Auscultation of the chest, particularly the contralateral side, should be done immediately. If absent or diminished breath sounds confirm the diagnosis, a chest tube should be inserted immediately. A large-bore intravenous catheter with needle may be inserted to release the tension pneumothorax if a chest tube is not immediately available.

The tension pneumothorax is usually on the contralateral side, because the high airway pressure required to inflate the hypoplastic lung may rupture the normal alveoli on the contralateral side, resulting in pneumothorax. Moreover, the ipsilateral chest usually already has a chest tube after surgery.

If there is no pneumothorax, or if deterioration is not improved after insertion of a chest tube, inferior vena cava compression (causing decreased venous return and decreased cardiac output) should be considered. The peritoneal cavity is often underdeveloped and unable to fully accommodate the returned abdominal organs, which increases the intraabdominal pressure. In this circumstance, the abdominal wound should be opened to relieve the compression on the vena cava and diaphragm. A Silastic patch may be used to cover the abdominal defect temporarily and the defect will be closed at a later time.

Gregory GA, ed. *Pediatric anesthesia*, 4th ed. New York: Churchill Livingstone, 2002:437.

C.8. Discuss fluid therapy in this patient.

Fluid therapy should be aimed to correct the preoperative deficit, provide maintenance fluid, and replace intraoperative evaporative, third space, and blood losses.

Kidneys are 80% to 90% mature by 1 month of age. Before that time, the infant cannot tolerate the extremes of renal stress. Neonates are obligate sodium losers; therefore, exogenous sodium should be supplied. In addition, neonates have decreased glycogen storage and are prone to hypoglycemia after brief periods of starvation. Therefore, glucose should also be provided. However, hyperglycemia may predispose the patient to intracranial hemorrhage and should be avoided. The preoperative fluid deficit may be evaluated by careful history taking, signs and symptoms of dehydration, urine output, and CVP monitoring. Maintenance fluids consisting of 5% dextrose in one-fourth to one-half strength saline are given at 4 mL/kg/hour. Intraoperative evaporative and third space losses are replaced with Ringer's lactate or saline at approximately 6 to 8 mL/kg/hour. Each milliliter of blood loss is replaced with 3 mL of Ringer's lactate or 1 mL of 5% albumin. Blood pressure, heart rate, urine output, CVP, hematocrit, and sodium and glucose levels are monitored following the fluid therapy.

Dierdorf SF, Krishna G. Anesthetic management of neonatal surgical emergencies. *Anesth Analg* 1981;60:204–214.

Stoelting RK, Dierdorf SF. *Anesthesia and co-existing disease*, 4th ed. New York: Churchill Livingstone, 2002:696–697.

C.9. At the conclusion of surgery, would you extubate the patient in the operating room?

No. The patient should not be extubated in the operating room because varying degrees of pulmonary dysfunction are always present postoperatively. The endotracheal tube should be left in place and the baby should be transported to the intensive care unit for further postoperative care.

D. Postoperative Management

D.1. What postoperative problems would you expect in this patient? What is the mortality rate in patients with CDH?

The postoperative course is often characterized by a "honeymoon" period of rapid improvement, followed by sudden deterioration with profound arterial hypoxemia, hypercapnia, and acidosis.

The mortality in patients with CDH varies from 30% to 60%. Factors affecting the mortality include the following:

- Pulmonary hypoplasia
- *Associated congenital defect.* Cardiovascular and central nervous systems

- *Inadequate preoperative preparation.* Hypothermia, acidosis, shock, and tension pneumothorax
- *Ineffective postoperative management.* Hemorrhage, tension pneumothorax, inferior vena cava compression, persistent fetal circulation, excessive suction on chest tube

Behrman RE, Kliegman RM, Jenson HB, eds. *Nelson textbook of pediatrics*, 17th ed. Philadelphia: WB Saunders, 2004:1353–1355.

Vacanti JP, Crone RK, Murphy JD, et al. The pulmonary hemodynamic response to perioperative anesthesia in the treatment of high-risk infants with congenital diaphragmatic hernia. *J Pediatr Surg* 1984;19:672–679.

Waldschmidt J, vonLengerke HG, Berlien P. Causes of death in operated neonates with diaphragmatic defects. *Prog Pediatr Surg* 1979;13:239.

D.2. The neonate's blood gas analyses improved right after surgery. However, 3 hours later, severe hypoxemia recurred in spite of ventilatory support with high inspired oxygen concentration. What are the possible causes? How should this patient be treated?

As discussed earlier, a tension pneumothorax should be considered and treated if it exists. In the absence of a tension pneumothorax, persistent hypoxemia suggests persistent pulmonary hypertension (PPH) with right-to-left shunting of venous blood. Recurrent pulmonary hypertension carries a high mortality. ECMO support should be continued or reestablished if already discontinued before surgery. If the infant cannot be weaned from ECMO after repair, options include discontinuing support or therapies such as NO or lung transplantation. High-frequency jet ventilation and oscillatory ventilation have had limited success in patients with CDH.

Behrman RE, Kliegman RM, Jenson HB, et al. eds. *Nelson textbook of pediatrics*, 17th ed. Philadelphia: WB Saunders, 2004:1353–1355.

Gregory GA, ed. *Pediatric anesthesia*, 4th ed. New York: Churchill Livingstone, 2002:437–438.

The Cardiovascular System

CHAPTER 7

Ischemic Heart Disease and Coronary Artery Bypass Grafting

FUN-SUN F. YAO • NIKOLAOS SKUBAS • MANUEL L. FONTES

A 57-YEAR-OLD MAN

with triple-vessel coronary artery disease (CAD) was scheduled for coronary artery bypass grafting (CABG). He had a myocardial infarction 7 months ago. He was taking nitroglycerin, digoxin, metoprolol, isosorbide dinitrate (Isordil), and nifedipine. His blood pressure (BP) was 120/80 mm Hg and his heart rate (HR) 60 per minute.

A. Medical Disease and Differential Diagnosis

1. What is triple-vessel CAD? Name the branches of the coronary arteries.
2. What are the indications for CABG?
3. What is percutaneous transluminal coronary angioplasty (PTCA)? Discuss its indications, contraindications, and results.
4. What are the results of coronary artery bypass surgery?

B. Preoperative Evaluation and Preparation

1. Which preoperative tests would you order?
2. How would you evaluate the patient's left ventricular function?
3. What are the three major determinants of myocardial oxygen consumption? How are they measured clinically?
4. Which factors determine myocardial oxygen supply?

5. Would you discontinue digoxin? Why? What is its half-life?

6. Would you discontinue the β-blocker (metropolol)? Why? What is its half-life? What is the role of β-adrenergic blockers in treating congestive heart failure (CHF)?

7. If the patient who is on metropolol develops hypotension intraoperatively, how would you manage it?

8. What is nifedipine? How does it work?

9. How would you premedicate the patient? Why?

C. Intraoperative Management

C.I. Before Cardiopulmonary Bypass

1. How do you monitor the patient?

2. What is Allen's test?

3. Why do you need multiple temperature monitoring?

4. How do you know that the tip of the pulmonary artery (PA) catheter is in the right ventricle (RV) or PA?

5. What is normal pulmonary artery occlusion pressure (PAOP)?

6. Is it necessary to monitor PA pressure for coronary artery operations?

7. What are the complications of PA catheterization?

8. What are the hemodynamic consequences of myocardial ischemia? How can you detect myocardial ischemia? Is PAOP a sensitive indicator of myocardial ischemia?

9. How would you monitor electrocardiogram (ECG)? Why V_5? If you do not have precordial leads in your ECG machine, how can you monitor the left ventricle (LV)?

10. Discuss the principles and clinical applications of intraoperative transesophageal two-dimensional echocardiography.

11. How would you induce anesthesia?

12. How would you maintain anesthesia?

13. What is the better anesthetic agent for this operation—an inhalation or intravenous agent?

14. What are the cardiovascular effects of halothane, enflurane, isoflurane, desflurane, sevoflurane, morphine, and fentanyl?

15. Is isoflurane dangerous for the patient with coronary artery disease (CAD)?

16. What is the cardiovascular effect of nitrous oxide?

17. What kind of muscle relaxant would you use? Why?

18. If ST-segment depression is seen during surgery, how would you treat it? What is the relation between perioperative myocardial ischemia and postoperative myocardial infarction?

19. Would you use prophylactic nitroglycerin during coronary artery bypass grafting (CABG) to prevent intraoperative myocardial ischemia or perioperative myocardial infarction?

20. How would you correct hypertension?

21. How would you treat hypotension?

22. What are the indications for intravenous metoprolol, labetalol, or esmolol during surgery? How much would you give? What are the relative contraindications?

23. How would you correct increased PAOP?

24. What should you do during sternal splitting?

25. Would you monitor PAOP continuously? Why?

26. Discuss autologous transfusion and blood conservation for cardiac surgery.

C.II. During Cardiopulmonary Bypass

1. What anticoagulant would you give before cardiopulmonary bypass (CPB)? How much would you give? What is its mechanism?

2. What is the half-life of heparin? How is it eliminated?

3. How do you monitor heparin dosage? What is the activated coagulation time (ACT) test?

4. What is total CPB? What is partial bypass?

5. What is the purpose of venting the LV? How can it be done?

6. How many types of oxygenators are there? What are the advantages of each type?

7. What kind of priming solution would you use? How much priming solution would you use? Would you prime with blood? Why?

8. What are the advantages and disadvantages of hemodilution?

9. What kind of pumps do you use? Are they pulsatile or not?

10. How do you monitor the patient during CPB?

11. How much BP would you keep during CPB? Why?

12. How would you treat hypotension during CPB?

13. How would you treat hypertension (a mean arterial pressure (MAP) of over 100 mm Hg)?

14. How do you prepare an intravenous infusion of sodium nitroprusside, nicardipine, and nitroglycerin? What are the usual doses? Which do you prefer to use?

15. How much pump flow would you maintain during CPB?

16. How would you adjust the pump flow during hypothermia?

17. How would you adjust the pump flow during hemodilution?

18. What are the advantages of hypothermia? Does hypothermia offer neuroprotection?

19. How does blood viscosity change during hypothermia and hemodilution?

20. What are the main causes of death associated with accidental hypothermia?

21. Would you give anesthesia during CPB? Why?

22. Would you give muscle relaxants during CPB? How is the action of muscle relaxant affected during CPB?

23. How do you know the patient is well perfused during CPB?

24. How much gas flow would you use for the oxygenator? What kind of gas would you use? Why?

25. What are the disadvantages of hypocapnia during CPB?

26. The arterial blood gases and electrolytes during CPB are pH, 7.36; $Paco_2$, 42 mm Hg; Pao_2, 449 mm Hg; CO_2 content, 24 mEq per L; Na, 128 mEq per L; K, 5.8 mEq per L; Ht, 20%. The patient's temperature is 27°C (80.6°F). At what temperature are blood gases measured? How would you correct the blood gases according to patient's body temperature? Would you treat the arterial blood gases at 37°C (98.6°F) or at patient's body temperature?

27. If the blood level of the venous reservoir is low, what would you replace it with? Blood or balanced salt solution?

28. How do you estimate the fluid balance during CPB?

29. How would you preserve the myocardium during CPB?

30. What is the cardioplegic solution? How much would you use?

31. For how long a period can the aorta be cross-clamped?
32. Why does urine become pink after 2 hours of CPB? What is the renal threshold for plasma hemoglobin?
33. At what temperature can the patient be weaned from CPB?
34. Why does it take longer to rewarm than to cool the patient by the pump oxygenator?
35. How would you defibrillate the heart internally during CPB?
36. Why is calcium chloride usually administered right before the patient comes off the pump?
37. If the HR is 40 beats per minute, what should you do?
38. How does the blood sugar level change during CPB? Why? Does hyperglycemia increase neurologic complications during CPB?
39. What are the effects of CPB on platelet and coagulation factors?
40. How would you prepare for termination of cardiopulmonary bypass (CPB)?
41. How would you decide the need for inotropic support?

C.III. After Cardiopulmonary Bypass

1. How would you reverse heparin? How much protamine would you use? What are the other drugs used to neutralize heparin?
2. What is the action mechanism of protamine?
3. What are the complications of too much protamine?
4. Why did the patient develop hypotension after protamine was administered? How do you treat and prevent this condition?
5. What are the indications for intraaortic balloon pump (IABP)?
6. What are the principles of IABP?
7. What are the complications of IABP?
8. Can pulmonary artery occlusion pressure (PAOP) represent left ventricular end-diastolic volume (LVEDV) after CABG?

D. Postoperative Management

1. What are the postoperative complications?
2. Would you reverse the muscle relaxants? Why?
3. When will you wean the patient from the respirator?
4. What criteria would you use in deciding when to wean the patient from the respirator?

A. Medical Disease and Differential Diagnosis

A.1. What is triple-vessel coronary artery disease (CAD)? Name the branches of the coronary arteries.

Triple-vessel CAD involves progressive arteriosclerosis of the major branches of the coronary arteries with eventual luminal obstruction and myocardial injury. The intimal disease is typically segmental but can be diffuse in severe cases. The coronary arteries are the following:

- The right coronary artery (RCA)
- The left anterior descending branch (LAD) of the left main
- The left circumflex branch (CFX) of the left main

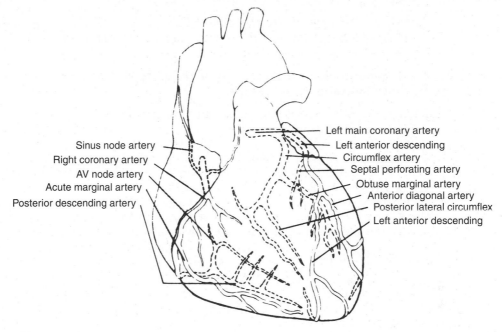

Figure 7.1 Branches of the coronary arteries.

The branches of coronary arteries are shown in Fig. 7.1. The LAD and CFX arise from the left main coronary artery. The sinus node is supplied by the RCA in approximately 50% to 60% of human beings and by the left CFX artery in the remaining 40% to 50%. The atrioventricular (AV) node is supplied by the RCA in 85% to 90% of humans and by the left CFX artery in the remaining 10% to 15%; therefore, the RCA is dominant in 85% to 90% of patients. The most common arteries for coronary bypass grafting are LAD, obtuse marginal (branch of CFX), and posterior descending (branch of RCA) arteries.

Braunwald E, Zipes DP, Libby P, eds. *Heart disease, a textbook of cardiovascular medicine*, 6th ed. Philadelphia: Elsevier Science, WB Saunders, 2005:430–434.

A.2. What are the indications for coronary artery bypass grafting (CABG)?

The indications for CABG are the need for improvement of the quality or duration of life. Patients whose angina is not controlled by medical treatment or who have unacceptable side-effects with such management should be considered for coronary revascularization.

The candidates for CABG are usually older patients with more diffuse CAD and decreased left ventricular function. The indications for CABG are:

- Unstable angina pectoris or episodes of prolonged myocardial ischemia
- Persistent angina pectoris, despite optimal medical therapy
- Repeated episodes of myocardial ischemia following myocardial infarction
- Prinzmetal's angina (variant angina) with coronary artery obstruction
- High-grade left main coronary artery obstruction, double- or triple-vessel obstruction, or proximal LAD artery obstruction
- Acute myocardial infarction, cardiogenic shock, intractable ventricular arrhythmias
- Stable angina pectoris that interferes with desired life style

Braunwald E, Zipes DP, Libby P, eds. *Heart disease, a textbook of cardiovascular medicine*, 6th ed. Philadelphia: Elsevier Science, WB Saunders, 2005:1281–1334.

A.3. What is percutaneous transluminal coronary angioplasty (PTCA)? Discuss its indications, contraindications, and results.

PTCA has developed rapidly since its introduction by Gruentzig in 1977. It is now an acceptable method of treating selected patients who have angina pectoris. This technique involves the passage of a small (3F) catheter into the involved coronary artery and through the stenosis. With the balloon portion of the catheter straddling the stenosis, inflations are performed that result in enlargement of the stenotic lumen. The luminal widening is achieved by a controlled injury involving, to a varying degree, plaque compression, intimal fissures, and medial stretching.

PTCA has re-defined who is candidate for elective surgical myocardial revascularization. The indications for PTCA have changed during the recent past. With the current available technology, PTCA is considered a therapeutic option in any individual with disabling ischemic symptoms despite good medical therapy and focal obstructive coronary disease regardless of cause. The indications for PTCA are as follows:

- Isolated discrete proximal single-vessel disease
- Proximal double-vessel disease
- Postcoronary artery bypass grafting with new stenotic lesions or stenosis at distal anastomosis
- Restenosis following PTCA
- Contraindications to CABG
- Coronary stenosis following cardiac transplantation
- Occluded vessels within the last 6 months and less than 15 mm in length
- Poststreptokinase therapy for revascularization

PTCA is contraindicated in the following:

- Left main CAD in which the distal vessels are not protected by at least one completely patent large collateral vessel
- Multivessel disease with severe diffuse arteriosclerosis
- Absence of a discrete obstructing lesion
- Absence of a formal cardiac surgical program within the institution

The results of PTCA are as follows: The primary success rate is approximately 90%. The primary weakness of the procedure is restenosis, at a rate of approximately 30%, 6 months after the procedure. Dilatation can be repeated with a 90% success rate. The artery tends to remain patent after the second angioplasty. With the introduction of coronary stents, which act as a metal scaffold, the restenosis rate after PTCA has been decreasing, and fewer patient require subsequent revascularization: 10% to 15% after stenting versus 25% to 35% after PTCA alone. The largest decrease in luminal diameter following stent placement is evident within the first 6 to 9 months after stent placement and is the result of proliferative neointimal tissue growth in response to the associated injury and inflammation. Recently, pharmacologic agents (sirolimus, an immunosuppressant, and paclitaxel, an antineoplastic) are coupled with polymers that elute or slowly release these inhibitors from the stent surface. The drug-eluting stents have reduced the need for target-lesion revascularization to an even lower rate, 4% to 6%.

However, the PTCA is a different therapeutic approach than CABG. PTCA is targeting the area of lesion only, whereas CABG bypass targets not only the existing, but future lesion areas. This may be the reason that, at least in the intermediate term, CABG is considered to be superior for patients with multivessel disease.

Diegeler et al. showed that, for isolated high-grade lesions of the LAD, CABG through a left anterior thoracotomy is as effective as PTCA with stent placement. Although stenting provided excellent short-term results with fewer periprocedural adverse events, CABG was superior with regard to the need for repeated intervention in the target vessel and freedom from angina at 6 months of follow-up.

Braunwald E, Zipes DP, Libby P, eds. *Heart disease, a textbook of cardiovascular medicine*, 6th ed. Philadelphia: WB Saunders, 2005:1308–1311.

Diegeler A, Thiele H, Falk V, et al. Comparison of stenting with minimally invasive bypass surgery for stenosis of the left anterior descending coronary artery. *N Engl J Med* 2002; 347:561–566.

Moliterno DJ. Healing achilles—sirolimus versus paclitaxel. *N Engl J Med* 2005;353:724–727.

A.4. What are the results of coronary artery bypass surgery?

Kuan et al. reported a perioperative myocardial infarction rate of 4% to 6%. The overall operative mortality rate of CABG at major medical centers is approximately 1%. Reoperation is associated with a higher operative mortality, approximately 2% to 3%. Rahimtoola et al. studied the status of patients who underwent CABG for unstable angina over a 10-year period. The 1-month mortality rate was 1.8%. The 5-year survival rate was 92% and the 10-year survival rate was 83%. CABG was repeated at a rate of 1% to 2% per year; 81% of patients were angina-free or had only mild angina. Loop et al. found that the 10-year survival rate among the group receiving the internal mammary artery graft, as compared with the group receiving the vein grafts (exclusive of hospital deaths), was 93.4% versus 88% for those with one-vessel disease; 90.0% versus 79.5% for those with two-vessel disease; and 82.6% versus 71.0% for those with three-vessel disease. At the end of the first 10 postoperative years, the patency of internal mammary artery grafts is 85% to 95%, whereas the patency of saphenous vein grafts is only 38% to 45%.

A systematic overview of the seven randomized trials that compared coronary bypass surgery with medical therapy between 1972 and 1984 yielded 2,649 patients. Patients undergoing CABG had a significantly lower mortality at 5, 7, and 10 years, but by 10 years 41% of the patients initially randomized to medical therapy had undergone CABG. Therefore, coronary bypass surgery prolongs survival in patients with significant left main CAD irrespective of symptoms, in patients with multivessel disease and impaired left ventricular function, and in patients with three-vessel disease that includes the proximal LAD coronary artery (irrespective of left ventricular function). Surgical therapy also has been demonstrated to prolong life in patients with two-vessel disease and left ventricular dysfunction, particularly in those with a critical stenosis of the proximal LAD coronary artery. Although no study has documented a survival benefit with surgical treatment in patients with single-vessel disease, there is some evidence that such patients who have impaired left ventricular function have a poor long-term survival rate with medical therapy alone. Such patients with angina and/or evidence of ischemia at a low or moderate level of exercise, especially those with obstruction of the proximal LAD coronary artery, may benefit from coronary revascularization by either angioplasty or bypass surgery.

Hannah et al. studied prospectively 37,212 patients who underwent CABG and 22,102 patients who underwent stenting, CABG was associated with a significantly higher likelihood of survival (hazard ratios for death 0.75 for two- and 0.64 for three-vessel CAD, compared with stenting). The CABG patients had significantly lower median ejection fractions, were more likely than patients who received stents to have had a myocardial infarction in the week before the procedure, had a significantly higher prevalence of numerous coexisting conditions and were significantly more likely to have three-vessel disease. However, stent implantation is associated with a much lower in-hospital mortality than CABG.

Braunwald E, Zipes DP, Libby P, eds. *Heart disease, a textbook of cardiovascular medicine*, 6th ed. Philadelphia: WB Saunders, 2001:1311–1328.

Haase J, Jung T, Storger H, et al. Long-term outcome after implantation of bare metal stents for the treatment of coronary artery disease: rationale for the clinical use of antiproliferative stent coatings. *J Interv Cardiol* 2003;16(6):469–473.

Hannah EL, Racz MJ, Walford G, et al. Long-term outcomes of coronary-artery bypass grafting versus stent implantation. *N Engl J Med* 2005;352:2174–2184.

Kandzari DE, Leon MB, Popma JJ, et al. ENDEAVOR III Investigators. Comparison of zotarolimus-eluting and sirolimus-eluting stents in patients with native coronary artery disease: a randomized controlled trial. *J Am Coll Cardiol* 2006;48(12):2440–2447

Loop FD, Lytle BW, Cosgrove DM, et al. Influence of the internal mammary artery graft on 10-year survival and other cardiac events. *N Engl J Med* 1986;314:1–6.

Lytle BW, Loop FD, Cosgrove DM, et al. Long-term (5 to 12 years) serial studies of internal mammary artery and saphenous vein coronary bypass grafts. *J Thorac Cardiovasc Surg* 1985;89:248–258.

Rahimtoola SH, Nanley D, Grunckemeier G, et al. Ten-year survival after coronary bypass surgery. *N Engl J Med* 1983;308:676.

B. Preoperative Evaluation and Preparation

B.1. Which preoperative tests would you order?

In addition to the routine systemic examinations of all organ systems, special attention should be paid to the cardiovascular status.

- Renal function—urinalysis, blood urea nitrogen (BUN), creatinine
- The routine evaluation of the hepatic function is not any more the standard, unless specifically indicated, that is, previous history of hepatitis or jaundice or the patient is drug abuser.
- Pulmonary function—chest x-ray film (absolutely indicated in reoperated sternotomies to investigate the proximity of the sternum to the anterior surface of the heart), baseline arterial blood gases, and spirometry if indicated.
- Hematologic function—complete blood count, prothrombin time (PT), partial thromboplastin time (PTT), platelets (platelet function if available and/or indicated)
- Metabolism—electrolytes and blood sugar
- Cardiovascular function—resting and exercise ECG (if a stress test was performed preoperatively), cardiac catheterization and coronary angiography, location and severity of coronary occlusion, echocardiography, and left ventricular function (from catheterization and/or echocardiography).

B.2. How would you evaluate the patient's left ventricular function?

- Medical history—presence or absence of myocardial infarction and angina
- Symptoms and clinical signs of left ventricular failure (dyspnea at rest or exercise, nocturnal orthopnea) and/or right heart failure (ascites, pitting edema, jugular vein distention)
- Cardiac catheterization, angiography, and echocardiography
  - Ejection fraction (normally ~65%)
  - Left ventricular end-diastolic pressure (LVEDP) or pulmonary artery occlusion pressure (PAOP: normal 6 to 15 mm Hg)
  - Left ventricular wall motion—normal (wall thickening of >30%), hypokinesia (wall thickening 10% to 30%), akinesia (wall thickening <10%), or dyskinesia (outward motion during systole) Fig. 7.2
  - Cardiac index (normal 2.2 to 3 L/minute/m^2)
- End-systolic pressure volume relation (ESPVR) from multiple pressure–volume loops

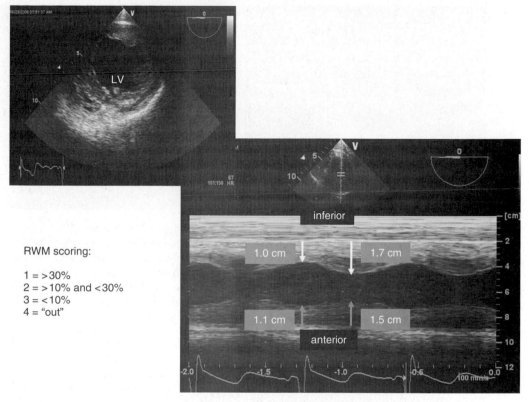

Figure 7.2   Echocardiographic evaluation of the left ventricle (LV). The transgastric mid-papillary short axis view of the left ventricle is shown in left. By placing a cursor line across the middle of the inferior (top of the image) and anterior (bottom of the image) segments of the left ventricular myocardium, the motion of the segments over time is shown in the image right. The percent wall thickening can be either visually estimated, or measured, between diastole and systole.

Abnormal regional wall motion (RWM) most commonly is the result of coronary artery disease (CAD), which interrupts perfusion to fairly well defined territories and hence results in abnormal motion in those segments. There is a gradation of wall motion abnormality that consists progressively of hypokinesis, akinesis, and subsequently dyskinesis in which a wall moves away from the center of the ventricle. Because wall thickening and endocardial motion are intrinsically tied, virtually all RWM abnormalities are expected initially to be associated with abnormalities of thickening as well as endocardial motion.

(See also Chapter 8, question A.3.)

Braunwald E, ed. *Heart disease, a textbook of cardiovascular medicine*, 6th ed. Philadelphia: WB Saunders, 2005:248–380.

Johnson B, Adi A, Licina MG, et al. Cardiac physiology. In: Kaplan JA, Reich DL, Lake CL, et al. eds. *Kaplan's cardiac anesthesia*. Philadelphia: WB Saunders, 2006:71–84.

B.3. What are the three major determinants of myocardial oxygen consumption? How are they measured clinically?

The three major determinants of myocardial oxygen consumption are myocardial wall tension, contractility, and HR.

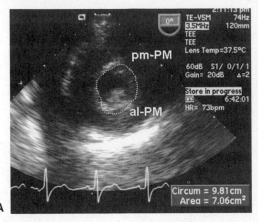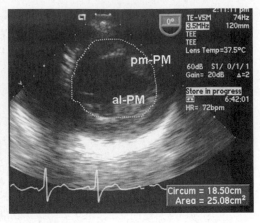

Figure 7.3 Echocardiographic evaluation of the systolic function of the left ventricle. The transgastric mid-papillary short axis view of the left ventricle is shown in systole **(A)** and diastole **(B)**. The endocardial border is traced (without including the endocardium of the two papillary muscles), and the end-systolic and end-diastolic areas are calculated. The percentage area change (fractional area change) is calculated as: FAC = (EDA − ESA)/EDA. The FAC correlates with, but does not substitute the percentage ejection fraction. al-PM, anterolateral papillary muscle; pm-PM, posteromedial papillary muscle.

Myocardial Wall Tension is estimated by the following:

- The Laplace equation states that the wall tension (T) is analogous to the diameter of the ventricle (R, radius) and the intracavitary pressure (P) and inversely proportional to the myocardial wall thickness (Th): $T = P \times R \div 2Th$
- Preload—LVEDV, LVEDP, left atrial pressure, or PAOP
- Afterload—systolic ventricular pressure or systolic BP if there is no aortic stenosis

Contractility is measured by the following:

- *Invasive techniques.* Maximal velocity of contraction (Vmax), dP/dt (pressure time indices of ventricle: how fast (dt) the intraventricular pressure (dP) develops), or left ventricular end-systolic pressure/volume ratio
- *Noninvasive technique.* Preejection period (PEP)/left ventricular ejection time (LVET), and global and regional ventricular wall motion by echocardiography (Fig. 7.3)

Braunwald E, ed. *Heart disease, a textbook of cardiovascular medicine*, 6th ed. Philadelphia: WB Saunders, 2005:1284.

O'Brien ERM, Nathan HJ. Coronary physiology and atherosclerosis. In: Kaplan JA, Reich DL, Lake CL, et al. eds. *Kaplan's cardiac anesthesia*. Philadelphia: WB Saunders, 2006:97–102.

B.4. Which factors determine myocardial oxygen supply?

Myocardial oxygen supply = coronary blood flow × arterial oxygen content

The coronary blood flow depends on the following:

- Aortic diastolic pressure (DAP)
- LVEDP

- Patency of coronary arteries
- Coronary vascular tone

And it can be determined by the formula:

Coronary blood flow $=$ coronary perfusion pressure $\div$ myocardial vascular resistance,

Or, $(DAP - LVEDP) \div$ myocardial vascular resistance

Arterial O_2 content is determined by the following equation:

$$CaO_2 \quad = 1.34 \times Hb \times O_2 \text{ saturation} + (0.0031 \times PaO_2)$$

O'Brien ERM, Nathan HJ. Coronary physiology and atherosclerosis. In: Kaplan JA, Reich DL, Lake CL, et al. eds. *Kaplan's cardiac anesthesia*. Philadelphia: Elsevier Science, WB Saunders, 2006:97–102.

B.5. Would you discontinue digoxin? Why? What is its half-life?

In order to prevent digitalis intoxication after CPB, digitalis preparations are usually discontinued one half-life (1.5 to 1.7 days for digoxin, 5 to 7 days for digitoxin) before surgery. Digitalis intoxication is quite possible, especially after CPB when acid-base and electrolytes are abnormal. If a digitalis-dependent patient is in CHF, digitalis is continued until the night before surgery. However, the predisposing factors to digitalis intoxication, especially hypopotassemia and hypercalcemia, have to be prevented.

Royster RL, Butterworth J, Groban L, et al. Cardiovascular pharmacology. In: Kaplan JA, Reich DL, Lake CL, et al. eds. *Kaplan's cardiac anesthesia*. Philadelphia: Elsevier Science, WB Saunders, 2006:249.

B.6. Would you discontinue the β-blocker (metoprolol)? Why? What is its half-life? What is the role of the β-adrenergic blockers in treating congestive heart failure (CHF)?

The β-blocker (metoprolol) should be continued not only up until surgery, but probably throughout the perioperative period. In patients with unstable angina, sudden withdrawal of β-blocker may produce an exacerbation of symptoms and may precipitate acute myocardial infarction. The dose of β-blocker does not need to be reduced before surgery for fear of bradycardia, hypotension, or difficulty in weaning from CPB. The half-life of oral propranolol is 3.4 to 6 hours and of metoprolol 3 hours. Both propranolol and metoprolol are metabolized in the liver. Propranolol disappears from the plasma and atria within 24 to 48 hours after discontinuing doses of 30 to 240 mg per day. Shand and Keats have shown that with a 0.5-mg dose of propranolol IV, blood levels as high as 50 ng per mL are obtained, but rapidly drop off to immeasurable levels within 5 to 10 minutes. No myocardial depression has been seen with these small intravenous doses. Current advanced cardiac life support (ACLS) guidelines suggest a 5 mg bolus of metoprolol at 5-minute intervals, and a 0.1 mg per kg bolus dose of propranolol divided into three equal doses at 2- to 3-minute intervals.

Reductions in HR with a β-blocker (propranolol or metoprolol) occur at lower serum levels than depression of myocardial contractility. Accordingly, as drug levels decrease after discontinuation of therapy, reductions in chronotropic response last longer than reductions in inotropy. This is an important concept in treating tachycardias in patients with significant ventricular dysfunction and CHF: a small dose is appropriate, and indicated, whereas a large dose may suppress even further the inotropic state.

Numerous studies have confirmed improvements in cardiac function, exercise capacity, and long-term survival in patients with heart failure resulting from myocardial infarction, hypertrophic cardiomyopathy, or idiopathic dilated cardiomyopathy with β-antagonists. β-Antagonists may also be of benefit in patients with diastolic dysfunction, secondary to hypertension.

Potential benefits of β-adrenergic blockade in heart failure include decreased HR and normalization of β-receptor function. Slower HRs improve diastolic function, by increasing the diastolic filling time and myocardial perfusion and by decreasing the myocardial oxygen consumption. β-Adrenergic receptors are down-regulated in heart failure. but their response is normalized by long-term β-blockade. Partial β-agonists may provide baseline sympathetic drive but act as antagonists against excessive sympathetic stimulation.

Royster RL, Butterworth J, Groban L, et al. Cardiovascular pharmacology. In: Kaplan JA, Reich DL, Lake CL, et al. eds. *Kaplan's cardiac anesthesia*. Philadelphia: WB Saunders, 2006:219–225.

B.7. If the patient who is on metoprolol develops hypotension intraoperatively, how would you manage it?

The more common causes of intraoperative hypotension, such as hypovolemia, deep anesthesia, and surgical manipulation, should be corrected first. There are no specific antagonists for metoprolol. In rare instances, it is necessary to administer atropine for bradycardia or epinephrine, isoproterenol, glucagon, calcium, or digitalis to counteract the negative inotropic state associated with β-blockade. Cardiogenic hypotension is usually associated with high PAOP and low BP.

Royster RL, Butterworth J, Groban L, et al. Cardiovascular pharmacology. In: Kaplan JA, Reich DL, Lake CL, et al. eds. *Kaplan's cardiac anesthesia*. Philadelphia: WB Saunders, 2006:219–225.

B.8. What is nifedipine? How does it work?

Nifedipine is a calcium channel blocker. The commonly used calcium channel blockers in the United States are nifedipine, verapamil, and diltiazem hydrochloride. Five classes of compounds have been examined: phenylalkylamines, dihydropyridines, benzothiazepines, diphenylpiperazines, and a diarylaminopropylamine. At present, verapamil (a phenylalkylamine); diltiazem (a benzothiazepine); nicardipine, nifedipine, isradipine, amlodipine, felodipine, and nimodipine (dihydropyridines); and bepridil (a diarylaminopropylamine ether) are approved for clinical use in the United States. They inhibit excitation—contraction coupling of myocardial and smooth muscle by blocking calcium influx at cellular membranes. This results in decreased myocardial contractility and vasodilation. Therefore, myocardial oxygen consumption is decreased. Calcium channel blockers are effective for the treatment of variant angina (Prinzmetal's angina), angina pectoris, and possibly acute myocardial infarction. (See also Chapter 18, question A.11.)

Although nitrates and β-adrenergic blockers are effective for angina, the calcium channel blockers are longer acting and may be used in the presence of chronic obstructive pulmonary disease and asthma. Calcium also plays a key role in cardiac electrical activity. The electrical activity of the sinoatrial (SA) and AV nodal cells are especially dependent on the calcium or "slow" current, whereas the remaining of the specialized conduction system is more dependent on the sodium or "fast" current. Verapamil has a more profound influence on the calcium current of the SA and AV nodes. This drug has been most useful in the treatment of supraventricular

Table 7.1   Relative Cardiovascular Effects of Calcium Channel Blockers.

	VERAPAMIL	DILTIAZEM	NIFEDIPINE
Antiarrhythmic	+++	++	−
Cardiac depression	++	+	+
Vasodilation	+	++	+++
Tachycardia	−	−	++

tachyarrhythmias, which are often caused by reentry through the AV node. In contrast, nifedipine has less influence on the SA node and no effect on AV conduction time. Therefore, nifedipine might be used when further suppression of AV conduction is undesirable. The relative cardiovascular effects of calcium channel blockers are shown in Table 7.1. Verapamil was found to profoundly depress the cardiovascular system during high concentrations of halothane, enflurane, or isoflurane anesthesia. However, because of a tendency for increased incidence of sinus arrest and bradycardia and more hemodynamic depression during enflurane anesthesia, Rogers et al. concluded that intravenous verapamil is better tolerated during low-dose isoflurane and halothane anesthesia than during comparable concentrations of enflurane anesthesia.

Curran MP, Robinson DM, Keating GM. Intravenous nicardipine: its use in the short-term treatment of hypertension and various other indications. *Drugs* 2006;66(13):1755–1782.

Gradman AH, Vivas Y. New drugs for hypertension: what do they offer? *Curr Hypertens Rep* 2006;8(5):425–432.

Royster RL, Butterworth J, Groban L, et al. Cardiovascular pharmacology. In: Kaplan JA, Reich DL, Lake CL, et al. eds. *Kaplan's cardiac anesthesia*. Philadelphia: WB Saunders, 2006:225–230.

B.9. How would you premedicate the patient? Why?

The patient should be sedated well, to prevent anxiety, which may precipitate angina. We usually administer a short acting benzodiazepine (midazolam 1 to 2 mg) IV as soon as basic monitoring is applied.

Although atropine or scopolamine is not contraindicated, atropine is not given at the New York Presbyterian Hospital-Cornell Medical Center because of the possibility of tachycardia, which will increase O_2 demand.

All antianginal and antihypertensive drugs are continued up to the time of surgery.

C. Intraoperative Management

C.I. Before Cardiopulmonary Bypass

C.I-1. How do you monitor the patient?

- ECG—simultaneous leads V_5 and II, multiple-lead ST-segment analysis if available
- Arterial line for BP and arterial blood gases
- PA catheter—pulmonary and central venous pressures (CVP), hemodynamic parameters (cardiac output, stroke volume, systemic and pulmonary vascular resistance)
- CVP line only—if the patient has good left ventricular function and no problems are expected
- Urine output
- Temperature—esophageal (or PA) and bladder (or rectal or tympanic or nasopharyngeal)

- Laboratory—arterial blood gases, electrolytes, hematocrit, ACT, and oxygen saturation of the mixed venous blood (Svo_2)
- Oxygen analyzer for inspired gas mixture
- End-tidal CO_2 analyzer
- Pulse oximeter for plethysmography (adequacy of peripheral pulse, pulse rate) and arterial oxygenation
- Transesophageal echocardiography (TEE) if not contraindicated (esophageal [stricture or stenosis, varices, Zenker's diverticulum] or stomach [recent history of bleeding, active ulcers] pathology)
- Cerebral oximeter especially for patients with high risks of postoperative neurologic outcomes, such as those undergoing hypothermic circulatory arrest.
- Bispectral index to ensure adequate level of unconsciousness and eliminate the risk of intraoperative awareness.

C.I-2. What is Allen's test?

The Allen's test is used to detect the presence of adequate collateral ulnar circulation. The radial and ulnar arteries are occluded by the examiner's hands. The patient is then asked to make a tight fist to empty the blood from the hand. The hand is held above the heart level to help venous drainage. If the patient is under anesthesia, the blood in the hand may be drained by a third person squeezing the hand. Then the fist is opened slowly and put down to the heart level. Only the ulnar compression is released and the flush of the hand is watched.

- Normal—less than 7 seconds (presence of adequate collateral connections between the superficial [ulnar] and deep [radial] palmar arches)
- Borderline—7 to 15 seconds
- Abnormal—greater than 15 seconds

A modified Allen's test may be done with a Doppler detector or a pulse oximeter. The results of Allen's test are abnormal in approximately 3% of young healthy individuals. However, Slogoff et al. studied the complications following radial artery cannulation in 1699 cardiovascular surgical patients. They concluded that in the absence of peripheral vascular disease, Allen's test is not a predictor of ischemia of the hand during or after radial artery cannulation, and that radial artery cannulation is a low-risk, high-benefit monitoring technique that deserves wide clinical use. However, in the current litigious setting and in the face of some evidence to the contrary, it is probably prudent to continue to perform Allen's test and document the results. Some authorities still consider the use of Allen's test as the standard of care.

Alastruey J, Parker KH, Peiro J, et al. Can the modified Allen's test always detect sufficient collateral flow in the hand? A computational study. *Comput Methods Biomech Biomed Engin* 2006;9(6):353–361.

Barbeau GR, Arsenault F, Dugas L, et al. Evaluation of the ulnopalmar arterial arches with pulse oximetry and plethysmography: comparison with the Allen's test in 1010 patients. *Am Heart J* 2004;147(3):489–493.

Cederholm I, Sorensen J, Carlsson C. Thrombosis following percutaneous radial artery cannulation. *Acta Anaesthesiol Scand* 1986;30:227.

Hildick-Smith D. Use of the Allen's test and transradial catheterization. *J Am Coll Cardiol* 2006;48(6):1287.

Reich DL, Mittnacht A, London M, et al. Monitoring of the heart and vascular system. In: Kaplan JA, Reich DL, Lake CL, et al. eds. *Kaplan's cardiac anesthesia*. Philadelphia: WB Saunders, 2006:388.

Slogoff S, Keats AS, Arlund C. On the safety of radial artery cannulation. *Anesthesiology* 1983;59:42.

C.I-3. Why do you need multiple temperature monitoring?

In many medical centers, measurement of two or more temperatures is a common practice. During cooling and rewarming, there is uneven distribution of body heat. Esophageal, nasopharyngeal, bladder or tympanic sites measure core temperature; the rectal site represents peripheral temperature. During cooling and rewarming by the extracorporeal circulation (ECC), the esophageal temperature changes rapidly, whereas the rectal temperature changes slowly. The opposite changes are witnessed during surface cooling or warming: the rectal temperature changes quickly, whereas the esophageal temperature changes slowly. In order to estimate the accurate temperature and to achieve even distribution of body heat, it is necessary to record both esophageal and rectal temperatures. However, bladder temperature monitoring through a urinary bladder catheter is quite convenient and popular, as it reflects a body temperature between esophageal and rectal temperature.

Temperatures are measured during cooling, to ensure that the organs most susceptible to potential hypoperfusion actually receive the protective effect of the desired hypothermia. In this regard, the brain is the organ mostly monitored nasopharyngeal, tympanic membrane and esophageal temperatures are the usually accepted best estimates of brain temperature, although they, at times, overestimate or underestimate the actual brain temperature. During rewarming, cerebral hyperthermia is often detected and should be avoided (by maintaining a gradient of 5°C between the arterial blood and brain, with the brain having the lower temperature) and corrected immediately, because it increases the cerebral oxygen consumption, and may exacerbate postoperative neuropsychologic dysfunction.

Gravlee GP, Davis RF, Karusz M, et al. *Cardiopulmonary bypass, principles and practice.* Philadelphia: Lippincott Williams & Wilkins, 2000:567–568.

Mora-Mangano CT, Chow JL, Kanevsky M. Cardiopulmonary bypass and the anesthesiologist. In: Kaplan JA, Reich DL, Lake CL, et al. eds. *Kaplan's cardiac anesthesia.* Philadelphia: WB Saunders, 2006:899–900.

C.I-4. How do you know that the tip of the pulmonary artery (PA) catheter is in the RV or PA?

There are three main differences in the pressure tracings, as shown in Fig. 7.4.

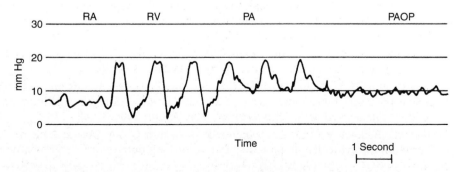

Figure 7.4 Pressure tracings of right atrium (RA), right ventricle (RV), pulmonary artery (PA), and pulmonary artery occlusion pressure (PAOP).

Diastolic Pressure Is Higher in PA than in RV, because the closed pulmonary valve maintains a diastolic gradient between the PA and the RV

- PA pressure—20–25/5–10 mm Hg
- RV pressure—20–25/0–5 mm Hg

Pressure Contour

- PA pressure tracing has a dicrotic notch, which is created by the closure of pulmonary valve, and the diastolic part is descending (decreasing).
- RV pressure tracing has a sharp drop and a plateau in early diastole, and the diastolic part is ascending (increasing).

Ventricular Filling

- In the late diastolic phase, PA pressure is decreasing, because of diastolic runoff in the pulmonary circulation, whereas the RV pressure is increasing, because of ventricular filling.

C.I-5. What is normal pulmonary artery occlusion pressure (PAOP)?

- Normal—4 to 12 mm Hg
- Borderline—13 to 17 mm Hg
- Heart failure—over 18 mm Hg

Braunwald E, Zipes DP, Libby P, eds. *Heart disease, a textbook of cardiovascular medicine*, 6th ed. Philadelphia: WB Saunders, 2005:409–411.

C.I-6. Is it necessary to monitor pulmonary artery (PA) pressure for coronary artery operations?

The indication to monitor PA pressure depends on the left ventricular function. Patients may be divided into two categories on the basis of left ventricular function. For patients who have good left ventricular function (ejection fractions >0.5 and normal ventricular wall motion), the CVP correlates well with the PAOP; therefore, pulmonary pressure monitoring may not be necessary for this group of patients. On the other hand, for patients with poor left ventricular function (ejection fractions <0.4 or ventricular dyssynergy), the CVP does not correlate with the PAOP; therefore, pulmonary pressure monitoring is indicated. Other indications for monitoring PA pressure include the presence of pulmonary hypertension, combined coronary stenosis and valvular disease, and complex cardiac lesions.

However, in a recent observational study of critically ill patients, after adjustment for treatment selection bias, monitoring PA pressure was associated with increased mortality and increased utilization of resources. The cause of this apparent lack of benefit is unclear. The result of this analysis should be confirmed in other studies. These findings justify reconsideration of a randomized controlled trial of right heart catheterization and may guide patient selection for such a study.

Connors AF, Speroff T, Dawson NV, et al. The effectiveness of right heart catheterization in initial care of critically ill patients. *JAMA* 1996;276:889–897.

Djaiani G, Karski J, Yudin M et al. Clinical outcomes in patients undergoing elective coronary artery bypass graft surgery with and without utilization of pulmonary artery catheter-generated data. *J Cardiothorac Vasc Anesth* 2006;20:307–310.

Fontes ML, Bellows W, Ngo L, et al. McSPI Research Group. Assessment of ventricular function in critically ill patients: limitations of pulmonary artery catheterization. *J Cardiothorac Vasc Anesth* 1999;13:1–8

Mangano DT. Monitoring pulmonary arterial pressure in coronary-artery disease. *Anesthesiology* 1980;53:364–369.

Vender JS. Editorial: Pulmonary artery catheter utilization: The use, misuse, or abuse. *J Cardiothorac Vasc Anesth* 2006;20:295–299.

C.I-7. What are the complications of PA catheterization?

From Venopuncture Sites (as for central venous pressure)

Common complications:

- Infection—sepsis
- Hematoma
- Air embolism
- Thrombosis
- Catheter shearing and embolization

Subclavian approach:

- Pneumothorax
- Hemothorax
- Hydrothorax

Internal jugular approach:

- Pneumothorax
- Neck hematoma from puncture of carotid artery
- Possible vagus nerve injury and brachial plexus injury
- Thoracic duct perforation from left side approach

The basilar or cephalic vein approach has fewer complications, but the failure rate is higher.

From Pulmonary Artery Catheter

Arrhythmias 1.5% to 11%, complete heart block, thromboembolism, pulmonary infarction from continuous wedging, massive hemorrhage from perforation of PA or right atrium (RA), failure to wedge, hemoptysis, intracardiac knotting, balloon rupture, endocardial thrombi, and tricuspid valve injury.

Fontes ML. *Complications of central venous cannulation. Problems in anesthesia.* Philadelphia: Lippincott Williams & Wilkins, 1998.

Murphy GS, Vender JS. Monitoring the anesthetized patient. In: Barash PG, Cullen BF, Stoelting RK, eds. *Clinical anesthesia*, 5th ed. Philadelphia: Lippincott Williams & Wilkins, 2006:678–679.

Reich DL, Mittnacht A, London M, et al. Monitoring of the heart and vascular system. In: Kaplan JA, Reich DL, Lake CL, et al. eds. *Kaplan's cardiac anesthesia*. Philadelphia: WB Saunders, 2006:404–406.

C.I-8. What are the hemodynamic consequences of myocardial ischemia? How can you detect myocardial ischemia? Is PAOP a sensitive indicator of myocardial ischemia?

For four decades following Tennant and Wiggers' classic observation on the effects of coronary occlusion on myocardial contraction, it was believed that transient severe ischemia caused either irreversible cardiac injury—that is, infarction—or prompt recovery. However, in the 1970s it became clear that after a brief episode of severe ischemia, prolonged myocardial dysfunction with gradual return of contractile activity occurred, a condition termed myocardial stunning. Alternatively, severe chronic ischemia can result in diminished contractile performance such as chronic regional wall motion (RWM) abnormalities (hibernation).

Acute myocardial ischemia affects systolic and diastolic pump function. Diastolic dysfunction usually manifests before systolic alterations in function. The immediate impact on ventricular compliance is related to the etiology of the ischemic event. Decreased myocardial oxygen supply is initially accompanied by an increase in compliance. In contrast, increased myocardial oxygen demand is associated with an immediate loss of ventricular compliance (e.g., the ventricle becomes stiffer). Therefore, the ventricle requires a higher filling pressure (end diastolic pressure [EDP]) to maintain a given stroke volume. A cascade of events occurs, that may include wall motion abnormalities, dysrhythmias, and conduction block. An 80% reduction of coronary blood flow causes akinesis, whereas a 95% decrease causes dyskinesis. If the ischemia becomes severe, the rise in EDP will lead to pulmonary edema (Fig. 7.5).

Although a number of sensitive techniques are available for detection of ischemia, such as magnetic resonance spectroscopy, radio-labeled lactate determinations, or direct measurement of end-diastolic pressure, these are impractical. The most popular and accepted sign of ischemia is ECG ST-segment changes. The ECG criteria for ischemia are horizontal or down-sloping ST-segment depression at least 0.1 mV at 0.06 second from J-point, up-sloping ST-segment depression at least 0.2 mV at 0.08 second from J-point, and ST-segment elevation at least 0.15 mV (1 mV = 10 mm). Other ECG signs of ischemia include inverted T waves and a new onset of arrhythmias or conduction abnormalities.

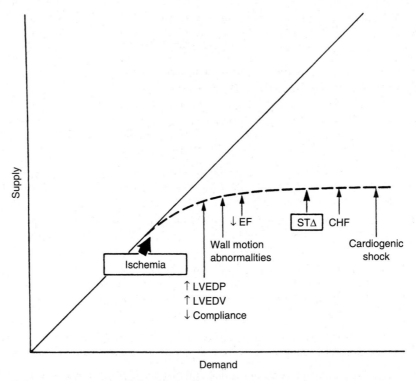

Figure 7.5 Hemodynamic consequences of myocardial ischemia. Ischemia occurs when demand exceeds supply. CHF, congestive heart failure; EF, ejection fraction; LVEDP, left ventricular end-diastolic pressure; LVEDV, left ventricular end-diastolic volume; ST, ST-segment changes. (From Barash PG. Monitoring myocardial oxygen balance: physiologic basis and clinical application. *ASA Refresher Courses in Anesthesiology* 1985;13:24, with permission.)

Regional wall motion abnormalities (RWMA), detected with two-dimensional echocardiography, have been shown to be the earliest and most sensitive sign of myocardial ischemia. RWMA are produced with just 25% decrease in coronary blood flow in the absence of ECG changes, whereas ECG signs of ischemia are apparent with a 50% decrease in coronary blood flow. During exercise, patients with CAD develop RWMA after 30 seconds, whereas ECG changes do not occur until after 90 seconds. Smith et al. found that RWMA was four times more sensitive than ECG ST-segment change in detecting intraoperative ischemia. Moreover, ST changes cannot be analyzed if the patient has conduction disturbances, such as bundle-branch block or ventricular paced rhythms. They have also found that patients experiencing persistent RWMA were more likely to have myocardial infarction than those having only transient changes. No patient without a new wall motion abnormality had myocardial infarction. Although TEE is the most sensitive monitor for myocardial ischemia, a recent study by Eisenberg et al. concludes that, routine monitoring for myocardial ischemia with TEE or 12-lead ECG during noncardiac surgery appears to have little incremental clinical value over preoperative clinical data and two-lead ECG monitoring, in identifying patients at high risk for perioperative ischemic outcome.

Measurement of PAOP has been suggested as an early and sensitive indicator of ischemia, to be used when the ECG is not diagnostic. Although acute increases in PAOP or development of V waves may reflect ischemia, the absence of a change in PAOP does not ensure the absence of ischemia. Haggmark et al. reported that the sensitivity, specificity, and predictive value (positive and negative) of PAOP abnormalities for ischemia ranged between 40% and 60%. In CABG patients, Lieberman et al. also found a low positive predictive value (24%) but a higher negative predictive value (85%); however, the PAOP was no better than CVP measurement, except in patients with moderate to severe preoperative ventricular dysfunction. Leung et al. found that 61% of TEE wall-motion abnormalities in CABG patients occurred without significant changes (>20% of control) in HR, systolic arterial pressure, or PA pressure. Only 10% of episodes were accompanied by 5 mm Hg or greater changes in PA pressure. Roizen et al. found that 11 out of 12 patients developed TEE wall-motion abnormalities when the aorta was cross-clamped above the supraceliac artery, but that PAOP remained normal (12 mm Hg) in 10 out of 12, with only 2 out of 12 having transient increases. Therefore, these studies question the value of PA catheterization and monitoring for detection of intraoperative ischemia.

Barash PG. Sequential monitoring of myocardial ischemia in the perioperative period. *ASA Annual Meeting Refresher Courses Lectures*, Park Ridge, IL. American Society of Anesthesiologists. 2002;233.

Ellis JE, Roizen MF, Mantha S, et al. Anesthesia for vascular surgery. In Barash PG, Cullen BF, Stoelting RK, eds. *Clinical anesthesia*, 5th ed. Philadelphia: Lippincott Williams & Wilkins, 2006:942–945.

Haggmark S, Hohner P, Ostman M, et al. Comparison of hemodynamic, electrocardiographic, mechanical, and metabolic indicators of intraoperative myocardial ischemia in vascular surgical patients with coronary artery disease. *Anesthesiology* 1989;70:19–25.

London M, Mittnacht A, Kaplan JA. Anesthesia for myocardial revascularization. In: Kaplan JA, Reich DL, Lake CL, et al. eds. *Kaplan's cardiac anesthesia*. Philadelphia: WB Saunders, 2006:627–628.

C.I-9. How would you monitor ECG? Why V₅? If you do not have precordial leads in your ECG machine, how can you monitor the LV?

Multiple-lead ECG monitoring provides the best clinically available method of detecting perioperative ischemia. Based primarily on results obtained from exercise treadmill testing, combining ECG leads II and V_5, can detect 96% of ischemic events, and the optimal leads for intraoperative myocardial ischemia. However, London et al. recently found that the standard combination of leads II and V_5 was only 80% sensitive, whereas combining leads V_4 and V_5 increased sensitivity to 90% in patients with known or suspected CAD undergoing noncardiac surgery with general anesthesia. The sensitivity increased to 96% by combining leads II, V_4, and V_5. If only one lead can be displayed, V_5 should be used because lead V_5 has the greatest sensitivity: 75% intraoperatively and 89% during exercise treadmill testing. See also Chapter 18, question C.3.

London MJ, Hollenberg M, Wong MG, et al. Intraoperative myocardial ischemia: localization by continuous 12-lead electrocardiography. *Anesthesiology* 1988;69:232–241.

C.I-10. Discuss the principles and clinical applications of intraoperative transesophageal two-dimensional echocardiography.

TEE is a well-established technique to visualize cardiac anatomy and function. Echocardiography is based on fundamental ultrasonic principles. Ultrasound is defined as sound above the upper threshold of human hearing (20,000 Hz). The ultrasound waves (1 to 7 MHz) are created by applying an alternating electric current of 500 to 1,500 pulses per second on an appropriate piezoelectric crystal. A short burst or pulse of high-frequency, low-intensity sound is then emitted and directed through the human body to detect boundaries between structures of different acoustic impedance. The ultrasound wave is partially reflected at the boundary of media with different acoustic impedance, a property that is primarily determined by the slight difference in density between different tissues. The transmission of pulsed-reflected ultrasound through the heart, with detection of the returning echoes detailing the position and movement of cardiac acoustic interfaces, is termed *cardiac ultrasound* or *echocardiography*. The difference between the M-mode and two-dimensional techniques is that the M-mode ultrasonic beam is aimed in one direction and therefore depicts only one dimension of the target structure in an image that does not resemble cardiac structure, whereas beam sweeps in an arc to give a panoramic view of the heart that results in cross-sectional images that are anatomically recognizable. Also see Chapter 8, question B.6.

Doppler echocardiography provides an alternative method for imaging blood flow by applying Doppler frequency shift analysis to echoes reflected by a moving target (red blood cells or cardiac tissue). The Doppler principle states that the frequency of the reflected ultrasound is different from the frequency of the emitted ultrasound. The shift in frequency is proportional to the speed of the moving target Color-coded Doppler flow imaging (color Doppler) simultaneously presents real-time images of intracardiac flow and structure in two dimensions: continuous color maps of flow superimposed on monochromatic cross-sectional echocardiograms. Color Doppler greatly improves the evaluation of valvular function and intracardiac shunts.

The clinical applications of intraoperative echocardiography are as follows:

- *Monitoring left ventricular filling and ejection.* When left ventricular short-axis cross-section is monitored at the level of the midpapillary muscles, TEE provides the anesthesiologist with a direct, semiquantitative method to assess left ventricular preload and ejection in real time, and guide the administration of fluids and inotropes.
- *Ischemic heart disease.* RWM abnormalities, such as hypokinesia, akinesia, and dyskinesia, are the earliest signs of myocardial ischemia (Figs. 7.2 and 7.3), as discussed in question C.I-8. Measurements of systolic wall thickening, another excellent sign of myocardial ischemia, are not reproducible because of a difficulty in delineating the epicardial border accurately in two-dimensional echocardiography. The impairment of the diastolic function can be qualitatively estimated and the filling pressures can be estimated using a combination of spectral Doppler measurements of the blood flow through the pulmonary veins and the mitral valve.
- *Valvular heart disease*
- *Air embolism.* In the left atrium, LV, and aorta, air embolism can be detected by TEE during open-heart surgery. Therefore, TEE can be used to help the surgeon evacuate air bubbles from the left heart before the heart ejects blood and air into the systemic circulation.

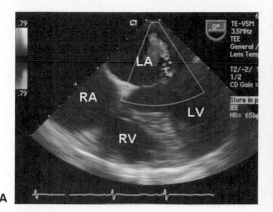 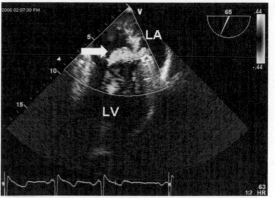

Figure 7.6 Color Doppler echocardiography. **A:** Superimposed on a two-dimensional image (here, the mid esophageal view), the relative velocities of the red blood cells from a selected area (triangle) are visualized. Timed to the ECG (on the bottom of the sector image), normal or abnormal blood flows can be viewed as they cross orifices. In this case, a small regurgitant jet originating from the mitral valve during systole is seen. The color of the jet displays velocity and direction, according to the scale, on the left side of the figure. The mitral regurgitation jet is moving upwards towards the left atrium (LA), and is colored red. **B:** In this mid-commissural view of the left ventricle (LV), the systolic mitral regurgitant jet, due to a prolapsing anterior leaflet (*arrow*), is directed anteriorly, inside the left atrium. RA, right atrium; RV, right ventricle.

- *Valvular regurgitation.* Valvular regurgitation can be determined intraoperatively by color Doppler echocardiography before and immediately after conservative valve repair (annuloplasty, commissurotomy), or valve replacement. The degree of valvular incompetency can be accurately measured using a combination of two-dimensional and Doppler techniques (Figs. 7.6 and 7.7) and the function of the repaired or replaced valve can be quantitatively evaluated.
- *Valvular stenosis.* Spectral Doppler echocardiography can be used intraoperatively to measure the pressure gradient across a valvular stenosis and calculate the area of the diseased valve.
- *Congenital heart disease.* TEE techniques allows a more aggressive approach to complex cardiac reconstructions because the surgeon has the ability to visualize the heart and evaluate adequacy of the surgical repair immediately after the operative procedure.
- *Thoracic aorta.* TEE can accurately diagnose thoracic aortic aneurysm, dissection, disruption, and atheromatosis. At the New York Presbyterian Hospital-Cornell Medical Center, we routinely use TEE for all patients to screen severe atheromatosis of the aortic arch and descending aorta. Epiaortic echocardiography is performed to examine the ascending aorta and arch, if severe atheromatosis is found in the descending aorta or arch. Severe atheromatosis of thoracic aorta is an independent predictor of postoperative neurologic outcome. The atheroma is graded as follows: grade I, normal to mild intimal thickening; grade II, severe intimal thickening; grade III, atheroma protruding less than 5 mm into the lumen; grade IV, atheroma protruding greater than 5 mm; and grade V, atheroma with a mobile component (Fig. 7.8).
- *Cardiac tumors.* Atrial myxoma can be easily diagnosed by TEE. Pre- and postoperative TEE with contrast can assess the presence and severity of mitral regurgitation secondary to valve damage from a ball-valve effect of the myxoma.
- *Other cardiac lesions.* Hypertrophic obstructive cardiomyopathy (HOCM) (idiopathic hypertrophic subaortic stenosis [IHSS]) can be identified by the combination of systolic anterior motion of the mitral valve (SAM) and left ventricular outflow obstruction. Cardiac tamponade caused by a pericardial effusion or hematoma can be detected.

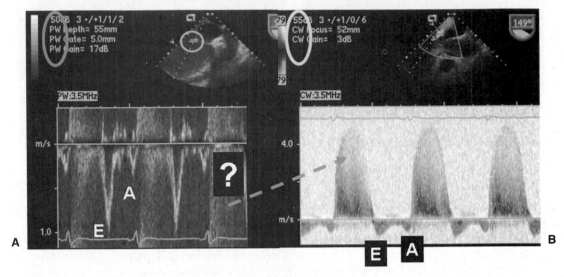

Figure 7.7 Doppler mode. **A:** A typical pulsed-wave (PW) Doppler velocity consists of a spectral recording of varying intensity, depending on the acoustic density of the reflected interface (the mass of blood cells). The most dense (or brightest) portion of the spectral tracing represents the velocity of most blood cells. The velocity is recorded from a specific site (white circle), and the maximum velocity recorded is limited (usually <1.5 m/s). In this PW Doppler spectrum, *E* represents the diastolic early filling, and *A* the diastolic late (due to atrial contraction) velocity. During systole, there is a broad signal (*question mark*), representing systolic flow through the mitral valve (probably mitral regurgitation). However, neither the direction, nor the peak velocity can be visualized. **B:** In contrast, continuous-wave (CW) Doppler records the velocities of all the red blood cells moving along the path of the sound beam. A CW Doppler recording always consists of a full spectral envelope with the outer border corresponding to the fastest moving blood cells. The site of origin of a high-velocity jet is inferred from the particular lesion that is being examined. The maximum velocity that can be recorded can be as high as 8 m/s. Here, the direction (from bottom to top, or from the left ventricle towards the left atrium) as well as, the maximum systolic velocity (~5 m/s) can be visualized, detailing the mitral regurgitation jet.

- *Neurosurgery.* TEE was found to be the most sensitive monitor to detect venous air embolism during neurosurgical operations in the sitting position. Patent foramen ovale and paradoxical air embolism can be detected by TEE.

Agricola E, Oppizzi M, Melisurgo G, et al. Transesophageal echocardiography: a complementary view of the heart. *Expert Rev Cardiovasc Ther* 2004;2(1):61–75.

Kahn RA, Shernan SK, Konstadt SN. Intraoperative echocardiography. In: Kaplan JA, Reich DL, Lake CL, et al. eds. *Kaplan's cardiac anesthesia*. Philadelphia: WB Saunders, 2006:437–488.

Kuhl HP, Hanrath P. The impact of transesophageal echocardiography on daily clinical practice. *Eur J Echocardiogr* 2004;5(6):455–468.

Shapira Y, Vaturi M, Weisenberg DE, et al. Impact of intraoperative transesophageal echocardiography in patients undergoing valve replacement. *Ann Thor Surg* 2004;78(2): 579–583.

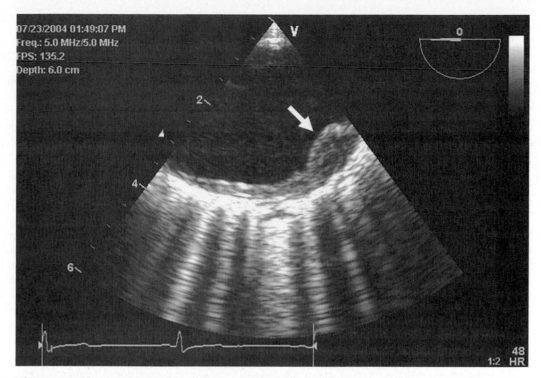

Figure 7.8 Atheromatous aortic disease. An echocardiographic picture of the short axis view of the descending thoracic aorta is shown. The anterior aortic wall is irregularly thickened, and a large atheroma (8 mm) is present at 5 o'clock (*arrow*). This is a grade IV atheroma.

Troianos CA, Konstadt S. Evaluation of mitral regurgitation. *Semin Cardiothorac Vasc Anesth* 2006;10(1):67–71.

C.I-11. How would you induce anesthesia?

Midazolam 1 to 2 mg is given as soon as the standard monitors are applied and the arterial line is inserted under local anesthesia. A smooth induction is essential to prevent hypotension, hypertension, and tachycardia. Different techniques may be used to achieve a smooth induction. For patients with good left ventricular function, anesthesia is induced with fentanyl, 5 to 10 μg per kg, and thiopental, 2 to 4 mg per kg. The patient is ventilated by mask with 100% oxygen. After administration of succinylcholine, 1 mg per kg, or pancuronium 0.1 mg per kg the trachea is intubated. Alternatively, anesthesia is induced with thiopental, 4 mg per kg, and deepened with fentanyl 5 to 10 μg per kg and 2.0% isoflurane for 3 to 5 minutes. When adequately anesthetized, the patient is given a muscle relaxant and intubated. If the patient has a history of hypertension or the initial systolic BP is over 150 mm Hg, fentanyl 10 μg per kg is usually required to blunt the intubation-associated hypertension and tachycardia. For patients with poor left ventricular function, potent inhalation agents such as, isoflurane, sevoflurane and desflurane are avoided during induction and maintenance of anesthesia. Additional midazolam 2 to 5 mg and less thiopental 1 to 2 mg per kg will be given for induction; however, in lieu of the increasing incidence of delirium in the elderly postoperatively, benzodiazepines should be avoided in patients older than 70 years. Alternatively, etomidate 0.2 mg per kg may be administered for induction.

See also Chapter 12, question C.6 for other measures to prevent tachycardia and hypertension at the time of intubation.

London M, Mittnacht A, Kaplan JA. Anesthesia for myocardial revascularization. In: Kaplan JA, Reich DL, Lake CL, et al. eds. *Kaplan's cardiac anesthesia*. Philadelphia: WB Saunders, 2006:605–609.

C.I-12. How would you maintain anesthesia?

Again, smooth anesthesia is essential to achieve a balance between myocardial oxygen demand and supply. Different agents and techniques may be used to accomplish the same goal. A combination of fentanyl (or another synthetic opioid) and isoflurane (or propofol) is a popular choice. After the patient is intubated, a mixture of 60% air and 40% oxygen is administered to keep the patient unconscious.

The depth of anesthesia must be titrated to meet the requirements of the varying intensities of surgical stimulation. Skin incision and sternal splitting are very painful. But the strongest stimulation is usually from sternal retraction with the self-retaining retractor. Fentanyl, 5 μg (0.1 mL) per kg, is given right before the skin incision. Another dose of fentanyl 5 μg per kg is usually given before sternotomy. Then fentanyl, 5 μg per kg, is given every 30 to 60 minutes to maintain anesthesia. Very high doses of fentanyl or sufentanil, have been successfully used for cardiac anesthesia. The possibility of oxygen toxicity from the use of 100% oxygen should also be kept in mind.

London M, Mittnacht A, Kaplan JA. Anesthesia for myocardial revascularization. In: Kaplan JA, Reich DL, Lake CL, et al. eds. *Kaplan's cardiac anesthesia*. Philadelphia: WB Saunders, 2006:605–619.

C.I-13. What is the better anesthetic agent for this operation—an inhalation or intravenous agent?

The choice of anesthetic agents is still debatable. Both inhalation, intravenous and combined agents have been used successfully. Both have advantages and disadvantages. Understanding the cardiovascular effects of each anesthetic agent and careful titration of each drug will improve the balance between myocardial oxygen demand and supply. Early detection and appropriate control of the major determinants of myocardial oxygen consumption (BP, HR, PAOP) are mandatory if myocardial ischemia is to be avoided. Another consideration is the desirability of early extubation. High-dose narcotic and large doses of sedatives and muscle relaxants should be avoided if early extubation is planned.

Three large-scale outcome studies of patients undergoing CABG surgery reported that anesthetic choice did not affect incidence of perioperative morbidity and mortality. However, studies do point towards a beneficial effect of volatile agents in preconditioning the myocardium against an ischemic injury.

Guarracino F, Landoni G, Tritapepe L, et al. Myocardial damage prevented by volatile anesthetics: a multicenter randomized controlled study. *J Cardiothorac Vasc Anesth* 2006; 20(4):477–483.

London M, Mittnacht A, Kaplan JA. Anesthesia for myocardial revascularization. In: Kaplan JA, Reich DL, Lake CL, et al. eds. *Kaplan's cardiac anesthesia*. Philadelphia: WB Saunders, 2006:609–614.

Slogoff S, Keats AS, Dear WE, et al. Steal-prone coronary anatomy and myocardial ischemia associated with four primary anesthetic agents in humans. *Anesth Analg* 1991;72:22–27.

Smul TM, Lange M, Redel A, et al. Desflurane-induced preconditioning against myocardial infarction is mediated by nitric oxide. *Anesthesiology* 2006;105(4):719–725.

Tuman KJ, McCarthy RJ, Spiess BD, et al. Does choice of anesthetic agent significantly affect outcome after coronary artery surgery? *Anesthesiology* 1989;70:189–198.

C.I-14. What are the cardiovascular effects of halothane, enflurane, isoflurane, desflurane, sevoflurane, morphine, and fentanyl?

In general, halothane, enflurane, isoflurane, desflurane, and sevoflurane produce a dose-related depression in ventricular function and vascular tonus. Halothane sensitizes the heart to catecholamine much more than enflurane, isoflurane, desflurane, and sevoflurane. Isoflurane and desflurane depress cardiac output to a lesser degree than does halothane or enflurane secondary to their greater vasodilating capacity. The HR changes least with halothane and increases most with desflurane. Isoflurane may cause tachycardia; the mechanism is unclear. Most studies suggest that halothane, enflurane, and isoflurane decrease coronary vascular resistance. Of these, isoflurane is the most potent coronary vasodilator.

All of the potent drugs decrease arterial pressure in a dose-related manner. The mechanism of BP decrease includes vasodilation, myocardial depression and decreased cardiac output, and decreased sympathetic nervous system tone. With halothane, decreased cardiac output is the predominant cause. Halothane also increases venous compliance, and in patients who have high sympathetic tone, such as those with heart failure, halothane decreases systemic vascular resistance. Enflurane causes both vasodilation and decreased myocardial contractility. With isoflurane and desflurane a low peripheral resistance is the major cause of hypotension. Evidence of the relatively greater myocardial depression with halothane and enflurane is the greater increase in right atrial pressure seen with these drugs than with isoflurane.

Narcotics such as morphine and fentanyl at their clinical dose have minimal cardiovascular effects. Both may cause bradycardia. Neither sensitizes the heart to catecholamine or depresses myocardial function. The cardiovascular effects of morphine depend on the dose used. Large doses of morphine sulfate have reportedly caused myocardial lactate production and reduction in coronary blood flow in animals. Sethna found that morphine sulfate, 0.25 mg per kg IV, did not produce a global myocardial ischemia in patients with CAD. High doses of morphine, 1 mg per kg, produce a significant decrease in arterial BP and systemic vascular resistance accompanied by an average 750% increase in plasma histamine. On the other hand, high doses of fentanyl, 50 μg per kg, do not produce any significant changes in BP, vascular resistance, and plasma histamine levels.

London M, Mittnacht A, Kaplan JA. Anesthesia for myocardial revascularization. In: Kaplan JA, Reich DL, Lake CL, et al. eds. *Kaplan's cardiac anesthesia*. Philadelphia: WB Saunders, 2006:607–614.

Malan TP, DiNardo JA, Isner RJ, et al. Cardiovascular effects of sevoflurane compared with those of isoflurane in volunteers. *Anesthesiology* 1995;83:918–928.

Sethna DH, Moffitt EA, Gray RJ, et al. Cardiovascular effects of morphine in patients with coronary artery disease. *Anesth Analg* 1982;61:109–114.

Skubas N, Lichtman AD, Shaarma A, et al. Anesthesia for cardiac surgery. In: Barash PG, Cullen BF, Stoelting RK, eds. *Clinical anesthesia*, 5th ed. Philadelphia: Lippincott Williams & Wilkins, 2006:916–919.

C.I-15. Is isoflurane dangerous for the patient with coronary artery disease (CAD)?

In patients with CAD, the use of isoflurane is still controversial. Reiz et al. reported that 1% isoflurane induced coronary vasodilation that was not related to normal autoregulation and that both decreased coronary perfusion pressure (systemic hypotension), and redistribution of myocardial blood flow (coronary steal) may contribute to development of regional myocardial ischemia. Another Reiz study, using 1.5 minimum alveolar concentration (MAC) isoflurane–nitrous oxide anesthesia, concluded that isoflurane may cause coronary steal with myocardial ischemia in patients with CAD. However, Smith et al. reported that the substitution of 0.5% to 1.12% isoflurane for 85 μg per kg of fentanyl did not result in an increased incidence of myocardial ischemia, as seen by ST-segment or segmental wall-motion changes in patients with CAD. Moreover, Tarnow et al. demonstrated that 0.5% isoflurane with 50% nitrous oxide improved the tolerance to pacing-induced myocardial ischemia in patients with significant CAD. Two large-scale prospective outcome studies by Slogoff et al. and Tuman et al. could find no evidence that the incidence of ischemia was increased by isoflurane in patients with CAD undergoing coronary artery bypass grafting (CABG) surgery. Furthermore, this finding held true even for patients with steal-prone coronary anatomy in the studies by Slogoff et al., Pulley et al., and Leung et al.

Several animal studies further confused this issue. Priebe proved that isoflurane was a myocardial depressant and a potent coronary vasodilator in the dog. Sill et al. demonstrated that high concentrations of isoflurane (1.5% and 2.5%) dilated intramyocardial arterioles rather than epicardial coronary arteries in the intact dog. Buffington et al. reported that isoflurane (1.2% to 1.5%) produced a decrease in collateral flow and a decrement in collateral zone contraction while enhancing flow in the normally perfused zone. They concluded that isoflurane was an arteriolar vasodilator and hence produced coronary steal in dogs with chronic coronary occlusion. On the contrary, Cason et al. found that in the dog, isoflurane or halothane at 0.5% MAC and 1.5 MAC had little effect on coronary vascular resistance, and ischemia was precipitated by tachycardia or hypotension rather than by coronary steal. Moreover, Davis and Frank demonstrated that isoflurane decreased myocardial infarct size after left anterior descending (LAD) coronary artery occlusion in dogs. In addition, Gilbert et al. reported greater coronary reserve in swine anesthetized with isoflurane versus halothane at 0.5 to 2.0 MAC. Recently, Hartman et al. demonstrated that adenosine but not isoflurane redistributed blood flow away from collateral-dependent myocardium in the presence of a coronary steal-prone anatomy in the chronically instrumented dog. They further found that reductions in myocardial perfusion during isoflurane anesthesia depend on systemic arterial pressure and that isoflurane did not produce coronary steal in this model of multivessel CAD. Furthermore, Cheng et al. found that neither isoflurane nor halothane as the sole anesthetic in clinical concentrations caused significant coronary vasodilation or coronary steal when the coronary perfusion pressure decreased from 55 to 30 mm Hg in a swine model of chronic coronary occlusion with collateral development.

On the basis of recent animal and recent clinical studies, we can conclude that isoflurane in clinical concentrations may be used safely in patients with CAD provided that hypotension and tachycardia are avoided.

Cheng DCH, Moyers JR, Knutson RM, et al. Dose-response relationship of isoflurane and halothane versus coronary perfusion pressures. Effects on flow redistribution in a collateralized chronic swine model. *Anesthesiology* 1992;76:113–122.

Gilbert M, Roberts SL, Blomberg RW, et al. Greater coronary reserve in swine anesthetized with isoflurane versus halothane. *Anesthesiology* 1985;63:A15.

Hartman JC, Kampine JP, Schmeling WT, et al. Steal-prone coronary circulation in chronically instrumented dogs: isoflurane versus adenosine. *Anesthesiology* 1991;74: 744–756.

Leung JM, Goehner P, O'Kelly BF, et al. Isoflurane anesthesia and myocardial ischemia: comparative risk versus sufentanil anesthesia in patients undergoing coronary artery bypass graft surgery. *Anesthesiology* 1991;74:838–847.

Lillehaug SL, Tinker JH. Why do "pure" vasodilators cause coronary steal when anesthetics don't (or seldom do)? (editorial). *Anesth Analg* 1991;73:681–682.

London M, Mittnacht A, Kaplan JA. Anesthesia for myocardial revascularization. In: Kaplan JA, Reich DL, Lake CL, et al. eds. *Kaplan's cardiac anesthesia*. Philadelphia: WB Saunders, 2006:609–614.

Priebe HJ. Differential effects of isoflurane on regional right and left ventricular performances and on coronary, systemic, and pulmonary hemodynamics in the dog. *Anesthesiology* 1987;66:262–272.

Pulley DD, Kirvassilis GV, Kelermenos N, et al. Regional and global myocardial circulatory and metabolic effects of isoflurane and halothane in patients with steal-prone coronary anatomy. *Anesthesiology* 1991;75:756–766.

Reiz S, Balfors E, Sorensen MB, et al. Isoflurane: a powerful coronary vasodilator in patients with coronary artery disease. *Anesthesiology* 1983;59:91–97.

Reiz S, Ostman M. Regional coronary hemodynamics during isoflurane-nitrous oxide anesthesia in patients with ischemic heart disease. *Anesth Analg* 1985;64:570–576.

Slogoff S, Keats AS, Dear WE, et al. Steal-prone coronary anatomy and myocardial ischemia associated with four primary anesthetic agents in humans. *Anesth Analg* 1991;72:22–27.

Tarnow J, Markschies-Hornung A, Schulte-Sasseu U. Isoflurane improves the tolerance to pacing-induced myocardial ischemia. *Anesthesiology* 1986;64:147–156.

Tuman KJ, McCarthy RJ, Spiess BD, et al. Does choice of anesthetic agent significantly affect outcome after coronary artery surgery? *Anesthesiology* 1989;70:189–198.

C.I-16. What is the cardiovascular effect of nitrous oxide?

Nitrous oxide is a weak central nervous system depressant. It has been generally considered to have minimal effects on other organ systems. Nitrous oxide has significant cardiovascular effects that may be depressant or stimulatory depending on the anesthetics with which it is combined. When high-dose fentanyl is used during coronary surgery, the effects of N_2O depend on the patient's cardiac function. Following the administration of 50% N_2O, there are no significant changes in any of the hemodynamic parameters in patients with normal left ventricular function (LVEDP <15 mm Hg). On the contrary, there is a significant decrease in cardiac index and stroke volume index in patients with left ventricular dysfunction (LVEDP >15 mm Hg). When added to other inhalation anesthetics, N_2O increases arterial pressure and systemic vascular resistance, suggesting that it has a vasoconstrictive action. Nitrous oxide increases pulmonary vascular resistance in patients with mitral stenosis and pulmonary hypertension.

The pulmonary vascular effects of nitrous oxide are also variable. Patients with elevated PA pressure may have further increases when nitrous oxide is added. Konstadt et al. did not corroborate these findings in patients with mitral valvular disease. A study in infants failed to show further increases of pulmonary vascular resistance with the addition of nitrous oxide.

The contribution of nitrous oxide to myocardial ischemia is controversial. Philbin et al. suggested that addition of nitrous oxide to anesthesia with high-dose fentanyl (100 μg/kg followed by 1 μg/kg/minute), or sufentanil (30 μg/kg followed by 0.3 μg/kg/minute), can produce clinically imperceptible regional myocardial ischemia in the areas supplied by stenotic coronary arteries of dogs. However, monitoring with two-dimensional TEE did not reveal myocardial ischemia in patients with CAD, when nitrous oxide was added to low-dose fentanyl (15 μg/kg followed by 0.2 μg/kg/minute), or high-dose sufentanil (20 μg/kg).

Clinically, nitrous oxide may be used before CPB if high-dose narcotics are not used and hypotension does not occur. However, after CPB, nitrous oxide should be avoided because of the possibility of expanding any air bubbles remaining in the coronary and cerebral circulation.

Balasaraswathi K, Kumar P, Rao TLK, et al. Left ventricular end-diastolic pressure (LVEDP) as an index for nitrous oxide use during coronary artery surgery. *Anesthesiology* 1981; 55:708–709.

Cahalan MK, Prakash O, Rulf EN, et al. Addition of nitrous oxide to fentanyl anesthesia does not induce myocardial ischemia in patients with ischemic heart disease. *Anesthesiology* 1987;67:925–929.

Messina AG, Yao FS, Canning H, et al. The effect of nitrous oxide on left ventricular pump performance and contractility with coronary artery disease: effect of preoperative ejection fraction. *Anesth Analg* 1993;77:954–962.

Philbin DM, Fox P, Drummond G, et al. Postsystolic shortening of canine left ventricle supplied by a stenotic coronary artery when nitrous oxide is added in the presence of narcotics. *Anesthesiology* 1985;62:166–174.

C.I-17. What kind of muscle relaxant would you use? Why?

We usually use pancuronium. When full paralyzing doses are given in a bolus, pancuronium generally produces tachycardia and hypertension caused by vagolytic effect and norepinephrine released from cardiac sympathetic nerves. Pancuronium is a better choice if hypotension (BP <80 mm Hg systolically) and bradycardia (HR <50/minute) are present. Theoretically, pancuronium may increase myocardial O_2 consumption caused by tachycardia and hypertension. Nevertheless, pancuronium is the most commonly used muscle relaxant for CABG. In practice, most patients with CAD receive β-adrenergic blocking agents, which can counteract the vagolytic effects of pancuronium. Also, the bradycardia associated with the popular narcotic anesthetic techniques can attenuate the tachycardia induced by pancuronium. Vecuronium and cisatracurium have no major cardiovascular effects, but their intermediate duration of action necessitates frequent administration of the relaxant. Pipecuronium and doxacurium are new long-acting, nondepolarizing muscle relaxants. They seem to have no hemodynamic side-effects associated with neuromuscular blockade. They can be used in large bolus doses.

London M, Mittnacht A, Kaplan JA. Anesthesia for myocardial revascularization. In: Kaplan JA, Reich DL, Lake CL, et al. eds. *Kaplan's cardiac anesthesia*. Philadelphia: WB Saunders, 2006:615–616.

C.I-18. If ST-segment depression is seen during surgery, how would you treat it? What is the relation between perioperative myocardial ischemia and postoperative myocardial infarction?

ST-segment depression indicates myocardial ischemia, either from increased O_2 demand or decreased O_2 supply. The treatment includes the following:

- *Increase O_2 supply.* Correct hypotension and hypoxemia.
- *Decrease O_2 demand.* Correct hypertension, tachycardia, and increased PAOP or CVP by deepening anesthesia or by using vasodilators and metoprolol or esmolol. All the major determinants of decreased O_2 demand have to be considered and corrected to their normal levels.

Gerson et al. (in experimental dogs) found that elevation of ST segments induced by occlusion of the coronary artery was less prominent with halothane than with a combination of nitroprusside and propranolol. These can be explained the effects of halothane on coronary vascular reserve and the known effects of nitroprusside (reduction of myocardial blood flow to ischemic myocardium).

If there are no obvious changes in BP, HR, and pulmonary wedge pressure, nitroglycerin is indicated if coronary spasm is suspected. Nitroglycerin may be given by intravenous drip. Sublingual nifedipine or intravenous nicardipine or diltiazem may also be given to relieve coronary spasm.

Slogoff and Keats reported that perioperative myocardial ischemia occurred in 37% of all patients undergoing CABG. They proved that perioperative myocardial infarction was almost three times as frequent in patients with ischemia (6.9%) compared with patients without ischemia (2.5%). Intraoperative tachycardia was associated with a higher incidence of myocardial ischemia and infarction. However, Knight et al. demonstrated that 42% of CABG patients had preoperative episodes of myocardial ischemia, 87% of which were clinically silent. They further found that anesthesia and surgery did not worsen the preoperative ischemic pattern. Furthermore, Slogoff and Keats in another study postulated that approximately 90% of new myocardial ischemia observed during anesthesia was the manifestation of silent ischemia observed in the patient before the operation and only 10% was related to anesthetic management. Therefore, the relation between intraoperative ischemia and postoperative outcome is still unsolved.

Gerson JI, Hickey RF, Bainton CR. Treatment of myocardial ischemia with halothane or nitroprusside-propranolol. *Anesth Analg* 1982;61:10–14.

Hill AB, Bowley CJ, Nahrwold ML, et al. Intranasal administration of nitroglycerin. *Anesthesiology* 1981;54:346–348.

Knight AA, Hollenberg M, London MJ, et al. Perioperative myocardial ischemia: importance of the preoperative ischemia pattern. *Anesthesiology* 1988;68:681–688.

Mangano DT. Perioperative cardiac morbidity. *Anesthesiology* 1990;72:153–184.

Slogoff S, Keats AS. Does perioperative myocardial ischemia lead to postoperative myocardial infarction. *Anesthesiology* 1985;62:107–114.

Slogoff S, Keats AS. Randomized trial of anesthetic agents on outcome of coronary artery bypass operations. *Anesthesiology* 1989;69:179–188.

C.I-19. Would you use prophylactic nitroglycerin during coronary artery bypass grafting (CABG) to prevent intraoperative myocardial ischemia or perioperative myocardial infarction?

No. It has been reported that prophylactic administration of nitroglycerin, 0.5 or 1.0 μg/kg/minute, during fentanyl anesthesia in patients undergoing CABG did not prevent myocardial ischemia or reduce the incidence of perioperative myocardial infarction.

Royster RL, Butterworth J, Groban L, et al. Cardiovascular pharmacology. In: Kaplan JA, Reich DL, Lake CL, et al. eds. *Kaplan's cardiac anesthesia*. Philadelphia: WB Saunders, 2006:213–219.

C.I-20. How would you correct hypertension?

Blood pressure = blood flow × resistance

Hypertension is usually due to inadequate depth of anesthesia. Occasionally it is due to fluid overloading. The treatment of hypertension includes the following:

- *Deepen the anesthesia.* Inhalation agents, such as halothane, enflurane, and isoflurane are more effective than narcotics because of their vasodilator effect.
- *Vasodilators.* when inhalation agents are not used.
  - Sodium nitroprusside produces more arteriolar dilation than venodilation. Dose: 10 to 100 μg per minute IV drip titration
  - Nicardipine. Dose 0.5 μg/kg/minute, titrated to effect.
  - Labetalol. Dose 5-mg increments, titrate to effect.
  - Nitroglycerin produces more venodilation than arteriolar dilation. Dose: 20 to 200 μg per minute IV drip titration, or bolus in 20 μg increments

See also Chapter 14, question C.10.

C.I-21. How would you treat hypotension?

Hypotension is usually caused by hypovolemia, deep anesthesia, bradycardia, or CHF. The treatments are as follows:

- Increase fluid infusion and put the patient in head-down position when CVP or PAOP is low.
- Lighten the level of anesthesia or use a vasoconstrictor: phenylephrine, 0.1 mg IV increments, to correct vasodilation produced by anesthesia.
- Atropine, 0.2 to 2.0 mg, for bradycardia, or isoproterenol, 1 mg per 100 mL D_5 W IV drip titration, rarely indicated
- Treat CHF when PAOP is high and TEE shows hypokinesia:
  - Lighten the level of anesthesia.
  - Restrict fluids.
  - Diuretics—furosemide (Lasix) 20 to 40 mg IV
  - Inotropes
    - $CaCl_2$ (0.5 to 1.0 g).
    - Epinephrine—2 to 8 μg per minute IV drip
    - Dobutamine or dopamine—5 to 20 μg/kg/minute IV drip
    - Amrinone—0.75 to 1.5 mg per kg, then 5 to 10 μg/kg/minute IV drip, or
    - Milrinone 0.05 mg per kg, then 0.5 to 0.7 μg/kg/minute IV drip
    - Norepinephrine if peripheral vascular resistance is low.
    - IABP

C.I-22. What are the indications for intravenous metoprolol, labetalol, or esmolol during surgery? How much would you give? What are the relative contraindications?

Indications

- ST-segment depression associated with tachycardia; no response to deepening the level of anesthesia
- Supraventricular tachycardia over 120 per minute
- Recurrent ventricular arrhythmias

Contraindications

- Asthma, reactive chronic obstructive pulmonary disease

However, esmolol is cardioselective and appears to have little effect on bronchial or vascular tone at doses that decrease HR in humans. It has been used successfully in low doses in patients with asthma. Esmolol is metabolized rapidly in the blood by an esterase located in the erythrocyte cytoplasm. Esmolol is a short-acting β-blocker with an elimination half-life of 9 minutes and a pharmacologic half-life of 10 to 20 minutes.

Dosage

- Metoprolol, 1- to 2-mg increments every 1 to 2 minutes, total dose 5 to 10 mg
- Esmolol, 10-mg increments up to 0.5 mg per kg followed by 50 to 300 μg/kg/minute IV drip.
- Labetalol, 5-mg increments, titrate to effect. Not indicated if BP is decreased.

Royster RL, Butterworth J, Groban L, et al. Cardiovascular pharmacology. In: Kaplan JA, Reich DL, Lake CL, et al. eds. *Kaplan's cardiac anesthesia*. Philadelphia: WB Saunders, 2006:219–225.

C.I-23. How would you correct increased pulmonary artery occlusion pressure (PAOP)?

It is important to treat the patient as a whole. All monitored parameters should be taken into account. Increased PAOP is usually due to a light level of anesthesia or CHF. Combining the readings of PAOP and BP will produce a differential diagnosis. Occasionally an increased PAOP with hypotension and low cardiac output is caused by hypertrophic obstructive cardiomyopathy (HOCM), also known as idiopathic hypertrophic subaortic stenosis (*IHSS*). HOCM can be diagnosed by TEE, which demonstrates systolic anterior motion (SAM) of mitral valve and left ventricular outflow obstruction, mitral regurgitation and usually good left ventricular contractility.

Inadequate Anesthesia: Increased PAOP with Hypertension

- Deepen the level of anesthesia with inhalation agents, such as isoflurane, halothane, or enflurane, which also have a vasodilator effect.
- Give a vasodilator. Nitroglycerin is a better venodilator than nitroprusside.

Congestive Heart Failure: Increased PAOP with Hypotension and Low Cardiac Output

- Lighten the level of anesthesia.
- Restrict fluids.
- Use arterial vasodilators.
- Give diuretics.
- Use inotropes.

HOCM (IHSS)

- β-Blocker and volatile agents to decrease HR and contractility
- Fluid loading to keep LV full and decrease left ventricle outflow tract (LVOT) obstruction
- Increase afterload to keep LV full

Reich DL, Mittnacht A, London M, et al. Monitoring of the heart and vascular system. In: Kaplan JA, Reich DL, Lake CL, et al. eds. *Kaplan's cardiac anesthesia*. Philadelphia: WB Saunders, 2006:399–403.

C.I-24. What should you do during sternal splitting?

Stop ventilation and deflate the lungs to prevent lung injury from the electric saw.

C.I-25. Would you monitor PAOP continuously? Why?

No, If the Swan-Ganz catheter balloon is inflated continuously, pulmonary infarction distal to the occlusion may ensue. Usually pulmonary artery diastolic pressure (PADP) is monitored continuously because the gradient between PADP and PAOP is small.

Skubas N, Lichtman AD, Shaarma A, et al. Anesthesia for cardiac surgery. In: Barash PG, Cullen BF, Stoelting RK, eds. *Clinical anesthesia*, 5th ed. Philadelphia: Lippincott Williams & Wilkins, 2006:916.

C.I-26. Discuss autologous transfusion and blood conservation for cardiac surgery.

Autologous transfusion is the collection and reinfusion of the patient's own blood or blood components. The realization that homologous blood is responsible for transmission of acquired immunodeficiency syndrome (AIDS), hepatitis, transfusion reaction, and autosensitization has led to increased interest in autologous transfusion and blood conservation. There are several options for autologous transfusion: preoperative autologous blood donation, preoperative use of erythropoietin, intraoperative normovolemic hemodilution, intraoperative plasmapheresis, pharmacologic treatment, and perioperative blood salvage.

Preoperative Autologous Blood Donation

Donations are appropriate for properly selected patients with stable CAD, stable valvular disease, and congenital heart disease. The risk of blood donation may be higher for patients with unstable angina or severe aortic stenosis; these patients are usually not considered good candidates for autologous blood donation. The patient should have a hemoglobin of greater than 11 g per dL to donate blood.

The optimal donation period begins 4 to 6 weeks before surgery, and the last donation is usually collected no later than 72 hours before surgery. Despite the potential benefits of the method, it is rarely used currently because of logistical reasons (multiple preoperative visits to the hospital, cost).

Preoperative Use of Erythropoietin

This is an established, efficacious but relatively expensive therapy to reduce blood transfusions. To optimize the hemoglobin response, oral or intravenous iron supplementation is recommended. The method is particularly indicated in anemic patients.

Intraoperative Normovolemic Hemodilution

This is the removal of blood through an arterial or venous catheter immediately after induction of anesthesia, before CPB or the administration of heparin. Depending on the patient's size and hematocrit, 500 to 1,000 mL of blood is collected into blood bags containing CPDA-1 anticoagulant and is kept at room temperature.

This blood is spared the rigors of CPB, including hemolysis, platelet destruction, and clotting factor degradation. The autologous blood is transfused after reversal of the heparin with protamine. It has been demonstrated that the effect of one unit of fresh whole blood on platelet aggregation after CPB is at least equal, if not superior, to the effect of 8 to 10 stored platelet units. However, if the patient's hematocrit is below 33% or the hemoglobin is below 11 g per dL, normovolemic hemodilution is not recommended because further decreasing the oxygen-carrying capacity may worsen myocardial ischemia. In addition, hemodilution during CPB will further decrease hematocrit to levels that require homologous blood transfusion. Normovolemic hemodilution should be performed cautiously in patients with critical left main coronary stenosis and aortic stenosis because sudden cardiac arrest has been observed during the procedure.

Intraoperative Plasmapheresis

Coagulopathy associated with hypothermia, shock, CPB, multiple transfusions, and the blood salvage technique, which removes clotting factors and platelets, often necessitates use of fresh-frozen plasma and platelet packs to control postoperative bleeding and clotting problems. Recently a plasma-collection system has been developed to salvage up to 1,000 mL of platelet-rich plasma before CPB. This technique does not cause hemodilution; therefore, it can be utilized in all patients, including those with anemia. The platelet-rich plasma can be stored at room temperature until transfused, usually after protamine reversal of the heparin. It is recommended that the collected product be placed on a rocker until infusion and that the pH be held constant.

Pharmacologic Treatment

The prophylactic use of aprotinin, ε-aminocaproic acid (EACA) and tranexamic acid reduces blood transfusions in cardiac surgery. Aprotinin inhibits a host of proteases, including trypsin, plasmin, kallikrein and factor XIIa activation of complement. The adult dose is 2 million kallikrein inhibition units (KIU) for the patient and bypass pump followed by 500,000 KIU per hour for 4 hours. The synthetic antifibrinolytics, EACA and tranexamic acid, bind to plasminogen and plasmin, thereby inhibiting binding of plasminogen at the lysine residues of fibrinogen. Effective antifibrinolysis requires a loading dose of 100 to 150 mg per kg for EACA or 10 mg per kg for tranexamic acid and a constant infusion for each at one-tenth the loading dose each hour.

Perioperative Blood Salvage

This is the collection and reinfusion of blood lost during and immediately after surgery. The posttransfusion survival of perioperatively-salvaged red cells has been shown to be comparable to that of allogeneic red cells. At the conclusion of CPB, all blood remaining in the oxygenator and bypass circuits should be salvaged and, if needed, infused. Blood salvaged intraoperatively may be transfused directly (unwashed) or processed (washed) before infusion. Commercially available equipment exists for each option. Blood collected by intraoperative salvage represents an excellent source of red-cell support. However, salvaged blood is deficient in coagulation factors and platelets.

Postoperative blood salvage is another technique of autologous blood transfusion utilizing blood lost following surgery. Blood salvaged following cardiac surgery is generally collected from mediastinal and chest drains and transfused without washing. Because it is usually defibrinated, it does not require anticoagulation before transfusion. Although dilute, the blood is sterile and contains viable red cells.

Drummond JC, Petrovich CT. Hemotherapy and hemostasis. In: Barash PG, Cullen BF, Stoelting RK, eds. *Clinical anesthesia*, 5th ed. Philadelphia: Lippincott Williams & Wilkins, 2006.217–219.

Gravlee GP, Davis RF, Utley JR. *Cardiopulmonary bypass, principles and practice*. Philadelphia: Lippincott Williams & Wilkins, 2000:536–542.

Lilly KJ, O'Gara PJ, Treanor PR, et al. Cardiopulmonary bypass: it's not the size, it's how you use it! Review of a comprehensive blood-conservation strategy. *J Extra Corpor Technol* 2006;36(3):263–268.

Shander A, Moskowitz D, Rijhwani TS. The safety and efficacy of "bloodless" cardiac surgery. *Semin Cardiothorac Vasc Anesth* 2005;9(1):53–63.

Spahn DR, Casutt M. Eliminating blood transfusions. New aspects and perspectives. *Anesthesiology* 2000;93:245–255.

Van der Linden P. Perioperative blood conservation strategies: an update for clinicians. *Can J Anaesth* 2006;50(6 Suppl):S1–S2.

C.II. *During Cardiopulmonary Bypass*

C.II-1. What anticoagulant would you give before CPB? How much would you give? What is its mechanism?

Heparin has been used conventionally in doses of 300 (200 to 400) units per kg of body weight, assuming an initial concentration of at least 2 to 4 units per mL of whole blood. Empirically, after 2 hours of the initial dose, subsequent doses of 1 mg per kg are given for each additional hour of bypass. Because there is marked individual variation, heparin doses are best monitored by the celite-ACT test.

Heparin acts indirectly by means of a plasma cofactor. The heparin cofactor, or antithrombin III, is an α_2-globulin and a protease inhibitor that neutralizes several activated clotting factors: XIIa, kallikrein, XIa, IXa, Xa, IIa, and XIIIa. Antithrombin III forms irreversible complexes with thrombin (IIa) and, as a result, both proteins are inactivated. Inhibition of thrombin and factor Xa accounts for most of the anticoagulant effect of heparin. Heparin increases the rates of the thrombin-antithrombin reaction at least 1,000-fold by serving as a catalytic template to which both the inhibitor and the protease bind. Heparin also binds to cofactor II, a glycoprotein of 65,000 Da that inactivates thrombin independently of antithrombin III. This reaction occurs more slowly and requires higher heparin concentrates than does thrombin inhibition through the heparin-AT III complex.

Spiess BD, Horrow J, Kaplan JA. Transfusion medicine and coagulation disorders. In: Kaplan JA, Reich DSN, Lake CL, et al. eds. *Kaplan's cardiac anesthesia*, 5th ed. Philadelphia: Elsevier Science, WB Saunders, 2006:948–951.

C.II-2. What is the half-life of heparin? How is it eliminated?

The biologic half-life of heparin varies with dosages and temperature. It has a remarkable individual variation. The average half-life is approximately 100 minutes in normothermic man for the initial doses of 300 units, increasing with higher doses and decreasing temperature. When 100, 400, or 800 units of heparin are given intravenously, the approximate half-life is 1, 2.5, and 5 hours respectively. Heparin concentrations decline progressively at all temperatures, but the rate of decline is delayed in proportion to the hypothermia.

The primary mechanism for heparin elimination remains uncertain. Heparin appears to be cleared and degraded primarily by the reticuloendothelial system; a small amount of heparin also appears in the urine.

Spiess BD, Horrow J, Kaplan JA. Transfusion medicine and coagulation disorders. In: Kaplan JA, Reich DSN, Lake CL, et al. eds. *Kaplan's cardiac anesthesia*, 5th ed. Philadelphia: Elsevier Science, WB Saunders, 2006:949.

C.II-3. How do you monitor heparin dosage? What is the activated coagulation time (ACT) test?

Heparin therapy can be assessed by the PTT, heparin assay, heparin-protamine titration, and the ACT test. The most convenient and practical method used to monitor heparin therapy in the operating room is the celite-ACT test. There is a very good correlation among the ACT, plasma heparin units, and thrombin time. After central venous injection of a heparin bolus, the onset of maximal ACT prolongation in the radial artery blood sample occurs within 1 minute. Previous work suggested that heparin action peaks 10 to 20 minutes after administration, but this finding probably represented an artifact from other factors prolonging the ACT such as hemodilution and hypothermia. Two milliliters of blood are put into a test tube containing celite to activate coagulation. Then the tube is kept at 37°C (98.6°F) and clot formation is watched for ACT. The normal control value of ACT is 105 to 167 seconds. A baseline value is determined before the administration of heparin, and the test is repeated 3 to 5 minutes after heparin is given and at intervals of 30 to 60 minutes thereafter. With the dose of heparin in milligrams per kilogram on the vertical axis and ACT in seconds on the horizontal axis, a dose-response curve can be plotted. ACT values are maintained at least twice the control value and should never decrease less than 300 seconds during normothermia. At the New York Presbyterian Hospital-Cornell Medical Center, we keep the ACT above 480 seconds.

Shore-Lesserson L. Coagulation monitoring. In: Kaplan JA, Reich DSN, Lake CL, et al. eds. *Kaplan's cardiac anesthesia*, 5th ed. Philadelphia: Elsevier Science, WB Saunders, 2006:558–559.

C.II-4. What is total cardiopulmonary bypass (CPB)? What is partial bypass?

Total bypass indicates that all the venous return from superior and inferior venae cavae, and the coronary sinus is drained to the oxygenator, and no blood is pumped by the RV to the lungs. The PA and systemic pressure tracings become nonpulsatile. Partial bypass means that some of the blood return is still pumped by both right and LVs. Some venous blood is drained to the oxygenator and pumped back to the arterial side. Femoral–femoral bypass is one example of partial CPB.

Gravlee GP, Davis RF, Kurusz M, et al. *Cardiopulmonary bypass, principles and practice*. Philadelphia: Lippincott Williams & Wilkins, 2000:552–553.

C.II-5. What is the purpose of venting the LV? How can it be done?

Although all the venous return is bypassed from the RV, 2% to 5% of cardiac output is draining to the LV. This represents the physiologic shunt from the bronchial, thebesian, and pleural veins. Other sources of blood flow to the left heart during CPB include aortic regurgitation from aortic insufficiency and extracardiac left-to-right shunts such as patent ductus arteriosus and Blalock-Taussig, Waterston, and Potts shunts. The left ventricular sump drain prevents overdistention of the LV, which may cause postpump heart failure. A suction needle inserted proximal to the aortic cross-clamp may serve the same purpose.

Venting of the LV can be accomplished by inserting a catheter to the following sites:

- Aortic root such as cardioplegia cannula for CABG
- Junction of the right superior pulmonary vein and the left atrium and advancing through the left atrium and mitral valve into the LV
- Apex of the LV
- PA or the left atrium only

Gravlee GP, Davis RF, Kurusz M, et al. *Cardiopulmonary bypass, principles and practice*. Philadelphia: Lippincott Williams & Wilkins, 2000:99–103.

C.II-6. How many types of oxygenators are there? What are the advantages of each type?

There are two basic types of oxygenators in terms of their interface with blood.

Direct Gas Interface
- Disk
- Vertical screen
- Bubble

Without Gas Interface
- Membrane—solid or microporous
- Fluid—fluid using fluorocarbon liquid

The disk and screen oxygenators are not disposable and have proven to be somewhat difficult to clean, prepare, and resterilize.

The bubble oxygenator has the advantages of simplicity, disposability, and relatively low cost. The disadvantages of gas interface oxygenators include the following:

- Protein denaturation
- Increased fragility of cells
- Susceptibility to hemolysis
- Denaturation of platelet membrane materials resulting in platelet aggregation, clumping
- Formation of air embolism
- Large priming volume
- Variable reservoir level resulting in potential shifts of blood volume between intracorporeal and extracorporeal circuit

The membrane oxygenator has become more popular, economical, and efficient, and less traumatic to blood. Its advantages include the following:

- Less trauma to blood components
- No defoaming
- Decreased complement activation
- Independent control of oxygen and carbon dioxide exchange
- Use of air–oxygen mixture without the risk of gaseous microemboli

However, the advantage of a membrane oxygenator for a short perfusion (<2 hours) is unclear, although lower plasma hemoglobin levels are present using membrane oxygenators.
The disadvantages of membrane oxygenators include the following:

- Expense
- Potential difficulty in eliminating all bubbles during priming
- Moderately large priming volume

The major differences in changes of clotting factors between the bubble and membrane oxygenators become apparent after 4 to 6 hours of ECC.

Gravlee GP, Davis RF, Kurusz M, et al. *Cardiopulmonary bypass, principles and practice*. Philadelphia: Lippincott Williams & Wilkins, 2000:55–58.

Skubas N, Lichtman AD, Shaarma A, et al. Anesthesia for cardiac surgery. In: Barash PG, Cullen BF, Stoelting RK, eds. *Clinical anesthesia*, 5th ed. Philadelphia: Lippincott Williams & Wilkins, 2006:910.

Wagner JA. Oxygenator anatomy and function. *J Cardiothorac Vasc Anesth* 1997;11:175–281.

C.II-7. What kind of priming solution would you use? How much priming solution would you use? When would you prime with blood? Why?

The usual priming solution for adults at the New York Presbyterian Hospital-Cornell Medical Center includes 1,400 mL of balanced salt solution (Normosol) 100 mL of 25% albumin and 200 mL of 20% mannitol. The priming volumes vary with the size of the oxygenators used and the tubing volume; most oxygenators for adult patients have priming volumes of 500 to 1,000 mL. In general, blood is added to the oxygenator if the patient is markedly anemic (prepump hematocrit below 30%) or if the priming volume is large in relation to the patient's blood volume, such as in pediatric patients. In order to maintain oxygen carrying capacity, the hematocrit is kept at levels above 18% to 20%. Mannitol has long been used as an osmotic diuretic in situations where hemolysis or diminished renal function is expected. Mannitol has been found to decrease the incidence of renal failure during hypotension by promoting osmotic diuresis and increasing renal blood flow by decreasing renal vascular resistance. Heparin, 3,000 to 10,000 units, is added to the prime depending on the size of the prime volume. This allows heparin to be distributed over the thrombogenic surfaces of the CPB circuit.

Gravlee GP, Davis RF, Kurusz M, et al. *Cardiopulmonary bypass, principles and practice.* Philadelphia: Lippincott Williams & Wilkins, 2000:191–193, 648.

C.II-8. What are the advantages and disadvantages of hemodilution?

Advantages of Hemodilution

- An increase in microcirculation due to a reduction of blood viscosity
- Decreased metabolic acidosis
- Increased urine output
- Reduced blood demands
- Reduced incidence of hepatitis, AIDS, or reactions from blood transfusions
- Reduced postoperative blood loss

Disadvantages of Hemodilution

- Decreased oxygen carrying capacity
- Postoperative extracellular fluid overload
- Possible pulmonary edema
- Hypotension from decreased viscosity and peripheral resistance
- Decreased concentration of calcium, magnesium, phosphate, and zinc

Gravlee GP, Davis RF, Kurusz M, et al. *Cardiopulmonary bypass, principles and practice.* Philadelphia: Lippincott Williams & Wilkins, 2000:186–194.

C.II-9. What kind of pumps do you use? Are they pulsatile or not?

There are three types of pumps available for modern CPB machines: the double-headed nonocclusive roller pump, the centrifugal blood pump, and the ventricular-type pneumatic or hydraulic pump. Only the first two types are in common use.

The roller pump is the most commonly used pump. It is driven by an afterload-independent motor. Once the pump speed is set, it will continue the forward displacement of the same blood volume (or even air volume) even if the resistance is increased by kinking or clamping the arterial line. This will result in the rupture of connections between sections of tubing. Some centers use pressure gauges on the arterial inflow line to avoid this type of disaster.

The centrifugal pump is a kinetic pump that operates on the constrained vortex principle. Blood is driven through the pump by centrifugal forces generated by a vortex in the pump. The advantages of centrifugal pumps are as follows:

- Less trauma to blood components than the roller pump.
- Less risk of increasing arterial line pressure because blood flow decreases when line resistance is increased.
- Inflow responsiveness—if a large quantity of air is introduced into the pump, cohesive forces will no longer exist between layers of blood and pumping will stop.
- Less risk of micro-air embolism because small, low-density air bubbles are trapped in the center of the vortex.

Ventricular-type pumps, although potentially more powerful, are rather cumbersome and have not been well accepted. This type of pump is mainly used for pulsatile bypass.

The first two types of pumps are nonpulsatile. Pulsatile pumps are commercially available now. Methods available to generate pulsatile flow include an indwelling IABP, an extracorporeal balloon, ventricular-type pumps, Keele pump, Polystan pulsatile pump, modified roller pumps, and modified centrifugal pumps. Some studies indicate that with prolonged perfusion, pulsatile flow appears to be more physiologic and superb for organ function; however, scientists are less certain that it is an important factor during short-term bypass. The differences between the two modes and a benefit for pulsatile perfusion are most clearly manifested in identifiable high-risk patient groups.

Gravlee GP, Davis RF, Kurusz M, et al. *Cardiopulmonary bypass, principles and practice*. Philadelphia: Lippincott Williams & Wilkins, 2000:37–47, 82–83.

Hornick P, Taylor K. Pulsatile and nonpulsatile perfusion: the continuing controversy. *J Cardiothorac Vasc Anesth* 1997;11:310–315.

C.II-10. How do you monitor the patient during cardiopulmonary bypass (CPB)?

Clinical Monitoring

- MAP should be kept between 50 and 100 mm Hg to maintain tissue perfusion. In hypertensive patients and in older patients, a higher MAP is frequently utilized—there is very little support for this in the literature.
- PA pressure should be low or zero to prevent overdistention of the LV.
- CVP should be low or zero to make sure there is no obstruction to venous return from the head (when monitored from a site proximal to the RA) or there is adequate drainage of blood to the CPB circuit (when monitored from inside the RA).
- Pump-flow rate should be adequate for tissue perfusion and oxygenation.
- Urine output should be maintained above 1 mL/kg/hour by adequate perfusion.
- ECG.
- Electroencephalogram (EEG) is used in patients in whom cerebral circulation problems may occur.
- Both rectal and esophageal temperatures are recorded.
- Anesthesia should be maintained at the appropriate level.
- Pupillary size should remain normal and equal.
- Transcranial Doppler (TCD) and/or TEE may be used to detect aortic and cerebral embolism.
- Cerebral oximeter to maintain adequate brain oxygen saturation (>40%).

Laboratory Monitoring at Least Once Every Hour

- Arterial blood gases are kept at normal range.
- Venous PO_2 should be 40 to 45 mm Hg.
- Hematocrit maintained between 20% and 30%.
- Electrolytes Na^+, K^+, ionized Ca^{2+}.
- ACT measured each hour and maintained above 400 to 480 seconds.
- Blood sugar probably should be kept below 250 mg per dL.

Gravlee GP, Davis RF, Kurusz M, et al. *Cardiopulmonary bypass, principles and practice*. Philadelphia: Lippincott Williams & Wilkins, 2000:555–569.

Mora-Mangano CT, Chow JL, Kanevsky M. Cardiopulmonary bypass and the anesthesiologist. In: Kaplan JA, Reich DSN, Lake CL, et al. eds. *Kaplan's cardiac anesthesia*, 5th ed. Philadelphia: Elsevier Science, WB Saunders, 2006:893–935.

Yao FS, Tseng CC, Trifiletti RR, et al. Neurologic complications following cardiac surgery is associated with cerebral desaturation. *Anesth Analg* 2000;90(45):76.

C.II-11. How much BP would you keep during CPB? Why?

Controversy continues over what constitutes adequate pressures while the patient is on bypass. The MAP is usually maintained at approximately 50 to 100 mm Hg to ensure adequate tissue perfusion. BP depends on cardiac output (pump flow) and total peripheral resistance (TPR). We believe that adequate cardiac output (pump flow) is more important for tissue perfusion than BP.

During hypothermic cardioplegia, higher systemic pressures (mean blood pressure >70 mm Hg) are often avoided because of increased noncoronary collateral blood flow into the heart through the pericardium and pulmonary venous drainage. Such collateral flow of relatively warm blood tends to wash the colder cardioplegic solution out of the heart and decreases the hypothermic protection against myocardial ischemia.

The range of cerebrovascular autoregulation during hypothermia is controversial. Although pooled data from clinical studies indicate a lower autoregulatory threshold of 20 to 30 mm Hg in patients without cerebrovascular disease or preexisting hypertension, other studies suggest a pressure-dependent cerebral circulation when MAP is less than 50 mm Hg. Until prospective studies clearly define the autoregulatory threshold under various clinical conditions, BP of less than 50 mm Hg should be regarded as potential physiologic trespass, which may compromise cerebral circulation. In patients with cerebrovascular disease or hypertension, higher perfusion pressure is recommended. For patients over 50 years of age, we recommend to keep MAP equal to the patient's age. For example, MAP is kept at approximately 70 mm Hg for patients 70 years old and 80 mm Hg for patients 80 years old.

We recently studied 248 patients randomized to either low MAP (50 to 70 mm Hg) or high MAP (80 to 100 mm Hg) during CPB and found an across-the-board improvement in combined cardiac and neurologic outcome with higher MAP. However, MAP had no significant effect on neurologic outcome, in those patients at low risk for cerebral embolization (normal to mild aortic atherosclerosis by TEE). Patients at high risk for adverse neurologic outcome (severe aortic atherosclerosis by TEE) had a significantly lower risk of worse neurologic outcome when randomized to higher MAP. More recently, widened pulse pressure was shown to be a better predictor of cerebral and renal ischemic outcomes over that of systolic or diastolic BP. Other recent data suggest that MAP during CPB is not a primary predictor of cognitive decline or stroke following cardiac surgery. However, there was an association among hypotension (<50 mm Hg) and age, and decline in spatial and figural memory. Therefore, we recommend maintenance of high MAP during CPB in patients with increased risk of neurologic outcome such as history of cerebrovascular accident (CVA) or transient ischemic attack (TIA), hypertension, carotid stenosis, advanced age, and severe aortic atherosclerosis detected by TEE.

With the recent introduction of noninvasive cerebral oximetry, the frontal cortex oxygen saturation can be monitored by near-infrared spectroscopy. The technique measures the oxygen saturation of the mixed arterial and venous blood in the brain cortex. Because the volume of blood is predominantly venous, it reflects the balance between oxygen supply and demand in the brain. Our study showed good correlation between brain oxygen saturations and neurologic and cognitive outcomes. The MAP should be kept at levels enough to maintain adequate cerebral oxygen saturations (at least 70% of baseline values or >40% saturation).

Aronson S, Fontes ML. Hypertension: a new look at an old problem. *Curr Opin Anesthesiol* 2006;19:59–64.

Fontes ML. New insights in hypertension. *ASA Refresher Course Anesthesiol* 2006;34:43–53.

Gold JP, Charlson ME, Williams-Russo P, et al. Improvement of outcomes after coronary artery bypass: a randomized trial comparing intraoperative high versus low mean arterial pressure. *J Thorac Cardiovasc Surg* 1995;110:1302–1311.

Gravlee GP, Davis RF, Kurusz M, et al. *Cardiopulmonary bypass, principles and practice*. Philadelphia: Lippincott Williams & Wilkins, 2000:557–561.

Hartman GS, Yao F, Bruefach M, et al. Cardiopulmonary bypass at high pressure reduces stroke incidence in patients with TEE diagnosed severe aortic atheromatous disease. *Anesthesiology* 1995;83:A141.

Murkin JM, Farrar JK, Tweed A, et al. Cerebral autoregulation and flow/metabolism coupling during cardiopulmonary bypass: the influence of $PaCO_2$. *Anesth Analg* 1987; 66:825.

Newman MF, Kramer DC, Croughwell ND, et al. Differential age effects of mean arterial pressure and rewarding cognitive dysfunction after cardiac surgery. *Anesth Analg* 1995; 81:236–242.

Yao FSF, Tseng CC, Boyd WC, et al. Cognitive dysfunction following cardiac surgery is associated with cerebral oxygen desaturation. *Anesthesiology* 1999;91(3A):A73.

Yao FSF, Tseng CC, Boyd WC, et al. Frontal lobe dysfunction following cardiac surgery is associated with cerebral oxygen desaturation. *Ann Thorac Surg* 1999;68:1464.

C.II-12. How would you treat hypotension during CPB?

Mean arterial pressure (MAP) = cardiac output (CO) × total peripheral resistance (TPR)

Hypotension may be caused by low cardiac output or low peripheral resistance. First, cardiac output should be corrected by increasing the pump-flow rate. Then, if the cardiac output is adequate, peripheral resistance can be raised by giving vasopressors. We use the primarily α-adrenergic vasopressor phenylephrine in increments of 0.5 mg to raise the MAP to 50 mm Hg. According to Poiseuille's law, low TPR usually is due to decreased viscosity or increased vascular diameter (vasodilation). During CPB using blood-free–priming solutions, total viscosity is reduced by hemodilution although plasma viscosity is increased by hypothermia. A short period of hypotension with a MAP of approximately 30 to 40 mm Hg is usually seen in the first 5 to 10 minutes of bypass. It is due to the following causes:

- Inadequate pump flow at the beginning of bypass
- Hypoxic vasodilation from initial perfusion with blood-free primes carrying no oxygen
- Vasodilation from vasoactive materials released because of the initial reaction of the serum proteins, blood cells, and platelets with the foreign surfaces of the heart-lung machine
- Decreased plasma levels of catecholamines by hemodilution
- Infusion of cardioplegic solution, which contains nitroglycerin

Balasaraswathi K, Glisson SN, El-Etr AA, et al. Effect of priming volume on serum catecholamine during cardiopulmonary bypass. *Can Anaesth Soc J* 1980;27:135–139.

Mora-Mangano CT, Chow JL, Kanevsky M. Cardiopulmonary bypass and the anesthesiologist. In: Kaplan JA, Reich DSN, Lake CL, et al. eds. *Kaplan's cardiac anesthesia*, 5th ed. Philadelphia: Elsevier Science, WB Saunders, 2006:895–897.

C.II-13. How would you treat hypertension (a MAP of over 100 mm Hg)?

Hypertension during bypass is usually the result of inadequate depth of anesthesia, which causes increased catecholamine output and increased vascular resistance. Pump-flow rate should not be reduced to lower the pressure. Low pump flow may cause tissue hypoxia although BP is high. The most effective treatment involves administering an inhalation agent such as isoflurane through the vaporizer in the heart–lung machine. Intravenous agents, such as sodium thiopental, diazepam, midazolam, and large doses of narcotics may be used, but they are frequently not effective and have to be supplemented with vasodilator drugs. One may use nitroprusside, nitroglycerin, or nicardipine.

C.II-14. How do you prepare an intravenous infusion of sodium nitroprusside, nicardipine, and nitroglycerin? What are the usual doses? Which do you prefer to use?

Intravenous solutions may be prepared by adding to 250 mL of 5% dextrose in water 50 mg of nitroglycerin or sodium nitroprusside, or 25 mg of nicardipine, to make a concentration of 200 μg per mL (nitroglycerin or nitroprusside) or 100 μg per mL nicardipine. The usual doses are nitroglycerin or nitroprusside 0.5 to 10 μg/kg/minute, or 0.05 μg/kg/minute nicardipine, determined by careful titration (Table 7.2). We prefer nitroglycerin or nicardipine infusion. Sodium nitroprusside dilates both arterial and venous smooth muscle. It is very effective in reducing both preload and afterload. It may cause cyanide and thiocyanate toxicity. Because nitroprusside dilates the intramyocardial arterioles, intracoronary steal may occur. The solution has to be covered with aluminum foil to prevent decomposition from exposure to light. Nitroglycerin primarily causes venodilation, resulting in reduction of preload and myocardial oxygen consumption. At larger doses and by the intravenous route, it has mild arteriolar dilation and reduces afterload. It has no known toxicity and does not produce intracoronary steal because it dilates epicardial arteries. It may redistribute blood flow to the subendocardium and increase collateral circulation through the myocardium. Nicardipine is a systemic and coronary arterial dilator. The afterload is decreased, while the preload is not affected. It may cause a slight increase in HR (reflex tachycardia).

Gerson JI, Allen FB, Seltzer JL, et al. Arterial and venous dilation by nitroprusside and nitroglycerin: is there a difference? *Anesth Analg* 1982;61:256–260.

Lawson NW, Johnson JO. Autonomic nervous system: physiology and pharmacology. In: Barash PG, Cullen BF, Stoelting RK, eds. *Clinical anesthesia*, 5th ed. Philadelphia: Lippincott Williams & Wilkins, 2006:327–330.

C.II-15. How much pump flow would you maintain during CPB?

The pump blood flow is equivalent to cardiac output and to supply tissue oxygenation. The normal average cardiac output for adults is 70 mL/kg/minute or 3.1 L/minute/m^2. Because of higher metabolism, pediatric patients need higher flow rates for each unit of body weight. Usually 70% of normal cardiac output is enough to maintain tissue oxygenation. When body surface is used, both pediatric and adult patients require about the same pump flow, 2.2 to 3.1 L/minute/m^2. In summary, at normothermia and normal hemoglobin levels, the pump flow is as follows:

Adults 50 to 70 mL/kg/min	or	2.2 to 3.1 L/min/m^2
Children 100 to 150 mL/kg/min	or	2.2 to 3.1 L/min/m^2

However, some perfusion teams use low flow (40 mL/kg/minute), low pressure (approximately 40 mm Hg) bypass quite successfully. This technique has the advantages of less bleeding through intracardiac collaterals, less trauma to blood cells and platelets, and lower fluid requirements, but it also has the potential for inadequate perfusion. Clinically, low-flow and low-pressure techniques are used in conjunction with hypothermia and hemodilution. Therefore, pump blood flow should be adjusted accordingly to match the oxygen supply with demand.

Gravlee GP, Davis RF, Kurusz M, et al. *Cardiopulmonary bypass, principles and practice*. Philadelphia: Lippincott Williams & Wilkins, 2000:560.

Table 7.2 Cardiac Anesthesia Intravenous Medications[a].

DRUG	AMOUNT TO ADD	TOTAL VOLUME WITH D_5 W	CONCENTRATION	DOSAGE RANGE
Amicar (EACA)	15 g	150 mL	1 mL = 100 mg 10 mL = 1 g	Load: 10 g over 1/2 hr Maintenance: 1 g/hr × 5 hr

Amiodarone	450 mg	250 mL	1 mL = 1.8 mg	Initial: 150 mg over 10 min
				Followed by: 1 mg/min × 6 hr
				  (360 mg). Then:
				  0.5 mg/min × 18 hr

Amrinone	500 mg	500 mL	1 gt = 17 μg 1 mL = 1 mg	Load: 0.75 mg/kg over 10 min Maintenance: 2–20 μg/kg/min
Aprotinin (regimen A, "full dose")	2,000,000 kIU	200 mL (premixed)	1 mL = 10,000 kIU	Test: 1 mL Load: 200 mL or 2,000,000 kIU Maintenance: 50 mL/hr or 500,000 kIU/hr
Dexamedetomadine			1 mL = 4 μg	Load: 1.0 μg/kg over 10 min Maintenance: 0.2–0.7 μg/kg/hr
Diltiazem	25 mg	100 mL	1 mL = 0.25 mg	Load: 0.1–0.15 mg/kg Maintenance: 0.5–0.25 μg/kg/min
Dobutamine	500 mg	250 mL	1 gt = 33.3 μg 1 mL = 2 mg	5–20 μg/kg/min
Dopamine	400 mg	250 mL (premixed)	1 gt = 26.6 μg 1 mL = 1.6 mg	Renal: 1–5 μg/kg/min β: 10 μg/kg/min α: 10–15 μg/kg/min
Epinephrine	2 mg	250 mL	8 gtt = 1 μg	2–8 μg/min
Esmolol	5 g	250 mL	1 gt = 333 μg 1 mL = 20 mg	50–300 μg/kg/min
Levophed	8 mg	250 mL	2 gtt = 1 μg	4–32 μg/min
Lidocaine	2 g	500 mL (premixed)	15 gtt = 1 mg 1 mL = 4 mg	1–4 mg/min
Metaraminol	200 mg	250 mL	1 mL = 7.5 μg	50–400 μg/min
Milrinone	20 mg	100 mL	3 gtt = 1 μg 1 mL = 200 μg	0.375–1 μg/kg/min
Nicardipine	25 mg	250 mL	1 gt = 1.66 μg	Loading dose: 5 mg/hr Maintenance: Increase by 2.5 mg/hr every 15 min Maximum amount: 15 mg/hr
Nitroprusside	50 mg	250 mL (premixed)	1 gt = 3.33 μg	1–10 μg/kg/min
Nitroglycerin	50 mg	250 mL (premixed)	1 gt = 3.33 μg	10–80 μg/min
Phenylephrine	20 mg	250 mL	19 gtt = 25 μg	25–125 μg/min
Procainamide	2 g	500 mL (premixed)	15 gtt = 1 mg 1 mL = 4 mg	Loading dose: 500–1,000 mg (20 mg/min) Dosage: 1–4 mg/min
Sodium bicarbonate	100 mEq	100 mL undiluted	1 mL = 1 mEq	1–3 mEq/kg/hr (titrate to pH)

Vasopressin	100 units	100 mL	1 mL = 1 unit	Initial dose: 0.04 U/min, 2.4 U/hr
				Titrate: 0.005–0.01 U/min
				  (0.3–0.6 mL/hr) every 10 min
				  to max of 0.1 U/min or 6 U/hr

[a] There are 60 guttae per milliliter (gtt/mL); therefore, gtt/min = mL/hr.
EACA: aminocaproic acid.

Kolkka R, Hilberman M. Neurological dysfunction following cardiac operation with low flow, low pressure cardiopulmonary bypass. *J Thorac Cardiovasc Surg* 1980;79:432–437.

Mora-Mangano CT, Chow JL, Kanevsky M. Cardiopulmonary bypass and the anesthesiologist. In: Kaplan JA, Reich DSN, Lake CL, et al. eds. *Kaplan's cardiac anesthesia*, 5th ed. Philadelphia: Elsevier Science, WB Saunders, 2006:898.

C.II-16. How would you adjust the pump flow during hypothermia?

Hypothermia decreases oxygen consumption. Therefore, the pump flow may be decreased proportionally if the blood oxygen content does not change. The oxygen consumption at different body temperatures is listed in the following text.

Temperature (°C)	37	32	30	28	25	20	10
O$_2$ Consumption (%)	100	60	50	40	25–30	20	10

Because the O$_2$ consumption at 30°C (86°F) is half of that at 37°C (98.6°F), the required pump flow at 30°C (86°F) is 50% of the flow at 37°C (98.6°F) (50 to 70 mL/kg/minute). Therefore, a pump flow of 25 to 35 mL/kg/minute is adequate for adults at 30°C (86°F), if there is no hemodilution. During profound hypothermia (10°C to 20°C [50°F to 68°F]) the patients usually can tolerate total circulatory arrest without pump support for approximately 60 to 90 minutes. The decrease in metabolism during hypothermia is not a linear process. From 37°C to 30°C (98.6°F to 86°F), the metabolism decreases approximately 7% by each degree centigrade. Below 30°C (86°F) the rate of metabolism decrease slows down. Usually every 7°C to 8°C (44.4°F to 46.4°F) decrease in temperature reduces oxygen consumption by 50%. Clinically, it has been demonstrated that pump flows as low as 30 mL/kg/minute or 1.2 L/minute/m^2 will not compromise whole-body oxygen delivery when moderate systemic hypothermia is employed.

C.II-17. How would you adjust the pump flow during hemodilution?

$$\text{Oxygen delivery} = \text{cardiac output} \times \text{arterial oxygen content}$$
$$\text{Arterial oxygen content} = 1.34 \times Hb \times O_2 \text{ saturation} + (0.003 \times Pa_{O_2})$$

Hemodilution reduces hemoglobin concentration and hence decreases oxygen content. In order to deliver the same amount of oxygen, the pump flow has to be increased accordingly during hemodilution. For example, if the hematocrit is diluted from 40% to 20% during CPB, the pump flow has to be doubled (increased by a factor of 40/20 = 2). Clinically, both hypothermia and hemodilution are applied simultaneously, so that the adjustment has to be done at the same time. For example, the pump flow for adults at a temperature of 30°C (86°F) and a hematocrit of 25% will be as follows:

$$50 \text{ to } 70 \text{ mL/kg/min} \times 50\% \times 40/25 = 40 \text{ to } 56 \text{ mL/kg/min}$$

C.II-18. What are the advantages of hypothermia? Does hypothermia offer neuroprotection?

Hypothermia decreases oxygen consumption and helps to preserve the function of tissues during a hypoxic or ischemic insult. Pump flow may be decreased during CPB with hypothermia.

Hypothermia has been shown to confer significant protection in the setting of transient, but not permanent, ischemia. The mechanism is unclear. The reduction in cerebral metabolic rate is believed to be less important when compared with the effect of hypothermia on the release of excitatory neurotransmitters, catecholamines, or other mediators of cellular injury. It is for this reason that mild hypothermia (33°C to 35°C [91.4°F to 95°F]) provides significant neuroprotection.

The effect of hypothermia during CPB on postoperative cognitive or neurologic function remains controversial. Animal models show profound reduction in infarct size and release of excitatory amino acid with minimal levels of hypothermia. However, clinical studies comparing normothermic and moderately hypothermic CPB have yielded conflicting results and did not produce evidence of protection from cognitive decline. This may relate to differences in defining normothermia. Many groups allow temperature to drift downwards during normothermic CPB, with temperature decreasing to below 34°C (93.2°F). Mclean in a recent study of this type showed no difference in cognitive or neurologic outcome between warm and moderately hypothermic groups. In actuality, this is a study of mild versus moderate hypothermia confirming the experimental animal data that as little as 2°C to 3°C (3.6°F to 5.4°F) of hypothermia markedly reduces excitatory amino acid release and neurologic injury compared to normothermia. The single large study comparing true normothermia with hypothermia during CPB showed a significantly greater incidence of focal neurologic injury in the warm group, supporting the beneficial role of hypothermia in neuroprotection. In addition, recent data showed that minimum CPB temperatures greater than 35°C (95°F) increased the incidence of perioperative stroke approximately fourfold (4.5% vs. 1.2%).

In this context, the avoidance of cerebral hyperthermia deserves comment. Hyperthermia as little as a 2°C (3.6°F) increase in temperature significantly worsens neurological outcomes. It has been demonstrated in a rat model, that following 10 minutes of ischemia during which temperature was increased from 35°C to 39°C (95°F to 102.2°F), the percentage of damaged neurons increased from 15% to 80%. This is clinically relevant because cerebral temperatures above 39°C (102.2°F) have been documented in patients during rewarming, a period when cerebral embolic risk is greatest. Therefore, hyperthermia should be carefully monitored and avoided.

Gravlee GP, Davis RF, Kurusz M, et al. *Cardiopulmonary bypass, principles and practice.* Philadelphia: Lippincott Williams & Wilkins, 2000:417–418.

Mclean RF, Wong BI. Normothermic versus hypothermic cardiopulmonary bypass: central nervous system outcomes. *J Cardiothorac Vasc Anesth* 1996;10:45–53.

Mora-Mangano CT, Chow JL, Kanevsky M. Cardiopulmonary bypass and the anesthesiologist. In: Kaplan JA, Reich DSN, Lake CL, et al. eds. *Kaplan's cardiac anesthesia*, 5th ed. Philadelphia: Elsevier Science, WB Saunders, 2006:899–890.

Yao FSF, Barbut D, Leon FJ, et al. Cerebral hyperthermia during cardiopulmonary bypass rewarming in patients undergoing cardiac surgery. *Anesthesiology* 1998;89(3A): A238.

C.II-19. How does blood viscosity change during hypothermia and hemodilution?

Blood viscosity varies inversely with temperature; a 2% increase occurs for every 1°C (1.8°F) decrease in temperature. At a hematocrit of 40%, a decrease in temperature from 37°C to 27°C (98.6°F to 80.6°F) increases viscosity by approximately 25%. Hemodilution with balanced salt solution will decrease blood viscosity. Decreasing the hematocrit from 40% to 20% at 27°C (80.6°F) decreases viscosity by approximately 40%. It has been recommended that the hematocrit be adjusted to the same numerical value as the core body temperature in°C if blood viscosity is to be kept approximately constant. For example, normal viscosity at 37°C (98.6°F) with hematocrit of 40% approximates that seen at 25°C (77°F) with hematocrit of 25%.

Gravlee GP, Davis RF, Kurusz M, et al. *Cardiopulmonary bypass, principles and practice.* Philadelphia: Lippincott Williams & Wilkins, 2000:561.

C.II-20. What are the main causes of death associated with accidental hypothermia?

Ventricular fibrillation and asystole are the major rhythm disturbances leading to cardiac arrest during hypothermia. In humans externally cooled for cardiac surgery, ventricular fibrillation generally occurs at 23°C (73°F) and asystole at 20°C (68°F). However, asystole and ventricular fibrillation have been reported at 21°C to 28°C (69.8°F to 82.4°F). Respiratory arrest usually accompanies cardiac arrest during accidental hypothermia.

Gravlee GP, Davis RF, Kurusz M, et al. *Cardiopulmonary bypass, principles and practice.* Philadelphia: Lippincott Williams & Wilkins, 2000:717.

Southwick FS, Dalglish PH. Recovery after prolonged asystolic cardiac arrest in profound hypothermia. *JAMA* 1980;243:1250–1253.

C.II-21. Would you give anesthesia during cardiopulmonary bypass (CPB)? Why?

Yes. Anesthesia is maintained with intermittent administration of intravenous barbiturates or benzodiazepines and narcotic or inhalation agents through the pump oxygenator to achieve unconsciousness and analgesia, to control BP, and to prevent shivering. Intravenous agents are diluted by the priming solution during CPB. Meanwhile, hypothermia itself produces anesthesia and prolongs the action duration of intravenous agents by decreasing hepatic metabolism and urinary excretion. Barbiturates may be of particular benefit for temporary focal lesions (gas emboli from bypass pump or open chamber) if metabolic suppression is not being achieved by hypothermia.

Gravlee GP, Davis RF, Kurusz M, et al. *Cardiopulmonary bypass, principles and practice.* Philadelphia: Lippincott Williams & Wilkins, 2000:189, 292.

Nussmeier NA, Arlund C, Slogoff S. Neuropsychiatric complications after cardiopulmonary bypass: cerebral protection by a barbiturate. *Anesthesiology* 1986;64:165–170.

Nussmeier NA, Fish KJ. Neuropsychological dysfunction after cardiopulmonary bypass: a comparison of two institutions. *J Cardiothorac Vasc Anesth* 1991;5:584–588.

Zaiden JR, Klochany A, Martin WM, et al. Effect of thiopental on neurologic outcome following coronary artery bypass grafting. *Anesthesiology* 1991;74:406–411.

C.II-22. Would you give muscle relaxants during CPB? How is the action of muscle relaxant affected during CPB?

Yes. Muscle relaxants are given to prevent diaphragmatic movement that interferes with surgery and to prevent shivering during hypothermia. Shivering may increase oxygen consumption to as high as 486% of normal. The effect of a muscle relaxant is altered by both hypothermia and hemodilution. The plasma concentration of muscle relaxants is diluted by the priming solution. Therefore, more relaxant is required to maintain the same degree of relaxation. Hypothermia was originally reported to decrease the effect of nondepolarizing relaxants, because decreased cholinesterase enzyme activity during hypothermia resulted in more acetylcholine accumulation to compete with the nondepolarizing relaxant. Contrary to the earlier reports, it is now established that less *d*-tubocurarine, atracurium, vecuronium, or pancuronium is needed to maintain muscle relaxation during hypothermia because hypothermia reduces renal and biliary excretions of both *d*-tubocurarine and pancuronium. Ham et al. reported that hypothermia in man does not affect *d*-tubocurarine pharmacokinetics or the sensitivity of the neuromuscular junction to *d*-tubocurarine. Hypothermia does prolong the onset of paralysis. Moreover, hypothermic CPB *per se* facilitates neuromuscular transmission at the electrochemical level, yet compromises mechanical contractility.

Modifications of partial neuromuscular blockade by hypothermic bypass are the result of muscle relaxation enhancing or interfering with the impact of hypothermia on normal neuromuscular transmission. The best way to monitor muscle relaxation is by using a peripheral nerve stimulator.

Buzello W, Pollmaecher T, Schluermann D, et al. The influence of hypothermia cardiopulmonary bypass on neuromuscular transmission in the absence of muscle relaxants. *Anesthesiology* 1986;4:279–281.

Buzello W, Schluermann D, Schindler M, et al. Hyperthermic cardiopulmonary bypass and neuromuscular blockade by pancuronium and vecuronium. *Anesthesiology* 1985;62: 201–204.

Gravlee GP, Davis RF, Kurusz M, et al. *Cardiopulmonary bypass, principles and practice*. Philadelphia: Lippincott Williams & Wilkins, 2000:279–293.

Grogan K, Nyhan D, Berkowitz DE. Pharmacology of anesthetic drugs. In: Kaplan JA, Reich DSN, Lake CL, et al. eds. *Kaplan's cardiac anesthesia*, 5th ed. Philadelphia: Elsevier Science, WB Saunders, 2006:202.

C.II-23. How do you know the patient is well perfused during CPB?

If the perfusion pressure is maintained between 50 mm Hg and 100 mm Hg, and the pump-flow rate is adequately maintained according to the degree of hypothermia and hemodilution, there should be adequate urine output, greater than 1 mL/kg/hour, no metabolic acidosis, and normal mixed venous oxygen tension of 40 to 45 mm Hg. However, cerebral perfusion is not routinely monitored and the autoregulation range of BP may be higher than the normal range in the elder and high-risk patients. Cerebral oximetry should be used for patients with increased risk for neurologic and cognitive outcomes. It is recommended to keep cerebral oxygen saturation over 40%.

Gravlee GP, Davis RF, Kurusz M, et al. *Cardiopulmonary bypass, principles and practice*. Philadelphia: Lippincott Williams & Wilkins, 2000:559–560.

Mora-Mangano CT, Chow JL, Kanevsky M. Cardiopulmonary bypass and the anesthesiologist. In: Kaplan JA, Reich DSN, Lake CL, et al. eds. *Kaplan's cardiac anesthesia*, 5th ed. Philadelphia: Elsevier Science, WB Saunders, 2006:895–898.

Yao FSF, Tseng CC, Boyd WC, et al. Neurological complications following cardiac surgery is associated with cerebral oxygen desaturation. *Anesth Analg* 2000;90:76.

Yao FS, Tseng CA, Ho CA, et al. Cerebral oxygen desaturation is associated with early postoperative neuropsychological dysfunction in patients undergoing cardiac surgery. *Cardiothorac Vasc Anesth* 2004;18:552–558.

C.II-24.   How much gas flow would you use for the oxygenator? What kind of gas would you use? Why?

Normal alveolar ventilation is 4 L per minute and pulmonary circulation is 5 L per minute. The $\dot{V}/\dot{Q}$ ratio is 0.8. The oxygenator is not as efficient as human lungs. We usually start with 2 L of gas for each liter of pump-flow rate, and then adjust the gas-flow rate according to blood $Paco_2$ and Pao_2. The gas flow may be decreased if the $Paco_2$ is low and the Pao_2 is too high. The ratio may be increased if the $Paco_2$ is over 40 mm Hg or the Pao_2 is under 100 mm Hg. In the past we used a mixture of 99% oxygen and 1% carbon dioxide for the bubble oxygenator. Because of low CO_2 production during hypothermia, high CO_2 elimination from high gas flow, and high CO_2 diffusion capacity, 1% CO_2 was added to oxygen to prevent severe hypocapnia. Because the routine use of membrane oxygenators oxygen-air mixtures, instead of 100% oxygen have been used. In a bubble oxygenator bubbles containing nitrogen may be slowly absorbed into the systemic circulation, increasing the risk of gaseous microemboli. In a membrane oxygenator this risk does not exist. Meanwhile, air-oxygen mixtures allow better control of oxygen tension during CPB. Because we use alpha-stat regulation for acid-base management, it is not necessary to add CO_2 to the ventilating gas during hypothermia to elevate $Paco_2$ and decrease the *pH*.

C.II-25.   What are the disadvantages of hypocapnia during CPB?

- Cerebral blood flow decreases approximately 2% to 4% for each mm Hg decrease in $Paco_2$ when $Paco_2$ is in the range of 20 mm Hg to 60 mm Hg, due to cerebral vasoconstriction. Cerebral oxygen saturation decreases approximately 1% for each mm Hg decrease in $Paco_2$
- Respiratory alkalosis shifts the oxygen dissociation curve to the left, which increases the O_2 affinity to hemoglobin and decreases the release of O_2 to the tissues.
- Hypokalemia occurs because alkalosis shifts the potassium intracellularly.
- Alkalosis decreases ionized calcium.

Smith AL, Wollman H. Cerebral blood flow and metabolism: effects of anesthetic drugs and techniques. *Anesthesiology* 1972;36:378–400.

Yao FSF, Tseng CC, Yu J, et al. Relationship between E TCO$_2$ and cerebral oxygen saturation. *Anesthesiology* 2000;93(3A):A320.

C.II-26.   The arterial blood gases and electrolytes during CPB are pH, 7.36; PaCO$_2$, 42 mm Hg; PaO$_2$, 449 mm Hg; CO$_2$ content, 24 mEq per L; Na, 128 mEq per L; K, 5.8 mEq per L; Ht, 20%. The patient's temperature is 27°C (80.6°F). At what temperature are blood gases measured? How would you correct the blood gases according to patient's body temperature? Would you treat the arterial blood gases at 37°C (98.6°F) or at patient's body temperature?

Blood gases are measured at a constant temperature of 37°C (98.6°F). They may be corrected according to body temperature. Each degree centigrade below 37°C (98.6°F) increases blood pH by 0.015. If pH is 7.40 at 37°C (98.6°F) *in vitro, in vivo* pH will be 7.55 at 27°C (80.6°F) body temperature $(7.40 + 0.015 \times [37 - 27] = 7.55)$. The pH increases at lower temperatures, because of increased Pka and decreased CO_2 tension from increased CO_2 blood solubility during hypothermia. *In vivo* Pao_2 is decreased because of increased oxygen solubility during hypothermia. At the New York Presbyterian Hospital-Cornell Medical Center, we measure blood gases at 37°C (98.6°F) and interpret at 37°C (98.6°F) without correcting them to body temperature. The normal values of blood gases at 37°C (98.6°F) are pH 7.40 ± 0.05, $Paco_2$ 40 ± 5, Pao_2 95 ± 5; During hypothermia, the normal values of blood gases are not the same as those at 37°C (98.6°F).

The same blood specimen has different PO_2 values when measured at different temperatures. Yet, the oxygen content remains unchanged. It is easier to calculate the oxygen content at 37°C (98.6°F) than at other temperatures where oxygen dissociation curves are shifted.

Optimal management of pH and $PaCO_2$ for patients undergoing hypothermic CPB remains controversial. The two strategies for interpreting blood gases are the pH-stat (temperature-corrected) method and the alpha-stat (temperature-uncorrected) method. The pH-stat strategy aims at keeping constant arterial pH at 7.40 and $PaCO_2$ at 40 mm Hg at any given temperature. A $PaCO_2$ of 60 mm Hg analyzed at 37°C (98.6°F) would be equivalent to a $PaCO_2$ of 40 mm Hg if "corrected" for a body temperature of 27°C (80.6°F). The alpha-stat strategy aims at keeping a constant ratio of $[OH^-] : [H^+]$ at approximately 16:1. This is based on the premise that the pH of blood is regulated to keep the state of dissociation of imidazole moiety (i.e., the alpha of imidazole) constant. Histidine, which contains the imidazole moiety, is an integral part of the active site of many enzyme systems. The function of enzyme systems has been shown to be optimal when the ratio of $[OH^-] : [H^+]$ is approximately 16:1. This ratio represents different pH values at different temperatures.

The differences between pH-stat and alpha-stat strategies are listed in Table 7.3. With the pH-stat strategy, the blood gas values are corrected to the patient's temperature; the patient is treated as if he were a hibernating animal. With the alpha-stat strategy, the blood gas values are not corrected regardless of the patient's actual temperature; the patient is treated as if he were a poikilotherm. Studies indicate that myocardial function is better preserved when the alpha-stat strategy is employed. Moreover, maintenance of cerebral blood flow autoregulation appears to remain intact with alpha-stat management, whereas flow becomes pressure dependent with pH-stat management. Therefore, most medical centers use alpha-stat management of blood gases during hypothermic CPB. However, Bashein et al. found no difference in neuropsychologic outcome between patients randomized to alpha-stat or pH-stat management.

However, more recent studies have shown less decline in cognitive performance when alpha-stat management is used, especially in cases with prolonged CPB times. This data may support an embolic threshold above which recognizable neurologic injury occurs.

During deep hypothermic circulatory (DHCA) both animal and clinical studies have shown that pH-stat is associated with better neurologic outcome probably because of increased cerebral blood flow, which provides better brain cooling and greater cellular oxygen availability. In summary, most recent outcome studies support the utilization of alpha-stat for adult CPB and pH-stat for children under DHCA.

Bashein G, Townes BD, Nessly ML, et al. A randomized study of carbon dioxide management during hypothermic cardiopulmonary bypass. *Anesthesiology* 1990;72:7–15.

Dahlbacka S, Heikkinen J, Kaakinen T, et al. pH-stat versus alpha-stat acid-base management strategy during hypothermic circulatory arrest combined with embolic brain injury. *Ann Thorac Surg* 2005;79(4):1316–1325.

Gravlee GP, Davis RF, Kurusz M, et al. *Cardiopulmonary bypass, principles and practice.* Philadelphia: Lippincott Williams & Wilkins, 2000:199–204.

Iglesias I, Murkin JM. Central nervous system dysfunction after cardiopulmonary bypass. In: Kaplan JA, Reich DSN, Lake CL, et al. eds. *Kaplan's cardiac anesthesia*, 5th ed. Philadelphia: Elsevier Science, WB Saunders, 2006:1116–1117.

Jonas RA. Hypothermia, circulatory arrest and the paediatric brain. *J Cardiothorac Vasc Anesth* 1996;10:6–74.

Murkin JM, Farrar JK, Tweed WA, et al. Cerebral autoregulation and flow/metabolism coupling during cardiopulmonary bypass: the influence of $PaCO_2$. *Anesth Analg* 1987;66: 825–832.

Table 7.3 Different Hypothermic Acid-Base Regulatory Strategies.

STRATEGY	AIM	TOTAL CO_2 CONTENT	pH AND $PaCO_2$ MAINTENANCE	INTRACELLULAR STATE	α-IMIDAZOLE AND BUFFERING	ENZYME STRUCTURE AND FUNCTION	CEREBRAL BLOOD FLOW AND COUPLING	EFFECT ON ISCHEMIC TISSUE
pH-stat	Constant pH	Increases	Normal corrected values	Acidotic (excess H^+)	Excess (+) charge	Altered and activity decreased	Flow close to normothermic	? Lessens hypothermic protection
					Buffering decreased		? Flow and metabolism uncoupled	
Alpha-stat	Constant OH^-/H^+	Constant	Normal uncorrected values	Neutral ($H^- = OH^-$)	Constant net charge	Normal and activity maximal	Flow decreases (appropriate)	? Allows full hypothermic protection
					Buffering constant		? Flow and metabolism coupled	

From Tinker JH, ed. *Cardiopulmonary bypass: current concepts and controversies.* Philadelphia: JB Lippincott Co., 1989:16, with permission.

Murkin JM, Martzke JS, Buchan AM, et al. A randomized study of the influence of perfusion technique and pH management strategy in 316 patients undergoing coronary artery bypass surgery. II. Neurologic and cognitive outcomes. *J Thorac Cardiovasc Surg* 1995; 110:349–362.

O'Dwyer C, Prough DS, Johnston WE. Determinants of cerebral perfusion during cardiopulmonary bypass. *J Cardiothorac Vasc Anesth* 1996;10:54–65.

Pokela M, Dahlbacka S, Biancari F, et al. pH-stat versus alpha-stat perfusion strategy during experimental hypothermic circulatory arrest: a microdialysis study. *Ann Thorac Surg* 2003;76(4):1215–1226.

Prough DS, Stump DA, Roy RC, et al. Response of cerebral blood flow to phenylephrine infusion during hypothermic cardiopulmonary bypass: influence of $PaCO_2$. *Anesthesiology* 1986;64:576–581.

Tallman RD. Acid-base regulation, alpha-stat, and the emperor's new clothes. *J Cardiothorac Vasc Anesth* 1997;11:282–288.

C.II-27. If the blood level of the venous reservoir is low, what would you replace it with? Blood or balanced salt solution?

We try to maintain a hematocrit of at least 18% to 20% during hemodilution. If the hematocrit decreases below 18% to 20%, blood is added to the CPB circuit. If the hematocrit is above 20%, a balanced salt solution (Normosol) is added to the oxygenator. However, hematocrit values in the range of 15% to 18% appear to be well tolerated clinically. When cerebral oxygen saturation (rSO_2) is less than 40%, we use packed red cells to improve oxygen carrying capacity. When rSO_2 is over 40%, it means the patient has acceptable cerebral oxygenation although hematocrit is below 18%.

Gravlee GP, Davis RF, Kurusz M, et al. *Cardiopulmonary bypass, principles and practice.* Philadelphia: Lippincott Williams & Wilkins, 2000:435–442.

Yao FSF, Tseng CC, Woo D, et al. Maintaining cerebral oxygen saturation during cardiac surgery decreased neurological complications. *Anesthesiology* 2001;95:A152.

C.II-28. How do you estimate the fluid balance during CPB?

During CPB, all intravenous lines are shut off. The intake includes cardioplegic solution, fluid or blood added to the oxygenator during CPB, and the decreased blood level in the oxygenator. The output includes urine and the increased blood level in the oxygenator.

C.II-29. How would you preserve the myocardium during CPB?

The most popular and effective method of protecting the myocardium is to reduce myocardial oxygen demand by hypothermia and cardioplegia. Hypothermia is induced by a combination of systemic blood cooling by heat exchangers in the oxygenator, local application of cold saline solution or iced slush to the external surface and chambers of the heart (if the heart is open), and infusion of cold cardioplegic solution through the aortic root, venous grafts, retrograde coronary sinus, or coronary ostium to the coronary arterial tree. The myocardial temperature may be decreased to 10°C to 15°C (50°F to 59°F).

In addition to inducing hypothermia and cardioplegia, one may take the following measures before aortic cross-clamping:

- Avoid tachycardia or increased contractility by discontinuing pacing at rapid rate and discontinuing inotropes if they were utilized.

- Initiating rapid arrest (asystole)
- Utilize proper venting methods and ensure adequate venous drainage to the pump to avoid ventricular distention, which decreases subendocardial blood supply.
- Prevent and treat ventricular fibrillation, which increases oxygen demand in normothermic myocardium.
- Maintain adequate coronary perfusion pressure of at least 50 mm Hg and greater than 70 mm Hg in the presence of severe coronary disease or left ventricular hypertrophy.

Gravlee GP, Davis RF, Kurusz M, et al. *Cardiopulmonary bypass, principles and practice.* Philadelphia: Lippincott Williams & Wilkins, 2000:228–250.

C.II-30. What is the cardioplegic solution? How much would you use?

Cardioplegic solution contains mainly high concentrations of potassium (10 to 30 mEq/L) or magnesium (160 mEq/L) to relax the heart. Flaccid cardioplegia itself reduces myocardial oxygen consumption and provides optimal conditions for surgery. Bicarbonate or tris(hydroxymethyl)-aminomethane (THAM) is usually added to raise the pH to levels between 7.40 and 7.80 to increase the intracellular shift of potassium and to decrease the metabolic acidosis from ischemia. Steroids, calcium, and procaine may be added to stabilize lysosomal and cell membranes. Glucose and insulin are added to provide energy and improve the intracellular shift of potassium. Nitroglycerin is added to dilate coronary vessels, resulting in better perfusion to the myocardium, including ischemic areas. At the New York Presbyterian Hospital-Cornell Medical Center, for crystalloid cardioplegia we add 20 mEq of potassium chloride and 10 mEq of sodium bicarbonate to 1,000 mL of 5% glucose in a 0.225% salt solution, resulting in a final pH of 7.83, potassium of 20 mEq per L, and osmolarity of 380 mOsm per L.

When blood cardioplegia is used, four parts of bypass blood are mixed with one part of cardioplegic solution. The composition of full-strength solution is as follows: 500 mL of 5% glucose in a 0.225% salt solution, 70 mEq of potassium chloride, 10 mEq of sodium bicarbonate, and 1 mg of nitroglycerin. Blood cardioplegia seems to have several advantages over crystalloid cardioplegia. The heart is arrested while being oxygenated, so that adenosine triphosphate (ATP) is not depleted before asystole. Repeated infusions provide a source of oxygen and glucose for continued metabolism and ATP repletion. Although little oxygen is released from hemoglobin during hypothermia, enough is probably dissolved in the plasma to sustain metabolism when reinfusion is performed every 30 minutes. Buffering capacity is improved because of the presence of the histidine buffering system present in red cells. Myocardial edema is reduced because of the osmolarity of blood. The risk of calcium paradox following ischemia is reduced and functional recovery is improved because of the physiologic calcium concentration provided by blood. The presence of red cell enzyme catalase may scavenge free radicals produced by ischemia. Capillary perfusion is improved and more homogeneous because of the presence of red cells. However, results of clinical studies in which blood cardioplegia was compared with crystalloid cardioplegia either detected no significant difference or showed that blood cardioplegia improved contractility late in the postoperative course. Multiple-dose cardioplegia is required for satisfactory results, whereas single-dose blood cardioplegia results in poor ventricular function.

Intermittent, continuous, or single infusions of cardioplegic solution have been used. Usually 300 to 600 ml of cold cardioplegic solution is needed to paralyze the myocardium and cool the myocardium to 10°C to 20°C (50°F to 68°F).

In the case of severe obstructive coronary lesions, antegrade infusion into the aortic root may cause maldistribution of the cardioplegia. Therefore, retrograde infusion through the coronary sinus into the coronary veins may be additionally employed to ensure homogeneous distribution of cardioplegia.

In the late 1980s and early 1990s warm cardioplegia with near-systemic normothermia was popular for better myocardial protection. However, one study identified a threefold increase in strokes in the "warm" patients. The technique is no longer popular.

Gravlee GP, Davis RF, Kurusz M, et al. *Cardiopulmonary bypass, principles and practice.* Philadelphia: Lippincott Williams & Wilkins, 2000:214–215, 228–250.

Mclean RF, Wong BI. Normothermic versus hypothermic cardiopulmonary bypass: central nervous system outcomes. *J Cardiothorac Vasc Anesth* 1996;10:45–53.

Shapiro N, Kirsh M, Jochim K, et al. Comparison of the effect of blood cardioplegia to crystalloid cardioplegia on myocardial contractility in man. *J Thorac Cardiovasc Surg* 1980;80:647.

C.II-31. For how long a period can the aorta be cross-clamped?

When cardio-protective strategies including intermittent hypothermic blood cardioplegia, initiation of rapid arrest and left ventricular venting are employed, the limits of "safe" ischemic time during aortic cross-clamping can be increased from as little as 15 to 45 minutes to as much as 240 minutes in animal models with normal ventricular function. However, many patients have preoperative ventricular dysfunction and the protection from hypothermic cardioplegia may not be optimal because of coronary artery obstruction. Clinically, the aorta may be safely cross-clamped for 60 to 120 minutes without perfusion. The shorter the cross-clamping time, the better the myocardial function will be.

Gravlee GP, Davis RF, Kurusz M, et al. *Cardiopulmonary bypass, principles and practice.* Philadelphia: Lippincott Williams & Wilkins, 2000:217.

Rosenkranz GR, Buckberg CD. Myocardial protection during surgical coronary reperfusion. *J Am Coll Cardiol* 1983;1:12354–11246.

C.II-32. Why does urine become pink after 2 hours of CPB? What is the renal threshold for plasma hemoglobin?

Pink urine is a sign of massive hemolysis. Hemolysis is mainly associated with the frothing, violent turbulence, acceleration, and shear forces of negative pressures generated by the suction apparatus and is associated to a lesser degree with the action of the pumps or with the gas-blood interface effects in the oxygenator. The renal threshold for hemoglobin is 100 to 150 mg per 100 mL. It is advisable to maintain a high output of alkaline urine to prevent possible tubular damage from acid hematin crystals, which are converted from hemoglobin.

Gravlee GP, Davis RF, Kurusz M, et al. *Cardiopulmonary bypass, principles and practice.* Philadelphia: Lippincott Williams & Wilkins, 2000:42, 59, 99.

C.II-33. At what temperature can the patient be weaned from CPB?

An esophageal or nasopharyngeal temperature of 37°C (98.6°F) and a rectal or bladder temperature at least 35°C (95°F) must be reached before the patient can come off the pump. After discontinuation of the pump, surface warming should be continued in pediatric patients to prevent hypothermia owing to redistribution of heat in the body. However, in adults the use of warming blankets and warmed humidified airway gases has not been found beneficial in preventing the expected temperature "afterdrop." Usually, esophageal or nasopharyngeal temperature will decrease and rectal or bladder temperature will increase during heat redistribution.

DiNardo JA, Schwartz MJ, eds. *Anesthesia for cardiac surgery*. Norwalk: Appleton & Lange, 1990:236.

Gravlee GP, Davis RF, Kurusz M, et al. *Cardiopulmonary bypass, principles and practice*. Philadelphia: Lippincott Williams & Wilkins, 2000:613–614.

C.II-34. Why does it take longer to rewarm than to cool the patient by the pump oxygenator?

It usually takes 5 to 10 minutes to cool the patient from 37°C to 25°C (98.6°F to 77°F) of average body temperature. It takes 20 to 40 minutes to rewarm the patient from 28°C to 35°C (82.4°F to 95°F). The speed of heat exchange by the bloodstream depends on the temperature gradient between venous blood and water in the heat exchanger, the pump blood-flow rate, and the water-flow rate of the heat exchanger. The initial venous blood temperature is 37°C (98.6°F) and the water temperature of the heat exchanger is 0°C to 4°C (32°F to 39.2°F) during cooling, creating a temperature gradient of 34°C to 37°C (93.2°F to 98.6°F). During rewarming, the water temperature is limited to 42°C (107.6°F) or less to prevent denaturation and destruction of blood proteins. The temperature gradient is limited to 10°C (18°F) or less to prevent gas embolism from a decrease of gas solubility in the blood associated with a sharp increase in temperature. The heat exchanger water flow does not differ much during cooling and rewarming. However, the pump blood flow is usually maintained to a very high level during the initial cooling because of low BP in the beginning of cooling. During rewarming, the pump blood flow is frequently maintained at a low level because the BP is usually high and the body temperature is still low. Rewarming may be accelerated by administering inhalation anesthetics, or employing vasodilators, to decrease vascular resistance and thereby increase pump flow to maintain the same BP. Because the increased vascular resistance is usually due to inadequate anesthesia during rewarming, we prefer inhalation anesthetics to vasodilators in patients with good ventricular function. In cases of poor ventricular function, inhalation agents are avoided because of the potential cardiac depression after CPB.

Gravlee GP, Davis RF, Kurusz M, et al. *Cardiopulmonary bypass, principles and practice*. Philadelphia: Lippincott Williams & Wilkins, 2000:567–568.

Stanley TH, Berman L, Green O, et al. Plasma catecholamine and cortisol responses to fentanyl-oxygen anesthesia for coronary artery operations. *Anesthesiology* 1980;53: 250–253.

C.II-35. How would you defibrillate the heart internally during CPB?

The heart is defibrillated internally by a DC defibrillator, with 5 to 10 watt-seconds (joules). If the heart remains in ventricular fibrillation, blood gases, electrolytes, and temperature are rechecked and lidocaine, 1 to 2 mg/kg, is administered before repeated DC defibrillation attempts. MAP is usually increased to 80 mm Hg. Occasionally, esmolol, metoprolol, and amiodarone are added to treat intractable ventricular fibrillation or tachycardia.

Shanewise JS, Hines RL, Kaplan JA. Discontinuing cardiopulmonary bypass. In: Kaplan JA, Reich DSN, Lake CL, et al. eds. *Kaplan's cardiac anesthesia*, 5th ed. Philadelphia: Elsevier Science, WB Saunders, 2006:1024–1025.

C.II-36. Why is calcium chloride usually administered right before the patient comes off the pump?

With hemodilution, the ionized calcium frequently falls to approximately 1.5 to 1.8 mEq/L (normal 2.2 to 2.6 mEq/L, 1.1 to 1.3 mmol/L or 4.5 to 5.6 mg/dL). Calcium chloride, 0.5 to 1.0 g, is frequently given to increase myocardial contractility and reverse potassium cardioplegia. Calcium increases the inotropic state of the myocardium and induces an increase in systemic vascular resistance that outlasts the inotropic effects. However, some believe that calcium administration is contraindicated at this time because of the compromised calcium hemostasis that accompanies the insult of aortic cross-clamping. Administration of calcium may exacerbate ischemic and reperfusion injury by causing accumulation of intracellular calcium. β-Blockers, on the other hand, increase intracellular calcium but also promote its reuptake into the sarcoplasmic reticulum and may be more appropriate in this setting. Therefore, use of calcium salts at the conclusion of bypass should be guided by determination of ionized calcium levels. Calcium salts should probably not be given to patients with good ventricular function in the absence of hypocalcemia or hyperkalemia because of the potential detrimental effects of iatrogenic hypercalcemia; whether this is true in patients with ventricular dysfunction is unknown.

Gravlee GP, Davis RF, Kurusz M, et al. *Cardiopulmonary bypass, principles and practice.* Philadelphia: Lippincott Williams & Wilkins, 2000:356–358, 629.

Shanewise JS, Hines RL, Kaplan JA. Discontinuing cardiopulmonary bypass. In: Kaplan JA, Reich DSN, Lake CL, et al. eds. *Kaplan's cardiac anesthesia*, 5th ed. Philadelphia: Elsevier Science, WB Saunders, 2006:1023–1024.

C.II-37. If the HR is 40 beats per minute, what should you do?

A temporary AV block at the end of bypass, because of potassium cardioplegia and ischemic insult during aortic cross-clamping. Although atropine may be theoretically administered to treat sinus or nodal bradycardia, more frequently, a temporary epicardial pacemaker is usually employed. Atrial pacing is preferred because of improved cardiac output when the atrial kick is preserved. Ventricular pacing is necessary if there is complete AV block. AV sequential pacing is indicated when ventricular pacing does not provide adequate cardiac output.

Shanewise JS, Hines RL, Kaplan JA. Discontinuing cardiopulmonary bypass. In: Kaplan JA, Reich DSN, Lake CL, et al. eds. *Kaplan's cardiac anesthesia*, 5th ed. Philadelphia: Elsevier Science, WB Saunders, 2006:1025.

C.II-38. How does the blood sugar level change during CPB? Why? Does hyperglycemia increase neurologic complications during CPB?

Blood sugar levels are elevated during perioperatively in patients undergoing cardiac surgery with use of CPB. Hyperglycemia is most profound during hypothermic CPB with approximately 100% of patients (diabetic and nondiabetic) achieving plasma glucose levels greater than 200 mg/dL. There are several reasons for this: first, the practice of making patients NPO (nothing by mouth) overnight induces a state of starvation, marked by peripheral resistance to insulin at the level of muscle and fatty tissues; therefore, allowing glucose uptake by the brain; second, sympathoadrenal activation in response to surgical stress, also tends to induce a diabetogenic state; third, active-cooling the body during bypass causes a profound reduction in insulin production, induces peripheral insulin resistance, and is associated with renal tubular impairment in glucose regulation; lastly, use of dextrose-containing cardioplegia, is a major contributor to intraoperative hyperglycemia. Of interest, postoperative hyperglycemia continues despite insulin administration and has been shown to remain above normal up to several weeks postoperatively. At the cellular level, the alterations in insulin receptor/resistance are very similar to that of type 2 diabetes. It is controversial as to whether hyperglycemia increases neurologic complications during CPB. Under conditions of limited cerebral oxygen delivery, anaerobic glucose oxidation becomes the primary method of ATP production, resulting in intracellular lactic acidosis. Hyperglycemia, by providing more glucose for anaerobic oxidation, increases the degree of intracellular acidosis, which, in numerous animal studies, correlates with the severity of subsequent injury. Although the deleterious effect of hyperglycemia in the face of both global and focal cerebral ischemia is generally accepted, a recent human study challenges these conclusions. Metz and Keats reported zero neurologic injury in a group of 54 patients undergoing CABG managed with glucose-containing fluids (glucose during bypass—approximately 700 ± 100 mg/dL) versus 1 stroke and 1 case of encephalopathy in 53 patients in whom glucose was avoided during CABG (glucose during bypass—approximately 200 ± 100 mg/dL). The authors contend that glucose does not affect neurologic outcome in the presence of a permanent focal lesion. Although provocative, this study can be faulted for (a) its lack of sensitive monitors of neurologic outcome and (b) its small sample size in relation to the occurrence rate of the event of interest. More recently, there are a number of reports that show a strong association between plasma glucose levels and postoperative morbidity and mortality. Based on these findings, "tight" glucose control is being recommended for all patients undergoing CPB. Achieving optimal glucose control during hypothermic CPB is nearly impossible; however, with use of continuous insulin infusion, plasma glucose levels can be best managed. Regarding the optimal range of glucose control, there continues to be some debate about maintaining plasma glucose below the threshold of 110 mg/dL. From both a practical point and safety issues (hypoglycemia), most would accept target plasma glucose of less than 140 mg per dL as being adequate.

Fontes ML, Koval KJ, Desvarieux T, et al. Epidemiology of hyperglycemia in non-diabetic patients undergoing hypothermic cardiopulmonary bypass. *Anesthesiology* 2006;105:A749.

Fontes ML, Skubas N, Girardi L, et al. Glucosuria during cardiopulmonary bypass: does hypothermia provide protection or a blow to the kidneys? *Anesth Analg* 2007;104.3CA81.

Gravlee GP, Davis RF, Kurusz M, et al. *Cardiopulmonary bypass, principles and practice.* Philadelphia: Lippincott Williams & Wilkins, 2000:414.

Grocott HP, Stafford-Smith M. Organ protection during cardiopulmonary bypass. In: Kaplan JA, Reich DSN, Lake CL, et al. eds. *Kaplan's cardiac anesthesia*, 5th ed. Philadelphia: Elsevier Science, WB Saunders, 2006:992–993.

Hindman B. Con: glucose primary solutions should not be used for cardiopulmonary bypass. *J Cardiothorac Vasc Anesth* 1995;9:605–606.

Lanier WL. Glucose management during cardiopulmonary bypass: cardiovascular and neurologic implications. *Anesth Analg* 1991;72:423–427.

Metz S. Pro: glucose priming solution should be used for cardiopulmonary bypass. *J Cardiothorac Vasc Anesth* 1995;9:603–604.

Metz S, Keats AS. Benefits of a glucose-containing priming solution for cardiopulmonary bypass. *Anesth Analg* 1991;72:428–434.

O'Dwyer C, Prough DS, Johnston WE. Determinants of cerebral perfusion during cardiopulmonary bypass. *J Cardiothorac Vasc Anesth* 1996;10:54–65.

Stanley TH, Berman L, Green O, et al. Plasma catecholamine and cortisol responses to fentanyl-oxygen anesthesia for coronary-artery operations. *Anesthesiology* 1980;53: 250–253.

Wass CT, Lanier WL. Glucose modulation of ischemic brain injury: review and clinical recommendations. *Mayo Clin Proc* 1996;71:801–812.

C.II-39. What are the effects of CPB on platelet and coagulation factors?

Platelet dysfunction and thrombocytopenia are found on and after CPB. Platelet dysfunction is the most common cause of a bleeding problem following CPB after heparin is reversed and surgical bleeding is controlled. Transient defects in platelet plug formation and aggregation are seen in all patients put on CPB. Generally, platelet function returns to near normal status 2 to 4 hours following CPB. The defects are exacerbated and prolonged by drugs such as aspirin and platelet glycoprotein GPIIb/IIIa inhibitors (clopidogrel, tirofiban), which inhibit platelet function.

Platelet counts fall more with the bubble-type oxygenator than with the membrane-type oxygenator, but rarely below the levels clinically required for hemostasis. Thrombocytopenia is mainly caused by hemodilution, aggregation, adhesion, and the adenosine diphosphate (ADP)-release reaction induced by the foreign surfaces and the blood-gas interface. Heparin may potentiate platelet aggregation and adhesions.

The level of coagulation factors decreases at the beginning of bypass because of hemodilution; surface absorption by the plastic, glass, and metal; and protein denaturation induced by the blood-gas interface. At the same time, the synthesis of clotting factors by the liver increases so that the concentration of clotting factors returns to normal within a period of hours. Membrane oxygenators cause few changes in clotting factors.

Gravlee GP, Davis RF, Kurusz M, et al. *Cardiopulmonary bypass, principles and practice.* Philadelphia: Lippincott Williams & Wilkins, 2000:497–500.

C.II-40. How would you prepare for termination of CPB?

Before termination of CPB, cardiac and pulmonary function must be optimized. To ensure that all-important steps are not inadvertently omitted, the patient and all monitors should be carefully checked. The mnemonic LAMPS for Laboratory data, Anesthesia machine, Monitors, Patient (Pump), and Support is one useful approach.

Laboratory Data

- Arterial pH, P_{CO_2}, P_{O_2} within normal limits
- Hematocrit—20% to 25%
- K^+ —4.0 to 5.5 mEq per L
- Ionized calcium 1.1 to 1.2 mmol per L
- Pump mixed venous O_2 saturation greater than 70%

Anesthesia/Machine

- Adequate anesthesia
- Anesthesia machine functional

Monitors

- ECG—stable rate and rhythm (use pacing if necessary)
- Systemic BP restored to normothermic levels
- PA catheter functional
- Transducers rezeroed and calibrated
- TEE out of freeze mode
- Nasopharyngeal/PA catheter temperature 36°C to 37°C (96.8°F to 98.6°F)
- Bladder/rectal temperature greater than 35°C (95°F)

Patient/Pump

- The heart—contractility, size, rhythm, and air removed
- The lungs—atelectasis re-expanded, fluid in thoracic cavities drained, ventilation reinstituted

Support

- Inotropes/vasopressors/vasodilators
- IABP if needed

Gravlee GP, Davis RF, Kurusz M, et al. *Cardiopulmonary bypass, principles and practice.* Philadelphia: Lippincott Williams & Wilkins, 2000:614.

Shanewise JS, Hines RL, Kaplan JA. Discontinuing cardiopulmonary bypass. In: Kaplan JA, Reich DSN, Lake CL, et al. eds. *Kaplan's cardiac anesthesia*, 5th ed. Philadelphia: Elsevier Science, WB Saunders, 2006:1023–1026.

C.II-41. How would you decide the need for inotropic support?

The need for inotropic support after CPB is usually assessed by the following (Fig. 7.9):

- Preoperative ventricular function (ejection fraction)
- Effectiveness of intraoperative myocardial protection
- Adequacy of surgical repair
- Duration of aortic cross-clamping and CPB
- Patient's age

If LVEF is predicted to be 25% to 35%, milrinone infusion may be added. Norepinephrine infusion is usually needed during milrinone therapy. Generally, intraaortic balloon pump is also employed when LVEF is predicted to be below 25%. The choice of vasoactive and cardioactive agents used is frequently center and/or physician specific and, in most cases, initiated as prophylaxis. Recent data suggests that this practice should be avoided because inotropic and vasopressors can have negative effects, which can result in both morbid and fatal events.

Gravlee GP, Davis RF, Kurusz M, et al. *Cardiopulmonary bypass, principles and practice.* Philadelphia: Lippincott Williams & Wilkins, 2000:617–618.

Shanewise JS, Hines RL, Kaplan JA. Discontinuing cardiopulmonary bypass. In: Kaplan JA, Reich DSN, Lake CL, et al. eds. *Kaplan's cardiac anesthesia*, 5th ed. Philadelphia: Elsevier Science, WB Saunders, 2006:1024–1034.

C.III. After Cardiopulmonary Bypass

C.III-1. How would you reverse heparin? How much protamine would you use? What are the other drugs used to neutralize heparin?

It has been recommended that 1.1 to 1.3 mg of protamine sulfate is needed to reverse each 100 units of remaining heparin calculated by ACT dose-response curve or protamine titration test. At the New York Presbyterian Hospital-Cornell Medical Center, we give 1.0 mg of protamine to reverse each 100 units or 1 mg of heparin initially administered. Only the initial dose of heparin is counted. The subsequently added dose of heparin, to keep the ACT level above 480 seconds, is not considered because of its metabolism and elimination. The ACT test is repeated 10 minutes after the administration of protamine. ACT usually returns to its control level. If the ACT is still prolonged, additional protamine is given according to the ACT dose-response curve. However,

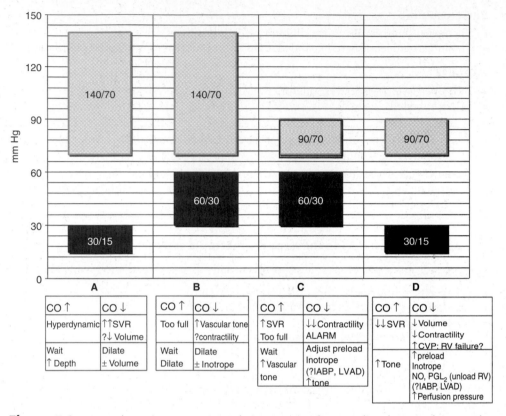

CO ↑	CO ↓	CO ↑	CO ↓	CO ↑	CO ↓	CO ↑	CO ↓
Hyperdynamic	↑↑SVR ?↓ Volume	Too full	↑Vascular tone ?contractility	↑SVR Too full	↓↓Contractility ALARM	↓↓SVR	↓ Volume ↓Contractility ↑CVP: RV failure?
Wait ↑ Depth	Dilate ± Volume	Wait Dilate	Dilate ± Inotrope	Wait ↑Vascular tone	Adjust preload Inotrope (?IABP, LVAD) ↑tone	↑Tone	↑preload Inotrope NO, PGL₂ (unload RV) (?IABP, LVAD) ↑Perfusion pressure

Figure 7.9 Hemodynamic management during weaning from cardiopulmonary bypass. The hemodynamic evaluation is performed by combining information from the systemic (light shade boxes) and pulmonary (black boxes) arterial pressures. **A:** a combination of elevated systemic arterial and low pulmonary arterial pressure suggests either a hyperdynamic cardiac function (if cardiac output is high) or a vasoconstrictive state (if the peripheral vascular resistance is high); **B:** if systemic hypertension is accompanied by pulmonary hypertension, then either the volume status is elevated (if cardiac output is high), or there is generalized vasoconstriction (if cardiac output is decreased). **C:** in case of systemic hypotension and pulmonary hypertension, the cardiac output may be high (systemic vasodilation) or low (depressed contractility, requiring immediate intervention). **D:** when both systemic and pulmonary pressures are decreased, there is either vasodilation (if the cardiac output is high) or hypovolemia or depressed contractility or right-sided failure are suspected (if cardiac output is decreased). The relative treatment for each hemodynamic derangement is shown in the table. CO, cardiac output; CVP, central venous pressure; IABP, intraaortic balloon pump; LVAD, left ventricular assist device; NO, nitric oxide; PGI₂, prostacyclin; RV, right ventricle; SVR, systemic vascular resistance ↑, increase; ↑↑, marked increase; ?, questionable.

the ACT is affected by dilution and by hypothermia; dose-response curves utilizing data obtained during hypothermia may be misleading. In addition, severe thrombocytopenia also prolongs the ACT because clot formation using the ACT depends on platelet phospholipids surface. Furthermore, because heparin rebound is possible, it may be optimal to administer protamine at two times following CPB: once after bypass and again 1 or 2 hours later to counteract heparin rebound.

Other drugs that have been used to neutralize heparin include platelet factor 4 (PF4), heparinase, protamine variants, polybrene, and toluidine blue. Human or recombinant PF4 has been used in animals and humans to reverse heparin and does not cause systemic arterial hypotension, or pulmonary hypertension, or changes in white blood cell count, platelet count, or complement levels. Heparinase neutralizes heparin by enzymatic cleavage of α-glycoside linkages at AT III binding site. Heparinase is an effective antagonist of heparin and has minimal effects on platelets, whereas protamine markedly inhibits platelets responsiveness. It appears to be a potential alternative to protamine.

Two protamine variants, so-called "designer protamines" are currently under investigation. The side effects of protamine such as hypotension and low cardiac output were significantly reduced by the protamine variants. Polybrene, also known as hexadimethrine bromide, at one time was commonly used, but it was withdrawn from clinical use because of suspected nephrotoxicity and production of pulmonary hypertension. Toluidine blue has also been used for heparin reversal, but it is less effective than protamine and is associated with methemoglobinemia.

Gravlee GP, Davis RF, Kurusz M, et al. *Cardiopulmonary bypass, principles and practice.* Philadelphia: Lippincott Williams & Wilkins, 2000:473–478.

Spiess BD, Horrow J, Kaplan JA. Transfusion medicine and coagulation disorders. In: Kaplan JA, Reich DSN, Lake CL, et al. eds. *Kaplan's cardiac anesthesia*, 5th ed. Philadelphia: Elsevier Science, WB Saunders, 2006:958–966.

C.III-2. What is the action mechanism of protamine?

Heparin is a strong organic acid (polyanion). Protamine is a strong organic base (polycation). They combine ionically to form a stable salt and lose their own anticoagulant activity. Protamine contains two active sites, one that neutralizes heparin and another that exerts a mild anticoagulant effect independent of heparin.

Gravlee GP, Davis RF, Kurusz M, et al. *Cardiopulmonary bypass, principles and practice.* Philadelphia: Lippincott Williams & Wilkins, 2000:471.

Spiess BD, Horrow J, Kaplan JA. Transfusion medicine and coagulation disorders. In: Kaplan JA, Reich DSN, Lake CL, et al. eds. *Kaplan's cardiac anesthesia*, 5th ed. Philadelphia: Elsevier Science, WB Saunders, 2006:959.

C.III-3. What are the complications of too much protamine?

Protamine itself is an anticoagulant. Protamine administered intravenously in the absence of heparin interacts with platelets and with many clotting proteins. Protamine induces transient thrombocytopenia in humans. Platelet aggregation is impaired by the protamine–heparin complex, but protamine alone has no deleterious effects. Protamine may bind to thrombin and inhibit thrombin's ability to convert fibrinogen to fibrin.

However, it has been shown that excess protamine minimally increases the Lee-White whole-blood coagulation time. After 600 mg for every 70 kg body weight of protamine, the clotting time increased from 6.7 minutes to 8.2 minutes in unheparinized volunteers; the PTT was not affected. In addition, the clotting time returned to baseline within 30 minutes. The results were similar in patients undergoing CPB. Therefore, protamine does inhibit coagulation *in vitro* and does minimally prolong clotting time in volunteers and in patients. However, the doses needed to achieve clinical anticoagulant effects are more than double those used routinely and greater than three to four times the dose shown to result in return of adequate coagulation. Because of protamine's apparent rapid disappearance and because small doses of heparin do exert an important clinical effect, it seems prudent not to withhold additional doses of protamine in moderation whenever a residual heparin effect is suspected. The danger in giving additional doses of protamine for continued bleeding is that the hemostatic defect may not be due to residual heparin. Therefore, the search for and correction of the real hemostatic defect may be delayed or forgotten.

Gravlee GP, Davis RF, Kurusz M, et al. *Cardiopulmonary bypass, principles and practice.* Philadelphia: Lippincott Williams & Wilkins, 2000:473.

Spiess BD, Horrow J, Kaplan JA. Transfusion medicine and coagulation disorders. In: Kaplan JA, Reich DSN, Lake CL, et al. eds. *Kaplan's cardiac anesthesia*, 5th ed. Philadelphia: Elsevier Science, WB Saunders, 2006:960.

C.III-4. Why did the patient develop hypotension after protamine was administered? How do you treat and prevent this condition?

Three different types of circulatory reactions to protamine reversal of heparin have been proposed by Horrow:

Type I: Systemic Hypotension from Rapid Injection: A Predictable Pharmacologic Reaction
Type II: Anaphylactic or Anaphylactoid Reaction
- Antibody-medicated
- Immediate anaphylactoid response without antibody involvement
- Delayed anaphylactoid response (? noncardiac pulmonary edema)

Type III: Catastrophic Pulmonary Vasoconstriction with Systemic Hypotension
However, etiologically there are only two types of reaction: (a) pharmacologic side-effect reactions and (b) idiosyncratic reactions. Therefore, an alternative classification was proposed by Moorman, Zapl, and Lowenstein as follows:
- Pharmacologic histamine release
- True anaphylaxis (IgE-mediated)
- Anaphylactoid reactions
  Pulmonary vasoconstriction
  Noncardiogenic pulmonary edema

Mild to moderate systemic hypotension from pharmacologic side-effects is almost always the reaction seen when protamine is given rapidly or is given to patients who are relatively hypovolemic and vasoconstricted. Because it can be elicited in most patients, it is classified as a pharmacologic side-effect, not an idiosyncratic reaction. This side-effect is possibly mediated by histamine and is characterized by venodilation, reduced cardiac filling pressures, and decreased vascular resistance. Mild cardiac depression by protamine is suggested but probably does not occur. This type of hypotension can be corrected by rapid volume administration from a CPB pump and phenylephrine in 0.1-mg increments. There have been many attempts to modify the hypotensive response (e.g., intraaortic or left atrial administration, protamine pretreatment), with little evidence of predictable success. Only slower rates of intravenous infusion over 5 to 10 minutes and simultaneous maintenance of an adequate blood volume have been shown to decrease the incidence of hypotension.

Anaphylactic or anaphylactoid reaction is uncommon and rarely seen in infants and children. The reaction varies from mild skin flushing and urticaria to severe vascular collapse. Systemic hypotension is usually accompanied by low pulmonary arterial pressure and low right-sided and left-sided filling pressures. This type of hypotension may be treated and prevented with rapid volume infusion and administration ofvasoconstrictors, antihistamines, and steroids. Diabetic patients taking NPH insulin may develop antibodies to protamine and would appear to be at increased risk. However, clinical reactions do not predictably occur in these patients. Suspected cross-sensitivity in cases of fish allergy or autosensitization in men after vasectomy do not seem to put most patients at increased risk.

Catastrophic pulmonary hypertension occurs in approximately 0.2% to 4.0% of patients. There are several-fold increases in PA pressure leading to right ventricular failure, elevated CVP, low flow across the pulmonary circuit, and low left atrial pressure. Elevated plasma levels of C5a anaphylatoxins and thromboxane are responsible for pulmonary vasoconstriction and accompanied bronchoconstriction. Treatment with isoproterenol, milrinone or amrinone is reasonable; epinephrine in 0.1-mg increments has been successfully used. If severe hypotension persists, the patient should be heparinized again and return back on bypass to maintain circulation. A recent study has shown that left ventricular infusion of protamine provides no protection from pulmonary hypertension and that histamine and platelet-activating factors are not involved in acute pulmonary vasoconstriction. Therefore, antihistamines and steroids may not be effective in preventing this reaction. However, it has been shown that the rate of intravenous protamine infusion in sheep is an important factor in the generation of sufficient mediators required to initiate a characteristic physiologic response, including pulmonary vasoconstriction and thromboxane B_2 generation. Slowing the rate of protamine infusion results in a proportional attenuation of the response (Figs. 7.10 and 7.11).

In conclusion, the treatment of hypotension after protamine administration depends on pulmonary arterial pressure. Hypotension with low pulmonary arterial pressure may be corrected with rapid volume infusion and vasoconstrictors, and hypotension with high pulmonary arterial pressure should be treated with inotropes that have a vasodilating effect. The only effective prevention is a slow infusion of diluted protamine solution.

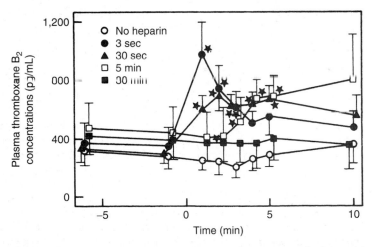

Figure 7.10 Plasma thromboxane B_2 concentrations before and after administration of protamine infused over 3 seconds, 30 seconds, 300 seconds, and 30 minutes. Heparin is injected at 5 minutes; protamine infusion is started at 0 minutes. Data points represent mean $\pm$ SE values; $n = 6$ in each group ($p < 0.05$ from unheparinized group). (From Morel DR, Costabella PMM, Pittet JF. Adverse cardiopulmonary effects and increased plasma thromboxane concentrations following the neutralization of heparin with protamine in awake sheep are infusion rate-dependent. *Anesthesiology* 1990;73:415–424, with permission.)

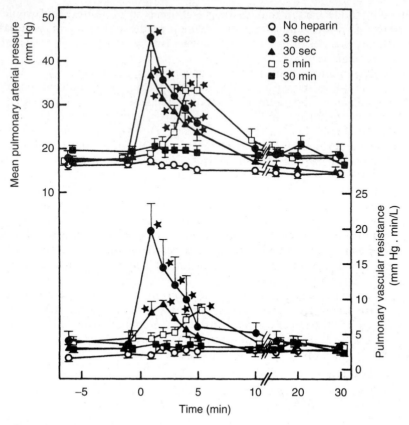

Figure 7.11 Pulmonary hemodynamics before and after administration of protamine infused over 3 seconds, 30 seconds, 300 seconds, and 30 minutes. Heparin is injected at 5 minutes; protamine infusion is started at 0 minutes. Data points represent mean ± SE values; $n = 6$ in each group ($p < 0.05$ from unheparinized group). (From Morel DR, Costabella PMM, Pittet JF. Adverse cardiopulmonary effects and increased plasma thromboxane concentrations following the neutralization of heparin with protamine in awake sheep are infusion rate-dependent. *Anesthesiology* 1990;73:415–424, with permission.)

Recently Yang developed a reactor device containing immobilized protamine (defined as a protamine bioreactor) that can be placed on the distal end of the extracorporeal CPB circuit. The protamine bioreactor binds and selectively removes heparin in the extracorporeal device before it is returned to the patient. The device successfully prevents protamine-induced complications in dogs. It is hoped that in the near future, the device can be used clinically to remove heparin without administration of protamine to the patients.

Coleman RN. Humoral mediators of catastrophic reactions associated with protamine neutralization. *Anesthesiology* 1987;66:595–596.

Gravlee GP, Davis RF, Kurusz M, et al. *Cardiopulmonary bypass, principles and practice.* Philadelphia: Lippincott Williams & Wilkins, 2000:480–488.

Habazettl H, Conzen PF, Vollmar B, et al. Pulmonary hypertension after heparin-protamine: roles of left-sided infusion, histamine and platelet activation factor. *Anesth Analg* 1990; 71:637–637.

Kien ND, Quam DD, Reitan JA, et al. Mechanism of hypotension following rapid infusion of protamine sulfate in anesthetized dogs. *J Cardiothorac Vasc Anesth* 1992;6:143–147.

Morel DR, Costabella PMM, Pittet JF. Adverse cardiopulmonary effects and increased plasma thromboxane concentrations following the neutralization of heparin with protamine in awake sheep are infusion rate-dependent. *Anesthesiology* 1990;73:415–424.

Spiess BD, Horrow J, Kaplan JA. Transfusion medicine and coagulation disorders. In: Kaplan JA, Reich DSN, Lake CL, et al. eds. *Kaplan's cardiac anesthesia*, 5th ed. Philadelphia: Elsevier Science, WB Saunders, 2006:960–965.

C.III-5. What are the indications for intraaortic balloon pump (IABP)?

IABP is primarily used for pump failure and myocardial ischemia that are not responsive to maximal pharmacologic support. The indications include the following:

Ischemic heart disease
- Cardiogenic shock
- Acute myocardial infarction complicated by
  ○ Mechanical defects: ventricular or septal rupture, acute mitral insufficiency, or ventricular aneurysm
  ○ Continued ischemic pain and extension of infarction
  ○ Refractory ventricular arrhythmias
- During cardiac catheterization
- Undergoing noncardiac surgery
- Failed PTCA and awaiting CABG

Cardiac surgery
- Before CPB and postoperatively
- After CPB: low output syndrome

Pulsatile CPB. Rare

Pediatric congenital heart disease. Rare

Neurosurgery. Temporarily increases total cerebral blood flow in specific circumstances.

Gravlee GP, Davis RF, Kurusz M, et al. *Cardiopulmonary bypass, principles and practice.* Philadelphia: Lippincott Williams & Wilkins, 2000:135–136.

Shanewise JS, Hines RL, Kaplan JA. Discontinuing cardiopulmonary bypass. In: Kaplan JA, Reich DSN, Lake CL, et al. eds. *Kaplan's cardiac anesthesia*, 5th ed. Philadelphia: Elsevier Science, WB Saunders, 2006:1034–1039.

Skubas N, Lichtman AD, Shaarma A, et al. Anesthesia for cardiac surgery. In: Barash PG, Cullen BF, Stoelting RK, eds. *Clinical anesthesia*, 5th ed. Philadelphia: Lippincott Williams & Wilkins, 2006:923.

C.III-6. What are the principles of IABP?

IABP counterpulsation is designed to increase the myocardial oxygen supply during diastole and to decrease myocardial oxygen demand during systole (Fig. 7.12). The balloon is inflated during diastole to increase the diastolic aortic pressure, resulting in increased coronary blood flow. The balloon should be inflated immediately following the closure of the aortic valve at the dicrotic notch of arterial tracing. The balloon is deflated just before the next systole to decrease the

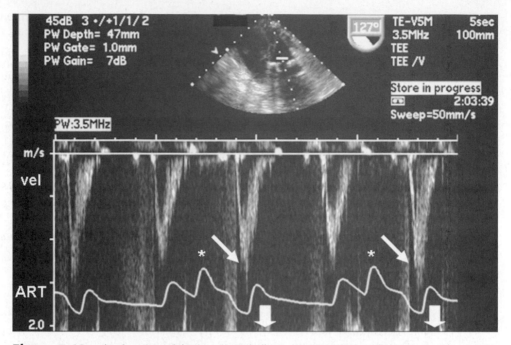

Figure 7.12 The function of the intraaortic balloon pump (IABP). In this patient with an IABP in place, the velocity (vel) of the blood flow, as it exits the left ventricle (LV), is recorded. The arterial waveform is shown in the following text. The IABP is set on a 1:2 ratio, that is, it inflates every other beat, in diastole (*asterisk*). The velocity (and the amount) of blood exiting the LV is increased (*arrow*) after the diastolic inflation of the IABP, because the LV is ejecting against lower systemic resistance. This is the reason, that the systolic arterial pressure following IABP inflation is lower (*down arrow*).

intraaortic pressure and afterload, resulting in decreased myocardial oxygen consumption. The cardiac output is increased because of increased coronary perfusion (diastolic augmentation) and decreased resistance (systolic unloading).

Gravlee GP, Davis RF, Kurusz M, et al. *Cardiopulmonary bypass, principles and practice*. Philadelphia: Lippincott Williams & Wilkins, 2000:135–136.

Shanewise JS, Hines RL, Kaplan JA. Discontinuing cardiopulmonary bypass. In: Kaplan JA, Reich DSN, Lake CL, et al. eds. *Kaplan's cardiac anesthesia*, 5th ed. Philadelphia: Elsevier Science, WB Saunders, 2006:1034.

Skubas N, Lichtman AD, Shaarma A, et al. Anesthesia for cardiac surgery. In: Barash PG, Cullen BF, Stoelting RK, eds. *Clinical anesthesia*, 5th ed. Philadelphia: Lippincott Williams & Wilkins, 2006:923.

C.III-7. What are the complications of intraaortic balloon pump (IABP)?

- Ischemia of the leg
- Dissection of the aorta
- Thrombus formation and embolization
- Renal artery occlusion
- Splenic, mesenteric, and spinal cord infarction

- Internal mammary occlusion
- Thrombocytopenia
- Infection
- Gas embolization
- Inability to place the IABP
- Retroperitoneal bleeding
- Arterial–venous fistula

Gravlee GP, Davis RF, Kurusz M, et al. *Cardiopulmonary bypass, principles and practice.* Philadelphia: Lippincott Williams & Wilkins, 2000:435–442.

Kaplan J, ed. *Cardiac anesthesia*, 4th ed. Philadelphia: WB Saunders, 1999:1201–1202.

Shanewise JS, Hines RL, Kaplan JA. Discontinuing cardiopulmonary bypass. In: Kaplan JA, Reich DSN, Lake CL, et al. eds. *Kaplan's cardiac anesthesia*, 5th ed. Philadelphia: Elsevier Science, WB Saunders, 2006:1036–1038.

Skubas N, Lichtman AD, Shaarma A, et al. Anesthesia for cardiac surgery. In: Barash PG, Cullen BF, Stoelting RK, eds. *Clinical anesthesia*, 5th ed. Philadelphia: Lippincott Williams & Wilkins, 2006:923.

C.III-8. Can pulmonary artery occlusion pressure (PAOP) represent left ventricular end-diastolic volume (LVEDV) after coronary artery bypass grafting (CABG)?

It has been demonstrated that in nonsurgical patients, there was a significant correlation between changes in PAOP and LVEDV. However, in patients during the first few hours after CABG there was a poor correlation between changes in PAOP and LVEDV. The poor correlation was not explained by changes in systemic or pulmonary vascular resistance. The altered ventricular pressure–volume relation may reflect acute changes in ventricular compliance. Although measurement of PAOP remains valuable in clinical management to avoid pulmonary edema, it cannot reliably be used as an index of left ventricular preload while attempting to optimize stroke volume. TEE can accurately assess LVEDV and cardiac contractility.

Harsen RM, Viquerat CE, Matthay MA, et al. Poor correlation between pulmonary arterial wedge pressure and left ventricular end-diastolic volume after coronary artery bypass graft surgery. *Anesthesiology* 1986;64:764–770.

Reich DL, Mittnacht A, London M, et al. Monitoring of the heart and vascular system. In: Kaplan JA, Reich DSN, Lake CL, et al. eds. *Kaplan's cardiac anesthesia*, 5th ed. Philadelphia: Elsevier Science, WB Saunders, 2006:399–401.

D. Postoperative Management

D.1. What are the postoperative complications?

Cardiovascular. Congestive heart failure, arrhythmias, low output syndrome, myocardial ischemia or infarction due to surgical manipulation, prolonged CPB and aortic cross-clamp (coronary ischemia), use of cardioplegic solution, and occlusion or kinking of grafts

Pulmonary. Pump lung or adult respiratory distress syndrome due to the following:
- Decreased blood flow to the lung during total CPB
- Collapsed alveoli during CPB, resulting in decreased surfactant and decreased distensibility

- Fluid overloading
- Hyperoxia during CPB
- Left ventricular failure
- Microemboli

Renal

- Polyuria from hemodilution and diuretics
- Oliguria from hypoperfusion

Hemorrhage

- Too much or too little protamine to reverse heparin
- Thrombocytopenia and decreased coagulation factors
- Disseminated intravascular coagulopathy
- Poor surgical hemostasis

Embolism. Due to air, destroyed or aggregated formed blood elements, fat, endogenous and exogenous debris

Neurologic. Functional changes in behavior, personality, or other brain functions; cerebral embolism

Hyperglycemia. Due to increased catecholamine levels

Hypopotassemia. Due to hemodilution and diuretics

Gravlee GP, Davis RF, Kurusz M, et al. *Cardiopulmonary bypass, principles and practice.* Philadelphia: Lippincott Williams & Wilkins, 2000:382, 403, 506, 628–629.

Levy JH, Tanaka K, Bailey JM, et al. Postoperative cardiovascular management. In: Kaplan JA, Reich DSN, Lake CL, et al. eds. *Kaplan's cardiac anesthesia*, 5th ed. Philadelphia: Elsevier Science, WB Saunders, 2006:1061–1086.

D.2. Would you reverse the muscle relaxants? Why?

No. Muscle relaxants are usually not reversed. When early extubation (fast-track) is planned, pancuronium is given 0.1 mg/kg for intubation and 0.05 to 0.1 mg/kg at the initiation of CPB. Patients should spontaneously recover from the effect of muscle relaxants 2 to 3 hours after surgery. We discourage the use of large doses of long-acting muscle relaxants which may cause recurarization even after reversal with neostigmine. Moreover, reversal with atropine and neostigmine may cause severe tachycardia or bradycardia in cardiac patients.

D.3. When will you wean the patient from the respirator?

Generally, the patient is weaned from the respirator the following morning after surgery. If the operative course is smooth and if the patient has good ventricular function, the patient may be weaned from the respirator early, usually 2 to 6 hours after surgery.

Early tracheal extubation (fast-track) after CABG surgery has cost benefits and improves resource use when compared with late tracheal extubation. Early tracheal extubation 1 to 6 hours after surgery reduces total cost per CABG surgery by 25% without increasing the rate or costs of complications in patients younger than 75 years.

Cheng DC, Havski J, Peniston C, et al. Early tracheal extubation after coronary artery graft surgery reduces costs and improves resource use. *Anesthesiology* 1996;85:1300–1310.

Higgins TL, Yared J-P. Postoperative respiratory care. In: Kaplan JA, Reich DSN, Lake CL, et al. eds. *Kaplan's cardiac anesthesia*, 5th ed. Philadelphia: Elsevier Science, WB Saunders, 2006:1097–1099.

D.4. What criteria would you use in deciding when to wean the patient from the respirator?

- Consciousness—awake and alert
- Stable vital signs
- Acceptable arterial blood gases—pH, 7.35 to 7.45; P_{O_2}, over 80 mm Hg with F_{IO_2}, 0.4; P_{CO_2}, 35 to 45 mm Hg
- Acceptable respiratory mechanics
  - Vital capacity greater than 10 to 15 mL/kg
  - Maximal inspiratory force—greater than 20 to 25 cm H_2O
- Hemostasis—less than 100 mL per hour of chest tube drainage
- Stable metabolic state—normal temperature and electrolytes

When the patient can satisfy the above criteria, the patient is put on continuous positive airway pressure (CPAP) of 5 cm H_2O with 50% oxygen. If the patient tolerates the CPAP well for 30 minutes and arterial blood gases are acceptable, the patient is extubated.

Higgins TL, Yared J-P. Postoperative respiratory care. In: Kaplan JA, Reich DSN, Lake CL, et al. eds. *Kaplan's cardiac anesthesia*, 5th ed. Philadelphia: Elsevier Science, WB Saunders, 2006:1097–1099.

CHAPTER 8

Valvular Heart Disease

GREGG S. HARTMAN • STEPHEN J. THOMAS

A 78-YEAR-OLD MAN

was admitted with increasing shortness of breath. He had chest pain in the past but was able to continue with normal activities. He had passed out twice in the past year. On physical examination, a loud systolic murmur could be heard at the left sternal border radiating to the neck. His vital signs were: blood pressure 150/90 mm Hg, heart rate 88 beats per minute and irregular. The electrocardiogram (ECG) showed sinus rhythm with atrial premature contractions and left ventricular hypertrophy (LVH) with strain. A transthoracic echocardiogram showed a hypertrophied left ventricle (LV) and Doppler examination demonstrated severe aortic stenosis (AS) with a gradient of 64 mm Hg, mild aortic insufficiency (AI), and moderate mitral regurgitation (MR). He was scheduled for aortic valve replacement (AVR) and possible mitral valve (MV) repair or mitral valve replacement (MVR).

A. Medical Disease and Differential Diagnosis

1. What are the major etiologies of AS, AI, mitral stenosis (MS), and MR?
2. What are the major changes in the loading conditions of the LV that result from the four different lesions? Why do they occur? What changes result from them?
3. What are pressure–volume (P–V) loops? What do the different inflection points represent?
4. What are representative P–V loops for the four valvular lesions?
5. Draw the pressure/time curves for the LV, left atrium, pulmonary artery (PA), and aorta (Ao) for a normal patient and for patients with each of the four valvular lesions.
6. What are the basic principles of echocardiography? What are M-mode, B-mode, and Doppler color modalities? How do transthoracic echocardiography (TTE) and transesophageal echocardiography (TEE) differ?
7. What are the three TEE vantage points for the comprehensive imaging of the LV? How are pressure gradients measured by echocardiography? How do the pressure gradients derived from Doppler echocardiography differ from those obtained in the catheterization laboratory by direct pressure measurement?
8. What are the echocardiographic and cardiac catheterization criteria for the four valvular lesions?

B. Preoperative Evaluation and Preparation

1. What are the presenting signs and symptoms of the four valvular lesions listed previously?
2. What is the New York Heart Association (NYHA) classification of heart failure?

3. Discuss the role of premedication for patients with the four different valvular lesions.

4. How would you premedicate the patient with severe aortic stenosis (AS) and mitral regurgitation (MR)?

C. Intraoperative Management

1. Outline the hemodynamic management goals for each of the four valvular lesions. What are the anesthetic goals with respect to heart rate and rhythm, preload, afterload, and contractility?

2. What are the hemodynamic goals for this patient with the combination of severe AS and MR?

3. How would you monitor this patient with severe AS and MR?

4. Should the patient have a PA catheter placed before induction?

5. Is a PA catheter with pacing capabilities indicated?

6. What anesthetic technique will you employ? Why?

7. What muscle relaxant would you use for this patient?

8. What are the usual transesophageal echocardiography (TEE) findings in a patient with AS/AI/MR? How do you grade the severity of AS by TEE? How do you quantify the severity of MR? What is the impact of AS on the severity of MR?

9. What special considerations particular to cardiopulmonary bypass (CPB) operations do you have for each of the four lesions? Focus on these concerns with respect to the induction and prebypass, bypass, and postbypass periods.

10. The patient cannot be weaned from bypass following an aortic valve replacement (AVR) and mitral valve replacement (MVR). What are the possible causes?

11. How would you diagnose right heart failure and pulmonary hypertension? How would you treat it?

12. What role does an intraaortic balloon pump (IABP) have in this setting?

13. How does the IABP work to benefit the failing heart?

14. What role does TEE play in the placement, timing, and demonstration of efficacy of an IABP?

15. How would you properly time the IABP cycle?

16. What are the contraindications to the use of an IABP?

D. Postoperative Management

1. In the intensive care unit (ICU) 4 hours later, the patient became hypotensive with a low cardiac output. How could you distinguish between cardiac tamponade and pump failure? How would the TEE images differ?

2. Would you extubate this patient early in the ICU? Why?

3. What are the advantages and disadvantages of early extubation?

A. Medical Disease and Differential Diagnosis

A.1. What are the major etiologies of AS, AI, MS, and MR?

AS occurs as a congenital lesion but more commonly as an acquired disease. Stenosis may develop on a previously normal valve following rheumatic fever (RF) or from progressive calcification. Congenitally bicuspid valves are also prone to calcification with eventual stenosis. Calcification of the leaflets can result in incomplete closure of the valve with associated insufficiency.

AI is usually an acquired disease. The most common causes include bacterial endocarditis and rheumatic heart disease. Annular dilation may result from diseases such as cystic medial necrosis and collagen disorders or following aortic dissections with resultant insufficiency. When occurring as a congenital lesion, aortic insufficiency (AI) rarely occurs in the absence of other cardiac abnormalities.

Mitral stenosis (MS) is almost always caused by rheumatic fever (RF), although only half of patients will have a history of an acute febrile illness. The inflammatory process of RF results in thickening of the leaflets and fusion of the commissures. Other rare causes include congenital stenosis and other systemic diseases including systemic lupus erythematosus and carcinoid. Pathophysiology similar to that seen with valvular MS can occur with obstructing left atrial (LA) tumors and cor triatriatum. MS commonly occurs in conjunction with other valvular heart disease; only 25% of patients present with isolated MS; approximately 40% have combined MS and mitral regurgitation (MR).

MR can result from defects in the leaflets, the annular ring or the supporting chordae, the papillary muscles, or any combination of these. Primary leaflet dysfunction occurs with RF but can also follow bacterial endocarditis, connective tissue disorders, and congenital malformations. Annular dilation can follow ventricular dysfunction and left ventricular dilation. MV prolapse and/or rupture of papillary muscles results in incomplete leaflet closure or coaptation with resultant MR. Left ventricular ischemia can affect papillary muscle contraction and is the cause of postischemic or postinfarction MR.

Hartman GS. *Management of patients with valvular heart disease*. Cleveland: International Anesthesia Research Society, 1994:141–151. 1994 IARS Review Course Lectures.

Schoen FJ. Cardiac valves and valvular pathology: update on function, disease, repair, and replacement. *Cardiovasc Pathol* 2005;14(4):189–194.

Thys DM, Hillel Z, Schwartz AJ, eds. *Textbook of cardiothoracic anesthesiology*. New York: McGraw-Hill, 2001:589–629.

A.2. What are the major changes in the loading of the left ventricle (LV) that result from the four different lesions? Why do they occur? What changes result from them?

Aortic stenosis (AS) represents a chronic systolic pressure load on the LV. This elevation increases wall tension in accordance with Laplace's law.

$$\text{Wall tension} = \frac{(\text{Pressure} \times \text{radius})}{(2 \times \text{Wall thickness})}$$

The ventricle undergoes parallel duplication of muscle fibers in an attempt to compensate for the increase in tension. This results in increased wall thickness or concentric (common center) hypertrophy and some decrease in radius thereby normalizing wall stress. If the MV remains competent, the major pressure overload occurs in the LV and little change in the other cardiac chambers results.

AI causes left ventricular diastolic volume overload resulting in eccentric (away from the center) hypertrophy and left ventricular dilation. Compliance, the relation between volume and pressure is altered only slightly because both end-systolic and end-diastolic volumes increase. Some concentric hypertrophy occurs as well secondary to the increase in wall stress resulting from an increase in left ventricular radius. The aortic diastolic pressure is lower with AI. Remember, the diastolic pressure is the pressure that must be exceeded by the work of the LV to open the aortic valve and result in ventricular ejection. Therefore, the increased volume work required to eject the additional blood (which flowed into the LV across the incompetent aortic valve during diastole) is reduced because the work can be performed against a lower outflow impedance (lower diastolic pressure). Stroke volume (SV) and ejection fraction (EF), therefore, may be preserved until late in the disease process. As with aortic stenosis (AS), the presence of a competent MV confines the changes to the LV. However, the left ventricular dilation that follows chronic AI may result in mitral annular dilation or alteration in chordae tendineae geometry with resultant mitral regurgitation (MR). Left atrial (LA) enlargement secondary to MR can, therefore, occur. It may also occur because of LA pressure overload as left ventricular end-diastolic pressures (LVEDPs) rise in the course of aortic insufficiency (AI).

Mitral stenosis (MS) results in a chronically underfilled left ventricle (LV) because of progressive obstruction to LA emptying. This chronic underloading condition can result in decreased left ventricular thickness and diminished contractile function (a "disuse atrophy" of sort). In addition, if the cause of the MS is rheumatic, myofibril damage may have occurred. Although the LV is pressure and volume *under*loaded, the left atrium is both pressure and volume *over*loaded. To maintain flow across the progressively narrowing mitral orifice, the pressure in the left atrium must be correspondingly increasing. Gorlin's equation for pressure gradient follows.

$$\text{Pressure gradient} = \left\{ \frac{\text{Flow rate}}{(K \times \text{valve area})} \right\}^2$$

It would predict that the pressure gradient increases by the square of any increase in flow rate or decrease in valve area. The elevations in LA pressure leads to hypertrophy and eventually dilation that predisposes to premature atrial contractions and subsequently atrial fibrillation. The loss of atrial contraction further diminishes forward flow across the stenotic mitral valve (MV). The elevations in LA pressure limit pulmonary venous flow with consequent pulmonary engorgement. The pulmonary vasculature undergoes reactive changes including intimal fibroelastosis inducing irreversible elevations in pulmonary vascular resistance. Right ventricular (RV) failure may develop because this chamber is poorly equipped to deal with the elevations in afterload (e.g., pulmonary hypertension). RV dilation combined with increased RV systolic pressures leads to tricuspid regurgitation.

MR results in volume overload of the LV. The outflow of the LV is divided between the high-pressure/low-compliance outflow tract of the arterial tree and the low-pressure/high-compliance outflow route across the incompetent MV into the left atrium. Although the volume work of the LV is increased, the high-compliance outflow route permits a large portion of this work to be performed at a low pressure; therefore, left ventricular wall tension is minimally increased if increased at all. As with AI, the volume overload results in marked left ventricular dilation and eccentric hypertrophy. In contrast, however, the left atrium is also volume overloaded and undergoes dilation. When the volume overload occurs slowly, the left atrium enlarges and minimal rises in pulmonary pressures result despite large regurgitant volumes. In contrast, the occurrence of acute MR, for example, an acute myocardial infarction with papillary muscle rupture, presents the left atrium with a sudden volume overload. Without the time to dilate, the LA pressure rapidly rises limiting pulmonary drainage with resultant pulmonary engorgement.

Hartman GS. *Management of patients with valvular heart disease*. Cleveland: International Anesthesia Research Society, 1994:141–151. 1994 IARS Review Course Lectures.

Schoen FJ. Cardiac valves and valvular pathology: update on function, disease, repair, and replacement. *Cardiovasc Pathol* 2005;14(4):189–194.

Thys DM, Hillel Z, Schwartz AJ, eds. *Textbook of cardiothoracic anesthesiology*. New York: McGraw-Hill, 2001:589–629.

Zipes DP, Libby P, Bonow RO, et al. eds. *Braunwald's heart disease: a textbook of cardiovascular medicine*, 7th ed. Philadelphia: WB Saunders, 2005:1553–1615.

A.3. What are pressure–volume (P–V) loops? What do the different inflection points represent?

The P–V loop analysis (Fig. 8.1) depicts the relation between left ventricular volume and left ventricular pressure during a single cardiac cycle. Opening and closing of the mitral and aortic valves are represented by the inflection points A, B, C, and D, respectively (Fig. 8.1). Moving from points A through D, AB depicts left ventricular filling, BC depicts isovolumetric contraction, CD shows left ventricular ejection, and DA shows isovolumetric relaxation. Point A coincides with opening of the mitral valve (MV) and represents left ventricular end-systolic volume and early diastolic pressure. Point B is closure of the MV and the end of diastolic pressure (LVEDP) and volume (left ventricular end-diastolic volume [LVEDV]). Point C represents the opening of the aortic valve and coincides with systemic, aortic diastolic pressure. Finally, point D is the closure of the aortic valve and represents left ventricular end-systolic pressure and volume, coinciding with the dicrotic notch in the aortic pressure tracing (Fig. 8.1). Left ventricular compliance is the relation between the change in pressure and change in volume of the chamber and is defined by the slope of the filling phase or segment AB. Preload is the P–V relation before the onset of contraction (LVEDP). Contractility may be illustrated by the slope of a line called the *end-systolic pressure–volume relation* (ESPVR). The ESPVR slope is created by connecting multiple points (D) from multiple P–V loops generated by changing the filling volume to the left ventricle (LV) (Fig. 8.2). Increased contractility results in a steeper line whereas diminished contractility results in a flatter relation. The P–V loop analysis permits illustration of stroke volume (SV) and ejection fraction (EF). SV is defined as difference in volume from the end of filling to the end of ejection (EDV–ESV), whereas EF is the ratio of stroke volume (SV) to total volume in the heart at peak

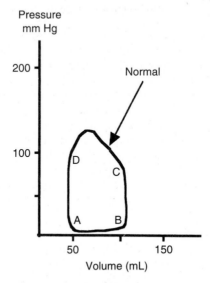

Figure 8.1 Normal pressure–volume loop and valve positions. *A*, mitral valve (MV) opening; *B*, MV closure; *C*, aortic valve (AV) opening; *D*, AV closure; *AB*, left ventricular filling; *BC*, isovolumetric contraction; *CD*, ejection; *DA*, isovolumetric relaxation.

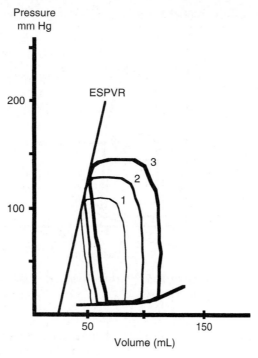

Figure 8.2 Contractility. ESPVR, end-systolic pressure–volume relations.

filling (SV/EDV). Therefore, the P–V loop analysis permits illustration of the volume-pressure relations and their changes with each of the four valvular lesions.

Hartman GS. *Management of patients with valvular heart disease*. Cleveland: International Anesthesia Research Society, 1994:141–151. 1994 IARS Review Course Lectures.

Sagawa K, Maugan L, Suga H, et al. *Cardiac contraction and the pressure-volume relationship*. New York: Oxford University Press, 1988.

Thomas SJ, Kramer JL, eds. *Manual of cardiac anesthesia*, 2nd ed. New York: Churchill Livingstone, 1993:81–127.

A.4. What are representative pressure–volume (P–V) loops for the four valvular lesions?

The hallmarks of aortic stenosis (AS) illustrated by the P–V loop analysis framework are a high left ventricular systolic pressure and an upward and counterclockwise rotation in the end-diastolic P–V relation (AB) indicative of decreased chamber compliance (Fig. 8.3). Stroke volume (SV) and ejection fraction (EF) are well preserved, but the ejection phase of the loop occurs at much higher pressures. This is permitted by an increase in contractility of a counterclockwise rotation of the end-systolic pressure–volume relation (ESPVR) line.

The schematic P–V loop for aortic insufficiency (AI) depicts the enlarged left ventricle (LV) of chronic AI. The minimal change in LVEDP despite the large volume overload is seen by the shift in the diastolic P–V curve to the right (A′B′) (Fig. 8.4). Low systemic diastolic pressures result in a brief isovolumetric phase (B′C′) and early complete ejection. The isovolumetric relaxation

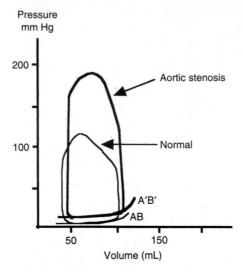

Figure 8.3 Pressure–volume loop of aortic stenosis.

phase is absent as the incompetent valve permits regurgitant filling of the LV from the Ao during diastole even before opening of the MV. In contrast, when acute AI occurs, the left ventricular compliance is unchanged. Rapid increases in left ventricular end-diastolic pressure (LVEDP) from volume overload along the unshifted left ventricular diastolic P–V curve (AB) rapidly lead to increased left atrial (LA) pressure and pulmonary congestion.

The P–V loop of MS illustrates hypovolemia, the cause of which cannot be determined from the loop alone (Fig. 8.5). Because the predominant impact of MS occurs proximal to the LV, the P–V analysis format is less useful.

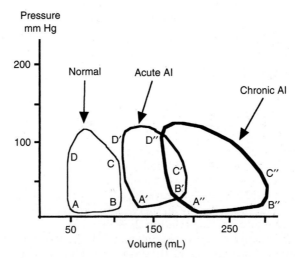

Figure 8.4 Pressure–volume loops of acute and chronic aortic insufficiency (AI).

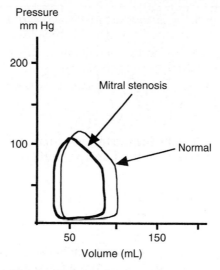

Figure 8.5 Pressure−volume loops of mitral stenosis.

In mitral regurgitation (MR), the diastolic P–V relation (line AB) is shifted to the right, as it is in chronic AI, consistent with a marked increase in compliance (Fig. 8.6). The isovolumetric phase (BC) is nearly absent because the left atrium generally serves as a low-pressure/high-compliance route for ejection because of the incompetent mitral valve (MV). Decreases in contractility are depicted by a decrease in the slope of the end-systolic-PV line (line through D). Nevertheless SV and EF are maintained because of this low-pressure LA vent.

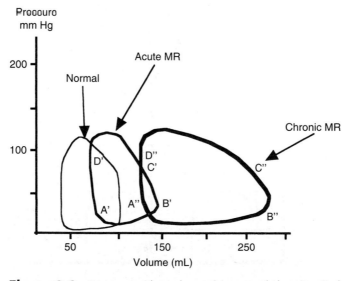

Figure 8.6 Pressure−volume loop of acute and chronic mitral regurgitation (MR).

Hartman GS. *Management of patients with valvular heart disease*. Cleveland: International Anesthesia Research Society, 1994:141–151. 1994 IARS Review Course Lectures.

Sagawa K, Maugan L, Suga H, et al. *Cardiac contraction and the pressure-volume relationship*. New York: Oxford University Press, 1988.

Thomas SJ, Kramer JL, eds. *Manual of cardiac anesthesia*, 2nd ed. New York: Churchill Livingstone, 1993:81–127.

A.5. Draw the pressure/time curves for the left ventricle (LV), left atrium, pulmonary artery (PA) and aorta (Ao) for normal patient and patients with each of the four valvular lesions.

Normal curves are shown in Fig. 8.7. The points A, B, C, and D correspond to the same points in the P–V loops.

Aortic stenosis

The additional systolic pressure work of AS can be seen in the left ventricular pressure tracing (Fig. 8.8). Elevations in left ventricular end-diastolic pressure (LVEDP) (point B) can be seen to diminish the perfusion gradient for coronary flow to the LV. The augmentation in left ventricular filling late in diastole secondary to atrial contraction (LA "kick" from sinus rhythm) is highlighted in the inset. Rising left ventricular diastolic pressures secondary to decreased compliance necessitate elevations in left atrial (LA) pressures to permit complete left ventricular volume

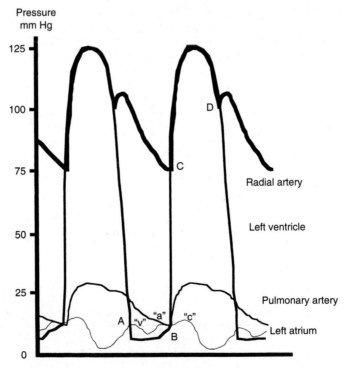

Figure 8.7 Pressure curves for the left ventricle, left atrium, pulmonary artery, and aorta in a healthy individual.

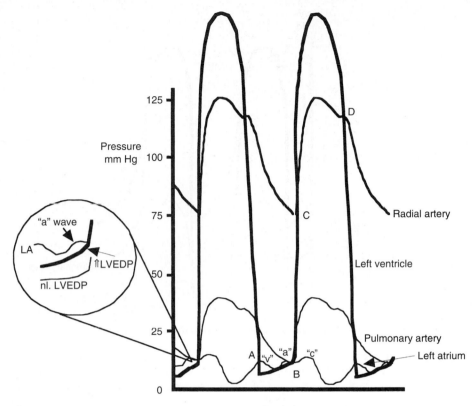

Figure 8.8 Pressure curves for the left ventricle, left atrium (LA), pulmonary artery, and aorta in patients with aortic stenosis. LVEDP, left ventricular end-diastolic pressure.

loading. Atrial systole provides this elevation in LA pressure synchronous with elevations in LVEDP while keeping LA pressures relatively low during the remaining cardiac cycle facilitating pulmonary venous drainage.

Aortic insufficiency

The rapid upstroke and rapid decline of arterial pressure indicate absence of aortic valve closure and low end-diastolic aortic pressure (Fig. 8.9). Elevations in the left ventricular end-diastolic volume (LVEDV) and LVEDP are typical of AI. The early increase in LVEDP can result in left ventricular pressures exceeding those of the left atrium during diastole with resultant premature closure of the MV.

Mitral stenosis

Elevations in pressure are seen in both the left atrial (LA) and pulmonary artery (PA) tracing with mitral stenosis (MS) (Fig. 8.10). The large gradient between LA and left ventricular pressures is highlighted in the inset. Chronic elevation in pulmonary volume induces changes in the luminary vascular bed and leads to pulmonary hypertension.

Mitral regurgitation

The hallmark of MR is the marked elevations of LA pressure during systole and the occurrence of a giant "cv" wave and elevated PA pressures (Fig. 8.11).

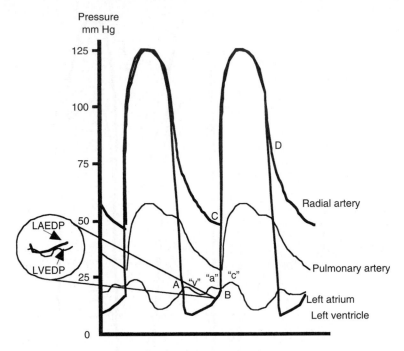

Figure 8.9 Pressure curves for the left ventricle, left atrium, pulmonary artery, and aorta in patients with aortic regurgitation. LAEDP, left atrium end-diastolic pressure; LVEDP, left ventricular end-diastolic pressure.

Hartman GS. *Management of patients with valvular heart disease*. Cleveland: International Anesthesia Research Society, 1994:141–151. 1994 IARS Review Course Lectures.

Kaplan JA, Reich DL, Konstadt SN, eds. *Cardiac anesthesia*, 4th ed. Philadelphia: WB Saunders, 1999:727–784.

A.6. What are the basic principles of echocardiography? What are M-mode, B-mode and Doppler color modalities? How do transthoracic echocardiography (TTE) and transesophageal echocardiography (TEE) differ?

Echocardiography is the use of sound waves to image structures and blood flow within the heart and great vessels. To image tissue, sound waves are emitted from a transducer at known speeds and constant intervals. The sound packets bounce off structures in their path and the reflected sound waves are received at the point of origin, either by a separate receiving crystal or by the same emitting transducer, which spends a portion of its time in this "listening" mode. The time it takes for the reflected waves to return to the crystal is measured, and because the velocity of sound in tissues is relatively constant, solving for distance can be easily accomplished.

$$\text{Distance} = {}^1\!/_2(\text{velocity} \times \text{time})$$

($^1\!/_2$ because the distance is traversed twice, once to the object and again on returning.)

In this manner, the spatial orientation of cardiac structures can be determined. The strength of the returning signal can be quantified as an amplitude, therefore "A" or amplitude mode

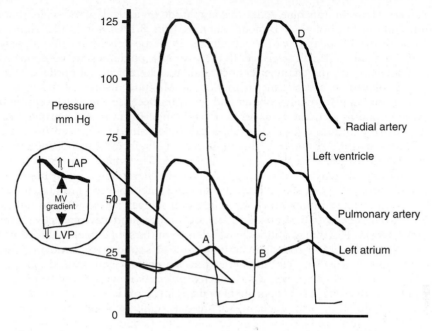

Figure 8.10 Pressure curves for the left ventricle, left atrium, pulmonary artery, and aorta in patients with mitral stenosis. LAP, left atrial pressure; LVP, left ventricular pressure; MV, mitral valve.

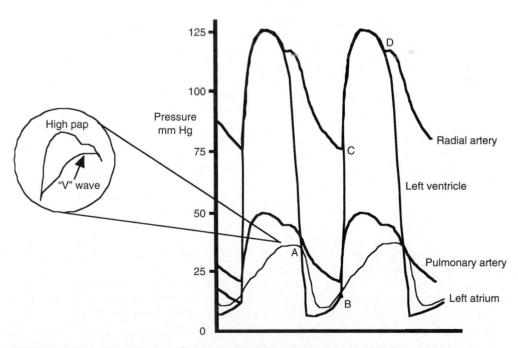

Figure 8.11 Pressure curves for the left ventricle, left atrium, pulmonary artery, and aorta in patients with mitral regurgitation. PAP, pulmonary artery pressure.

(Fig. 8.12B). The echo machine codes this amplitude on a black/white scale, thereby converting the amplitude to brightness or B-mode scanning (Fig. 8.12C). Fig. 8.12D shows this "ice-pick" view through the LV of the heart. Each change in tissue density results in some sound waves being reflected and hence an interface. In this example, bold lines are seen at the epicardial, the endocardial-chamber, the chamber-endocardial, and the epicardial borders. If these amplitude bars are displayed in a real time, a motion or M-mode display results (Fig. 8.12E). These images were difficult to reliably obtain and interpret because the views represent a linear slice without surrounding structural images for referencing. However, if the probe is rocked back and forth repetitively, multiple M-mode images can be obtained in a given instant and, therefore, a two-dimensional image formed. This rapid rocking back and forth of the ultrasound beam is performed electronically in a phased-array transducer. The images derived in this manner appear as a "cine-x-ray" display of myocardial movement. Therefore, echocardiography can provide information about the size, shape, location, and movement of myocardial structures.

In addition to determining how long it takes for a given sound wave to return and, thereby, deriving the distance from the transducer, contact of the sound wave packet with the reflecting object (tissue, blood cells, air) will alter the wavelength of the sound packet according to the Doppler principle. When the object coming in contact with the sound wave is moving toward the source of the ultrasound, the reflected ultrasound wavelengths are compressed (shorter) or of higher pitch. The opposite occurs when the contacted object is moving away from the sound source. These shifts in frequency are proportional to the velocity of the contacted structure and, thereby, the speed and direction of the encountered object (usually of blood flow) can be calculated. This velocity information can be displayed on a color map (Doppler color flow) or on a time/velocity scale (spectral Doppler display). Doppler-derived blood flow velocity information can determine laminar and turbulent flow patterns, regurgitant or stenotic lesions, congenital anomalies and can permit quantification of pressure gradients. Using the modified Bernoulli equation ($\Delta P = 4\,v^2$), determination of a blood flow velocity permits the estimation of pressure gradients.

Simply, the greater the velocity of blood flow the higher the pressure gradient. Only the component of blood flow parallel to the Doppler beam will be analyzed. The Doppler equation: $V = c\,(F_S - F_T)/2\,F_T\,(\cos\theta)$, contains the cosine of the angle of incidence between the ultrasound beam and the moving object. Because the cosine of 90 degrees is zero, blood flow that is perpendicular to the ultrasound beam will not have any Doppler shift and, therefore, will not be represented in the color display. For this reason, it is important to choose an ultrasound "window" in which the expected blood flow direction is most parallel to the ultrasound.

TTE uses imaging points or "acoustic windows" obtained with the transducer hand held on the chest wall. It is simple and importantly noninvasive. Most standard echocardiograms are obtained from this position. However, during cardiac surgery, the chest wall is in the sterile field and, therefore, unavailable. The esophagus lies immediately adjacent to the heart outside of the operative field and, therefore, affords an excellent imaging vantage point. In 1976, Yasu Oka from the Albert Einstein College of Medicine developed a practical method of intraoperative imaging. He mounted an ultrasound crystal on the end of a gastroscope and, thereby, obtained images of the heart during surgery. This has been refined considerably since. transesophageal echocardiography (TEE) has become the standard of care for heart surgery at many institutions. The close proximity of the probe to the heart affords excellent resolution. The probe is not in the operative field hence surgery is unhindered and sterility is not an issue. Though mildly invasive, the risk of esophageal injury in the anesthetized state is very low.

Intraoperative TEE is beneficial for quantification of cardiac contractility, for determination of the severity of regurgitant and stenotic valvular disease, for the detection of intracardiac shunts and the occurrence of dissections, and as a guide for catheter placement.

Perrino AC, Reeves ST, eds. *A practical approach to transesophageal echocardiography.* Philadelphia: Lippincott Williams & Wilkins, 2003:3–94.

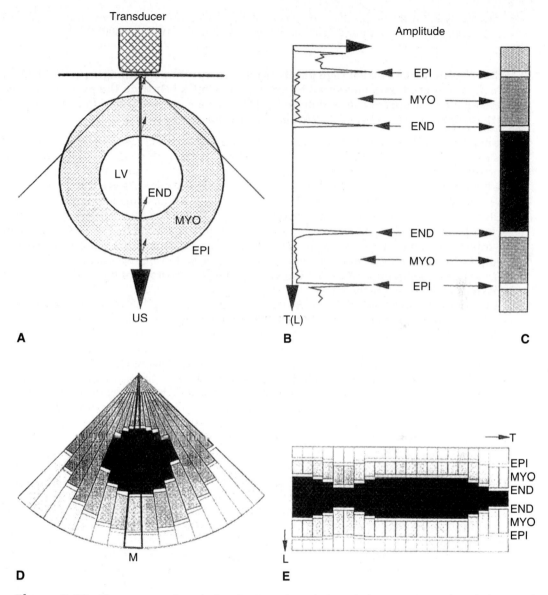

Figure 8.12 The process of producing the B-mode and M-mode images. **A:** A pulse of ultrasound is emitted into the object, and the backscattered echo is received by the same transducer. **B:** The received acoustic signal is converted to the electric signal (A-mode). **C:** The amplitude is modulated into brightness (B-mode). **D:** As subsequent pulses of ultrasound are emitted with the sequentially changing angles and the obtained one-dimensional B-mode images are compounded according to the direction of each ultrasound emission, the first frame of the sector-shaped image is formed. **E:** When the ultrasound is repeatedly transmitted in one direction, a series of one-dimensional B-mode images is obtained. As these are arranged against time, an M-mode image is obtained. (From Okay Y, Goldiner PL, eds. *Transesophageal echocardiography.* Philadelphia: JB Lippincott Co, 1992:12, with permission.) LV, left ventricle; END, endocardium; EPI, epicardium; US, ultrasound; T, time; L, length; M, motion.

Savage RM, Aronson S, eds. *Comprehensive textbook of intraoperative transesophageal echocardiography*. Philadelphia: Lippincott Williams & Wilkins, 2005:3–61.

A.7. **What are the three TEE vantage points for the comprehensive imaging of the LV? How are pressure gradients measured by echocardiography? How do the pressure gradients derived from Doppler echocardiography differ from those obtained in the catheterization laboratory by direct pressure measurement?**

The heart has two main axes, the longitudinal axis running from the base to the apex and the short axis perpendicular to that. Because the ultrasound beam can be thought of as a two-dimensional structure, multiple scan planes are required to completely image a three-dimensional structure. The left ventricle (LV) may be divided into 16 segments, 6 at the basal level, 6 at the midpapillary level, and 4 at the apical level (Fig. 8.13). By moving the transesophageal echocardiography (TEE) probe in the esophagus and by rotation of the crystal within the transducer tip, the LV can be imaged from three acoustic windows. These are the midesophageal four-chamber, the transgastric short axis, and the transgastric two-chamber view. Normal ventricular motion requires that the wall segment move centrally with systole and similarly undergo thickening along this axis during contraction. Function is usually quantified as normal; mild, moderate, and severe hypokinesis; akinesis; and dyskinesis.

In addition to function, TEE permits the determination of wall thickness and chamber size, important parameters in understanding the pathophysiology of valvular heart disease.

As mentioned previously, pressure gradients are derived through analysis of the Doppler profiles of blood flow. A commonly determined echocardiography gradient is that which is present from the LV to the aorta (Ao) in the setting of aortic stenosis (AS). To obtain the change in blood flow velocity across the aortic valve with TEE, the probe is advanced far into the stomach and sharply anteflexed and left deflected to obtain the window from the apex of the heart (deep transgastric long axis) and align the ultrasound beam most parallel to the path of blood flow. From this window, the continuous wave Doppler cursor is directed across the left ventricular outflow tract and aortic valve. An example of such a spectral Doppler display is seen in Fig. 8.14. The large increase in blood flow velocity in this display occurs at the narrowest point along its path, which in this case is the aortic valve. Using the modified Bernoulli equation mentioned previously, a gradient is calculated (100 mm Hg in the example). This represents the maximum instantaneous pressure difference between the LV and the Ao. AS is also quantified at the time of catheterization by measuring the pressures from within the LV and the Ao as a rapid response pressure transducer catheter is withdrawn from the LV back to the Ao across the stenotic valve. The standard reported gradient is the difference between the maximum left ventricular and Ao pressures. Fig. 8.15 illustrates that these peaks are not simultaneous events. Therefore, Doppler-derived AS gradients are usually higher than those derived at the time of left heart catheterization.

Perrino AC, Reeves ST, eds. *A practical approach to transesophageal echocardiography*. Philadelphia: Lippincott Williams & Wilkins, 2003:77–130.

Savage RM, Aronson S, eds. *Comprehensive textbook of intraoperative transesophageal echocardiography*. Philadelphia: Lippincott Williams & Wilkins, 2005:65–102.

Shanewise JS, Cheung AT, Aronson S, et al. ASE/SCA guidelines for performing a comprehensive multiplane transesophageal echocardiography examination: recommendations of the American Society of Echocardiography and the Society of Cardiovascular Anesthesiologists task force for certification in perioperative transesophageal echocardiography. *Anesth Analg* 1999;89:870–884.

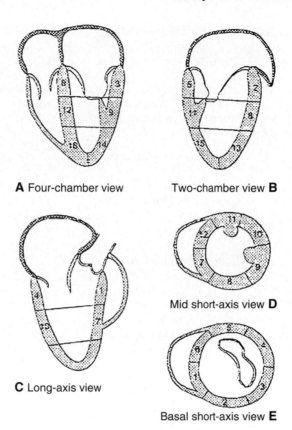

A Four-chamber view   Two-chamber view **B**

C Long-axis view

Mid short-axis view **D**

Basal short-axis view **E**

Basal segments	Mid segments	Apical segments
1 = Basal anteroseptal	7 = Mid anteroseptal	13 = Apical anterior
2 = Basal anterior	8 = Mid anterior	14 = Apical lateral
3 = Basal lateral	9 = Mid lateral	15 = Apical inferior
4 = Basal posterior	10 = Mid posterior	16 = Apical septal
5 = Basal inferior	11 = Mid inferior	
6 = Basal septal	12 = Mid septal	

Figure 8.13 Sixteen-segment model of the left ventricle. **A:** Four-chamber views show the three septal and three lateral segments. **B:** Two-chamber views show the three anterior and three inferior segments. **C:** Long-axis views show the two anteroseptal and two posterior segments. **D:** Mid short-axis views show all six segments at the mid level. **E:** Basal short-axis views show all six segments at the basal level. (From Shanewise JS, Cheung AT, Aronson S, et al. eds. ASE/SCA guidelines for performing a comprehensive intraoperative multiplane transesophageal echocardiography examination: recommendations of the American Society of Echocardiography council for intraoperative echocardiography and the Society of Cardiovascular Anesthesiologists task force for certification in perioperative transesophageal echocardiography. *Anesth Analg* 1999,89:870–884, with permission.)

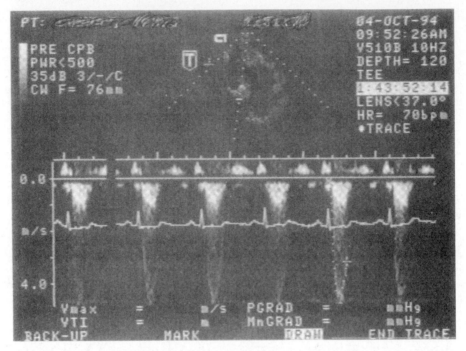

Figure 8.14 Continuous wave Doppler across the aortic valve in the deep transgastric apical view from a patient with severe aortic stenosis.

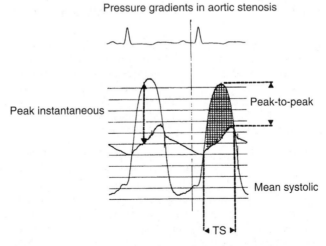

Figure 8.15 Pressure gradients in severe aortic stenosis are measured during systole as the difference between aortic and left ventricular pressures displayed using a 0- to 200-mm Hg scale. The peak instantaneous gradient is the maximum gradient noted; the peak-to-peak gradient is the difference between peak left ventricular and aortic pressures. The mean systolic gradient is the average of all systolic pressure gradients noted during systolic ejection (TS). (From Nanda NC, ed. *Doppler echocardiography.* Philadelphia: Lea & Febiger, 1993:130, with permission.)

A.8. What are the echocardiographic and cardiac catheterization criteria for the four valvular lesions?

The TEE severity scales of the various valvular lesions are summarized in Table 8.1.

Aortic stenosis

Echocardiographic criteria for AS include two-dimensional images demonstrating limited aortic valve opening and motion and left ventricular concentric hypertrophy. Doppler examination will reveal a turbulent, high-velocity jet across the aortic valve and color flow Doppler will demonstrate a turbulent, mosaic-appearing color map. The gradient across the aortic valve measured at cardiac catheterization is different from that measured by echocardiography as mentioned previously. Quantification of this Doppler-derived pressure gradient again relies on the modified Bernoulli equation.

$$\text{Pressure gradient} = 4\, v^2$$

where v = velocity (m/second), pressure (mm Hg)

Because flow is an important determinant of pressure gradients, both these catheterization and Doppler-derived values are interpreted along with cardiac output. Calculations permit the determination of a valve area. Severe AS is present when the gradient exceeds 75 mm Hg and/or the valve area is less than $0.8\ \text{cm}^2$.

Table 8.1   The Transesophageal Echocardiography Severity Scales of Valvular Lesions.

	SEVERITY SCALES			
	NORMAL	**MILD**	**MODERATE**	**SEVERE**
MEASUREMENT	**0**	**1+**	**2+** **3+**	**4+**
MS				
MVA (cm^2)	4.0–6.0	1.5–2.5	1.0–1.5	<1.0
Mean pressure gradient (mm Hg)	<2	2.0–6.0	6.0–12.0	>12
AS				
AVA (cm^2)	2.5–3.5	1.2–2.0	0.8–1.1	<0.8
Peak pressure gradient (mm Hg)	<10	16–34	35–75	>75
MR				
Jet length/LA length	0	<1/3	1/3–2/3	>2/3
Jet area/LA area	0	<1/3	1/3–2/3	>2/3
Jet area (cm^2)	0	<3	3.0–6.0	>6
Pulmonary vein Doppler	S wave≫D wave	Blunting S wave	S < D S≪D	Systolic reversal of flow
AI				
Jet width/LVOT width	0	<1/4	1/4–1/2 1/2–2/3	>2/3
Jet length (pressure dependent)	0	to middle of AML	to tip of AML to PM	beyond PM

AI, aortic insufficiency; AML, anterior mitral leaflet; AS, aortic stenosis; AVA, aortic valve area; LA, left atrial; LVOT, left ventricular outflow tract; MR, mitral regurgitation; MS, mitral stenosis; MVA, mitral valve area; PM, papillary muscle.

Aortic insufficiency

Catheterization criteria for aortic insufficiency (AI) rely on the qualitative estimation of the regurgitation volume and an estimation of left ventricular size and EF. Similar quantification can be made from Doppler color echocardiography derived data. A commonly used echocardiographic criteria compares the width of the regurgitant jet at the level of the valve to the width of the left ventricular outflow tract. A ratio of greater than 0.66 corresponds with severe AI.

Mitral stenosis

The severity of mitral stenosis (MS) can be obtained by the direct measurement of a diastolic gradient between the left atrium and ventricle at the time of cardiac catheterization. However, this requires a transatrial puncture, a procedure largely replaced by echocardiographic techniques. Echocardiographic diagnosis is based on gradient estimation by Doppler and by measuring the rate of decay in the pressure with the time spent in diastole (pressure half-time). The MV area in cm^2 can be derived from an empirical formula wherein the MV area equals 220 divided by this pressure half-time (Hatle constant). Severe MS is present when the end-diastolic gradient exceeds 12 mm Hg corresponding to a valve area of less than 1.0 cm^2.

Mitral regurgitation

In the presence of mitral regurgitation (MR), ventriculography will demonstrate the reflux of dye from the LV into the left atrium. Severe MR is diagnosed when dye refluxes into the pulmonary veins. Color Doppler echocardiography permits similar quantification. Estimation relies on an estimation of regurgitant jet volume as compared with the left atrium and through analysis of pulmonary venous flow profiles.

In every case, color Doppler echocardiography is often useful in identifying the cause of the valvular lesion, its extent of involvement within and around the valve, and the associated hemodynamic changes. Therefore, for many valvular lesions, it may be sufficient for the diagnosis. Catheterization, however, is often performed to assess the presence of concomitant coronary artery disease, especially in patients of advanced age.

Quinones M, Otto C, Stoddard M, et al. Recommendations for quantification of Doppler echocardiography: a report of from the Doppler quantification task force of the nomenclature and standard's committee of the American Society of Echocardiography. *J Am Soc Echocardiogr* 2002;15:167–180.

Schoen FJ. Cardiac valves and valvular pathology: update on function, disease, repair, and replacement. *Cardiovasc Pathol* 2005;14:189–194.

Weyman AE, ed. *Principles and practice of echocardiography*, 2nd ed. Philadelphia: Lea & Febiger, 1994:391–574.

Zipes DP, Libby P, Bonow RO, et al. eds. *Braunwald's heart disease: a textbook of cardiovascular medicine*, 7th ed. Philadelphia: WB Saunders, 2005:1553–1615.

B. Preoperative Evaluation and Preparation

B.1. What are the presenting signs and symptoms of the four valvular lesions listed previously?

See Table 8.2.

Table 8.2   The Signs and Symptoms for the Various Valvular Lesions.

LESION	SIGNS AND SYMPTOMS
AS	Angina, syncope, dyspnea/CHF
AI	
Chronic	Fatigability, dyspnea
Acute	Severe pulmonary edema, CHF
MS	Pulmonary congestion, AFib
MR	
Chronic	DOE, PND, AFib
Acute	Severe pulmonary edema, CHF

AFib, atrial fibrillation; AI, aortic insufficiency; AS, aortic stenosis; CHF, congestive heart failure; DOE, dyspnea on exertion; MR, mitral regurgitation; MS, mitral stenosis; PND, paroxysmal nocturnal dyspnea.

Aortic stenosis

The triad of angina, syncope, and congestive heart failure represent the progression of symptoms associated with AS. These symptoms correlate directly with mortality; the 50% survival data for these symptoms are 5, 3, and 2 years from the onset of these symptoms, respectively. Angina results from both increased demand for and a decrease in supply of coronary blood flow. Increased muscle mass from left ventricular hypertrophy and the high energy requirements to generate increased (high) systolic pressure combine to increase demands for coronary blood flow. In addition, insufficient supply secondary to decreased perfusion gradients and a decrease in coronary vasculature relative to the large amount of myocardium sum to diminish relative myocardial blood supply. Therefore, up to one third of patients with aortic stenosis can have angina in the absence of significant coronary artery disease.

Aortic insufficiency

Patients with AI have variable clinical presentations, primarily depending on the rapidity with which the left ventricular volume overload develops. When the volume increase occurs gradually as in chronic AI, there is usually a long asymptomatic period. The onset of the symptoms of fatigability and dyspnea signals either reduced cardiac output or increased left ventricular end-diastolic pressure (LVEDP) indicative of impairment of left ventricular contractile function. When aortic insufficiency occurs acutely, the ventricular compliance is unchanged; increased left ventricular diastolic volumes from regurgitant flow, therefore, lead to rapid rises in LVEDP and the clinical picture of congestive failure.

Mitral stenosis

Mitral stenosis (MS) is a slowly progressive obstruction to flow across the MV with gradual increase in left atrial (LA) pressure and volume. Symptoms of pulmonary congestion result from elevations in LA pressures and *not* from poor left ventricular systolic function. Atrial fibrillation develops secondary to atrial dilation.

Mitral regurgitation

The time course for the development of mitral regurgitation determines the severity of the symptoms. When the volume of regurgitant flow from the left ventricle to the left atrium increases gradually, the left atrium compensates by gradual dilatation. In contrast, the onset of acute mitral regurgitation can lead to rapid increases in LA pressures and severe pulmonary congestion and congestive heart failure.

Hartman GS. *Management of patients with valvular heart disease*. Cleveland: International Anesthesia Research Society, 1994:141–151. 1994 IARS Review Course Lectures.

Thomas SJ, Kramer JL, eds. *Manual of cardiac anesthesia*, 2nd ed. New York: Churchill Livingstone, 1993:81–127.

Zipes DP, Libby P, Bonow RO, et al. eds. *Braunwald's heart disease: a textbook of cardiovascular medicine*, 7th ed. Philadelphia: WB Saunders, 2005:1553–1615.

B.2. What is the New York Heart Association (NYHA) classification of heart failure?

The NYHA heart failure classification is based on the amount of symptoms, specifically dyspnea and fatigue. The various classes are listed in the following:

Class I. No symptoms
Class II. Symptoms with ordinary activity
Class III. Symptoms with less than ordinary activity
Class IV. Symptoms at rest

Criteria Committee of the New York Heart Association. *Diseases of the heart and blood vessels (Nomenclature and criteria for diagnosis)*, 6th ed. Boston: Little, Brown and Company, 1964.

B.3. Discuss the role of premedication for patients with the four different valvular lesions.

The role of premedication is to allay the anxiety of the impending surgical procedure thereby controlling the sympathetic outflow that may accompany the stress response. However, acute changes in heart rate, venous return, and systemic resistance can have particularly profound effects on patients with valvular heart disease.

Patients with aortic stenosis (AS) may benefit from premedication by preventing unnecessary increases in heart rate. Concern however must be taken to ensure adequate venous return and preservation of sinus mechanism (see later).

Patients with aortic insufficiency (AI) can similarly benefit from premedication because any increases in afterload, which may accompany sympathetic stimulation, can increase regurgitant volume. Drug doses should be adjusted based on the severity of debilitation and degree of systemic hypoperfusion.

Patients with mitral stenosis (MS) should be premedicated with caution. Elevations in carbon dioxide resulting from narcotic-induced hypoventilation can dramatically elevate pulmonary pressures further compromising right ventricle output. Conversely venodilation may excessively diminish filling pressures.

Patients with mitral regurgitation (MR) can respond similarly to those with MS, particularly when pulmonary hypertension is present. However, elevations in systemic pressure from stress can also compromise forward left ventricular output. Proper premedication can be delivered by careful dose selection and the provision of supplemental oxygen.

Hartman GS. *Management of patients with valvular heart disease*. Cleveland: International Anesthesia Research Society, 1994:141–151. 1994 IARS Review Course Lectures.

Thomas SJ, Kramer JL, eds. *Manual of cardiac anesthesia*, 2nd ed. New York: Churchill Livingstone, 1993:81–127.

B.4. How would you premedicate the patient with severe AS and MR?

Premedication of a patient with severe AS and MR must be approached with caution. The patient should receive supplemental oxygen. A light premedication could be provided with small doses of benzodiazepines by mouth. However, I would prefer to titrate in small intravenous doses of sedation while the patient was under the closely monitored situation of the operating room or holding area and with inspired oxygen supplementation. In this setting, incremental doses of midazolam (0.5 mg intravenously) would be administered. It is important to remember that there may be significant delay in the onset of effect of intravenous medications secondary to pooling in the pulmonary and left atrial systems. Adequate waiting periods must be observed between each aliquot to avoid inadvertent overdose with ensuing respiratory depression, pulmonary hypertension, systemic hypotension, and right heart failure. In the elderly; however, use of benzodiazepines has been linked to postoperative delirium, which can be quite severe and difficult to treat as well as increase length of stay and resource utilization.

C. Intraoperative Management

C.1. Outline the hemodynamic management goals for each of the four valvular lesions. What are the anesthetic goals with respect to heart rate and rhythm, preload, afterload, and contractility?

Table 8.3 summarizes the hemodynamic goals with respect to heart rate and rhythm, afterload, and contractility.

Aortic stenosis

Patients with aortic stenosis (AS) need the left ventricular filling obtained through a well-timed atrial contraction. Similarly, left ventricular hypertrophy renders the ventricle stiff and adequate preload is required. Reducing vascular tone will do little to relieve the fixed afterload increases from a stenotic valve but rather lower diastolic coronary perfusion gradients and should be avoided. Patients with AS experiencing angina may require the administration of an α-agonist such as phenylephrine rather than nitroglycerin to increase coronary perfusion pressure.

Aortic insufficiency

The severity of aortic insufficiency (AI) is determined by the size of the regurgitant orifice, the pressure gradient between the aorta and left ventricle during diastole, and the time spent in that phase of the cardiac cycle. Elevated heart rates decrease the time spent in diastole and can lead to a decrease in heart size. Afterload reduction can lessen the regurgitant driving forces but therapeutic maneuvers to accomplish this may be limited by resulting systemic hypotension.

Table 8.3 The Hemodynamic Goals for the Various Valvular Lesions.

	HEMODYNAMIC GOALS			
LESIONS	**HR AND RHYTHM**	**PRELOAD**	**AFTERLOAD**	**CONTRACTILITY**
AS	60–70, sinus	Full	Maintain	—
AI	80–90	Maintain	Lower	May need support
MS	60–70	Full	—	—
MR	80–90, sinus if possible	Maintain	Lower	May need support

HR, heart rate (beats/min); AI, aortic insufficiency; AS, aortic stenosis; MR, mitral regurgitation; MS, mitral stenosis.

Mitral stenosis

Patients with mitral stenosis (MS) can swiftly deteriorate in the setting of rapid heart rates. The decreased filling time necessitates the marked elevation of left atrial (LA) pressures and pulmonary edema can rapidly ensue. Whereas left ventricle (LV) contractility is generally preserve in mitral stenosis, use of β-blockade does result in decreased right ventricular (RV) contractility, which in the setting of pulmonary hypertension can further compromise the cardiac output and systemic blood pressure. However, the loss in RV contractility is more than offset by the beneficial effects of the reduction of heart rate. Slower heart rates permit adequate time for transfer of blood from the left atrium to the LV across the stenotic mitral valve (MV) to occur. In addition, the pressure gradient across the MV is also reduced; thereby lowering left atrial pressure and diminishing pulmonary congestion. Because there is some variability in the individual response, the use of short-acting β-blockers such as esmolol is prudent because an adverse response should be evanescent.

Mitral regurgitation

Patients with mitral regurgitation (MR) can rapidly deteriorate with marked increases in systemic blood pressure and afterload. As with other volume overload lesions such as aortic insufficiency (AI), slightly rapid heart rates (80 to 90 beats/minute) should result in smaller left ventricular volumes. This may lessen any component of MR secondary to annular dilation or chordal malalignment. Importantly, tachycardia should be avoided in patients with ischemic MR.

C.2. What are the hemodynamic goals for this patient with the combination of severe AS and MR?

In the patient with combined aortic stenosis (AS) and MR, the situation is more complex than when only a singular valvular lesion is present. Careful examination of the hemodynamic goals for each of the two lesions will reveal that therapy beneficial to patients with AS may exacerbate the severity of the MR. Early aggressive intervention is the key to these combined lesions. There usually exists less of a margin for error because minor hemodynamic aberrations can rapidly lead to cardiac collapse. A good rule of thumb is to prioritize the management based on the character of the present symptoms. Patients with AS and MR who present with syncope or angina are best managed for their AS, whereas patients with dyspnea and pulmonary edema are best managed for their congestive symptoms. It is prudent to maintain the patient's own usual hemodynamics and avoid physiologic trespass. Transesophageal echocardiography (TEE) evaluation of left ventricular performance can be helpful in separating pulmonary congestion secondary to left heart failure from that secondary to poor diastolic left ventricular compliance.

Hartman GS. *Management of patients with valvular heart disease.* Cleveland: International Anesthesia Research Society, 1994:141–151. 1994 IARS Review Course Lectures.

Thomas SJ, Kramer JL, eds. *Manual of cardiac anesthesia*, 2nd ed. New York: Churchill Livingstone, 1993:81–127.

C.3. How would you monitor this patient with severe AS and MR?

In addition to the standard American Society of Anesthesiologists (ASA) recommended monitors, the patient would have a radial artery and a pulmonary artery (PA) catheter. Following induction of anesthesia and endotracheal intubation, a TEE probe would be inserted to confirm the valvular pathology and to assess ventricular function. Following valve replacement, the TEE would be used to check for adequacy of valvular function and the absence of paravalvular leaks and to assess postbypass ventricular function.

Practice guidelines for perioperative transesophageal echocardiography. A report by the American Society of Anesthesiologists and the Society of Cardiovascular Anesthesiologist Task Force on transesophageal echocardiography. *Anesthesiology* 1996;84: 986–1006.

C.4. Should the patient have a pulmonary artery (PA) catheter placed before induction?

Volume status may be particularly difficult to assess in patients with valvular heart disease yet of critical importance in the management of these patients. Patients with stenotic lesions depend on adequate filling pressures for diastolic filling of the ventricle. Patients with the volume overload lesions of aortic insufficiency (AI) and mitral regurgitation (MR) can benefit from the careful reductions in pulmonary pressure guided by the simultaneous assessment of cardiac performance. In these capacities, the PA catheter is useful. Patients with current hemodynamic stability, without severe respiratory distress, can be safely anesthetized before placement of the PA catheter. In all, there is no evidence that use of the PA catheter improves outcome in the setting of surgery.

Practice guidelines for pulmonary artery catheterization: an updated report by the American Society of Anesthesiologists task force on pulmonary artery catheterization. *Anesthesiology* 2003;99:4.

C.5. Is a PA catheter with pacing capabilities indicated?

Patients with aortic stenosis (AS) can become severely compromised with the loss of atrial kick or the presence of slow junctional rhythms. Patients with AI or MR can experience left ventricular dilation in the setting of slow heart rates. In such cases, a PA catheter with atrial and ventricular pacing capacity can be useful in this setting. In patients with intact conduction systems, rate manipulation can often be achieved pharmacologically. Transesophageal atrial pacing is another option; transthoracic pacing elicits a ventricular response only and does not permit atrial stimulation. Transthoracic pacing is indicated when the ability to rapidly open the pericardium and obtain epicardial pacing is limited. This occurs in the setting of reoperations or with patients having a history of inflammatory pericardial disease. Pacing will be limited to capture of the ventricle alone. The loss of atrial contraction can lead to underfilling and hemodynamic compromise in patients dependent on the added volume from atrial systole. One of the other pacing modalities is best in this setting.

Maisel WH, Epstein AE. The role of cardiac pacing: American College of Chest Physicians guidelines for the prevention and management of postoperative atrial fibrillation after cardiac surgery. *Chest* 2005;128(Suppl 2):36S–38S.

Risk SC, Brandon D, D'Ambra M, et al. Indications for the use of pacing pulmonary artery catheters in cardiac surgery. *J Cardiothorac Vasc Anesth* 1992;6:275–279.

C.6. What anesthetic technique would you employ? Why?

For the patient undergoing cardiopulmonary bypass (CPB) and aortic valve replacement (AVR), general anesthesia with endotracheal intubation is the obvious choice. Both narcotics and inhalation anesthetics can be safely administered. When prolonged postoperative ventilation is anticipated, a high-dose narcotic anesthetic has numerous advantages. Recent anesthetic technique for cardiac surgery has focused on the use of techniques permitting earlier extubation, so-called fast-tracking. Anesthetic combinations using smaller total narcotic doses, inhalation anesthetics, and short-acting intravenous sedatives such as propofol are gaining popularity. For uncomplicated valve replacements with good ventricular function, the advantages of early extubation can be safely achieved. In complicated cases with longer bypass periods, poor ventricular function, or postbypass bleeding, the hemodynamic stability of a high-dose narcotic technique may be advantageous.

DiNardo JA. *Anesthesia for cardiac surgery*, 2nd ed. Stamford: Appleton & Lange, 1998: 109–140.

Howie MB, Black HA, Romanelli VA, et al. A comparison of isoflurane versus fentanyl as primary anesthetics for mitral surgery. *Anesth Analg* 1996;83:941–948.

Tuman KJ, McCarthy RJ, Spiess BD, et al. Comparison of anesthetic techniques in patients undergoing heart valve replacement. *J Cardiothorac Anesth* 1990;4:159–167.

C.7. What muscle relaxant would you use for this patient?

Muscle relaxants can alter hemodynamics both from the effects of histamine release including vasodilatation and bronchospasm and through effects on rhythm. Although slowing of heart rates usually benefits the patient with angina, it may have severe consequences in patients with valvular heart disease. The typical high-dose narcotic anesthesia usually results in bradycardia secondary to the vagotonic actions. Pancuronium-mediated increases in heart rate usually offset these actions and result in a stable heart rate.

Certainly the newly released long-duration relaxants doxacurium and pipe-curonium have the potential for minimal effects on hemodynamics. However, as outlined previously, the potential side effect of one agent may be rationally used to counter the adverse effect of another. Hemodynamically "neutral" relaxants such as vecuronium, rocuronium, or *cis*-atracurium could be used but their intermediate duration of action offers little if any advantage in this setting.

Therefore, it is important to choose that combination of agents that will promote hemodynamic stability in a particular patient with his or her unique hemodynamic presentation. In this patient, I would use pancuronium in conjunction with the high-dose narcotic anesthetic.

Fleming N. Con: the choice of muscle relaxants is not important in cardiac surgery. *J Cardiothorac Vasc Anesth* 1995;9:768–771.

Hudson RJ, Thomson IR. Pro: the choice of muscle relaxants is important in cardiac surgery. *J Cardiothorac Vasc Anesth* 1995;9:768–771.

Thys DM, Hillel Z, Schwartz AJ, eds. *Textbook of cardiothoracic anesthesiology*. New York: McGraw-Hill, 2001:589–629.

C.8. What are the usual TEE findings in a patient with AS/AI/MR? How do you grade the severity of AS by TEE? How do you quantify the severity of MR? What is the impact of AS on the severity of MR?

The severity of aortic stenosis is usually stated in terms of aortic valve area (AVA). Normal AVA is 2.5 to 3.5 cm^2. Moderate stenosis is when the AVA is within the range of 0.8 to 1.2 cm^2 and severe stenosis when the AVA is less than 0.8 cm^2. A patient with a large peak pressure gradient (usually more than 75 mm Hg) in the absence of excessively high cardiac output is usually considered to have severe AS as well. In the setting of low cardiac outputs, the pressure gradient may not be that great (20 to 30 mm Hg), and determination of AVA is required. This can be accomplished with echocardiography.

Mitral regurgitation (MR) is graded by the amount of blood regurgitated backward into the left atrium during systole. Doppler color flow permits quantification of this flow. Common methods for MR quantification include the depth of MR jet extent into the left atrium (25% mild MR, 25% to 75% moderate MR, and more than 75% severe MR). Other methods of quantification include calculation of the area of the regurgitant jet by planimetry, by comparison of the MR jet area to the area of the left atrium, and by analysis of pulmonary vein flow profiles. It is important to remember that the amount of regurgitant blood flow in the setting of MR is determined by the amount of time spent in systole, the size of the defect in the mitral valve (MV), and the pressure gradient across the defect. Therefore, MR severity by Doppler color flow is load dependent. The lower pressure of the anesthetic state can often mask more severe degrees of MR seen when the patient is under his or her usual hemodynamic conditions.

The left ventricular pressures are increased in the setting of aortic stenosis (AS). Therefore, the gradient across the MV is increased often leading to more severe MR. Following replacement of the stenotic aortic valve and elimination of the outflow tract obstruction, left ventricular pressures are markedly reduced. Moderate levels of MR without major structural defects in the MV apparatus usually revert to minimal or certainly less severe levels following reduction in the left ventricular outflow obstruction.

Carabello BA, Crawford FA Jr. Valvular heart disease. *N Engl J Med* 1997;337:32–41.

Spain MG, Smith MD, Grayburn PA, et al. Quantitative assessment of mitral regurgitation by Doppler color flow imaging. Angiographic and hemodynamic correlations. *J Am Coll Cardiol* 1989;13:585–590.

C.9. What special considerations particular to cardiopulmonary bypass (CPB) operations do you have for each of the four lesions? Focus on these concerns with respect to the induction and prebypass, bypass, and postbypass periods.

Aortic stenosis

Critical to the management of a patient with AS is the avoidance of hypotension. Low blood pressure can initiate a cascade of events leading to cardiac arrest. Hypotension decreases the gradient for coronary perfusion with resultant ischemia. Ischemia leads to diminished cardiac output and decreased blood pressure further compromising coronary perfusion. The occurrence of cardiac arrest in a patient with AS is particularly catastrophic because closed chest cardiac massage will provide little gradient for blood flow across a stenotic aortic valve.

Patients with AS are particularly dependent on their atrial kick for adequate ventricular filling volume and can rapidly become hypotensive and ischemic following the onset of supraventricular tachycardia (SVT) or atrial fibrillation. These rhythms are not uncommon during atrial cannulation. Therefore, it is of particular importance that every preparation for the initiation of CPB be made before atrial manipulation. Increased muscle mass of ventricular hypertrophy can be more difficult to adequately protect with cardioplegia. Careful attention to surface cooling, myocardial temperature measurement, and/or the use of retrograde cardioplegia can be helpful. Following aortic valve replacement (AVR), hypertension from left ventricular output now unopposed by any valvular lesion can result in stress on suture lines and excessive bleeding. It is important to remember that the compliance of the left ventricle is unchanged by surgery and still critically dependent on adequate preload and sinus rhythm.

Aortic insufficiency

Patients undergoing AVR for aortic insufficiency (AI) can often present difficult management decisions. The usual treatment measures for hypotension (α-agonist) may have deleterious effects by increasing regurgitant volume. The use of combined α- and β-agonists (ephedrine, epinephrine, or infusions of dopamine or dobutamine) may be required. Although it would serve to lessen regurgitant volume, afterload reduction is beneficial in only a subset of patients with AI. Those patients with elevated left ventricular end-diastolic pressure (LVEDP), reduced ejection fractions, diminished cardiac output, and systemic hypertension usually benefit from afterload reduction. In contrast, those patients without the previously mentioned constellation may experience a decrease in forward cardiac output secondary to diminished preload from reduced venous return. Systemic hypotension usually limits the utility in the acute setting. The presence of aortic insufficiency (AI) makes initiation of cardiopulmonary bypass a critical period. Periods of bradycardia or ventricular fibrillation can lead to rapid volume overload of the LV through the incompetent aortic valve. Pacing, electrical defibrillation, and/or cross-clamping should be performed to prevent ventricular distention. Similarly, myocardial protection is compromised by AI. Generation of adequate root pressures is usually not obtainable; hence delivery of cardioplegia requires aortotomy and cannulation of the coronary ostia. Use of retrograde cardioplegia is advantageous. Following aortic valve replacement (AVR), the ventricle no longer has the lower pressure/impedance outflow afforded by the low aortic diastolic pressure. Inotropic support is often required. As with aortic stenosis (AS), the presence of an aortic suture line necessitates rapid response to hypertension to avoid bleeding and dissection.

Mitral stenosis

Patients undergoing mitral valve replacement (MVR) for mitral stenosis (MS) are particularly challenging. Marked elevations in pulmonary vascular resistance can be present with associated right heart failure. Stasis in the left atrium necessitates the careful echocardiographic examination for the presence of atrial thrombi. Manipulation of the heart before cross-clamping should be avoided. Following replacement, the chronically under filled, under worked LV may be unable to handle the new volume load. Inotropic support is often required for RV failure and occasionally to improve LV function. Afterload reduction and improved systemic perfusion through an IABP may be beneficial.

Mitral regurgitation

Similarly, patients with mitral regurgitation (MR) may have pulmonary hypertension and right heart failure. In contrast to aortic insufficiency (AI), almost all patients with MR can be greatly benefited by afterload reduction, both pharmacologically and/or through an intraaortic balloon pump. Diminution of left ventricular systolic pressure through afterload reduction decreases the pressure gradient from the left ventricle to the left atrium during systole with resultant decreased regurgitant volume.

Prebypass assessment can be misleading. Preserved ejection fractions and elevated stroke volumes may mask marked left ventricular systolic dysfunction. It should be remembered that much of the left ventricular volume is ejected into the low-pressure/impedance outflow path of the left atrium. This route is no longer available after valve replacement. Following MVR, dysfunctional ventricles may be unable to provide adequate forward flow into the systemic circuit with its elevated vascular resistance and usually necessitate the use of inotropic support.

Patients previously in atrial fibrillation without marked atrial enlargement often revert to or can be converted to sinus rhythm following valve replacement. The capacity of maintaining a person in sinus rhythm dramatically decreases when the diameter of the atrium is more than 5 cm.

Hartman GS. *Management of patients with valvular heart disease*. Cleveland: International Anesthesia Research Society, 1994:141–151. 1994 IARS Review Course Lectures.

Kaplan JA, Reich DL, Konstadt SN, eds. *Cardiac anesthesia*, 4th ed. Philadelphia: WB Saunders, 1999:727–784.

Thys DM, Hillel Z, Schwartz AJ, eds. *Textbook of cardiothoracic anesthesiology*. New York: McGraw-Hill, 2001:589–629.

C.10. The patient cannot be weaned from cardiopulmonary bypass (CPB) following an AVR and MVR. What are the possible causes?

The adequacy of myocardial preservation should be considered. Left ventricular hypertrophy (LVH) without or with accompanying coronary artery disease increases myocardial oxygen demands. Prolonged cross-clamp time necessitated by dual valve replacement can lead to inadequate and/or nonhomogeneous myocardial protection. In addition, there may be residual cardioplegia present within the myocardium. Therefore, some degree of postbypass left ventricular dysfunction can be anticipated. Inotropic support may be required. It is important to remember that although the obstruction to left ventricular ejection is acutely relieved by replacement of the stenotic valve, left ventricular compliance is largely unchanged. Adequate preload still depends on sinus rhythm and sufficient left ventricular filling pressures (pulmonary artery occlusion pressure [PAOP] or left ventricular end-diastolic pressure [LVEDP]). Elevations in pulmonary vascular resistance may render estimation of left atrial (LA) pressure through the pulmonary artery (PA) catheter inaccurate. In this setting, placement of an LA catheter is indicated. TEE may prove invaluable in identifying surgically correctable causes for inability to wean from CPB. Evaluation of left ventricular filling and contractility can help resolve the situation of low cardiac output and high filling pressures. A small underfilled left ventricle (LV) with hyperdynamic contractility and a dilated, overfilled, hypokinetic LV can both give the same hemodynamic parameters but obviously require different pharmacologic interventions. Abnormal valve seating may compromise flow into the coronary ostia and return to bypass with valve repositioning and/or coronary artery bypass grafting may be indicated. Similarly, perivalvular leaks or aortic dissections can be readily identified.

Thomas SJ, Kramer JL, eds. *Manual of cardiac anesthesia*, 2nd ed. New York: Churchill Livingstone, 1993:81–127.

Thys DM, Hillel Z, Schwartz AJ, eds. *Textbook of cardiothoracic anesthesiology*. New York: McGraw-Hill, 2001:589–629.

C.11. How would you diagnose right heart failure and pulmonary hypertension? How would you treat it?

Right heart failure is diagnosed by the elevations in right-sided filling pressures, specifically central venous pressure (CVP). Careful examination is required to rule out tricuspid insufficiency as the cause of the CVP elevation. A high CVP indicates the inability of the right heart to adequately propel the venous return volume into the pulmonary circulation. Elevation in the PA pressures is indicative of pulmonary hypertension. The combination of high CVP and high PA pressures indicates severe right heart failure. This scenario can be difficult to manage. Attempts to elevate systemic perfusion pressure with α-agonists can worsen pulmonary hypertension. Administration of vasodilators to lower pulmonary pressures results in systemic hypotension. In this setting, it is often prudent to return to cardiopulmonary bypass, relieve ventricular distention, and improve myocardial perfusion. During this "rest period," adjustments in inotropic therapy, ventilation, and cardiac rhythm can be instituted. Optimization of acid-base status and hemoglobin concentration should also be performed. Separation from bypass can then be reattempted.

Typical inotropic agents effective in this setting are those with high degrees of β-adrenergic potency. Commonly employed agents include dobutamine, epinephrine, and/or the phosphodiesterase-III (PDE-III) inhibitors amrinone and milrinone. It is not uncommon to require the administration of α-agonists to counteract the systemic vasodilating effects of prostaglandin E_1 and the PDE-III agents. Some selective pulmonary vasodilating action and systemic vasoconstricting effects can often be achieved by administration of pulmonary vasodilating agents such as prostaglandin E_1 through the right-sided access (CVP or PA catheter) and infusion of the α-agonists through the LA line. Therefore, the vasoconstriction of the pulmonary arterial bed can be minimized.

Nitric oxide (NO) is a potent, inhaled pulmonary vasodilator. Its half-life in the systemic circulation is extremely short permitting its administration to the pulmonary vasculature with minimal systemic hypotensive effects. NO can selectively and effectively dilate the pulmonary vasculature. The exact method of delivery, scavenging of waste gases, and high cost remain as obstacles to its clinical application.

Body SC, Hartigan PM, Shernan SK, et al. Nitric oxide: delivery, measurement, and clinical application. *J Cardiothorac Vasc Anesth* 1995;9:748–763.

Kieler-Jensen N, Houltz E, Ricksten SE. A comparison of prostacyclin and sodium nitroprusside for the treatment of heart failure after cardiac surgery. *J Cardiothorac Vasc Anesth* 1995;9:641–646.

Savage RM, Aronson S, eds. Assessment of the right ventricle. In: *Comprehensive textbook of intraoperative transesophageal echocardiography*. Philadelphia: Lippincott Williams & Wilkins, 2005:147–155.

C.12. What role does an intraaortic balloon pump (IABP) have in this setting?

An IABP may be useful, because unlike any pharmacologic maneuver it is capable of increasing mean pressure during diastole critical for coronary perfusion while lowering afterload to systolic left ventricular ejection. Myocardial dysfunction secondary to inadequate protection during bypass can be reduced by decreased afterload and augmentation of diastolic pressures through IABP counterpulsation.

C.13. How does the IABP work to benefit the failing heart?

An IABP is a catheter with a large balloon (40 to 60 mL) at its tip. It is positioned in the thoracic Ao distal to the left subclavian artery origin and proximal to the take-off of the renal vessels. It is timed to inflate during diastole to increase diastolic perfusion pressure to the coronary arteries, great vessels, and major abdominal organs and to deflate just before systole to decrease afterload thereby increasing forward cardiac output. It is the unique modality, which can improve coronary perfusion pressures while reducing myocardial oxygen demand.

Baskett RJ, Ghali WA, Maitland A, et al. The intraaortic balloon pump in cardiac surgery. *Ann Thorac Surg* 2002;74(4):1276–1287.

Cheung AT, Savino JS, Weiss SJ. Beat-to-beat augmentation of left ventricular function by intraaortic counterpulsation. *Anesthesiology* 1996;84:545–554.

C.14. What role does transesophageal echocardiography (TEE) play in the placement, timing, and demonstration of efficacy of an IABP?

The thoracic Ao and aortic arch can be clearly imaged by TEE. Imaging of the take-off of the left subclavian artery facilitates optimal positioning of the IABP. In addition, before insertion the Ao can be evaluated for dissection or the presence of severe atheromatous disease, both contraindications to IABP insertion. TEE can demonstrate the efficacy of an IABP by showing enhanced ventricular emptying during systole and filling during diastole.

C.15. How would you properly time its cycle?

Inflation should occur just following the dicrotic notch and deflation before the upstroke in the aortic pressure curve. Augmentation in diastolic and mean pressures with a reduction in systolic pressure should follow its proper function.

C.16. What are the contraindications to the use of an IABP?

The most common contraindications are severe AI and severe aortic disease, atheromatous, aneurysmal, or a dissection. Although often listed as absolute contraindications, there are reports of the effective use of IABP in these settings.

Sanfelippo PM, Baker NH, Ewy HG, et al. Experience with intraaortic balloon counterpulsation. *Ann Thorac Surg* 1986;41:36–41.

D. Postoperative Management

D.1. In the intensive care unit (ICU) 4 hours later, the patient became hypotensive with a low cardiac output. How could you distinguish between cardiac tamponade and pump failure? How would the transesophageal echocardiography (TEE) images differ?

The differentiation between cardiac tamponade and primary pump failure in the immediate postbypass-ICU setting can be difficult. Elevations in filling pressures, systemic hypotension, and low cardiac output are consistent with both diagnoses. The classic teaching of equalization of cardiac pressures seen in a "fluid" tamponade may not be present as areas of focal compression from clot can markedly reduce filling of only one chamber. Echocardiography can be beneficial in this setting by permitting visualization of chamber volume and function. The transesophageal approach has particular advantage over TTE in the postoperative setting in which the usual transthoracic window may be obscured by dressings and drainage tubing. Focal compression of the cardiac chambers from a clot or pericardial effusion can readily be distinguished from a volume-overloaded, failing heart with poor myocardial contractility. When the diagnosis is not clear, however, surgical reexploration may be indicated.

Bommer WJ, Follette D, Pollock M, et al. Tamponade in patients undergoing cardiac surgery: a clinical-echocardiographic diagnosis. *Am Heart J* 1995;130:1216–1223.

D.2. Would you extubate this patient early in the ICU? Why?

No. This patient has undergone a double valve replacement. In this more complex procedure, coagulopathy and postoperative bleeding, hypothermia from incomplete and nonuniform rewarming, and pulmonary hypertension are not uncommon occurrences in the immediate postoperative period. Sedation, paralysis, and mechanical ventilation can reduce the oxygen requirements during this early phase of recovery, minimize pulmonary hypertension secondary to hypercarbia, and permit reestablishment of core temperatures.

Cheng DCH. Pro: early extubation after cardiac surgery decreases intensive care unit stay and cost. *J Cardiothorac Vasc Anesth* 1995;9:460–464.

Guenther CR. Con: early extubation after cardiac surgery decreases intensive care unit stay and cost. *J Cardiothorac Vasc Anesth* 1995;9:465–467.

D.3. What are the advantages and disadvantages of early extubation?

The advantages of early extubation are both medical and financial. Early extubation can lessen the adverse sequelae from prolonged endotracheal intubation including epithelial damage, decreased ciliary motility, and diminished mobilization of secretions. Positive pressure ventilation can have adverse effects on venous return. However, the overwhelming drive toward early extubation is cost and patient comfort. Early extubation can decrease cost by decreasing ICU staff requirements, decreasing the cost of sedatives, lessening the duration of ICU stays, and improving operating room use by lessening cancellation of cases secondary to blocked ICU beds.

The potential advantages of early extubation, both financial and physiologic, must be weighed against the potential disadvantages of early extubation. The potential for respiratory compromise leading to hypoxemia, hypercarbia, ischemia, and the potential for infarction and neurologic injury is real. Any savings realized from early extubation can be rapidly lost by one adverse event. Success relies on careful integration of all players in the care of the cardiac surgery patient, from the management of intraoperative anesthetic techniques to the organization of the ICU and staff and the provision of postoperative analgesia. Equally important to the success of an early extubation program is appropriate patient selection.

Cheng DCH. Pro: early extubation after cardiac surgery decreases intensive care unit stay and cost. *J Cardiothorac Vasc Anesth* 1995;9:460–464.

Guenther CR. Con: early extubation after cardiac surgery decreases intensive care unit stay and cost. *J Cardiothorac Vasc Anesth* 1995;9:465–467.

CHAPTER 9

Pacemakers and Implantable Cardioverter-Defibrillators

Alan Cheng • Fun-Sun F. Yao

A 70-YEAR-OLD MAN

was scheduled for urgent open cholecystectomy. He underwent a permanent pacemaker (PPM) implantation 5 years ago for sick sinus syndrome. The pacemaker was upgraded to an implantable cardioverter-defibrillator (ICD) with dual-chamber pacing function 6 months ago due to episodes of ventricular tachycardia (VT). His blood pressure was 120/80 mm Hg, heart rate was regular at 70 beats per minute.

A. Medical Disease and Differential Diagnosis

1. What are the indications for PPMs?
2. What is sick sinus syndrome?
3. How would you diagnose first-, second-, and third-degree atrioventricular (AV) block, right bundle branch block (RBBB) with left anterior fascicular hemiblock, and left posterior fascicular hemiblock?
4. Is it necessary to insert a temporary pacemaker before general anesthesia for an asymptomatic patient with bifascicular block?
5. What are the three-letter and five-letter identification codes of the North American Society of Pacing and Electrophysiology (NASPE) and British Pacing and Electrophysiology Group (BPEG) generic (NBG) code for pacemaker classification?
6. How many modes of pacing are available in modern day PPMs? How do they work?
7. The patient was mechanically hyperventilated during surgery and his pacemaker gradually increased his heart rate. What feature of the PPM is accounting for this?
8. What are the advantages and disadvantages of atrial pacing only?
9. What are the indications for and complications associated with AV sequential PPMs?
10. How would you know if the patient's PPM was atrially, ventricularly, or AV sequentially pacing?
11. What is the maximum amount of energy that a modern day PPM can provide in terms of pulse amplitude and pulse width?
12. During a PPM implantation, what are the acceptable values for modern day pacemaker leads in terms of pacing thresholds, amplitude of sensed R waves, and resistance?
13. What is a biventricular PPM or cardiac resynchronization therapy (CRT) device? What are the indications for such a device?

14. What are the usual life spans of PPMs and ICDs?
15. What is an ICD? How does it work?
16. What are the indications for ICDs?
17. What is the North American Society of Pacing and Electrophysiology (NASPE) and British Pacing and Electrophysiology Group (BPEG) generic defibrillator (NBD) code?

B. Preoperative Evaluation and Preparation

1. How would you preoperatively evaluate the patient described earlier?
2. How do you determine whether the patient has a cardiac rhythm management device (CRMD) and define what type of CRMD?
3. How do you determine whether the patient is dependent on pacing function of the CRMD?
4. How do you know if the implanted PPM or ICD is working?
5. What information would you like to obtain from interrogating this device?
6. How do you preoperatively prepare the patient for surgery and anesthesia?
7. Would you recommend reprogramming this device to asynchronously pace before surgery?
8. Would you reprogram the ICD preoperatively?

C. Intraoperative Management

1. How would you monitor this patient?
2. What drugs and equipment would you like to have on hand in the operating room?
3. How would you set up the transcutaneous external pacer and defibrillator?
4. Had this patient's ICD been implanted the day before surgery, would you consider avoiding certain inhalational gases for anesthesia?
5. Electromagnetic interference (EMI) from cautery during the case results in significant noise on your cardiac monitor. You recall that EMI can also inhibit pacing function from the pacemaker. In this pacemaker-dependent patient, how can you determine whether inappropriate inhibition of the pacemaker is occurring?
6. What are the potential responses of pacemakers and ICDs to electrocautery?
7. How would you prevent the effects of EMI on the pacemaker or ICD from the electrocautery?
8. What are the effects of a magnet over pacemakers and ICDs?
9. In the middle of surgery, the patient developed ventricular tachycardia. What would you do?
10. What precautions should be taken when a patient with a CRMD is undergoing extracorporeal shock wave lithotripsy (ESWL)?
11. Is electroconvulsive therapy (ECT) contraindicated in patients with pacemakers or ICDs?
12. Is magnetic resonance imaging (MRI) contraindicated in patients with a CRMD?
13. What are the precautions during radiofrequency ablation for a patient with a CRMD?

D. Postoperative Management

1. How would you monitor this patient in the post–anesthesia care unit?
2. How would you confirm that the CRMD is functioning properly after surgery?
3. What types of environmental EMIs may temporarily affect the function of a PPM?

A. Medical Disease and Differential Diagnosis

A.1. What are the indications for permanent pacemakers (PPMs)?

Artificial pacing is generally indicated for the treatment of symptomatic bradycardia of any origin. The two major indications for permanent pacing are failure of impulse formation and failure of cardiac conduction. Clinically, sick sinus syndrome and complete heart block are the most common indications for pacemakers. The following types of arrhythmias are common indications for pacemakers:

- Sinoatrial (SA) node—sick sinus syndrome, tachy-brady arrhythmia, symptomatic sinus bradycardia, hypersensitive carotid sinus syndrome, or vasovagal syncope
- Atrioventricular (AV) node—second-degree block or third-degree AV block
- Trifascicular block or bifascicular block with prolonged infranodal conduction
- Right bundle branch block (RBBB) and left anterior hemiblock with hemodynamic symptoms
- RBBB and left posterior hemiblock with hemodynamic symptoms
- Alternating left bundle branch block (LBBB) and RBBB
- High-risk patients with congenital long Q-T syndrome or those with documented sustained pause-dependent ventricular tachycardia
- Syncope without an electrocardiogram (ECG) diagnosis
- Cardiomyopathy—patients with medically refractory hypertrophic obstructive cardiomyopathy or decompensated heart failure in patients with dilated cardiomyopathy despite optimal medical therapy (e.g., biventricular pacing)

Atlee JL, Bernstein AD. Cardiac rhythm management devices (part I). *Anesthesiology* 2001; 95:1265–1280.

Kusumoto FM, Goldschlager N. Cardiac pacing. *N Engl J Med* 1996;334:89–98.

Salukhe TV, Dob D. Pacemakers and defibrillators: anesthetic implications. *Br J Anesth* 2004; 93:95–104.

Zipes DP, Libby P, Bonow RO, et al. eds. *Braunwald's heart disease, a textbook of cardiovascular medicine*, 6th ed. Philadelphia: WB Saunders, 2005:767–787.

A.2. What is sick sinus syndrome?

Sick sinus syndrome describes an array of clinical disorders due to irreversible sinus node dysfunction. This may be manifested by episodes of sinus arrest, sinus pause or bradycardia secondary to inadequate sinus node automaticity. As a result, episodes of tachyarrhythmias from ectopic atrial foci can occur as well. Twenty-four–hour Holter monitoring is necessary to make a diagnosis. When episodes of tachycardia and bradycardia coexist, it is often referred to as *tachy-brady* syndrome. This is one of the most common indications for pacemakers and is characterized by the following:

- Unexpected persistent severe sinus bradycardia
- Episodes of sinus arrest or exit block
- Paroxysmal or chronic atrial fibrillation or atrial flutter
- Alteration of paroxysms of rapid regular or irregular atrial tachyarrhythmias and periods of slow atrial and ventricular rates (tachy-brady syndrome)
- Slow return to sinus rhythm following cardioversion
- Lack of increase in sinus rate above 90 per minute following intravenous administration of 1.5 to 2.0 mg atropine

Ferrer MI. The sick sinus syndrome. *Circulation* 1973;47:635–641.

Mangrum JM, DiMarco JP. The evaluation and management of bradycardia. *N Engl J Med* 2000;342:703–709.

Zipes DP, Libby P, Bonow RO, et al. eds. *Braunwald's heart disease, a textbook of cardiovascular medicine*, 6th ed. Philadelphia: WB Saunders, 2005:767–787.

A.3. How would you diagnose first-, second-, and third-degree atrioventricular (AV) block, right bundle branch block (RBBB) with left anterior fascicular hemiblock, and left posterior fascicular hemiblock?

First-degree AV block is characterized by a PR interval of greater than 0.20 seconds. Second-degree AV block is subdivided into two types. Mobitz type I, or Wenckebach block, is characterized by a progressively lengthening PR interval, which occurs until a P-wave is not conducted down the AV node and a QRS complex is dropped. The site of block is typically in the AV node. Mobitz type II block is characterized by a loss of AV conduction with no progressive lengthening of the PR interval prior to the sudden dropping of the QRS complex. The site of block is typically below the AV node and within the His-Purkinje system. Third-degree AV block, also called complete heart block, occurs when all electrical activity from the atrium fails to progress into the Purkinje system. The site of block can lie either in the AV node or the His-Purkinje system. The atrial and ventricular contractions have no relation with each other. The QRS complex is normal in complete AV nodal block. The QRS complex with complete infranodal block is frequently wide, and the ventricular rate is slow, averaging 40 beats per minute. RBBB with left anterior hemiblock is indicated when the electrocardiogram shows RBBB and left axis deviation in the absence of an inferior myocardial infarction (MI). Complete RBBB with right axis deviation is indicative of RBBB and left posteroinferior hemiblock in the absence of a lateral MI or evidence of right heart failure.

Zipes DP, Libby P, Bonow RO, et al. eds. *Braunwald's heart disease, a textbook of cardiovascular medicine*, 6th ed. Philadelphia: WB Saunders, 2005:767–787.

A.4. Is it necessary to insert a temporary pacemaker before general anesthesia for an asymptomatic patient with bifascicular block?

Only a small minority of patients with bifascicular block develops transient or established complete heart block and require implantation of a permanent pacemaker (PPM). The risk of progression to complete heart block in asymptomatic patients is very small and such patients do not require a PPM; therefore, it is not necessary to insert a temporary pacemaker before general anesthesia. However, it is advisable to have an external pacemaker available in the operating room.

Berg GR, Kotler MN. The significance of bilateral bundle branch block in the preoperative patient. *Chest* 1971;59:62–67.

Gauss A, Hubner C, Radermaker P, et al. Perioperative risk of bradyarrhythmias with asymptomatic chronic bifascicular block or left bundle block. does an additional first degree atrioventricular block make any difference? *Anesthesiology* 1998;88:679–687.

Trohman RG, Kim MH, Pinski SL. Cardiac pacing: the state of the art. *Lancet* 2004;364: 1701–1719.

Zipes DP, Libby P, Bonow RO, et al. eds. *Braunwald's heart disease, a textbook of cardiovascular medicine*, 6th ed. Philadelphia: WB Saunders, 2005:767–787.

Table 9.1   The NASPE/BPEG Generic (NBG) Pacemaker Identification Code.

LETTER I CHAMBER(S) PACED	LETTER II CHAMBER(S) SENSED	LETTER III MODE OF RESPONSE	LETTER IV PROGRAMMABILITY RATE MODULATION	LETTER V ANTITACHYARRHYTHMIA FUNCTION(S)
O = None	O = None	O = None	O = None	O = None
A = Atrium	A = Atrium	T = Triggered	P = Single programmable	P = Pacing
V = Ventricle	V = Ventricle	I = Inhibited	M = Multi-programmable	S = Shock
D = Dual(A + V)	D = Dual(A + V)	D = Dual(T + I)	C = Communicating	D = Dual(P + S)
			R = Rate modulation	

BPEG. British Pacing and Electrophysiology Group; NASPE, North American Society of Pacing and Electrophysiology; NBG, North American and British Generic.

A.5. What are the three-letter and five-letter identification codes of the North American Society of Pacing and Electrophysiology (NASPE) and British Pacing and Electrophysiology Group (BPEG) generic (NBG) code for pacemaker classification?

With the growing complexity of pacing modes and location and function of cardiac pacing leads, difficulties with terminology became apparent. In the 1970s, the Intersociety Commission for Heart Disease Resources (ICHD) suggested a classification code, which is now widely accepted. The original nomenclature involved a three-letter identification code, as shown in the first three columns of Table 9.1. In 1980, this code was extended to five letters; the last two letters can be deleted when not applicable. In 1987, the NASPE (now known as the *Heart Rhythm Society*) and BPEG adopted a new five-letter code to describe the operation of implantable pacemakers (Table 9.1). The five-letter code is also called the *NBG* pacemaker code. The first letter describes the chamber(s) that the pacemaker can pace, the second letter describes the chamber(s) that it senses, and the third letter describes the response of the pacemaker to sensed intrinsic activity. The last two letters describe additional features such as rate responsiveness that are commonly omitted when not used. For example, a VVI pacing mode paces in the ventricle, can sense intrinsic activity in the ventricle and inhibits pacing when it senses intrinsic activity. A VOO pacing mode paces in the ventricle but does not sense intrinsic activity nor does it inhibit pacing—it simply paces regardless of the heart's electrical activity.

American Society of Anesthesiologists Task Force on Perioperative Management of Patients with Cardiac Rhythm Management Devices. Practice advisory for the perioperative management of patients with cardiac rhythm management devices: pacemakers and implantable cardioverter–defibrillators. A report by the American Society of Anesthesiologists task force on perioperative management of patients with cardiac rhythm management devices. *Anesthesiology* 2005;103:186–198.

Zipes DP, Libby P, Bonow RO, et al. eds. *Braunwald's heart disease, a textbook of cardiovascular medicine*, 6th ed. Philadelphia: WB Saunders, 2005:767–787.

A.6. How many modes of pacing are available in modern day permanent pacemakers (PPMs)? How do they work?

Modern day pacemakers are programmable into one of three modes of pacing: asynchronous pacing, single-chamber demand pacing, and dual-chamber atrioventricular (AV) sequential demand pacing.

Asynchronous or fixed-rate (e.g., AOO, VOO, DOO [see question A.5 for details]) modes pace at a preset rate that is independent of the inherent heart rate. They can be atrial, ventricular, or dual chamber. Competition and ventricular fibrillation (VF) are the potential complications when normal heart rate reappears. VF can theoretically occur because the pacing spike can potentially be delivered during ventricular repolarization, resulting in an R on T phenomenon. This, however, is very rare.

Single-chamber demand pacing (e.g., AAI, VVI) paces at a preset rate only when the spontaneous heart rate drops below the preset rate. The ventricular-inhibited pacer is the most popular type and is suppressed by normal electrical activity of the QRS complex. For example, if this patient's device was programmed to VVI 70 beats per minute, the device would pace in the ventricle only when the native ventricular rate fell below 70 beats per minute. Once the native ventricular rate resumed above 70 beats per minute, the device would sense this activity and inhibit further pacing. Single-chamber demand pacing in the atrium functions in a similar way but is rarely used alone in the United States.

Dual-chamber AV sequential pacing requires two pacemaker leads, one in the right atrium and one in the right ventricle. The atrium is stimulated to contract first; then, after an adjustable PR interval, the ventricle is stimulated to contract. For example, if this patient's device was programmed to DDD 70 beats per minute with a PR interval (AKA: AV delay) of 200 ms, the device would begin pacing the atrium first if the intrinsic sinus rate fell below 70 beats per minute. After the atrium has been paced, the device will wait for 200 ms to sense intrinsic ventricular activity. If it does not see intrinsic activity within 200 ms, it will then pace in the ventricle as well. DDD pacemakers can also pace in the ventricle in response to intrinsic atrial activity. For example, if the intrinsic atrial rate was 80 beats per minute, the device would inhibit pacing in the atrium because the base rate was set to 70 beats per minute. But because it is a dual-chamber device capable of sensing and pacing in both chambers, it will wait 200 ms from the time of the intrinsic atrial activity and watch for intrinsic ventricular activity as well. If it does not see intrinsic ventricular activity occurring within 200 ms from the intrinsic atrial activity, it will then pace in the ventricle.

Programmable pacemakers have been widely used since 1980. Pacing rate, pulse duration, voltage output, and R-wave sensitivity are the most common programmable functions. Refractory periods, PR intervals, mode of pacing, hysteresis, and atrial tracking rate can be programmed in modern pacemakers.

Zipes DP, Libby P, Bonow RO, et al. eds. *Braunwald's heart disease, a textbook of cardiovascular medicine*, 6th ed. Philadelphia: WB Saunders, 2005:767–787.

A.7. The patient was mechanically hyperventilated during surgery and his pacemaker gradually increased his heart rate. What feature of the permanent pacemaker (PPM) is accounting for this?

All modern day pacemakers have the ability to adjust the pacing rate according to the patient's level of activity in an effort to obtain a more physiologic response to exercise. This is known as *rate-response* (adaptive) pacing and is denoted by an "R" in the fourth position of the NBG coding schema. Various activity-detecting systems have been developed in years past to create a reliable rate-responsive pacemaker. They included muscle movement, respiratory rate, minute ventilation, central venous temperature, QT interval, myocardial contractility (dp/dt), oxygen saturation and pH in mixed venous blood, and ventricular depolarization gradient. Nowadays, PPMs used in the United States rely on sensors of motion (Medtronic, St. Jude Medical, Guidant-Boston Scientific) or sensors of changes in minute ventilation (Medtronic, Guidant-Boston Scientific). Because of the latter phenomenon, patients undergoing general anesthesia who are subjected to mechanical hyperventilation (e.g., neurosurgery) can experience an increase in the rate of pacing. As a result, most device manufacturers recommend disabling the rate-responsive features before surgery. If reprogramming the device is not readily available, a magnet may be placed over the pacemaker site to temporarily convert it to asynchronous pacing. Most properly functioning pacemakers within the United States respond to magnets in this way.

Zipes DP, Libby P, Bonow RO, et al. eds. *Braunwald's heart disease, a textbook of cardiovascular medicine*, 6th ed. Philadelphia: WB Saunders, 2005:767–787.

A.8. What are the advantages and disadvantages of atrial pacing only?

Atrial pacing only increases cardiac output by 26% over the cardiac output of ventricular pacing only because atrial contraction contributes to approximately 15% to 25% of the diastolic filling of the ventricle. It has been shown that coronary blood flow increases and coronary resistance decreases during atrial pacing only. Atrial pacing has also been shown to reduce the incidence of atrial fibrillation. Atrial pacing only is seldomly used in the United States and often is implanted with the addition of a ventricular pacing lead in the event of atrioventricular (AV) block.

Healey JS, Toff WD, Lamas GA, et al. Cardiovascular outcomes with atrial-based pacing compared with ventricular pacing: meta-analysis of randomized trials, using individual patient data. *Circulation* 2006;114:11–17.

Yoshida S, Ganz W, Donoso R, et al. Coronary hemodynamics during successive elevation of heart rate by pacing in subjects with angina pectoris. *Circulation* 1971;44:1062–1071.

A.9. What are the indications for and complications associated with atrioventricular (AV) sequential permanent pacemakers (PPMs)?

When ventricular pacing alone cannot maintain adequate cardiac output and atrial pacing alone is not justified, as in complete AV block, AV sequential pacing is indicated. Because of the success of atrial transvenous leads, bioengineering advances such as thinner polyurethane insulation and improved device programmability, the indications for dual-chamber pacing have broadened. It can be used for sick sinus syndrome and all degrees of heart block. PPMs programmed to DDD pacing are the ultimate form of physiologic pacing. Programmable features include the mode of pacing, the AV delay, the maximum atrial rate that the ventricle will follow (atrial tracking), and the minimum atrial rate for sensing at which atrial pacing commences. The major advantage of such pacing is the ability to increase the cardiac output by 200% to 300% under extreme stress and a reduced incidence of atrial fibrillation development. Historically, the major disadvantage of DDD pacing has been the possibility of pacemaker-mediated tachycardia. More recently, another disadvantage recognized has been the development of ventricular dyssynchrony (see question A.13) due to ventricular pacing. Long-term follow-up of patients with dual-chamber pacemakers demonstrated reductions in left ventricular ejection fractions when compared to atrial pacing alone, especially in the setting of preexisting left ventricular dysfunction.

Nielsen JC Bottcher M, Nielsen TT, et al. Regional myocardial blood flow in patients with sick sinus syndrome randomized to long-term single chamber atrial or dual chamber pacing—effect of pacing mode and rate. *J Am Coll Cardiol* 2000;35:1453–1461.

Zipes DP, Libby P, Bonow RO, et al. eds. *Braunwald's heart disease, a textbook of cardiovascular medicine*, 6th ed. Philadelphia: WB Saunders, 2005:767–787.

A.10. How would you know if the patient's permanent pacemaker (PPM) was atrially, ventricularly, or atrioventricular (AV) sequentially pacing?

In atrial pacing, an electrical spike appears before the P wave and the QRS complex is usually normal. In ventricular pacing, the electrical spike is followed immediately by a widened QRS complex. In AV sequential pacing, there are two spikes, one before the P wave and another preceding the QRS complex.

Zipes DP, Libby P, Bonow RO, et al. eds. *Braunwald's heart disease, a textbook of cardiovascular medicine*, 6th ed. Philadelphia: WB Saunders, 2005:767–787.

A.11. What is the maximum amount of energy that a modern day permanent pacemaker can provide in terms of pulse amplitude and pulse width?

In order to successfully pace the heart, PPM must provide enough energy to allow for cardiac depolarization. Energy is a direct function of the amount of voltage produced (pulse amplitude) and the duration of time the voltage is delivered (pulse width). Although small variations exist among all modern day PPMs, the maximum pulse amplitude or output of stimulation usually is 7.5 volts (V). The maximum pulse width or the duration of stimulation is usually 1.5 msec.

Zipes DP, Libby P, Bonow RO, et al. eds. *Braunwald's heart disease, a textbook of cardiovascular medicine*, 6th ed. Philadelphia: WB Saunders, 2005:767–787.

A.12. During a new permanent pacemaker implantation, what are the acceptable values for modern day pacemaker leads in terms of pacing thresholds, amplitude of sensed R waves, and resistance?

Because current PPMs have a maximal pacing output of 7.5 V at 1.5 msec, the pacing threshold cannot exceed the previously mentioned values. In fact, fluctuations in the pacing threshold can occur during the first few weeks after a pacing lead has been implanted. There is an initial sharp rise in the pacing threshold during the first 2 weeks because of tissue reaction around the tip of the electrode despite the presence of steroid embedded at the tip. Then it falls to two to three times the acute level from the scar formation. As a result, all device manufacturers recommend that the pacing output be at least two times the voltage of the threshold value or three times the pulse width of the threshold value. In the chronic state, pacing thresholds remain essentially at the same level in 80% of patients. For Ventricular lead, the intrinsic R waves should be at least 5 to 6 mV in amplitude to allow for proper sensing by the PPM because most modern day PPM have preset sensitivity settings approximately 2.0 to 3.0 mV. Impedance should be between 250 and 1,300 ohms. In atrial lead implantation, the acceptable sensing P wave values are at least 1.5 to 2.0 mV, and pacing threshold is 0.6 to 2.0 V.

Bonow RO, Zipes DP, Libby P, et al. eds. *Braunwald's Heart disease, a textbook of cardiovascular medicine*, 6th ed. Philadelphia: WB Saunders, 2005:767–787.

A.13. What is a biventricular permanent pacemaker (PPM) or cardiac resynchronization therapy (CRT) device? What are the indications for such a device?

It has long been recognized that individuals with interventricular conduction abnormalities, specifically left bundle branch block (LBBB) conduction patterns, have a predilection toward impaired left ventricular systolic function. In fact, the most common ventricular conduction delay seen in patients with congestive heart failure is LBBB. On a mechanistic level, individuals with LBBB demonstrate ventricular dyssynchrony, a phenomenon whereby the left ventricle contracts in a stepwise process. Unlike normal individuals where the left ventricular septum and the left ventricular lateral free wall contract nearly simultaneously, patients with LBBB have a delay in the activation of the left lateral free wall. As a result, there is marked impairment in left ventricular systolic function and increased myocardial work and oxygen consumption. One approach to correct this dyssynchrony is to "resynchronize" the heart through the use of a biventricular pacemaker/implantable cardioverter-defibrillator. These devices are capable of pacing both the left ventricular septum (through a pacemaker lead in the right ventricle) and the left ventricular lateral free wall simultaneously (through a pacemaker lead in the coronary sinus), therefore allowing for activation of the entire left ventricle at the same time.

Candidates for implantation of a biventricular device include individuals with severe cardiomyopathy (EF <= 35%), and LBBB with New York Heart Association (NYHA) class III or class IV symptoms despite optimal medical therapy.

Nesser HJ, Breithardt O-A, Khandheria BK, et al. Established and evolving indications for cardiac resynchronization. *Heart* 2004;90:vi5–vi9.

A.14. What are the usual life spans of permanent pacemakers (PPMs) and implantable cardioverter-defibrillators (ICDs)?

The lithium-powered pacemakers can last 5 to 10 years for dual-chamber pacing and 7 to 12 years for single-chamber pacing. The silver-vanadium oxide batteries used in ICDs typically last for 5 to 8 years.

Atlee JL, Bernstein AD. Cardiac rhythm management devices (part I). *Anesthesiology* 2001; 95:1265–1280.

Zipes DP, Libby P, Bonow RO, et al. eds. *Braunwald's heart disease, a textbook of cardiovascular medicine*, 6th ed. Philadelphia: WB Saunders, 2005:767–802.

A.15. What is an implantable cardioverter-defibrillator (ICD)? How does it work?

An ICD system consists of a pulse generator and leads for tachyarrhythmia detection and therapy. ICDs provide antitachycardia and antibradycardia pacing; synchronized (cardioversion) or nonsynchronized (defibrillation) shocks; telemetry; and diagnostics, including stored event electrograms and history logs. Essentially, the pulse generator is a self-powered computer within a hermetically sealed titanium casing (can). One or two (in series) 3.2 V lithium–silver vanadium oxide batteries with high power density are used to power the pulse generator, circuitry, and aluminum electrolytic storage capacitors. Most ICD designs use two capacitors in series to achieve a maximum voltage for defibrillation. A major challenge in ICD design is the large range of voltages that must be controlled in a very small package. Therapeutic defibrillatory shocks approach 850 V in modern day devices.

Modern ICDs use transvenous lead systems for sensing, pacing, and shocks. Epicardial leads are still used in infants and small children. Ventricular demand pacing for bradycardia is a standard feature of all single-chamber ICDs. Dual-chamber ICDs have all the capabilities of dual-chamber pacemakers, including rate-adaptive pacing and automatic mode switching. However the response to magnet differs. See section C.8.

Current ICDs have many programmable features, but essentially they measure each cardiac R-R interval and categorize the rate as normal, too fast (short R-R interval) or too slow. When the device detects a sufficient number of short R-R intervals within a period of time (all programmable), it will declare a tachycardia episode. The internal computer will decide between antitachycardia pacing (less energy use, better tolerated by patient) and shock based on its programmed algorithm. If shock is chosen, an internal capacitor is charged which take approximately 5 to 13 seconds. Most devices are programmed to reconfirm ventricular tachycardia (VT) or ventricular fibrillation (VF) after charging to prevent inappropriate shock therapy. Typically, ICDs deliver no more than six shocks per episode. Once a shock is delivered, the ICD will redetect to determine whether or not the shock successfully terminated the arrhythmia. A tachycardia episode is considered terminated when sinus rhythm has been restored for a certain period of time (varies with manufacturer).

Atlee JL, Bernstein AD. Cardiac rhythm management devices (part I). *Anesthesiology* 2001; 95:1265–1280.

Fuster V, Alexander RW, O'Rooke RA, eds. *Hurst's the heart*, 11th ed. New York: McGraw-Hill, 2004:989–1000.

Zipes DP, Libby P, Bonow RO, et al. eds. *Braunwald's heart disease, a textbook of cardiovascular medicine*, 6th ed. Philadelphia: WB Saunders, 2005:787–802.

A.16. What are the indications for implantable cardioverter-defibrillators (ICDs)?

Initially ICDs were indicated for hemodynamically significant ventricular tachycardia (VT) or ventricular fibrillation (VF). Newer indications include the following and continue to evolve:

- Cardiac arrest resulting from VT/VF not resulting from a transient or reversible cause
- Spontaneous sustained VT with structural heart disease
- Syncope of undetermined origin with clinically relevant, hemodynamically significant sustained VT or VF induced at electrophysiology study (EPS)
- Ischemic cardiomyopathy (EF ≤30%) without a recent myocardial infarction (within the last 4 weeks) or revascularization in the past 3 months.
- Ischemic or nonischemic dilated cardiomyopathy (EF ≤35%) with New York Heart Association (NYHA) class II or III heart failure symptoms stable for the past 9 months.
- Brugada syndrome—right bundle branch block (RBBB) and ST segment elevation leads V_1 to V_3
- Arrhythmogenic right ventricular dysplasia
- Long and short Q-T syndrome
- Hypertrophic obstructive cardiomyopathy

Goldberger Z, Lampert R. Implantable cardioverter-defibrillators: expanding indications and technologies. *JAMA* 2006;295:809–818.

Zipes DP, Libby P, Bonow RO, et al. eds. *Braunwald's heart disease, a textbook of cardiovascular medicine*, 6th ed. Philadelphia: WB Saunders, 2005:787–802.

A.17. What is the North American Society of Pacing and Electrophysiology (NASPE)/British Pacing and Electrophysiology Group (BPEG) generic defibrillator (NBD) code?

Like pacemakers, implantable cardioverter-defibrillators (ICDs) have a generic code to indicate lead placement and function. The NBD code is shown in Table 9.2. However, the most robust form of identification, called the "label form," replaces the fourth letter of the NBD with the appropriate generic pacemaker code.

Table 9.2   NASPE/BPEG Generic Defibrillator (NBD) Code.

LETTER I SHOCK CHAMBER(S)	LETTER II ANTITACHYCARDIA PACING CHAMBER(S)	LETTER III TACHYCARDIA DETECTION	LETTER IV ANTIBRADYCARDIA PACING CHAMBER(S)
O = None	O = None	E = Electrogram	O = None
A = Atrium	A = Atrium	H = Hemodynamic	A = Atrium
V = Ventricle	V = Ventricle	(not yet available)	V = Ventricle
D = Dual(A + V)	D = Dual(A + V)		D = Dual(A + V)

BPEG, British Pacing and Electrophysiology Group; NASPE, North American Society of Pacing and Electrophysiology; NBG, North American and British Generic.

> American Society of Anesthesiologists Task Force on Perioperative Management of Patients with Cardiac Rhythm Management Devices. Practice advisory for the perioperative management of patients with cardiac rhythm management devices: pacemakers and implantable cardioverter–defibrillators. A report by the American Society of Anesthesiologists task force on perioperative management of patients with cardiac rhythm management devices. *Anesthesiology* 2005;103:186–198.

B. Preoperative Evaluation and Preparation

B.1. How would you preoperatively evaluate the patient described earlier?

Preoperative evaluation should include the routine systemic workup, paying particular attention to cardiovascular disorders. The systemic routine includes complete blood count, urinalysis, coagulation screening with prothrombin time and partial thromboplastin time, serum electrolytes, blood urea nitrogen (BUN), blood sugar, chest x-ray film, and electrocardiogram. Special attention should be paid to the history, symptoms, and signs of myocardial infarction (MI), congestive heart failure, and arrhythmia. Serum electrolytes, especially potassium level, must be in the normal range. For the patient with a cardiac rhythm management device (CRMD), preoperative evaluation should include the following:

- Establish whether a patient has a CRMD
- Define the type of CRMD
- Determine dependency on pacing function of the CRMD
- Determine CRMD function

> American Society of Anesthesiologists Task Force on Perioperative Management of Patients with Cardiac Rhythm Management Devices. Practice advisory for the perioperative management of patients with cardiac rhythm management devices: pacemakers and implantable cardioverter–defibrillators. A report by the American Society of Anesthesiologists task force on perioperative management of patients with cardiac rhythm management devices. *Anesthesiology* 2005;103:186–198.
>
> Salukhe TV, Dob D. Pacemakers and defibrillators: anesthetic implications. *Br J Anesth* 2004; 93:95–104.

B.2. How do you determine whether the patient has a cardiac rhythm management device (CRMD) and define what type of CRMD?

Determining whether a patient has a CRMD should be based on (a) a focused history including but not limited to the patient interview, medical records review, review of available chest x-ray films, electrocardiogram, or any available monitor or rhythm strip information and (b) a focused physical examination (checking for scars, palpating for device).

Defining the type of device is accomplished by (a) obtaining the manufacturer's identification card from the patient or other source, (b) ordering chest x-ray studies if no other data are available, or (c) referring to supplemental resources (e.g., manufacturers' databases, pacemaker clinic records, consultation with a cardiologist).

American Society of Anesthesiologists Task Force on Perioperative Management of Patients with Cardiac Rhythm Management Devices. Practice advisory for the perioperative management of patients with cardiac rhythm management devices: pacemakers and implantable cardioverter–defibrillators. A report by the American Society of Anesthesiologists task force on perioperative management of patients with cardiac rhythm management devices. *Anesthesiology* 2005;103:186–198.

B.3. How do you determine whether the patient is dependent on pacing function of the cardiac rhythm management device (CRMD)?

CRMD dependency for pacemaking function may be determined by one or more of the following: (a) a verbal history or an indication in the medical record that the patient has experienced a bradyarrhythmia that has caused syncope or other symptoms requiring CRMD implantation, (b) a history of successful atrioventricular nodal ablation that resulted in CRMD placement, or (c) a CRMD evaluation that shows no evidence of spontaneous ventricular activity when the pacemaking function of the CRMD is programmed to VVI pacing mode at the lowest programmable rate. The electrocardiogram will show pacing spikes if the patient is dependent on the pacing function.

American Society of Anesthesiologists Task Force on Perioperative Management of Patients with Cardiac Rhythm Management Devices. Practice advisory for the perioperative management of patients with cardiac rhythm management devices: pacemakers and implantable cardioverter–defibrillators. A report by the American Society of Anesthesiologists task force on perioperative management of patients with cardiac rhythm management devices. *Anesthesiology* 2005;103:186–198.

B.4. How do you know if the implanted permanent pacemaker (PPM) or implantable cardioverter-defibrillator (ICD) is working?

The cardiac rhythm management device (CRMD) function is ideally assessed by interrogating the device. If interrogating the device is not an option, one can slow the intrinsic heart rate to a rate below that of the pacemaker by carotid massage or a Valsalva maneuver. Carotid massage to slow the heart rate should be used cautiously because it could result in an arteriosclerotic plaque embolizing to the cerebral circulation. If the rate does not slow down enough for the pacemaker to take over the ventricle, device can be tested by placing a magnet over it to convert it to a fixed-rate pacing mode. In this mode, one will see pacing spikes march through the rhythm strip with no regard for the intrinsic electrical activity of the heart. The rate at which the pacemaker will pace in the presence of a magnet varies among device manufacturers and is dependent on the battery life.

American Society of Anesthesiologists Task Force on Perioperative Management of Patients with Cardiac Rhythm Management Devices. Practice advisory for the perioperative management of patients with cardiac rhythm management devices: pacemakers and implantable cardioverter–defibrillators. A report by the American Society of Anesthesiologists task force on perioperative management of patients with cardiac rhythm management devices. *Anesthesiology* 2005;103:186–198.

B.5. What information would you like to obtain from interrogating his device?

Device interrogations provide information on the status and current programmed settings of a permanent pacemaker (PPM) or implantable cardioverter-defibrillator (ICD). The important primary information for anesthesiologists include (a) battery life, (b) programmed pacing mode such as VVIR, DDDR, (c) pacemaker dependency, (d) intrinsic rhythm, (e) magnet rate and rhythm (f) prior recorded arrhythmic events, and (g) pacemaker lead parameters (including pacing threshold, ability to sense intrinsic activity, and lead impedance).

Zipes DP, Libby P, Bonow RO, et al. eds. *Braunwald's heart disease, a textbook of cardiovascular medicine*, 6th ed. Philadelphia: WB Saunders, 2005:767–787.

B.6. How do you preoperatively prepare the patient for surgery and anesthesia?

Preparation for patient safety and proper maintenance of the device during a procedure includes the following:

- Determining whether electromagnetic interference (EMI) is likely to occur during the planned procedure;
- Determining whether reprogramming the cardiac rhythm management device (CRMD) pacemaking function to an asynchronous pacing mode or disabling any special algorithms, including rate-adaptive functions, is needed;
- Suspending antitachyarrhythmia functions if present;
- Advising the surgeon performing the procedure to consider use of a bipolar electrocautery system or ultrasonic (harmonic) scalpel to minimize potential adverse effects of EMI on the pulse generator or leads;
- Assuring the availability of temporary pacing and defibrillation equipment; and
- Evaluating the possible effects of anesthetic techniques on CRMD function and patient-CRMD interactions.

American Society of Anesthesiologists Task Force on Perioperative Management of Patients with Cardiac Rhythm Management Devices. Practice advisory for the perioperative management of patients with cardiac rhythm management devices: pacemakers and implantable cardioverter–defibrillators. A report by the American Society of Anesthesiologists task force on perioperative management of patients with cardiac rhythm management devices. *Anesthesiology* 2005;103:186–198.

B.7. Would you recommend reprogramming this device to asynchronously pace before surgery?

The patient has an implantable cardioverter-defibrillator (ICD) with dual-chamber pacing because of sick sinus syndrome and ventricular tachycardia. I would recommend reprogramming the device to asynchronous pacing mode before surgery for the following reasons:

- Electrocautery during surgery may inhibit pacing function
- The patient may become pacemaker dependent during abdominal surgery
- A magnet cannot convert the pacemaker in an ICD system to asynchronous mode pacing. A magnet placed over an ICD only disables tachycardia detection and therapy of the ICD. This is true of all devices used in the United States. One notable exception are ICDs manufactured by ELA Medical (Cedex, France) which, in the presence of a magnet, will not only disable tachycardia detection therapy but also convert pacing to a fixed rate at 96 beats per minute.

American Society of Anesthesiologists Task Force on Perioperative Management of Patients with Cardiac Rhythm Management Devices. Practice advisory for the perioperative management of patients with cardiac rhythm management devices: pacemakers and implantable cardioverter–defibrillators. A report by the American Society of Anesthesiologists task force on perioperative management of patients with cardiac rhythm management devices. *Anesthesiology* 2005;103:186–198.

B.8. Would you reprogram the implantable cardioverter-defibrillator (ICD) preoperatively?

The ICD can be reprogrammed to disable the antitachycardia function before surgery in the operating room where a defibrillator is readily available. Alternatively, a magnet can be placed over the ICD to disable the antitachycardia function in the operating room. The advantage of placing a magnet on an ICD is that the magnet can be easily removed and the antitachycardia function is quickly enabled in case of ventricular tachycardia (VT)/ventricular fibrillation (VF) during surgery.

Zipes DP, Libby P, Bonow RO, et al. eds. *Braunwald's heart disease, a textbook of cardiovascular medicine*, 6th ed. Philadelphia: WB Saunders, 2005:787–802.

C. Intraoperative Management

C.1. How would you monitor this patient?

Intraoperative monitoring should include both continuous electrocardiogram (ECG) and continuous peripheral pulse monitorings. Peripheral pulse can be monitored by palpation of the pulse, auscultation of heart sounds, pulse plethysmography or oximetry, a tracing of arterial wave form, or ultrasound peripheral pulse monitoring.

Arterial line and central venous pressure or pulmonary artery pressure monitoring may be used only if the patient has poor ventricular function. The "artifact filter" on the ECG monitor should be disabled in order to detect the pacing spikes. The ECG monitor should be set in diagnostic mode instead of monitoring mode.

American Society of Anesthesiologists Task Force on Perioperative Management of Patients with Cardiac Rhythm Management Devices. Practice advisory for the perioperative management of patients with cardiac rhythm management devices: pacemakers and implantable cardioverter–defibrillators. A report by the American Society of Anesthesiologists task force on perioperative management of patients with cardiac rhythm management devices. *Anesthesiology* 2005;103:186–198.

C.2. What drugs and equipment would you like to have on hand in the operating room?

A complete array of drugs and equipment must be immediately available for cardiopulmonary resuscitation. The minimal requirements include, electrocardiograph (ECG) monitor, a transcutaneous external pacing and DC defibrillator, and the usual drugs for resuscitation.

Atlee JL, Bernstein AD. Cardiac rhythm management devices (part I). *Anesthesiology* 2001; 95:1265–1280.

Zipes DP, Libby P, Bonow RO, et al. eds. *Braunwald's heart disease, a textbook of cardiovascular medicine*, 6th ed. Philadelphia: WB Saunders, 2005:767–787.

C.3. How would you set up the transcutaneous external pacer and defibrillator?

We prefer using defibrillating electrodes such as Zoll Pads to paddles because the electrodes can be placed before surgery at the desirable positions and connected to a defibrillator/pacemaker readily available for pacing and defibrillation. The electrodes should be placed as far (more than 6 in. or 15 cm) from a cardiac rhythm management device (CRMD) as possible. The electrodes are positioned perpendicular to the CRMD system. There are three recommended electrode placements:

- *Anteroposterior placement.* The right arm (RA) electrode placed under the left scapula and the left leg (LL) electrode at apex of the heart (as shown in Fig. 9.1).
- *Apex-anterior placement.* The RA electrode placed under the right clavicle and the LL electrode at the apex of the heart (Fig. 9.2A).
- *Apex-posterior placement.* The RA electrode placed over the right scapula and the LL electrode at the apex of the heart (Fig. 9.2B).

It is important to remember that the presence of a CRMD should not deter standard resuscitation efforts.

Stone KR, McPherson CA. Assessment and management of patients with pacemakers and implantable cardioverter defibrillator. *Crit Care Med* 2004;32(Suppl):S155–S165.

C.4. Had this patient's implantable cardioverter-defibrillator (ICD) been implanted the day before surgery, would you consider avoiding certain inhalational gases for anesthesia?

It has been reported that nitrous oxide could cause pacemaker malfunction by increasing gas in the prepectoral pacemaker pocket. Despite air evacuation with antibiotic solution before closure of the prepectoral pocket, a small amount of air remains entrapped in the pocket. In general, this small amount of air should have no clinical significance. However, nitrous oxide is 35 times more soluble in blood than nitrogen. When nitrous oxide is used for anesthesia, the amount of nitrous oxide diffused from blood to the air pocket is much more than the amount of nitrogen diffused from the air pocket to blood. Therefore, this causes an expansion of the gas in the pocket, which leads to loss of anodal contact and pacing system malfunction. It is advisable not to use nitrous oxide in a patient with a newly implanted pacemaker.

Lamas GA, Rebecca GS, Braunwald NS, et al. Pacemaker malfunction after nitrous oxide anesthesia. *Am J Cardiol* 1985;56:995.

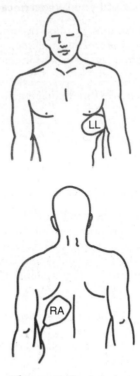

Figure 9.1 Anterior–posterior placement of defibrillating electrodes. The right arm (RA) electrode is placed under the left scapula and the left leg (LL) electrode is placed at the apex of the heart.

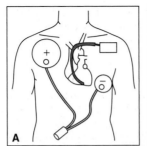
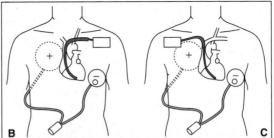

Figure 9.2 Placement of defibrillating electrodes. **A:** Apex—anterior placement with both pads placed anteriorly. **B and C:** Apex—posterior placement are shown with the device in the left prepectoral region **(B)** and the right pectoral region **(C)**. (Reprinted with permission from Ellenbogen KA, Kay GN, Wilkoff BL, eds. *Clinical cardiac pacing and defibrillation*. 2nd ed, Philadelphia: Saunders, 2000;944.)

C.5. Electromagnetic interference (EMI) from electro cautery during the case results in significant noise on your cardiac monitor. You recall that EMI can also inhibit pacing function from the permanent pacemaker (PPM). In this pacemaker-dependent patient, how can you determine whether inappropriate inhibition of the PPM is occurring?

During electrocautery, the electrocardiogram is frequently useless because of interference. The best monitor available to determine if inhibition is taking place is a hand on the pulse. The precordial or esophageal stethoscope, pulse oximeter, or blood pressure is also acceptable.

American Society of Anesthesiologists Task Force on Perioperative Management of Patients with Cardiac Rhythm Management Devices. Practice advisory for the perioperative management of patients with cardiac rhythm management devices: pacemakers and implantable cardioverter–defibrillators. A report by the American Society of Anesthesiologists task force on perioperative management of patients with cardiac rhythm management devices. *Anesthesiology* 2005;103:186–198.

C.6. What are the potential responses of pacemakers and implantable cardioverter-defibrillators (ICDs) to electrocautery?

The responses of pacemakers to electrocautery or other electromagnetic interference include the following:

- Inhibition of pacing
- Asynchronous pacing
- Reset to Backup mode
- Myocardial burns, rare
- Ventricular fibrillation (VF), rare

The responses of ICDs include the following:

- Inhibition of pacing
- Asynchronous pacing
- Inappropriate tachy therapy
- Inhibition of tachy therapy

Salukhe TV, Dob D. Pacemakers and defibrillators: anesthetic implications. *Br J Anesth* 2004;93:95–104.

Stone KR, McPherson CA. Assessment and management of patients with pacemakers and implantable cardioverter defibrillator. *Crit Care Med* 2004;32(suppl):S155–S165.

C.7. How would you prevent the effects of electromagnetic interference (EMI) on the pacemaker or implantable cardioverter-defibrillator (ICD) from the electrocautery?

The safest way to prevent intraoperative EMI response is appropriate reprogramming. The following precautions should be taken to minimize the effects of electrocautery:

- Place the cautery grounding plate as close to the operative site and as far from the cardiac rhythm management device (CRMD) as possible to make sure that the current pathway does not pass through or near the CRMD system. For some cases, the grounding plate might need to be placed on a site different from the thigh (e.g., the superior posterior aspect of the shoulder contralateral to the CRMD generator position for a head and neck case).

- Do not use cautery within 15 cm of the pacemaker as it may interfere with the battery circuitry. If in contact with a break in the insulation of the electrode, it may cauterize the myocardium at the electrode tip rendering it insensitive to pacing impulses.
- Limit cautery use to 1-second bursts every 10 seconds to prevent repetitive asystolic periods.
- If the pacemaker is inhibited by the cautery, place a high-powered magnet over the demand nonprogrammable pacemaker to convert it to fixed-rate mode.
- Using bipolar electrocautery forceps or ultrasonic (harmonic) scalpel reduces electromagnetic interference.

American Society of Anesthesiologists Task Force on Perioperative Management of Patients with Cardiac Rhythm Management Devices. Practice advisory for the perioperative management of patients with cardiac rhythm management devices: pacemakers and implantable cardioverter–defibrillators. A report by the American Society of Anesthesiologists task force on perioperative management of patients with cardiac rhythm management devices. *Anesthesiology* 2005;103:186–198.

Salukhe TV, Dob D. Pacemakers and defibrillators: anesthetic implications. *Br J Anesth* 2004;93:95–104.

Stone KR, McPherson CA. Assessment and management of patients with pacemakers and implantable cardioverter defibrillator. *Crit Care Med* 2004;32(suppl):S155–S165.

C.8. What are the effects of a magnet over pacemakers and implantable cardioverter-defibrillators (ICDs)?

The effect of placing a magnet over a pacemaker or ICD can vary quite considerably depending on the device manufacturer, model and individual programmed modes. This information may be obtained by consulting the device manufacturer's representative. Most pacemakers will switch to a fixed-rate pacing mode when a magnet is placed. However, the response of a pacemaker to a magnet placement may also include the following:

- Asynchronous pacing without rate responsiveness
- No response
- Brief (10 to 100 beats) asynchronous pacing
- Continuous or transient loss of pacing

The response of an ICD to a magnet placement is different from the response of a pacemaker. Magnets will disable tachyarrhythmia detection and therapy which, except in some Guidant-Boston Scientific devices, are reenabled when the magnet is removed. Magnets generally will, with a few exceptions, not affect the pacing mode or rate of ICDs. Therefore the pacemaker in an ICD can be inappropriately inhibited by electrocautery even when a magnet is placed.

It is important to remember that some Guidant-Boston Scientific ICDs are permanently disabled when a magnet is placed for more than 30 seconds. The ICD will not be reactivated when the magnet is removed. To reactivate the Guidant-Boston Scientific ICDs, the magnet has to be reapplied over the ICD for more than 30 seconds and then removed. If a magnet is to be used during surgery, the magnet effects should be tested in the operating room before surgery to ensure that the desired effects will occur during surgery.

Salukhe TV, Dob D. Pacemakers and defibrillators: anesthetic implications. *Br J Anesth* 2004;93:95–104.

Stone KR, McPherson CA. Assessment and management of patients with pacemakers and implantable cardioverter defibrillator. *Crit Care Med* 2004;32(suppl):S155–S165.

C.9. In the middle of surgery, the patient developed ventricular tachycardia. What would you do?

For a patient with an implantable cardioverter-defibrillator (ICD) and magnet-disabled therapies:

- Advise the surgeon performing the procedure to terminate all sources of electromagnetic interference (EMI).
- Remove the magnet to reenable antitachycardia therapies.
- Observe the patient and the monitors for appropriate cardiac rhythm management device (CRMD) therapy. This can be delayed for as long as 10 to 12 seconds as the ICD is charging up.
- If the activities mentioned in the preceding text do not restore ICD function, proceed with emergency external defibrillation or cardioversion.

For a patient with an ICD and programming-disabled therapies:

- Advise individual performing the procedure to terminate all sources of EMI while magnet is removed.
- Reenable therapies through programming if the programmer is immediately available and ready to be used.
- Observe the patient and the monitors for appropriate CRMD therapy.
- If the activities mentioned in the preceding text do not restore ICD function, proceed with emergency external defibrillation or cardioversion.

For external defibrillation (see also question C.3):

- Position defibrillation/cardioversion pads or paddles as far as possible from the CRMD generator.
- Position defibrillation/cardioversion pads or paddles perpendicular to the major axis of the CRMD to the extent possible by placing them in an anteroposterior location.
- If it is technically impossible to place the pads or paddles in locations that help to protect the CRMD, defibrillate/cardiovert the patient in the quickest possible way and be prepared to provide pacing through other routes.
- Use a clinically appropriate energy output.

American Society of Anesthesiologists Task Force on Perioperative Management of Patients with Cardiac Rhythm Management Devices. Practice advisory for the perioperative management of patients with cardiac rhythm management devices: pacemakers and implantable cardioverter–defibrillators. A report by the American Society of Anesthesiologists task force on perioperative management of patients with cardiac rhythm management devices. *Anesthesiology* 2005;103:186–198.

C.10. What precautions should be taken when a patient with a cardiac rhythm management device (CRMD) is undergoing extracorporeal shock wave lithotripsy (ESWL)?

ESWL is no longer contraindicated for patients with pacemakers. The only exception to this general statement is the abdominally placed pacemaker generators. Because these generators are in the blast path of the shock wave, such patients should not be treated with ESWL. However, most transvenous pacemaker generators are placed in a pectoral location that is at a safe distance from the blast path. Consider preoperative disabling of atrial pacing if the lithotripsy system triggers on the R wave.

Although most pacemakers are not affected by ESWL, sometimes it may cause pacemaker malfunctions that include the following:

- Switching to magnet mode
- Reaching upper rate limit

- Pacing irregularity
- Oversensing of asynchronous shocks
- Damage to rate-sensing piezoelectric crystal
- Intermittent inhibition of ventricular output in dual-chamber pacemaker
- Electromagnetic interference

There may be a rate increase in a rate-response (adaptive) pacemaker after ESWL shocks. Therefore, special precautions should be taken preoperatively. The type of pacemaker, indications for its placement, degree of patient dependence, and pacemaker programmability must be determined before lithotripsy. A dedicated pacemaker programmer should be available in the lithotripsy suite should pacemaker malfunction be caused by the shock waves. In addition, an alternative means of pacing, such as transcutaneous pacing, should also be available in case the pacemaker becomes permanently damaged. Low-energy shock waves (<16 kV) should be used initially; then the energy level is gradually increased while pacemaker function is monitored carefully.

It is best to disable tachycardia detection of an ICD during ESWL and to thoroughly test the ICD following the procedure.

American Society of Anesthesiologists Task Force on Perioperative Management of Patients with Cardiac Rhythm Management Devices. Practice advisory for the perioperative management of patients with cardiac rhythm management devices: pacemakers and implantable cardioverter–defibrillators. A report by the American Society of Anesthesiologists task force on perioperative management of patients with cardiac rhythm management devices. *Anesthesiology* 2005;103:186–198.

Atlee JL, Bernstein AD. Cardiac rhythm management devices (part I). *Anesthesiology* 2001; 95:1265–1280.

C.11. Is electroconvulsive therapy (ECT) contraindicated in patients with pacemakers or implantable cardioverter-defibrillators (ICDs)?

It is advisable to consult with the ordering physician, the patient's cardiologist, a cardiac rhythm management device (CRMD) service or the device manufacturer. ECT appears safe for patients with pacemakers because little current flows within the heart due to the high impedance of body tissues. However, the seizure and succinylcholine fasciculations may generate sufficient myopotentials for pacemaker inhibition (unipolar devices) or ventricular tracking (adaptive-rate devices). Therefore, it is advisable to program the pacemaker to nonsensing (asynchronous) mode for pacemaker-dependent patients. An external pacemaker should also be available. All ICDs should be programmed so that tachycardia detection is disabled before ECT and reprogrammed to its original programmed parameters afterwards.

American Society of Anesthesiologists Task Force on Perioperative Management of Patients with Cardiac Rhythm Management Devices. Practice advisory for the perioperative management of patients with cardiac rhythm management devices: pacemakers and implantable cardioverter–defibrillators. A report by the American Society of Anesthesiologists task force on perioperative management of patients with cardiac rhythm management devices. *Anesthesiology* 2005;103:186–198.

Atlee JL, Bernstein AD. Cardiac rhythm management devices (part I). *Anesthesiology* 2001; 95:1265–1280.

Stone KR, McPherson CA. Assessment and management of patients with pacemakers and implantable cardioverter defibrillator. *Crit Care Med* 2004;32(suppl):S155–S165.

C.12. Is magnetic resonance imaging (MRI) contraindicated in patients with a cardiac rhythm management device (CRMD)?

MRI is generally contraindicated in patients with a CRMD. If MRI must be performed, consult with the ordering physician, the patient's cardiologist, the diagnostic radiologist and the CRMD manufacturer. MRI can cause rapid pacing, inhibition, resetting of DDD pacemakers, and transient reed switch malfunction with asynchronous pacing. Serious malfunction with no output or rapid pacing may occur because pulsed energy from MRI can enter the lead by capacitive coupling and cause rapid ventricular pacing. Recent studies suggest that MRI may be safe, at least with some models of pacemakers or implantable cardioverter-defibrillators (ICDs), provided the CRMD generator and leads are not inside the magnet bore. When an MRI is considered absolutely essential, it is reasonable to program the pacemaker to its lowest voltage and pulse width or to OOO mode, provided the patient has an adequate underlying rhythm. The pulse waveform should be closely monitored in pacemaker-dependent patients and an external pacemaker and defibrillator should be available. Device function must be checked after MRI.

American Society of Anesthesiologists Task Force on Perioperative Management of Patients with Cardiac Rhythm Management Devices. Practice advisory for the perioperative management of patients with cardiac rhythm management devices: pacemakers and implantable cardioverter–defibrillators. A report by the American Society of Anesthesiologists task force on perioperative management of patients with cardiac rhythm management devices. *Anesthesiology* 2005;103:186–198.

Atlee JL, Berstein AD. Cardiac rhythm management devices (part I). *Anesthesiology* 2001; 95:1265–1280.

Salukhe TV, Dob D. Pacemakers and Defibrillators: anesthetic implications. *Br J Anesth* 2004;93:95–104.

C.13. What are the precautions during radiofrequency ablation for a patient with a cardiac rhythm management device (CRMD)?

- Avoid contact of radiofrequency catheter with the CRMD generator and leads
- Radiofrequency current path far away from the CRMD generator and leads
- Discuss these concerns with the operator

American Society of Anesthesiologists Task Force on Perioperative Management of Patients with Cardiac Rhythm Management Devices. Practice advisory for the perioperative management of patients with cardiac rhythm management devices: pacemakers and implantable cardioverter–defibrillators. A report by the American Society of Anesthesiologists task force on perioperative management of patients with cardiac rhythm management devices. *Anesthesiology* 2005;103:186–198.

D. Postoperative Management

D.1. How would you monitor this patient in the post–anesthesia care unit?

Cardiac rate and rhythm should be continuously monitored throughout the immediate postoperative period. Backup pacing capability and cardioversion-defibrillation equipment should be immediately available at all times.

American Society of Anesthesiologists Task Force on Perioperative Management of Patients with Cardiac Rhythm Management Devices. Practice advisory for the perioperative management of patients with cardiac rhythm management devices: pacemakers and implantable cardioverter–defibrillators. A report by the American Society of Anesthesiologists task force on perioperative management of patients with cardiac rhythm management devices. *Anesthesiology* 2005;103:186–198.

D.2. How would you confirm that the cardiac rhythm management device (CRMD) is functioning properly after surgery?

Postoperative interrogation and restoration of CRMD function are basic elements of postoperative management. The CRMD first should be interrogated to assess postoperative device functions. If interrogation determines that CRMD settings are inappropriate, the device should be reprogrammed to appropriate settings. For an implantable cardioverter-defibrillator (ICD), all antitachyarrhythmic therapies should be restored. Consultation with an electrophysiologist or pacemaker—ICD service may be necessary.

American Society of Anesthesiologists Task Force on Perioperative Management of Patients with Cardiac Rhythm Management Devices. Practice advisory for the perioperative management of patients with cardiac rhythm management devices: pacemakers and implantable cardioverter–defibrillators. A report by the American Society of Anesthesiologists task force on perioperative management of patients with cardiac rhythm management devices. *Anesthesiology* 2005;103:186–198.

D.3. What types of environmental electromagnetic interferences (EMIs) may temporarily affect the function of a permanent pacemaker (PPM)?

- Microwave oven—the patient with the older generation of pacemaker should not approach within 3 feet of an operating microwave oven. However, a modern pacemaker system can easily reject the interference.
- Diathermy—contraindicated
- Electrocautery—do not use within 15 cm of the implanted pulse generator.
- Electric razor—do not use on the skin area over the implant site.
- Amateur radio transmitting equipment—linear power amplifiers are contraindicated.
- Power transmission lines—high-voltage electric fields produced by 765 kV power lines should be avoided.
- Arc welding—contraindicated
- Telephone transformer—contraindicated.
- Cellular phones—analog cellular phones are safe; however, digital cellular phones should not be placed over the pacemaker.
- Radiofrequency catheter ablation of arrhythmias potentially can produce similar disturbances of pacemaker behavior caused by electrocautery and can produce upper rate pacing in a minute ventilation-driven DDDR pacemaker.
- Magnetic resonance imaging (MRI)—generally contraindicated.
- Radiation therapy—this can damage pacemaker electronics and can cause unpredictable transient or permanent malfunction including runaway behavior. The effect is cumulative and similar whether the dose is given at one time or spread over several treatments. Given a sufficiently high cumulative absorbed dose, all pulse generators will fail catastrophically. Appropriate shielding of the pulse generator during radiation therapy is mandatory.

In some cases, the pacemaker may need to be repositioned before initiating radiation therapy.

Zipes DP, Libby P, Bonow RO, et al. eds. *Braunwald's heart disease, a textbook of cardiovascular medicine*, 6th ed. Philadelphia: WB Saunders, 2005:767–787.

CHAPTER 10

Thoracoabdominal Aortic Aneurysms

MANU SETHI • CHARLES D. COLLARD • MANUEL L. FONTES

A 67-YEAR-OLD WOMAN

presents for evaluation and surgical treatment of a thoracoabdominal aortic aneurysm (TAAA). The patient's past medical history is significant for a type III aortic dissection 8 years ago, hypertension, chronic obstructive pulmonary disease (COPD), smoking (one pack/day), and chronic renal insufficiency. The patient currently complains of intermittent back pain. Computed tomography (CT) reveals a 9-cm TAAA originating just distal to the left subclavian artery that extends to the iliac bifurcation. Chest x-ray shows thoracic aortic aneurysmal dilation, with displacement of the left bronchial mainstem. Echocardiogram shows concentric left ventricular hypertrophy and a normal ejection fraction. The laboratory findings show hemoglobin 9.3 g per dL, hematocrit 37%, blood urea nitrogen (BUN) 22 mg per dL, and creatinine 1.9 mg per dL.

A. Medical Disease and Differential Diagnosis

1. What are the causes of aortic aneurysms?
2. How are "dissecting aortic aneurysms" classified?
3. How are **thoracoabdominal aortic aneurysms (TAAAs)** classified?
4. Describe the natural history, medical management, and timing of surgical intervention for TAAAs.

B. Preoperative Evaluation and Preparation

1. How should TAAAs be surgically evaluated?
2. Describe the anesthetic evaluation of the patient scheduled for TAAA repair.
3. Describe the spinal cord blood supply.
4. What coexisting diseases commonly accompany TAAAs?
5. What factors are associated with an increased risk of TAAA rupture?

C. Intraoperative Management

1. What hemodynamic monitors should be used for the patient undergoing TAAA repair?
2. What blood bank support is necessary?
3. What type of anticoagulation is used for TAAA repair? What can be done to minimize blood transfusion?

4. Describe the surgical approach to TAAA repair.
5. How would you induce the patient for TAAA repair?
6. What major organ systems are threatened during TAAA repair?
7. What strategies are used for spinal cord protection?
8. How do you detect spinal cord ischemia?
9. What strategies are used for mesenteric and renal preservation?
10. Describe the pathophysiology of aortic clamping and unclamping.

D. Postoperative Management

1. What are the potential complications of TAAA repair?

E. Anesthesia for Endovascular TAAA Repair

1. Which patients are candidates for endovascular TAAA repair?
2. What are the surgical steps for endovascular TAAA repair?
3. What are some of the anesthetic considerations for endovascular TAAA repair?
4. What are the potential complications of endovascular TAAA repair?

A. Medical Disease and Differential Diagnosis

A.1. What are the causes of aortic aneurysms?

A true aneurysm is defined as a localized dilation of the aorta, 50% over the normal diameter, which includes all three-vessel layers (i.e., the intima, media, and adventitia). Causes of aortic aneurysms include the following:

- *Atherosclerosis.* Atherosclerosis is the predominant etiology of descending thoracic aortic aneurysms, affecting the medial wall diffusely, thereby diminishing the cushioning property of the aorta. With medial necrosis and subsequent remodeling, which is nonhomogeneous, segments of the aortic wall become weakened and prone to dilation as well as rupture.
- *Aortic dissection.* Chronic aortic dissections often dilate over time and are at high risk for aneurysm formation. Aortic dissections and aneurysms often coexist, in particular, in older patients suffering from hypertension and atherosclerosis.
- *Collagen vascular diseases*
  a. *Marfan syndrome.* Marfan syndrome is an autosomal dominant disorder classically associated with cystic medial degeneration in young patients. Both the amount and organization of elastin are decreased in patients with Marfan syndrome.
  b. *Ehlers-Danlos syndrome.* Ehlers-Danlos syndrome is a heterogeneous group of heritable connective tissue disorders, characterized by articular hypermobility, skin extensibility, and tissue fragility.
- *Familial thoracic aortic aneurysm syndrome.* Cystic medial degeneration is also seen in patients with ascending thoracic aortic aneurysms who do not have overt connective tissue disorders. When familial, they are now referred to as the familial thoracic aortic aneurysm syndrome.
- *Trauma*
- *Bicuspid aortic valve.* Many ascending thoracic aortic aneurysms are associated with a bicuspid aortic valve. Cystic medial degeneration is often seen in these cases. Cardiologists should routinely image the ascending aorta in patients with a bicuspid aortic valve, as 50% will develop aortic dilatation.
- *Turner's syndrome.* Turner's syndrome is associated with multiple cardiovascular anomalies, including a bicuspid aortic valve (30%) and aortic coarctation. Thoracic aortic aneurysms are not uncommon, and typically involve the ascending aorta. It has been recommended that all

women with Turner's syndrome undergo a complete cardiac evaluation at least every 5 years to detect potential aneurysm formation.

- *Inflammation*
  a. Takayasu arteritis
  b. Polyarteritis
- *Infection*
  a. Bacterial
  b. Viral
  c. Spirochete
  d. Fungal

Isselbacher EM. Thoracic and abdominal aortic aneurysms. *Circulation* 2005;111:816.

Johnston KW, Rutherford RB, Tilson MD, et al. Suggested standards for reporting on arterial aneurysms. Subcommittee on Reporting Standards for Arterial Aneurysms, Ad Hoc Committee on Reporting Standards, Society for Vascular Surgery and North American Chapter, International Society for Cardiovascular Surgery. *J Vasc Surg* 1991;13: 452.

Kaplan JA, Reich DL, Konstadt SN, eds. *Cardiac anesthesia*, 5th ed. Philadelphia: WB Saunders, 2006.

Kouchoukos NT, Dougenis D. Surgery of the thoracic aorta. *N Engl J Med* 1997;336: 1876–1889.

A.2. How are "dissecting aortic aneurysms" classified?

The term *dissecting aneurysm* is a misnomer, because the condition is not an aneurysm but an *aortic dissection* (i.e., a dissection of the aortic wall). Aortic dissections result from cystic medial necrosis (i.e., mucoid and cystic degeneration of elastin fibers within the aortic media). Currently, there are several aortic dissection classification systems. The DeBakey classification system classifies aortic dissections by their site of origin and distal extension (Fig.10.1).

- Type I dissection begins in the ascending aorta near the aortic valve and extends throughout the aorta down to the common iliac arteries. Type I aortic dissections are common.
- Type II dissection is limited to the ascending aorta. Type II dissections are common in patients with Marfan syndrome; however, the rarest form of dissection.
- Type IIIa dissection begins distal to the left subclavian artery and ends in the descending thoracic aorta. Its localized nature makes it accessible to surgical excision if needed.
- Type IIIb dissection begins distal the left subclavian artery and extends into the abdominal aorta. Type IIIb dissections rarely require surgical intervention.

In contrast, the Stanford classification system classifies aortic dissections into two types based on their clinical course and surgical significance:

- A type A dissection originates in the ascending aorta and includes DeBakey's type I and type II dissections.
- A type B dissection originates in the descending aorta and is equivalent to DeBakey's type III dissection. Type B dissections may dissect retrograde into the aortic arch or ascending aorta.

Crawford ES. The diagnosis and management of aortic dissection. *JAMA* 1990;264: 2537–2541.

Daily PO, Trueblood H, Stinson E, et al. Management of acute aortic dissections. *Ann Thorac Surg* 1990;10:237–247.

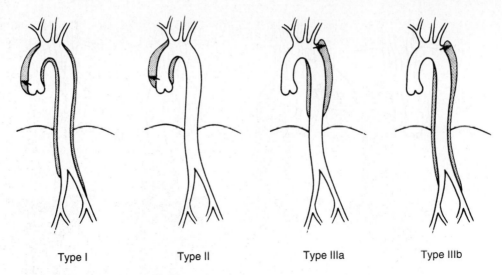

Type I   Type II   Type IIIa   Type IIIb

Figure 10.1 The DeBakey classification system.

DeBakey ME, Cooley DA, Crawford ES, et al. Aneurysms of the thoracic aorta. *J Thorac Surg* 1958;36:393–420.

O'Connor CJ, Rothenberg DM. Anesthetic considerations for descending thoracic aortic surgery: Part I. *J Cardiothorac Vasc Anesth* 1995;9:581–588.

Schwartz SI, ed. *Principles of surgery*, 6th ed. New York: McGraw-Hill, 1994:915–916.

A.3. How are thoracoabdominal aortic aneurysms (TAAAs) classified?

Crawford described four TAAA types (Fig. 10.2):

- Type I TAAA originates below the left subclavian artery and extends to the celiac axis and mesenteric arteries.
- Type II TAAA involves the same areas as type I, but extends caudally to include the infrarenal aorta. This type is associated with prolonged surgical times and worse overall outcomes.
- Type III TAAA begins in the lower descending thoracic aorta (T6) and involves the remainder of the aorta.
- Type IV TAAA begins at the diaphragm and involves the entire abdominal aorta.

Crawford ES, Crawford JL, Safi HJ, et al. Thoracoabdominal aneurysms: preoperative and intraoperative factors determining immediate and long-term results in 605 patients. *J Vasc Surg* 1986;3:389–404.

A.4. Describe the natural history, medical management and timing of surgical intervention for thoracoabdominal aortic aneurysms (TAAAs).

Both the etiology and location of an aneurysm may affect its growth rate and propensity for dissection or rupture. Surgical intervention is performed when the aneurysm is large enough to be considered at significant risk for rupture. The mean rate of growth for all thoracic aneurysms is 0.1 cm per year. The rate of growth is greater for descending versus ascending aorta aneurysms,

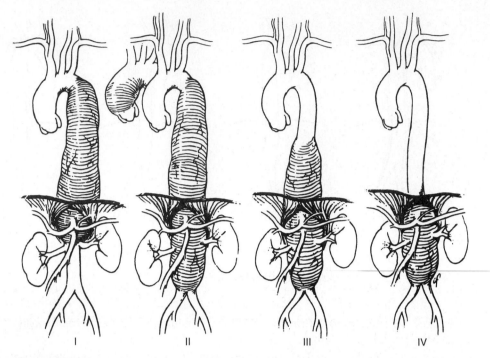

Figure 10.2 The Crawford thoracoabdominal aortic aneurysm (TAAA) classification system.

for dissected versus nondissected aneurysms, and for in patients with Marfan syndrome. The initial size is an important predictor of the rate of thoracic aneurysm growth. With regards to aneurysm size and the risk of rupture or dissection, the annual rate is 2% for aneurysms less than 5 cm, 3% for aneurysms 5 to 5.9 cm, and 7% for aneurysms 6 cm or more in diameter.

Medical therapy to slow aneurysm growth or to reduce the risk of dissection or rupture has met with limited success. Long-term β-blocker therapy has been shown to significantly slow the rate of aortic dilatation and to lower mortality. The goal of antihypertensive therapy is to maintain systolic blood pressure (BP) between 105 and 120 mm Hg. Patients should be followed with serial imaging studies for surveillance. A second imaging study should be obtained 6 months after initial diagnosis. If the aneurysm is unchanged in size, it is then reasonable to obtain an imaging study annually in most cases, excepting patients with Marfan syndrome or acute aortitis. Should there be a significant increase in aneurysm size between studies, the study interval should be decreased to 3 or 6 months.

The optimal timing of surgical repair of thoracic aortic aneurysms depends both on the aneurysm size and the patient's associated comorbidities. For most ascending thoracic aortic aneurysms, surgery is indicated at a diameter of 5.5 cm or more. The threshold for surgery is raised to 6 cm or more for patients with an increased operative risk (e.g., the elderly or those with comorbidities). Conversely, among patients who are at increased risk of aortic dissection or rupture (e.g., Marfan syndrome or bicuspid aortic valve), aortic repair is recommended earlier (5 cm or smaller). Indeed, when patients with a bicuspid aortic valve require valve replacement surgery, the recommendation is for prophylactic replacement of the ascending aorta if its diameter is 4 cm or more. In general, for most descending thoracic aortic aneurysms, surgery is recommended at an aortic diameter 6 cm or more.

Davies RR, Goldstein LJ, Coady MA, et al. Yearly rupture or dissection rates for thoracic aortic aneurysms: simple prediction based on size. *Ann Thorac Surg* 2002;73: 17–28.

Devereux RB, Roman MJ. Aortic disease in Marfan's syndrome. *N Engl J Med* 1999;340: 1358–1359.

Isselbacher EM. Thoracic and abdominal aortic aneurysms. *Circulation* 2005;111:816.

B. Preoperative Evaluation and Preparation

B.1. How should thoracoabdominal aortic aneurysms (TAAAs) be surgically evaluated?

Preoperative assessment of the patient for elective TAAA repair requires a fine balance between the risks of aneurysm rupture vs. surgical morbidity. Most surgeons agree that a TAAA measuring 6 cm or more with a growth rate greater than 1 cm per year warrants surgical correction as a result of increased risk of rupture. The mortality of TAAA repair ranges from 3% to 23%. The incidence of spinal cord injury is 3% to 18%, with long-term survival being shorter in patients who suffer postoperative paraplegia or paraparesis. In one report, the 5-year survival rate for patients with spinal cord injury was 44%, whereas it was 62% for those without spinal cord injury. Spinal cord injury is caused by inadequate blood flow to the spinal cord during or after surgery. The period of cross clamping is most vulnerable as well as immediate period following declamping, whereby reperfusion injury can occur.

Once the decision has been made to proceed with surgical repair, a comprehensive radiographic evaluation of the aorta is necessary for operative planning. Studies may include helical computed tomography (CT), contrast arteriography, and magnetic resonance (MR) angiography. All iodinated contrast studies should be performed well in advance of the planned procedure to avoid contrast-related renal dysfunction. Patients with baseline renal insufficiency may receive *N*-acetylcysteine to reduce the risk of contrast-related nephropathy and progressive renal failure. Preoperative assessment of the aneurysm anatomy and of the major branches is critical to surgical planning. Surgeons must decide to use a clamp-and-sew technique versus a distal aortic perfusion technique. Factors determining this decision include the expected difficulty of aortic exposure and completing the proximal aortic anastomosis.

Unfortunately, the studies used to assess the aneurysm vasculature are imperfect with respect to delineating the spinal cord blood supply. CT angiography and MR angiography detect the artery of Adamkiewicz in only 50% to 80% of patients. This is significant as the risk of postoperative paraplegia is 5% if the artery of Adamkiewicz is identified preoperatively and reimplanted, whereas it is as high as 50% if the artery is not identified and reattached.

Kieffer E, Ricard T, Chiras J, et al. Preoperative spinal cord arteriography in aneurysmal disease of the descending thoracic and thoracoabdominal aorta: preliminary results in 45 patients. *Ann Vasc Surg* 1987;3:34–46.

Levine WC, Lee JJ, Black JH, et al. Thoracoabdominal aneurysm repair: anesthetic management. *Int Anesth Clin* 2005;43:39–60.

Svensson LG, Crawford ES, Hess KR, et al. Experience with 1509 patients undergoing thoracoabdominal aortic operations. *J Vasc Surg* 1993;17:357–370.

Tabayashi K. Spinal cord protection during thoracoabdominal aneurysm repair. *Surg Today* 2005;35:1–6.

B.2. Describe the anesthetic evaluation of the patient scheduled for thoracoabdominal aortic aneurysm (TAAA) repair.

The preoperative assessment of a patient undergoing TAAA repair requires a thorough multisystem evaluation. Over 50% of patients are symptomatic at presentation. These include back pain, epigastric pain, hoarseness related to left recurrent laryngeal nerve palsy, shortness of breath, cough, and hemoptysis.

Hypertension (70% to 90%) and coronary artery disease (CAD) (50%) are common in this patient population. Hemodynamic stress placed on the heart by proximal aortic cross-clamping mandates a thorough preoperative cardiac evaluation. Adequate knowledge of preoperative ventricular function, valvular function, and coronary anatomy can guide hemodynamic management and surgical decision making. The elective patient with clinical symptoms or electrocardiogram (ECG) signs of myocardial ischemia should undergo stress testing and, if necessary, coronary angiography. Angioplasty or coronary artery bypass graft surgery should be performed in patients with clinically significant CAD. The risk of perioperative cardiac morbidity and mortality is approximately 12% to 15%. Recent studies have shown that perioperative β-blockade may minimize this risk. Therefore, β-blocker therapy should be initiated early and continued throughout the perioperative period.

Postoperative respiratory failure is the leading cause of mortality in patients undergoing TAAA repair. Pulmonary function must be carefully evaluated as one-lung ventilation is essential for surgical repair of type I, II, and III aneurysms. As a large aneurysm can distort the left mainstem bronchus, the chest x-ray and computed tomography scan may give vital information regarding double lumen endotracheal tube placement. Patients actively smoking should be advised to quit smoking at least 2 weeks before surgery. Those showing good response to bronchodilators should be started on the same preoperatively to optimize pulmonary function. Patients with poor diffusing capacity or severe chronic obstructive pulmonary disease may require the use of cardiopulmonary bypass for TAAA repair as they may not be able to tolerate one-lung ventilation.

Among patients presenting for surgical correction of TAAA, 13% to 24% have baseline renal insufficiency (serum creatinine>1.5 mg/dL), primarily related to hypertension, diabetes, and atherosclerotic disease. As type II, III, and IV thoracoabdominal aneurysms involve the visceral and juxtarenal aorta, renovascular disease is often encountered. Preoperative renal insufficiency is associated with an increased risk of postoperative renal failure, which in turn, is associated with increased mortality. Therefore, baseline renal function should be assessed.

Kaplan JA, Reich DL, Konstadt SN, eds. *Cardiac anesthesia*, 5th ed. Philadelphia: WB Saunders, 2006.

Kouchoukos NT, Dougenis D. Surgery of the thoracic aorta. *N Engl J Med* 1997;336: 1876–1889.

Levine WC, Lee JJ, Black JH, et al. Thoracoabdominal aneurysm repair: anesthetic management. *Int Anesth Clin* 2005;43:39–60.

B.3. Describe the spinal cord blood supply.

The spinal cord has a system of longitudinal and transverse arteries. Anatomic studies have shown that the most important longitudinal arteries are a single anterior spinal artery supplying 75% of the cord and a pair of posterior spinal arteries supplying 25% of the cord. The territory supplied by the anterior spinal artery is divided into three functionally distinct levels: cervicodorsal, midthoracic, and thoracolumbar. The cervicodorsal region receives its blood supply from the vertebral, subclavian, thyrocervical, and costocervical arteries. The midthoracic region is supplied by a meager left or right intercostal artery arising between the fourth and the ninth thoracic vertebrae. The thoracolumbar region of the anterior spinal artery receives its blood supply mainly from one of the intercostal arteries called the *arteria radicularis magna* (ARM) or the artery of Adamkiewicz. It arises at the level of T5-8 in 15%, T9-12 in 60%, L1 in 14%, and L2 in 10% of patients. The ARM is often involved in the surgical repair.

The anterior spinal artery is smaller above than below the entry of the ARM. Resistance to blood flow is 51 times greater going "up" the anterior spinal artery. Therefore, distal aortic perfusion during thoracic aortic cross-clamping protects the spinal cord below the ARM, but has minimal impact above it. This is why paraplegia still occurs in approximately 2% to 15% of patients having thoracic aortic surgery with distal aortic perfusion. However, reimplantation of intercostal arteries during surgery reduces the incidence of neurologic injury.

Bromage PR. *Epidural anesthesia*. Philadelphia: WB Saunders, 1978:50–54.

DiChiro G, Fried LC, Doppman JL. Experimental spinal angiography. *Br J Radiol* 1970;43: 19–30.

Kaplan JA, Reich DL, Konstadt SN, eds. *Cardiac anesthesia*, 5th ed. Philadelphia: WB Saunders, 2006.

Miller RD, ed. *Anesthesia*, 6th ed. Philadelphia: Churchill Livingstone, 2005.

Piccone W, DeLaria GA, Najafi H. Descending thoracic aneurysms. In: Bergan JJ, Yao JST, eds. *Aortic surgery*. Philadelphia: WB Saunders, 1989:249.

Svensson LG, Richards E, Coull A, et al. Relationship of spinal cord blood flow to vascular anatomy during thoracic aortic cross-clamping and shunting. *J Thorac Cardiovasc Surg* 1986;91:71–78.

B.4. What coexisting diseases commonly accompany thoracic aortic aneurysms?

The preoperative assessment of a patient undergoing thoracoabdominal aortic aneurysm (TAAA) repair requires a thorough multisystem evaluation. Because TAAAs are more common in the elderly, the frequency of comorbid disease is high. Hypertension, coronary artery disease, chronic obstructive pulmonary disease (COPD), diabetes and renal insufficiency are common in this patient population.

Cambria RP, Clouse WD, Davison JK, et al. Thoracoabdominal aneurysm repair: results with 337 operations performed over a 15-year interval. *Ann Surg* 2002;236:471–479.

Svensson LG, Crawford ES, Hess KR, et al. Experience with 1509 patients undergoing thoracoabdominal aortic operations. *J Vasc Surg* 1993;17:357–368, discussion 368–370.

Svensson LG, Hess KR, Coselli JS, et al. A prospective study of respiratory failure after high-risk surgery on the thoracoabdominal aorta. *J Vasc Surg* 1991;14:271–282.

B.5. What factors are associated with an increased risk of thoracoabdominal aortic aneurysm rupture?

Both aneurysm size and rate of expansion are predictors of rupture. The annual rupture rate is 2% for aneurysms less than 5 cm, 3% for aneurysms 5 to 5.9 cm, and 7% for aneurysms 6 cm or more in diameter. Therefore, the risk of rupture rises significantly when thoracic aneurysms reach a 6 cm size. Certain concomitant diseases also predict an increased risk of rupture, such as smoking, chronic obstructive pulmonary disease (COPD), advancing age, pain, and renal failure. Hypertension, although correlating with aneurysm development, has not been conclusively shown to increase the risk of rupture.

Dapunt OE, Galla JD, Sadeghi AM, et al. The natural history of thoracic aortic aneurysms. *J Thorac Cardiovasc Surg* 1994;107:1323–1333.

Davies RR, Goldstein LJ, Coady MA, et al. Yearly rupture or dissection rates for thoracic aortic aneurysms: simple prediction based on size. *Ann Thorac Surg* 2002;73:17–28.

Griepp RB, Ergin MA, Galla JD, et al. Natural history of descending thoracic and thoracoabdominal aneurysms. *Ann Thorac Surg* 1999;67:1927–1930.

Juvonen T, Ergin MA, Galla JD, et al. Prospective study of the natural history of thoracic aortic aneurysms. *Ann Thorac Surg* 1997;63:1533–1544.

C. Intraoperative Management

C.1. What hemodynamic monitors should be used for the patient undergoing thoracoabdominal aortic aneurysm (TAAA) repair?

Although the anesthetic management for TAAA repair varies amongst institutions, invasive hemodynamic monitoring, a double lumen endotracheal tube for one-lung ventilation, and rapid volume infusers are standard. Large bore peripheral IV's and central venous access are essential, as the potential for rapid intraoperative blood loss is significant. A rapid infusing system capable of heating and delivering fluids up to 500 mL per minute should be immediately available. An arterial line is usually placed in the upper extremity. During type I and II aneurysm repairs, the arterial line should be placed in the right radial artery as the proximal aortic cross-clamp may disrupt left subclavian arterial blood flow. If left-heart bypass or a shunt is planned, a femoral arterial line may also be inserted to monitor distal aortic perfusion pressure. Transesophageal echocardiography (TEE) is also often used to monitor heart function and volume status. Similarly, a pulmonary arterial catheter may be useful for monitoring intraoperative hemodynamics and for postoperative management.

Levine WC, Lee JJ, Black JH, et al. Thoracoabdominal aneurysm repair: anesthetic management. *Int Anesth Clin* 2005;43:39–60.

C.2. What blood bank support is necessary?

Thoracoabdominal aortic aneurysm repair is associated with the potential for massive blood loss. As such, early and timely communication with the blood bank is necessary to ensure that adequate quantities of packed red blood cells (pRBCs), fresh frozen plasma, and platelets are available. Five to ten units of pRBCs should be immediately available in the operating room, with a similar number of units available in the blood bank.

Kaplan JA, Reich DL, Konstadt SN, eds. *Cardiac anesthesia*, 5th ed. Philadelphia: WB Saunders, 2006.

C.3. What type of anticoagulation is used for thoracoabdominal aortic aneurysm (TAAA) repair? What can be done to minimize blood transfusion?

Heparin (100 U/kg) is typically administered 5 minutes before aortic cross-clamp placement. Unlike full cardiopulmonary bbypass (CPB), a reduced dose of heparin may be used for left-heart bypass. Autologous blood can be collected from the patient before or during (i.e., hemodilution) surgery. Use of blood salvaging techniques, such as the "cell saver," can also limit homologous red cell transfusion. However, cell saving techniques may wash out valuable plasma clotting factors and platelets, resulting in a dilutional coagulopathy and thrombocytopenia. Additionally, if heparin is used as an anticoagulant in the cell saver, additional protamine sulfate may need to be administered. Although antifibrinolytic therapy may be used to minimize blood loss, several studies have suggested that antifibrinolytic therapy is of limited efficacy in the setting of TAAA repair.

Kaplan JA, Reich DL, Konstadt SN, eds. *Cardiac anesthesia*, 5th ed. Philadelphia: WB Saunders, 2006.

Shore-Lesserson L, Bodian C, Vela-Cantos F, et al. Antifibrinolytic use and bleeding during surgery on the descending thoracic aorta: a multivariate analysis. *J Cardiothorac Vasc Anesth* 2005;19:453–458.

C.4. Describe the surgical approach to thoracoabdominal aortic aneurysm repair.

- *Position.* The surgical approach is typically through the left chest, with the patient in a partial right lateral decubitus position and the hips almost supine to allow femoral cannulation.
- *Incision.* The incision is tailored to complement the aneurysm extent. For types II, III, or IV, a thoracoabdominal incision is made from the symphysis pubis, extending midline to the umbilicus, curving straight into the costal cartilage and into a posterolateral thoracotomy incision. For types I and V, a modified thoracoabdominal incision is used, where the incision extends from the umbilicus to the chest and exposes the upper abdominal aorta. In this manner, an aortic cross can be applied either above or below the renal arteries.
- *Cannulation for left heart bypass.* Left atrial to femoral artery bypass is often used in patients with significant myocardial dysfunction or other systemic disease, and in patients with extensive aneurysms that would require prolonged aortic cross clamping. Typically, an outflow cannula is placed in the left atrium, and blood is shunted through a centrifugal pump to an inflow cannula in the right femoral artery. Unlike cardiopulmonary bypass (CPB), left heart bypass requires reduced heparinization, that is, 100 U per kg of heparin approximately 5 minutes before cannulation. Potential advantage of left heart bypass include improved perfusion of the lower extremities and possibly of the anterior spinal artery through collateral vessels, while the proximal aorta is cross-clamped. Left heart bypass therefore minimizes the development of acidosis in the lower extremities, which in turn improves hemodynamic stability upon release of the aortic cross clamp. Left-heart bypass is typically initiated at a rate of 500 mL per minute, and once the proximal aortic clamp is placed, the flows are adjusted to maintain the proximal aortic pressure above 90 mm Hg or distal mean pressure of approximately 70 mm Hg.
- *Proximal aortic anastomosis.* In type I and II repairs, the proximal thoracic aorta distal to the left subclavian is dissected away from the esophagus in order to prevent esophageal aortic fistula. Following placement of the proximal aortic clamp, a second clamp is placed at the sixth or eighth intercostal space of the mid-descending aorta. An appropriately sized Dacron graft is then sutured proximally to the descending thoracic aorta and checked for hemostasis. Once the proximal anastomosis is completed, the mid-descending thoracic clamp is moved to the infrarenal abdominal aorta. In type II aneurysms, left heart bypass is stopped and the aneurysm is opened. The celiac axis, superior mesenteric artery (SMA), and renal arteries are then identified and perfused with special catheters in order to protect the mesentery. The catheters perfusing the kidneys are typically passed through an ice-bath, maintaining the renal artery temperature below 15°C (59°F). Where feasible, reattachment of patent segmental intercostal and lumbar arteries in the T8 to L1 region is then performed. Intercostal arteries

in the T4-8 region are usually ligated if they exhibit excessive retrograde bleeding, indicating good collateral circulation. If the intercostal arteries between T8 and L1 are occluded by intimal atherosclerosis, patent intercostal arteries in the T4-8 region may be reattached to preserve circulation.

- *Visceral aortic anastomoses.* The visceral aortic anastomoses are evaluated intraoperatively. If the celiac axis, SMA, and renal arteries are close together, a single patch may be used to anastomose the viscera to the graft. Frequently, the left renal artery is pushed more caudad and is reattached with a bypass graft. Once the anastomoses are complete, visceral perfusion is stopped and the cannulas removed. The patient is then placed in a head down position, the aortic graft flushed proximally, and then the aortic cross clamp slowly released. The clamp is then moved to the abdominal aortic graft distal to visceral anastomoses.
- *Distal aortic anastomosis.* The graft is now cut to the appropriate length and is sutured to the infrarenal aorta. Before the completion of the distal anastomosis, the graft is flushed proximally and the aorta distally. The lower clamp is slowly released to restore the pulsatile flow to the viscera. Any patent lumbar arteries are usually ligated.
- *Other techniques.* Other techniques include the "clamp and sew" technique and use of CPB with deep hypothermic circulatory arrest (DHCA). The clamp and sew technique involves clamping the proximal descending thoracic aorta and replacing the aneurysm with a graft. The distal anastomosis to the lower abdominal aorta is then performed without a clamp, allowing the distal aorta to decompress. Although this technique avoids the need for full heparinization, it imposes a time limit on the surgeon as there is no pump to support distal or collateral perfusion. CPB with DHCA is used when the proximal aorta cannot be clamped without disrupting cerebral blood flow. Advantages of this technique include lack of hemodynamic changes with aortic clamping and unclamping, a bloodless surgical field, and organ protection because of low temperatures. Disadvantages include the need for full heparinization and the potential neurological risks of DHCA.

Coselli JS, LeMaire SA. Left heart bypass reduces paraplegia rates after thoracoabdominal aortic aneurysm repair. *Ann Thorac Surg* 1999;67:1931–1934.

Coselli JS, LeMaire SA, Figueiredo LP, et al. Paraplegia after thoracoabdominal aortic aneurysm repair: Is dissection a risk factor? *Ann Thorac Surg* 1997;63:28–36.

Kaplan JA, Reich DL, Konstadt SN, eds. *Cardiac anesthesia*, 5th ed. Philadelphia: WB Saunders, 2006.

O'Conner CJ, Rothenberg DM. Anesthetic considerations for descending thoracic aortic surgery: Part II. *J Cardiothorac Vasc Anesth* 1995;9:734–747.

Safi HJ. How I do it: thoracoabdominal aortic aneurysm graft replacement. *Cardiovas Surg* 1999;7:607–613.

C.5. How would you induce the patient for thoracoabdominal aortic aneurysm repair?

The goal of anesthetic induction is to avoid anything that will increase the risk of aneurysm rupture, whereas at the same time, maintaining adequate end-organ perfusion. In general, the systolic blood pressure (BP) should be kept between 105 to 115 mm Hg, the heart rate between 60 to 80 bpm, and the cardiac index between 2 to 2.5 L/minute/m^2. Short acting agents such as nitroglycerin, nicardipine or esmolol are ideal for hemodynamic control. Use of nitroprusside is discouraged because it has been associated with a higher risk of neurological complications. If motor evoked potentials (MEPs) are being monitored, either succinylcholine or a short acting nondepolarizing agent such as *cis*-atracurium may be used to facilitate tracheal intubation.

Anesthetic maintenance may be achieved using a low concentration of an inhalation agent, combined with an infusion of propofol or short acting narcotic (e.g., sufentanil, remifentanil). If MEPs are not being monitored, the patient may be fully paralyzed, and inhalation agents with intermittent narcotics used.

Hensley FA, Martin DE, Gravlee GP, eds. *A practical approach to cardiac anesthesia*, 3rd ed. Philadelphia: Lippincott Williams & Wilkins, 2003:617–647.

C.6. What major organ systems are threatened during thoracoabdominal aortic aneurysm repair?

The most significant threat to organ function and survival is the aortic cross clamp duration. The aortic cross clamp time is in turn related to the surgeon, surgical technique, and aneurysm type.

- *Spinal cord.* Prolonged spinal cord ischemia can result in paraplegia or paraparesis. Factors contributing to spinal cord ischemia include the duration of the aortic cross-clamp, preexisting cord ischemia, and variability in the spinal arterial supply.
- *Kidneys and visceral mesentery.* Ischemia of the kidneys can result in renal dysfunction or failure. Bowel ischemia can lead to an increase in intestinal permeability and sepsis.
- *Lungs.* The lung parenchyma is subjected to manipulation, compression, and retraction throughout the surgery. Much of this manipulation occurs after the patient is anticoagulated. Tracheobronchial bleeding can significantly complicate perioperative ventilation.
- *Heart.* Alterations in preload, afterload, and oxygen carrying capacity subject the heart to profound alterations in myocardial oxygen delivery and consumption. These factors, along with intraoperative acidosis, hypocalcemia, and hypokalemia, can all negatively affect myocardial contractility and conduction. It is critical to assess these patients preoperatively for coronary disease given the many concomitant risk factors shared in patients with aortic disease and ischemic heart disease. In the setting of severe multivessel disease, it is common to perform coronary revascularization first, followed by thoracoabdominal surgery a few months later.

O'Conner CJ, Rothenberg DM. Anesthetic considerations for descending thoracic aortic surgery: Part I. *J Cardiothorac Vasc Anesth* 1995;9:581–588.

O'Conner CJ, Rothenberg DM. Anesthetic considerations for descending thoracic aortic surgery: Part II. *J Cardiothorac Vasc Anesth* 1995;9:734–747.

C.7. What strategies are used for spinal cord protection?

Although type I and II thoracoabdominal aortic aneurysms (TAAAs) carry the greatest risk of injury, neurologic deficits can be seen with all types. Further, the risk of spinal cord injury increases with the duration of aortic clamping, with cross clamp times exceeding 60 minutes being associated with substantial risk; however, as little as 30 minutes of ischemia can increase the risk of paralysis. In general, there are two strategies to decrease the incidence and severity of spinal cord injury: (a) maintenance of spinal cord blood flow and (b) use of neuroprotective adjuncts to attenuate the excitatory and inflammatory mechanisms that contribute to ischemic injury.

- *Preoperative identification of the arteria radicularis magna (ARM).* The risk of paraplegia is 5% if the ARM is identified preoperatively and reimplanted, whereas it is reported to be as high as 50% if it is not identified and reattached. However, postoperative paraplegia cannot always be prevented even if the ARM is identified and reimplanted.
- *Distal aortic perfusion/left heart bypass.* Left heart bypass has the advantage of allowing mesenteric perfusion during the proximal clamp phase, minimizing myocardial hemodynamic

stress by reducing preload and reducing time pressure on the surgeon to complete the proximal anastomosis. To minimize spinal cord injury, the distal aortic perfusion pressure should be 60 mm Hg or more. The risks of paraplegia are 2.2%, 2.3%, and 5.8% with left heart bypass, passive shunts (e.g., Gott shunt) and the "clamp and sew" technique, respectively; nevertheless, there can be significant differences in outcomes amongst centers and amongst surgeons.

- *Reattachment of the intercostal arteries.* Reattachment of patent segmental intercostal and lumbar arteries in the T8 to L1 region is performed whenever feasible. This may require local end-arterectomy of the artery's origin. Intercostals in the T4–8 zone are typically oversewn, unless situated so as to be easily preserved in a beveled proximal aortic anastomosis in type I, II, or III TAAAs.

- *Hypothermia.* Passive cooling (34°C to 35°C [93.2°F to 95°F]) is used to limit ischemic damage by reducing the tissue metabolic rate, which decreases the loss of intracellular adenosine 5'-triphosphate (ATP) stores and lactic acid production. The precise temperature, however, to maximize this protective effect while minimizing related complications such as cardiac dysrhythmias and coagulopathy, is not well defined. After completing all anastomosis, effort is made to warm-up the patient so as to limit shivering and coagulopathy.

- *Placement of a cerebrospinal fluid (CSF) drain.* Spinal cord perfusion pressure (SCPP) = MAP - CSF pressure. Although mean arterial pressure (MAP) minimally changes from central aorta to the periphery, there is concern over utilizing this modified estimation of SCPP. This is particularly worrisome in patients with systolic hypertension, which comprise most patients with aortic aneurysms, whereby the MAP may be overestimated. Nevertheless, evidence derived from animal models suggests that decreasing the CSF pressure to 10 mm Hg or more during aortic clamping enhances spinal cord perfusion and decreases the risk of injury. Therefore, a passive CSF drain is often used in the immediate perioperative period to keep the CSF pressure between 10 mm Hg and 12 mm Hg in patients at high risk for paraplegia (type I, II, and III TAAAs). Critically important is the rate and amount of volume removed. Excessive CSF drainage could cause cerebral hemorrhage consequent to massive intracranial fluid shifts or, more plausibly, from tearing of cerebral bridging. Recently, Darlik et al., reported a 3.5% incidence of subdural hematoma associated with TAAA surgery utilizing CSF drain. Of 230 patients, 8 were diagnosed with this complication that resulted in 50% surgical mortality. The result of a multivariate analysis identified CSF drain in excess of 690 ± 79 mL to be an independent predictor of a subdural hemorrhage. Similarly, Settepani et al., reported on two rare cases of intracerebellar hematoma that was related to CSF drainage following thoracoabdominal aortic repair. Other reported side effects of CSF drainage include meningitis and iatrogenic paraplegia.

- *Neuroprotective agents.* Several pharmacological agents have been evaluated, both experimentally and in the clinical setting, to determine their protective effects against spinal cord injury. However, further clinical study of all of these agents is still necessary.
  a. Free radical scavengers (e.g., superoxide dismutase)
  b. Barbiturates
  c. Steroids
  d. CSF drainage combined with intrathecal papaverine
  e. Opioid antagonists (e.g., naloxone)
  f. Amide local anesthetics

- *Somatosensory evoked potentials (SSEPs) and Motor Evoked Potentials (MEPs).* Evoked potentials are used to continuously monitor spinal cord perfusion. SSEPs monitor the function of the spinal dorsal columns. The posterior tibial nerve is stimulated and the somatosensory cortex response recorded. However, the spinal cord dorsal columns are supplied by the posterior spinal arteries. Therefore, SSEPs may fail to detect ischemia in the anterior spinal cord. SSEP tracings may also be adversely altered by anesthetic agents, hypothermia, and neuromuscular blockade. In contrast to SSEPs, MEPs monitor the function of the corticospinal tract and anterior horn motor neurons. The motor cortex is stimulated and the anterior tibial muscle response recorded. Some surgeons do a 5-minute clamp test while monitoring the MEP. If the MEP levels decrease, distal aortic perfusion is increased to keep the mean distal aortic perfusion pressure greater than 60 mm Hg.

In summary, a multi-modality approach for spinal cord protection during TAAA repair is currently used by most institutions (e.g., left heart bypass, CSF drainage, aggressive intercostal artery reconstruction, MEP monitoring).

Azizzadeh A, Huynh TT, Miller CC, et al. Postoperative risk factors for delayed neurologic deficit after thoracic and thoracoabdominal aortic aneurysm repair: a case control study. *J Vasc Surg* 2003;37:750–754.

Berger J, Rijkov N, Girardi L, et al. Retrograde cerebral perfusion: report of a fatal complication from a subarachnoid venous hemorrhage during thoracoabdominal surgery. *J Cardiothorac Vasc Anesth* 2005;19:650–653.

Dardik A. Subdural hematoma after thoracoabdominal aortic aneurysm repair: an underreported complication of spinal fluid drainage? *J Vasc Surg* 2002;36:47–50.

Tabayashi K. Spinal cord protection during thoracoabdominal aneurysm repair. *Surg Today* 2005;35:1–6.

Levine WC, Lee JJ, Black JH, et al. Thoracoabdominal aneurysm repair: anesthetic management. *Int Anesth Clin* 2005;43:39–60.

Ueki R, Okutani R, Sasaki K, et al. Subarachnoid venous hemorrhage in a patient with retrograde cerebral perfusion during surgery for a thoracic aortic aneurysm. *J Anesth* 2000;14:218–220.

C.8. How do you detect spinal cord ischemia?

Evoked potentials may be used to monitor and detect spinal cord ischemia. Specifically, spinal cord ischemia is indicated by increases in latency and/or decreases in amplitude of evoked potential tracing. Two varieties of evoked potentials are commonly used. Somatosensory evoked potentials (SSEPs) travel through the dorsal root ganglia to the posterior columns of the spinal cord. The potentials continue along the lemniscal pathways on to the thalamus and the cortex. Comparison of the latency and amplitude of the potentials, tested minutes apart, define the degree of change in the SSEP. Loss of SSEP signals for longer than 14 to 30 minutes has been shown to be associated with an increased risk of postoperative neurologic deficit. In addition to ischemia, evoked potentials may be also altered by changes in temperature, anesthetic depth, and blood flow. As changes in blood flow through the anterior spinal artery are not reflected in the posterior columns, it is possible to develop postoperative paralysis despite normal intraoperative SSEPs. In contrast, motor evoked potentials (MEPs) monitor areas of the cord supplied by the anterior spinal artery. However, to properly assess MEPs, patients must be partial paralyzed and only lightly anesthetized. Both of these requirements are suboptimal anesthetic options for a thoracoabdominal aortic aneurysm repair.

Coles JC, Wilson GJ, Sima AF, et al. Intraoperative detection of spinal cord ischemia using somatosensory cortical evoked potentials during thoracic aortic occlusion. *Ann Thorac Surg* 1982;34:299–306.

Cunningham JN Jr, Laschinger JC, Spencer FC. Monitoring of somatosensory evoked potentials during procedures on the thoracoabdominal aorta: clinical observations and results. *J Thorac Cardiovasc Surg* 1987;94:275–285.

Ginsbury HH, Shetter AG, Raudzens PA, et al. Postoperative paraplegia with preserved intraoperative somatosensory evoked potentials. *J Neurosurg* 1985;63:296–300.

Grundy BL. Intraoperative monitoring of sensory-evoked potentials. *Anesthesiology* 1983;58:72–87.

Meylaerts SA, Jacobs MJ, van Iterson V, et al. Comparison of transcranial motor evoked potentials and somatosensory evoked potentials during thoracoabdominal aortic aneurysm repair. *Ann Surg* 1999;230:742–749.

C.9. What strategies are used for mesenteric and renal preservation?

- *Mesenteric protection.* Visceral ischemia has been implicated as an important cause of coagulopathy. Although the exact mechanism of coagulopathy remains uncertain, some studies have suggested that altered intestinal permeability with bacterial translocation may be responsible. Others studies have implicated hepatic ischemia with primary fibrinolysis. Several strategies exist for mesenteric protection. Most surgeons electively perfuse the distal aorta during the proximal aortic anastomosis. Once the proximal anastomosis is completed, the aortic clamp is moved distally to the infrarenal aorta. At this point the surgeon has two options. One is to maintain distal aortic perfusion while the intercostals, celiac axis, and superior mesenteric artery (SMA) are reconstructed, whereas the other is to discontinue distal aortic perfusion and open the aneurysm. When this approach is selected, perfusion catheters may be directly placed into the celiac axis, SMA, and renal arteries. These vessels are then perfused with blood from the centrifugal pump while the proximal intercostals are reconstructed, thereby reducing the mesentery ischemic time.
- *Renal protection.* Renal perfusion may be maintained through the use of distal aortic perfusion during the proximal aortic anastomosis. Continuous dopamine or fenoldopam infusion may also be useful. When the aneurysm is open, the kidneys may be continuously perfused with iced saline containing methylprednisolone and mannitol through catheters placed in the renal arteries.

Levine WC, Lee JJ, Black JH, et al. Thoracoabdominal aneurysm repair: anesthetic management. *Int Anesth Clin* 2005;43:39–60.

Schepens M, Dossche K, Morshuis W, et al. Introduction of adjuncts and their influence on changing results in 402 consecutive thoracoabdominal aortic aneurysm repairs. *Eur J Cardiothorac Surg* 2004;25:701–707.

C.10. Describe the pathophysiology of aortic clamping and unclamping.

Response to aortic cross-clamping

- *Hemodynamics.* Arterial hypertension is the most dramatic and consistent component of the hemodynamic response to aortic cross-clamping, and is attributed to a sudden increase in afterload. During supraceliac aortic cross-clamping, venous capacitance below the clamp decreases, expelling blood from the splanchnic and nonsplanchnic vascular beds toward the heart. Preload therefore acutely increases, as manifested by increases in central filling pressures (e.g., central venous pressure, pulmonary artery occlusion pressure), left ventricular end-diastolic area, and cardiac output. Over time, with increasing duration of aortic cross-clamp, systemic vascular resistance increases and cardiac output decreases. In contrast, infraceliac aortic cross-clamping has minimal impact on arterial and myocardial filling pressures.
- *Total body oxygen consumption.* Oxygen consumption below the aortic cross clamp decreases, while oxygen uptake in tissues above the clamp increases.

- *Coronary blood flow.* Aortic cross-clamping is acutely associated with substantial increases in myocardial preload and afterload, both of which increase myocardial oxygen demand.
- *Tissue perfusion distal to the aortic cross clamp.* Aortic pressure below the cross-clamp is directly dependent on proximal aortic pressure. Blood flow distal to the cross clamp does not increase when preload (fluid infusion) and cardiac output are increased.

Response to Aortic Unclamping

- *Hemodynamics.* The primary hemodynamic response to aortic cross clamp removal is hypotension. Hypotension is due to the following: (a) central hypovolemia caused by blood volume redistribution to the lower extremities; (b) hypoxia-mediated vasodilation with increased venous capacity; and (c) release of vasoactive and myocardial-depressant metabolites from ischemic tissues. Hypotension may be minimized by gradual release of the aortic cross clamp, administration of fluid and vasoactive drugs before unclamping, reducing the depth of anesthesia, and by minimizing the cross-clamp time.
- *Hypoxemia.* Following cross-clamp release, a large volume of desaturated blood returns to the heart from hypoperfused tissues below the cross-clamp. However, the transit time through the pulmonary circulation may be inadequate for hemoglobin to fully saturate. The result is temporary systemic hypoxemia.
- *Metabolic.* Glucose regulation can be difficult because of preexisting diabetes in many of these patients, as well as the surgical stress response. Massive transfusions are accompanied by hyperkalemia and hypocalcemia.
- *Acidosis.* Aortic cross-clamping results in increased lactate production in hypoperfused tissues below the clamp. Removal of the aortic cross-clamp may therefore result in an acute metabolic acidosis that may increase ventricular irritability, decrease myocardial contractility, and cause profound vasodilatation. In cases of "clamp-and-sew" technique, it is highly recommended to begin sodium bicarbonate infusion before aortic clamping at 1 to 2 mEq/kg/hour and to begin to administer up to several amps of sodium bicarbonate with release of the cross clamp to overcome the profound academia. Such liberal use of sodium bicarbonate may reflect institutional practices, and its role in treating this form of metabolic acidosis has been debated.

Gelman S. The pathophysiology of aortic cross-clamping and unclamping. *Anesthesiology* 1995;82:1026–1057.

D. Postoperative Management

D.1. What are the potential complications of Thoracoabdominal Aortic Aneurysm repair?

Morbidity and mortality are significantly higher in the elderly and in patients undergoing TAAA reoperation. Postoperative complications may include the following:

- *Myocardial infarction (MI).* The incidence of perioperative MI is 7% to 13%.
- *Respiratory failure.* The likelihood of respiratory complications is increased in surgeries with thoracic and abdominal incision. Respiratory failure occurs in up to 20% of patients following TAAA repair. Many of these patients have preexisting pulmonary disease, which may be worsened by the traumatic sequelae of one-lung ventilation. The release of vasoactive substances from the ischemic lower extremities and lung hypoperfusion may also lead to interstitial edema. The risk of respiratory failure is increased in the elderly and in patients with a history of chronic obstructive pulmonary disease, smoking, or cardiac or renal failure.

- *Renal failure.* The incidence of renal failure is 3% to 14% after TAAA repair. A cross-clamp duration greater than 30 minutes is the major determinant of postoperative renal dysfunction. Other risk factors for postoperative renal failure include age more than 50 years, coronary artery disease, diabetes, an elevated preoperative creatinine, and massive transfusion.
- *Bleeding.* The incidence of reoperation for bleeding is 3% to 5%. Causes of bleeding include heparinization, thrombocytopenia, hypothermia, acidosis, factor deficiency, disseminated intravascular coagulation, and chronic hepatic or renal failure
- *Spinal cord injury.* The incidence of paraplegia following TAAA repair is 2% to 40%, and depends on the aneurysm type, surgical technique, and ischemic duration. Paraplegia is increased significantly with emergency surgery and cross-clamp times greater than 30 minutes. Spinal cord injury presents as loss of motor function and sensation.
- *Stroke.* The incidence of stroke following TAAA repair is 9.6%.

Acher CW, Wynn MM, Hoch JR, et al. Cardiac function is a risk factor for paralysis in thoracoabdominal aortic replacement. *J Vasc Surg* 1998;27:821–830.

Cambria RP, Davison KJ, Zannetti S, et al. Thoracoabdominal aneurysm repair. Perspective over a decade with the clamp-and-sew technique. *Ann Surg* 1997;226:294–305.

Godet G, Fleron MH, Vicaut E, et al. Risk factors for acute postoperative renal failure in thoracic or thoracoabdominal aortic surgery: a prospective study. *Anesth Analg* 1997;85: 1227–1232.

LeMaire SA, Miller CC III, Conklin LD, et al. A new predictive model for adverse outcomes after elective thoracoabdominal aortic aneurysm repair. *Ann Thorac Surg* 2001;71: 1233–1238.

E. Anesthesia for Endovascular thoracoabdominal aortic aneurysm (TAAA) Repair

E.1. Which patients are candidates for endovascular thoracoabdominal aortic aneurysm (TAAA) repair?

Endovascular TAAA repair is an alternative to conventional surgical repair. Advantages of endovascular repair include the following: (a) it is less invasive; (b) local or regional anesthesia may be used; (c) the aorta is only briefly occluded; (d) there is minimal hemodynamic and metabolic stress; (e) the patient can ambulate and be discharged earlier; and (f) reduced hospital costs. Not all patients are candidates for endovascular repair. Patient selection must take into account the surgical risk attached with "open repair" in patients with significant comorbidity. Further, the proximal aneurysm neck must be at least 15 mm in length, and the maximum aneurysm diameter should be no larger than the largest available endograft. The distal attachment site must also be nonaneurysmal and of sufficient length to accommodate the graft. Finally, there must be at least one large, straight iliac artery that can be used as a conduit for graft delivery. After these considerations, approximately 40% to 60% of patients presenting for endovascular repair are candidates for treatment. However, there are few long-term outcome data comparing endovascular repair to other medical and surgical options.

Bergeron P, De Chaumaray T, Gay J, et al. Endovascular treatment of thoracic aortic aneurysms. *J Cardiovasc Surg* 2003;44:349–361.

Kahn RA, Moskowitz DM, Marin M, et al. Anesthetic considerations for endovascular aortic repair. *Mt Sinai J Med* 2002;69:57–67.

E.2. What are the surgical steps for endovascular thoracoabdominal aortic aneurysm (TAAA) repair?

The most common point of access is the femoral artery. A small horizontal incision is made in the inguinal fold and common femoral artery is exposed. Alternatively, a percutaneous approach from the left or right humeral artery may be used, especially when the supraaortic vessels need to be imaged. A puncture is made in the femoral artery and a guide wire inserted and advanced into the thoracic aorta. A 7 French introducer is then placed over the guide wire. An optional 7 French introducer may also be placed through the contralateral femoral artery to permit arteriography of the TAAA. The ascension of the delivery system follows removal of the 7F introducer. Once the stent-graft is properly positioned, it is then deployed. If graft extension is needed, one or more complementary stent-grafts may be deployed, with overlap of at least 2 cm between grafts. Finally, there is a global angiographic check for any endoleaks, with additional balloon inflation or cuff extension being performed as necessary to complete sealing. The delivery system is then removed and the arteriotomy site closed. For aortic dissections, the endoluminal graft is deployed in the true channel, covering the proximal dissection entry site. Intraoperative transesophageal echocardiography (TEE) is extremely helpful in confirming exclusion of the false channel.

Bergeron P, De Chaumaray T, Gay J, et al. Endovascular treatment of thoracic aortic aneurysms. *J Cardiovasc Surg* 2003;44:349–361.

E.3. What are some of the anesthetic considerations for endovascular thoracoabdominal aortic aneurysm (TAAA) repair?

The preoperative workup of the patient scheduled for endovascular TAAA repair does not differ from that of the patient scheduled for open repair. Large bore central venous access and a right radial arterial line are recommended. Depending on the aneurysm extent, a cerebrospinal fluid (CSF) drain may also be useful. Either general or regional anesthesia may be used. General anesthesia with tracheal intubation offers the advantage of having the airway already secured in the event of aneurysm rupture. However, regional anesthesia (i.e., continuous spinal, single shot spinal, continuous epidural or local anesthesia with monitored anesthesia care [MAC]) may be used. Patients undergoing endovascular grafting under general anesthesia have been found to require more vasopressor support, have a significantly higher fluid balance, and to have an increased duration of surgery and intensive care unit (ICU) stay. Regional anesthesia therefore offers an attractive alternative as it is associated with less cardiodepression and catecholamine release, and permits early postoperative ambulation.

The critical phase is during device deployment. Older generation devices are balloon based devices with a large cross-sectional area. As such, these devices are predisposed to distal migration as a result of forward aortic blood flow. Device malposition secondary to inadvertent migration may result either in occlusion of major arterial branches or incomplete aneurysm exclusion. Induced hypotension may therefore be used to reduce device migration. One method is to administer high-dose adenosine to temporarily induce asystole. General anesthesia with the airway secured may be preferable in these patients. Newer generation endografts are either thermally or mechanically activated during proximal graft deployment. Therefore, they tend not to migrate and induced hypotension is generally not required.

Kahn RA, Moskowitz DM, Marin M, et al. Anesthetic considerations for endovascular aortic repair. *Mt Sinai J Med* 2002;69:57–67.

Lippmann M, Lingam K, Rubin S, et al. Anesthesia for endovascular repair of abdominal and thoracic aortic aneurysms: a review article. *J Cardiovasc Surg* 2003;44:443–451.

E.4. What are the potential complications of endovascular thoracoabdominal aortic aneurysm (TAAA) repair?

- *Hypotension.* The differential diagnosis of acute hypotension after stent deployment includes aortic rupture, allergic reaction to IV contrast dye, adenosine side effect, or sympathetic nerve blockade if regional anesthesia is being used. Because of the possibility of acute intraoperative aneurysm rupture, the anesthesiologist must always be prepared for rapid volume resuscitation, including large bore IVs, central venous access, arterial line, and vasoactive agents.
- *Spinal cord ischemia.* The incidence of postoperative neurological injury after endovascular TAAA repair is similar to that of open repair. Risk factors for paraplegia include the length of the deployed endograft and a history of previous repair. Patients requiring longer grafts presumably are at a higher risk of spinal cord injury because a greater number of intercostal arteries are excluded. Cerebrospinal fluid drainage, avoidance of hypotension, and steroid administration are recommended in patients at high risk of spinal cord injury.
- *Postimplantation syndrome.* This commonly observed postoperative syndrome is characterized by fever, elevated C-reactive protein levels and leukocytosis. It is usually mild and self-limiting, lasting from 2 to 10 days. Treatment is with nonsteroidal antiinflammatory agents.

Kahn RA, Moskowitz DM, Marin M, et al. Anesthetic considerations for endovascular aortic repair. *Mt Sinai J Med* 2002;69:57–67.

CHAPTER 11

Abdominal Aortic Aneurysm Repair

LORI A. RUBIN

THE PATIENT WAS A 76-YEAR-OLD MAN

with a 6.0-cm infrarenal aortic aneurysm discovered on routine physical examination and confirmed with abdominal computed tomography (CT) scan. He was a former smoker and complained of dyspnea on exertion and claudication. His electrocardiogram (ECG) showed Q waves in leads II, III, and avF, chest x-ray film displayed mild hyperinflation of the lung fields, and his hematocrit was 46%. His baseline serum creatinine was 1.9 mg per dL.

A. Medical Disease and Differential Diagnosis

  1. What are the major causes of morbidity and mortality in the patient with an abdominal aortic aneurysm (AAA)?
  2. What other diseases are commonly found in patients with aortic aneurysms?
  3. What is the incidence of morbidity and mortality in these patients if they undergo elective surgical repair? What is the natural history of the disease without surgical repair?
  4. What should be done for smaller aortic aneurysms?
  5. What is the risk of perioperative myocardial infarction in patients with ischemic heart disease? By which means can we reduce the risk of further ischemic events in these patients?
  6. Does the morbidity and mortality of elective repair of an aortic aneurysm differ significantly from that of an emergency repair?

B. Preoperative Evaluation and Preparation

  1. Which preoperative laboratory tests would you require for this patient?
  2. Was this patient's preoperative electrocardiogram (ECG) significant? Would you wish to pursue further preoperative cardiac workup? What tests would you request, and what would they tell you?
  3. Is it necessary to evaluate this patient's pulmonary status?
  4. Preoperative arterial blood gas measurement showed pH 7.38, P_{CO_2} 45 mm Hg, and P_{O_2} 68 mm Hg on room air. What was the significance of this result?
  5. How would you measure creatinine clearance in this patient, and why is it an important value in this case?

6. Describe the blood flow to the spinal cord. What is its relevance to surgery of the abdominal aorta?

7. How do you detect spinal cord ischemia?

8. What are the various surgical approaches to repair an AAA? How does the choice of surgical technique affect the anesthetic management?

9. How would you premedicate this patient?

C. Intraoperative Management

1. Would you use an arterial line? What are the complications of an arterial line placement?

2. What various monitors are available for detecting myocardial ischemia? Is a pulmonary artery catheter (PAC) helpful in assessing myocardial ischemia?

3. What additional monitors would you employ?

4. How would you anesthetize this patient for an open repair of the aorta? What techniques could be used for an endovascular aortic aneurysm repair? What are the various anesthetic techniques that can be employed for this surgery?

5. This patient is to be heparinized intraoperatively and anticoagulation is to be continued postoperatively. Is this a contraindication to the preoperative placement of either an epidural or intraspinal catheter?

6. What are your plans for fluid and blood replacement during surgery?

7. What are the hemodynamic changes of aortic cross-clamp placement? What efforts can be made to minimize these changes both before and during cross-clamping? If the patient develops ST-segment depressions with a rising pulmonary artery occlusion pressure (PAOP) during cross-clamp, what maneuvers should be taken?

8. Because this case involves an infrarenal aneurysm, is renal blood flow affected with the placement of the cross-clamp? If an endovascular repair is chosen what are the risks to kidneys? Are there any treatment maneuvers that can be taken to minimize these risks in either type of repair?

9. What are the hemodynamic consequences of aortic cross-clamp removal? What can be done to minimize the effects of removing the aortic cross-clamp? If the systemic blood pressure remains depressed after removal of the cross-clamp, what is the differential diagnosis? How would you define and correct the problem?

D. Postoperative Management

1. What are the parameters used to extubate this patient?

2. What are the anticipated changes in postoperative pulmonary function in these patients? How does the surgical technique affect postoperative pulmonary function? Are there any postoperative maneuvers that can maximize respiratory parameters?

3. How would you control postoperative pain? What are the alternatives in the management of this patient's postoperative pain?

A. Medical Disease and Differential Diagnosis

A.1. What are the major causes of morbidity and mortality in the patient with an abdominal aortic aneurysm (AAA)?

Myocardial infarction is the single most common cause of early morbidity in AAA resection patients, accounting for approximately 55% of perioperative deaths. Of all patients who suffer a perioperative myocardial infarction, 70% will not survive. Other postoperative complications include bleeding, renal insufficiency, pulmonary infections and insufficiency, cerebrovascular accidents, hepatic failure, and paraplegia resulting from spinal cord ischemia. However, these events account for less than 1% of the total number of deaths from this operation. Risk factors affecting postoperative mortality are the presence of coronary artery disease (CAD), serum creatinine of greater than 1.2 mg per dL, blood urea nitrogen (BUN) greater than 40 mg per dL, age older than 60 years, emergency surgery, and indicators of poor liver function. Postoperative complications also increase with increasing transfusion requirements and are more likely with emergency surgery on the abdominal aorta.

Barash PG, Cullen BF, Stoelting RK, eds. *Clinical anesthesia*, 5th ed. Philadelphia: Lippincott Williams & Wilkins, 2006:938.

Dieke JT, Cali RF, Hertzer NR, et al. Complications of abdominal aortic reconstruction: an analysis of perioperative risk factors in 557 patients. *Ann Surg* 1983;197:49–56.

A.2. What other diseases are commonly found in patients with aortic aneurysms?

The major pathologic cause of aneurysmal disease is atherosclerosis. In addition to peripheral vascular disease (PVD), this population has a high incidence of coronary artery (50% to 70%), cerebrovascular, and renal disease. Commonly, these patients also suffer from hypertension, diabetes mellitus, and pulmonary disease. Patients with diffuse aortoiliac disease are more likely to be smokers and have hypertension, diabetes, and/or hypercholesterolemia, which contributes to their vascular disease. The previous risk factors, combined with advanced age (>60), are often exacerbated by the extreme physiologic changes during aneurysmal surgery.

Barash PG, Cullen BF, Stoelting RK, eds. *Clinical anesthesia*, 5th ed. Philadelphia: Lippincott Williams & Wilkins, 2006:945–946, 954–960.

DeBakey ME. Changing concepts in vascular surgery. *J Cardiovasc Surg* 1986;27:367–409.

A.3. What is the incidence of morbidity and mortality in these patients if they undergo elective surgical repair? What is the natural history of the disease without surgical repair?

Morbidity in this patient group is most commonly due to cardiovascular, pulmonary, and renal complications. Perioperative mortality for elective open abdominal aortic aneurysm (AAA) repair is 2% to 5%. Increased postoperative mortality was associated with older age, elevated serum creatinine, and lower forced expiratory volume in 1 second (FEV_1). The major cause of mortality in the nonsurgically treated patient is rupture with mortality of up to 80%. In one study, resection of the aneurysm doubled life expectancy. The incidence of rupture within 5 years of diagnosis of an AAA is 80%. The incidence of rupture increases with aneurysmal size: 25% for lesions of 4 to 7 cm in diameter, 45% for lesions 7 to 10 cm, and 60% for lesions larger than 10 cm. Patients with aneurysm greater than 5 cm should have surgical consideration.

After 10 years, graft patency is worse for patients with disease in more distal vessels, as is survival rate, which is 28% in patients with isolated aortoiliac disease and increases to 41% in patients with femoral, popliteal or tibial disease.

Brady AR, Fowkes FG, Greenhalgh RM, et al. Risk factors for postoperative death following elective surgical repair of abdominal aortic aneurysm: results from the UK small aneurysm trial. *Br J Surg* 2000;87(6):742–749.

Roizen MF, ed. *Anesthesia for vascular surgery*. New York: Churchill Livingstone, 1990: 12–13, 253.

A.4. What should be done for smaller aortic aneurysms?

Physical examination and screening, either by abdominal ultrasound or computed tomography (CT) scan uncovers many patients with aortic aneurysms less that 5.5 cm in diameter. One study compared patients with smaller aneurysms that were followed until they reached 5.5 cm or enlarged by 0.7 cm in 6 months, 1.0 cm in 1 year, or were symptomatic from their aneurysm. When patients were randomized to immediate repair or were followed closely, the mortality was the same. Ultimately, the patients that were monitored had their aneurysm repaired but were delayed by 4 years. Therefore, watchful waiting is suggested for aneurysms that are relatively small.

Lederle FA, Wilson SE, Johnson GR, et al. Immediate repair compared with surveillance of small abdominal aortic aneurysms. *N Engl J Med* 2002;346(19):1437–1444.

A.5. What is the risk of perioperative myocardial infarction in patients with ischemic heart disease? By which means can we reduce the risk of further ischemic events in these patients?

A retrospective analysis confirmed that cardiac mortality is high for patients who undergo vascular surgery and experience postoperative myocardial ischemia. Key factors that determine perioperative morbidity and mortality rates include the stress of surgery (aortic, peripheral vascular, emergency surgery), increased blood loss, poor preoperative cardiac functional status, congestive heart failure, low ejection fraction, known coronary artery disease (CAD), and preoperative history of coronary bypass grafting.

The occurrence of a recent myocardial infarction is an important independent predictor of perioperative morbidity and mortality. In a group of patients studied prospectively for perioperative reinfarction by Rao et al., the statistical rate of reinfarction was related to the length of time since the initial myocardial infarction, decreasing to less than 2% if the infarction occurred more than 6 months earlier. Patients were monitored with pulmonary artery (PA) catheters and arterial lines and were aggressively treated and monitored in an intensive care unit (ICU) setting for 3 to 4 days postoperatively. Currently, the acute care for myocardial infarction has improved and subsequent risk stratification with noninvasive testing allows for a more tailored approach to the timing of surgery in these patients. If bare-metal coronary stenting is performed a wait of at least 6 weeks is required due to the use of antiplatelet drugs during this period. Because of concern that late stent thrombosis may develop in patients treated with drug-eluting stents, most authors had recommended this combine antiplatelet therapy for 6 months maybe up to a year. One study suggests that coronary artery bypass grafting or coronary stenting before surgery usually will not decrease morbidity and mortality.

In most studies, the morbidity following a perioperative myocardial infarction approaches 50%. Fleisher and Barash suggest that risk after a myocardial infarction may be best linked to the ongoing risk of ischemia. Patients who have survived a non–Q wave infarction are potentially at great risk of further ischemia. Badner et al. reported a 17% post–posterior myocardial infarction (PMI) mortality rate after noncardiac surgery. The mortality rate was higher if the ST-segment and T-wave changes occurred intraoperatively. These patients should be evaluated by symptom-limited exercise testing and/or cardiac catheterization.

The prevention of perioperative myocardial ischemia is the focus of the anesthesiologist regardless of the technique they have chosen. The basic goal is to reduce myocardial oxygen demand by avoiding tachycardia and hypertension, while increasing oxygen supply by preventing hypotension and anemia. Oxygen demand on the left ventricle is dependent on heart rate, contractility, and the ventricular loading conditions. Of the three, the increase in heart rate is the most important of the factors that we can control. Left ventricular preload and afterload also affect oxygen demand by end-diastolic and systolic wall tension. Other factors, such as coronary collateral flow, hematocrit, blood rheology, and coronary collateral blood flow may also influence myocardial ischemia.

β-Adrenergic antagonists are a well-established group of drugs effective in the prevention of myocardial ischemia. It has been demonstrated that perioperative β-blockade provides benefit in preventing cardiac morbidity and mortality in higher risk patients. Ideally therapy should be started a week before surgery, continued into the perioperative period and titrated to a heart rate of less than 65 beats per minute. Atenolol has been shown to protect against reinfarction and to reduce mortality in the immediate and remote perioperative periods. The mechanism of action is related to decreases in heart rate and myocardial contractility, counteracting the deleterious effects of sympathetic stimulation. In addition, this class of drugs has antiarrhythmic qualities. Nitrates reduce myocardial oxygen demand by decreasing preload and by dilating large epicardial coronary arteries and collateral conduit vessels. However, the benefit of nitroglycerin prophylaxis intraoperatively has not been proven. Statins, α-blockers, and angiotensin-converting enzyme (ACE) inhibitors may also be beneficial, and should be continued if part of the patient's prior regime (also see Chapter 15, question A.9).

Auer J, Berent R, Weber T, et al. Risk of non cardiac surgery in month following placement of a drug-eluting stent. Letter to the editor. *J Am Coll Cardiol* 2004;43:713.

Badner NH, Knill RL, Brown JE, et al. Myocardial infarction after noncardiac surgery. *Anesthesiology* 1998;88:572–578.

Devereaux PJ, Beattie WS, Choi PT, et al. How strong is the evidence for the use of perioperative beta blockers in non-cardiac surgery? Systematic review and meta-analysis of randomized controlled trials. *Br Med J* 2005;331:313–321.

Fleischer LA. Editorial: Perioperative β-blocker: how best to translate evidence into practice. *Anesth Analg* 2007;104:1–3.

Fleisher LA, Beckman JA, Freeman WK, et al. ACC/AHA guideline update for perioperative cardiovascular evaluation for noncardiac surgery: focus update on perioperative Beta-blocker therapy. A report of the American College of Cardiology/American Heart Association task force on practice guidelines. *J Am Coll Cardiol* 2006;47: 1–12.

Levine G, Morton K, Berger P, et al. Management of patients undergoing percutaneous coronary revascularization. *Ann Intern Med* 2003;139:123–136.

Lindenauer PK, Pekow P, Wang K, et al. Perioperative beta-blockade therapy and mortality after major noncardiac surgery. *N Engl J Med* 2005;353(4):349–360.

London MJ. Con: Beta-blockers are indicated for all adults at increased risk undergoing noncardiac surgery. *Anesth Aanalg* 2007;104:9–12.

Mangano DT. Perioperative cardiac morbidity. *Anesthesiology* 1990;72:153–184.

McFalls EO, Ward HB, Moritz TE, et al. Coronary-artery revascularization before elective major vascular surgery. *N Eng J Med* 2004;351:2795–2804.

Poldermans D, Boersma E, Bax JJ, et al. The Efficacy of bisoprolol on perioperative mortality and myocardial infarction in high risk patients undergoing vascular surgery. *N Eng J Med* 1999;341(24):1789–1794.

Rao TL, Jacobs KH, El-Etr AA. Reinfarction following anesthesia in patients with myocardial infarction. *Anesthesiology* 1983;59:499–505.

Satler L. Recommendations regarding stent selection in relation to the timing of non cardiac surgery post percutaneous coronary intervention. Editorial comment. *Cath and Cardiovascular Interventions* 2004;63:146–147.

Schouten O, Bax JJ, Dunkelgrun M, et al. Pro: Beta-blockers are indicated for patients at risk for cardiac complications undergoing noncardiac surgery. *Anesth Analg* 2007;104:8–10.

Sprung J, Abdelmalak B, Gottlieb A, et al. Analysis of risk factors for myocardial infarction and cardiac mortality after major vascular surgery. *Anesthesiology* 2000;93:129–140.

A.6. Does the morbidity and mortality of elective repair of an aortic aneurysm differ significantly from that of an emergency repair?

Overall mortality for a ruptured aortic aneurysm is greater than 50%. One study showed an overall survival rate of 19.8% as compared with an elective surgical survival rate of 95%. The worst prognosis occurred in patients older than 80 years; a systolic blood pressure of less than 80 mm Hg on admission; a prior history of hypertension, angina, or previous myocardial infarction; and an operating time of greater than 4 hours. Other factors include a systolic blood pressure less than 100 mm Hg at the end of surgery, and blood loss greater than 11,000 mL. Retroperitoneal rupture was more likely to be associated with survival. Elective surgical intervention is indicated if the aneurysm changes rapidly or if its diameter is greater than 6 cm.

Ingoldby CJ, Wuyanto R, Mitchell JE. Impact of vascular surgery on community mortality from ruptured aortic aneurysms. *Br J Surg* 1986;73:551–553.

Lambert ME, Baguley P, Charlesworth D. Ruptured abdominal aortic aneurysms. *J Cardiovasc Surg* 1986;27:256–261.

B. Preoperative Evaluation and Preparation

B.1. Which preoperative laboratory tests would you require for this patient?

The patient should have the following laboratory tests as part of the preoperative evaluation: complete blood count and platelet count, serum electrolytes, blood urea nitrogen (BUN), creatinine, coagulation profile. Arterial blood gas may be useful. Clues to chronic hypercarbia may be gleaned from the serum bicarbonate value. Chest x-ray film, bedside spirometry, urinalysis and electrocardiogram (ECG) should be obtained. Preoperative laboratory tests should be defined by positive findings on history and physical examination.

Barash PG, Cullen BF, Stoelting RK, eds. *Clinical anesthesia*, 5th ed. Philadelphia: Lippincott Williams & Wilkins, 2006:954–960.

B.2. Was this patient's preoperative electrocardiogram (ECG) significant? Would you wish to pursue further preoperative cardiac workup? What tests would you request, and what would they tell you?

The patient's preoperative ECG was consistent with a prior inferior wall myocardial infarction. Patients having a history of a prior myocardial infarction or a history of angina in conjunction with an abnormal ECG have a fivefold increase in postoperative mortality when compared with those that have no clinical indication of coronary artery disease (CAD). His history of claudication suggests peripheral vascular disease (PVD). Patients with PVD have a fourfold increase in risk for myocardial infarction and a two to three times greater risk of stroke than those without PVD. If this patient's dyspnea on exertion is a symptom of CHF, this would significantly increase the perioperative morbidity. This increased risk may be altered by measurement and maintenance of normal hemodynamics with a pulmonary artery (PA) catheter. In selected patients with severe or unstable cardiac ischemia, prior myocardial revascularization may be indicated.

When coronary angiography was performed on 1,000 patients undergoing elective peripheral vascular surgery it was revealed that more than half of the patients had significant CAD (>50% stenosis) and 33% had severe stenosis (>70%). Of the asymptomatic patients with no history or electrocardiographic evidence of ischemic heart disease, 15% had severe CAD and 22% of these seemingly normal patients had impaired left ventricular function. Hertzer et al. found that only 8% of patients undergoing elective vascular surgery had normal coronary arteries.

A comparison of this patient's current ECG with a prior ECG may aid in assessing the timing of the previous infarction if the history alone is not helpful. In 2002 updated guidelines were published by the American Heart Association and the American College of Cardiology (AHA/ACC) for the preoperative assessment of patients undergoing noncardiac surgery. It suggests incorporating clinical history, exercise tolerance, and surgical risk when deciding further testing. The proposed algorithm for patients undergoing surgical procedures associated with a high risk of perioperative myocardial ischemia is shown in Fig. 11.1. Many vascular surgery patients are unable to undergo exercise stress testing because of limitations presented by their cardiac, pulmonary, or PVD. A dipyridamole-thallium stress test or a dobutamine stress echocardiogram are pharmacologic tests to assess ischemic potential. Dipyridamole causes vasodilation of normal coronary arteries. This results in a "steal" of blood flow from the area beyond a coronary stenosis. Blood flow redistributes as the drug dissipates. Boucher et al. found that redistribution is predictive of a 20-fold increase in postoperative ischemic events in patients undergoing peripheral vascular surgery. Those without redistribution had no perioperative cardiac events.

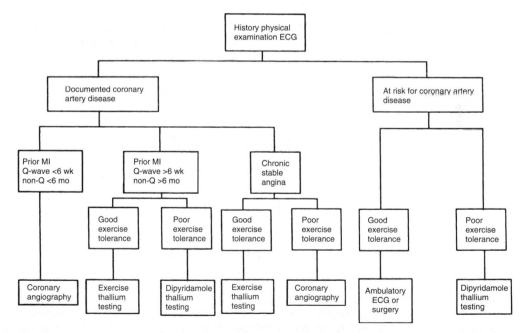

Figure 11.1 Proposed algorithm for patients undergoing surgical procedures associated with a high risk of perioperative myocardial ischemia (i.e., abdominal aortic aneurysm [AAA] resection). In these patients, further cardiovascular evaluation to delineate the extent of coronary artery disease (CAD) is warranted if the information obtained influences clinical care (see text). ECG, echocardiogram.

However, recent study by Poldermans et al. concluded that cardiac testing can safely be omitted in intermediate-risk patients undergoing major vascular surgery, provided that β-blockers aiming at tight heart rate control (below the ischemic threshold) are prescribed (also see Chapter 15, question B.2).

Boucher CA, Brewster DC, Darling RC, et al. Determination of cardiac risk by dipyridamole-thallium imaging before peripheral vascular surgery. *N Engl J Med* 1985;312:389–394.

Eagle KA, Berger PB, Calkins H, et al. ACC/AHA guideline update for perioperative cardio-vascular evaluation for noncardiac surgery—executive summary. *Anesth Analg* 2002; 94:1052–1064.

Eagle KA, Brundage BH, Chaitman BR, et al. Guidelines for perioperative cardiovascular evaluation for noncardiac surgery. Report of the American College of Cardiology/American Heart Association Task Force on Practice Guidelines (Committee on Perioperative Cardiovascular Evaluation for Noncardiac Surgery). *J Am Coll Cardiol* 1996;274:910–948.

Goldman L. Cardiac risk in non-cardiac surgery: an update. *Anesth Analg* 1995;80:810–820.

Hertzer NR, Beven EG, Young JR, et al. Coronary artery disease in peripheral vascular patients. A classification of 1000 coronary angiograms and results of surgical management. *Ann Surg* 1984;199:223–233.

Poldermans D, Bax JJ, Schouten O, et al. Should major vascular surgery be delayed because of perioperative cardiac testing in intermediate-risk patients receiving beta-blocker therapy with tight heart rate control? *J Am Coll Cardiol* 2006;48:964–969.

Sirrek CC, Watson DD, Smith WH, et al. Dipyridamole thallium-201 imaging versus dobutamine echocardiography for the evaluation of coronary artery disease in patients unable to exercise. *Am J Cardiol* 1993;72:1257–1262.

Whittemore AD, Clowes AW, Hechtman HB, et al. Aortic aneurysm repair: reduced operative mortality associated with maintenance of optimal cardiac performance. *Ann Surg* 1980;192:414–421.

B.3. Is it necessary to evaluate this patient's pulmonary status?

An assessment of pulmonary function should include an arterial blood gas analysis and spirometry. Arterial blood gas measurement evaluates the patient's ability to oxygenate and ventilate. Preoperative spirometry evaluates baseline forced vital capacity (FVC) and forced expiratory volume in 1 second (FEV_1). Maximum midexpiratory flow rate (MMEFR) is an effort-independent value and a sensitive index of small airway obstruction. Peak expiratory flow rate (PEFR) is related to the FEV_1 and MMEFR, although it is often less reproducible.

This patient was a two pack per day smoker with dyspnea on exertion and the anticipated surgery required an upper abdominal incision. These factors affect his baseline pulmonary function and presage postoperative ventilatory problems. A vital capacity (VC) less than 50% of predicted, or less than 2 L total, is an indicator of increased risk because a VC at least three times tidal volume is necessary for an effective cough. FEV_1 less than 2 L, maximum breathing capacity (MBC) less than 50% of predicted, and MMEFR less than 50% of predicted are also values associated with increased risk.

These tests should be performed before and after bronchodilator therapy to assess reversibility of airway obstruction. A 15% improvement is considered a positive response. Discontinuation of smoking for 48 hours preoperatively increases oxygen tissue availability and, if stopped 4 to 6 weeks before surgery, may decrease postoperative complications. Pulmonary function tests should be viewed as a management tool to optimize preoperative pulmonary function not as a means to assess risk, because they do not predict postoperative pulmonary complications.

Barash PG, Cullen BF, Stoelting RK, eds. *Clinical anesthesia*, 5th ed. Philadelphia: Lippincott Williams & Wilkins, 2006:954–960.

Gass GD, Olsen GN. Clinical significance of PFT: preoperative pulmonary testing to predict postoperative morbidity and mortality. *Chest* 1986;89:127–135.

Tisi GM. Preoperative identification and evaluation of the patient with lung disease. *Med Clin North Am* 1987;71:399–412.

Warner DO. Preventing postoperative pulmonary complications. The role of the anesthesiologist. *Anesthesiology* 2000;92:1467–1472.

B.4. Preoperative arterial blood gas measurement showed pH 7.38, PCO_2 45 mm Hg, and PO_2 68 mm Hg on room air. What was the significance of this result?

The normal value for PaO_2 in young adults ranges from 85 to 100 mm Hg with an average of approximately 95 mm Hg. This value falls steadily with aging to an average PO_2 of 80 mm Hg at age 60. A method of estimating the expected PaO_2 is 100–(age in years ÷ 3). The normal $PaCO_2$ is 37 to 43 mm Hg and is unaffected by aging. For every 10 mm Hg increase in $PaCO_2$, pH decreases by 0.08. For every 10 mm Hg decrease in $PaCO_2$, pH increases by 0.1.

The main causes of hypoxemia in arterial blood are hypoventilation, diffusion impairment, shunting, and ventilation/perfusion ($\dot{V}/\dot{Q}$) mismatch. The major causes of hypercarbia or carbon dioxide (CO_2) retention are hypoventilation and $\dot{V}/\dot{Q}$ mismatch. Not all $\dot{V}/\dot{Q}$ mismatches cause increases in arterial CO_2 because the chemoreceptors can recognize increasing CO_2 tension and cause an increase in ventilation. This, however, will not lead to a normalization of the hypoxemia caused by $\dot{V}/\dot{Q}$ imbalances.

The assessment of this patient's blood gas analysis reveals moderate hypoxemia with a high normal CO_2 tension. The pH is consistent with the CO_2. The most likely reason for this patient's blood gas abnormalities is $\dot{V}/\dot{Q}$ mismatches secondary to the many years of smoking. It is also likely that the patient has developed some obstructive lung disease with resultant $\dot{V}/\dot{Q}$ mismatches.

Lumb AB. *Nunn's applied respiratory physiology*, 6th ed. London: Butterworth-Heinemann, 2005:110–131.

West JB. *Respiratory physiology*, 7th ed. Baltimore: Lippincott Williams & Wilkins, 2005: 42–47, 55–72.

B.5. How would you measure creatinine clearance in this patient and why is it an important value in this case?

Preoperative renal dysfunction indicates potential postoperative impairment. Despite maximal medical management, including hemodialysis, acute renal failure (ARF) after aortic reconstruction carries a mortality of greater than 30% postoperatively. Maintenance of intravascular volume and adequate blood pressure is the best means of avoiding postoperative renal failure. This complication is more likely in patients requiring a suprarenal cross-clamp.

Operative mortality is 19% when aortic reconstruction is performed on patients with a creatinine greater than 2 mg per dL, but mortality is only 4.6% if the levels are lower. Therefore, if the creatinine is greater than 2 mg per dL, reversible factors, such as renal stenosis, should be investigated. The most direct measurement of glomerular filtration rate (GFR) is the measurement of creatinine clearance. Although blood urea nitrogen (BUN) and serum creatinine are related to renal function, they are altered by such nonrenal factors as protein metabolism, diet, liver dysfunction, or skeletal muscle mass. A 24-hour collection of urine is measured, and the following equation is used to calculate GFR: GFR = U × V/P where U, urine concentration of creatinine (mg/dL); V, volume of urine measured (mL/minute); P, plasma concentration of creatinine (mg/dL). A 2-hour sample collected through a Foley catheter correlates well with the 24-hour sample.

Diehl JT, Cali RF, Hertzer NR, et al. Complications of abdominal aortic reconstruction: an analysis of perioperative risk factors in 557 patients. *Ann Surg* 1983;197:49–56.

Miller DC, Myer BD. Pathophysiology and prevention of acute renal failure associated with thoracoabdominal or abdominal aortic surgery. *J Vasc Surg* 1987;5:518–523.

Ostri P, Mouritsen L, Jorgensen B, et al. Renal function following aneurysmectomy of the abdominal aorta. *J Cardiovasc Surg* 1986;27:714–718.

Sladen RN, Endo E, Harrison T. Two hour versus 22 hour creatinine clearance in critically ill patients. *Anesthesiology* 1987;67:1013–1016.

B.6. Describe the blood flow to the spinal cord. What is its relevance to surgery on the abdominal aorta?

The spinal cord has a system of longitudinal arteries and a system of transverse arteries as shown in Fig. 11.2. Anatomic studies have shown that the most important longitudinal arteries are a single anterior spinal artery supplying 75% of the cord and a pair of posterior spinal arteries supplying 25% of the cord. Although in humans the anterior spinal artery is a continuous vessel, modern anatomy has emphasized the importance of the reinforcing transverse arteries rather than the meager longitudinal vessels. The territory supplied by the anterior spinal artery is divided into three functionally distinct levels: cervicodorsal, intermediate or midthoracic, and thoracolumbar. The cervicodorsal region receives its blood supply from the vertebral, subclavian, thyrocervical, and costocervical arteries. The midthoracic region is supplied by a meager left or right intercostal artery arising between the fourth and the ninth thoracic vertebrae. The thoracolumbar region of the anterior spinal artery receives its blood supply mainly from one of the intercostal arteries called the arteria radicularis magna or the artery of Adamkiewicz. It arises at the level of T5-8 in 15%, T9-12 in 60%, L1 in 14%, and L2 in 10% of patients. The arteria radicularis magna is often involved in the surgical repair.

The anterior spinal artery is smaller above than below the entry of the arteria radicularis magna. Resistance to blood flow is 51.7 times greater going up the anterior spinal artery as compared with coming down the artery. Therefore, distal aortic perfusion during thoracic aortic cross-clamping protects the spinal cord below the arteria radicularis magna but not above it. This is why paraplegia still occurs in approximately 2% to 15% of patients having thoracic aortic surgery with distal aortic perfusion. However, reimplantation of intercostal arteries during surgery has been shown to reduce the incidence of neurologic injury.

Spinal cord ischemia can develop during aortic cross-clamping as a result of one of two mechanisms: Decreased blood flow through critical intercostal arteries (important in infrarenal cross-clamping) and hypotension in the aorta distal to the cross-clamp, leading to a "steal" phenomenon through the collateral circulation to the distal aorta (important in thoracic cross-clamping). There are many strategies to prevent spinal cord ischemia: moderate hypothermia (local and systemic), cerebrospinal fluid (CSF) drainage, and femoral–femoral bypass. The only definitive methods of preservation are fast surgery and maintenance of adequate cardiac output.

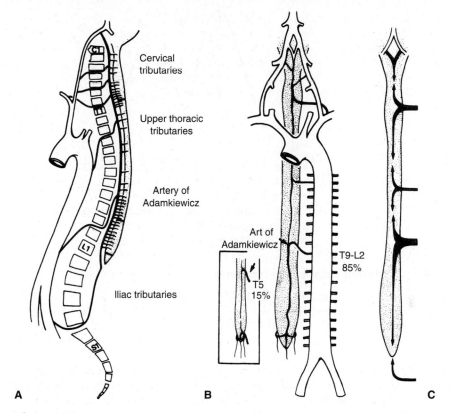

Cervical tributaries

Upper thoracic tributaries

Artery of Adamkiewicz

Iliac tributaries

Art of Adamkiewicz

T5
15%

T9-L2
85%

A

B

C

Figure 11.2 Diagram to show components of the anterior spinal artery. **A:** lateral view. **B:** Anteroposterior view showing origins of artery of Adamkiewicz. **C:** Schematic representation of direction and volume of flow from nutrient vessels supplying the anterior spinal artery. Size of arrows is proportional to flow contribution. (From Bromage PR. *Epidural anesthesia*. Philadelphia: WB Saunders, 1978:50–54, with permission.)

Bromage PR. *Epidural anesthesia*. Philadelphia: WB Saunders, 1978:50–54.

Ling E, Arellano R. Systematic overview of the evidence supporting the use of cerebrospinal fluid drainage in thoracoabdominal aneurysm surgery for prevention of paraplegia. *Anesthesiology* 2000;93:1115–1122.

Miller RD, ed. *Miller's anesthesia*, 6th ed. Philadelphia: Churchill Livingstone, 2005: 2086–2088.

Piccone W, DeLaria GA, Najafi H. Descending thoracic aneurysms. In: Bergan JJ, Yao JST, eds. *Aortic surgery*. Philadelphia: WB Saunders, 1989:249.

Richenbacher J, Landolt AM, Theiler K. *Applied anatomy of the back*. Berlin: Springer-Verlag New York, 1985:268–280.

Svensson LG, Richards E, Coull A, et al. Relationship of spinal cord blood flow to vascular anatomy during thoracic aortic cross-clamping and shunting. *J Thorac Cardiovasc Surg* 1986;91:71–78.

Williams GM, Perler BA, Burdick JF, et al. Angiographic localization of spinal cord blood supply and its relationship to postoperative paraplegia. *J Vasc Surg* 1991;13:23–33.

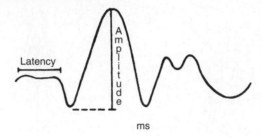

Figure 11.3 Typical somatosensory evoked potential trace. (From Cunningham JN Jr, Laschinger JC, Merkin HA, et al. Measurement of spinal cord ischemia during operations upon the thoracic aorta: initial clinical experience. *Ann Surg* 1982;196:285–296, with permission.)

B.7. How do you detect spinal cord ischemia?

Evoked potential is used in thoracoabdominal surgery to detect spinal cord ischemia. Two varieties of evoked potential are used in thoracoabdominal aortic aneurysm (TAAA) repair. somatosensory evoked potentials (SSEPs) travel through the dorsal root ganglia to the posterior columns of the spinal cord. The potentials continue along the lemniscal pathways on to the thalamus and the cortex. Comparison of the latency and amplitude of the potentials, tested minutes apart, define the degree of change in the SSEP. Temperature, anesthetic depth, and changes in blood flow can alter the evoked potentials. Changes in blood flow through the anterior spinal artery are not reflected in the posterior columns. It is possible, therefore, to have paralysis with normal SSEPs.

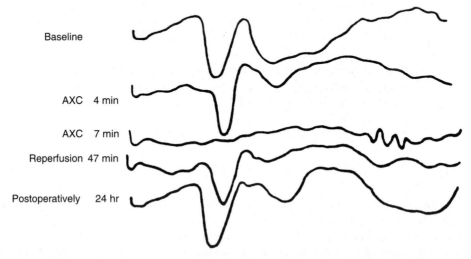

Figure 11.4 Somatosensory evoked potential response to aortic cross-clamping (AXC). (From Cunningham JN Jr, Laschinger JC, Merkin HA, et al. Measurement of spinal cord ischemia during operations upon the thoracic aorta: initial clinical experience. *Ann Surg* 1982;196:285–296, with permission.)

Ischemia of the spinal cord is indicated by increases in latency and/or decreases in amplitude of evoked potential tracing. The typical SSEP trace is shown in Fig. 11.3, and its response to aortic cross-clamping is shown in Fig. 11.4. The latency increases as early as 4 minutes following aortic cross-clamping, with progress to cessation of spinal cord conduction within 7 minutes of cross-clamping. Return of spinal cord conduction occurs 47 minutes following distal aortic reperfusion, with return to normal spinal cord conduction within 24 hours after operation. It has been shown that the loss of SSEP signals for longer than 14 to 30 minutes was associated with postoperative neurologic deficit.

Motor evoked potentials (MEPs) do monitor areas of the cord supplied by the anterior spinal artery. To assess MEPs, patients require partial paralysis and light plane of anesthesia. Both of these requirements are suboptimal anesthetic options for a TAAA repair.

Finally, the signal-to-noise ratio of evoked potentials make interpretation of the data in the operating room more difficult and less reliable.

Coles JC, Wilson GJ, Sima AF, et al. Intraoperative detection of spinal cord ischemia using somatosensory cortical evoked potentials during thoracic aortic occlusion. *Ann Thorac Surg* 1982;34:299–306.

Cunningham JN Jr, Laschinger JC, Spencer FC. Monitoring of somatosensory evoked potentials during procedures on the thoracoabdominal aorta: clinical observations and results. *J Thorac Cardiovasc Surg* 1987;94:275–285.

Ginsbury HH, Shetter AG, Raudzens PA, et al. Postoperative paraplegia with preserved intraoperative somatosensory evoked potentials. *J Neurosurg* 1985;63:296–300.

Grundy BL. Intraoperative monitoring of sensory-evoked potentials. *Anesthesiology* 1983;58: 72–87.

Meylaerts SA, Jacobs MJ, van Iterson V, et al. Comparison of transcranial motor evoked potentials and somatosensory evoked potentials during thoracoabdominal aortic aneurysm repair. *Ann Surg* 1999;230:742–749.

Miller RD, ed. *Miller's anesthesia*, 6th ed. Philadelphia: Churchill Livingstone, 2005:1211–1212, 1527–1530.

B.8. What are the various surgical approaches to repair an abdominal aortic aneurysm (AAA)? How does the choice of surgical technique affect the anesthetic management?

The classic approach to the abdominal aorta is through a vertical anterior midline incision with a transperitoneal approach to the retroperitoneal space. This gives access to all major arteries in the abdomen and pelvis. A transverse abdominal incision (supraumbilical) is also adequate for a transperitoneal approach. Although the entry is slower, there is less pain and pulmonary impairment postoperatively. The transperitoneal approach, with the necessary exposure of the abdominal organs, causes major heat and fluid loss and prolonged postoperative ileus.

The retroperitoneal approach is performed through a left flank incision with the patient in the right lateral decubitus position. In some studies, this approach has been shown to have less respiratory and wound complications, less postoperative ileus, less blood loss, lower fluid requirements, and earlier discharge from the hospital. Monitoring and line placement must take the lateral position into consideration.

A less invasive approach to aortic aneurysm repair is endovascular aortic stent-graft surgery. Half of the patients for aneurysm repair are candidates for endovascular repair. Shorter length of stay for patients relative to open repair is one clear advantage as well as a shortened recovery period. Due to the cost of the stents and imaging equipment this does not necessarily translate to overall cost savings. It is necessary to have a sufficient distance below the renal arteries to fix the graft and common femoral arteries or iliac arteries of sufficient caliber to accommodate placement of the stent. Successful aneurysm exclusion has been achieved in 50% to 90% of selected cases. Problems of the procedure include vessel perforation, inability to seal the aneurysm (endoleaks), and inability to advance the device past the iliac artery, ultimately necessitating the conversion to an open repair. Some of these patients may require a second noninvasive procedure as endoleaks requiring repair occur in up to 15% of patients. This highlights the importance of close follow up in these patients. When compared with open abdominal repair, the endovascular group sustained 60% less blood loss, were extubated sooner, and spent fewer days in the intensive care unit (ICU) and the hospital in total. Currently, overall mortality of the procedures appears similar, and when using the Eagle criteria as a predictor of adverse cardiac events for patients undergoing major vascular surgery, it appears that a history of CHF and Q waves on electrocardiogram (ECG) were predictive of cardiac events (6% in the open repair group vs. 4.8% in the endovascular group).

Debate exists over the advantages of general anesthesia compared with regional anesthesia or combined approaches for the management of patients with coronary artery disease (CAD). Meticulous control of heart rate and blood pressure are the goals of any method chosen. Regional anesthesia has the potential to decrease coronary perfusion pressure as sympathetic tone is diminished, and general anesthesia risk increases in sympathetic stimulation with intubation and emergence. Regional anesthesia may decrease hypercoagulability and thrombotic events in patients undergoing vascular surgery. Postoperatively, the epidural may be used to prevent the sympathetic stimulation created by postoperative pain.

The goals for the management of patients with CAD should include prevention and control of the effects of sympathetic nervous system stimulation by using β-blockers, narcotics, or volatile anesthetics during the perioperative period. Preservation of coronary perfusion pressure should be meticulously maintained. Myocardial contractility and heart rate should not be increased, as this will increase oxygen demand.

Baler AB. Retrospective review of 100 cases of endoluminal aortic stent-graft surgery from an anaesthetic perspective. *Anaesth Intensive Care* 1997;25:378–384.

Ballard JL, Yonemoto H, Killeen JD. Cost-effective aortic exposure: a retroperitoneal experience. *Ann Vasc Surg* 2001;14(1):54–58.

De Virgilio C, Bui H, Donayre C, et al. Endovascular vs open abdominal aortic aneurysm repair: a comparison of cardiac morbidity and mortality. *Arch Surg* 1999;134:947–951.

DeVirgilio C, Romero L, Donayre C, et al. Endovascular aortic aneurysm repair with general versus local anesthesia: a comparison of cardiopulmonary morbidity and mortality rates. *J Vasc Surg* 2002;36:988–991.

Quinones-Baldrich WJ, Garner C, Caswell D, et al. Endovascular, transperitoneal, and retroperitoneal abdominal aortic aneurysm repair: results and costs. *J Vasc Surg* 1999; 30:59–67.

Sampram ES, Karafa MT, Mascha EJ. Nature, frequency and predictors of secondary procedures after endovascular repair of abdominal aortic aneurysm. *J Vasc Surg* 2003; 37:930–937.

Warltier DC, Pagel PS, Dersten JR. Approaches to the prevention of perioperative myocardial ischemia. *Anesthesiology* 2000;92:253–259.

Zarin CK, White RA, Schwarten D, et al. AneuRx stent graft versus open surgical repair of abdominal aortic aneurysms: multicenter prospective clinical trial. *J Vasc Surg* 1999; 29:292–308.

B.9. How would you premedicate this patient?

The most common problem a patient faces in presentation to the operating room is anxiety. The method to relieve anxiety needs to be individualized for each patient with the preference of their anesthesiologist. Any drugs that are given should keep the goals of the induction and surgery in mind and minimize side effects that maybe deleterious. For this reason we would suggest a low-dose anxiolytic as sufficient premedication for most patients. The remainder of preoperative medications can be given intravenously after arrival in the operating room. Oral medication, if given, maybe taken with a sip of water 1 hour before the procedure. In addition, psychologic preparation for surgery is an important preoperative task for the anesthesiologist.

Additional pharmacologic regimens should be tailored to the specific needs of the patient. Various medications and combinations have been used, including narcotics, anticholinergics, barbiturates, and benzodiazepines. No single agent or combination has been demonstrated to be greatly superior to others. Certainly respiratory depressants should be avoided in patients who are at risk to develop hypoventilation (e.g., after carotid repair or chronic CO_2 retention). In high risk patients, such as diabetics, the risk of aspiration should be kept in mind and prophylaxis considered.

Barash PG, Cullen BF, Stoelting RK, eds. *Clinical anesthesia*, 5th ed. Philadelphia: Lippincott Williams & Wilkins, 2006:489–498.

Lineberger CK. Optimizing the patient for vascular surgery. In: Kaplan JA, Lake CL, Murray MJ, eds. *Vascular anesthesia*, 2nd ed. Philadelphia: Churchill Livingstone, 2004: 118–120.

C. Intraoperative Management

C.1. Would you use an arterial line? What are the complications of an arterial line placement?

Arterial pressure monitoring is exceedingly important in this case, from induction of anesthesia through emergence. For patients without coronary or cerebral artery disease, the arterial line can be placed after induction. However, because this patient has coronary artery disease (CAD), an arterial line is important for blood pressure management during induction and should be placed before institution of anesthesia.

Vascular insufficiency and infection are the two major complications of arterial line placement. Catheter size and duration of cannulation are implicated in vascular occlusion. The causes of most vascular injuries are embolic. Radial artery cannulation is a low-risk, high-benefit method used to closely monitor blood pressure in this patient with labile blood pressure, who also requires frequent sampling of arterial blood gases, hematocrits, and level of anticoagulation.

Bedford RF. Radial arterial function following percutaneous cannulation with 18 and 20 gauge catheters. *Anesthesiology* 1977;47:37–39.

Bedford RF, Wollman H. Complications of radial artery cannulation: an objective prospective study in man. *Anesthesiology* 1973;38:228–236.

Slogoff S, Keats AS, Arkind C. On the safety of radial artery cannulation. *Anesthesiology* 1983;59:42–47.

C.2. What various monitors are available for detecting myocardial ischemia? Is a pulmonary artery (PA) catheter helpful in determining the occurrence of ischemia?

Monitoring of the patient undergoing aortic reconstruction surgery should be aimed at preserving myocardial, pulmonary, and renal function as well as maintaining intravascular volume. Therefore, it is mandatory, particularly in the patient with known coronary artery disease (CAD), to monitor for myocardial ischemia. Monitoring of the V_5 lead as well as lead II, of the electrocardiogram (ECG) for ST-segment changes is the most common intraoperative assessment of myocardial ischemia. However, in some studies, this alone was insufficient to recognize from 40% to 75% of intraoperative ischemic events as detected by wall-motion abnormalities seen with a two-dimensional transesophageal echocardiogram.

Monitoring the PA pressure tracing for the appearance of V waves and increasing pulmonary artery occlusion pressure (PAOP) with decreasing cardiac output are other relatively insensitive means of detecting intraoperative myocardial ischemia. As with the ECG, wall-motion abnormality changes associated with early ischemia as detected by transesophageal echocardiography (TEE) are found far earlier than the appearance of V waves or changes in PAOP.

A microcomputer-based ECG reader (ST-segment trend monitor) has also been advocated as a monitor of myocardial ischemia. These systems can pick up more subtle changes in ST segments than by simple observation. Multilead ECG systems are most helpful. The most sensitive means for monitoring patients to determine the development of myocardial ischemia at its earliest presentation is, in fact, wall-motion dyskinesis demonstrated by two-dimensional TEE. As yet, no improvement in outcome has been demonstrated by the use of these monitors.

Barash PG, Cullen BF, Stoelting RK, eds. *Clinical anesthesia*, 5th ed. Philadelphia: Lippincott Williams & Wilkins, 2006:942–945.

Kalman PG, Wellwood MR, Weisel RD, et al. Cardiac dysfunction during abdominal aortic operation: the limitations of pulmonary wedge pressures. *J Vasc Surg* 1986;3:773–781.

Kotrly KJ, Kotter GS, Mortara D, et al. Intraoperative detection of myocardial ischemia with an ST segment trend monitoring system. *Anesth Analg* 1984;63:343–345.

Mangano DT. Perioperative cardiac morbidity. *Anesthesiology* 1990;72:153–184.

C.3. What additional monitors would you employ?

A monitor of central venous pressures (CVP) is recommended to determine volume status in these patients. The choice of monitor, CVP or pulmonary artery (PA) catheter, can be based on the level of aortic cross-clamping and the severity of the patient's underlying cardiac disease. The CVP is informative only if it is very low or very high. Because the right side of the heart is usually a compliant system, large changes in intravascular volume can occur without significant changes in the CVP. The pulmonary artery occlusion pressure (PAOP) may provide better information about intravascular volume status. In addition, the PA catheter allows for the simple measurement of cardiac output, which is exceedingly helpful during aortic cross-clamp in the patient with left ventricular dysfunction. In this situation particularly, CVP is not an accurate reflection of left-sided pressures reflected by the PAOP. This is also true of the patient with severe pulmonary disease.

Another useful measure of intravascular volume status, as well as renal blood flow, is the collection of urine through a Foley catheter. Urine output will diminish with decreasing glomerular filtration caused by decreased renal blood flow.

SSEPs during aortic reconstruction surgery monitor spinal cord function. For thoracic aortic surgery, SSEPs remain stable if the distal aortic pressure is maintained above 60 mm Hg. At lower pressures, SSEPs disappear gradually. In one study, paraplegia occurred in five of six patients whose SSEPs remained absent for more than 30 minutes. Patients should be monitored for SSEP changes if they are at higher risk of spinal cord ischemia. SSEPs are changed or lost with aortic cross-clamp most commonly in those patients who are already at increased risk for neurologic complications. Higher (especially thoracic) or prolonged cross-clamp placement also places the patient at increased risk for development of spinal cord ischemia. With a conduction block in place, as in epidural or spinal anesthesia, SSEPs will be ablated (also see question B.7).

These patients can undergo tremendous heat and insensible fluid loss as a result of the enormous surface area of the bowel exposed to room air. Therefore, body temperature should be monitored and aggressively maintained. Forced hot air thermal blankets are contraindicated on the lower extremities when an aortic cross-clamp is applied but may be used on the upper body along with fluid warmers to maintain temperature.

Ansley DM, Ramsay JG, Whalley DG, et al. The relationship between central venous pressure and pulmonary capillary wedge pressure during aortic surgery. *Can J Anaesth* 1987;34:594–600.

Barash PG, Cullen BF, Stoelting RK, eds. *Clinical anesthesia*, 5th ed. Philadelphia: Lippincott Williams & Wilkins, 2006:960, 963–966.

Bush H Jr, Hydo LU, Fischer E, et al. Hypothermia during elective abdominal aortic aneurysm repair: the high price of avoidable morbidity. *J Vasc Surg* 1995;21:392–402.

Nuwer MR. *Evoked potential monitoring in the operating room*. New York: Raven Press, 1986:93–95.

ASA Task Force on PA catheterization. Practice guidelines for PA catheterization. A report by the ASA Task Force on PA catheterization. *Anesthesiology* 1993;78:380–394.

Teplick R. Measuring central vascular pressures: a surprisingly complex problem. *Anesthesiology* 1987;67:289–291.

C.4. How would you anesthetize this patient for an open repair of the aorta? What techniques could be used for an endovascular aortic aneurysm repair? Discuss the various anesthetic techniques that can be employed for this surgery?

All anesthetic techniques have been used and advocated for abdominal aortic surgery. Pure general anesthesia, combined general and regional techniques, and pure regional anesthesia have all been described. Outcome studies seem to indicate no particular difference with technique or agents used. Benefits and problems can be argued from any side and a case made for each technique and agent selected. Tailoring the anesthetic administered to the individual patient is the single most important approach. In some, an inhalational technique may be indicated. In others, an opiate or mixed technique would better serve the patient's medical problems. The most important goals in the anesthetic management of patients undergoing aortic reconstruction include protection of myocardial and renal function. As long as these goals are met, the actual technique is probably less important. In patients with ischemic heart disease a slow heart rate is exceedingly beneficial. The anesthetic should be constructed with this goal in mind. Combined regional (epidural) and general anesthesia techniques usually involve an additional fluid requirement of up to 2 L per case. This can be offset by the concomitant use of an α agonist for vasoconstriction. The placement of an epidural catheter may also be of benefit in the postoperative management of the patient.

Anesthesia for endoluminal repair has ranged from general, general combined with epidural anesthesia, or lumbar epidural with sedation. Considerations for choice of anesthesia include the need to have the patient remain perfectly still for an extended period, the need for intravenous anticoagulation (heparin), the possibility of massive blood loss, and prevention of heat loss. It is important to keep blood pressure low during the time of balloon occlusion of the aorta to prevent distal migration of the stent. If neuraxial techniques are used the coagulation status must be carefully monitored throughout.

Baler AB. Retrospective review of 100 cases of endoluminal aortic stent-graft surgery from an anaesthetic perspective. *Anaesth Intensive Care* 1997;25:378–384.

Baron JF, Coriat P, Mundler O, et al. Left ventricular global and regional function during lumbar epidural anesthesia in patients with and without angina pectoris: influence of volume loading. *Anesthesiology* 1987;66:621–627.

Gamulin Z, Forster A, Simonet F, et al. Effects of renal sympathetic blockade on renal hemodynamics in patients undergoing major aortic abdominal surgery. *Anesthesiology* 1986;65:688–692.

Liu S, Carpenter RL, Neal JM. Epidural anesthesia and analgesia. Their role in postoperative outcome. *Anesthesiology* 1995;82:1474–1506.

Norris EJ, Beattie C, Perler BA, et al. Double-masked randomized trial comparing alternate combinations of intraoperative anesthesia and postoperative analgesia in abdominal aortic surgery. *Anesthesiology* 2001;95:1054–1067.

Yaeger MP, Chaimberg KH. Anesthetic techniques for major vascular surgery. In: Kaplan JA, Lake CL, Murray MJ, eds. *Vascular anesthesia*, 2nd ed. Philadelphia: Churchill Livingstone, 2004:165–186.

C.5. This patient is to be heparinized intraoperatively and anticoagulation is to be continued postoperatively. Is this a contraindication to the preoperative placement of either an epidural or intraspinal catheter?

There is concern that placement of an epidural catheter in a patient to be anticoagulated increases the risk of an epidural hematoma and a subsequent neurologic deficit. For those cases in which there is significant risk of spinal cord ischemia, the diagnostic confusion of epidural hematoma versus cord ischemia may preclude the placement of an epidural catheter. However, an epidural catheter can be placed with a relative degree of confidence in patients who are not anticoagulated at the time of the puncture but who will be anticoagulated later, with careful maintenance of the partial thromboplastin time (PTT) at 1.5 to 2 times the control value. Removal of the catheter should occur when the PTT is normalized.

Low molecular weight heparins (LMWHs) pose the potential for increased risk of epidural hematoma. Needle placement should occur 10 to 12 hours after the last dose of LMWH. If higher doses have been used (enoxaparin 1 mg/kg twice daily), delay should be 24 hours. It is currently recommended that indwelling catheters be removed before LMWH thromboprophylaxis, and the first administered dose given 2 hours after the catheter is removed.

Fibrinolytic and thrombolytic drugs are at high risk of adverse neuraxial bleeding during spinal or epidural anesthesia and should be avoided within 10 days of puncture of noncompressible vessels. Combinations of anticoagulants and antiplatelet drugs increase the risk of hemorrhagic complications perioperatively. Neurologic testing of sensory and motor function should be routinely performed on patients with indwelling catheters undergoing simultaneous anticoagulation. Analgesic solutions should be tailored to minimize sensory and motor changes.

Rao TLK, El-Etr AA. Anticoagulation following placement of epidural and subarachnoid catheters: an evaluation of neurologic sequelae. *Anesthesiology* 1981;55:618–620.

Horlocker TT, Wedel DJ, Benzon H. Regional anesthesia in the anticoagulated patient: defining the risks (second ASRA consensus conference on neuraxial anesthesia and anticoagulation). *Reg Anesth Pain Med* 2003;28:173–197.

Vandermeulen EP, Van Aken H, Vermylen J. Anticoagulants and spinal-epidural anesthesia. *Anesth Analg* 1994;79:1165–1177.

C.6. What are your plans for fluid and blood replacement during surgery?

Fluid replacement should be aimed at maintaining the patient's intravascular filling pressures. The use of a pulmonary artery catheter (PAC) simplifies this matter greatly. In most patients, crystalloid fluid should be isotonic. All preoperative fluid deficits must be accounted for early in the procedure (e.g., half the deficit in the first hour, half the remainder in the second hour, etc.); one must also watch the hourly fluid requirement for the weight of the patient (which takes into account the urine output and the usual insensible loss from skin and lungs) and the insensible loss from the large abdominal incision. Additional third-space loss from surgical trauma ranges from 3 to 5 mL/kg/hour for small incisions to 8 to 10 mL/kg/hour for large incisions (as in abdominal aortic aneurysm [AAA] repair). Blood loss should be replaced milliliter for milliliter with blood or colloid, or in a 3:1 ratio with crystalloid. There is data to suggest that patients may do better when crystalloid is limited to maintenance and colloid is used for hemodynamic stability and blood loss replacement. This approach should be weighed against the danger of prerenal damage to the kidneys and the need to keep urine output in excess of 0.5 mL/Kg/hour.

The concurrent use of an autotransfuser (e.g., Cell Saver) decreases the need for homologous blood transfusions. Transfusions have been shown to cause a clinically significant depression of immune function. With the hemodynamic changes associated with aortic cross-clamping, it is vital to maintain adequate intravascular volume to ensure adequate renal perfusion and normotension after removal of the cross-clamp.

Barash PG, Cullen BF, Stoelting RK, eds. *Clinical anesthesia*, 5th ed. Philadelphia: Lippincott Williams & Wilkins, 2006:954–966.

Joshi GP. Intraoperative fluid restriction improved outcome after major elective gastrointestinal surgery. *Anesth Analg* 2005;101:601–605.

Keane RM, Munster AM, Birmingham W, et al. Suppression of lymphocyte function after aortic reconstruction. Use of non-immunosuppressive anesthesia. *Arch Surg* 1982;117: 1133–1135.

C.7. What are the hemodynamic changes of aortic cross-clamp placement? What efforts can be made to minimize these changes both before and during cross-clamping? If the patient develops ST-segment depressions with a rising pulmonary artery occlusion pressure (PAOP) during cross-clamp, what maneuvers should be taken?

The systemic hemodynamic response to aortic cross-clamping is shown in Fig. 11.5.

Arterial hypertension is the most dramatic and consistent result of the application of an aortic cross-clamp. This is easily envisioned as a result of a sudden increase in afterload resulting in increased left ventricular end-diastolic wall stress and systemic arterial pressure. Usually these changes are accompanied by decreased cardiac output. Some of these changes may also be due to redistribution of blood volume from the venous vasculature to the upper part of the body. All of the previously stated factors are more profound in the case of a supraceliac or thoracic cross-clamp placement. Variations in blood volume status or splanchnic vascular tone are effected by the depth of anesthesia, type of anesthesia, and the extent of fluid load, which affect the pattern of blood volume redistribution.

A sudden increase in afterload can lead to left ventricular failure, particularly in the patient with a left ventricular dysfunction. Ideally, the patient should have lower filling pressures for the half hour before cross-clamp placement. This helps to minimize these responses to cross-clamp

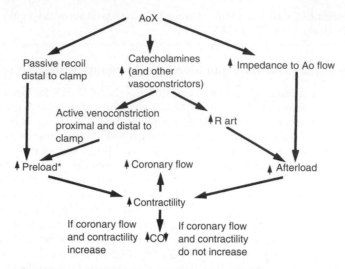

Figure 11.5 Systemic hemodynamic response to aortic cross-clamping. Preload does not necessarily increase. If during infrarenal aortic cross-clamping blood volume shifts into the splanchnic vasculature, preload does not increase (Fig. 13.1). *Different patterns are possible. Ao, aortic; AoX, aortic cross-clamping; CO, cardiac output; R art, arterial resistance; ↑ and ↓, increase and decrease, respectively. (From Gelman S. The pathophysiology of aortic cross-clamping, and unclamping. *Anesthesiology* 1995;82:1026–1060, with permission.)

placement. The pulmonary artery (PA) catheter is helpful in accurately assessing and maintaining the preclamp values for the left side of the heart. A potent inhalational agent and/or an intravenous vasodilator such as nicardipine is used to return afterload to near normal. This also helps increase the cardiac output and decrease stress on the left ventricle. If this is insufficient to reverse the left ventricular failure, the addition of an inotrope such as dopamine may be necessary.

The increase in afterload may also result in myocardial ischemia. Ischemia, reflected as a rising PAOP and ST-segment depressions, can be managed with intravenous nitroglycerin, a potent dilator of the capacitance vessels. This drug is used to decrease left ventricular end-diastolic volume (LVEDV) and left ventricular end-diastolic pressure (LVEDP). By decreasing LVEDP, one also decreases the transluminal pressure in the coronary vasculature. Blood flow to the myocardium is thereby increased.

Gelman S. The pathophysiology of aortic cross-clamping and unclamping. *Anesthesiology* 1995;82:1026–1060.

C.8. Because this case involves an infrarenal aneurysm, is renal blood flow affected with the placement of the cross-clamp? If an endovascular repair is chosen what are the risks to kidneys? Are there any treatment maneuvers that can be taken to minimize these risks in either type of repair?

ARF after aortic aneurysm repair is associated with a mortality of greater than 30%. Decreased renal function is observed in many patients after aortic cross-clamping, even when the clamp is placed distal to the renal arteries. Although it is clear that a suprarenal cross-clamp will decrease renal blood flow up to 80%, an infrarenal cross-clamp also causes a decrease in renal cortical blood flow with an associated decrease in GFR. The degree of decrease in urine output does not correlate with the decrease in GFR nor does it predict postoperative renal failure. The most dangerous complication of alteration in renal blood flow is acute tubular necrosis (ATN) and ARF.

The maintenance of cardiac output and adequate circulating blood volume is of prime importance in sustaining renal blood flow and in the prevention of renal failure. Low-dose dopamine (2 to 3 μg/kg/minute) increases renal blood flow and may improve urine output, although decreased incidence of postoperative renal failure has not been proven. In addition, renal protection may be provided by the administration of mannitol (0.25 g/kg). The use of mannitol attenuates the reduction of renal cortical blood flow before, during, and after renal ischemia, causes a concurrent increase in glomerular ultrafiltration pressure, which increases the GFR, and is a hydroxyl free radical scavenger. Other drugs that are used are fenoldopam and furosemide. Strong clinical evidence is currently lacking for any of these measures.

During endovascular repair the use of radiocontrast material may cause further insult to the kidneys. There are studies suggesting that the use of a bicarbonate infusion or pretreatment with *N*-acetylcysteine maybe protective. It is prudent to minimize the use of nonionic contrast or to use gadolinium dimeglumine, if possible, for imaging.

Alpert RA, Roizen MF, Hamilton WK, et al. Intraoperative urinary output does not predict postoperative renal function in patients undergoing abdominal aortic revascularization. *Surgery* 1984;95:707–710.

Gamulin Z, Forster A, Morel D, et al. Effects of infrarenal aortic cross-clamping on renal hemodynamics in humans. *Anesthesiology* 1984;61:394–399.

Miller DC, Myers BD. Pathophysiology and prevention of acute renal failure associated with thoracoabdominal or abdominal aortic surgery. *J Vasc Surg* 1987;5:518–523.

Merten GJ, Burgess WP, Gray JV, et al. Prevention of contrast-induced nephropathy with sodium bicarbonate: a randomized clinical trial. *JAMA* 2004;291(19):2328–2334.

Paul MD, Mazer CD, Byrick RJ, et al. Influence of mannitol and dopamine on renal function during elective infrarenal aortic clamping in man. *Am J Nephrol* 1986;6:427–434.

Youngberg JA, Lake CL, Roizen MF, et al. *Cardiac, vascular, and thoracic anesthesia.* New York: Churchill Livingstone, 2000:557–559.

C.9. **What are the hemodynamic consequences of aortic cross-clamp removal? What can be done to minimize the effects of removing the aortic cross-clamp? If the systemic blood pressure remains depressed after removal of the cross-clamp, what is the differential diagnosis? How would you define and correct the problem?**

The hemodynamic response to aortic unclamping is shown in Fig. 11.6.

During cross-clamping, blood flow to the lower extremities is grossly diminished. Metabolism switches from aerobic to anaerobic as ischemia develops. This results in maximal vasodilation and lactic acid production. When the cross-clamp is released, systemic vascular resistance and arterial blood pressure decreases dramatically. Reactive hyperemia is a consequence of unclamping. This may be the result of arterial relaxation (myogenic mechanism), an accumulation of vasodilating substances below the occlusion, or anoxic relaxation of smooth muscles. Peripheral vasodilation can result in relative volume depletion and hypotension. Vasodilation may become systemic as the lactic acid is washed out of the extremities into the central circulation. This condition is sometimes known as *declamping shock.*

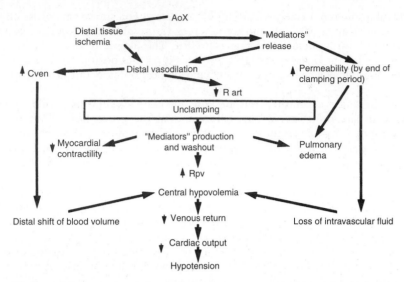

Figure 11.6 Systemic hemodynamic response to aortic unclamping. AoX, aortic cross-clamping; Cven, venous capacitance; R art, arterial resistance; Rpv, pulmonary vascular resistance; ↑ and ↓, increase and decrease, respectively. (From Gelman S. The pathophysiology of aortic cross-clamping and unclamping. *Anesthesiology* 1995;82:1026–1060, with permission.)

To minimize the hypotensive response, volume loading in the period before cross-clamp release is suggested to raise filling pressures to slightly above normal. Vasodilators such as nicardipine and nitroglycerin during this period allow additional volume loading with maintenance of filling pressures. In addition, gradual release of the clamp allows time for adjustments in volume, administration of pressors, and sodium bicarbonate replacement.

Sometimes, even in the face of adequate volume loading, the blood pressure remains low following cross-clamp removal. The more cephalad the cross-clamp placement, the greater the incidence of this problem. In this situation it is advisable to ask the surgeon to reapply the aortic cross-clamp in various degrees depending on the severity of the hypotension. This allows more time for correction of blood volume or acidosis.

Other causes of sustained hypotension in the face of adequate management include a continued site of hemorrhage and myocardial ischemia and/or failure. Measurement of filling pressures would help in this differentiation. Ischemia or failure would have elevated filling pressures with hypotension, whereas hemorrhage would naturally have low filling pressures.

Eklof B, Neglen P, Thomson D. Temporary incomplete ischemia of the legs induced by aortic clamping in man: effects on central hemodynamics and skeletal muscle metabolism by adrenergic block. *Ann Surg* 1981;193:89–98.

Gelman S. The pathophysiology of aortic cross-clamping and unclamping. *Anesthesiology* 1995;82:1026–1060.

Reiz S, Peter T, Rais O. Hemodynamic and cardiometabolic effects of infrarenal aortic and common iliac artery declamping in man: an approach to optimal volume loading. *Acta Anesth Scand* 1979;23:579–586.

D. Postoperative Management

D.1. What are the parameters used to extubate this patient?

When a patient is awake and alert, the common criteria used for extubation include the following:

- Vital capacity (VC) greater than 15 mL per kg
- pH greater than 7.30 PaO_2 greater than 60 mm Hg at FIO_2 less than 50%
- $PaCO_2$ less than 50 mm Hg
- Maximal negative inspiratory force greater than–20 cm H_2O
- Stable hemodynamic status
- Respiratory rate less than 30 breaths per minute

For shorter cases with minimal fluid shifts, the patient can be extubated in the immediate postoperative period. For longer cases or instances of large fluid replacement, extubation should be delayed until the hemodynamics are stabilized and temperature is normalized.

Stoelting RK, Dierdorf SF, McCammon RL, eds. *Anesthesia and co-existing diseases*, 4th ed. New York: Churchill Livingstone, 2002:408–424.

D.2. What are the anticipated changes in postoperative pulmonary function in these patients? How does the surgical technique affect postoperative pulmonary function? Are there any postoperative maneuvers that can maximize respiratory parameters?

The transabdominal approach to the aorta involves an upper abdominal incision. Total lung capacity (TLC) and its subdivisions decrease after upper abdominal surgery. Vital capacity (VC) decreases 25% to 50% and returns to normal in 1 to 2 weeks, and residual volume (RV) increases 13%. Functional residual capacity (FRC) declines 30% and recovers over 3 to 4 days. Expiratory reserve volume (ERV) declines 20% after lower abdominal surgery and up to 60% after upper abdominal and thoracic incisions. Tidal volume decreases 20% on the first postoperative day and gradually returns to normal. The retroperitoneal approach to the aorta involves a flank incision, which leads to far less respiratory compromise.

In a series of adult men undergoing abdominal surgery, postoperative pulmonary complications occurred more frequently than cardiac complications (9.6% vs. 5.7%) and were associated with significantly greater length of hospitalization. Many of these complications are related to disruption of the normal activity of the respiratory muscles, from the beginning of the anesthetic to the postoperative period. In addition, the effects of surgical trauma are most pronounced after upper abdominal surgery. Lower abdominal and thoracic incisions impact the respiratory muscles to a lesser degree. This occurs through surgical disruption of the respiratory muscles, postoperative pain, and abdominal contents preventing normal movement of the diaphragm. The resulting respiratory pattern is that of shallow rapid breaths without sighs.

Although regional anesthetic techniques have the potential to improve pain and reflex inhibition of respiratory muscles, they may also significantly alter postoperative respiratory muscle function. The overall effect of postoperative regional analgesia on the pattern of breathing may be complex, but it is thought that epidural analgesia may decrease the risk for postoperative pulmonary complications. Ambulation and control of postoperative pain diminish splinting and help maximize respiratory parameters. Maneuvers to encourage deep breathing are of proven benefit.

Barash PG, Cullen BF, Stoelting RK, eds. *Clinical anesthesia*, 5th ed. Philadelphia: Lippincott Williams & Wilkins, 2006:1422–1429, 810.

Warner DO. Preventing postoperative pulmonary complications. The role of the anesthesiologist. *Anesthesiology* 2000;92:1467–1472.

D.3. How would you control postoperative pain? What are the alternatives in the management of this patient's postoperative pain?

The goal of effective postoperative pain relief is to produce a high quality of pain control with the fewest number of side effects and complications. Neuraxial analgesia in the immediate postoperative period is the preferred method of pain management in this high-risk patient population. The ideal opiate, its concentration, and combination with local anesthetic have yet to be defined. (For suggested protocols see Table 11.1.) Alternatively, intravenous narcotics administered by a patient-controlled analgesia (PCA) pump is another choice for pain control.

Complications of the epidural route of analgesia include dural puncture, epidural hematoma, and epidural abscess. The risk of epidural hematoma is small in patients receiving appropriate doses of anticoagulation postoperatively but is prohibitively high in patients receiving thrombolytic treatment or LMWHs. Consideration should be taken at the timing of both insertion and removal of the catheter. The risk of complications are similar whether the catheter is placed at the thoracic or lumbar level. Other complications include pruritus, nausea, urinary retention, and delayed respiratory depression. The latter is less than 1% when epidural morphine is used, similar to the oral and parenteral route. Difficulty ambulating and orthostatic hypotension are minimized when catheters are placed in the thoracic region with low infusion rates and bupivacaine concentrations less than 0.08%.

Alternatively, a systemic narcotic analgesic can be used. These are most commonly administered by a PCA pump allowing the patient to titrate their narcotic needs. The modified infusion pumps are able to administer infusions of narcotics, small preprogrammed bolus doses on patient demand, and larger bolus doses by prescription. This allows patients to titrate their

Table 11.1 Epidural Opioid/Bupivacaine Combinations Administered by Continuous Infusion[a].

DRUG COMBINATIONS	SOLUTION[b] (%)	BOLUS DOSE OF BUPIVACAINE (%)	BASAL INFUSION[c]	BREAKTHROUGH DOSES	INCREMENTS IN BREAKTHROUGH[d]
Morphine	0.01		6–8 mL/hr	1–2 mL every 10–15 min	1 mL of the solution
Bupivacaine[e]	0.05–0.1	0.5–0.25			
Hydromorphone	0.0025–0.005		6–8 mL/hr	1–3 mL every 10–15 min	1 mL of the solution
Bupivacaine[f]	0.05–0.1	0.5–0.25			
Fentanyl	0.001		0.1–0.15 mL/kg/hr	1–1.5 mL every 10–15 min	1 mL of the solution
Bupivacaine[g]	0.05–0.1	0.5–0.25			
Sufentanil	0.0001		0.1–0.2 mL/kg/hr	1–1.5 mL every 10–15 min	1 mL of the solution
Bupivacaine[h]	0.05–0.1	0.5–0.25			

[a]Catheter insertion site is the dermatome corresponding to the middle of the surgical incision. Administer a bolus dose of 0.5% bupivacaine or 2% lidocaine to establish surgical anesthesia, or 0.25% bupivacaine to induce postoperative analgesia in 5-mL aliquots.

[b]Due to infectious control, a total volume of 150 mL is recommended.

[c]Initial basal infusion rates will depend on the age, general condition, and weight of the patient.

[d]If analgesia is inadequate after 1 hr, increase the breakthrough dose by the recommended amount. If analgesia is inadequate after one additional hour, decrease the lockout interval by 5 min.

[e]Prepare this solution by mixing 75–150 mg of bupivacaine with 15 mg of preservative-free morphine in a total volume of 150 mL of preservative-free normal saline.

[f]Prepare this solution by mixing 75–150 mg of bupivacaine with 3.75–7.5 mg of hydromorphone in a total volume of 150 mL of preservative-free normal saline.

[g]Prepare this solution by mixing 75–150 mg of bupivacaine with 1,500 μg of fentanyl in a total volume of 150 mL of preservative-free normal saline.

[h]Prepare this solution by mixing 75–150 mg of bupivacaine with 150–300 μg of sufentanil in a total volume of 150 mL of preservative-free normal saline.

From de Leon-Casasola OA, Lema MJ: Postoperative epidural opioid analgesia: What are the choices? *Anesth Analg* 1996;83:867–875. with permission.

narcotic doses to need while avoiding the toxic side effects that result from high peak serum levels (also see Chapter 32).

Barash PG, Cullen BF, Stoelting RK, eds. *Clinical anesthesia*, 5th ed. Philadelphia: Lippincott Williams & Wilkins, 2006:1405–1440.

de Leon-Casasola OA, Lema MJ. Postoperative epidural opioid analgesia: what are the choices? *Anesth Analg* 1996;83:867–875.

Liu S, Carpenter RL, Neal JM. Epidural anesthesia and analgesia. Their role in postoperative outcome. *Anesthesiology* 1995;82:1474–1506.

Mann C, Pouzeratte Y, Boccara G, et al. Comparison of intravenous or epidural patient-controlled analgesia in the elderly after major abdominal surgery. *Anesthesiology* 2000;92:433–441.

Yeager M, Glass DD, Neff RK, et al. Epidural anesthesia and analgesia in high-risk surgical patients. *Anesthesiology* 1987;66:729–736.

CHAPTER 12

Hypertension

MANUEL L. FONTES • FUN-SUN F. YAO

A 70-YEAR-OLD MAN

with cholelithiasis was scheduled for a cholecystectomy. His blood pressure (BP) was 230/120 mm Hg; pulse 60 beats per minute. Hematocrit was 38%; serum sodium, 140 mEq per L; and serum potassium, 2.7 mEq per L. His medications included propranolol and hydrochlorothiazide.

A. Medical Disease and Differential Diagnosis

1. Define hypertension and classify its severity.
2. What is the prevalence of hypertension?
3. What is the general classification of hypertension? Enumerate the causes of each type of hypertension.
4. What are the clinical patterns of hypertension encountered?
5. What is the pathophysiology of essential hypertension?
6. What is the pathophysiology of isolated systolic hypertension (ISH) and of pulse pressure hypertension (PPH)?
7. What are the end-organ damages caused by long-standing hypertension?
8. Are hypertensive patients at an increased risk of perioperative cardiac morbidity?
9. Perioperative cerebral and renal complications are mostly associated with which subtype of hypertension?
10. Would you employ a controlled hypotensive technique for hypertensive patients? How much would you safely lower the blood pressure (BP)?
11. What is the mechanism of action of antihypertensive drugs?
12. Does the choice of antihypertensive therapy influence hemodynamic responses to induction, laryngoscopy, and intubation?
13. Does chronic angiotensin-converting enzyme (ACE) inhibition influence anesthetic induction?

B. Preoperative Evaluation and Preparation

1. How would you evaluate this patient preoperatively?
2. Would you postpone the surgery? Why? What BP would you like the patient to achieve before surgery?
3. Should all or any of the chronic medications be discontinued before the operation?
4. Should hypokalemia be treated before anesthesia? Why?
5. Should hypomagnesemia be treated before anesthesia? Why?

6. Does an asymptomatic carotid bruit increase the risk in these patients?
7. The surgery was postponed for 6 weeks. The patient has been on propranolol, captopril, hydrochlorothiazide, and KCl. His BP was 160/95 mm Hg and potassium 4.0 mEq per L. How would you premedicate this patient?
8. If the patient is an untreated hypertensive patient with BP 170/100 mm Hg, would you pretreat the patient preoperatively with an antihypertensive agent?

C. **Intraoperative Management**
1. How would you monitor this patient?
2. What are the anesthetic goals for hypertensive patients?
3. How would you induce anesthesia for the hypertensive patient?
4. How does tracheal intubation produce hypertension?
5. What happens to the left ventricular ejection fraction during and immediately following intubation?
6. What other measures can prevent hypertension and tachycardia at the time of intubation?
7. After induction and intubation, the BP went down to 70/40 mm Hg. What would you do?
8. What is your choice of agents for maintenance of anesthesia? Why?
9. How would you manage fluid therapy for hypertensive patients?
10. During the surgery, BP went up to 220/120 mm Hg. How would you treat the hypertension?
11. What could you do to prevent hypertension during extubation and emergence?
12. Would you consider regional anesthesia for this patient?

D. **Postoperative Management**
1. The patient developed hypertension BP 210/110 mm Hg in the postanesthesia care unit. What would you do?

A. Medical Disease and Differential Diagnosis

A.1. Define hypertension and classify its severity.

True systemic hypertension can be diagnosed when there is an increase in arterial pressure above accepted normal pressure for age, sex, and race. According to the latest classification and characterization of blood pressure (BP) by the Joint National Committee on Evaluation, Detection, and Prevention of High Blood Pressure, an optimal BP for adults is less than 120 mm Hg systolic with a diastolic of less than 80 mm Hg. Table 12.1 shows the categories of BP for optimal, normal and high normal as well as the three stages of hypertension. The accepted upper limits of normal BP in pediatric are as follows:

Adolescent	100/75 mm Hg
Early childhood	85/55 mm Hg
Infant	70/45 mm Hg

It is important to note that newer classification of hypertension define and specify hypertension according to systolic and to diastolic hypertension each representing different pathophysiologic processes. Systolic hypertension is a marker of macrovascular disease and large arterial stiffening (atherosclerosis) and diastolic hypertension is a consequence of microvascular disease involving typically vessels less than 1 mm in size (arteriosclerosis).

Table 12.1 Categories of Blood Pressure and Subtypes of Hypertension.

CATEGORY	BLOOD PRESSURE (MM HG)	
	SYSTOLIC	DIASTOLIC
Optimal	<120	<80
Normal	<130	<85
High normal	130–139	85–89
Hypertension		
Stage 1	140–159	90–99
Stage 2	160–179	100–109
Stage 3	>180	>110
ISH	>140	<90
PPH	(Pulse pressure > 65 mm Hg)	

ISH, isolated systolic hypertension; PPH, pulse pressure hypertension.

Aronson S, Fontes ML. Hypertension: a new look at an old problem. *Curr Opin Anesth* 2006;19:59–64.

Fontes ML. New insights in hypertension. *ASA Refresher Courses Anesthesiol* 2006;34:43–53.

Zipes DP, Libby P, Bonow RO, et al. eds. *Heart disease*, 7th ed. Philadelphia: WB Saunders, 2005:961–964.

A.2. What is the prevalence of hypertension?

The prevalence of hypertension depends on both the racial composition of the population and the criteria used to define hypertension. In a white suburban population like that in the Framingham Study, nearly one fifth have blood pressure (BP) greater than 160/95 mm Hg, and almost one half have BP greater than 140/90 mm Hg. A higher prevalence has been found in the nonwhite population. The frequency increases with the age of the population with nearly two thirds of hypertensive patients being older than 50 years. The subtype of hypertension is also influenced by age. Younger individuals suffer from diastolic hypertension and combined systolic and diastolic hypertension whereas older persons predominantly experience systolic hypertension. The number of hypertensive persons in the United States in 1983 was estimated to be 57.7 million—more than double the estimate made in 1960 to 1962. Currently, approximately 70 million Americans suffer from hypertension.

Aronson S, Fontes ML. Hypertension: a new look at an old problem. *Curr Opin Anesth* 2006;19:59–64.

Franklin SS, Larson MG, Khan SA, et al. Does the relation of blood pressure to coronary heart disease risk change with aging? The Framingham Heart Study. *Circulation* 2001; 1031:1245–1249.

Kasper DL, Braunwald E, Fauci AS, et al. eds. *Harrison's principles of internal medicine*, 16th ed. New York: McGraw-Hill, 2005:1463–1467.

Zipes DP, Libby P, Bonow RO, et al. eds. *Heart disease*, 7th ed. Philadelphia: WB Saunders, 2005:963–964.

Table 12.2   Classification of Hypertension.

Systolic and diastolic hypertension
- Essential
- Renal
- Endocrine
- Neurogenic
- Miscellaneous

Systolic hypertension with wide pulse pressure
- Increased cardiac output
- Rigidity of aorta

A.3. What is the general classification of hypertension? Enumerate the causes of each type of hypertension.

Hypertension is classified according to its subtypes: systolic, diastolic, and pulse pressure (Table 12.2). Historically, only diastolic hypertension—essential hypertension—was recognized but more recently there has been increasing emphasis and recognition of systolic hypertension, namely, *isolated systolic hypertension* (ISH). ISH is the most common subtype of hypertension affecting predominantly individuals older than 60 years of age. In fact, approximately 70% of hypertensive patients have ISH with approximately half of these individuals having very wide pulse pressure (>65 mm Hg) or *pulse pressure hypertension* (PPH). *Isolated diastolic hypertension* (IDH) is most prevalent in individuals younger than 50 years and is an important marker of coronary heart disease and mortality in this age group. Some hypertensive patients have both systolic and diastolic hypertension categorized as *combined systolic and diastolic hypertension*. The ranges of systolic, diastolic, and pulse pressure that define each subtype of hypertension are presented in Table 12.1.

Etiology of hypertension

- *Essential hypertension.* Unknown etiology
- *Renal.* Acute and chronic glomerulonephritis, chronic pyelonephritis, polycystic kidney, diabetic nephropathy, hydronephrosis, renovascular stenosis, renin-producing tumors, primary sodium retention
- *Endocrine.* Adrenal—Cushing's syndrome, primary aldosteronism, congenital adrenal hyperplasia, pheochromocytoma, acromegaly, hypothyroidism, carcinoid, hyperthyroidism, oral contraceptives, corticosteroids
- *Neurogenic.* Psychogenic, increased intracranial pressure, spinal cord section, familial dysautonomia, lead poisoning, Guillain-Barré syndrome, sleep apnea
- *Miscellaneous.* Coarctation of aorta, increased intravascular volume, pregnancy-induced hypertension, polyarteritis nodosa, acute porphyria, hypercalcemia, alcohol and drug use, acute stress including surgery

Benetos A, Thomas F, Safar ME. Should diastolic and systolic blood pressure be considered for cardiovascular risk evaluation: a study in middle-aged men and women. *J Am Coll Cardiol* 2001;37:163–168.

Franklin SS, Khan SA, Wong ND, et al. Is pulse pressure useful in predicting risk for coronary heart disease? The Framingham Heart Study. *Circulation* 1999;100:353–360.

Kannel WB. Cardiovascular hazards of components of blood pressure. *J Hypertens* 2002;20:395–397.

Kasper DL, Braunwald E, Fauci AS, et al. eds. *Harrison's principles of internal medicine*, 16th ed. New York: McGraw-Hill, 2005:1463–1467.

Sesso HD, Stampfer MJ, Rosner B, et al. Systolic and diastolic blood pressure, pulse pressure, and mean arterial pressure as predictors of cardiovascular disease risk in men. *Hypertension* 2000;36:801–807.

Zipes DP, Libby P, Bonow RO, et al. eds. *Heart disease*, 7th ed. Philadelphia: WB Saunders, 2005:963–964.

A.4. What are the clinical patterns of hypertension encountered?

- "Vasoconstricted" hypertension—in medical patient with chronic renovascular hypertension, characterized by diastolic hypertension and systemic vascular resistant with normal or even decreased cardiac output and heart rate.
- "Hyperdynamic" hypertension—in postoperative surgical patient, characterized by acute systolic hypertension; widened pulse pressure; and increased cardiac output, heart rate, and systemic vascular resistant.

Sladen RN. Perioperative hypertension. *IARS review course lectures*. Cleveland: International Anesthesia Research Society, 2002:100–114.

A.5. What is the pathophysiology of essential hypertension?

The underlying mechanism of essential hypertension is unknown. A variety of abnormalities including heredity, fetal undernutrition, abnormal sympathetic nervous system (SNS) activity, cell membrane defects, renal retention of excess salt, microcirculatory alterations, endothelial cell dysfunction, hyperinsulinemia secondary to insulin resistance, vascular hypertrophy, and altered renin–angiotensin system regulation are implicated. There is increasing evidence that "local renin–angiotensin" paracrine factors may be involved in the development of hypertension. However, characteristic hemodynamic changes are present as follows:

- Increased systemic vascular resistance (SVR) with normal cardiac output
- Markedly increased sympathetic response to stress such as endotracheal intubation
- A greater increase in blood pressure (BP) with vasoconstriction and a greater decrease in BP with vasodilation because of the increased thickening of arterial wall and high ratio of wall thickness to internal diameter

The higher the level of BP, the more likely that various cardiovascular diseases will develop prematurely through acceleration of arteriosclerosis. If untreated, approximately 50% of hypertensive patients die of coronary heart disease or congestive heart failure (CHF), approximately 33% of stroke, and 10% to 15% of renal failure.

Kasper DL, Braunwald E, Fauci AS, et al. eds. *Harrison's principles of internal medicine*, 16th ed. New York: McGraw-Hill, 2005:1465–1475.

Zipes DP, Libby P, Bonow RO, et al. eds. *Heart disease*, 7th ed. Philadelphia: WB Saunders, 2005:968–973.

A.6. What is the pathophysiology of Isolated Systolic hypertension (ISH) and of pulse pressure hypertension (PPH)?

ISH is a manifestation of atherosclerotic disease involving predominantly the aorta and its major branches. Both ISH and PPH reflect arterial stiffening and represent the pulsatile component of blood pressure (BP) whereas the mean arterial pressure (MAP) represent the static state. Systole, then, is directly influenced by the ventricular contractile state, the ejected volume, heart rate, and, importantly, compliance of the aorta and pulse wave velocity. With increasing age and factors such as diabetes, smoking, increased cholesterol as well as some genetic factors, compliance of the aorta diminishes markedly (Fig.12.1). The net result is stiffening of the arterial tree and inability to absorb the pulsatile load, causing the systolic pressure to rise sharply. Pulse wave velocity has gained much attention lately because it may be a richer substrate for characterizing the physiology of blood flow and pressure. Under normal physiologic conditions, the ejected blood volume is transmitted peripherally as a propagated wave. After reaching the periphery, in particular, at the bifurcation sites, a reflected wave or a retrograde wave is generated, which travels toward the aortic valve. Arrival of this wave generally coincides with the beginning of diastole, thereby augmenting the diastolic pressure. However, with stiffening of the aorta as occurs with aging, both the propagated and the reflected waves travel much more rapidly, and early return of the reflected arterial wave during late systole augments the systolic component, effectively increasing afterload. The ensuing loss of diastolic augmentation results in a disproportionate increase in the systolic blood pressure with a lower diastolic blood pressure—a hallmark of isolated systolic hypertension and of pulse pressure hypertension.

Mechanistically, pulse pressure is also an index of the stiffness of conduit vessels and the rate of pressure wave propagation and reflection within the arterial tree. Approximately half of patients with ISH also have wide pulse pressure; however, both individuals who are normotensive (systolic, 140 mm Hg) with a low diastolic pressure or persons with combined systolic and diastolic hypertension (systolic >140 mm Hg and diastolic >90 mm Hg) can have wide pulse pressure (normal values being ≤40 mm Hg).

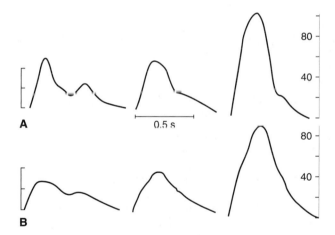

Figure 12.1 Change in amplitude and contour of the upper limb **(A)** and ascending aortic **(B)** pressure wave with age, as recorded in three female members of a family: at age 18 **(left)**, at age 48 **(center)**, and 97 years **(right)**. Upper limb pulse pressure was just more than twice as high in the old compared with the young subject (102 vs. 46 mm Hg), whereas aortic pulse pressure was more than three times higher (104 vs. 27 mm Hg). (From O'Rourke MF, Nichols WW. Aortic diameter, aortic stiffness, and wave reflection increase with age and isolated systolic hypertension. *Hypertension* 2005;45(4):652–628 with permission.)

Dart AM, Kingwell BA. Pulse pressure-a review of mechanism and clinical relevance. *J Am Coll Cardiol* 2001;37:975–984.

Franklin SS. Systolic blood pressure: it's time to take control. *Am J Hypertens* 2004;17: 49S–54S.

Laurent S, Boutouyrie P, Benetos A. Pathophysiology of hypertension in the elderly. *Am J Geriatr Cardiol* 2002;11:34–39.

O'Rourke MF, Nichols WW. Aortic diameter, aortic stiffness, and wave reflection increase with age and isolated systolic hypertension. *Hypertension* 2005;45(4):652–658.

Safer ME, Levy BI, Struijker-Boudier H. Current perspective on arterial stiffness and pulse pressure in hypertension and cardiovascular disease. *Circulation* 2003;107:2864–2869.

Schiffrin EL. Vascular stiffening and arterial compliance. Implications for systolic blood pressure. *Am J Hypertens* 2004;17:39S–48S.

A.7. What are the end-organ damages caused by long-standing hypertension?

The end-organ damages caused by long-standing hypertension are as follows:

Cardiac involvement:
Left ventricular hypertrophy
Angina or myocardial infarction
Arrhythmias
Congestive failure
Eye involvement:
Vascular changes in the fundus reflect hypertensive retinopathy and arteriosclerotic retinopathy
Renal involvement:
Nephropathy
Cerebral involvement:
Stroke or transient ischemic attack

Complications of hypertension to vascular disease probably involve three interrelated processes: pulsatile flow, endothelial cell dysfunction, and smooth muscle cell hypertrophy. These three interrelated processes are probably responsible for the arteriolar and arterial sclerosis that is the usual consequence of long-standing hypertension. Large vessels such as the aorta may be directly affected and be at risk for aneurysms and dissection. As discussed previously, the consequences of long-standing hypertension need be addressed according to the subtypes of hypertension; for, the associated risks for cerebral, cardiac, and renal vascular complications differ according to systolic, diastolic, and pulse pressure hypertension. For example, diastolic hypertension being a better predictor of coronary heart disease in younger patients, whereas systolic and pulse pressure being associated with greater risk of stroke, coronary heart disease and mortality in persons older than 60 years.

Aronson S, Fontes ML. Hypertension: a new look at an old problem. *Curr Opin Anesth* 2006;19:59–64.

Braunwald E. *Heart disease*, 6th ed. Philadelphia: WB Saunders, 2001:950–955.

Franklin SS. Systolic blood pressure: it's time to take control. *Am J Hypertens* 2004;17: 49S–54S.

A.8. Are hypertensive patients at an increased risk for perioperative cardiac morbidity?

Hypertensive patients are at increased risk for coronary artery disease, silent myocardial ischemia, congestive heart failure (CHF), and stroke. However, whether preoperative hypertension is predictive of perioperative major cardiac morbidity remains controversial. Some investigators have shown that patients with untreated, poorly controlled, or labile preoperative hypertension are at increased risk for perioperative blood pressure (BP) lability, dysrhythmias, myocardial ischemia, and transient neurologic complications. Some suggested that preoperative hypertension predicted perioperative myocardial infarction (MI). However, Goldman and Caldera demonstrated that mild-to-moderate hypertension did not increase the risk of major morbid events. Instead, preoperative hypertension may predict several intermediates of outcome, such as BP lability and myocardial ischemia. The controversy may be due to the wide variability in the hypertensive population. Hypertension may affect perioperative morbidity through the extent of end-organ damage and not the manifestation of the disease itself. Left ventricular hypertrophy, which signifies long-standing poorly controlled hypertension, can increase the risk of myocardial ischemia from imbalances of myocardial oxygen supply and demand regardless of the presence or absence of coronary artery disease.

Isolated systolic hypertension (ISH) (systolic BP >140 mm Hg and diastolic BP <90 mm Hg) has been identified as a risk factor for cardiovascular complications in the general population and treatment reduces the future risk of stroke. More recently, Aronson and Fontes found that amongst the various component of BP, preoperative pulse pressure was independently and significantly associated with postoperative stroke, renal failure, and mortality in patients undergoing coronary artery bypass. Neither ISH nor isolated diastolic hypertension were predictive of vascular complications. This finding is consistent with results of longitudinal studies finding that increase in pulse pressure is a better predictor of major vascular complications than either systolic or diastolic BP. Interestingly, rises in pulse pressure as few as 10 mm Hg in both normotensive and hypertensive individuals is associated with 20% or more increase risk of renal, coronary, and cerebral events.

Aronson S, Fontes ML. Hypertension: a new look at an old problem. *Curr Opin Anesth* 2006;19:59–64.

Casadei B, Abuzeid H. Is there a strong rationale for deferring elective surgery in patients with poorly controlled hypertension? *J Hypertens* 2005;23(1):19–22.

Fleisher LA. Preoperative evaluation of the patient with hypertension. *JAMA* 2002;287: 2043–2046.

Foëx P, Prys-Roberts C. Anaesthesia and the hypertensive patient. *Br J Anaesth* 1974;46:575.

Goldman L. Cardiac risk in noncardiac surgery: an update. *Anesth Analg* 1995;80:810–820.

Goldman L, Caldera DL. Risks of general anesthesia and elective operation in the hypertensive patient. *Anesthesiology* 1979;50:285–292.

Hollenberg M, Mangano DT, Browner WS, et al. Predictors of postoperative myocardial ischemia in patient undergoing noncardiac surgery. *JAMA* 1992;268:205–209.

Mangano DT. Perioperative cardiac morbidity. *Anesthesiology* 1990;72:153–184.

A.9. Perioperative cerebral and renal complications are mostly associated with which subtype of hypertension?

Both systolic hypertension and high pulse pressure are strongly associated with risk for perioperative cerebrovascular accidents and acute renal failure. The brain and the kidneys as well as the heart differ from most organs in that they receive large amount of blood flow and have very low resistance. As such, the pulsatile load (pulse pressure) tends to be very high. Over a period of many years of poorly or untreated hypertension, endothelial injury and vascular remodeling changes can promote both arteriosclerosis and atherosclerosis, which are known risk factors for cerebral and renal vascular complications. The pulsatile stress can also cause dislodgment of plaques from the aorta and its major branches resulting in embolic stroke.

In hypertensive patients, autoregulation of cerebral blood flow is reset to a higher range than normal, and although it protects the brain against sudden increases in pressure, it makes it more vulnerable to hypotension. Therefore, when blood pressure (BP) is lowered acutely, hypertensive patients will show signs of cerebral ischemia at a higher level of BP than normotensive patients.

Hypertension may accelerate cognitive decline with age. Hypertension, particularly systolic, is a major risk factor for initial and recurrent stroke and for transient ischemia attacks caused by extracranial atherosclerosis.

Chronic renal insufficiency is a common sequela of hypertension. Patients with hypertension should have a measurement of baseline serum creatinine. In the original Cardiac Risk Index, an elevated serum creatinine level (>3.0 mg/dL [>265.2 μmol/L]) was one of the independent risk factors for perioperative cardiovascular morbidity and mortality. This has been confirmed in the revised Cardiac Risk Index, in which a preoperative serum creatinine level greater than 2.0 mg per dL (176.8 μmol/L) was one of six independent factors that predicted increased cardiovascular risk.

Davis BR, Vogt T, Frost PH, et al. Risk factors for stroke and type of stroke in persons with isolated systolic hypertension. *Stroke* 1998;29:1333.

Finnerty FA, Witkin L, Fazekas JF. Cerebral hemodynamics during cerebral ischemia induced by acute hypotension. *J Clin Invest* 1955;34:1227.

Fontes ML. New insights in hypertension. *ASA Refresher Courses Anesthesiol* 2006;34: 43–53.

Fontes ML, Garwood S, Aronson S. Renal pathophysiology. In: Hemmings H, Hopkins P, eds. *Foundation of anesthesia: basic and clinical sciences*, 2nd ed, Elsevier Science, London 2006, 699–708.

Goldman L, Caldera DL. Risks of general anesthesia and elective operation in the hypertensive patient. *Anesthesiology* 1979;50:285.

Goldman L, Caldera DL, Nussbaum SR, et al. Multifactorial index of cardiac risk in noncardiac surgical procedures. *N Engl J Med* 1977;297:845–850.

Lee TH, Marcantonio ER, Mangione CM, et al. Derivation and prospective validation of a simple index for prediction of cardiac risk of major noncardiac surgery. *Circulation* 1999;100:1043–1049.

Strangaard S, Olsen J, Skinhof E, et al. Autoregulation of brain circulation in severe arterial hypertension. *Br Med J* 1973;3:507.

A.10. Would you employ a controlled hypotensive technique for hypertensive patients? How much would you safely lower the blood pressure (BP)?

Uncontrolled or untreated severe hypertension is a contraindication to controlled hypotension. However, controlled hypotension may be used with caution in treated hypertensive patients. Because cerebral autoregulation is shifted to the right with chronic hypertension, the lower limit of controlled hypotension should be higher for hypertensive patients. However, with long-term treatment, the autoregulation curve shifts leftward to approach that in normals. Strangaard found that the lower limit of autoregulation was 113 mm Hg in severe untreated or uncontrolled hypertensives; 96 mm Hg in formerly severe, now-treated hypertensives; and

73 mm Hg in normotensive patients. The lowest level of mean BP tolerated without symptoms of hypoperfusion was 65 mm Hg in severe hypertensives, 53 mm Hg in treated hypertensives, and 43 mm Hg in normal patients. However, although the autoregulation may shift toward normal with treatment, in many patients the autoregulation did not shift toward normal even after 12 months of treatment. Because one cannot measure patients' autoregulation, a useful clinical guide is that a 25% decrease in mean arterial pressure (MAP) reaches the lower limit of autoregulation and a 55% decrease in MAP reaches symptomatic cerebral hypoperfusion. Another suggested rule is that the systolic pressure of controlled hypotension should not be lower than the diastolic pressure of the patient's usual pressure.

Recently, noninvasive cerebral oximeter using near-infrared spectroscopy may be used to monitor the oxygen saturations of cerebral cortex. The values of cerebral oxygen saturations correspond with those of a mixture of 85% jugular venous O_2 saturation and 15% of arterial O_2 saturation. It reflects the balance between cerebral O_2 delivery and O_2 demand. In a steady state of anesthesia, the cerebral O_2 demand does not change significantly. Therefore, cerebral O_2 saturations will not decrease until the BP falls below its autoregulation range. Therefore, the cerebral oximeter may be employed to determine the lower limit of autoregulation and to ensure adequate cerebral oxygenation.

It should be mentioned that neither the threshold for upper nor lower limits of systolic and diastolic BP have been established. Frequently these limits have been chosen arbitrarily and the relation of perioperative hypertension to outcomes has been inconsistent amongst the studies that have addressed this question. In part, the limitation comes from grouping all types of hypertension together. Moreover, available vasoactive agents are not selective in lowering or raising systolic BP and diastolic BP without a concomitant increase or fall in the other component. Undermining the broad-based reliance on systolic BP and diastolic BP are a number of studies in humans over the past several decades that clearly show that both morbidity and mortality do not always linearly correlate with rises or fall in BP. In individuals with demonstrable coronary disease, namely, those with previous infarcts, coronary mortality was significantly related to diastolic pressure in a U shape configuration—occurring more frequently in those with very high or very low diastolic BP. Unfortunately, the emphasis on BP management perioperatively has been to control the systolic component with no attention paid to the diastolic component. This is particularly concerning in patients with isolated systolic hypertension and with very wide pulse pressure where the diastolic BP is already critically low. By reducing the systolic component, further lowering of the diastolic BP can result in ischemic complications in most sensitive vascular beds such as the brain, the heart, and the kidneys. Lastly, it is critical to recognize that peripheral arterial pressures do not necessarily reflect central pressures with exception of the MAP. In a subset of hypertensive individuals, both the systolic and the pulse pressures are grossly higher peripherally as compared to central aortic pressures, such that lowering of the peripheral BP may result in critical reduction in perfusion pressure.

Fontes ML, Garwood S, Aronson S. Renal pathophysiology. In: Hemmings H, Hopkins P, eds. *Foundation of anesthesia: basic and clinical sciences*, 2nd ed. London: Elsevier Science, 2006:699–708.

Lindop MJ. Complications and morbidity of controlled hypotension. *Br J Anaesth* 1975; 47:799.

Mitchell GF. Pulse pressure arterial compliance and cardiovascular morbidity and mortality: review article. *Curr Opin Nephrol Hypertens* 1999;8:335–342.

Murray MJ. Perioperative hypertension. *ASA Annual Refresher Course Lectures*. Park Ridge: American Society of Anesthesiologists, 2002:512.

Strangaard S. Autoregulation of cerebral blood flow in hypertension patients. *Circulation* 1976;53:720–727.

Yao FS, Tseng CA, Ho CA, et al. Cerebral oxygen desaturation is associated with early postoperative neuropsychological dysfunction in patients undergoing cardiac surgery. *J Cardiothorac Vasc Anesth* 2004;18:552–558.

A.11. What is the mechanism of action of antihypertensive drugs?

Antihypertensive drugs are categorized by their mechanism of action as follows.

Diuretics

They include thiazides (e.g., hydrochlorothiazide), loop diuretics (e.g., furosemide, ethacrynic acid), and potassium-sparing agents (e.g., spironolactone, triamterene). All diuretics initially lower the blood pressure (BP) by increasing urinary sodium excretion and by reducing plasma volume, extracellular fluid volume, and cardiac output. Within 6 to 8 weeks, the cardiac output returned to normal. The lowered BP is related to a fall in peripheral resistance. Diuretics may cause hypokalemia, hypomagnesemia, hyperuricemia, hyperlipidemia, hypercalcemia, and hyperglycemia. For patients with ST-segment changes and evidence of pulmonary edema and hypertension or with increased intracranial cerebral pressure and hypertension, intravenous furosemide may be appropriate.

Antiadrenergic agents

- *Centrally acting drugs*. Clonidine, dexmedetomidine and mivazerol. These drugs and their metabolites are primarily α_2 receptor agonists. Stimulation of α_2 receptors in the vasomotor centers of the brain reduces sympathetic outflow.
- *Peripherally acting drugs*
  - α-Receptor blockers
  - α_1 and α_2 Receptors—phenoxybenzamine (Dibenzyline), phentolamine (Regitine)
  - α_1 Receptor—prazosin (Minipress), doxazosin (Cardura)
    By blocking α-mediated vasoconstriction, these drugs induce a fall in peripheral resistance with both arteriolar and venous dilation.
  - β-Receptor blockers—atenolol (Tenormin), metoprolol (Lopressor), nadol (Corgard), pindolol (Visken), propranolol (Inderal), esmolol (Brevibloc). These drugs lower the BP by decreasing heart rate, contractility, cardiac output, and renin levels. BP is decreased without reflex tachycardia or widening of the pulse pressure. They also have antiarrhythmic activity and suppress both ventricular and supraventricular ectopic rhythms.
  - α- and β-Receptor blockers—labetalol (Trandate)
- Endothelin Receptor Antagonist—act on endothelin A and B receptors to block the effect of endothelin-1, which is the most potent vasoconstrictor that is secreted primarily from vascular smooth muscle and endothelial cells. Bosentan (receptor A and B antagonist) and sitaxsentan (receptor A antagonist) are examples of a few of this class of agents used in the management of pulmonary hypertension and less so for hypertension-related heart failure

Direct vasodilators

They include hydralazine, nitroprusside, nitroglycerin, and calcium channel blockers. These drugs directly relax the smooth muscle of resistance and capacitance vessels to different degrees.

Dopaminergic agonists

Dopaminergic agonists (DAs) are classified into DA_1 and DA_2 subtypes.

Stimulation of DA_1 receptors causes vasodilation, and inhibition of active sodium transport in the proximal tubule, leading to natriuresis.

Stimulation of DA_2 receptors inhibits norepinephrine release and promotes peripheral vasodilation.

Table 12.3 Cardiovascular Effects of Calcium Channel Blockers.

	VERAPAMIL	DILTIAZEM	NIFEDIPINE	NICARDIPINE
Heart rate	↓	↓	↑−	↑−
Nodal conduction	↓↓	↓	↓ or −	− or −
Myocardial depression	↑↑	↑	− or	−
Vasodilation	↑	↑	↑↑	↑↑

↑↑, more increase; ↓↓, more decrease; ↑, increase; ↓, decrease;−, no change.

Fenoldopam, dopamine receptor (DA_1 selective) agonist, a systemic and renal vasodilator, offers significant advantages as a parenterally administered agent for the management of BP in hypertensive emergencies and in the perioperative setting. Parenteral fenoldopam has a rapid onset and offset of effect, with an elimination half-time of approximately 10 minutes. Prepared in concentration of 10 mg in 250 mL (40 μg/mL), the recommended starting dose is 0.05 μg/kg/minute. This should be titrated to effect by 0.025 μg/kg/minute every 10 to 15 minutes, to a maximum dose of 0.5 to 0.8 μg/kg/minute. The drug should not be administered in boluses; the incidence of reflex tachycardia is related to rapidity of upward titration. Unlike dopamine, it has no β- or α-adrenergic activity and increasing doses result in increasing vasodilation without tachycardia or tachyarrhythmias.

Calcium channel blockers

The cardiovascular effects of calcium antagonists are listed in Table 12.3. These drugs decrease BP mainly by peripheral vasodilation. Renin and aldosterone secretion may be reduced as well.

Angiotensin-converting enzyme inhibitors

They include captopril, enalapril, lisinopril, quinapril, and ramipril. The renin–angiotensin system may be inhibited in four ways as shown in Fig. 12.2. These drugs inhibit the conversion of the inactive decapeptide angiotensin I to the active octapeptide angiotensin II. Lower levels of angiotensin II may decrease BP by reducing angiotensin II–induced vasoconstriction and by decreasing aldosterone synthesis. Angiotensin-converting enzyme (ACE) inhibitors also retard the degradation of a potent vasodilator (bradykinin), alter prostaglandin production (most notably with captopril), and can modify the activity of the adrenergic nervous system.

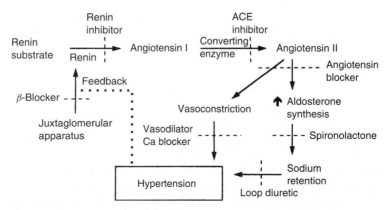

Figure 12.2 The renin–angiotensin system and the mechanism of action of antihypertensive drugs. ACE, angiotensin-converting enzyme.

ACE inhibitors provide predominantly arterial vasodilation and have become primary therapy for the treatment of CHF by afterload reduction. Cardiac output is increased without excessive decrease in preload, with a favorable effect on survival.

Angiotensin II receptor blockers

Angiotensin II receptor antagonists or blockers (ARBs), represent the third class that antagonizes the renin–angiotensin–aldosterone system. Blockade of the action of angiotensin II leads to elevations in plasma levels of renin, angiotensin I, and angiotensin II. However, this build-up of precursors does not overwhelm the receptor blockade, as evidenced by a persistent fall in both BP and plasma aldosterone levels. There are several possible differences between ACE inhibitors and angiotensin II receptor antagonists. These include the following:

- Angiotensin-converting enzyme is a kininase. Therefore, inhibiting this enzyme, which normally degrades bradykinin, with an ACE inhibitor leads to increased kinin levels, an effect not seen with an angiotensin II receptor antagonist. High bradykinin levels may also provide additional vasodilation and other benefits not observed with angiotensin II receptor antagonists.
- ACE inhibitors, by decreasing angiotensin II production, reduce the effect of both AT_1 and AT_2 receptors; only the former are inhibited by the angiotensin II receptor blockers. Chronic stimulation of the AT_2 receptor may be beneficial.
- In the heart, kidney, and perhaps the blood vessels, the production of angiotensin II may be catalyzed by enzymes other than angiotensin-converting enzyme, such as chymase. The effect of the angiotensin II produced by this reaction can be inhibited by the angiotensin II receptor antagonists but not by ACE inhibitors.

There is evidence that ARBs are more effective in treating isolated systolic hypertension (ISH) and pulse pressure hypertension (PPH) particularly in combination with ACE inhibitors and with endothelin receptor blockers.

Other vasodilators

They include brain natriuretic peptides such as nesiritide that is primarily used in acute exacerbation of heart failure to improve forward flow and reduce symptoms and signs of heart failure. There has been recent controversy about the clinical efficacy of these agents. Importantly, there have been several reports suggesting that the renal outcome is worsened in patients receiving nisiritide.

Benigni A, Remuzzi G. Endothelin antagonists. *Lancet* 1999;353:133.

Bornstein N, Silvestrelli G, Caso V. Arterial hypertension and stroke prevention: an update. *Clin Exp Hypertens* 2006;28(3–4):317–326.

Burnier M, Brunner HR. Angiotensin II receptor antagonists. *Lancet* 2000;355:637.

Huang XR, Chen WY, Truong LD. Chymase is upregulated in diabetic nephropathy: implications for an alternative pathway of angiotensin II-mediated diabetic renal and vascular disease. *J Am Soc Nephrol* 2003;14:1952.

Kasper DL, Braunwald E, Fauci AS, et al. eds. *Harrison's principles of internal medicine*, 16th ed. New York: McGraw-Hill, 2005:1470–1480.

Murray MJ. Perioperative hypertension. *ASA Annual Refresher Course Lectures*. Park Ridge: American Society of Anesthesiologists, 2002:512.

Oparil S, Aronson S, Deeb GM, et al. Fenoldopam: a new parenteral antihypertensive: consensus roundtable on the management of perioperative hypertension and hypertensive crisis. *Am J Hypertens* 1999;12:653–664.

Rousso P, Buclin T, Nussberger J, et al. Effects of a dual inhibitor of angiotensin-converting enzyme and neutral endopeptides, MDL 100240 on endocrine and renal functions in healthy volunteers. *J Hypertens* 1999;17:427.

Tsouli SG, Liberopoulos EN, Kiortsis DN. Combined treatment with angiotensin-converting enzyme inhibitors and angiotensin II receptor blockers: a review of the current evidence. *J Cardiovasc Pharmacol Ther* 2006;11:1–15.

Zipes DP, Libby P, Bonow RO, et al. eds. *Heart disease*, 7th ed. Philadelphia: WB Saunders, 2005:994–1005.

A.12. Does the choice of antihypertensive therapy influence hemodynamic responses to induction, laryngoscopy, and intubation?

The pressor responses to induction, laryngoscopy, and intubation differ little whether patients with mild-to-moderate hypertension receive a β-blocker, a calcium channel blocker, an ACE inhibitor, or a diuretic. Even changes of a similar magnitude are also observed in untreated hypertensive patients. On the other hand, hypotensive responses may be magnified in those patients with poorly controlled hypertension following induction—generally due to a reduced intravascular volume in the face of increased vascular sympathetic tone. As mentioned previously, attention should be directed not only to the systolic but also to pulse and diastolic pressures.

Sear JW, Jewkes C, Teller JC, et al. Does the choice of antihypertensive therapy influence haemodynamic responses to induction, laryngoscopy and intubation? *Br J Anaesth* 1994;73:303–308.

A.13. Does chronic angiotensin-converting enzyme (ACE) inhibition influence anesthetic induction?

Coriat et al. reported that, in hypertensive patients chronically treated with ACE inhibitors, therapy until the day of surgery is a major factor influencing blood pressure (BP) responsiveness to anesthetic induction for vascular surgery. If enalapril (a long-acting ACE inhibitor) treatment is continued, a very low plasma-converting enzyme activity will be observed and an exaggerated hypotensive response may occur at induction. If captopril (a short-acting ACE inhibitor) treatment is continued, the magnitude of the decrease in BP in response to induction, although lower than with enalapril, is enhanced compared with that noted in patients in whom captopril had been stopped. All of the hypotensive episodes in patients who received ACE inhibitors until the day of surgery were easily corrected by administration of an α agonist. The temporary withdrawal of these two ACE inhibitors attenuated the hypotensive response to induction but did not lead to an abnormal BP response to induction and intubation. However, recently Ryckwaert and Colson reported that ACE inhibitor treatment in patients with infarction-induced myocardial dysfunction does not increase the incidence of severe hypotension after induction of anesthesia. In all, the overwhelming opinion is to continue all antihypertensive medication including the day of surgery and resumption of such therapy postoperatively. A number of studies have shown an improvement in outcome when therapy is continued versus a worsening in outcome when either ACE inhibitors or β blockers have been withdrawn.

Coriat P, Richter C, Douraki T, et al. Influence of chronic angiotensin-converting enzyme inhibition on anesthetic induction. *Anesthesiology* 1994;81:299–307.

Kwapisz MM, Muller M, Schindler E, et al. The effect of intravenous quinaprilat on plasma cytokines and hemodynamic variables during cardiac surgery. *J Cardiothorac Vasc Anesth* 2004;18:53–58.

Licker M, Schweizer A, Hohn L, et al. Chronic angiotensin converting inhibition does not influence renal hemodynamic and function during cardiac surgery. *Can J Anaesth* 1999;46:626–634.

Ryckwaert F, Colson P. Hemodynamic effects of anesthesia in patients with ischemic heart failure chronically treated with angiotensin-converting enzyme inhibitors. *Anesth Analg* 1997;84:945–949.

Wallace A, Fontes ML, Mathew J, et al. Association of different patterns of use of anti-ischemic agents on mortality and morbidity after coronary artery bypass surgery. *Anesthesiology* 2003:A255.

B. Preoperative Evaluation and Preparation

B.1. How would you evaluate this patient preoperatively?

In addition to the routine systemic preoperative physical and history, special attention should be paid to the following: etiology and severity of hypertension, the subtype of hypertension, current therapy, and the end-organ damage by chronic hypertension.

The underlying cause of hypertension should be clear. Surgical mortality is relatively high in patients with renovascular hypertension. Moreover, failure to diagnose a pheochromocytoma preoperatively, albeit a rare finding, may prove fatal, because anesthetic agents are well known to precipitate a crisis in such patients. Meanwhile, the severity of hypertension alters anesthetic risk.

Antihypertensive drugs have different anesthetic implications. Diuretics frequently cause chronic hypokalemia and hypomagnesemia, which may increase the risk of arrhythmia. Therefore, serum electrolytes should be checked preoperatively.

The presence of target-organ damage in the brain, heart, and kidney signifies long-standing, poorly controlled hypertension. Unfortunately, markers of organ damage become demonstrable only after significant end-organ damage has occurred.

For cardiac evaluation, electrocardiogram (ECG) and chest x-ray film serve as minimal tests. The echocardiogram will be helpful. Left ventricular hypertrophy (LVH) can increase the risk of perioperative myocardial ischemia from imbalances of myocardial oxygen supply and demand regardless of the presence or absence of coronary artery disease. There is a very high correlation between LVH and isolated systolic hypertension (ISH) and pulse pressure hypertension (PPH)—uncertain which comes first. Some authorities believe that hypertensive patients without evidence of LVH or other risk factors are at a lower perioperative cardiac risk and do not require further evaluation for most operations. Patients with severe hypertension are also at increased risk for congestive heart failure (CHF) and pulmonary edema.

For renal evaluation, urinalysis, serum creatinine, and blood urea nitrogen should be measured to define the presence and extent of renal parenchymal disease. If chronic renal failure exists, hyperkalemia and elevated plasma volume may be of concern.

For cerebrovascular evaluation, a history of cerebrovascular accidents (CVAs) and transient ischemic attacks (TIAs) and the presence of hypertensive retinopathy should be looked for.

Barash PG, Cullen BF, Stoelting RK, eds. *Clinical anesthesia*, 5th ed. Philadelphia: Lippincott Williams & Wilkins, 2006:481–489.

Fleisher LA. Preoperative evaluation of the patient with hypertension. *JAMA* 2002;287: 2043–2046.

Fleisher LA, Barash PH. Preoperative cardiac evaluation for noncardiac surgery. *Anesth Analg* 1992;74:586–598.

B.2. Would you postpone the surgery? Why? What blood pressure (BP) would you like the patient to achieve before surgery?

Yes. I would postpone the elective surgery because the BP was 230/120 mm Hg. In general, elective surgery should be delayed for patients with severe hypertension (diastolic BP >115 mm Hg) or with severe isolated systolic hypertension (ISH) (systolic BP >200 mm Hg) until the BP is below 180/110 mm Hg. If time permits, the BP should be lowered over 6 to 8 weeks to less than 140/90 mm Hg. Acute control within several hours is inadvisable before elective surgery, because this practice may put the cerebral or other circulations at risk for ischemia.

In moderate hypertensive patients with severe end-organ involvement, preoperative BP should be normalized as much as possible, although in asymptomatic patients with mild-to-moderate hypertension (diastolic BP <110 mm Hg), elective surgery may proceed without increased cardiovascular risks. Goldman et al. found that patients with mild and moderate hypertension were not at increased risk of vascular complications unless they had other risks of coronary heart disease. In all, the thresholds being recommended apply only in part to today's surgical population. Most hypertensive patients presenting for surgery are elderly patients who suffer almost exclusively from ISH and pulse pressure hypertension (PPH). It is uncertain what acute changes in BP preoperatively will have on outcome giving that the pathologic changes are chronic and unlikely to normalize with treatment.

Fleisher LA. Preoperative evaluation of the patient with hypertension. *JAMA* 2002;287: 2043–2046.

Fleisher LA, Barash PH. Preoperative cardiac evaluation for noncardiac surgery. *Anesth Analg* 1992;74:586–598.

Fontes ML. New insights in hypertension. *ASA Refresher Courses Anesthesiol* 2006;34:43–53.

Murray MJ. Perioperative hypertension. *ASA Annual Refresher Course Lectures*. Park Ridge: American Society of Anesthesiologists, 2002:512.

B.3. Should all or any of the chronic medications be discontinued before the operation?

Current opinion generally favors continuation of antihypertensive medications, especially β-blockers, up to the time of surgery. There is concern that acute withdrawal of these medications may precipitate ischemic myocardial events. Because β-blockade does not impair the hemodynamic response to hemorrhage and does not adversely affect responses to hypoxia, the medications should be continued. The withdrawal syndrome is characterized by an enhanced sensitivity to sympathetic stimulation and has been attributed to various factors, including sympathetic overactivity and increased triiodothyronine levels, but most probably it is a result of increased β-receptor density.

The safety of β-blockers and their benefits (prevention of hypertensive responses, dysrhythmias, and myocardial ischemia) have been long established. Similarly, treatment with calcium channel blockers, angiotensin-converting enzyme (ACE) inhibitors, and diuretics can be maintained. Indeed, the responses to induction of anesthesia, laryngoscopy, and intubation differ little whether patients receive a β-blocker, a calcium channel blocker, an ACE inhibitor, or a diuretic. However, Coriat et al. reported that maintenance of ACE inhibitor therapy until the day of surgery might increase the probability of hypotension at induction and that the hypotensive episodes were easily corrected by ephedrine infusion.

Withdrawal of clonidine has been associated with rebound hypertension.

Barash PG, Cullen BF, Stoelting RK, eds. *Clinical anesthesia*, 5th ed. Philadelphia: Lippincott–Raven Publishers, 2006:497.

Coriat P, Richters C, Douraki T, et al. Influence of chronic angiotensin-converting enzyme inhibition on anesthetic induction. *Anesthesiology* 1994;81:299–307.

Fleisher LA. Preoperative evaluation of the patient with hypertension. *JAMA* 2002;287: 2043–2046.

Prichard BN, Walder RJ. The syndrome associated with the withdrawal of beta-adrenergic receptor blocking drugs. *Br J Clin Pharmacol* 1982;13 (Suppl 2):337S–343S.

Sear JW, Jewkes C, Tellez JC, et al. Does the choice of antihypertensive therapy influence haemodynamic responses to induction, laryngoscopy and intubation? *Br J Anaesth* 1994;73:303–308.

Sladen RN. Perioperative hypertension. *IARS review course lectures*, Cleveland: International Anesthesia Research Society, 2002:100–114.

Stoelting RK, Diedorf SF. *Anesthesia and co-existing disease*, 4th ed. New York: Churchill Livingstone, 2002:99–103.

B.4.   Should hypokalemia be treated before anesthesia? Why?

Hypokalemia is a frequent finding in hypertensive patients treated with the diuretic thiazides. It is important to maintain normal electrolyte balance in patients with heart or coronary artery disease. A low value of potassium (3.0 to 3.5 mEq/L) in these patients may cause arrhythmias, increase sensitivity to digitalis, and depress neuromuscular function. In patients without risk of cardiac complications of surgery and anesthesia, this modest reduction (3.0 to 3.5 mEq/L) should not prompt postponement of surgery or immediate potassium replacement. Patients with more severe potassium depletion ($\leq$2.9 mEq/L) should be treated. For those patients, at least 1 week before surgery supplemental potassium should be given if renal function is not impaired. In surgical emergencies, potassium may be given at a rate not to exceed 0.5 mEq per kg of body weight per hour. Administration should be stopped during surgery and restarted postoperatively, depending on serial potassium determinations. Vitez et al. concluded that chronic hypokalemia *per se* is not associated with a higher incidence of intraoperative arrhythmia.

Barash PG, Cullen BF, Stoelting RK, eds. *Clinical anesthesia*, 5th ed. Philadelphia: Lippincott Williams & Wilkins, 2006:195–196.

McGovern B. Hypokalemia and cardiac arrhythmias [Editorial]. *Anesthesiology* 1985;63:127.

Stoelting RK, Diedorf SF. *Anesthesia and co-existing disease*, 4th ed. New York: Churchill Livingstone, 2002:99–103.

Vitez TS, Soper LE, Wong KC, et al. Chronic hypokalemia and intraoperative dysrhythmias. *Anesthesiology* 1985;63:130–133.

B.5.   Should hypomagnesemia be treated before anesthesia? Why?

The normal level of magnesium is between 1.5 and 2.5 mEq per L. Magnesium ion is essential for the proper function of most enzyme systems. Depletion is characterized by neuromuscular and central nervous system hyperexcitability. These signs are similar to those of calcium deficiency. Cardiovascular abnormalities include coronary artery spasm, cardiac failure, and dysrhythmias. When severe, hypomagnesemia may induce seizures, confusion, and coma. Replacement should be done only in cases of severe depletion. Magnesium should not be given to the oliguric patient and should be given very carefully to patients with renal insufficiency. Small intravenous doses should be used, with careful observation for toxicity (lethargy, weakness, and loss of deep tendon reflexes).

Barash PG, Cullen BF, Stoelting RK, eds. *Clinical anesthesia*, 5th ed. Philadelphia: Lippincott Williams & Wilkins, 2006:203–204.

B.6. Does an asymptomatic carotid bruit increase the risk in these patients?

Yes. The incidence of stroke is increased in such patients, although the stroke may not be thrombotic or related to the carotid artery in which the bruit was heard. Bruits are general predictors of vascular disease and may be predictors of perioperative strokes.

De Feo M, Renzulli A, Onorati F, et al. The risk of stroke following CABG: one possible strategy to reduce it. *Int J Cardiol* 2005;98(2):261–266.

Wolf P, Kannel WB, Sorlie P, et al. Asymptomatic carotid bruit and the risk of stroke: the Framingham study. *JAMA* 1981;245:1442.

Yatsu FM, Hart RG. Asymptomatic carotid bruit and stenosis: a reappraisal. *Curr Concepts Cerebrovascular Dis* 1982;17:21.

B.7. The surgery was postponed for 6 weeks. The patient has been on propranolol, captopril, hydrochlorothiazide, and KCl. His blood pressure (BP) was 160/95 mm Hg and potassium was 4.0 mEq per L. How would you premedicate this patient?

Because half or more of hypertensive patients still have elevated BP despite treatment, the anesthesiologist should determine the anxiety level of the patient. With this knowledge, the premedication with diazepam, lorazepam, or midazolam can be regulated to have the patient arrive in the operating room sedated. However, due to a high occurrence of delirium in the elderly receiving benzodiazepines, Premedication with such agents are being discouraged. This will help to prevent a starting BP well above the optimal level. All the antihypertensive medications are continued up to the day of surgery.

Cavaliere F, D'Ambrosio F, Volpe C, et al. Postoperative delirium. *Current Drug Targets* 2005;6(7):807–814.

Lepouse C, Lautner CA, Liu L, et al. Emergence delirium in adults in the post-anaesthesia care unit. *Br J Anaesth* 2006;96(6):747–753.

Wallace AW, Galindez D, Salahieh A, et al. Effect of clonidine on cardiovascular morbidity and mortality after noncardiac surgery. *Anesthesiology* 2004;101(2):284–293.

B.8. If the patient is an untreated hypertensive patient with blood pressure (BP) 170/100 mm Hg, would you pretreat the patient preoperatively with an antihypertensive agent?

Yes. The preoperative administration of clonidine, β-blockers, or angiotensin-converting enzyme (ACE) inhibitors has been advocated to reduce the intraoperative hemodynamic lability and myocardial ischemia in hypertensive patients. Clonidine, a central α_2 agonist, decreases sympathetic outflow and reduces plasma catecholamines, aldosterone levels, and renin activity. A single dose of clonidine, 5 μg per kg orally, 2 hours before surgery significantly decreases anesthetic requirements and hemodynamic lability in patients with mild-to-moderate hypertension. However, preoperative clonidine did not decrease BP lability during aortic operation. Perioperative use of clonidine has also been shown to have short and long-term benefits related to cardiac morbidity and survival.

The best treatment may be cardioselective β-blocker therapy. A single small oral dose of a β-adrenergic blocking agent such as labetalol, atenolol, or oxprenolol given preoperatively to untreated, asymptomatic, mildly hypertensive patients effectively attenuated tachycardia with tracheal intubation and emergence. The incidence of myocardial ischemia was reduced from 28% in the control group to 2% in the β-blocker groups. An oral-dose ACE inhibitor such as enalapril given preoperatively also attenuates the hemodynamic responses to intubation and surgical stimulation.

Engelman E, Lipszyc M, Gilbart E. Effects of clonidine on anesthetic drug requirements and hemodynamic response during aortic surgery. *Anesthesiology* 1989;71:178–187.

Fleisher LA. Preoperative evaluation of the patient with hypertension. *JAMA* 2002;287: 2043–2046.

Ghignone M, Calvillo O, Quintin L. Anesthesia and hypertension: the effect of clonidine on perioperative hemodynamics and isoflurane requirements. *Anesthesiology* 1987; 67:3–10.

Stone JG, Foex P, Sear JW, et al. Myocardial ischemia in untreated hypertensive patients: effect of a single small oral dose of a beta-adrenergic blocking agent. *Anesthesiology* 1988;68:495–500.

Wallace AW, Galindez D, Salahieh A, et al. Effect of clonidine on cardiovascular morbidity and mortality after noncardiac surgery. *Anesthesiology* 2004;101(2):284–293.

Yeates AP. Anaesthesia and angiotensin-converting enzyme inhibitors. *Anaesthesia* 1988; 43:935–939.

C. Intraoperative Management

C.1. How would you monitor this patient?

- *Electrocardiogram (ECG).* Simultaneous leads V_5 and II, multiple lead ST analysis, if possible, are essential because hypertensive patients are at increased risk for myocardial ischemia regardless of the presence or absence of coronary disease.
- *Blood pressure (BP).* A continuous monitoring of BP is essential because of lability of BP in these patients. Direct intraarterial measurement of BP permits beat-to-beat observation. However, noninvasive automatic sphygmomanometric techniques are usually sufficient.
- *Pulmonary artery catheter (PAC).* for those hypertensive patients with a history of congestive heart failure (CHF) or a recent myocardial infarction (MI), a PAC may be extremely helpful in managing fluid replacement and monitoring ventricular function. Of note, there is a strong correlation between hypertension and left ventricular hypertrophy (LVH), which results in poor ventricular compliance reflected by elevated pulmonary artery occlusion pressure (PAOP) in the face of low or normal ventricular volumes and normal contractility. Presence of CHF in hypertensive patients is frequently a marker of diastolic dysfunction and NOT systolic dysfunction.
- *Pulse oximeter.* This should be used to monitor peripheral blood flow and oxygenation.
- *End-tidal CO_2 analyzer.* This monitor will help maintain normocarbia.
- Temperature

C.2. What are the anesthetic goals for hypertensive patients?

The anesthetic goal is to minimize wide lability of blood pressure (BP) in response to anesthetic and surgical stimuli to prevent the following:

- Myocardial ischemia from tachycardia or less common from either hypertension or hypotension
- Cerebral hypoperfusion from hypotension
- Cerebral hemorrhage and hypertensive encephalopathy resulting from hypertension or embolic stroke from rupture of plagues either locally or from the aorta and the neck vessels.
- Renal failure from renal hypoperfusion

Particular attention to diastolic BP is strongly recommended while attempting to reduce systolic BP. It is unfortunate that clinical practice perioperatively hinges on manipulation of the systolic BP without attention to the diastolic component. This is particularly troublesome in most elderly patients who suffer from isolated systolic hypertension (ISH) and/or wide pulse pressure. In both subtypes of hypertension, the already lower diastolic pressure can easily be reduced further—predisposing to myocardial hypoperfusion and ischemia.

Recently, Lee et al. showed that patients with wide pulse pressure have an increased risk for thrombogenesis marked by elevated levels of D-dimers, von Willebrand factor, and platelet activation. This along with extensive atherosclerotic disease of the aorta, carotid, and renal arteries, which is also common in patients with ISH, provide a pathophysiologic basis for the increase incidence of perioperative stroke, myocardial infarction (MI), and renal dysfunction observed in hypertensive patients.

Lastly, careful control of the hemodynamic responses to noxious stimuli such as endotracheal intubation, surgical incision and manipulation, and emergence from anesthesia is essential in the hypertensive patient.

Lee KW, Blann AD, Lip GY. High pulse pressure and nondipping circadian blood pressure in patients with coronary artery disease: relationship to thrombogenesis and endothelial damage/dysfunction. *Am J Health* 2005;18:104–115.

Lovett JK, Howard SC, Rothwell PM. Pulse pressure is independently associated with carotid plaque ulceration. *J Hypertens* 2003;21:1669–1676.

Stoelting RK, Diedorf SF. *Anesthesia and co-existing disease*, 4th ed. New York: Churchill Livingstone, 2002:99–103.

C.3. How would you induce anesthesia for the hypertensive patient?

While the patient is being preoxygenated, fentanyl, 7 to 8 μg per kg, is given slowly to achieve drowsiness. Then, either thiopental in 50-mg increments or propofol in 30 to 50 mg increments is titrated to produce unconsciousness, followed by succinylcholine, 1 mg per kg, or nondepolarizing muscle relaxants to facilitate tracheal intubation.

All anesthetic agents are acceptable with the possible exception of ketamine, which may produce significant hypertension and tachycardia. However, deeper anesthesia with potent inhalation agents to attenuate tachycardia and hypertension should be done with caution because of higher incidence of hypotension arising from both vasodilation and cardiac depression.

Martin DE, Rosenberg H, Aukburg SJ, et al. Low-dose fentanyl blunts circulatory responses to tracheal intubation. *Anesth Analg* 1982;61:680.

C.4. How does tracheal intubation produce hypertension?

Translaryngeal intubation of the trachea stimulates laryngeal and tracheal receptors, resulting in marked increase in the elaboration of sympathomimetic amines. This sympathetic stimulation results in tachycardia and a rise in blood pressure (BP). In normotensive patients, this rise is approximately 20 to 25 mm Hg; it is much greater in hypertensive patients. This increase in BP results from vasoconstriction, because of unopposed α stimulation in hypertensive patients taking β-blocking drugs.

Prys-Roberts C, Greene LT, Meloche R, et al. Studies of anaesthesia in relation to hypertension. II: haemodynamic consequences of induction and endotracheal intubation. *Br J Anaesth* 1971;43:531.

C.5. What happens to the left ventricular ejection fraction during and immediately following intubation?

During and immediately following intubation associated with tachycardia and hypertension, there is a decrease in the left ventricular ejection fraction. This is particularly marked in patients with coronary artery disease. Nevertheless, such hemodynamic perturbations can be anticipated and treated accordingly with β blockade, narcotic, and titration of hypnotic and/or inhalation agents.

Giles RW, Berger JH, Barash PG, et al. Continuous monitoring of left ventricular performance with the computerized nuclear probe during laryngoscopy and intubation before coronary artery bypass surgery. *Am J Cardiol* 1982;50:735.

C.6. What other measures can prevent hypertension and tachycardia at the time of intubation?

The rise in blood pressure (BP) and heart rate occurs approximately 14 seconds after the start of laryngoscopy and becomes maximal after 30 to 45 seconds of direct laryngoscopy. If possible, laryngoscopy time should be 15 seconds or less to minimize BP elevation. Simultaneous administration of fentanyl, 7 to 8 μg per kg with the induction dose of thiopental or propofol can blunt the cardiovascular response to tracheal intubation. Other measures are described as follows:

- Lidocaine, 1.5 mg per kg is given 2 minutes before intubation.
- Esmolol, up to 2 mg per kg, appears to be especially effective in providing consistent and reliable protection against hypertension and tachycardia with intubation. It is easy to titrate and does not exacerbate postintubation hypotension because of its short duration of action.
- Labetalol, 0.15 to 0.45 mg per kg is comparable to esmolol 1.5 to 4.5 mg per kg in attenuating hemodynamic effects. However, the half-lives of intravenous esmolol and labetalol are 9 minutes and 5 hours, respectively. Additionally, labetalol has minimal effects on heart rate and through its action on α receptors, it acts similar to a vasodilator, particularly with chronic use.
- Nicardipine, 1 mg intravenously 2 minutes before tracheal intubation maintained hemodynamic stability during the intraoperative period. Both doses of 0.015 and 0.03 mg per kg attenuated BP but not heart rate responses during emergence and extubation. Greater BP control occurred with the larger nicardipine dose of 0.03 mg per kg.

It is important to remember that all the previously mentioned doses are used with a single agent only. If a combination of different agents or anesthetics is used, doses should be decreased accordingly. Otherwise, severe hypotension may ensue.

Anthony LK, Cindy M, Carol JT, et al. Comparison of nicardipine versus placebo to control hemodynamic responses during emergence and extubation. *J Cardiothorac Vasc Anesth* 2001;15:704–709.

Barash PG, Cullen BF, Stoelting RK, eds. *Clinical anesthesia*, 5th ed. Philadelphia: Lippincott-Raven Publishers, 2006:330–331.

Cucchiara RF, Benefiel DJ, Matteo RS, et al. Evaluation of esmolol in controlling increases in heart rate and blood pressure during endotracheal intubation in patients undergoing carotid endarterectomy. *Anesthesiology* 1986;65:528–531.

Gold MI, Sacks DJ, Grosnoff DB, et al. Use of esmolol during anesthesia to treat tachycardia and hypertension. *Anesth Analg* 1989;68:101–104.

Helfman SM, Gold MI, Delisser EA, et al. Which drug prevents tachycardia and hypertension associated with tracheal intubation: lidocaine, fentanyl, or esmolol? *Anesth Analg* 1991;72:482–486.

Kapnoudhis P, Vaghadia H, Jenkins LC, et al. Esmolol versus fentanyl for preventing haemodynamic response to intubation in cardiovascular disease. *Can J Anaesth* 1990; 37:S145.

Martin DE, Rosenberg H, Aukburg SJ, et al. Low-dose fentanyl blunts circulatory responses to tracheal intubation. *Anesth Analg* 1982;61:680.

Sladen RN. Perioperative hypertension. *IARS review course lectures*. Cleveland: International Anesthesia Research Society, 2002:100–114.

Song D, Singh H, White PF, et al. Optimal dose of nicardipine for maintenance of hemo-dynamic stability after tracheal intubation and skin incision. *Anesth Analg* 1997;85: 1247–1511.

Stoelting RK. Blood pressure and heart rate changes during short-duration laryngoscopy for tracheal intubation: influence of viscous or intravenous lidocaine. *Anesth Analg* 1978;57:197.

Stoelting RK, Diedorf SF. *Anesthesia and co-existing disease*, 4th ed. New York: Churchill Livingstone, 2002:99–103.

C.7. After induction and intubation, the blood pressure (BP) went down to 70/40 mm Hg. What would you do?

Hypotension after induction of anesthesia is usually due to combination of vasodilation, hypovolemia, and cardiac depression. Vasodilation can be caused by inducing agents such as thiopental, propofol, diazepam, or midazolam; moderate to high doses of narcotics; and potent inhalation agents. Hypertensive patients are in relative hypovolemia because of chronic vasoconstriction and/or diuretic therapy. Preoperative bowel preparation and nothing by mouth further contribute to hypovolemia. Barbiturates, benzodiazepines, and inhalation agents can cause a mild-to-moderate degree of cardiac depression.

Hypotension after induction of anesthesia usually can be easily corrected by volume replacement and simultaneous titration of vasopressors such as ephedrine 5 to 10 mg or phenylephrine in 0.1-mg increments.

Coriat P, Richters C, Douraki T, et al. Influence of chronic angiotensin-converting enzyme inhibition on anesthetic induction. *Anesthesiology* 1994;81:299–307.

C.8. What is your choice of agents for maintenance of anesthesia? Why?

I would use low to moderate doses of fentanyl and isoflurane for maintenance of anesthesia. No particular anesthetic technique or specific drug combinations have been demonstrated to be superior to others in hypertensive patients. Potent inhalation anesthetics or narcotics should be titrated to the desired level of central nervous system depression while the blood pressure (BP) is monitored continuously.

Narcotics and nitrous oxide provide an anesthetic with less overall lability of BP, but commonly intraoperative hypertension is difficult to control by moderate doses of narcotics. High doses of narcotics are not suitable for early extubation. Likewise, use of nitrous oxide is debatable in open cholecystectomy given its propensity to increase bowel distension—the severity being related to higher concentration of nitrous oxide and to longer duration of use. This concern is less pertinent for laparoscopic cholecystectomy whereby insufflation of gas to pressurize the abdomen should counteract the distensible property of nitrous oxide (also see Chapter 39, question C.8).

Potent inhalation agents provide greater control of hypertension but seem to produce less stability. Isoflurane, desflurane, and sevoflurane possess the advantage of more peripheral vasodilation and less cardiac depression. Enflurane may be least useful in patients receiving β-blockers because of the potential for greater cardiac depression than is observed with halothane or isoflurane. The combination of nitrous oxide and low to moderate doses of narcotics and potent inhalation agents may provide the most stable intraoperative course.

Akca O, Lenhardt R, Fleischmann E, et al. Nitrous oxide increases the incidence of bowel distension in patients undergoing elective colon resection. *Acta Anaesthesiol Scand* 2004;48(7):894–898.

Stoelting RK, Diedorf SF. *Anesthesia and co-existing disease*, 4th ed. New York: Churchill Livingstone, 2002:99–103.

Taylor E, Feinstein R, White PF. Anesthesia for laparoscopic cholecystectomy. Is nitrous oxide contraindicated? *Anesthesiology* 1992;76(4):541–543.

C.9. How would you manage fluid therapy for hypertensive patients?

Patients with essential hypertension are usually hypovolemic because of vasoconstriction and diuretic therapy. Hydration of the hypertensive patient should be started before induction of anesthesia to minimize the "roller-coaster" often seen with hypertension. However, overhydration should be avoided because it may contribute to postoperative hypertension when the vasodilating effects of anesthetics are gone. Therefore, careful estimation of fluid intake and output is essential. Foley catheter and central venous pressure monitor are indicated for major surgery with extensive fluid exchange.

As discussed previously, presence of left ventricular hypertrophy (LVH) in hypertensive patients shifts the left ventricular compliance curve upwardly and leftwardly such that for the same ventricular volume, a higher left ventricular diastolic pressure is attained as compared to a non-hypertrophied ventricle. When managing these patients with a Pulmonary artery catheter (PAC), higher pulmonary artery occlusion pressure (PAOP) (sometimes >20 mm Hg) is necessary to achieve normovolemia. Cardiac output must also be checked frequently during volume challenges.

Fontes ML, Bellows W, Ngo L, et al. McSPI Research Group. Assessment of ventricular function in critically ill patients: limitations of pulmonary artery catheterization. *J Cardiothorac Vasc Anesth* 1999;13:1–8.

Fontes ML, Hines RH. Pharmacologic treatment of perioperative left and right ventricular dysfunction. In: Kaplan JA, Reich DSN, Konstadt SN, eds. *Cardiac anesthesia*, 4th ed. Philadelphia: Grune & Stratton, 1999:1155–1191.

Murray MJ. Perioperative hypertension. *ASA annual refresher course lectures*. EMPH-Park Ridge: American Society of Anesthesiologists, 2002:512.

Table 12.4 Intraoperative Control of Hypertension.

Anesthetics
 Narcotics, inhalation agents, butorphanol, lidocaine
Antihypertensives
 Adrenergic blockers
  α-Blocker: phentolamine
  β-Blocker: propranolol, metoprolol
  α- and β-blocker: labetalol
 Calcium channel blockers
  Diltiazem, nicardipine, verapamil
 ACE inhibitors
  Enalapril
 Direct vasodilators
  Hydralazine, nitroglycerin, nitroprusside
 Dopaminergic agonists
  Fenoldopam

ACE, angiotensin-converting enzyme.

C.10. During the surgery, blood pressure (BP) went up to 220/120 mm Hg. How would you treat the hypertension?

Intraoperative control of hypertension is outlined in Table 12.4. Severe hypertension that occurs during a surgical procedure is most frequently due to inadequate anesthesia. Inadequate blockade of sensory input from the surgical procedure stimulates the elaboration of sympathomimetic amines, resulting in hypertension and tachycardia. If a potent inhalation anesthetic is being used, the level of anesthesia should be deepened by increasing the inspired concentration of the anesthetic. A narcotic may not control the rise in BP, and it may be necessary to switch to a potent inhalation anesthetic.

Hydralazine, 5-mg increments, may be titrated to decrease BP safely with little chance of excessive reduction. The onset of action is in 10 to 15 minutes with 1 to 2 hours duration.

Labetalol, 5- to 10-mg increments, is very useful in controlling hypertension and tachycardia. It makes the most sense to use β-blockers after a significant rise in BP because these agents act directly to antagonize the effects of the catecholamines. Although other agents may lower the BP, it is highly possible that the excessive availability of both norepinephrine and epinephrine will continue to exert their effects at the receptor site—compromising tissue perfusion from microcirculatory vasoconstriction. This view may explain the broad antiischemic effects of perioperative β-blockers on the brain, the heart, and the kidneys.

Rarely, continuous infusion of nicardipine, nitroglycerin, or nitroprusside, direct arteriolar vasodilators, is needed to control hypertension during anesthesia.

Lindenauer PK, Pekow P, Wang K. Perioperative beta-blocker therapy and mortality after major noncardiac surgery. *N Eng J Med* 2005;353(4):349–361.

Maggio PM, Taheri PA. Perioperative issues: myocardial ischemia and protection-beta-blockade. *Surg Oncol Clin N Am* 2005;85(6):1091–1102.

Passamonti E, Pirelli S. Reducing risk of cardiovascular events in noncardiac surgery. *Expert Opin Pharmacother* 2005;6(9):1507–1515.

Sladen RN. Perioperative hypertension. *IARS review course lectures*. Cleveland: International Anesthesia Research Society, 2002:100–114.

Stoelting RK, Diedorf SF. *Anesthesia and co-existing disease*, 4th ed. New York: Churchill Livingstone, 2002:99–103.

C.11. What could you do to prevent hypertension during extubation and emergence?

Intraoperative hypertension can be controlled either by adequate anesthesia with moderate to high doses of narcotics or inhalation agents or by antihypertensive agents listed in question A.11. It is logical to use anesthetic agents to prevent hypertension during induction and intubation and to use antihypertensive agents during extubation and emergence, because the patient has to be awakened at the end of surgery. The alternative measures listed in question C.6 may be applied to prevent hypertension. Our preference is to give lower doses of preventive medications such as 1 mg per kg of lidocaine or esmolol or 0.1 mg per kg of labetalol, 2 minutes before extubation. If BP goes over desired levels after extubation, additional doses may be titrated to control BP.

Mikawa K, Nishina K, Maekawa N, et al. Attenuation of cardiovascular responses to tracheal extubation: verapamil versus diltiazem. *Anesth Analg* 1996;82:1205–1210.

Nishina K, Mikawa K, Maekawa N, et al. Attenuation of cardiovascular responses to tracheal extubation with diltiazem. *Anesth Analg* 1995;80:1217–1222.

C.12. Would you consider regional anesthesia for this patient?

Certainly, regional anesthesia can avoid marked increases in sympathetic tone and hemodynamic changes that occur with intubation and extubation. Spinal or epidural anesthesia may be used for lower abdominal surgery. For cholecystectomy, higher levels of regional anesthesia are needed and may compromise respiratory function. Meanwhile, prolonged surgery can cause anxiety and irritability that may induce hypertension and tachycardia.

Stoelting RK, Diedorf SF. *Anesthesia and co-existing disease*, 4th ed. New York: Churchill Livingstone, 2002:99–103.

D. Postoperative Management

D.1. The patient developed hypertension, blood pressure (BP) 210/110 mm Hg in the postanesthesia care unit. What would you do?

The management of postoperative hypertension depends on the etiology of the hypertension, the clinical scenario, and the level of hypertension. First, the cause of hypertension should be determined and treated accordingly. Hypertension *per se* should also be treated by an antihypertensive agent. The causes of postoperative hypertension include pain, emergence excitement, hypoxemia, hypercarbia, reaction to endotracheal tube, full bladder, hypothermia, relative hypervolemia from intraoperative administration of excess fluid, and chronic medication and withdrawal. The most common cause of postoperative hypertension is incisional pain. As the patient awakens, pain triggers an outpouring of catecholamines. The extreme lability of BP in many hypertensive patients makes this rapid increase critical to control. Depending on the cause of hypertension, intravenous analgesics and antihypertensives or diuretics should be titrated to control hypertension. If both tachycardia and hypertension occurred postoperatively, calcium channel blockers such as verapamil, diltiazem, or nicardipine and β-blocking agents such as propranolol, esmolol, labetalol, or metoprolol are preferred agents. Hypertension resulting from pain can be preventable or attenuated by asking the surgeon to inject a long-lasting local anesthetic along the incision or to perform a local nerve block.

Barash PG, Cullen BF, Stoelting RK, eds. *Clinical anesthesia*, 5th ed. Philadelphia: Lippincott Williams & Wilkins, 2006:330.

Davis RF. Acute postoperative hypertension. *ASA refresher courses in anesthesiology*. Park Ridge: American Society of Anesthesiologists, 1989:17:59–70.

Gal TJ, Cooperman LH. Hypertension in the immediate postoperative period. *Br J Anesth* 1975;47:70.

CHAPTER 13

Cardiac Tamponade

Manuel L. Fontes • Nikolaos Skubas • James Osorio

A 69-YEAR-OLD WOMAN

was presented with shortness of breath, inability to lie supine, oliguria, and overt weakness, 4 days following two-vessel coronary artery bypass graft (CABG) procedure and replacement of a mitral valve. On examination, she appeared anxious and diaphoretic with the following vital signs: respiratory rate 38 breaths per minute, heart rate (HR) 120 beats per minute (normal sinus rhythm [NSR]), and systemic blood pressure 115/66 mm Hg. A pulmonary artery catheter (PAC) was placed and revealed: pulmonary artery (PA) pressures 55/15 mm Hg; pulmonary artery occlusion pressure (PAOP) 14 mm Hg; central venous pressure (CVP) 23 mm Hg; and a cardiac output (CO) of 2.7 L per minute. Both the prothrombin and the partial thromboplastin times (PTTs) were elevated.

A. Medical Disease and Differential Diagnosis

1. What is the differential diagnosis of low cardiac output (CO) postoperatively?
2. What is cardiac tamponade? Enumerate the common etiologies.
3. What is the difference between acute and delayed cardiac tamponade?
4. How is postcardiotomy cardiac tamponade diagnosed?
5. What is regional cardiac tamponade?
6. What is pulsus paradoxus? What is Kussmaul's sign?
7. Describe ventricular interaction in cardiac tamponade.
8. How is coronary blood flow affected in cardiac tamponade?
9. What are the electrocardiographic abnormalities associated with cardiac tamponade?
10. What roentgenographic and echocardiogram findings are noted in cardiac tamponade?
11. What is in the differential diagnosis of postcardiopulmonary bypass (post-CPB) bleeding?
12. What is the mechanism of action of low molecular weight heparin (LMWH)?
13. Describe the advantages of LMWH therapy over standard heparin therapy.
14. What is heparin-induced thrombocytopenia (HIT)? How is the diagnosis made?
15. What is the therapy for HIT?
16. Can HIT be caused by LMWH?
17. What is the mechanism of heparin antagonism by protamine?
18. What is "heparin rebound"?
19. How does warfarin affect the coagulation system? What is the therapy for reversing its effect?

20. What do the following measure: prothrombin time (PT), activated partial thromboplastin time (aPTT), thrombin time, activated clotting time (ACT), and bleeding time?
21. How is the anticoagulant effect of LMWH monitored?
22. What is a thromboelastograph? What is a Sonoclot?
23. How does desmopressin aid hemostasis?
24. What is fibrinolysis?
25. What is aminocaproic acid? What is tranexamic acid?
26. What is aprotinin?

B. Preoperative Evaluation and Preparation

1. Interpret the hemodynamic findings of this patient.
2. How would you treat the low output status of this patient?
3. How would you evaluate this patient's coagulation status?
4. What do fresh frozen plasma (FFP) and cryoprecipitate contain?
5. What are the indications for transfusing FFP, platelet concentrate, and cryoprecipitate?
6. What are the complications associated with blood component transfusions?
7. What is the risk of acquiring human immunodeficiency virus (HIV) from blood exposure?
8. In what situation might aminocaproic acid improve hemostasis?
9. Assuming that the patient has cardiac tamponade, how would you prepare this patient for surgery?
10. What premedication would you prescribe?

C. Intraoperative Management

1. How would you monitor this patient during transport to the operating room? What emergency drugs would you bring with you?
2. In this patient, what hemodynamic effects would occur from intravenous induction with ketamine, thiopental, fentanyl, propofol, etomidate, or midazolam?
3. Describe the induction process for cardiac tamponade.
4. Following induction and intubation, the systemic blood pressure decreased to 55/30 mm Hg. Describe the clinical events accounting for this perturbation and the management steps required for resuscitation.
5. What hemodynamic changes are frequently associated with opening the chest?
6. What is myocardial stunning? What is myocardial hibernation?

D. Postoperative Management

1. How would you manage hypertension in the intensive care unit (ICU)?
2. When would it be appropriate to extubate this patient?

A. Medical Disease and Differential Diagnosis

A.1. What is the differential diagnosis of low cardiac output (CO) postoperatively?

Cardiac output is the product of stroke volume (SV) and heart rate (HR) (CO = HR × SV). Therefore, a low output state can occur when SV and/or HR decrease. Fast heart rates, of either ventricular or atrial origin (i.e., atrial fibrillation) can also cause a low output state, because the diastolic filling time is decreased and/or the atrial contribution to the ventricular filling is reduced or abolished. Because SV is the difference between left ventricular end-diastolic volume (LVEDV) and left ventricular end-systolic volume (LVESV), The etiology of a reduced SV can be more accurately determined by exploring whether there has been a change in the preload (LVEDV), the afterload, and/or the contractile state of the left ventricle. Either too much preload (that may cause ventricular over-distention and systolic dysfunction) or too little preload can lower the cardiac output. Myocardial contractility can be compromised by either direct causes (myocardial ischemia, myocardial infarction, myocardial stunning, or myocardial hibernation) and/or by indirect causes (mechanical factors as in cardiac tamponade, pulmonary embolism; pharmacologic agents; and by toxins, namely, inflammatory cytokines and bacterial endotoxins). A combination of different hemodynamic disturbances can coexist in the same patient. For example, a patient can have both a decrease in contractility and a reduced preload to account for the low output state. Therefore, correcting one problem alone may not produce the optimal hemodynamic condition.

Ghobashy A, Fontes M, Hines R. Cardiogenic shock. In: Murray MJ, Coursin DB, Pearl RG, et al. eds. *Critical care medicine: perioperative management*, 2nd ed. Philadelphia: Lippincott Williams & Wilkins, 2002.

Johnson B, Adi A, Licina MG, et al. Cardiac physiology. In: Kaplan JA, Reich DSN, Lake CL, et al. eds. *Kaplan's cardiac anesthesia*, 5th ed. Philadelphia: WB Saunders, 2006:71–89.

A.2. What is cardiac tamponade? Enumerate the common etiologies.

Cardiac tamponade is defined as significant extrinsic compression of the heart by accumulating intrapericardial blood and clots (postcardiotomy, chamber perforation, dissecting aortic aneurysm, trauma, anticoagulant therapy), exudative effusions (malignant states, infective pericarditis, idiopathic pericarditis), nonexudative effusions (uremia, systemic lupus erythematosus, rheumatoid arthritis, idiopathic, radiation), and air. Irrespective of the actual volume, if the intrapericardial pressure is increased enough, globally or regionally, the risk of cardiac tamponade exists. How significant cardiac tamponade is, depends on whether the definition is clinical or physiologic. Cardiac tamponade is a pathophysiologic continuum that, on one extreme may be clinically insignificant whereas, on the other extreme presents as a life-threatening condition requiring emergent surgical attention. Clinical tamponade is frequently associated with marked increase in pericardial pressure relative to atrial and ventricular intracardiac pressures such that, stroke volume (SV) progressively declines resulting in systemic hypotension and cardiogenic shock.

Fowler NO, Gabel M, Buncher CR. Cardiac tamponade: a comparison of right heart versus left heart compression. *J Am Coll Cardiol* 1988;12:187.

Oliver WC Jr, Nuttall GA. Uncommon cardiac diseases. In: Kaplan JA, Reich DSN, Lake CL, et al. eds. *Kaplan's cardiac anesthesia*, 5th ed. Philadelphia: WB Saunders, 2006:800–802.

Spodlick D. Pathophysiology of cardiac tamponade. *Chest* 1998;113:1372–1378.

Whittington J, Borrows L, Skubas N, et al. Pericardial diseases. In: Mathew J, Ayoub C, eds. *Clinical manual and review of transesophageal echocardiography*. New York: McGraw-Hill, 2005.

A.3. What is the difference between acute and delayed cardiac tamponade?

In the setting of cardiac surgery, acute cardiac tamponade can occur over minutes, hours, or after a few days postoperatively. The reported incidence of acute cardiac tamponade is 0.5% to 5.8%. In the typical patient, a significant chest tube output (>200 mL/hour) in the immediate postoperative period, with or without hemodynamic signs of inadequate CO, is a sign of an increased amount of blood around the heart. Alternatively, the chest tubes may become clogged by blood clots impeding mediastinal drainage, and the clinical picture of cardiac tamponade develops sooner. Delayed tamponade has been arbitrarily defined as cardiac tamponade occurring 5 to 7 days after pericardiotomy. The incidence is 0.3% to 2.6%. It is often misdiagnosed because of a low index of suspicion and because the clinical signs and symptoms can be comparable to those of congestive heart failure, pulmonary embolism, and generalized fatigue (i.e., failure to thrive postoperatively). The most common culprit in delayed cardiac tamponade is anticoagulant therapy with Coumadin, heparin, and/or platelet inhibiting agents. However, a pericardial effusion after cardiac surgery is common. Using echocardiography, Weitzman et al. evaluated 122 consecutive patients postoperatively and demonstrated that most of them, 103/122 (84%) had pericardial effusions (PE). Generally, effusions reach their maximum size by the 10th postoperative day and regress spontaneously thereafter.

D'Cruz IA, Overton DH, Pai GH. Pericardial complications of cardiac surgery: emphasis on the diagnostic role of echocardiography. *J Card Surg* 1992;7:257–268.

Nelson RM, Jeson CB, Smoot WM. Pericardial tamponade following open-heart surgery. *J Thorac Cardiovasc Surg* 1969;58:510–516.

Weitzman LB, Tinker WC, Kronzon I, et al. The incidence and natural history of pericardial effusions after cardiac surgery: an echocardiographic study. *Circulation* 1984;69: 506.

A.4.   How is postcardiotomy cardiac tamponade diagnosed?

The diagnosis of cardiac tamponade following cardiac surgery is often difficult to make and requires a high degree of clinical suspicion, physical examination, proficient knowledge of pulmonary artery catheter (PAC) derived measurements, and diagnostic tools such as echocardiography and chest radiography. Often, the diagnosis is made in the operating room, whereby evacuation of clot and blood from the mediastinum is associated with a drastic improvement in hemodynamics (Fig. 13.1). Relying on one modality alone for diagnosis can lead to inaccurate management decisions and increase patient morbidity. For example, the PAC is an important device for monitoring cardiac function; however, its measures can be misleading postcardiotomy, unless the clinician is aware of its limitations. The classical teaching of equalization of diastolic blood pressures in cardiac tamponade (central venous pressure [CVP] = pulmonary artery diastolic pressure [PAD] = pulmonary artery occlusion pressure [PAOP]) is infrequently observed postoperatively, because the previously transected pericardium is left open. As such, blood or clot or both, do not distribute homogeneously around the heart to produce equalization of pericardial diastolic pressures. Generally, the CVP is elevated but the PAD and the PAOP can be normal, elevated, or, in some cases, reduced. With significant compression of the right heart, reduced blood flow to the pulmonary artery (PA) and to the left heart can yield low left-sided heart pressures that would be inconsistent with "classical" tamponade physiology. Russo et al. found that only 33% of patients with the diagnosis of postoperative cardiac tamponade had right heart catheterization findings that reflected equalization of diastolic blood pressures. Overall, 90% of patients with postcardiotomy cardiac tamponade had either atypical clinical, hemodynamic, and/or echocardiographic findings. Therefore, the diagnosis of postoperative cardiac tamponade should be considered every time hemodynamic deterioration is encountered, particularly when reduction in cardiac output or blood pressure or both, are not readily responsive to conventional management. Furthermore, in delayed tamponade, the complaints tend to be vague and invasive hemodynamic data (i.e., PAC) is usually not available, to allow prompt diagnosis of tamponade. Whenever the patient is not progressing as expected postoperatively, and signs of end-organ dysfunction (fall in urine output and/or increase blood urea nitrogen [BUN] and creatinine) are present, an echocardiogram should be obtained to rule out cardiac tamponade.

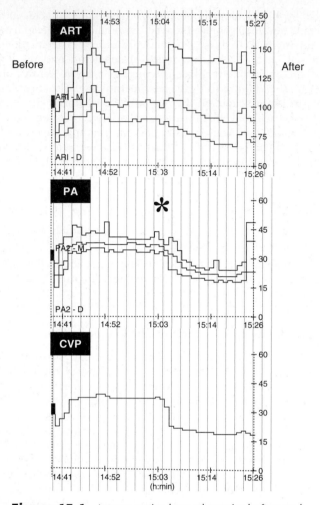

Figure 13.1 Intraoperative hemodynamics before and after evacuation of pericardial fluid. Arterial blood pressure (ART), pulmonary artery pressure (PA) and central venous pressure (CVP) are shown during chest exploration for cardiac tamponade. Notice the elevated diastolic PA and CVP at the beginning of the anesthetic (left hand of the pressure trends). There is equalization of CVP and diastolic PA pressure, suggesting global pericardial effusion. As soon as the chest was opened and the pericardial collection was evacuated (*asterisk*), the ART increased abruptly and the pulse pressure widened, although both PA and CVP immediately decreased to normal levels. Taking into consideration that ART increased whereas CVP decreased after evacuation of the pericardial collection, one can assume that the cardiac output has increased.

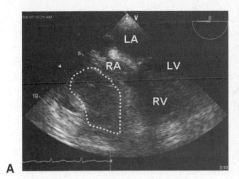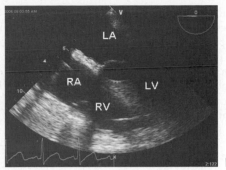

Figure 13.2 Regional, acute pericardial effusion. The heart is viewed in the mid esophageal four chamber view at 0 degree rotation, before **(A)** and after **(B)** evacuation of a loculated pericardial clot. The pericardial collection (*dotted line*) is around the right atrium (RA), almost obliterating its cavity (compared with the size of RA after evacuation). The collection is partially compressing the cavity of the right ventricle (RV). LA, left atrium; LV, left ventricle.

Russo A, O'Connor W, Waxman H. Atypical presentations and echocardiographic findings in patients with cardiac tamponade occurring early and late after cardiac surgery. *Chest* 1993;104:71–78.

Spodlick D. Pathophysiology of cardiac tamponade. *Chest* 1998;113:1372–1378.

A.5. What is regional cardiac tamponade?

Regional cardiac tamponade occurs when one or more cardiac chambers (and not necessary the entire heart) become compressed by blood or blood clot or both, thereby compromising heart function (Figs. 13.2 and 13.3). Postcardiotomy, the diastolic regional collapse of the right atrium (RA) or the right ventricle (RV) is the most common echocardiographic finding in "early" cardiac tamponade. Postoperatively, a right atrial hematoma often becomes localized around the anterior

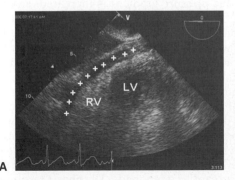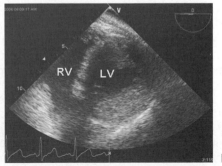

Figure 13.3 Pericardial effusion. The heart is viewed in the transgastric mid papillary short axis view, before **(A)** and after **(B)** the evacuation of a posterior pericardial collection (*asterisks*). Notice the increase in cavity size of the left ventricle (LV) and reappearance of the cavity of the right ventricle (RV) after evacuation of the pericardial collection.

and lateral walls, whereas clots are more commonly found behind the left atrium, where they become encysted in the oblique sinus. Selective compression of the right heart by hematoma becomes less prominent in "delayed" tamponade, as the right heart becomes adherent or tethered to the anterior chest wall. As discussed in the previous answer, the diagnosis of tamponade is often misdiagnosed, because the classical features of tamponade are often absent, and blood and blood clots are unevenly distributed around the heart. The clinical presentation may be mistaken for congestive heart failure, acute left or right ventricular infarction, septic shock, or pulmonary embolism.

Chuttani K, Pandian NG, Mohanty PK, et al. Left ventricular diastolic collapse. An echocardiographic sign of regional cardiac tamponade. *Circulation* 1991;83:1999–2006.

Fowler NO, Gabel M. Regional cardiac tamponade: a hemodynamic study. *J Am Coll Cardiol* 1987;10:164–169.

Hutchins GM. Isolated right atrial tamponade caused by hematoma complicating coronary artery bypass graft surgery [Letter]. *Arch Pathol Lab Med* 1980;104:612–614.

Jadhav P, Asirvatham S, Craven P, et al. Unusual presentation of late regional cardiac tamponade after aortic surgery. *Am J Cardiac Imaging* 1996;10:204–206.

Kochar GS, Jocab LE, Holter MN. Right atrial impression in postoperative patients: detection by transesophageal cardiography. *J Am Coll Cardiol* 1990;16:511–516.

Russo A, O'Connor W, Waxman H. Atypical presentations and echocardiographic findings in patients with cardiac tamponade occurring early and late after cardiac surgery. *Chest* 1993;104:71–78.

Sandifer DP, Gonzalez JL. Refractory postoperative hypoxemia associated with regional cardiac tamponade and patent foramen ovale. *Crit Care Med* 1997;25:1608–1611.

A.6. What is pulsus paradoxus? What is Kussmaul's sign?

The right heart fills from blood entering the chest cavity due to a pressure gradient between the extrathoracic vasculature (superior and inferior vena cava systems) and intrathoracic chambers (the right atrium [RA] and right ventricle [RV]). The left heart fills with blood moved by a pressure gradient between the intrathoracic, intrapulmonary vasculature (the pulmonary veins) and the intrathoracic, extrapulmonary left atrium and ventricle. Normally, during spontaneous inspiration, the extrathoracic to intrathoracic pressure gradient is increased, and the filling of the right heart is slightly larger than the filling of the left heart. In the latter, the decreased intrapulmonary pressure during inspiration will cause a relative "pooling" of the blood in the lungs and decreases the filling gradient. That causes an, inspiratory fall of less than 10 mm Hg in the arterial systolic pressure along with an accompanying inspiratory fall in the venous pressure. A paradoxical pulse differs from the normal situation in two aspects: (a) the inspiratory fall of the arterial pressure exceeds 10 mm Hg and (b) the inspiratory venous pressure remains steady or increases (Kussmaul's sign), instead of decreasing. Echocardiographic studies of patients with cardiac tamponade by D'Cruz et al. described phasic respiratory changes whereby both left ventricular dimensions and mitral valve excursion decreased during inspiration. In contrast, right ventricular dimensions increased in association with a shifting of the interventricular septum toward the left ventricle. That is, the right heart filling is done at the expense of the left. Of importance, pulsus paradoxus is not unique to cardiac tamponade. The phasic respiratory changes in ventricular dimensions with exaggerated decrease in systemic systolic arterial pressure during inspiration can be present in a variety of clinical conditions, whereby the inspiratory decrease of the intrapleural pressure is profound. This physiologic process is often present in respiratory distress, airway obstruction, chronic obstructive pulmonary disease (COPD), and pulmonary embolism. A prominent feature of cardiac tamponade, pulsus paradoxus, may not be present at all in patients with chest wall trauma, neuromuscular disease, and pneumothorax, because these patients cannot generate sufficient negative intrapleural pressure during inspiration to produce the typical changes in chamber dimension and the fall in left ventricular stroke volume. Similarly, those who are receiving positive pressure mechanical ventilation (early postoperative period) and patients with severe aortic regurgitation do not exhibit pulsus paradoxus.

D'Cruz IA, Overton DH, Pai GH. Pericardial complications of cardiac surgery: emphasis on the diagnostic role of echocardiography. *J Card Surg* 1992;7:257–268.

Frey B, Freezer N. Diagnostic value and pathophysiologic basis of pulsus paradoxus in infants and children with respiratory disease. *Pediatr Pulmonol* 2001;31:138–143.

Jay GD, Onuma K, Davis R, et al. Analysis of physician ability in the measurement of pulsus paradoxus by sphygmomanometry. *Chest* 2000;118:348–352.

McGregor M. Pulsus paradoxus. *N Engl J Med* 1979;301:480.

Tsang TS, Barnes ME, Hayes SN, et al. Clinical and echocardiographic characteristics of significant pericardial effusions following cardiothoracic surgery and outcomes of echo-guided pericardiocentesis for management: Mayo Clinic experience, 1979–1998. *Chest* 1999;116:322–331.

A.7. Describe the ventricular interaction in cardiac tamponade.

Ventricular interaction is extremely important for the maintenance of adequate cardiac performance. Under normal conditions, the average stroke volume (SV) of the right ventricle (RV) equals the SV of the left ventricle; however, cyclical respiratory differences in left and right ventricular SV do occur. One should keep in mind that the pressure gradients which fill the two ventricles are not the same: the RV fills with systemic blood that returns through an extrathoracic to intrathoracic gradient, whereas the left ventricle fills with pulmonary blood, which resides inside the lungs. During inspiration, the generated negative intrapleural pressure facilitates blood return to the right heart, whereas blood return to the left heart is diminished for the following reasons: (a) lung expansion increases its reservoir for blood and (b) the increase in right ventricular filling causes the interventricular septum to "bulge" leftwardly, thereby reducing left ventricular dimensions and altering its compliance and filling (ventricular interaction). During exhalation, the reverse process occurs. In the case of cardiac tamponade, the ventricular interaction is augmented, and involves not only the interventricular septum but also other chambers depending on the etiology of the tamponade (fluid vs. clot, regional vs. global tamponade). Fundamentally, as intrapericardial content increases, it will reach a point whereby the parietal pericardium cannot stretch to accommodate the rising pressure. Because of the fixed space within the pericardium, the cardiac chamber dimensions become smaller as the pericardial contents increase. First, the thin-walled and more compliant atria progressively gets compressed, followed by the RV, and lastly by the left ventricle. Overall, the physiology of ventricular interaction in clinical cardiac tamponade becomes complex, as the pressure–volume relation of mediastinal and chest structure alters with each heartbeat and from respiratory and neuroendocrine influences.

Spodlick D. Pathophysiology of cardiac tamponade. *Chest* 1998;113:1372–1378.

A.8. How is coronary blood flow affected in cardiac tamponade?

In the absence of coronary artery disease, coronary blood flow is reduced in cardiac tamponade, but this reduction is not sufficient to add an ischemic insult to the heart, because there is a proportionate decrease in (a) ventricular preload (underfilled heart) and (b) ventricular afterload. Consequently, both myocardial work and oxygen consumption are reduced. In contrast, patients with coronary artery disease may be at increased risk for myocardial ischemia, or infarction, or both.

Reddy PS, Curtiss EL, Otoole JD, et al. Cardiac tamponade; hemodynamic observation in man. *Circulation* 1978;58:265–272.

Spodlick DH. Threshold of pericardial constraint: the pericardial reserve volume and auxiliary pericardial functions. *J Am Coll Cardiol* 1985;6:296–299.

A.9. What are the electrocardiographic abnormalities associated with cardiac tamponade?

Electrocardiographic changes may occur in the setting of cardiac tamponade. These include nonspecific ST-T wave abnormalities, low voltage QRS complex, signs of myocardial ischemia and pericarditis, and *electrical alternans* (Fig. 13.4). The latter is seen in patients with large effusions and is characterized by beat-to-beat shifts in electrical axis. This beat-to-beat alteration may be due to increased distance between the heart and the chest wall resulting in a "pendulum" like motion of the heart. However, it has been shown that with minimal amount of pericardial fluid removal, the presence of electrical alternans can be abolished while the pericardial space remains enlarged. Therefore, the electrocardiographic change of electrical alternans may reflect

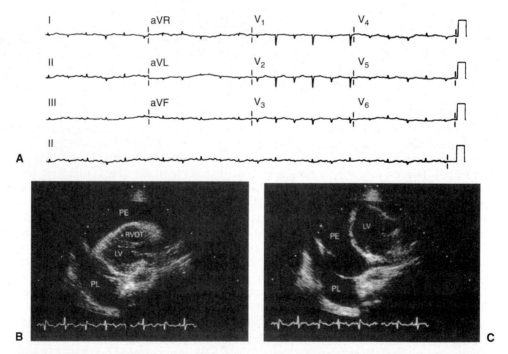

Figure 13.4 Depiction of electrical alternans in a patient with cardiac tamponade **(A)**. The images demonstrate significant pericardial effusions (PE) obtained during transthoracic echocardiography. Note the image of the left ventricle (LV) during systole **(B)** and diastole **(C)**. PL, pleural effusion; RVOT, right ventricular outflow tract. (From Longo MJ, Jaffe CC. Images in clinical medicine. Electrical alternans. *N Engl J Med* 1999;341:2060, with permission.)

a hemodynamic pathology rather than an anatomic abnormality. This finding, although sensitive for cardiac tamponade, is not very specific (very few patients with tamponade present with electrical alternans).

Fox JJ, McHarg JL, Gilmour RF Jr. Ionic mechanism of electrical alternans. *Am J Physiol Heart Circ Physiol* 2002;282:H516–H530.

Kosta E, Kronzon I. Electrical alternans in cardiac tamponade. *Echocardiography* 2000; 17(6 Pt 1):575–576.

Kronzon I, Cohen M, Winer H. Contribution of echocardiography to the understanding of the pathophysiology of cardiac tamponade. *J Am Coll Cardiol* 1983;1:1180–1182.

Longo MJ, Jaffe CC. Images in clinical medicine. Electrical alternans. *N Engl J Med* 1999; 341:2060.

A.10. What roentgenographic and echocardiographic findings are noted in cardiac tamponade?

On standard anterior-posterior chest roentgenography, the cardiac silhouette may appear normal in size or extremely enlarged, depending on the acuity and chronicity of the tamponade process. Normally, the pericardial fluid amounts to 15 to 25 mL. Acute tamponade physiology can arise with as little as 150 mL of effusion, whereas chronic effusions may exceed 1,000 mL before clinical signs and symptoms of cardiac tamponade become evident. In the latter case, on chest x-ray film, the cardiac silhouette will appear "widened" with or without features, such as obscuring of the pulmonary vessels at the hilum, and a globular or "water bottle" configuration of the heart.

Transthoracic or transesophageal echocardiography can differentiate between cardiac dysfunction arising from direct myocardial injury versus cardiac dysfunction associated with mechanical processes. Pericardial effusions (PE) can be readily seen and semi-quantitated. Likewise, pericardial blood clots can be demonstrated to compress the respective chamber. Additional echocardiographic signs observed in tamponade include (a) diminished left ventricular dimension and mitral valve excursion during inspiration, (b) shifting of the interventricular septum toward the left ventricle, (c) changes in transvalvular (mitral and aortic) flow characteristics seen by Doppler techniques, (d) diastolic posterior motion of the right ventricular wall, and (e) in some cases, a systolic notch on the right ventricular epicardium (Figs. 13.2 and 13.3). Although many of the findings of both x-ray film and echocardiogram can be suggestive of cardiac tamponade, not a single sign is 100% sensitive and specific.

Oliver WC Jr, Nutall GA. Uncommon cardiac diseases. In: Kaplan JA, Reich DSN, Lake CL, et al. eds. *Kaplan's cardiac anesthesia*, 5th ed. Philadelphia: WB Saunders, 2006:801.

Singh SM, Wann LS, Schuchard GH, et al. Right ventricular and right atrial collapse in patients with cardiac tamponade. *Circulation* 1984;70:996.

Whittington J, Borrows L, Skubas N, et al. Pericardial diseases. In: Mathew J, Ayoub C, eds. *Clinical manual and review of transesophageal echocardiography*, New York: McGraw-Hill, 2005.

A.11. What is in the differential diagnosis of postcardiopulmonary bypass (post-CPB) bleeding?

Significant bleeding following cardiac surgery requiring surgical exploration "bring-back" occurs in approximately 3% of cases. Often, the source of bleeding cannot be ascertained and its etiology is ascribed to a coagulation defect. Procedures that require cardiopulmonary bypass (CPB) are

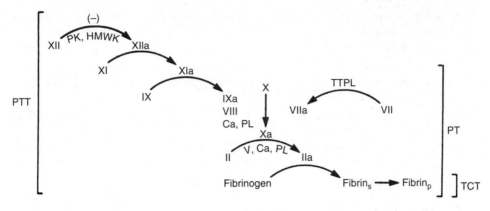

Figure 13.5 The coagulation cascade, illustrating the coagulation factors required for various screening tests. HMWK, high molecular weight kininogen; PK, prekallikrein; PL, phospholipid by platelets; PT, prothrombin time; PTT, partial thromboplastin time; TCT, thrombin clotting time; TTPL, tissue thromboplastin; fibrins, fibrin single standards; fibrinp, fibrin polymer. (From Coleman RW, Hirsch J, Marder VJ, et al., eds. Hemostasis and thrombosis: basic principles and clinical practice. 2nd ed. Philadelphia: JB Lippincott, 1987:1052, with permission.)

known to adversely affect the hemostatic mechanisms including vascular endothelium, fibrinolytic and coagulation factors, platelet, plasminogen, and inflammatory pathways (Fig. 13.5). Under normal settings, these systems (and others yet unknown) act in concert and in opposition with one another (a) to prevent bleeding by promoting clot formation at the site of endothelial injury (procoagulant effects) and (b) to prevent or destroy clot formation (anticoagulant effects—either directly or indirectly through inhibitory mediators). Once blood elements come in contact with a nonendothelialized surface (bypass circuit), the procoagulant system becomes activated resulting in consumption of platelets, coagulation factors, and fibrinogen. The potential for postoperative bleeding will depend on the degree of activation and preexisting levels of the procoagulants as well as other factors such as the duration of CPB, systemic hypothermia, comorbid states (renal and liver insufficiency), type of surgery (reoperation, circulatory arrest, combined procedures), and prior or current treatment with anticoagulant (platelet inhibitors, Coumadin, heparin).

Platelets play an important role in the coagulation process. Once activated, they secrete several types of granules. Granules, containing peptides such as fibrinogen, thrombospondin, factors V and VIII, and β-thromboglobulin, are reduced in both number and content during CPB. Of greater importance is the loss of several membrane glycoproteins (IIb-IIIa) that interact with fibrinogen and other cellular elements allowing for platelet conjugation and propagation of clot formation. Overall, postcardiotomy bleeding is due to (a) a qualitative and a quantitative platelet defect, (b) factor deficiency, and (c) surgical bleeding. The latter can arise from either venous or arterial sources that were undetected before closure of the chest. Attentive and meticulous effort to surgical hemostasis can significantly reduce the incidence of bring-backs.

Despotis GJ, Avidan MS, Hogue CW Jr. Mechanisms and attenuation of hemostatic activation during extracorporeal circulation. *Ann Thorac Surg* 2001;72:S1821–S1831.

Kojima T, Gando S, Morimoto Y, et al. Systematic elucidation of effects of tranexamic acid on fibrinolysis and bleeding during and after cardiopulmonary bypass surgery. *Thromb Res* 2001;104:301–307.

Levy JH. Pharmacologic preservation of the hemostatic system during cardiac surgery. *Ann Thorac Surg* 2001;72:S1814–S1820.

Spiess BD, Horrow J, Kaplan JA. Transfusion medicine and coagulation disorders. In: Kaplan JA, Reich DSN, Lake CL, et al. eds. *Kaplan's cardiac anesthesia*, 5th ed. Philadelphia: WB Saunders, 2006:966–968.

A.12. What is the mechanism of action of low molecular weight heparin (LMWH)?

The unfractionated heparin exerts its anticoagulant activity through antithrombin III (ATIII). ATIII inhibits thrombin (factor IIa), and factors IXa and Xa. Unfractionated heparin accelerates the formation of ATIII-IIa complex by 2,000 folds (and that requires the simultaneous binding of unfractionated heparin of at least 18 saccharide units-length to both ATIII and IIa), and the formation of ATIII-Xa by 1,200 folds. LMWHs are fragments of unfractionated heparin produced by controlled enzymatic or chemical depolymerization processes yielding chains having molecular weight of 6,000 to 7,000 daltons. LMWHs consist of 8–16 saccharide units and inhibits factor Xa preferentially. This inhibition requires only that LMWH binds to ATIII, and the latter interacts with factor Xa, without the interaction between LMWH and factor Xa being necessary. LMWH has greater inhibitory effect on factor Xa, whereas unfractionated heparin exerts an equipotent effect against both thrombin and factor Xa. The activated partial thromboplastin time (aPTT) monitors the anti-IIa activity more closely than the anti-Xa activity. Lastly, both LMWH and unfractionated heparin cause release of tissue factor pathway inhibitor from vascular endothelium, which then forms a complex with and inhibits factor Xa. This complex in turn inactivates factor VIIa.

Clark SC, Vitale N, Zacharias J, et al. Effect of low molecular weight heparin (fragmin) on bleeding after cardiac surgery. *Ann Thorac Surg* 2000;69:762–765.

Gohlke-Barwolf C. Anticoagulation in valvar heart disease: new aspects and management during non-cardiac surgery. *Heart* 2000;84:567–572.

Harenberg J. Pharmacology of low molecular weight heparins. *Semin Thomb Hemost* 1990; 16:12–18.

Spiess BD, Horrow J, Kaplan JA. Transfusion medicine and coagulation disorders. In: Kaplan JA, Reich DSN, Lake CL, et al. eds. *Kaplan's cardiac anesthesia*, 5th ed. Philadelphia: WB Saunders, 2006:949–950, 956–957.

Weitz JI. Drug therapy: low molecular weight heparins. *N Engl J Med* 1997;337:688–698.

A.13. Describe the advantages of low molecular weight heparin (LMWH) over standard heparin therapy.

There are several clinical and pharmacologic advantages of LMWH over unfractionated heparin. The plasma half-life of LMWH is two to four times longer than unfractionated heparin, which undergoes a dose-dependent elimination by the liver and the kidneys. A significant amount of unfractionated heparin is bound to plasma proteins, vascular endothelium, and macrophages resulting in less bioavailability and an unpredictable anticoagulant effect. Consequently, careful laboratory monitoring is required. Additional benefits of LMWH over unfractionated heparin include less bleeding (less platelet inhibition and decreased propensity for increased microvascular permeability). Several clinical trials have improved the efficacy and safety of LMWH over unfractionated heparin. Of note, LMWH is not recommended in the setting of renal failure. The anticoagulant activity of LMWH may be measured by assaying factor Xa levels. There are, many different types of LMWH available in the market, each having slightly different pharmacologic effects (bioavailability, anticoagulant effect). Our understanding of the anticoagulant mechanism of LMWH continues to evolve, and, although its indications continue to broaden, there may be safety concerns that ought not to be dismissed.

Alban S, Gastpar R. Plasma levels of total and free tissue factor pathway inhibitor (TFPI) as individual pharmacological parameters of various heparins. *Thromb Haemost* 2001;85:824–829.

Cohen AT, Bailey CS, Alikhan R, et al. Extended thromboprophylaxis with low molecular weight heparin reduces symptomatic venous thromboembolism following lower limb arthroplasty—a meta-analysis. *Thromb Haemost* 2001;85:940–941.

Huse DM, Cummins G, Taylor DC, et al. Outpatient treatment of venous thromboembolism with low-molecular-weight heparin: an economic evaluation. *Am J Manag Care* 2002;8(Suppl 1):S10–S16.

Kleinschmidt K, Charles R. Pharmacology of low molecular weight heparins [Review]. *Emerg Med Clin North Am* 2001;19:1025–1049.

A.14. What is heparin-induced thrombocytopenia (HIT)? How is the diagnosis made?

Heparin normally binds to platelet membranes at GPIb and other receptor sites, and aggregates normal platelets by releasing adenosine diphosphate (ADP). HIT is a serious complication of heparin therapy that is predominantly immune-mediated by a binary complex formed between heparin and platelet factor 4 (PF4). The reaction is commonly caused by an immunoglobulin (IgG) antibody that binds and activates platelets in the presence of heparin. Other immunoglobulins may also potentiate HIT.

HIT exists in two forms. A benign form of HIT, type I, is observed in approximately 10% to 20% of patients receiving unfractionated heparin. This mild form of thrombocytopenia (rarely <100,000/μL) occurs after 1 to 4 days of therapy with heparin, is due to proaggregatory effects of heparin on platelets and generally improves despite continuing heparin administration. In contrast, HIT type II, is a life-threatening condition that develops 5 to 10 days after initiating heparin therapy and is associated with devastating thromboembolic processes (most commonly arterial thrombosis resulting in limb ischemia, cerebrovascular events, and myocardial infarction), from activated platelets that adhere, aggregate and form platelet ("white") clots. The platelet count falls to less than 50,000 per μL and in severe cases to less than 5,000 per μL. The incidence of HIT in patients receiving full-dose heparin ranges between 0% and 30%. Although there is no randomized prospective study looking at the true incidence of HIT, the expected incidence is estimated to be less than 5%. Those patients who have had a previous exposure to heparin (recent and in some cases remote history) *may* develop HIT earlier after institution of heparin therapy as compared with those with no previous exposure. The frequency of HIT is also higher in patients receiving porcine mucosal heparin compared with bovine lung heparin.

The diagnosis of HIT should be entertained in any patient with a significant fall in platelet count while on heparin therapy (<150,000/μL or a 50% or greater decrease in platelet count after 5 days of heparin therapy). The definitive diagnosis requires the following steps: (a) thrombocytopenia while on heparin, (b) exclusion of other etiology of thrombocytopenia, (c) improvement in platelet count following cessation of heparin therapy, and (d) presence of heparin-dependent platelet antibody by an *in vitro* test. In most cases, the diagnosis is made on clinical findings.

Gerotziafas GT, Elalamy I, Lecrubier C, et al. The role of platelet factor 4 in platelet aggregation induced by the antibodies implicated in heparin-induced thrombocytopenia. *Blood Coagul Fibrinolysis* 2001;12:511–520.

Shea SI, Sands JJ, Nudo SA, et al. Frequency of anti-heparin-platelet factor 4 antibodies in hemodialysis patients and correlation with recurrent vascular access thrombosis. *Am J Hematol* 2002;69:72–73.

Spiess BD, Horrow J, Kaplan JA. Transfusion medicine and coagulation disorders. In: Kaplan JA, Reich DSN, Lake CL, et al. eds. *Kaplan's cardiac anesthesia*, 5th ed. Philadelphia: WB Saunders, 2006:953–955.

Warkentin TE, Greinacher A. Heparin-induced thrombocytopenia and cardiac surgery. *Ann Thorac Surg* 2003;76:2121–2131.

A.15. What is the therapy for heparin-induced thrombocytopenia (HIT)?

Because HIT type II is a potentially lethal condition, the most effective therapy is discontinuation of heparin. The thrombocytopenia should improve progressively. Although tempting, the need for platelet transfusion is discouraged because bleeding occurs infrequently and vascular thrombosis may be potentiated. Several anticoagulants have been recommended for use in HIT, as heparin replacement. These include direct thrombin inhibitors (hirudin, argatroban), low molecular weight heparin (LMWH), LMW heparinoid, ancrod, and antiplatelet agents). Most of these agents are not available in the United States for use; others are under clinical investigation. Hirudin has been extensively used in Europe with demonstrable benefit and safety. The LMWH have been shown to have cross reactivity with unfractionated heparin approaching 100% (by C-serotonin release or heparin-induced platelet aggregation [HIPA] assays) and should not be used in the setting of HIT unless there are demonstrable negative cross reactivity assays with standard heparin. The ancrod is a defibrinogenating agent (not available in the United States) extracted from the Malayan pit viper and is immunologically distinct from heparin. It acts by cleaving fibrinopeptide A from fibrinogen and its activity can be measured by assaying for plasma fibrinogen concentration. Lastly, in the setting of HIT, a synthetic analogue of prostacyclin (iloprost—a potent inhibitor of platelet activation) has been used successfully during cardiac surgery to inactivate platelets and prevent further reduction of platelet count.

Cheng-Lai A. Cardiovascular drug highlight: hirudin. *Heart Dis J Cardiovasc Med* 1999;1:41–49.

Deitcher SR, Carman TL. Heparin-induced thrombocytopenia: natural history, diagnosis, and management. *Vasc Med* 2001;6:113–119.

Koster A, Meyer O, Fischer T, et al. One-year experience with the platelet glycoprotein IIb/IIIa antagonist tirofiban and heparin during cardiopulmonary bypass in patients with heparin-induced thrombocytopenia type II. *J Thorac Cardiovasc Surg* 2001;122:1254–1255.

Robitaille D, Carrier M, Cartier R, et al. Successful management strategy for mechanical assistance and heart transplantation in patients suffering from heparin-induced thrombocytopenia type II. *J Heart Lung Transplant* 2001;20:1237–1240.

Spiess BD, Horrow J, Kaplan JA. Transfusion medicine and coagulation disorders. In: Kaplan JA, Reich DSN, Lake CL, et al. eds. *Kaplan's cardiac anesthesia*, 5th ed. Philadelphia: WB Saunders, 2006:955.

Warkentin TE, Dunn GL, Cybulsky IJ. Off-pump coronary artery bypass grafting for acute heparin-induced thrombocytopenia. *Ann Thorac Surg* 2001;72:1730–1732.

A.16. Can heparin-induced thrombocytopenia (HIT) be caused by low molecular weight heparin (LMWH)?

Based on confirmed laboratory tests, the prevalence of HIT is 2% for patients receiving unfractionated heparin. Although LMWHs can also induce thrombocytopenia, they may be acceptable alternatives for patients who develop HIT from unfractionated heparin, but reactivity of the particular LMWH with the patient's platelets should be confirmed *in vitro*.

Fabris F, Luzzatto G, Stefani PM, et al. Heparin-induced thrombocytopenia [Review]. *Haematologica* 2000;85:72–81.

Kleinschmidt K, Charles R. Pharmacology of low molecular weight heparins. *Emerg Med Clin North Am* 2001;19:1025–1049.

Shore-Lesserson L. Coagulation monitoring. In: Kaplan JA, Reich DSN, Lake CL, et al. eds. *Kaplan's cardiac anesthesia*, 5th ed. Philadelphia: WB Saunders, 2006:560–561.

Warkentin TE, Sheppard JA, Horsewood P, et al. Impact of the patient population on the risk for heparin-induced thrombocytopenia. *Blood* 2000;96:1703–1708.

A.17. What is the mechanism of heparin antagonism by protamine?

Heparin is a large molecule consisting of chains of alternating residues of D-glucosamine and uronic acid. It is highly negatively charged, whereas protamine is mostly positively charged. The two combine irreversibly to form a heparin-protamine complex that does not have the ability to bind to thrombin or factor Xa. Once neutralized, the complex of heparin and protamine is eliminated.

Carr JA, Silverman N. The heparin-protamine interaction. *J Vasc Surg* 1999;40(5):659–666.

Kimmel SE, Sekeres M, Berlin JA, et al. Mortality and adverse events after protamine administration in patients undergoing cardiopulmonary bypass. *Anesth Analg* 2002; 94:1402–1408.

Park KW. Protamine and protamine reactions. *Int Anesthesiol Clin* 2004;42(3):135–145.

A.18. What is "heparin rebound"?

The activated clotting time (ACT) is used to confirm the adequacy of heparin neutralization by protamine. The reappearance of circulating heparin several hours after its neutralization by protamine is called heparin rebound and is usually incriminated for clinical bleeding occurring after cardiac surgery. The concept of heparin rebound following protamine reversal may be explained by sequestration of heparin in tissues that are poorly perfused (i.e., fat) late release of heparin by endothelial cells, and more rapid clearance of protamine in relation to heparin (as heparin is mobilized back into circulation it can inhibit thrombin formation and predispose to post-CPB bleeding). Studies in which 1 mg of protamine is given per 100 units of heparin (total dose) found no evidence of heparin rebound.

Spiess BD, Horrow J, Kaplan JA. Transfusion medicine and coagulation disorders. In: Kaplan JA, Reich DSN, Lake CL, et al. eds. *Kaplan's cardiac anesthesia*, 5th ed. Philadelphia: WB Saunders, 2006:952.

Subramaniam P, Skillington P, Tatoulis J. Heparin-rebound in the early postoperative phase following cardiopulmonary bypass. *Aust N Z J Surg* 1995;65:331–333.

Woodman RC, Harker LA. Bleeding complications associated with cardiopulmonary bypass. *Blood* 1990;76:1680.

A.19. How does warfarin affect the coagulation system? What is the therapy for reversing its effect?

Warfarin (Coumadin) remains the most commonly used anticoagulant agent in the outpatient setting (atrial fibrillation, prosthetic valves and devices). Its predominant pharmacodynamic effect is inhibition of synthesis of vitamin K-dependent factors (II, VII, IX, and X) in the liver and its clinical efficacy is monitored by measuring the prothrombin time (PT) or more specifically, the international normalized ratio (INR). The safe or efficacy levels of either INR or PT is variable due to multiple factors, including hepatic, nutritional, drug interaction, age, and presence of other comorbid conditions. On average, it takes several days of therapy to achieve the desired INR (2 to 4); consequently, administration of either low molecular weight heparin (LMWH) or unfractionated heparin may be necessary for initiating anticoagulation. Complications occur either because of inadequate anticoagulation (thrombosis) or because of excessive anticoagulation (bleeding and hemorrhage). To reverse its effect, warfarin should be discontinued several days (>3 days) to allow levels of the aforementioned factors to normalize. Acute reversal is achieved with fresh frozen plasma (FFP). Administration of vitamin K is often necessary to accelerate the synthetic process.

Erban S. Initiation of warfarin therapy: recommendations and clinical pearls. *J Thromb Thrombolysis* 1999;7:145–148.

Henderson MC, White RH. Anticoagulation in the elderly. *Curr Opin Pulm Med* 2001;7: 365–370.

Horton JD, Bushwick BM. Warfarin therapy: evolving strategies in anticoagulation. *Am Fam Physician* 2002;65:172.

Jacobs LG. Warfarin pharmacology, clinical management, and evaluation of hemorrhagic risk for the elderly. *Clin Geriatr Med* 2006;22(1):17–32, vii–viii.

Keller C, Matzdorff AC, Kemkes-Matthes B. Pharmacology of warfarin and clinical implication. *Semin Thromb Hemost* 1999;25:13–16.

A.20. What do the following measure: prothrombin time (PT), activated partial thromboplastin time (aPTT), thrombin time, activated clotting time (ACT), bleeding time?

Prothrombin time

Prothrombin time (PT) measures the activity of the "extrinsic" pathway: factors I (fibrinogen), II (prothrombin), V, VII, and X (Fig. 13.5). Deficiencies of factors V, VII, and X (50% of normal) significantly prolong the PT. The concentrations of fibrinogen and prothrombin required to prolong the PT are much lower. The activity of three of the four vitamin K-dependent factors (II, VII, IX, and X) are measured by the PT. Normal values are less than 12 seconds.

Activated partial thromboplastin time

aPTT measures the activity of the "intrinsic" pathway: factors XII, XI, IX, VIII, V, X, prothrombin, and fibrinogen (Fig. 13.5). The aPTT is prolonged when the concentration of these factors is less than 20% to 30%. Normal values are 25 to 40 seconds.

Thrombin time

Thrombin time measures the conversion of fibrinogen to fibrin by thrombin—the final step in the coagulation cascade (Fig. 13.5). The thrombin time is decreased in the presence of low concentrations of fibrinogen and thrombin. Heparin prolongs the thrombin time, whereas warfarin has little effect. Normal values are less than 10 seconds.

Activated clotting time

ACT measures the overall function of the coagulation system. It is used primarily to measure the adequacy of heparinization during CPB and protamine reversal of heparin following CPB. Prolonged ACTs may be due to heparin, low levels of coagulation factors, or thrombocytopenia. It is not particularly specific for platelet or factor deficiencies. Normal values are 110 to 140 seconds.

Bleeding time

Bleeding time measures platelet activity, including both platelet number and aggregation. The bleeding time becomes prolonged with platelet counts less than 50,000 per μL and in the presence of inhibitors of platelet aggregation such as aspirin. Normal values are less than 5 minutes. The bleeding time has not been shown to be predictive of postoperative bleeding and is no longer performed as a routine preoperatively.

Barrowcliffe TW, Cattaneo M, Podda GM, et al. New approaches for measuring coagulation. *Haemophilia* 2006;12(Suppl 3):76–81.

Drummond JC, Petrovich CT. Hemotherapy and hemostasis. In: Barash PG, Cullen BF, Stoelting RK, eds. *Clinical anesthesia,* 5th ed. Philadelphia: Lippincott, Williams & Wilkins, 2006:228–229.

Sconce EA, Kamali F. Appraisal of current vitamin K dosing algorithms for the reversal of over-anticoagulation with warfarin: the need for a more tailored dosing regimen. *Eur J Haematol* 2006;77(6):457–462.

Owens CD, Belkin M. Thrombosis and coagulation: operative management of the anticoagulated patient. *Surg Clin North Am* 2006;85(6):1179–1189.

A.21. How is the anticoagulant effect of low molecular weight heparin (LMWH) monitored?

There is no evidence that monitoring of LMWH dosage improves the clinical efficacy. In contrast, any overdose increases the risk of hemorrhage. Because the kidneys play a significant role in the elimination of LMWH, therapeutic use of these agents should be monitored with an anti–factor Xa assay, especially in patients who have renal insufficiency, are elderly, and have clinical conditions that increase the risk of bleeding.

Boneu B, de Moerloose P. How and when to monitor a patient treated with low molecular weight heparin? *Semin Thromb Hemost* 2001;27:519–522.

A.22. What is a thromboelastograph? What is a Sonoclot?

The thromboelastograph is an instrument that measures the development of viscoelastic strength of the blood clot over time. A rotating piston is suspended in a cuvette filled with heated blood. As clot formation proceeds, the rotation of the piston is affected and characteristic curves are generated (Fig. 13.6). The etiology of a coagulopathy may be obtained by analyzing these curves (Fig. 13.7). The Sonoclot similarly measures the development of clot viscoelastic strength. The Sonoclot piston moves vertically and measures the impedance to vibration at the tip of the probe. Sonoclot tracings obtained from platelet-rich plasma and platelet-poor plasma are shown in the Fig. 13.8.

Forestier F, Belisle S, Contant C, et al. Reproducibility and interchangeability of the thromboelastograph, Sonoclot and Hemochron activated coagulation time in cardiac surgery. *Can J Anaesth* 2001;48:902–910.

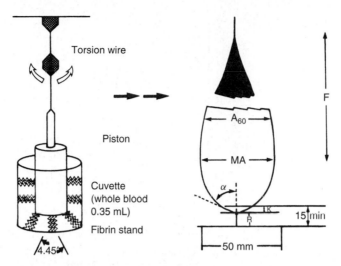

Figure 13.6 Production of normal thromboelastogram and measured parameters. R, reaction time, 7 to 14 minutes; K value, 3 to 7 minutes; α, clot formation rate, 40 degrees to 60 degrees; MA, maximum amplitude, 50 to 60 mm; A_{60}/ MA, amplitude 60 minutes after MA; whole blood clot lysis index, greater than 0.85; F, whole blood clot lysis time, greater than 300 minutes. (From Tumen KJ, Spiess BD, McCarthy RJ, et al. Effects of progressive blood loss on coagulation as measured by thromboelastography. Anesth Analg 1987;66:856–863.)

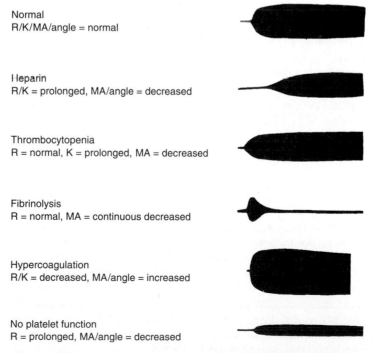

Normal
R/K/MA/angle = normal

Heparin
R/K = prolonged, MA/angle = decreased

Thrombocytopenia
R = normal, K = prolonged, MA = decreased

Fibrinolysis
R = normal, MA = continuous decreased

Hypercoagulation
R/K = decreased, MA/angle = increased

No platelet function
R = prolonged, MA/angle = decreased

Figure 13.7 Qualitative analysis of thromboelastograms.

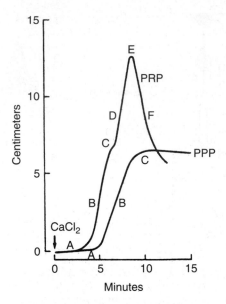

Figure 13.8 Sonoclot tracings of platelet-rich plasma (PRP) and platelet-poor plasma (PPP). *A*, lag period; *B*, primary wave; *C*, shoulder; *D*, secondary wave; *E*, peak; *F*, downward wave. (From Saleem A, Blifeld C, Saleh SA, et al. Viscoelastic measurement of clot formation: a new test of platelet function. *Ann Clin Lab Sci* 1983;13:115, with permission.)

Shore-Lesserson L. Coagulation monitoring. In: Kaplan JA, Reich DSN, Lake CL, et al. eds. *Kaplan's cardiac anesthesia*, 5th ed. Philadelphia: WB Saunders, 2006:573–577.

Vig S, Chitolie A, Bevan DH, et al. Thromboelastography: a reliable test. *Blood Coagul Fibrinolysis* 2001;12:555–561.

A.23. How does desmopressin aid hemostasis?

Desmopressin (1-deamino-8-D-arginine vasopressin [DDAVP]) is a vasopressin analog with more potency, longer lasting antidiuretic activity and much less vasoconstriction than the parent compound. Desmopressin increases von Willebrand's factor and factor VII activity in plasma. The von Willebrand's factor is found in subendothelial tissue, is released from platelets, and is in part responsible for platelet adhesion to damaged blood vessels. DDAVP was initially shown to significantly decrease postoperative bleeding. Although its routine use is not recommended, DDAVP may be beneficial in patients with end-stage renal disease, to increase von Willebrand's factor, that is decreased in those patients. The optimal dose of DDAVP is 0.3 μ per kg.

Spiess BD, Horrow J, Kaplan JA. Transfusion medicine and coagulation disorders. In: Kaplan JA, Reich DSN, Lake CL, et al. eds. *Kaplan's cardiac anesthesia*, 5th ed. Philadelphia: WB Saunders, 2006:969–970.

Kondo NI, Maddi R, Ewenstein BM, et al. Anticoagulation and hemostasis in cardiac surgical patients. *J Card Surg* 1994;9:443–461.

A.24. What is fibrinolysis?

Fibrinolysis is fibrin breakdown in thrombi. Plasmin, derived from plasminogen, is the enzyme involved in this process. Physiologic fibrinolysis involves clot remodeling and removal during the healing process. Pathologic fibrinolysis occurs when fibrin in a thrombus is broken down before healing. Although elevated concentrations of plasminogen activators are found during CPB, their half-lives are very short after bypass. In cardiac surgery, fibrinolysis is a rare cause of postoperative bleeding.

Spiess BD, Horrow J, Kaplan JA. Transfusion medicine and coagulation disorders. In: Kaplan JA, Reich DSN, Lake CL, et al. eds. *Kaplan's cardiac anesthesia*, 5th ed. Philadelphia: WB Saunders, 2006:947.

A.25. What is aminocaproic acid? What is tranexamic acid?

ε-Aminocaproic acid (Amicar) and tranexamic acid are analogues of lysine. Their primary mechanism of action is inhibition of plasminogen and plasmin, resulting in less breakdown of fibrinogen, fibrin (fibrinolysis), and other clotting components. These antifibrinolytic agents have been effective in treating coagulopathy in the setting of heart surgery, portocaval shunts, hematologic disorders such as aplastic anemia, abruptio placentae, hepatic cirrhosis, and neoplastic diseases.

Compared with placebo, use of tranexamic acid or aminocaproic acid in cardiac surgery has been shown to reduce blood loss by 30% to 49% as well as reduce homologous blood transfusion. Considering the low cost associated with aminocaproic acid therapy (<$12), many cardiac surgical centers use this agent routinely for uncomplicated open-heart procedures.

The standard intravenous preparation and dosage for cardiac surgery include 5 to 10 g of aminocaproic acid diluted and infused over 1 hour, followed by a continuous infusion at a rate of 1 g per hour. Higher infusion rates may be used. There are several adverse events that include thrombosis (early graft closure, myocardial ischemia and infarction), agranulocytosis, leukopenia, and thrombocytopenia. Although rare, bradycardia and mild reduction in blood pressure have also been reported.

Levi M, Cromheecke ME, de Jonge E, et al. Pharmacological strategies to decrease excessive blood loss in cardiac surgery: a meta-analysis of clinically relevant endpoints. *Lancet* 1999;354:1940–1947.

Spiess BD, Horrow J, Kaplan JA. Transfusion medicine and coagulation disorders. In: Kaplan JA, Reich DSN, Lake CL, et al. eds. *Kaplan's cardiac anesthesia*, 5th ed. Philadelphia: WB Saunders, 2006:970–971.

A.26. What is aprotinin?

Aprotinin is a complex polypeptide molecule belonging to the family of serine protease inhibitors that is extracted from bovine lung. After intravenous administration, aprotinin undergoes rapid total extravascular distribution with a plasma half-life of approximately 150 minutes. It is filtered by the glomeruli and reabsorbed by the proximal tubules. The terminal half-life is approximately 10 hours. The basis for its efficacy is not fully understood but consists of a

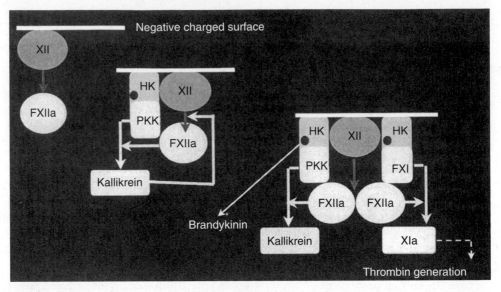

Figure 13.9 Contact activation and the role of the kallikrein system. XII, factor 12; XIIa, activated factor 12; XI, factor 11; XIa, activated factor 11; HK, high molecular weight kininogen; PKK, prekallikrein. (From slide set no. 3 tryaslol slide library [online]. Bayer, 2000. Available at http://www.trasylol.com/slides.htm, with permission.)

complex activation-interaction of the following systems: kallikrein resulting in kinin generation, complement and inflammatory pathways, coagulation (intrinsic and extrinsic), fibrinolytic, angiotensin, and others not yet determined (Fig. 13.9). Initial contact between blood elements and the nonendothelialized surface of the CPB circuit promote contact activation of both humoral and cellular inflammatory processes. The coagulation system may be the first to be activated by contact generating factor XIIa from factor XII, which then interacts with prekallikrein and high molecular weight kininogen (HMWK) to form kallikrein as well as promote the activation of the other coagulation factors. Once activated, kallikrein functions to stimulate and accelerate the generation of bradykinin from HMWK, factor XIIa, angiotensin, and complement activation. Factor XIIa, in turn, also interacts with fibrinogen to produce plasmin (Fig. 13.10).

Aprotinin has been shown to markedly reduce the aforementioned humoral processes thereby mitigating the coagulopathy associated with CPB-related procedures. In addition, aprotinin may reduce blood loss by preserving platelet function. The mechanism of this relates to preservation of platelet surface glycoproteins (IIb/IIIa), which is necessary for platelet-fibrinogen interaction and clot formation. The antiinflammatory properties of aprotinin (both cellular and humoral) have been shown in animal and in some human studies; however, clinical outcome trials addressing this effect have not been conducted. Clinical trials comparing Aprotinin to placebo and/or to Amicar have consistently shown greater efficacy related to reduction in blood loss and transfusions of blood elements.

Concerns regarding prothrombotic potentials, including myocardial infarction and renal dysfunction, have been controversial. However, Mangano et al. showed that there is a significant increased risk of cardiac and renal morbidity and mortality when aprotinin is used as antifibronolytic in patients undergoing coronary bypass surgery. In contrast, use of the other antifibrinolytics (Amicar and transamanic acid) do not appear to have nephrotoxic or myocardial ischemic effects. Consequently, the use of aprotinin in coronary bypass surgery has markedly

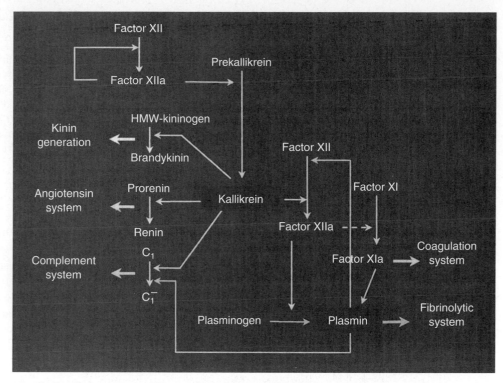

Figure 13.10 Involvement of the various components of coagulation including the coagulation factors, kallikrein system, complement activation, kinin generation, angiotensin system, and the fibrinolytic system. C_1, complement; HMW, high molecular weight. (From slide set no. 3 tryaslol slide library [online]. Bayer, 2000. Available at http://www.trasylol.com/slides.htm, with permission.)

decreased in the United States. Rarely, if aprotinin is used in patients with protein C or S deficiency, they may experience life-threatening thrombotic events shortly after protamine neutralization of heparin. In summary, the routine use of aprotinin in cardiac surgery is not recommended. On the other hand, aprotinin may be beneficial in high-risk patients undergoing procedures such as complex valvular replacements, reoperation, aortic surgery requiring deep hypothermic circulatory arrest, and in patients with bleeding disorders or belonging to the Jehovah's Witness religious group.

Another important aspect of aprotinin use is the type of reagent used to monitor adequacy of heparinization (activated clotting time [ACT]). Because aprotinin is a serine protease inhibitor, it interacts with antithrombin III to inhibit the action of all intrinsic and common pathway factors resulting in prolongation of measures of coagulation such as ACT. Kaolin absorbs approximately 98% of aprotinin and any intrinsic antithrombin effect that aprotinin has is eliminated. Therefore, kaolin-ACT is the recommended agent to monitor anticoagulation during CPB when aprotinin is used (ACT should be >480 seconds). If celite-ACT is used, the ACT value should be more than 750 seconds before initiation of CPB.

Aprotinin has a fair safety profile but serious anaphylaxis or shock can occur. This risk is increased in patients who are reexposed to aprotinin within 6 weeks. Most of the cases reported occurred within 200 days of exposure. It is recommended that a test dose of 1 mL be given, when possible, before cannulation for instituting bypass. Whether use of histamine antagonists or steroid lessens the incidence of aprotinin-associated anaphylaxis is not known.

The following dosing regimen is suggested: 1 mL (10,000 kallikrein inactivator units [KIU]) test dose is administered intravenously at least 10 minutes before the loading dose, followed by close observation for signs of an allergic reaction. Before initiation of CPB, a loading dose of 2 million KIU should then be given over 20 to 30 minutes. An additional 2 million KIU dose is added to the priming solution. The maintenance dose is a constant infusion of 500,000 KIU per hour for the duration of surgery. It may be beneficial and cost effective to continue the infusion of the remaining amount of the drug while the patient is transferred and recovering in the intensive care unit (ICU). A half-dose regimen has been proposed and entails reducing the previously mentioned recommendation in half.

Abe K, Moriya H, Landis RC, et al. The antithrombotic and antiinflammatory mechanisms of action of aprotinin. *Ann Thorac Surg* 2001;72:2169–2175.

Dobkowski WB, Murkin JM. A risk-benefit assessment of aprotinin in cardiac surgical procedures. *Drug Saf* 1998;18:21–41.

Karkouti K, Beattie WS, Dattilo KM, et al. A propensity score case-control comparison of aprotinin and tranexamic acid in high-transfusion-risk cardiac surgery. *Transfusion* 2006;46(3):327–338.

Mangano DT, Tudor IC, Dietzel C. Multicenter Study of Perioperative Ischemia Research Group. Ischemia Research and Education Foundation. The risk associated with aprotinin in cardiac surgery. Multicenter Study. *N Engl J Med* 2006;354(4):353–365.

Murkin JM. Attenuation of neurologic injury during cardiac surgery. *Ann Thorac Surg* 2001;72:S1838–S1844.

Spiess BD, Horrow J, Kaplan JA. Transfusion medicine and coagulation disorders. In: Kaplan JA, Reich DSN, Lake CL, et al. eds. *Kaplan's cardiac anesthesia*, 5th ed. Philadelphia: WB Saunders, 2006:971–972.

B. Preoperative Evaluation and Preparation

B.1. Interpret the hemodynamic findings of this patient.

The patient has an adequate blood pressure; however, this appears to be maintained through compensatory mechanisms, including an increase in both arterial resistance (systemic vascular resistance [SVR]) and heart rate (HR). The pulmonary artery (PA) systolic pressure is consistent with pulmonary hypertension arising most likely from either chronic mitral valvular disease (stenosis or insufficiency) or decreased compliance of the left ventricle (as it may occur in ischemia). Both the PAD and the PAOP suggest that the left ventricular end-diastolic pressure—a correlate of left ventricular preload—is within the normal limits. Keep in mind, that pressure measurements do not correlate with volume status unless the compliance of the chamber (the relation between pressure and volume in diastole) is constant. Therefore, a PAOP of 14 mm Hg could represent hypovolemia, normovolemia, or hypervolemia, depending on the compliance of the left ventricle (decreased, normal, or increased, respectively). A CVP of 23 mm Hg is suggestive of right ventricular or biventricular dysfunction, tricuspid stenosis or insufficiency, or obstruction and compression of the right atrium (RA). The cardiac output (CO) is inadequate. The derived stroke volume (SV) of 22 mL (CO/HR), combined with the other derangements (elevated CVP strongly reflect right heart dysfunction: the right heart cannot advance the volume to the left side. Taking into consideration of the patient's overall presentation (physical examination and laboratory findings), the differential diagnosis includes right ventricular ischemia and/or infarction, pulmonary embolism, atrial or ventricular septal defect causing volume overload of the right ventricle (RV) (most likely left-to-right), and cardiac tamponade. An echocardiogram should be performed to assist in the diagnostic process and clinical management.

Fontes ML, Bellows W, Ngo L, et al. McSPI Research Group. Assessment of ventricular function in critically ill patients: limitations of pulmonary artery catheterization. *J Cardiothorac Vasc Anesth* 1999;13:1–8.

B.2. How would you treat the low output status of this patient?

Although the heart rate (HR) is increased, it may be unwise to attempt to normalize it before correcting the stroke volume (SV). The latter is a function of the preload (end-diastolic volume [EDV]), the afterload (the afterload-dependent end-systolic volume [ESV] that remains inside the left ventricle at the end of systole), and the contractile status of the myocardium. Whereas the preload of the right heart may be excessive (CVP = 23 mm Hg), the preload of the left heart may not be adequate despite a PAOP of 14 mm Hg. While waiting for the echocardiogram to be performed, a fluid bolus can be attempted. If there is a positive response (i.e., the blood pressure and or the cardiac output increase), additional fluid bolus can be administered until the limit of the preload reserve has been reached (operating on the flat end portion of the Frank Starling's curve). In the setting of right ventricular failure, it is customary to fluid load the patient maintaining the CVP in the 1920s. It is important to note that fluid challenge alone will not improve cardiac performance without addressing the contractility and the afterload that, in this patient, appear to be deranged. Because there is no knowledge of the exact etiology of the low output state, it would be rational to institute inotropic support With regard to the afterload, both systemic and pulmonary afterload are elevated. On the right side, pulmonary artery (PA) hypertension can be improved with nitroglycerin or nitroprusside but the associated systemic hypotension would prohibit their use. In fact, most vasodilators with the exception of nitric oxide would compromise the systemic pressures. At the same time, if the compliance of the right ventricle (RV) is presumed to be decreased, then the increased CVP does not necessarily correlate with adequate preload of the RV. Alternatively, an inotrope that has vasodilatory properties (phosphodiesterase inhibitors: milrinone or amrinone, or dobutamine) would be a better choice. In summary, a rational management of the hemodynamic findings presented would include administering fluid (crystalloid or blood products as indicated), prescribing inotropic support, obtaining an echocardiogram, and addressing the other systemic complications (pulmonary, renal, and coagulation).

Ghobashy A, Fontes ML, Hines RL. Cardiogenic shock. In: Murray MJ, Coursin DB, Pearl RG, et al. eds. *Critical care medicine: perioperative management*, 2nd ed. Philadelphia: Lippincott Williams & Wilkins, 2002.

Levy JH, Tanaka K, Bailey JM, et al. Postoperative cardiovascular management. In: Kaplan JA, Reich DSN, Lake CL, et al. eds. *Kaplan's cardiac anesthesia*, 5th ed. Philadelphia: WB Saunders, 2006:1061–1086.

B.3. How would you evaluate this patient's coagulation status?

A complete blood cell count and a complete coagulation panel should be performed. Assuming that both the hematocrit and the platelet function are adequate, attention should be directed to the elevated PT and the activated partial thromboplastin time (aPTT). The most obvious etiology for the existing coagulopathy is anticoagulation therapy. The patient has a prosthetic valve and it would be appropriate to surmise that she has been taking anticoagulants. The most common agent to be used 4 days after surgery is warfarin (Coumadin). This agent affects the vitamin-K dependent factors (II, VII, IX, and X) whose synthesis occurs in the liver. Measuring the PT and or the international normalized ratio (INR) assesses the status of its anticoagulant effect. Why is the aPTT also elevated? This coagulation measure reflects the function of the following factors: V, VIII, IX, X, XI, XII, prothrombin, and fibrinogen. It can also be presumed that the elevated aPTT is due to anticoagulant therapy (e.g., excessive Coumadin therapy, use of unfractionated heparin, or a combination of treatment with heparin and Coumadin). The latter approach is standard practice in cardiac surgery for patients requiring prolonged anticoagulation (e.g., valvular replacement) and can account for elevations of both the PT and the aPTT. Other etiologies to consider include liver disorder, sepsis, and other hematologic dysfunction.

Keller C, Matzdorff AC, Kemkes-Matthes B. Pharmacology of warfarin and clinical implication. *Semin Thromb Hemost* 1999;25:13–16.

Spiess BD, Horrow J, Kaplan JA. Transfusion medicine and coagulation disorders. In: Kaplan JA, Reich DSN, Lake CL, et al. eds. *Kaplan's cardiac anesthesia*, 5th ed. Philadelphia: WB Saunders, 2006:947, 966–968.

B.4. What do fresh frozen plasma (FFP) and cryoprecipitate contain?

FFP contains the labile factors V and VIII as well as the stable coagulation factors (II, VII, IX, X, XI). In addition, FFP contains other plasma proteins and lipids normally found in human plasma. Cryoprecipitate is derived by thawing FFP at 4°C (39.2°F). It contains factors VIII and XIII, von Willebrand's factor, and fibrinogen.

Drummond JC, Petrovich CT. Hemotherapy and hemostasis. In: Barash PG, Cullen BF, Stoelting RK, eds. *Clinical anesthesia*, 5th ed. Philadelphia: Lippincott Williams & Wilkins, 2006:221.

B.5. What are the indications for transfusing fresh frozen plasma (FFP), platelet concentrate, and cryoprecipitate?

Blood usually coagulates appropriately when coagulation factor concentrations are at least 20% to 30% of normal and when fibrinogen levels are greater than 75 mg per dL. Although laboratory values such as PT and partial thromboplastin time (PTT) may be abnormal, The American Society of Anesthesiologist Task Force on Blood Component Therapy discourages conventional use of FFP for perioperative treatment of bleeding because there are few clinical circumstances whereby coagulopathy arises from factor deficiency. Although massive blood replacement can produce prolongation of PT and/or PTT, the task force states that a true dilutional coagulopathy does not ordinarily occur until more than 100% of the patient's blood volume has been replaced. It supports the use of FFP in patients having vascular bleeding with PT and PTT values greater than 1.5 times the laboratory's normal value. FFP should be administrated in doses calculated to achieve a minimum of 30% of plasma factor concentration (i.e., 10 to 15 mL/kg of FFP).

Recommended indications for FFP:
- Replacement of factor deficiencies
- Reversal of Coumadin effect
- Massive blood transfusions

- Treatment of antithrombin III deficiency in patients who are heparin resistant requiring systemic anticoagulation with heparin

In 1994 the College of American Pathologists recommended platelet transfusions after CPB in patients with normal coagulation values and platelet count below 100,000 per μL when major unexplained bleeding occurs. Transfusion of one platelet concentrate will increase the platelet count by approximately 5000 to 10,000 per μL in the average adult. The usual therapeutic dose is one platelet concentrate per 10-kg body weight.

Platelet concentrate is indicated in the following:
- Active bleeding associated with thrombocytopenia
- Massive blood transfusions

The American Society of Anesthesiologist's Task Force on Blood Component Therapy recommends the administration of cryoprecipitate for

- Prophylaxis in nonbleeding perioperative or peripartum patients with congenital fibrinogen deficiencies or von Willebrand's disease unresponsive to 1-deamino-8-D-arginine vasopressin (DDAVP) (whenever possible, these decisions should be made in consultation with the patient's hematologist)
- Bleeding patients with von Willebrand's disease
- Correction of microvascular bleeding in massively transfused patients with fibrinogen concentrations less than 80 to 100 mg per dL

One unit of cryoprecipitate per 10-kg body weight raises plasma fibrinogen concentration approximately 50 mg per dL in the absence of continued consumption or massive bleeding. Bleeding following cardiac surgery without demonstrable abnormalities of coagulation is not considered to be an indication for transfusion of FFP, platelets, or cryoprecipitate.

Dietrich W, Luth JU, Kormann J, et al. Intraoperative blood requirements and allogeneic blood transfusion in cardioanesthesia. Data analysis of 7729 patients in 12 cardiac surgical clinics. *Anaesthesist* 1999;48:876–883.

Kakkar N, Kaur R, Dhanoa J. Improvement in fresh frozen plasma transfusion practice: results of an outcome audit. *Transfus Med* 2004;14(3):231–235.

Napolitano LM. Current status of blood component therapy in surgical critical care. *Curr Opin Crit Care* 2004;10(5):311–317.

Nuttall GA, Stehling LC, Beighley CM, et al. American Society of Anesthesiologists Committee on Transfusion Medicine. Current transfusion practices of members of the American society of anesthesiologists: a survey. *Anesthesiology* 2003;99(6):1433–1443.

Stover EP, Siegel LC, Parks R, et al. Institutions of the Multicenter Study of Perioperative Ischemia Research Group. Variability in transfusion practice for coronary artery bypass surgery persists despite national consensus guidelines: a 24-institution study. Institutions of the Multicenter Study of Perioperative Ischemia Research Group. *Anesthesiology* 1998;88:327–333.

Wilhelmi M, Franke U, Cohnert T, et al. Coronary artery bypass grafting surgery without the routine application of blood products: is it feasible? *Eur J Cardiothorac Surg* 2001;19:657–661.

B.6. What are the complications associated with blood component transfusions?

Complications associated with transfusions of blood elements include transmission of infectious agents (e.g., hepatitis, human immunodeficiency virus [HIV] infection), hemolytic and nonhemolytic transfusion reactions, immunosuppression, anaphylactic or anaphylactoid reactions, and alloimmunization to platelet-specific antigens and the Rh antigen (resulting from erythrocyte contamination because they are stored at room temperature). Platelets in particular may contain proliferating bacteria. Finally, in the immunosuppressed, graft-versus-host effects may occur following platelet transfusion.

Ford SA, Kam PC, Baldo BA, et al. Anaphylactic or anaphylactoid reactions in patients undergoing cardiac surgery. *J Cardiothorac Vasc Anesth* 2001;15:684–688.

Frere MC, Rapaille A, Bouillenne C, et al. Analysis of 516 reports of reactions after the transfusion of labile blood products. *Transfus Clin Biol* 2001;8;333–342.

Lacritz EM, Sullen GA, Aberle-Grasse J. Estimated risk of transmission of the human immunodeficiency virus by screened blood in the United States. *N Engl J Med* 1995;333: 1721–1725.

Nightingale SD. Department of Health and Human Services Advisory Committee on Blood Safety and Availability. Universal WBC reduction. *Transfusion* 2001;41:1306–1309.

B.7. What is the risk of acquiring human immunodeficiency virus (HIV) from blood exposure?

The risk of HIV infection in the United States is 1/1,500,000 to 1/2,000,000 per unit transfused. However, with the implementation of donor screening tests for HIV-1 antigen, there is an expectation of preventing up to 25% of the window period cases (the period between viral infection and its detection by tests for the presence of antibodies). Perhaps the immunoviral agent most transmitted by blood transfusion is cytomegalovirus.

Drummond JC, Petrovich CT. Hemotherapy and hemostasis. In: Barash PG, Cullen BF, Stoelting RK, eds. *Clinical anesthesia*, 5th ed. Philadelphia: Lippincott Williams & Wilkins, 2006:209–210.

Goodnough LT, Brecher ME, Kanter MH, et al. Transfusion medicine: first of 2 parts—blood transfusion. *N Engl J Med* 1999;340:438–447.

Napolitano LM. Current status of blood component therapy in surgical critical care. *Curr Opin Crit Care* 2004;10(5):311–317.

Lacritz EM, Sullen GA, Aberle-Grasse J, et al. Estimated risk of transmission of the human immunodeficiency virus by screened blood in the United States. *N Engl J Med* 1995;333:1721–1725.

Lowe KC, Farrell K, Ferguson EM, et al. Current perceived risks of transfusion in the UK and relevance to the future acceptance of blood substitutes. *Artif Cells Blood Substit Immobil Biotechnol* 2001;29:179–189.

Reine NJ. Infection and blood transfusion: a guide to donor screening. *Clin Tech Small Anim Pract* 2004;19(2):68–74.

B.8. In what situation might aminocaproic acid improve hemostasis?

ε-Aminocaproic acid (EACA) inhibits plasminogen activation by binding to plasminogen. It inhibits primary fibrinolysis, which is caused by excessive plasminogen activation by endogenous plasminogen activators (e.g., urokinase, tissue-type plasminogen activator) occasionally seen in urinary tract bleeding and subarachnoid hemorrhage from an intracranial aneurysm. Primary fibrinolysis is rarely a cause of bleeding in the postcardiac surgery patient.

Butterworth J, James RL, Lin YA, et al. Gender does not influence epsilon-aminocaproic acid concentrations in adults undergoing cardiopulmonary bypass. *Anesth Analg* 2001;92:1384–1390.

Chauhan S, Kumar BA, Rao BH, et al. Efficacy of aprotinin, epsilon aminocaproic acid, or combination in cyanotic heart disease. *Ann Thorac Surg* 2000;70:1308–1312.

Ray MJ, O'Brien MF. Comparison of epsilon aminocaproic acid and low-dose aprotinin in cardiopulmonary bypass: efficiency, safety and cost. *Ann Thorac Surg* 2001;71:838–843.

B.9. Assuming that the patient has cardiac tamponade, how would you prepare this patient for surgery?

As with any patient undergoing surgery, the following steps should be taken: first, a complete review of the patient's history, physical examination, and laboratory findings are mandated; second, key areas of concern should be identified and appropriate steps taken to address them; third, an anesthetic plan that is tailored to cardiac tamponade is devised; last, communication with the respective medical (surgeons, nurses, perfusionist, blood bank) and paramedical staff to ensure readiness and teamwork. The patient's presentation suggests that she is in some degree of respiratory distress. Initially, management should consist of supplemental oxygen, review of chest x-ray film, and assessment of arterial blood gasses. Shortness of breath and the inability to lie supine are frequent symptoms in patients having cardiac tamponade physiology, and every effort should be made to provide comfort and lessen the associated emotional stress. Positive pressure ventilation should be avoided at all cost unless the clinical picture indicates that the patient will have a cardiac arrest. The persistent oliguria most likely reflects prerenal or renal (acute tubular necrosis) process secondary to reduced cardiac output and the associated vasoconstrictive state. As described in the previous answer, optimization of hemodynamics should also improve the renal function. Whereas some may administer diuretics in this setting, such management is strongly discouraged. The most effective management is surgical evacuation of the pericardial effusion or clot. The hematologic issues include elevated PT and activated partial thromboplastin time (aPTT), blood loss, and the potential for further blood loss perioperatively. The coagulopathy should be corrected appropriately, the patient's hematocrit and platelets should be checked and treated accordingly, and sufficient blood (four to six units) will be required in the operating room before commencing surgery.

Ghobashy A, Fontes ML, Hines RL. Cardiogenic shock. In: Murray MJ, Coursin DB, Pearl RG, et al. eds. *Critical care medicine: perioperative management*, 2nd ed. Philadelphia: Lippincott Williams & Wilkins, 2002.

Levy JH, Tanaka K, Bailey JM, et al. Postoperative cardiovascular management. In: Kaplan JA, Reich DSN, Lake CL, et al. eds. *Kaplan's cardiac anesthesia*, 5th ed. Philadelphia: WB Saunders, 2006:1079–1080.

B.10. What premedication would you prescribe?

None. Although it is important to reduce the emotional stress preoperatively, it would be unwise to administer any type of anxiolytic in the setting of cardiac tamponade. The most effective approach is communication with the patient. Often, the physical appearance and the hemodynamics can be misguiding and catastrophic consequences can arise from premedicating these patients. A state of marked sympathoadrenal activation is supporting perfusion to vital organs. By partially blocking this compensatory effect with an anxiolytic, cardiovascular collapse may ensue, and most efforts to resuscitate the patient would probably fail. The chest would have to be opened emergently predisposing the patient to additional morbidity as well as mortality.

C. Intraoperative Management

C.1. How would you monitor this patient during transport to the operating room? What emergency drugs would you bring with you?

The patient must be under astute observation and the vital signs must be continuously assessed, including invasive monitoring of systemic blood pressure, electrocardiogram, and oxygen saturation. In addition, emergency cardioactive and vasoactive drugs should be available during transport:

- Oxygen: increase the FIO_2 as needed. All necessary equipment for intubation should be present (laryngoscope and several blades, bag-mask units, and adult-size endotracheal tube)
- DC cardioversion unit: in case of tachyarrhythmias
- Phenylephrine: dose: bolus, 0.1 to 0.5 mg; infusion, 25 to 125 μg per minute
- Epinephrine: dose 0.01 to 0.1 μg/kg/minute
- Calcium chloride: dose 2 to 4 mg per kg
- Lidocaine: 1 to 2 mg per kg
- Atropine: 0.01 mg per kg

C.2. In this patient, what hemodynamic effects would occur from intravenous induction with ketamine, thiopental, fentanyl, propofol, etomidate, or midazolam?

Ketamine

After intravenous administration, ketamine (1 mg/kg) has a rapid onset of action and achieves a peak plasma concentration in less than 1 minute. It also possesses a short duration of action. After the initial dose, patients may remain unconscious for 10 to 15 minutes, but the analgesic effect (somatic greater than visceral) persists for an additional 30 minutes or longer. Some of the hemodynamic effects of ketamine may include small increases in blood pressure, heart rate, cardiac output, and myocardial oxygen demand. This response is mediated by a direct central sympathetic stimulation and by inhibition of norepinephrine uptake into the postganglionic sympathetic nerve endings. Ketamine has also been shown to have intrinsic depressant properties on the myocardium. In clinical conditions whereby norepinephrine stores are reduced, and in the presence of preexisting cardiac dysfunction (mechanical or myocardial), administration of ketamine can produce hemodynamic depression.

Thiopental

Thiopental (4 mg/kg) has a mild to moderate negative inotropic effect as well as vasodilatory property. The hemodynamic response relates to the dose, coexisting diseases (hypertension, ventricular dysfunction), age, intravascular volume, and intactness of autonomic sympathetic responses. Generally, doses of 1 to 2 mg per kg do not cause significant hemodynamic disturbance; however, in patients with cardiac tamponade, thiopental should not be used for induction. These patients are, literally, on the "edge" of cardiovascular collapse.

Fentanyl

Fentanyl does not possess any depressant effects on myocardial contractility but because of its vagotonic effect (decreases in HR) and mild sympatholytic effect (central sympathetic outflow), blood pressure may decrease. This response may be more profound in shock or preshock states, and when fentanyl is used concomitantly with other induction agents (benzodiazepines, thiopental, propofol).

Propofol

Propofol produces very similar effects as thiopental. It can cause significant reduction in systemic pressures (>30%), and there have been several reports of cardiovascular arrest in both adults and children following inductions with propofol. Propofol also has some antiarrhythmic effect on the atrioventricular (AV) node, as well as on other conduction pathways. It should be used with caution when other agents that slow down AV nodal conduction are present (calcium channel blockers, β-blockers, digoxin). As with thiopental, the use of propofol for induction in cardiac tamponade is strongly disfavored.

Etomidate

Etomidate has a very favorable hemodynamic profile and is the preferred agent to be used during induction when cardiovascular collapse is anticipated. With an induction dose (0.2 to 0.3 mg/kg), etomidate may cause a slight decrease in mean arterial pressure but such changes are not attributable to myocardial depression, as is typical of propofol and sodium thiopental. Pain at the injection site and involuntary muscle movements are the most common adverse events noted with etomidate. It also appears to reduce seizure threshold and enhance its duration when used during electroconvulsion therapy.

Midazolam

Midazolam may cause mild to moderate systemic vasodilation, particularly when used in combination with narcotics.

Overall, of the agents discussed, etomidate would be the preferred agent for induction followed by ketamine, and/or fentanyl; whereas, thiopental and propofol would be the least desired.

White PF, Romero G. Nonopioid intravenous anesthesia. In: Barash PG, Cullen BF, Stoelting RK, eds. *Clinical anesthesia*, 5th ed. Philadelphia: Lippincott Williams & Wilkins, 2006:334–352.

C.3. Describe the induction process for cardiac tamponade.

The patient should have standard monitors placed as well as invasive monitors, including indwelling arterial access for beat-to-beat monitoring of systemic arterial pressures and for obtaining blood gases. This patient has a pulmonary artery catheter (PAC) *in situ*; however, its usefulness in this setting remains debatable. The actual induction should proceed ONLY in the presence of a surgical team that is ready and gowned and after the patient has been completely prepared and draped. The choice of induction agents is limited to narcotics, muscle relaxant (depolarizing or nondepolarizing), and either etomidate or ketamine. Regardless of the induction technique, the anesthesiologist should expect, and be prepared to manage, ensuing circulatory collapse.

Levy JH, Tanaka K, Bailey JM, et al. Postoperative cardiovascular management. In: Kaplan JA, Reich DSN, Lake CL, et al. eds. *Kaplan's cardiac anesthesia*, 5th ed. Philadelphia: WB Saunders, 2006:1079–1080.

C.4. Following induction and intubation, the systemic blood pressure decreased to 55/30 mm Hg. Describe the clinical events accounting for this perturbation, and the management steps required for resuscitation.

Cardiac tamponade is caused by significant pericardial pressure from accumulating pericardial contents (fluid, blood, and blood clots) that impede chamber filing resulting in a low CO state. The precipitous fall in blood pressure observed with induction can be accounted for by the following: first; most induction agents will have negative hemodynamic effects that are either direct or indirect; second, sympatholysis reduces arterial resistance as well as chronotropy and inotropy of the heart; third, the physiologic consequences of switching from negative pressure ventilation to positive pressure ventilation will further reduce cardiac filling by increasing intrathoracic pressure and afterload; and lastly, placing the patient in a supine position will also compromise atrial and ventricular preload (i.e., hydrostatic effects, loss of diaphragmatic motion, and mediastinal structures weighing on the heart).

The management of hypotension will require use of vasoactive drugs, cardioactive drugs, and/or fluid challenge. Reducing inspiratory positive pressure (i.e., lowering tidal volume or switching from ventilator-delivered breaths to hand ventilation) may also improve the hemodynamic status, by facilitating filling. These would be merely temporizing measures; surgical relief of tamponade would be the definitive treatment of this problem.

Levy JH, Tanaka K, Bailey JM, et al. Postoperative cardiovascular management. In: Kaplan JA, Reich DSN, Lake CL, et al. eds. *Kaplan's cardiac anesthesia*, 5th ed. Philadelphia: WB Saunders, 2006:1079–1080.

C.5. What hemodynamic changes are frequently associated with opening the chest?

Chest opening normalizes the pressure relation between the pericardium and the heart chambers, therefore relieving the tamponade and its hemodynamic effects. Unless the myocardium has suffered injury or is stunned, the expected hemodynamic changes include drastic improvement in both blood pressure and stroke volume. Most of the vasoactive and cardioactive agents being administered can be quickly weaned. In addition, oxygenation, acid-base status, and renal function (urine output) tend to improve significantly.

C.6. What is myocardial stunning? What is myocardial hibernation?

The myocardium can exhibit segmental dysfunction or a generalized decrease in function related to injury (i.e., ischemia and infarction). It has also been noted that myocardial function can be coupled or uncoupled with tissue perfusion. For example, following a period of oxygen deprivation and restoration of flow, the affected myocardium can resume normal function, or have diminished function, or no function (dysfunction). The term myocardial stunning represents a state of uncoupling between function and flow whereby myocardial flow is normal but function is diminished or absent. In the setting of cardiac surgery, myocardial stunning can be a cause of ventricular dysfunction that generally resolves within the first 6 to 8 hours post-CPB. During this period, inotropic support has been shown to be effective. Myocardial hibernation, on the other hand, is a myocardial process that manifests after weeks or months and denotes a condition whereby both myocardial function and flow are reduced (perfusion and function are coupled). Perhaps this is an adaptive process, that allows the myocytes to lower their metabolic activity and oxygen consumption, to survive during states of oxygen deprivation. The definitive diagnosis of stunning and hibernation may be difficult to make, because regional myocardial blood flow is difficult to assess or quantify clinically. Therefore, most cases of stunning and hibernation require a retrospective analysis. First, segmental myocardial dysfunction must be established; second, myocardial blood flow should be restored by revascularization (surgical, pharmacologic, or angioplasty/stenting); and third, improvement of regional function should follow revascularization.

D'Ancona G, Donias HW, Bergsland J, et al. Myocardial stunning after off-pump coronary artery bypass grafting: safeguards and pitfalls. *Ann Thorac Surg* 2001;72:2182–2183.

Grocott HP, Stafford-Smith M. Organ protection during cardiopulmonary bypass. In: Kaplan JA, Reich DSN, Lake CL, et al. eds. *Kaplan's cardiac anesthesia*, 5th ed. Philadelphia: WB Saunders, 2006:1004.

Lorusso R, La Canna G, Ceconi C, et al. Long-term results of coronary artery bypass grafting procedure in the presence of left ventricular dysfunction and hibernating myocardium. *Eur J Cardiothorac Surg* 2001;20:937–948.

Shah BR, Velazquez E, Shaw LK, et al. Revascularization improves survival in ischemic cardiomyopathy regardless of electrocardiographic criteria for prior small-to-medium myocardial infarcts. *Am Heart J* 2002;143:111–117.

Watzinger N, Saeed M, Wendland MF, et al. Myocardial viability: magnetic resonance assessment of functional reserve and tissue characterization. *J Cardiovasc Magn Reson* 2001;3:195–208.

D. Postoperative Management

D.1. How would you manage hypertension in the intensive care unit (ICU)?

The management of hypertension depends on its etiology. Rather than administering antihypertensive agents indiscriminately, the clinician should exclude the following conditions as causality of hypertension: hypoxemia, hypercarbia, acid-base derangements, and pain. The occurrence of hypertension is a common phenomenon during the first several hours in the ICU. In most cases, the etiology is uncertain and probably represents a state of marked sympathoadrenal activation. Once correctable causes of hypertension have been addressed, antihypertensive therapy can be achieved with a variety of agents. Most often, sodium nitroprusside is used because of its potent effect and titratability. Because the underlying mechanism of the hypertension involves endogenous release of norepinephrine (with minimal epinephrine), the most rational agents to use are the β-blockers. Labetalol antagonizes both α- and β-adrenergic receptors and is an effective antihypertensive agent. Alternatively, metoprolol, atenolol, esmolol, or propranolol can be used particularly if the hypertension is associated with tachycardia. Unfortunately, these agents are used infrequently because of theoretical concerns of myocardial depression and bradycardia. Current cardiology practice strongly endorses the use of β-blockers in the setting of moderate and severe ventricular dysfunction. In addition, the cardioprotective effects of β-blockers have been shown in several perioperative trials whereby the incidence of myocardial injury and mortality (up to 2 years postoperatively) are significantly reduced in patients treated perioperatively with β-blockers.

Kotlyar E, Macdonald PS, Keogh AM, et al. Optimization of left ventricular function with carvedilol before high-risk cardiac surgery. *J Heart Lung Transplant* 2001;20:1129–1131.

Leslie J, Brister N, Levy JH, et al. Treatment of postoperative hypertension after coronary artery bypass surgery. Double-blind comparison of intravenous isradipine and sodium nitroprusside. *Circulation* 1994;90(5 Pt 2):II256–II261.

Lucas WJ, Boysen PG. Antihypertensive agents following cardiac surgery. *Crit Care Med* 1997;25:1770–1771.

D.2. When would it be appropriate to extubate this patient?

The timing of extubation depends on the following:

- Clinical stability (stable hemodynamics without need for significant inotropic or vasoactive support)

- Intact neurologic function (alertness and ability to comprehend and execute simple verbal commands)
- Adequate pulmonary function (acceptable arterial blood gases and acid-base status and adequate weaning parameters—tidal volume, respiratory rate, vital capacity, and inspiratory effort)
- Normal body temperature and neuromuscular function (reverse paralysis if necessary)
- Normal coagulation (bleeding <s60 mL/hour and normalization of coagulation parameters)

Following relief of tamponade, most patients can be extubated as early as possible assuming that the previously listed criteria have been met.

CHAPTER 14

Heart Transplantation and Subsequent Noncardiac Surgery

DAVY C.H. CHENG • JEFF T. GRANTON

A 41-YEAR-OLD MAN

with a history of idiopathic dilated cardiomyopathy is admitted to the cardiac care unit in a quaternary cardiac center for potential heart transplantation assessment. He has known systolic dysfunction, with an ejection fraction of less than 25% on transthoracic echocardiogram. Recurrent ventricular arrhythmias necessitated insertion of an implantable cardioverter defibrillator (ICD). Right heart catheterization revealed a pulmonary vascular resistance of 4 Wood units. Recently, his symptoms have been worsening and progressed to New York Heart Association (NYHA) class IV. During this hospital admission his clinical status continued to deteriorate necessitating the initiation of inotropic support and the insertion of an intraaortic balloon pump (IABP). He is subsequently placed on the transplant list, with high priority. However, due to further deterioration, consideration is being given to the insertion of a left ventricular assist device (LVAD) to maintain adequate end-organ perfusion while waiting for a donor heart to become available.

A. Medical Disease and Differential Diagnosis

1. What are the common diagnoses requiring adult heart transplantation?
2. What are the criteria and contraindications for recipient selection?
3. What are the criteria for donor heart selection?
4. What are the principles of perioperative donor management?
5. What are the risk factors associated with posttransplant mortality?
6. What is the sequence of surgical anastomoses in heart transplantation?
7. When is combined heart/lung transplant indicated? What are the important differences?
8. What are the medical and surgical alternatives to cardiac transplantation?
9. What is the role for ventricular assist devices (VADs) in these patients?
10. What are the considerations in anesthetizing patients for left ventricular assist device (LVAD) insertion?

B. Perioperative Evaluation and Preparation

Three weeks after insertion of a left ventricular assist device (LVAD), a donor heart becomes available.

1. How would you assess this patient preoperatively?
2. How would you premedicate this patient? Why?

C. Intraoperative Management

1. What anesthetic equipment and monitors would you set up? Why?
2. What is the role of transesophageal echocardiography (TEE)?
3. Describe the induction and maintenance of anesthesia.
4. How would you manage this patient during cardiopulmonary bypass (CPB)?

D. Postoperative Management

1. What are the early postoperative complications?
2. What are the mechanisms of right heart failure?
3. How would you treat right heart failure following heart transplantation?
4. How does inhaled nitric oxide (NO) work as a selective pulmonary vasodilator?
5. What is the pathophysiology of the denervated heart?
6. What are the common cardiac dysrhythmias following heart transplant?
7. What are the causes of posttransplant bleeding?
8. How would you treat posttransplant bleeding?
9. What are the causes of early graft failure?
10. How would you manage this patient in the intensive care unit?

E. Subsequent Noncardiac Surgery

The patient recovers successfully following heart transplant. However, 2 years postoperatively he fractures his left radius after a fall and then presents for open reduction and internal fixation of the fracture.

1. How would you monitor this patient?
2. What type of anesthetic is best for the heart-transplanted patient?
3. Which anesthetic technique would you give this patient?
4. Do you need to use a muscarinic antagonist with cholinesterase inhibitors to reverse the muscle relaxant in heart-transplanted patients?
5. What are the anesthetic implications for heart-transplanted patients?
6. What is the significant implication of the denervated heart?
7. What is the significance of allograft rejection?
8. What is the significance of infection in these patients?
9. What are the significant implications of drug interactions?
10. What is cardiac allograft vasculopathy (CAV)? Why is this important?
11. What is the significant implication of posttransplant hypertension?
12. What is the significant implication of renal dysfunction?
13. Is ambulatory surgery appropriate for heart-transplant recipients?

A. Medical Disease and Differential Diagnosis

A.1. What are the common diagnoses requiring adult heart transplantation?

Heart transplantation is now considered a viable treatment option for selected patients with end-stage heart disease. At present, more than 4,000 heart transplants are done annually worldwide.

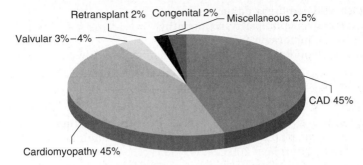

Figure 14.1   Indications for adult heart transplant. CAD, coronary artery disease.

The indications for adult heart transplant, as reported to the Registry of the International Society for Heart and Lung Transplantation in the overall Registry experience (1982 to 2004), are shown in Fig. 14.1. Ischemic coronary artery disease (**CAD**) (45%) and cardiomyopathy (45%) represent the most frequent causes for transplantation.

Taylor DO, Edwards LB, Boucek MM, et al. Registry of the International Society for Heart and Lung Transplantation: twenty-second official adult heart transplant report—2005. *J Heart Lung Transplant* 2005;24:945–955.

A.2.   What are the criteria and contraindications for recipient selection?

It should be noted that indications/contraindications can be flexible and can vary from center to center.
Criteria include the following:

- End-stage heart disease (New York Heart Association [NYHA] class III to IV) not responsive to medical management
- Physiologic age less than 65. However, in 2004, 8.3% of heart recipients were more or equal to 65 years of age.
- Maximal oxygen uptake less or equal to 14 mL/kg/minute (VO$_2$max) on a metabolic stress test. However, patients with VO$_2$max of 14 to 18 mL/kg/minute are more controversial. If these patients have other criteria that increase their potential mortality (very low ejection fraction, arrhythmia, hyponatremia), they may have greater consideration.

Contraindications

- Absolute
    a. Neoplasm, with the exception of skin
    b. Acquired immunodeficiency syndrome (AIDS)
    c. Multi-system lupus erythematosus or sarcoid
    d. Fixed pulmonary hypertension: pulmonary vascular resistance greater than 400 dyne/second/cm^5 (5 Wood units)
    e. Any systemic illness that would limit survival despite transplant
- Relative
    a. Age over 65
    b. Peripheral vascular disease, carotid stenosis (depending on severity)
    c. Human immunodeficiency virus (HIV), hepatitis B
    d. Severe pulmonary disease

e. Diabetes with end-organ damage
   ○ Neuropathy, nephropathy, retinopathy
f. Psychosocial impairments
   ○ Drug or alcohol addiction, smoking, mental defect, history of noncompliance

Steinman TI, Becker BN, Frost AE, et al. Guidelines for the referral and management of patients eligible for solid organ transplantation. *Transplantation* 2001;71:1189–1204.

Taylor DO, Edwards LB, Boucek MM, et al. Registry of the International Society for Heart and Lung Transplantation: twenty-second official adult heart transplant report—2005. *J Heart Lung Transplant* 2005;24:945–955.

A.3. What are the criteria for donor heart selection?

The limiting factor in heart transplantation is the shortage of donor organs. In the United States there are approximately 40,000 potential recipients from infancy to age 65, with approximately 2,500 donor hearts per year. Following establishment of brain death, organ harvest may be considered for the purpose of donation. The donor should not have sustained prolonged cardiac arrest, severe chest trauma, intracardiac injections, septicemia, or excessive inotropic support. In all cases, a careful clinical examination of the potential donor is undertaken to rule out coronary artery atherosclerosis and contractile dysfunction—investigations may include angiography and echocardiography. The use of coronary angiography would be dictated by patient age, sex, and risk factors. Generally a contrast ventriculogram is avoided to reduce the risk of nephrotoxicity.

Transplantation can proceed with mild left ventricular hypertrophy (LVH), however, wall thickness greater than 13 mm or electrocardiogram (ECG) criteria for LVH would make transplantation unadvisable. Generally severe congenital or valvular abnormalities would preclude donation, with the exception of abnormalities in which "bench" repair can be undertaken before transplant.

ABO compatibility is important, as mismatch may result in hyperacute rejection. The donor body weight should be within 20% of that of the recipient. However, in the case of a small donor matching with body mass index (BMI) or height is more accurate than using weight. Preferably donor heart ischemic time should be less than 4 hours. Prolonged ischemic time may contribute to early allograft failure; however, techniques to allow improved tolerance of ischemia may be on the horizon.

The use of non–heart-beating donors (NHBD) has been used successfully for nonthoracic organ transplantation. There is evidence that this approach may also be applicable to heart transplantation. However, at present there are a number of ethical, technical, and logistic hurdles regarding the use of NHBD for heart transplantation.

Jhaveri R, Tardiff B, Stanley TE III. Anesthesia for heart and heart—lung transplantation. *Anesthesiol Clin North America* 1994;12:729–747.

Livi U, Caforio ALP. Heart donor management and expansion of current donor selection criteria. *J Heart Lung Transplant* 2000;19:S43–S48.

Steinman TI, Becker BN, Frost AE, et al. Guidelines for the referral and management of patients eligible for solid organ transplantation. *Transplantation* 2001;71:1189–1204.

A.4. What are the principles of perioperative donor management?

The goals of management are to maintain euvolemia, achieve relatively normal afterload and optimize cardiac output (CO) without excessive use of inotropic medications, in particular β agonists. Unfortunately, the brain dead patient can often become extraordinarily unstable and achieving hemodynamic stability can be a challenge. In addition, the treatment modalities to support certain end organs for harvest are often at odds with each other. The onset of diabetes insipidus needs to be considered when excessive urine output (>300 mL/hour) is observed and treated promptly with desmopressin (1-deamino-8-D-arginine vasopressin [DDAVP]). As a result of dysfunction of the hypothalamic-pituitary system, it is suggested that hormonal replacement therapy be undertaken in patients with ejection fractions less than 45% or hemodynamic instability. This includes the use of triiodothyronine (T_3), arginine vasopressin, and methylprednisolone. In addition, adequate glycemic control should be achieved.

Van Bakel AB, Pitzer S, Drake P, et al. Early hormonal therapy stabilizes hemodynamics during donor procurement. *Transplant Proc* 2004;36:2573–2578.

Zaroff JG, Rosengard BR, Armstrong WR, et al. Consensus conference report. maximizing use of organs recovered from the cadaver donor: cardiac recommendations. *Circulation* 2002;106:836–841.

A.5.   What are the risk factors associated with posttransplant mortality?

Overall survival at 1 year is 83%. Having congenital heart disease as the indication for transplant is a powerful predictor of postoperative 1-year mortality. In addition, the requirement of extracorporeal circulatory support, dialysis, preoperative mechanical ventilation, coronary artery disease (CAD) as the indication for transplant and being hospitalized immediately before transplant all are risk factors for 1-year mortality. Mortality during the first year is 1.4 times the next 4 years combined, so risk factors associated with 1-year mortality are powerful predictors of 5-year mortality. For those that have survived after 1 year, previous transplant, stroke before transplant, allograft vasculopathy during first year posttransplant, treatment for rejection in year 1, treatment of infection before discharge, human leukocyte antigen (HLA) mismatches, recipient age, donor age and recipient weight are risk factors for 5-year mortality.

The most common causes of death are the following:

- Within 30 days posttransplant
  - Graft failure, multiorgan failure, non–cytomegalovirus (CMV) infection
- From 31 to 365 days posttransplant
  - Non–CMV infection, graft failure, acute rejection
- After 5 years
  - Allograft vasculopathy, late graft failures, malignancies, non–CMV infections

Taylor DO, Edwards LB, Boucek MM, et al. Registry of the International Society for Heart and Lung Transplantation: twenty-second official adult heart transplant report—2005. *J Heart Lung Transplant* 2005;24:945–955.

A.6.   What is the sequence of surgical anastomoses in heart transplantation?

The heart is excised transecting the great vessels and leaving cuffs of both left and right atria to minimize the number of anastomoses that need to be performed. The donor heart is prepared by creating a left atrial and right atrial (or superior vena cava [SVC] and inferior vena cava [IVC]) cuff. The sinoatrial node is preserved. Following atrial (or caval) anastomoses, the aortic anastomosis is often performed before the pulmonary artery to allow for earlier removal of the aortic cross-clamp.

Gallagher RC, Kormos RL. Heart transplantation. In: Makowka L, ed. *Handbook of transplantation management*. Austin: RG Landes Co, 1991:254.

A.7. When is combined heart/lung transplant indicated? What are the important differences?

Congenital cardiac disease is the most common indication for combined heart/lung transplant. Other indications include primary pulmonary hypertension, cystic fibrosis, α_1-antitrypsin deficiency and other forms of lung disease, such as emphysema and idiopathic pulmonary fibrosis. The procedure is performed through a transverse thoracotomy incision and the donor heart/lungs are transplanted *en bloc*. Important postoperative problems include bleeding and reperfusion lung injury that may require nitric oxide (NO) or occasionally extracorporeal membrane oxygenation (ECMO). Survival following heart/lung transplant is 63%, 43%, and 28% at 1, 5, and 10 years respectively.

Trulock EP, Edwards LB, Taylor DO, et al. Registry of the International Society for Heart and Lung Transplantation: twenty-second official adult lung and heart—lung transplant report—2005. *J Heart Lung Transplant* 2005;24:956–967.

A.8. What are the medical and surgical alternatives to cardiac transplantation?

An ongoing worldwide shortage of donor hearts has meant increased pressure to medically manage patients with end-stage cardiac failure. As heart failure progresses patients may respond to a variety of medications. Angiotensin converting enzyme (ACE) inhibitors have been shown to improve symptoms and decrease mortality in patients with heart failure. Patients with severe forms of heart failure may also benefit from a low-dose aldosterone antagonist (spironolactone), with attention paid to potential hyperkalemia. β-Blockade with carvedilol, sustained release metoprolol or bisoprolol has been shown to reduce the risk of death. In addition, patients with advanced heart failure may reduce their risk of sudden cardiac death by the insertion of an implantable cardioverter defibrillator (ICD). Furthermore, ICD implantation can be combined with cardiac resynchronization therapy (biventricular pacing), which has been shown to improve functional class and survival in advanced heart failure, once patients have also achieved optimal medical management. Increasingly, ventricular assist device (VAD) implantation or semiimplantable pericorporeal devices are also finding a role in the management of these patients.

Hunt SA, Antman EM, Smith SC, et al. ACC/AHA 2005 guideline update for the diagnosis and management of chronic heart failure in the adult—summary article. *Circulation* 2005;112:1825–1852.

A.9. What is the role for ventricular assist devices (VADs) in these patients?

Semi-implantable/pericorporeal devices can be used, commonly following cardiac surgery, as a temporizing measure; in this setting they can either allow myocardial recovery *(bridge-to-recovery)* or alternatively, allow definitive VAD implantation at a later stage *(bridge-to-bridge)*. These approaches are commonly taken in patients where there is a good chance of spontaneous recovery of cardiac function.

Where transplantation is ultimately indicated LVAD (left ventricular assist device) or BiVAD (biventricular assist device) implantation may be undertaken *(bridge-to-transplant)*. VAD support may allow for end-organ recovery to take place while awaiting a donor organ. These patients can be switched from transplant ineligible to eligible with a potential reduction in posttransplant morbidity and mortality.

Williams M, Oz M, Mancini D. Cardiac assist devices for end—stage heart failure. *Heart Dis* 2001;3:109–115.

A.10. What are the considerations in anesthetizing patients for left ventricular device (LVAD) insertion?

Significant cardiac abnormalities, for example, aortic insufficiency, patent foramen ovale, should be identified preoperatively and, if necessary, addressed at the time of surgery. Bleeding is a major problem in the perioperative management of these patients and adequate amounts of blood and blood products should be available. Many centers routinely give antifibrinolytics before LVAD implantation. Transesophageal echocardiography (TEE) is mandatory for LVAD insertion to assess for patent foramen ovale, to ensure aortic valve competence, assess adequate left ventricular decompression and to monitor right ventricular function. Inadequate right-sided heart function is a potential complication after LVAD insertion and can be treated with phosphodiesterase inhibitors and inhaled nitric oxide. Vasopressin and/or norepinephrine may be required to maintain adequate systemic vascular resistance postcardiopulmonary bypass.

Mets B. Anesthesia for left ventricular assist device placement. *J Cardiothorac Vasc Anesth* 2000;14:316–326.

Nussmeier NA, Probert CB, Hirsch D, et al. Anesthetic management for implantation of the Jarvik 2000™ left ventricular assist system. *Anesth Analg* 2003;97:964–971.

Williams M, Oz M, Mancini D. Cardiac assist devices for end—stage heart failure. *Heart Dis* 2001;3:109–115.

B. Perioperative Evaluation and Preparation

Three weeks after insertion of a left ventricular assist device (LVAD), a donor heart becomes available.

B.1. How would you assess this patient preoperatively?

Prospective transplant candidates have usually been fully preoperatively evaluated by a multidisciplinary team including cardiology, pulmonology, and surgery, as well as anesthesia. In case of subsequent deterioration, however, the anesthesiologist should review the recipient's current cardiac status including medications and level of mechanical support, with particular attention to hemodynamic parameters and reversibility of elevated pulmonary vascular resistance (PVR). Pertinent anesthetic history, concomitant diseases and fasting status must also be ascertained. Baseline electrolytes, urea, creatinine, blood glucose, international normalized ratio (INR)/prothrombin time (PTT), complete blood count should be obtained. In addition, specific preoperative investigations need to be reviewed such as pulmonary function tests, electrocardiogram (ECG) and chest radiograph.

There are typically two types of patients presenting for heart transplantation. The first type of patient is relatively compensated, requiring possible intravenous inotropic support or may even be ambulatory in a nonhospital setting. The second type is moribund and decompensated, requiring mechanical ventilation and/or mechanical circulatory support. At the time of transplant

47.9% of patients are on intravenous inotropes, 20.6% have a left ventricular assist device, 5.7% have an intraaortic balloon pump (IABP), and 2.5% are mechanically ventilated. Only 0.4% requires extracorporeal membrane oxygenation (ECMO) before transplant. Recipients who have undergone prior cardiac surgery need to be identified as this will increase the surgical time to achieve cardiopulmonary bypass (CPB) due to adhesions and bleeding. Many centers will treat these patients with antifibrinolytics to attenuate the risks of bleeding. Large bore intravenous access must be secured and cross-matched blood should be readily available in the operating room before the commencement of surgery.

Taylor DO, Edwards LB, Boucek MM, et al. Registry of the International Society for Heart and Lung Transplantation: twenty-second official adult heart transplant report—2005. *J Heart Lung Transplant* 2005;24:945–955.

B.2. How would you premedicate this patient? Why?

Patients should be transported to the operating room with oxygen supplementation. Premedication, if any, should be limited to H_2 receptor antagonists, rather than narcotic or sedative drugs. With minimal cardiac reserve, sedation may blunt the patient's respiratory and sympathetic drive and can lead to hypoxemia, hypercapnia, and even hypotension. Antibiotic prophylaxis is often achieved with 1 to 2 g of cephazolin.

Jhaveri R, Tardiff B, Stanley TE III. Anesthesia for heart and heart—lung transplantation. *Anesthesiol Clin North America* 1994;12:729–747.

C. Intraoperative Management

C.1. What anesthetic equipment and monitors would you set up? Why?

Anesthetic equipment includes a ventilator with air mixture capability, airway and intubation set-up, fluid/blood warmer, extracorporeal bypass machine with membrane oxygenator and nitric oxide (NO) delivery and monitoring system. The patient is taken to the operating room breathing supplemental oxygen. Monitors include a 5-lead electrocardiogram (ECG), digital pulse oximeter, noninvasive blood pressure cuff, capnography, urinary catheter, temperature probe(s), and peripheral nerve stimulator. All invasive lines are placed with meticulous attention to aseptic technique and titrated sedation. A no. 14-g intravenous line and a no. 20-g radial arterial catheter for continuous blood pressure monitoring are inserted. Routinely a pulmonary arterial (PA) catheter is inserted through the right internal jugular vein for pre-CPB, post-CPB, and postoperative measurement of pulmonary arterial pressure, pulmonary vascular resistance (PVR), and cardiac output (CO). The PA catheter is withdrawn back to approximately 20 cm position in a 80-cm sterile sleeve before cardiectomy. Transesophageal echocardiography (TEE) is also very useful in the intraoperative management of the pre- and posttransplant periods. Finally a bispectral index monitor (BIS) maybe applied before induction.

C.2. What is the role of transesophageal echocardiography (TEE)?

In addition to its potential role in assessment of the donor heart before harvesting, TEE may also be of benefit in the immediate posttransplant period. The echocardiographer can provide feedback to the surgeon and anesthesiologist regarding overall function of the transplanted heart. In particular, wall motion abnormalities, end diastolic volume and valvular function can be assessed. Of particular interest are right ventricular (RV) function and an assessment of pulmonary artery pressures. TEE may also be useful in the assessment of surgical anastomosis, by an echocardiographer with advanced training. Specifically, the main pulmonary artery anastomosis should be evaluated for stenosis. The long axis view of the left atrium is composed of recipient and donor tissue and may appear large. If excessive tissue is present, acquired cor triatriatum may develop due to an unfolding of redundant tissue.

Bryan AJ, Barzilai B, Kouchoukos NT. Transesophageal echocardiography and adult cardiac operations. *Ann Thorac Surg* 1995;59:773–779.

Couture R, Carrier M. Transesophageal echocardiography. In: Denault AY, Couture P, Buithieu J, et al. eds. *A perioperative transdisciplinary approach*. Taylor & Francis Group, 2005:471–480.

Suriani RJ. Transesophageal echocardiography during organ transplantation. *J Cardiothorac Vasc Anesth* 1998;12:686–694.

C.3. Describe the induction and maintenance of anesthesia.

It is important to time the anesthesia induction and surgery carefully to achieve cardiopulmonary bypass (CPB) at the time of donor heart arrival in order to minimize ischemia time, particularly for a resternotomy patient. Prompt securing of the airway may be required, as the recipient is not always properly fasted for transplantation surgery, however, a rapid induction needs to be balanced against the risk of hemodynamic compromise. The patient is anesthetized with midazolam and fentanyl or sufentanil titrated based on hemodynamic status and level of consciousness. Muscle relaxation may be achieved with pancuronium, rocuronium, cisatracurium, or vecuronium. Succinylcholine is not usually used because of concern of bradycardia during induction, as blood pressure in pre–heart-transplant recipients is often heart rate dependent. Maintenance phase is achieved through the use of a balance anesthetic technique. Volatile agents (sevoflurane or isoflurane) are combined with fentanyl or sufentanil, midazolam and muscle relaxation as required. Nitrous oxide is generally avoided, due to its effects on pulmonary vascular resistance (PVR).

Many centers routinely infuse aprotinin 2 million KIU (kallikrein inhibitor unit) after a test dose (10 to 50,000 KIU) before CPB, followed by 2 million KIU added to the CPB prime and 2 million KIU over 4 hours to prevent postoperative bleeding. However, a viable alternative may be tranexamic acid (50 to 100 mg/kg). At present, controversy exists regarding the association of aprotinin and postoperative renal dysfunction.

Karkouti K, Beattie SW, Dattilo KM, et al. A propensity score case—control comparison of aprotinin and tranexamic acid in high—transfusion—risk cardiac surgery. *Transfusion* 2006;46:327–338.

Mangano DT, Tudor IC, Dietzel C. The risk associated with aprotinin in cardiac surgery. *N Engl J Med* 2006;354:353–365.

C.4. How would you manage this patient during cardiopulmonary bypass (CPB)?

The anesthetic management of CPB in these patients is not different from that in nontransplant patients, except that rewarming is usually prolonged because of the profound cooling of the donor heart and the prolonged ischemic time. Early in the perfusion, mixed venous oxygen desaturation and metabolic acidosis must be corrected. The fluid balance, hematocrit, electrolyte composition and serum glucose must be closely monitored. During CPB, anesthesia maintenance is achieved by narcotic supplementation, an inhalational agent and/or benzodiazepine. Once cardiac rhythm has been established and anastomosis of the pulmonary artery is completed, the patient is placed in a head-down position for air evacuation from the left side of the heart. An isoproterenol infusion (1 to 5 μg/minute) may be considered to improve contractility and to increase heart rate to approximately 90 to 110 beats per minute. If necessary the heart may be externally paced through epicardial leads.

D. Postoperative Management

D.1. What are the early postoperative complications?

The early postoperative complications include:

- Right heart failure/pulmonary hypertension
- Denervated heart
- Bleeding
- Early graft failure

D.2. What are the mechanisms of right heart failure?

Right-sided heart failure is an important cause of posttransplant morbidity and mortality. It has a diverse number of causes related to both increases in flow and resistance across the pulmonary vascular bed. One prime cause is long standing elevation in left ventricular pressure leading to an increase in pulmonary pressure and vasoconstriction. This pulmonary vasoconstriction may become fixed over time, compromising right ventricular (RV) function after transplant. However, a normal preoperative pulmonary vascular resistance (PVR) does not rule out the potential for RV failure posttransplant. Poor organ preservation and cardiopulmonary bypass (CPB) can also have deleterious effects of graft ventricular function.

Stobierska-Dzierzek B, Awad H, Michler RE. The evolving management of acute right—sided heart failure in cardiac transplant recipients. *J Am Coll Cardiol* 2001;38: 923–931.

D.3. How would you treat right heart failure following heart transplantation?

Right ventricular (RV) failure can lead to dilation, ischemia and poor contractility. This can result in a shift of the ventricular septum to the left, with a reduction in left ventricular filling and reduced cardiac output (CO). Basic therapeutic goals are to maintain adequate coronary perfusion, optimize oxygen delivery, prevent further distention of the right ventricle by judicious use of fluids, minimizing myocardial oxygen consumption and reduce pulmonary vascular resistance (PVR) to decrease RV afterload.

Phosphodiesterase inhibitors, such as milrinone, which have systemic and pulmonary vasodilatory effects in addition to positive inotropy, are particularly useful. Prostacyclin (PGI$_2$), prostaglandin E$_1$, isoproterenol (1 to 5 μg/minute), dobutamine and nitrates have also been used with success to treat transient increases in PVR. However, vasodilator use can often be accompanied by arterial hypotension, requiring the administration of vasopressors to maintain adequate coronary perfusion. Inhaled nitric oxide (NO) is also widely used as a selective pulmonary vasodilator, in severe pulmonary hypertension and RV failure. It should be remembered that simple management goals of avoiding hypoxia, hypercarbia, and excessive positive end-expiratory pressure (PEEP) will help avoid elevated PVR.

In severe cases of refractory RV failure posttransplant, right ventricular assist device (RVAD) has been successfully used. Extracorporeal membrane oxygenation (ECMO) is also a potential option in refractory cases.

Stobierska-Dzierzek B, Awad H, Michler RE. The evolving management of acute right—sided heart failure in cardiac transplant recipients. *J Am Coll Cardiol* 2001;38: 923–931.

D.4. How does inhaled nitric oxide (NO) work as a selective pulmonary vasodilator?

The advantage of inhaled NO as a pulmonary vasodilator lies mainly in the fact that its smooth muscle relaxant effect is limited to the pulmonary vasculature—the half-life *in vivo* of inhaled NO is only a few seconds. Therefore it has little effect on the systemic circulation, unlike intravenous vasodilators such as nitroprusside, nitroglycerin, prostaglandins and calcium channel blockers. Furthermore, inhaled NO selectively causes vasodilation in ventilated lung units, therefore decreasing $\dot{V}/\dot{Q}$ mismatch and shunt. Inhaled NO (1 to 20 ppm) can result in significant decreases in pulmonary artery pressure, pulmonary vascular resistance (PVR), and central venous pressure (CVP), while increasing mean arterial pressure (MAP), cardiac output (CO), and arterial oxygenation (PaO_2). In addition, a transesophageal echocardiography (TEE) documented alteration of the ventricular septal shift with a significant reduction in right ventricular (RV) chamber and tricuspid valvular annulus size can be seen.

Girard C, Durand PG, Vedrinne C, et al. Inhaled nitric oxide for right ventricular failure after heart transplantation. *J Cardiothorac Vasc Anesth* 1993;7:481–485.

Konstadt S. Nitric oxide: has it progressed from molecule of the year to wonder drug of the decade? *J Cardiothorac Vasc Anesth* 1995;9(6):625–626.

D.5. What is the pathophysiology of the denervated heart?

Following cardiac transplantation, the cardiac plexus is interrupted and the heart is denervated. The recipient atrium remains innervated but hemodynamically unimportant, whereas the donor atrium is denervated and is responsible for the electrophysiological responses of the transplanted heart. The electrocardiogram (ECG) often contains two P waves. The denervated heart retains its intrinsic control mechanisms which include the Frank-Starling mechanism and intact α- and β-adrenoreceptor responses to circulating catecholamines. This denervated heart lacks the ability to respond acutely to hypovolemia or hypotension with reflex tachycardia, but responds to stress primarily by an increase in stroke volume. This reflects dependence of the sinus node on direct stimulation by endogenously released catecholamines and the absence of control through neural mechanisms. This is why heart transplanted patients are said to be "preload dependent." Interesting, however, some studies have demonstrated reinnervation within a year after transplantation. This has lead to symptoms of angina pectoris when ischemia develops in the transplanted heart.

Cheng DCH, Ong DD. Anaesthesia for non—cardiac surgery in heart transplanted patients. *Can J Anaesth* 1993;40:981–986.

Kobashigawa JA. Postoperative management following heart transplantation. *Transplant Proc* 1999;31:2038–2046.

D.6. What are the common cardiac dysrhythmias following heart transplant?

Cardiac dysrhythmias may occur due to lack of vagal tone or other aspects of the denervated heart. The sinus node may have an increased refractory period and atrial conduction may be prolonged. Therefore, first-degree atrioventricular (AV) block is common. It has been reported that 18% to 27% of orthotopic heart transplant patients develop prolonged (>24 hours) bradyarrhythmias within 5 days of transplantation. Arrhythmia occurrences are potentially associated with prolonged donor heart ischemic time, elevated pulmonary arterial pressure, and a lower ejection fraction.

Miyamoto Y, Curtiss EI, Kormos RL, et al. Bradyarrhythmia after heart transplantation. Incidence, time course, and outcome. *Circulation* 1990;82:313–317.

D.7. What are the causes of posttransplant bleeding?

Perioperative bleeding is a significant cause of mortality following heart transplantation. The causes of posttransplant bleeding are anastomosis leaks, bronchial artery injury and coagulopathy. Immediately before weaning from bypass, with the heart filled, the posterior anastomosis is carefully checked again by the surgeon for "water-tightness" because leaks in this area are more difficult and riskier to repair later. Patients with pulmonary hypertension develop enlarged bronchial vessels that are particularly liable to bleed if meticulous hemostasis has not been achieved. Coagulopathy, or what some term "medical bleeding," often results from a combination of mechanisms, including inadequate heparin reversal, dilution of platelets and coagulation factors, hypothermia and cardiopulmonary bypasses effect on fibrinolysis, platelet function and factor activation. In addition, those patients with a ventricular assist device (VAD) in place before transplant are at particular risk of perioperative hemorrhage.

Bourge RC, Naftel DC, Costanzo-Nordin MR, et al. Pre—transplantation risk factors for death after heart transplantation: a multi—institutional study. *J Heart Lung Transplant* 1993;12:549–562.

Wegner JA, DiNardo JA, Arabia FA, et al. Blood loss and transfusion requirements in patients implanted with a mechanical circulatory support device undergoing cardiac transplantation. *J Heart Lung Transplant* 2000;19:504–506.

D.8. How would you treat posttransplant bleeding?

Prevention of potential causes of bleeding is key. The use of antifibrinolytics (aprotinin or tranexamic acid) is strongly encouraged, in particular if redo sternotomy is to be undertaken. Avoidance of excessive crystalloid in the prebypass period may reduce the dilutional component of coagulopathy. Maintaining normothermia with forced air warming devices and fluid warmers is also imperative. When bleeding is evident in the postoperative period the judicious use of packed red blood cells, fresh frozen plasma and platelets is a starting point. If hemorrhage is not responsive to conservative measures, disseminated intravascular coagulopathy must be ruled out. If serum fibrinogen is low (<0.8 to 1.0 g/L) then the use of cryoprecipitate should be entertained. Desmopressin (0.3 μg/kg) may also have a role in refractory cases. Finally, recombinant factor VII has been used successfully to treat hemorrhage in cardiac transplant patients. However, the risk of thrombosis needs to be weighed against the risk of ongoing bleeding and consultation with a hematologist would be advisable before administration.

It should always be remembered that bleeding which is excessive and not clearly secondary to coagulopathy warrants surgical reexploration.

Kogan A, Berman M, Kassif Y, et al. Use of recombinant factor VII to control bleeding in a patient supported by right ventricular assist device after heart transplantation. *J Heart Lung Transplant* 2005;24:347–349.

D.9. What are the causes of early graft failure?

Graft failure (primary and nonspecific) is the most common (40%) cause of death in the first 30 days after heart transplant. Causes include biventricular failure (unknown cause), right ventricular (RV) failure (often due to high pulmonary vascular resistance [PVR]), flow limiting coronary stenosis, and hyperacute rejection.

Luckraz H, Goddard M, Charman SC, et al. Early mortality after cardiac transplantation: should we do better? *J Heart Lung Transplant* 2005;24:401–405.

D.10. How would you manage this patient in the intensive care unit?

Within the first 30 days, posttransplant graft failure (primary and nonspecific), multiorgan failure and non–cytomegalovirus (CMV) infection are the most common causes of death at 40%, 14%, and 13% respectively. Early management goals include prevention of infection and rejection, treatment of bleeding and dysrhythmias, and cardiovascular support. If possible, one should aim to wean the patient from the ventilator and extubate within 24 hours. In order to facilitate oxygenation and weaning, strict supervision of fluid balance and body weight is required. Immunosuppression is often achieved with a cocktail of medications including, steroids (methylprednisolone then prednisone), calcineurin inhibitors (tacrolimus, cyclosporine) and antiproliferative agents (mycophenolate mofetil, azathioprine). Some centers also use induction therapy with antilymphocyte antibody such as OKT3 or IL-2 receptor antibodies. Secondary to immunosuppression patients are often covered prophylactically with ganciclovir or valganciclor (CMV prophylaxis) and trimethoprim/sulfamethoxazole (toxoplasma and *Pneumocystis carinii* prophylaxis).

Taylor DO. Cardiac transplantation: drug regimens for the 21st century. *Ann Thorac Surg* 2003;75:S72–S78.

Taylor DO, Edwards LB, Boucek MM, et al. Registry of the International Society for Heart and Lung Transplantation: twenty-second official adult heart transplant report—2005. *J Heart Lung Transplant* 2005;24:945–955.

E. Subsequent Noncardiac Surgery

The patient recovers successfully following heart transplant. However, 2 years postoperatively he fractures his left radius after a fall. He presents for open reduction and internal fixation of the fracture.

E.1. How would you monitor this patient?

This patient should have similar monitoring requirements for nontransplant patients undergoing similar procedures. Patients who require invasive monitoring do so in keeping with a particular procedure, for example, arterial line for thoracotomy and open lung biopsy, central venous pressure (CVP) monitor for small bowel resection, or because the patient is unstable preoperatively. Smooth and safe anesthesia is contingent upon careful preoperative assessment that may reduce the need for invasive monitoring with all its attendant risks. Adequate preload must be attained preoperatively and intravascular volume status maintained intraoperatively because these patients are "preload dependent." Monitors in the case mentioned earlier would include, an electrocardiogram (ECG), noninvasive blood pressure cuff, capnometer, oxygen saturation probe and if general anesthetic was delivered a temperature probe and neuromuscular stimulator would be applied.

Cheng DCH, Ong DD. Anaesthesia for non—cardiac surgery in heart transplanted patients. *Can J Anaesth* 1993;40:981–986.

E.2. What type of anesthetic is best for the heart-transplanted patient?

In a series of 86 heart-transplanted recipients, 18 returned for 32 noncardiac surgical procedures. The breakdown included, 18 neurolept-anesthesia cases, 12 general anesthesia cases with a combination of N_2O/O_2/narcotic/relaxant and low doses of volatile agents, and 2 spinals The patients had normal requirements of intravenous and inhalational agents, muscle relaxants, and local anesthetics. There was no prolonged action of any anesthetic agents. This indicates that the choice of general, neuroleptic or spinal anesthesia does not affect postoperative outcome in heart-transplanted recipients undergoing subsequent noncardiac surgery.

Cheng DCH, Ong DD. Anaesthesia for non—cardiac surgery in heart transplanted patients. *Can J Anaesth* 1993;40:981–986.

E.3. Which anesthetic technique would you give this patient?

This patient could safely receive general anesthesia or regional blockade of his brachial plexus for the upcoming surgery.

E.4. Do you need to use a muscarinic antagonist with cholinesterase inhibitors to reverse the muscle relaxant in heart-transplanted patients?

Although it does not compromise other hemodynamic parameters, neostigmine has been shown to produce a dose dependent decrease in heart rate in heart-transplanted patients. In remote transplanted patients (>6 months), a muscarinic antagonist should be administered simultaneously with cholinesterase inhibitors to block the cardiac and muscarinic side effects, as slow development of cardiac reinnervation may be possible.

Ashary N, Kaye AD, Hegazi AR, et al. Anesthetic considerations in the patient with a heart transplant. *Heart Dis* 2002;4:191–198.

Backman SB, Fox GS, Stein RD, et al. Neostigmine decreases heart rate in heart transplant patients. *Can J Anaesth* 1996;43:373–378.

Wilson RF, Christensen BV, Olivari MT, et al. Evidence for structural sympathetic reinnervation after orthotopic cardiac transplantation in humans. *Circulation* 1991;83: 1210–1221.

E.5. What are the anesthetic implications for heart-transplanted patients?

The anesthetic implications for heart-transplanted patients include the following:

- Denervated heart
- Allograft rejection
- Infection due to immunosuppression
- Drug interaction
- Allograft coronary artery disease (CAD)
- Hypertension
- Renal dysfunction

Ashary N, Kaye AD, Hegazi AR, et al. Anesthetic considerations in the patient with a heart transplant. *Heart Dis* 2002;4:191–198.

Cheng DCH, Ong DD. Anaesthesia for non—cardiac surgery in heart transplanted patients. *Can J Anaesth* 1993;40:981–986.

E.6.   What is the significant implication of the denervated heart?

The denervated heart retains its intrinsic control mechanisms which include: Frank-Starling mechanism, impulse formation and conductivity and responsiveness to circulating cate-cholamines in the from of increased heart rate and contractility. But the normal respiratory variations or response to carotid sinus massage and Valsalva maneuvers are absent. At rest the heart rate reflects the intrinsic rate of depolarization at the donor sinoatrial node, and in the absence of any vagal tone, is faster than normal at approximately 90 to 100 beats per minute. The heart rate shows minimal response to drugs such as muscle relaxants (pancuronium), anti-cholinergics (atropine, glycopyrrolate and scopolamine), cholinesterase inhibitors (neostigmine, edrophonium, pyridostigmine, physostigmine), digoxin, nifedipine, phenylephrine, or nitroprus-side, but will respond to isoproterenol, ephedrine, dopamine, and glucagon.

Cardiac dysrhythmias may occur in heart-transplanted patients. First-degree atrioventricular (AV) block is common. Dual AV nodal pathways are frequently observed, but reentry dysrhythmias are rare. Bradyarrhythmic therapy in these patients should be a direct β-adrenergic stimulating agent (epinephrine, isoproterenol). Glucagon is also useful as a positive chronotrope and inotrope. Medications used to treat tachyarrhythmias (calcium channel blockers, β-blockers) need to be used with caution due to their negative inotropic effects.

Ashary N, Kaye AD, Hegazi AR, et al. Anesthetic considerations in the patient with a heart transplant. *Heart Dis* 2002;4:191–198.

Stein KL, Darby JM, Grenvik A. Intensive care of the cardiac transplant recipient. *J Cardiothorac Anesth* 1998;2:543–553.

E.7.   What is the significance of allograft rejection?

Most rejection episodes occur in the first 6 months posttransplant. These patients can present with fever, malaise, arrhythmias, and shortness of breath. Hemodynamic compromise is considered a late sign of rejection. The gold standard for diagnosis is endomyocardial biopsy. Rejection episodes are primarily treated with steroids, however, more severe forms may require more aggressive immunosuppression with OKT3, cyclophosphamide or plasmapheresis.

Kobashigawa JA. Postoperative management following heart transplantation. *Transplant Proc* 1999;31:2038–2046.

E.8.   What is the significance of infection in these patients?

Immunosuppressive drugs are continued indefinitely in heart-transplanted patients and infection remains a major cause of death, with 10% of mortality 5 years posttransplant secondary to non–cytomegalovirus (CMV) infections. It is most prevalent in the first several weeks after transplantation when immunosuppressive therapy is most intense. Early postoperative bacterial infections (e.g., mediastinitis) and opportunistic infections (e.g., CMV, *P. carinii*, toxoplasma) are of great concern. Invasive monitoring techniques and all forms of instrumentation should be kept to the minimum consistent with safe anesthesia. Attention to aseptic technique should be paramount. Intubation through the orotracheal route is preferable to the nasotracheal route because the latter is associated with infection by diphtheroids and staphylococcal organisms from the nasopharynx and skin.

Shaw IH, Kirk AJB, Conacher ID. Anaesthesia for patients with transplanted hearts and lungs undergoing non—cardiac surgery. *Br J Anaesth* 1991;67:772–778.

Taylor DO, Edwards LB, Boucek MM, et al. Registry of the International Society for Heart and Lung Transplantation: twenty-second official adult heart transplant report—2005. *J Heart Lung Transplant* 2005;24:945–955.

E.9. What are the significant implications of drug interactions?

Chronic steroid treatment may result in an abnormal stress response, so patients should receive perioperative steroid coverage. Azathioprine has been reported to antagonize the competitive neuromuscular blocking drugs by its phosphodiesterase inhibiting properties, therefore larger doses of relaxants may be required. In experimental animals, cyclosporine infusions have been shown to potentiate the neuromuscular blocking effects of atracurium and vecuronium, and single doses of cyclosporine may result in increased duration of action of both barbiturates and narcotics.

Ashary N, Kaye AD, Hegazi AR, et al. Anesthetic considerations in the patient with a heart transplant. *Heart Dis* 2002;4:191–198.

Cirella VN, Pantuck CB, Lee YJ, et al. Effects of cyclosporine on anesthetic action. *Anesth Analg* 1987;66:703–706.

E.10. What is cardiac allograft vasculopathy (CAV)? Why is this important?

The transplanted heart is vulnerable to an accelerated process of coronary atherosclerosis called CAV. Within a year of transplant 7.0% of recipients will have developed CAV. At 9.5 years posttransplant only 47% of recipients are free of angiographic evidence of CAV. It is characterized by concentric intimal proliferation and diffuse narrowing along the coronary vessel. Diagnosis is accomplished by coronary angiography. The etiology is likely multifactorial. Risk factors for CAV less than 3 years posttransplant include donor hypertension, infection immediately after transplant, recipient age, donor age and recipient body mass index (BMI). It appears donor history of diabetes and cerebrovascular accident as cause of brain death are risk factors for development of late CAV.

Kobashigawa JA. Postoperative management following heart transplantation. *Transplant Proc* 1999;31:2038–2046.

Taylor DO, Edwards LB, Boucek MM, et al. Registry of the International Society for Heart and Lung Transplantation: twenty-second official adult heart transplant report—2005. *J Heart Lung Transplant* 2005;24:945–955.

E.11. What is the significant implication of posttransplant hypertension?

At present, 72.6% to 76.8% of patients have developed hypertension within 1 year posttransplantation. Cyclosporine is often cited as a causative factor. Current therapy may consist of a calcium channel blocker, such as diltiazem. However, care must be taken, as diltiazem may increase cyclosporine serum levels. Nifedipine has a tendency to cause significant vasodilatation and may be poorly tolerated in these patients. When necessary, an angiotensin converting enzyme (ACE) inhibitor may be added. Because cardiac responsiveness during exercise is dependent on circulating catecholamines, β-blockers are often avoided after heart transplantation.

Kobashigawa JA. Postoperative management following heart transplantation. *Transplant Proc* 1999;31:2038–2046.

Rudas L, Pflugfelder PW, Kostuk WJ. Comparison of hemodynamic responses during dynamic exercise in the upright and supine postures after orthotopic cardiac transplantation. *J Am Coll Cardiol* 1990;16:1367–1373.

Taylor DO, Edwards LB, Boucek MM, et al. Registry of the International Society for Heart and Lung Transplantation: twenty-second official adult heart transplant report—2005. *J Heart Lung Transplant* 2005;24:945–955.

E.12. What is the significant implication of renal dysfunction?

Renal dysfunction is found in 31.7% of recipients within 1 year and by 9.5 years only 60% are free of significant renal dysfunction. Due to the nephrotoxic effects of cyclosporine, serum creatinine concentrations gradually increase after cardiac transplantation, but generally plateau approximately 170 to 180 mmol/L. Anesthetic drugs that are excreted mainly by renal clearance should be avoided if renal function is compromised. Also one needs to be mindful of medications that may further compromise renal function, such as nonsteroid antiinflammatory drugs (NSAIDs).

Kobashigawa JA. Postoperative management following heart transplantation. *Transplant Proc* 1999;31:2038–2046.

Miller LW. Long—term complications of cardiac transplantation. *Prog Cardiovasc Dis* 1991; 33:229–282.

Taylor DO, Edwards LB, Boucek MM, et al. Registry of the International Society for Heart and Lung Transplantation: twenty-second official adult heart transplant report—2005. *J Heart Lung Transplant* 2005;24:945–955.

E.13. Is ambulatory surgery appropriate for heart-transplant recipients?

Unfortunately there is a paucity of evidence supporting either the safety or harm of ambulatory surgery in heart-transplant recipients. In addition, the choice of anesthetic technique seems to have no influence on outcome. Regardless, these patients should be seen in preadmission clinics before the day of surgery and have appropriate screening tests done preoperatively, including but not limited to, an assessment of renal function, electrocardiogram (ECG) and an accurate blood pressure measurement. They should also be evaluated by the cardiology transplant service and if any concern is raised further testing should be undertaken, such as dobutamine stress echocardiography, coronary angiography or endomyocardial biopsy. Recommendations should also be obtained regarding perioperative antibiotic prophylaxis and immunosuppression.

Bryson GL, Chung F, Finegan BA, et al. Patient selection in ambulatory anesthesia—an evidence—based review: part I. *Can J Anaesth* 2004;51:768–781.

CHAPTER 15

Ischemic Heart Disease and Noncardiac Surgery

MARBELIA GONZALEZ • J. PATRICIO ESCANDON • PAUL G. BARASH

A 72-YEAR-OLD MAN

is scheduled for right hemicolectomy for colon cancer. Past history reveals a myocardial infarction (MI) 5 months ago and placement of a right coronary artery stent. He also has diabetes mellitus type 2. He is treated with atenolol, diltiazem, glyburide, losartan and an occasional sublingual nitroglycerin (NTG).

A. Medical Disease and Differential Diagnosis

1. What are the preoperative predictors for perioperative cardiac morbidity (PCM)?
2. What is the New York Heart Association (NYHA) classification of heart failure?
3. What is the specific activity scale (SAS) of cardiac function?
4. What are the determinants of myocardial oxygen demand? How are they measured clinically?
5. What factors determine myocardial oxygen supply?
6. What is the mechanism of perioperative myocardial ischemia?
7. What is the incidence of perioperative reinfarction for noncardiac surgery?
8. Based on his MI, would you recommend that the surgery be postponed for a certain period of time? If so, why?
9. State the perioperative medical therapy you would employ to reduce the incidence of myocardial ischemia?
10. Would the patient have increased risk for perioperative major cardiac complications if the patient's preoperative electrocardiogram (ECG) shows right bundle branch block (RBBB)/left bundle branch block (LBBB)?
11. Would you recommend that this elective colectomy be postponed, if the patient underwent placement of a coronary artery bare metal stent 3 weeks ago and is taking aspirin and clopidogrel (Plavix)?

B. Preoperative Evaluation and Preparation

1. How would you evaluate the patient's cardiac condition? What laboratory tests would you like to order?
2. Would you recommend further cardiac testing or coronary revascularization before surgery?
3. How would you classify the cardiac risk according to the type of surgery?

   4. Are patients with a Q-wave infarction at greater risk of perioperative reinfarction than those with a non–Q-wave infarction?
   5. What is the role of the exercise or pharmacologic stress test for this patient?
   6. Would you discontinue any medication before surgery?
   7. How would you premedicate this patient?
   8. Is there a role for α_2 agonist in premedication?

C. Intraoperative Management

   1. What are the intraoperative predictors for perioperative cardiac morbidity (PCM)?
   2. How would you monitor the patient in the operating room?
   3. What ECG leads would you monitor? Why V_5?
   4. Would you use a pulmonary artery catheter (PAC)?
   5. Would you use transesophageal echocardiography (TEE) as a monitor?
   6. Is regional anesthesia better than general anesthesia for patients with cardiac disease?
   7. How would you induce general anesthesia?
   8. Would you induce anesthesia with etomidate? Why?
   9. What is the best choice of anesthetic agents for maintenance of anesthesia? Why?
   10. What muscle relaxant would you choose? Why?
   11. You notice a new 3-mm ST-segment depression in lead V_5. How would you treat it?
   12. Would you give prophylactic intravenous nitroglycerin to prevent myocardial ischemia?
   13. What is the significance of tight control of the heart rate intraoperatively?
   14. When would you extubate the trachea in this patient? What could you do to prevent hypertension and tachycardia during extubation and emergence?

D. Postoperative Management

   1. What are the postoperative predictors of PCM?
   2. How would you control postoperative pain?
   3. Is postoperative anemia associated with adverse cardiac outcome?
   4. Is postoperative hypothermia associated with postoperative myocardial ischemia?
   5. How would you make a diagnosis of perioperative myocardial infarction (PMI)?
   6. How would you manage the patient with a suspected PMI?

A. Medical Disease and Differential Diagnosis

A.1. What are the preoperative predictors for perioperative cardiac morbidity (PCM)?

Perioperative myocardial infarction (PMI) is one of the most important predictors of short and long-term mortality and morbidity associated with noncardiac surgery. Therefore, the prevention of PMI relates to improvement in the postoperative outcome. Numerous risk indices and predictors for PCM have been published over the last 30 years.

In 1999, Lee et al. revised the Goldman Cardiac Risk Index, utilizing six independent predictors of cardiac risk:

- High-risk type of surgery
- History of ischemic heart disease
- History of congestive heart failure (CHF)
- History of cerebrovascular disease
- Preoperative treatment of diabetes mellitus with insulin
- Preoperative serum creatinine greater than 2.0 mg per dL

They concluded that the rate of major cardiac complications (myocardial infarction [MI], pulmonary edema, ventricular fibrillation, and primary cardiac arrest) with 0, 1, 2, and more than or equal to 3 predictors were 0.5%, 1.3%, 4%, and 9%, respectively.

According to the 2002 American College of Cardiology (ACC) and American Heart Association (AHA) guideline update on perioperative cardiovascular evaluation (ACC/AHA guidelines), clinical predictors of PCM are categorized into major, intermediate, and minor factors as follows:

Major predictors

- Unstable coronary syndromes
  - Acute (MI $\leq$7 days before examination) or recent MI (>7 days but $\leq$1 month) with evidence of important ischemic risk by clinical symptoms or noninvasive study. Notice that the traditional 3 and 6 months interval had been avoided,
- Unstable or severe angina (Canadian class III: Marked limitation of ordinary physical activity. Walking one to two blocks on the level and climbing one flight of stairs in normal conditions and at normal pace and class IV: Inability to carry on any physical activity without discomfort—anginal syndrome may be present at rest).
- Decompensated heart failure
- Significant arrhythmias
  - High-grade atrioventricular block
  - Symptomatic ventricular arrhythmias in the presence of underlying heart disease
  - Supraventricular arrhythmias with uncontrolled ventricular rate
- Severe valvular disease

Intermediate predictors

- Mild angina pectoris (Canadian class I: Ordinary physical activity, such as walking and climbing stairs, does not cause angina; angina is with strenuous or rapid or prolonged exertion at work or recreation. Class II: Slight limitations to ordinary activity. Walking or climbing stairs rapidly; walking uphill; walking or stair climbing after meals, or in cold, or in wind, or under emotional stress, or only during the few hours after awakening. Walking more than two blocks on the level and climbing more than one flight of ordinary stairs at a normal pace and in normal conditions.)
- Previous MI by history or pathologic Q waves
- Compensated or prior heart failure
- Diabetes mellitus (particularly insulin-dependent)
- Renal insufficiency

Minor predictors

- Advanced age
- Abnormal electrocardiogram (ECG) (left ventricular [LV] hypertrophy, left bundle branch block [LBBB], ST-T abnormalities)
- Rhythm other than sinus (e.g., atrial fibrillation)
- Low functional capacity (e.g., inability to climb one flight of stairs while carrying a bag of groceries)
- History of stroke
- Uncontrolled systemic hypertension

Eagle KA, Berger PB, Calkins H, et al. ACC/AHA guideline update for perioperative cardiovascular evaluation for noncardiac surgery—executive summary. A report of the American College of Cardiology/American Heart Association Task Force on practice guidelines. *Anesth Analg* 2002;94:1052–1064.

Lee TH, Marcantonio RE, Mangione CM, et al. Derivation and prospective validation of a simple index for prediction of cardiac risk of major noncardiac surgery. *Circulation* 1999;100:1043–1049.

Mangano DT. Perioperative cardiac morbidity. *Anesthesiology* 1990;72:153–184.

Mangano DT, Browner WS, Hollenberg M, et al. Association of perioperative myocardial ischemia with cardiac morbidity and mortality in men undergoing noncardiac surgery. *N Engl J Med* 1990;323:1781–1788.

A.2. What is the New York Heart Association (NYHA) classification of heart failure?

Large number of studies have listed congestive heart failure (CHF) as a condition that correlates with perioperative morbidity and mortality. CHF can be corrected or optimized before surgery. The impact of CHF on perioperative morbidity and mortality is often underestimated. The incidence of CHF doubles with each decade between 45 and 75 years.

The NYHA classification of heart failure is determined by severity of symptoms including dyspnea and fatigue.

- *Class I.* No symptoms
- *Class II.* Symptoms with ordinary activity
- *Class III.* Symptoms with less than ordinary activity
- *Class IV.* Symptoms at rest

Bristow M, Lowe B. Management of heart failure. In: Zipes DP, Libby P, Braunwald E, et al. eds. *Braunwald's heart disease: a textbook of cardiovascular medicine*, 7th ed. Philadelphia: WB Saunders, 2005:603–610.

The Criteria Committee of the New York Heart Association. *Diseases of the heart and blood vessels: nomenclature and criteria for diagnosis*, 9th ed. Boston: Little Brown and Company, 1994.

Hunt SA, Baker DW, Chin MH, et al. ACC/AHA guidelines for the evaluation and management of chronic heart failure in the adult: executive summary. A report of the American College of Cardiology/American Heart Association task force on practice guidelines (Committee to revise the 1995 guidelines for the evaluation and management of heart failure) developed in collaboration with the International Society for Heart and Lung Transplantation endorsed by the Heart Failure Society of America. *J Am Coll Cardiol* 2001;38:2101–2112.

A.3. What is the specific activity scale (SAS) of cardiac function?

SAS was developed in the 1980s as a tool used to measure functional status. It has a very good interobserver reliability and also good correlation with treadmill exercise time.

- *Class I.* Can carry at least 24 lb up eight steps; carry objects that are at least 80 lb; shovel snow; spade soil; jog/walk 5 mph; ski; or play basketball, football, squash, or handball.
- *Class II.* Can carry anything up a flight of eight steps without stopping, have sexual intercourse without stopping, garden, rake, weed, roller skate, dance, or walk at a rate of 4-mph on level ground.
- *Class III.* Can shower without stopping, strip and make bed, mop floors, hang washed clothes, clean windows, walk 2.5 mph, bowl, play golf (walk and carry clubs), push power lawn mower, or dress without stopping because of symptoms.
- *Class IV.* Can do none of the previous or have symptoms at rest.

Das P, Remington H, Chambers J. Exercise testing to stratify risk in aortic stenosis. *Eur Heart J* 2005;26:1309–1313.

Goldman L. Cardiac risk in noncardiac surgery: an update. *Anesth Analg* 1995;80:810–820.

A.4. What are the determinants of myocardial oxygen demand? How are they measured clinically?

The three major determinants are myocardial left ventricular (LV) wall tension (LV preload and afterload), cardiac contractility and heart rate.

A.5. What factors determine myocardial oxygen supply?

The factors include cardiac output, arterial oxygen content, heart rate, aortic diastolic pressure, left ventricular (LV) end-diastolic pressure, patency of coronary arteries and coronary vascular tone.

A.6. What is the mechanism of perioperative myocardial ischemia?

Myocardial ischemia occurs whenever myocardial oxygen supply does not match myocardial oxygen demand. Intraoperative ischemia can be precipitated by increases in myocardial oxygen demand caused by tachycardia, hypertension, anemia, stress, sympathomimetic drugs, or discontinuation of β-blockers. However, as many as 50% or more of the ischemic episodes may be unrelated to the indices of oxygen demand, suggesting decreased oxygen supply as the primary cause. Potential etiologies for decreased supply include external factors, such as hypotension, tachycardia, increased filling pressures, anemia, hypoxemia, and decreased cardiac output. In addition, internal factors such as acute coronary artery thrombosis and spasm also may play a role, although no data are available for determining their importance in the perioperative setting.

Perioperative myocardial infarction (PMI) is one of the most important predictors of short- and long-term morbidity and mortality associated with noncardiac surgery. Unfortunately, the exact nature of PMI remains an area of uncertainty and a subject of debate and controversy. The interaction between morphologic and functional factors is unpredictable. There is pathologic and angiographic evidence that the etiology of PMI resembles that in the nonsurgical setting. In PMI, acute plaque disruption and hemorrhage in the infarct-related coronary artery seems to be common, but the severity of underlying coronary artery stenosis does not necessarily predict the infarct territory. The high incidence of histologically-confirmed transmural infarctions seems to be contradictory to the electrocardiogram (ECG) finding of almost exclusively non–Q-wave PMIs. On the other hand, the presence of subendocardial PMIs is consistent with a myocardial oxygen supply/demand mismatch being the main trigger of myocardial injury. However, myocardial oxygen supply/demand mismatch and plaque rupture are not mutually exclusive mechanisms, and myocardial infarctions (MIs) may develop by different mechanisms at different locations in the same patient.

Most PMIs (>80%) occur early after surgery (0 to 72 hours), are asymptomatic, of the non–Q-wave type (60% to 100%), and are commonly preceded by ST-segment depression rather than ST-segment elevation. Long duration (single duration >20 to 30 minutes or cumulative duration >1 to 2 hours intraoperatively or postoperatively) rather than just the presence of postoperative ST-segment depression, seems to be the important factor associated with adverse cardiac outcome.

Landesberg's review of PMIs summarizes pathophysiology as follows:

- Ischemia occurs (67%) at the end of anesthesia or immediately after the surgery, during a period characterized by high sympathetic output, hypercoagulability, hypertension, and tachycardia. Ischemia in this period is usually silent, with only ST-segment depression as marker. And in at least one third of the patients this ST depression goes unnoticed.

- Patients with prolonged ST depression may present with troponin elevation, half of them asymptomatic. In this population, the diagnosis of PMI will be missed if troponins were not requested. The elevation may start within the first 8 hours postsurgery.
- Because the increase in troponin occurs during or shortly after prolonged ST-depression–type ischemia, without sudden conversion to ST elevation, it is assumed that PMI is most likely the consequence of stress-induced ischemia and not because of plaque rupture, however, the two mechanisms are not mutually exclusive.
- In approximately 50% of the patients who die secondary to a PMI, no plaque rupture or thrombosis was found in their coronary arteries at autopsy, despite their extensive coronary artery disease (CAD). The peak incidence of cardiac death in these patients is in the first 3 postoperative days, which corresponds to the peak incidence of prolonged, stress-induced, ST-depression–type PMI. The other 50% of patients with PMI, in whom plaque rupture or coronary thrombosis is detected, the timing of death is evenly distributed in the postoperative period, with no special correlation to the end of surgery (Fig. 15.1).

Landesberg G. Pathophysiology of perioperative myocardial infarction: facts and perspectives. *J Cardiothorac Vasc Anesth* 2003;17:90–100.

Mangano DT. Perioperative cardiac morbidity. *Anesthesiology* 1990;72:153–184.

Priebe HJ. Perioperative myocardial infarction—aetiology and prevention. *Br J Anaesth* 2005;95:3–19.

Slogoff S, Keats A. Myocardial ischemia revisited. *Anesthesiology* 2006;105:214–216.

A.7. What is the incidence of perioperative reinfarction for noncardiac surgery?

Previously, risk assessment for noncardiac surgery of patients with coronary artery disease (CAD) was based upon the time interval between the myocardial infarction (MI) and surgery. However, with improvements in perioperative care, this difference has become blurred. The importance

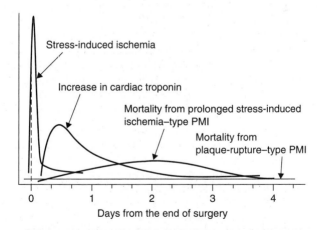

Figure 15.1 The time sequence of perioperative ischemia, infarction, and cardiac death after noncardiac surgery. PMI, perioperative myocardial infarction. (Reprinted with permission from Landesberg G. Pathophysiology of perioperative myocardial infarction: facts and perspectives. *J Cardiothorac Vasc Anesth* 2003;17:90–100.)

of the timing of the MI in relation to the proposed surgical procedure may no longer be valid in the era of thrombolytics, angioplasty, and risk stratification. Although many patients with a history of a MI may continue to have myocardium at risk, others may not. If a stress test does not indicate residual myocardium at risk, the likelihood of reinfarction is low. There is no data available to quote a perioperative reinfarction rate related to the age of the MI; despite this, statements contained in the current American Heart Association/American College of Cardiology (AHA/ACC) guidelines for perioperative cardiovascular evaluation confers a higher risk if the MI is at least 1 month old.

Landesberg states that mortality after PMI is 10% to 15%, similar to the in-hospital mortality after nonsurgical non–Q-wave infarction. This is in contrast to older data showing a higher (50%) mortality after PMI.

Eagle KA, Berger PB, Calkins H, et al. ACC/AHA guideline update for perioperative cardiovascular evaluation for noncardiac surgery—executive summary. A report of the American College of Cardiology/American Heart Association Task Force on practice guidelines. *Anesth Analg* 2002;94:1052–1064.

Landesberg G. Pathophysiology of perioperative myocardial infarction: facts and perspectives. *J Cardiothorac Vasc Anesth* 2003;17:90–100.

Rao TLK, Jacobs KH, El-Etr AA. Reinfarction following anesthesia in patients with myocardial infarction. *Anesthesiology* 1983;59:499–505.

Slogoff S, Keats A. Myocardial ischemia revisited. *Anesthesiology* 2006;105:214–216.

A.8. Based on his myocardial infarction (MI), would you recommend that the surgery be postponed for a certain period of time? If so, why?

The arbitrary delaying of a surgical procedure is not supported by American College of Cardiology/American Heart Association (ACC/AHA) guidelines. According to these guidelines an acute MI ($\leq$7 days before the preoperative evaluation) or recent MI (>7 days but $\leq$1 month) with evidence of important ischemic risk by clinical symptoms or noninvasive study is a major predictor of perioperative cardiac morbidity (PCM). Therefore, the separation of the interval of MI to operation into the traditional 3- and 6-month intervals has been avoided. Current management of MI provides for risk stratification during convalescence period. If a recent stress test does not indicate residual myocardium at risk, the likelihood of reinfarction after noncardiac surgery is low. Although there are no adequate clinical trials on which to base firm recommendations, it appears reasonable to wait 4 to 6 weeks after MI to perform elective surgery, due to the decrease in incidence of fatal arrhythmias and ventricular rupture after this period of time.

Eagle KA, Berger PB, Calkins H, et al. ACC/AHA guideline update for perioperative cardiovascular evaluation for noncardiac surgery—executive summary. A report of the American College of Cardiology/American Heart Association Task Force on practice guidelines. *Anesth Analg* 2002;94:1052–1064.

A.9. State the perioperative medical therapy you would employ to reduce the incidence of myocardial ischemia?

β-adrenergic antagonists (Esmolol, Atenolol, Metoprolol, Bisoprolol)

This drug class:

- Reduces myocardial oxygen consumption

- Improves coronary blood flow
  - Prolonged diastolic perfusion period
  - Improved collateral flow
  - Increased flow to ischemic areas
- Improves supply/demand ratio
- Stabilizes cellular membranes
- Improves oxygen dissociation from hemoglobin
- Inhibits platelet aggregation

β-Blockers suppress perioperative tachycardia and appear most efficacious in preventing perioperative myocardial ischemia. They are well tolerated by most surgical patients and may reduce long-term cardiac events.

Since 1980s evidence suggests tachycardia as a major determinant of perioperative ischemia and its relation with the occurrence of myocardial infarction (MI) in the postoperative period.

Slogoff et al. found that perioperative myocardial infarction (PMI) presented more frequently in patients that sustained ischemia independent of the time of occurrence. Ischemia was significantly related to tachycardia but not hypertension or hypotension and was frequently seen in the absence of any hemodynamic abnormalities. Also they advocated the perioperative use of β-blockers to prevent ischemia. Were the authors having a vision of what the present is? Today, their revisited myocardial ischemia article is a summary of what is very much in vogue regarding myocardial ischemia prevention and emphasizes perioperative myocardial ischemia relation to perioperative management instead of patient selection.

Mangano et al. reported a beneficial effect of atenolol in a randomized double-blind, placebo-controlled trial on overall survival and cardiovascular morbidity in noncardiac surgery patients with or at risk for coronary artery disease (CAD). Poldermans et al. reported that the β-blocker, bisoprolol, reduced the perioperative incidence of death from cardiac causes and nonfatal MI in vascular surgical patients with known CAD. Bisoprolol, started before noncardiac surgery (30 days), can substantially reduce perioperative cardiac complications in all but the highest-risk patients. Questions remain as to whether these findings extend to all types of β-blockers,

The American College of Cardiology/American Heart Association (ACC/AHA) guidelines on perioperative β-blocker therapy were revised in 2006. These recommendations identify the following groups of patients who are candidates for perioperative β-blockade:

- Patients undergoing vascular surgery with or without evidence of preoperative ischemia and with or without high- or intermediate-risk factors.
- Patients receiving chronic β-blocker therapy.
- Patients with high- or intermediate-risk factors undergoing intermediate- or high-risk surgery.
- Patients undergoing vascular surgery even if they have low-risk factors.

When possible, the evidence suggests, that β-blocker therapy should be started several days or weeks before the surgery, to achieve a heart rate between 50 and 60 beats per minute and should continue during the intra- and postoperative period to maintain a heart rate less than 80 beats per minute. The AHA/ACC guidelines on β-blocker therapy clearly specify that the literature is at best conflicting and that more randomized trials are necessary.

In a recent article, Feringa et al. found a significant reduction of cardiac events in patients with high dose of β-blockers compared to patients with low or no β-blockers use. They attributed their results to tight heart rate control and the reduction of absolute heart rate changes during the perioperative period.

There is newly published evidence that questions the strength of the results presented in the trials supporting the use of β-blockers in the perioperative period. Since the appearance of the initial reports on the beneficial effects of β-blockers others have found different results. Two larger randomized trials on the effect of metoprolol in patients undergoing vascular surgery [metoprolol after vascular surgery (MAVS trial) and in diabetic patients undergoing major noncardiac surgery diabetic postoperative mortality and morbidity (DIPOM trial)], and a small trial in patients undergoing infrarenal vascular surgery [perioperative beta-blockade (POBBLE trial)]. These trials challenge the widely held belief that nearly all patients scheduled for noncardiac surgery benefit from perioperative β-blockade

Indeed, Devereaux et al. in a review meta-analysis of the literature in 2005 found no statistically significant benefits in the use of β-blockers. The authors felt that the data was insufficient to draw conclusions and that caution should be exerted regarding the perioperative use of β-blockers.

The use of β-blockers remains controversial; perioperative cardiac events still occur despite its use.

α_2-adrenergic agonist (Clonidine)

The ACC/AHA guidelines mention the potential benefits on PMI reduction with the use of this drug class. Their benefits had been reviewed by two meta-analysis and only one randomized trial. The meta-analysis has shown the reduction of MI/ischemia in vascular patients, but not in all patient groups. However, a recent randomized trial suggests that using perioperative transdermal/oral clonidine reduced perioperative ischemia and mortality. There are no prospective trials comparing the two forms of adrenergic modulation (β-blockers vs. α_2 agonists).

Nitrovasodilators (Nitroglycerin, Isosorbide dinitrate)

Nitrates are associated with the following:

- Decreased left ventricular (LV) preload (low dose)
  - Systemic venous dilation
  - Pulmonary arterial bed dilation
  - Pulmonary vein dilation
  - Decreased LV filling pressure
  - Decrease in LV diastolic compressive forces
  - Decreased LV diastolic chamber size
- Decreased LV afterload (high dose)
  - Decreased systolic pressure
  - Decreased systemic vascular resistance
  - Decreased aortic impedance
- Coronary circulation
  - Coronary artery and arteriolar dilation (high dose)
  - Spasm reversal or prevention
  - Stenosis dilation
  - Increased collateral flow
  - Improvement of regional subendocardial ischemia

Nitroglycerin, one of the oldest antianginal therapies, has had very few trials in noncardiac surgery to evaluate its role in perioperative ischemia reduction. One meta-analysis suggests that nitrates do not reduce perioperative cardiac events. However, a recent meta-analysis published in Cochrane database has suggested that nitrates show an improvement in perioperative ischemia over placebo. Auerbach and Goldman recommend continuing antianginal medications during the perioperative period. However, the use of prophylactic intravenous nitroglycerin is not recommended.

Calcium channel blockers (Verapamil, Diltiazem, Nifedipine, Nicardipine)

Calcium channel blockers reduce myocardial oxygen demand by depression of myocardial contractility and dilation of coronary and collateral vessels, which improves blood flow. However, its most important effects may be the prevention of sympathetically mediated coronary vasoconstriction.

Calcium channel blockers interact with the L-type calcium channel and are composed of drugs from five classes: (a) the 1,4-dihydropyridine (DHP) derivatives, represented by nifedipine, nicardipine, nimodipine, and nitrendipine; (b) the phenylalkylamines, represented by verapamil; (c) the benzodiazepines, represented by diltiazem; (d) the diarylaminopropylamine ester, represented by bepridil; and (e) diphenylpiperazine.

Due to the initial experience with nifedipine, increase incidence of MI, there has been reluctance to use this drug class. A meta-analysis by Stevens showed no reduction in cardiac events, however, another meta-analysis in 2003 found a reduction of ischemia, MI and postoperative supraventricular tachycardia. The effects were mostly secondary to the use of diltiazem, and the use of dihydropyridine was associated with ischemia. Currently there are no recommendations for the prophylactic use of calcium channels blockers.

Antiplatelet and antithrombotic agents (Aspirin, Dipyridamole, Ticlopidine, Clopidogrel)

Aspirin (acetylsalicylic acid) inhibits platelet aggregation by blocking the production of thromboxane A_2 through a covalent acetylation of a serine residue near the active site of cyclooxygenase. This enzyme produces the cyclic endoperoxide precursor of thromboxane A_2. Acute withdrawal of aspirin may increase the risk of acute coronary syndrome at 8 to 10 days after discontinuation. However, if continued during the perioperative period, aspirin may increase the risk of bleeding. The ACC/AHA guidelines do not make reference to the use of this class of drugs to prevent PMI. However, there are two large randomized trials suggesting that the use of low-dose aspirin may reduce the incidence of thromboembolic events without increasing bleeding or blood transfusion. Given the limited amount of trials, Goldman states that it is difficult to make evidence-based recommendation regarding the perioperative use of antiplatelets therapy.

Statins

Noncontrolled studies and one randomized trial suggest a 30% reduction in perioperative cardiac events when patients were treated with statins. Although the usefulness of this drug group has been validated in acute coronary syndromes, there is not enough evidence that supports its use other than on a long-term basis.

Auerbach A, Goldman L. Assessing and reducing the cardiac risk of non-cardiac surgery. *Circulation* 2006;113:1361–1376.

Beattie WS. Evidence-based perioperative risk reduction. *Can J Anaesth* 2005; 52(Suppl 1):R3.

Boersma E, Poldermans D, Bax JJ, et al. Predictors of cardiac events after major vascular surgery: role of clinical characteristics, dobutamine echocardiography, and beta-blocker therapy. *JAMA* 2001;285(14):1865–1873.

Brady AR, Gibbs JS, Greenhalgh RM, et al. Perioperative beta-blockade (POBBLE) for patients undergoing infrarenal vascular surgery: results of a randomized double-blind controlled trial. *J Vasc Surg* 2005;41:602–609.

Burger W, Chemnitius JM, Kneissl GD, et al. Low-dose aspirin for secondary cardiovascular prevention: cardiovascular risks after its perioperative withdrawal versus bleeding risks with its continuation: review and meta-analysis. *J Intern Med* 2005;257:399–414.

Devereaux PJ, Beattie WS, Choi PT, et al. How strong is the evidence for the use of perioperative beta blockers in non-cardiac surgery? Systematic review and meta-analysis of randomized controlled trials. *Br Med J* 2005;331:313–321.

Feringa H, Bax J, Boersma E, et al. High dose beta-blockers and tight heart rate control reduce myocardial ischemia and troponin T release in vascular surgery patients. *Circulation* 2006;114:344–349.

Fleisher LA, Beckman JA, Freeman WK, et al. ACC/AHA guideline update for perioperative cardiovascular evaluation for noncardiac surgery: focus update on perioperative Beta-blocker therapy. A report of the American College of Cardiology/American Heart Association Task Force on practice guidelines. *J Am Coll Cardiol* 2006;47: 1–12.

Kertai MD, Boersma E, Westerhout CM, et al. A combination of statins and betablockers is independently associated with a reduction in the incidence of perioperative mortality and nonfatal myocardial infarction in patients undergoing abdominal aortic aneurysm surgery. *Eur J Vasc Endovasc Surg* 2004;28:343–352.

Lindenauer PK, Pekow P, Wang K, et al. Lipid-lowering therapy and in-hospital mortality following major noncardiac surgery. *JAMA* 2004;291:2092–2099.

Mangano DT, Layug EL, Wallace A, et al. Effect of atenolol on mortality and cardiovascular morbidity after non cardiac surgery. *N Engl J Med* 1996;335:1713–1720.

O'Neil-Callahan K, Katsimaglis G, Tepper MR, et al. Statins decrease perioperative cardiac complications in patients undergoing noncardiac vascular surgery: the statins for risk reduction in surgery (StaRRS) study. *J Am Coll Cardiol* 2005;45:336–342.

Poldermans D, Bax JJ, Kertai MD, et al. Statins are associated with a reduced incidence of perioperative mortality in patients undergoing major noncardiac vascular surgery. *Circulation* 2003;107:1848–1851.

Poldermans D, Boersma E, Bax JJ, et al. The effect of bisoprolol on perioperative mortality and myocardial infarction in high-risk patients undergoing vascular surgery. *N Engl J Med* 1999;341:1789–1794.

Prevention of pulmonary embolism and deep vein thrombosis with low dose aspirin: pulmonary embolism prevention (PEP) trial. *Lancet* 2000;355:1295–1302.

Robless P, Mikhailidis DP, Stansby G. Systematic review of antiplatelet therapy for the prevention of myocardial infarction, stroke or vascular death in patients with peripheral vascular disease. *Br J Surg* 2001;88:787–800.

Royster R, Zvara D. Anti-ischemic drug therapy. In: Kaplan J, Reich DL, Konstadt SN, eds. *Cardiac anesthesia*, 4th ed. Philadelphia: WB Saunders, 1999:95–123.

Schwartz GG, Olsson AG, Ezekowitz MD, et al. Effects of atorvastatin on early recurrent ischemic events in acute coronary syndromes: the MIRACL study: a randomized controlled trial. *JAMA* 2001;285:1711–1718.

Slogoff S, Keats A. Myocardial ischemia revisited. *Anesthesiology* 2006;105:214–216.

Stevens RD, Burri H, Tramer MR. Pharmacologic myocardial protection in patients undergoing noncardiac surgery: a quantitative systematic review. *Anesth Analg* 2003;97: 623–633.

Taylor DW, Ferguson GC, Barrnett HJ, et al. Low-dose and high-dose acetylsalicylic acid for patients undergoing carotid endarterectomy: a randomized controlled trial. ASA and carotid endarterectomy (ACE) trial collaborators. *Lancet* 1999;353:2179–2184.

Wallace AW, Galindez D, Salahieh A, et al. Effect of clonidine on cardiovascular morbidity and mortality after noncardiac surgery. *Anesthesiology* 2004;101:284–293.

Wetterslev J, Juul AB. Benefits and harms of perioperative beta-blockade. *Best Pract Res Clin Anesthesiol* 2006;20:285–302.

Wijeysundera DN, Naik JS, Beattie WS. Alpha-2 adrenergic agonists to prevent perioperative cardiovascular complications: a meta-analysis. *Am J Med* 2003;114:742–752.

A.10. Would the patient have increased risk for perioperative major cardiac complications if the patient's preoperative electrocardiogram (ECG) shows right bundle branch block (RBBB)/left bundle branch block (LBBB)?

A retrospective, cohort-controlled study of all noncardiac, nonophthalmologic, adult patients showed that the presence of RBBB or LBBB was not associated with a higher incidence of postoperative cardiac complications. Nevertheless, the patients with LBBB may not tolerate certain stress of perioperative noncardiac complications, such as severe sepsis. The presence of LBBB or RBBB may alert the clinician to the possibility of occult coronary artery disease (CAD) or impaired left ventricular (LV) function.

Alternatively, in men, but not in women, LBBB was associated with a significantly greater prevalence of cardiac enlargement and congestive heart failure (CHF) than RBBB. The Framingham Study concluded that in an ambulatory population, men with LBBB were more likely to have or subsequently develop advanced cardiovascular abnormalities than were men with RBBB. In women, however, the clinical scenarios that correlate with the two conduction abnormalities are similar.

The American College of Cardiology/American Heart Association (ACC/AHA) recommends careful evaluation for underlying cardiopulmonary disease, drug toxicity or metabolic abnormality. Frequent premature ventricular complexes (PVCs) or nonsustained ventricular tachycardia (VT) have not been associated with increased risk of myocardial infarction (MI) or cardiac death

---

Dorman T, Breslow M, Pronovost PJ, et al. Bundle-branch block as a risk factor in noncardiac surgery. *Arch Intern Med* 2000;160:1149–1152.

Schneider JF, Thomas HE, Sorlie P, et al. Comparative features of newly acquired left and right bundle branch block in the general population: the Framingham study. *Am J Cardiol* 1981;47:931–940.

A.11. Would you recommend that this elective colectomy be postponed, if the patient underwent placement of a coronary artery bare metal stent 3 weeks ago and is taking aspirin and clopidogrel (Plavix)?

Current recommendations for the antiplatelet therapy after percutaneous coronary intervention (PCI) with stenting (bare metal stents) is that patients should take aspirin and other platelet inhibitor (ticlopidine, clopidogrel) for at least a full 6 to 8 weeks to prevent restenosis and allow reendothelialization of the stent to be completed. Therefore, it is prudent to postpone the elective surgery until finishing the recommended antiplatelet therapy course. Kaluza et al. reported that perioperative discontinuation of antiplatelet therapy within 4 weeks of PCI with stenting actually increases the risks of stent thrombosis and subsequent catastrophic cardiac complications.

The role of preoperative coronary revascularization has been controversial for many years. Few randomized clinical trials and many small size studies have reported conflicting results. Some literature supports revascularization arguing that high-risk cardiac patients who have had PCI performed up to 18 months preoperatively have a lower incidence of perioperative cardiac morbidity (PCM) following vascular surgery. However, McFalls et al. published a randomized study where they concluded that coronary revascularization before vascular surgery does not significantly alter the long-term cardiovascular outcome in patients with stable cardiac symptoms.

The American College of Cardiology/American Heart Association (ACC/AHA) state that the indications for coronary artery bypass grafting (CABG) and PCI should be the same as in the nonsurgical settings. These interventions are rarely indicated to "get a patient through" noncardiac surgery.

In contemporary practice coronary stent thrombosis is a rare event. However, its association with high-mortality morbidity has important implications. Prevention of the stent thrombosis is key. There is uncertainty regarding how much time should pass between PCI, interrupting the antiplatelet therapy and noncardiac surgery. Delaying surgery for at least 4 to 8 weeks after PCI to allow healing of the vessel injury is recommended but still controversial. Patients treated with bare metal stents should receive 6 to 8 weeks of clopidogrel in addition to aspirin to prevent stent thrombosis. Because of concern that late stent thrombosis may develop in patients treated with drug-eluting stents, most authors had recommended this combine antiplatelet therapy for 6 months maybe up to a year.

Auer J, Berent R, Weber T, et al. Risk of non cardiac surgery in month following placement of a drug-eluting stent. Letter to the editor. *J Am Coll Cardiol* 2004;43:713.

Eagle KA, Berger PB, Calkins H, et al. ACC/AHA guideline update for perioperative cardiovascular evaluation for noncardiac surgery—executive summary. A report of the American College of Cardiology/American Heart Association Task Force on practice guidelines. *Anesth Analg* 2002;94:1052–1064.

Gottlieb A, Banoub M, Sprung J, et al. Perioperative cardiovascular morbidity in patients with coronary artery disease undergoing vascular surgery after percutaneous transluminal coronary angioplasty. *J Cardiothorac Vasc Anesth* 1998;12:501–506.

Kaluza GL, Joseph J, Lee JR, et al. Catastrophic outcomes of noncardiac surgery soon after coronary stenting. *J Am Coll Cardiol* 2000;35:1288–1294.

Levine G, Morton K, Berger P, et al. Management of patients undergoing percutaneous coronary revascularization. *Ann Intern Med* 2003;139:123–136.

Satler L. Recommendations regarding stent selection in relation to the timing of non cardiac surgery post percutaneous coronary intervention (editorial comment). *Catheter Cardiovasc Interv* 2004;63:146–147.

B. Preoperative Evaluation and Preparation

B.1. How would you evaluate the patient's cardiac condition? What laboratory tests would you like to order?

The initial history, physical examination, and electrocardiographic assessment should focus on identification of potentially serious cardiac disorders, including coronary artery disease (CAD) (e.g., prior myocardial infarction [MI], angina pectoris), congestive heart failure (CHF), and electrical instability (e.g., symptomatic arrhythmias).

In addition to identifying the presence of preexisting manifested heart disease, it is essential to define disease severity, stability, and prior treatment. Other factors that help determine cardiac risk include functional capacity, age, comorbid conditions (e.g., diabetes mellitus, peripheral vascular disease, renal dysfunction, chronic pulmonary disease), and type of surgery (vascular procedures and prolonged, complicated thoracic, abdominal, and head and neck procedures considered higher risk).

This patient is an insulin-dependent diabetic. Diabetes is associated with a two- to fourfold increase in the risk of developing CAD. The risk of a MI in patients with diabetes and no evidence of CAD match that of patients without diabetes who have had a previous MI. In patients with CAD and diabetes the mortality rate can be up to 70% in 10 years. In addition, patients will have a worse outcome for any CAD manifestation.

The preoperative workup varies according to the presence or absence of clinical indicators of underlying CAD:

- Exercise tolerance—poor exercise tolerance has been associated by some with twofold higher odds for postoperative complications. Lee, however, did not find an independent association of functional status with increased risk.

- Evaluation of the presence or absence of any coronary syndrome/symptoms after coronary revascularization.
- Determination of stress test results post-MI/revascularization and establishment of new symptoms since coronary revascularization.

For this patient, the preoperative laboratory workup should include a hemoglobin/hematocrit, prothrombin time, partial thromboplastin time, electrolytes, creatinine and blood urea nitrogen.

Di Carli M, Hachamovitch R. Should we screen for occult coronary artery disease among asymptomatic patients with diabetes? *J Am Coll Cardiol* 2005;45:50–53.

Eagle KA, Berger PB, Calkins H, et al. ACC/AHA guideline update for perioperative cardiovascular evaluation for noncardiac surgery—executive summary. A report of the American College of Cardiology/American Heart Association Task Force on practice guidelines. *Anesth Analg* 2002;94:1052–1064.

Fleisher L, Eagle K. Lowering cardiac risk in non-cardiac surgery. *N Engl J Med* 2001; 345:1677–1682.

Haffner SM, Lehto S, Ronnemaa T, et al. Mortality from coronary heart disease in subjects with type 2 diabetes and in nondiabetic subjects with and without prior myocardial infarction. *N Engl J Med* 1998;339:229–234.

B.2. Would you recommend further cardiac testing or coronary revascularization before surgery?

Successful perioperative evaluation and treatment of cardiac patients undergoing noncardiac surgery requires careful teamwork and communication between patient, primary care physician, anesthesiologist, and surgeon. In general, indications for further cardiac testing and treatment are the same as those in the nonoperative setting, but their timing is dependent on such factors as the urgency of noncardiac surgery, the patient's risk factors, and specific surgical considerations. Preoperative testing should be limited to circumstances in which the results will affect patient treatment and outcomes. A conservative approach to the use of expensive tests and treatments is recommended. Coronary revascularization before noncardiac surgery to enable the patient to "get through" the noncardiac procedure is inappropriate. However, in a high-risk subset of patients: Left main disease, severe multivessel disease, severe aortic stenosis, and ejection fraction of less than 20% revascularization/valve replacement may be indicated. Currently, there is overwhelming agreement that aggressive medical management to provide myocardial protection during the perioperative period is a very important element in the reduction of perioperative cardiovascular complications.

Several studies have suggested that a stepwise approach to the assessment of coronary artery disease (CAD) is both efficacious and cost effective. The patient sustained a myocardial infarction (MI) 5 months ago managed with a bare metal stent and was scheduled for an intermediate-risk procedure, hemicolectomy. If the patient has more than 4 mets of physical activity, without chest pain or shortness of breath (SOB), if no new cardiac symptoms are present since the revascularization and the resting ECG showed no changes compared to 5 months ago the patient is cleared for anesthesia and surgery. If any of these factors are positive then exercise thallium imaging or dipyridamole-thallium imaging (if unable to exercise) or stress dobutamine echo is performed. If the ischemic area is small, surgery is permissible with recommended aggressive medical therapy management. If the ischemic area is moderate to large, with a suspicion of new coronary stenosis, coronary revascularization after cardiac catheterization is recommended before the planned surgery.

An alternative view: McFalls et al. demonstrated the lack of benefit of perioperative revascularization of patients with significant but stable CAD, this will render the stress test and its low positive predictive value nonuseful in this patient. Considering the patient as high risk given all his comorbidities and adopting an aggressive perioperative medical treatment with β-blockers, α_2-blockers, statins and angiotensin inhibitors, as well as perioperative biochemical ischemia markers, would be the alternative plan recommended.

Eagle KA, Berger PB, Calkins H, et al. ACC/AHA guideline update for perioperative cardiovascular evaluation for noncardiac surgery—executive summary. A report of the American College of Cardiology/American Heart Association Task Force on practice guidelines. *Anesth Analg* 2002;94:1052–1064.

Fleisher LA, Eagle KA. Lowering cardiac risk in s surgery. *N Engl J Med* 2001;345:1677–1682.

McFalls EO, Ward HB, Moritz TE, et al. Coronary artery revascularization before elective major vascular surgery. *N Engl J Med* 2004;351:2795–2804.

Slogoff S, Keats A. Myocardial ischemia revisited. *Anesthesiology* 2006;105:214–216.

B.3. How would you classify the cardiac risk according to the type of surgery?

Surgery-specific cardiac risk of noncardiac surgery is related to two important factors: the type of surgery and the degree of hemodynamic stress associated with the procedure(s). The duration and intensity of coronary and myocardial stressors can be helpful in estimating the likelihood of perioperative cardiac events, particularly for emergency surgery. Surgery-specific risk for noncardiac surgery can be stratified as high, intermediate, and low.

- *High-risk* surgery (cardiac risk often >5%) includes major emergency surgery, particularly in the elderly; aortic and other major vascular surgery; peripheral vascular surgery; and anticipated prolonged procedures associated with large fluid shifts and/or blood loss.
- *Intermediate-risk* (cardiac risk generally <5%) procedures include carotid endarterectomy, head and neck surgery, intraperitoneal and intrathoracic, orthopedic, and prostate surgery.
- *Low-risk* (cardiac risk generally <1%) procedures include endoscopic and superficial procedures, cataract surgery, and breast surgery.

Eagle KA, Berger PB, Calkins H, et al. ACC/AHA guideline update for perioperative cardiovascular evaluation for noncardiac surgery—executive summary. A report of the American College of Cardiology/American Heart Association Task Force on practice guidelines. *Anesth Analg* 2002;94:1052–1064.

B.4. Are patients with a Q-wave infarction at greater risk of perioperative reinfarction than those with a non–Q-wave infarction?

Studies indicate that individuals who survive a non–Q-wave infarction are at greater risk of reinfarction than those who survive a Q-wave infarction. Patients who have not had a transmural wall infarction have a less extensive infarction and lower in-hospital mortality, however, they have a larger degree of jeopardized or susceptible myocardium leading to a higher incidence of reinfarction or recurrent angina. In distinction to patients with complicated Q-wave infarctions who frequently do not survive the immediate postinfarction period but have a lower rate of reinfarction than non–Q-wave myocardial infarction (MI) after this period. Theoretically, patients who have had a solitary coronary artery lesion and sustained a transmural infarction may be considered at a significantly lower risk for reinfarction as the area that was at risk of ischemia is already necrotic. Although their risk of reinfarction may be low, there may be an increased risk of dysrhythmias because of the necrotic myocardium. It is important to remember (a) that the distinction between the Q- and non–Q-wave MI is an electrocardiographic classification and does not necessarily correlate with the pathologic findings of transmural and subendocardial infarctions and (b) that there is overlap especially with the use of thrombolytic therapy.

Antman EM, Braunwald E. ST-elevation myocardial infarction: pathology, pathophysiology and clinical features. In: Zipes D, Libby P, Bonow R, et al. eds. *Braunwald's heart disease, a textbook of cardiovascular medicine*, 7th ed. Philadelphia: WB Saunders, 2005: 1141–1166.

Fleisher LA, Barash PG. Preoperative cardiac evaluation for noncardiac surgery: a functional approach. *Anesth Analg* 1992;74:586–598.

Landesberg G. Pathophysiology of perioperative myocardial infarction: facts and perspectives. *J Cardiothorac Vasc Anesth* 2003;17:90–100.

Priebe HJ. Perioperative myocardial infarction—aetiology and prevention. *Br J Anaesth* 2005;95:3–19.

B.5. What is the role of exercise or pharmacologic stress test for this patient?

The aim of functional cardiovascular testing is to elicit evidence of CAD by subjecting the heart to physiologic stress. The American College of Cardiology/American Heart Association (ACC/AHA) guidelines suggest that the best test for preoperative cardiac risk stratification is an exercise ECG. That recommendation is based on all but the highest-risk patients.

As with clinical risk assessment, noninvasive diagnostic testing must be used judiciously. Effective testing should be accurate, add useful information to the overall risk assessment, and avoid unnecessary delays in surgery. Noninvasive tests of myocardial perfusion are classified by the type of stress applied to elicit transient and reversible ischemia or by the mode of detecting the ischemic area. Stress can be applied by exercise (e.g., treadmill, sitting or supine bicycle, or handgrip), by a pharmacologic agent that increases chronotropy and inotropy (e.g., dobutamine, atropine), or by a pharmacologic agent that can cause redistribution of coronary blood flow (e.g., dipyridamole, adenosine). A significant fraction of the high-risk population cannot exercise to an adequate level and will require pharmacologic stress testing. During a stress test, an ischemic event might be suggested or detected by the patient's reporting of symptoms, appropriate ECG changes (horizontal or down-sloping ST-segment depression of 0.1 mV or ST elevation of 0.15 mV in two contiguous leads, reversible wall motion abnormalities on echocardiography, or reversible perfusion defects on radionuclide imaging with thallium or technetium.

The ACC/AHA Task Force reviewed the literature and determined that dipyridamole-thallium and dobutamine stress echocardiography before vascular surgery predict PMI or death, with a positive predictive value of only 12% to 14% and a negative predictive value of 88% and 94% respectively. The low positive predictive value is expected because stress tests are designed to discover fixed coronary artery stenosis that exceed 70%. However, at least 50% of PMIs are due to plaque rupture, and it is often the noncritical, nonischemia producing lesions that rupture.

Selection of the noninvasive stress test should be based primarily on patient characteristics, local availability, and expertise in interpretation. Because of simplicity, lower cost, and widespread familiarity with performance and interpretation, the standard low-level exercise ECG stress test remains the most reasonable test in patients who are able to exercise and have a resting ECG that is interpretable for ST-segment shifts. Patients with an ECG pattern that would interfere with interpretation of the ST segment (left bundle branch block [LBBB]) should have an exercise test with imaging. Patients who are unable to exercise should have a pharmacologic stress test with imaging.

Dobutamine stress echocardiography is the preferred test if there is an additional question regarding valvular function or left ventricular (LV) dysfunction.

Akhtar S, Silverman D. Assessment and management of patients with ischemic heart disease. *Crit Care Med* 2004;32(suppl):S126–S136.

Beattie WS. Evidence-base perioperative risk reduction. *Can J Anaesth* 2005;52(Suppl 1):R3.

Eagle KA, Berger PB, Calkins H, et al. ACC/AHA guideline update for perioperative cardiovascular evaluation for noncardiac surgery—executive summary. A report of the American College of Cardiology/American Heart Association Task Force on practice guidelines. *Anesth Analg* 2002;94:1052–1064.

Lustik S, Eichelberger J, Chhibber K. Preoperative stress testing: new guidelines. *J Clin Anesth* 2004;14:375–380.

Park K. Preoperative cardiac evaluation. *Anesthesiol Clin North America* 2004;22:199–208.

B.6. Would you discontinue any medication before surgery?

Patients with CAD are usually on a variety of medications. All antianginal drugs, especially β-blockers, should be continued up to the time of surgery. Sudden withdrawal of antianginal drugs may produce rebound tachycardia and hypertension that may precipitate acute myocardial ischemia or infarction.

Current management of hypertensive patients suggests the continuation of antihypertensive therapy up to the day of surgery. However, a number of investigators advocate the discontinuation of antihypertensive drugs from the class of angiotensin 2 receptor antagonist and angiotensin-converting enzyme inhibitors. Tuman et al. in the 1990s and recently Bertrand et al. demonstrated the higher incidence of hypotension postinduction of general anesthesia in patients chronically receiving these drugs. Additionally, it was demonstrated that hypotension was less responsive to the conventional treatment with vasopressors such as phenylephrine and ephedrine.

Bertrand M, Godet G, Meersschaert K, et al. Should the angiotensin 2 antagonists be discontinued before surgery? *Anesth Analg* 2001;92:26–30.

Eagle KA, Berger PB, Calkins H, et al. ACC/AHA guideline update for perioperative cardiovascular evaluation for noncardiac surgery—executive summary. A report of the American College of Cardiology/American Heart Association Task Force on practice guidelines. *Anesth Analg* 2002;94:1052–1064.

Tuman KJ, McCarthy RJ, O'Connor CJ, et al. Angiotensin-converting enzyme inhibitors increase vasoconstrictor requirements after cardiopulmonary bypass. *Anesth Analg* 1995; 88:7–17.

B.7. How would you premedicate this patient?

The patient with ischemic heart disease should be adequately sedated before surgery to avoid anxiety-induced tachycardia and hypertension that may cause adverse myocardial ischemic events. Appropriate doses of a benzodiazepine may be given with the antianginal medications.

B.8. Is there a role for α_2 agonist in premedication?

α_2 agonists stimulate prejunctional receptors and decrease norepinephrine release from prejunctional terminals, thereby decreasing noradrenergic central nervous system transmission, producing sedation, anxiolysis, and analgesia. Studies have shown that clonidine as a premedication reduces hypertension, tachycardia, and norepinephrine levels in patients undergoing aortic reconstruction. Clonidine also suppresses the normal postoperative increase in fibrinogen levels and antagonizes epinephrine-induced platelet aggregation. It has also been shown to decrease intraoperative myocardial ischemia. The more selective α_2 agonists, dexmedetomidine and mivazerol (IV form only available in Europe), may also reduce postoperative myocardial ischemia events in high-risk patients.

Eagle KA, Berger PB, Calkins H, et al. ACC/AHA guideline update for perioperative cardiovascular evaluation for noncardiac surgery—executive summary. A report of the American College of Cardiology/American Heart Association Task Force on practice guidelines. *Anesth Analg* 2002;94:1052–1064.

Wallace AW, Galindez D, Salahieh A, et al. Effect of clonidine on cardiovascular morbidity and mortality after non-cardiac surgery. *Anesthesiology* 2004;101:284–293.

Wjeysundera DN, Beattie WS, Naik JS. Alpha -2 adrenergic agonist to prevent perioperative cardiovascular complications: a meta-analysis. *Am J Med* 2003;114:742–752.

C. Intraoperative Management

C.1. What are the intraoperative predictors for perioperative cardiac morbidity (PCM)?

Intraoperative predictors

Among the classic intraoperative predictors for PCM emergency surgery, major vascular surgery, and prolonged (more than 3 hours) thoracic or upper abdominal surgery appear to be independent predictors, whereas choice of anesthesia does not. Among the dynamic predictors, both hypotension and tachycardia predict PCM. Preoperative hypertension remains a controversial predictor. Most myocardial infarctions (MIs) occur early after surgery and are commonly associated with ST-segment depression. Prolonged duration of myocardial ischemia (>20 to 30 minutes or cumulative duration of >1 to 2 hours) seems to be the important factor associated with adverse cardiac outcome. Although left ventricular (LV) end-diastolic pressure is a sensitive measure of ischemia, studies report that pulmonary capillary wedge pressure (PCWP) is an insensitive indicator. Other factors associated with poor outcome are: increased intraoperative bleeding/large quantity of blood transfusions and poor preoperative cardiac functional status.

Bui H, Haukoos J, Donayre C, et al. Predictors of cardiac morbidity and mortality in patients undergoing endovascular repair of the thoracic aorta. *Ann Vasc Surg* 2004;18(1):22–25.

Mangano DT. Perioperative cardiac morbidity. *Anesthesiology* 1990;72:153–184.

Priebe HJ. Perioperative myocardial infarction—aetiology and prevention. *Br J Anaesth* 2005;95:3–19.

Sprung J, Abdelmalak B, Gottlieb A, et al. Analysis of risk factors for myocardial infarction and cardiac mortality after major vascular surgery. *Anesthesiology* 2000;93(1):129–140.

C.2. How would you monitor the patient in the operating room?

The patient should be monitored using the following ASA standard guidelines:

- *ECG*—simultaneous leads V_5 and II
- *Blood pressure*—noninvasive automatic Doppler sphygmotonometer and an invasive arterial catheter
- *Capnography*—to determine continual end-tidal CO_2 analysis.

- *Pulse oximetry*—to assess arterial oxygenation
- *Oxygen analyzer*—to determine inspired fraction of oxygen.
- *Availability of esophageal/bladder temperature probe*—to determine temperature changes.

In addition to these monitors, this patient will also required the monitoring of urine output with a Foley catheter

---

American Society of Anesthesiologists. *ASA standards for basic anesthetic monitoring*. ASA House of Delegates, Oct. 2005.

C.3. What ECG leads would you monitor? Why V₅?

ECG ST-segment changes are most commonly used for detection of intraoperative myocardial ischemia. Multiple-lead ECG monitoring provides the best clinically available method of detecting perioperative ischemia, primarily by combining leads II, V_3, V_4, and V_5 (II/V_5 detection of 80%, II/V_4, V_5 detection of 96%).

Landesberg et al. were able to correlate the duration of ischemia observed in the ST-segment analysis of a continuously monitoring 12-lead ECG throughout the perioperative period with the incidence of perioperative myocardial infarction (PMI). He also found that ischemia is transient even in patients who will develop an infarct.

Certain prerequisites must be met to use the ECG effectively:

- The diagnostic mode allows detection of ST-segment changes that are filtered out by the monitoring mode.
- The number of ECG leads and their location affects detection of ischemic events.
- Immediate availability of a hard copy of the ECG leads for more detailed analysis.
- Studies have reported that even trained observers recognize only 15% to 40% of electrocardiographic ischemic events displayed on oscilloscope.
- The introduction of ST-segment trending helps as an early warning detection system but should not replace examination of the ECG printout.

Barash P. Monitoring myocardial ischemia in the perioperative period. *ASA annual refresher course lectures*. Park Ridge: American Society of Anesthesiologists, 2006:213.

Landesberg G. Pathophysiology of perioperative myocardial infarction: facts and perspectives. *J Cardiothorac Vasc Anesth* 2003;17:90–100.

Landesberg G, Mosseri M, Wolf Y, et al. The probability of detecting perioperative myocardial ischemia in vascular surgery by continuous 12-lead ECG. *Anesthesiology* 2002;96:264–270.

London MJ, Hollenberg M, Wong MG, et al. Intraoperative myocardial ischemia: localization by continuous 12-lead electrocardiography. *Anesthesiology* 1988;69:232–241.

C.4. Would you use a pulmonary artery catheter (PAC)?

A recently published meta-analysis of randomized controlled trials showed that the use of PAC neither increased mortality or conferred any benefits to critically ill patients.

A number of studies report that PAC is an insensitive monitor for myocardial ischemia and should not be inserted with this as a primary indication.

Eagle KA, Berger PB, Calkins H, et al. ACC/AHA guideline update for perioperative cardiovascular evaluation for noncardiac surgery—executive summary. A report of the

American College of Cardiology/American Heart Association Task Force on practice guidelines. *Anesth Analg* 2002;94:1052–1064.

Shah MR, Hasselblad V, Stevenson L, et al. Impact of pulmonary artery catheter in critically ill patients: meta-analysis of randomized control trials. *JAMA* 2005;294(13):1664–1670.

C.5. Would you use transesophageal echocardiography (TEE) as a monitor?

TEE is a very sensitive diagnostic method of new onset myocardial ischemia. However, its role as a intraoperative monitor of myocardial perfusion is not supported by many investigators.

The echocardiographic diagnosis of myocardial ischemia is based on the development of new regional wall motion abnormalities (RWMAs), decreased systolic wall thickening, and ventricular dilation. Usually, a cross-sectional view (deep transgastric short axis), of the left ventricle (LV) is imaged because this view displays the myocardial perfusion territories of the three major coronary arteries. TEE was found to be twice as predictive as ECG in identifying coronary artery bypass grafting (CABG) patients who have an myocardial infarction (MI). In CABG patients postbypass RWMAs were related to adverse clinical outcome.

However, preintubation events are missed. Real-time intraoperative analysis of the TEE image is associated with a decreased accuracy of interpretation. The examination could divert the anesthesiologist's attention from more important clinical details. Despite numerous reports extolling the virtues of TEE as an ischemia monitor, Hollenberg et al. demonstrated little incremental value over the 12-lead ECG.

As presented by many authors, myocardial ischemia occurs frequently at the end of the surgery when tachycardia and hypertension appear as part of the emergence of general anesthesia. During this period TEE use will not be feasible.

The American Society of Anesthesiologists and the Society of Cardiovascular Anesthesiologists Task Force in 1996 published a practice guideline for perioperative echocardiography. In these guidelines the use of TEE as a monitor of ischemia has a class II or III indication, meaning there is weak/little scientific evidence or expert support. However, its use has acquired more validity when ECG monitoring cannot provide accurate information, such as conduction abnormalities. Similarly, TEE use loses validity when clinical factors as preexisting ventricular dysfunction limit the accuracy of wall motion interpretations.

American Society of Anesthesiologists and the Society of Cardiovascular Anesthesiologists Task Force on Transesophageal Echocardiography. Practice guidelines for perioperative transesophageal echocardiography. A report by the American Society of Anesthesiologists and the Society of Cardiovascular Anesthesiologists Task Force on transesophageal echocardiography. *Anesthesiology* 1996;84:986–1006.

Barash PG. Sequential monitoring of myocardial ischemia in the perioperative period. *ASA annual refresher course lectures*. Park Ridge: American Society of Anesthesiologists, 2006:213.

Comunale ME, Body SC, Ley C, et al. The concordance of intraoperative left ventricular wall motion abnormalities and electrocardiographic ST segment changes: association with coronary revascularization. *Anesthesiology* 1998;88:945–954.

Eagle KA, Berger PB, Calkins H, et al. ACC/AHA guideline update for perioperative cardiovascular evaluation for noncardiac surgery—executive summary. A report of the American College of Cardiology/American Heart Association Task Force on practice guidelines. *Anesth Analg* 2002;94:1052–1064.

Hollenberg MJ, London MJ, Leung JM, et al. Monitoring myocardial ischemia during noncardiac surgery: a technology assessment of TEE and 12-lead ECG. *JAMA* 1992;268: 210–216.

Miller JP, Lambert S, Shapiro WA, et al. The adequacy of basic intra-operative transesophageal echocardiography performed by experienced anesthesiologists. *Anesth Analg* 2001;92:1102–1110.

Wenger MB, Herndon OW, Gaba DM. The effect of electronic record keeping and transesophageal echocardiography on task distribution, workload, and vigilance during cardiac anesthesia. *Anesthesiology* 1997;87:144–155.

C.6. Is regional anesthesia better than general anesthesia for patients with cardiac disease?

A number of studies in patients with cardiac disease have compared the effects of regional versus general anesthetics on the incidence of perioperative infarction, dysrhythmias, and congestive heart failure (CHF). No distinct advantage is apparent between them when considering perioperative cardiac morbidity (PCM) and mortality in peripheral vascular surgery. There is some evidence to support regional anesthesia over general anesthesia in an effort to optimize graft patency if the regional technique is extended into the postoperative period to provide neuraxial analgesia. The choice of technique does not appear to affect mortality in patients requiring hip fracture surgery, although Urwin et al. reported in a recent meta-analysis a decreased 1-month mortality and incidence of thromboembolic complications in patients receiving regional anesthesia for hip fracture repair. Epidural anesthesia has also been shown to promote quicker return of bowel function postoperatively when the catheter has been sited at T12 or higher. Anastomotic (colon/bowel) breakdown in patients with epidural anesthesia/analgesia (secondary to hyperperistalsis) has rarely been reported. Most studies tend to show quicker return of bowel function when local anesthetics alone are administered epidurally. In summary, no one technique demonstrates a consistent advantage.

The American College of Cardiology/American Heart Association (ACC/AHA) guidelines recommends that the choice of anesthesia is best left to the discretion of the anesthesia care team, which will consider the need for postoperative ventilation; pulmonary/neuromuscular comorbidities; cardiovascular effects, including myocardial depression; sympathetic blockade consequences; and dermatomal level of the procedure.

Bode RH Jr, Lewis KP, Zarich SW, et al. Cardiac outcome after peripheral vascular surgery: comparison of general and regional anesthesia. *Anesthesiology* 1996;84:3–13.

Breen P, Park K. General anesthesia versus regional anesthesia. *Int Anesthesiol Clin* 2002; 40(1):61–71.

Go AS, Browner WS. Cardiac outcomes after regional or general anesthesia, do we have the answer? *Anesthesiology* 1996;84:1–2.

Norris EJ, Beattie C, Perler BA, et al. Double-masked randomized trial comparing alternate combinations of intraoperative anesthesia and postoperative analgesia in abdominal aortic surgery. *Anesthesiology* 2001;95:1054–1067.

Urwin SC, Parker MJ, Griffiths R. General versus regional anaesthesia for hip fracture surgery: a meta-analysis of randomized trials. *Br J Anaesth* 2000;84:450–455.

C.7. How would you induce general anesthesia?

It is essential to prevent hypotension, hypertension, and tachycardia, which can precipitate myocardial ischemia. Different induction techniques may be employed to achieve this goal. For example, while the patient is being preoxygenated, fentanyl is given slowly to achieve drowsiness and to attenuate the sympathetic response to direct laryngoscopy and intubation of the trachea. Then using lower doses of thiopental, propofol or etomidate unconsciousness is achieved. Succinylcholine or an intermediate duration nondepolarizing relaxant is administered to facilitate tracheal intubation. A few minutes before intubation the use of a short acting β-blocker (esmolol) could help to further attenuate the sympathetic response to intubation if necessary. For this patient a high-dose fentanyl technique is not recommended because prolonged postoperative mechanical ventilation is not indicated.

Priebe HJ. Perioperative myocardial infarction—aetiology and prevention. *Br J Anaesth* 2005;95:3–19.

C.8. Would you induce anesthesia with etomidate? Why?

Although etomidate has a negative inotropic effect on failing and nonfailing human heart muscle in doses that exceed the clinical dose, it appears to have a better hemodynamic profile than other commonly used induction agents, especially in the setting of coronary heart disease; with an induction dose of 0.2 to 0.3 mg per kg there are minimal changes in heart rate, stroke volume or cardiac output, and the blood pressure may decrease up to 15% because of decrease of systemic vascular resistance. Thiopental at equivalent doses of 3 to 5 mg per kg can produce an increase in heart rate 10% to 36% which could be potentially deleterious. Etomidate does suppress adrenocortical function, cause myoclonus, and prolong duration of seizure when used for electroconvulsive therapy (ECT).

Fuchs-Buder T, Sparr HJ, Ziegenfuss T, et al. Thiopental or etomidate for rapid sequence induction with rocuronium. *Br J Anaesth* 1998;80:504–506.

Haessler R, Madler C, Klasing S, et al. Propofol/fentanyl versus etomidate/fentanyl for the induction of anesthesia in patients with aortic insufficiency and coronary artery disease. *J Cardiothorac Vasc Anesth* 1992;6:173–180.

Reves JG, Glass PS, Lubarsky D, et al. Intravenous non-opioids anesthetics. In: Miller RD, ed: *Miller's anesthesia*, 6th ed. Philadelphia: Churchill Livingstone, 2005:317–378.

Sprung J, Ogletree-Hughes ML, Moravec CS, et al. The effects of etomidate on the contractility of failing and nonfailing human heart muscle. *Anesth Analg* 2000;91:68–75.

Stoelting Robert K. *Pharmacology and physiology in anesthetic practice*, 4th ed. Philadelphia: Lippincott Williams & Wilkins, 2005:155–179.

C.9. What is the best choice of anesthetic agents for maintenance of anesthesia? Why?

There appears to be no one best myocardial protective agent or technique. The knowledge of physiologic and pharmacologic effects of anesthetic agents in patients with cardiac disease will allow flexibility in their selection. The use of inhalation versus narcotic anesthesia in patients with cardiac disease is still debated, although the cardiovascular effects of both techniques and the physiologic differences between them are well documented. However, most outcome studies have not demonstrated a difference between the techniques. Studies of more than 3,000 noncardiac surgical patients with CAD have concluded that anesthetic type does not affect outcome.

Inhalation anesthetics are thought to possess ischemic preconditioning properties. Most investigations of anesthetic ischemic preconditioning have been done in cardiac anesthesia, but maybe there are potential effects in the high-risk cardiac patients having noncardiac surgery. The use of nitrous oxide in patients with history of CAD has been questioned since the early 1990s when animal and human studies showed the increase in peripheral vascular resistance (PVR), diastolic dysfunction, and subsequently myocardial ischemia. Batner et al. demonstrated the increase on homocysteine plasma levels of patients during carotid endarterectomy when nitrous oxide was administered and the correlation of those levels with increase incidence of myocardial ischemia.

The objectives during maintenance are not dissimilar to any other patient: amnesia, unconsciousness and analgesia. These goals are constrained by the hemodynamic effect of each agent in order to provide heart rate control, coronary pressure perfusion, and effects on left ventricular (LV) function. The preferred anesthetic technique will be a balanced anesthetic approach: opioids, with low/moderate doses of volatile anesthetics and benzodiazepines. If the plan is extubate the trachea at the end of surgery a high-dose/longer-acting narcotics should be avoided.

Badner NH, Beattie WS, Freeman D, et al. Nitrous oxide-induced increased homocysteine concentrations are associated with increased postoperative myocardial ischemia in patients undergoing carotid endarterectomy. *Anesth Analg* 2000;91(5):1073–1079.

Beattie WS. Evidence-based perioperative risk reduction. *Can J Anaesth* 2005; 52(Suppl 1):R3.

Eagle KA, Berger PB, Calkins H, et al. ACC/AHA guideline update for perioperative cardiovascular evaluation for noncardiac surgery—executive summary. A report of the American College of Cardiology/American Heart Association Task Force on practice guidelines. *Anesth Analg* 2002;94:1052–1064.

Rao TK, Jacobs KH, El-Etr AA. Reinfarction following anesthesia in patients with myocardial infarction. *Anesthesiology* 1983;59:499–505.

Tuman KJ, McCarthy RJ, Spiess BD, et al. Does choice of anesthetic agent significantly affect outcome after coronary artery surgery? *Anesthesiology* 1989;70:189–198.

C.10. What muscle relaxant would you choose? Why?

The hemodynamic goals are to avoid hypotension, tachycardia, and hypertension. Intermediate-acting neuromuscular blocking agents such as vecuronium, cisatracurium, and rocuronium can be used safely because they produce minimally significant cardiovascular changes. A peripheral nerve stimulator should be used to monitor the degree of blockade.

Fleming N. Con: the choice of muscle relaxants is not important in cardiac surgery. *J Cardiothorac Vasc Anesth* 1995;9:772–774.

Hudson RJ, Thomson IR. Pro: the choice of muscle relaxants is important in cardiac surgery. *J Cardiothorac Vasc Anesth* 1995;9:768–771.

C.11. You notice a new 3-mm ST-segment depression in lead V_5. How would you treat it?

ST-segment depression can be an indicator of myocardial ischemia. Initial efforts should be focused on a determination of its etiology. Management of ischemia should include pharmacologic manipulation of the determinants of myocardial oxygen supply and demand.

The crucial aspect of such management includes the following:

- Heart rate control and adequate coronary perfusion pressure. Heart rate control can be achieved by the use of β-blockers, caution should be exerted in patients with known contraindications. Calcium channel blockers have also improved mortality after myocardial infarction (MI). The use of this drug class could play an important role if coronary spasm is suspected.

- Avoidance of hypotension and use of vasopressors to sustain coronary perfusion pressure.
- The use of nitrates is advocated as long as it does not compromise coronary perfusion pressure. Nitrates decrease myocardial oxygen demand by decreasing preload and intracavitary pressure. In addition, it increases the ratio of endocardial to epicardial blood flow.
- Oxygen delivery should be increased by correcting anemia, and increasing the fraction of inspired oxygen.
- Oxygen demand could be also reduced by correction of hypothermia and/or shivering if present.
- Secondary therapies should consider the use, if feasible, of antiplatelet therapy such as aspirin. If necessary even consideration of the use of heparin intraoperative as long as not surgically contraindicated.

Eagle KA, Berger PB, Calkins H, et al. ACC/AHA guideline update for perioperative cardiovascular evaluation for noncardiac surgery—executive summary. A report of the American College of Cardiology/American Heart Association Task Force on practice guidelines. *Anesth Analg* 2002;94:1052–1064.

Nyhan D, Johns R. Anesthesia for cardiac surgery procedures. In: Miller RD, ed. *Miller's anesthesia*, 6th ed. Philadelphia: Churchill Livingstone, 2005:1946–1954.

Priebe HJ. Perioperative myocardial infarction—aetiology and prevention. *Br J Anaesth* 2005;95:3–19.

C.12. Would you give prophylactic intravenous nitroglycerin to prevent myocardial ischemia?

There are no randomized data that support the use of prophylactic intraoperative intravenous nitroglycerin (NTG) in patients at high risk. NTG should be used only when ischemia is detected and the hemodynamic effects of other agents in use are considered.

Beattie WS. Evidence-based perioperative risk reduction. *Can J Anaesth* 2005; 52(Suppl 1):R3.

Eagle KA, Berger PB, Calkins H, et al. ACC/AHA guideline update for perioperative cardiovascular evaluation for noncardiac surgery—executive summary. A report of the American College of Cardiology/American Heart Association Task Force on practice guidelines. *Anesth Analg* 2002;94:1052–1064.

C.13. What is the significance of tight control of the heart rate intraoperatively?

Numerous studies have shown that intraoperative tachycardia could cause myocardial ischemia. Therefore, tight control of heart rate intraoperatively could significantly reduce the risk of perioperative myocardial events. Multiple reviews document how the duration of tachycardia is directly proportional associated with troponin elevation in the perioperative period.

Slogoff et al. in the 1980s were able to correlate tachycardia with the occurrence of intraoperative myocardial ischemia.

Raby et al. demonstrated that by identifying the high-risk patients, whose preoperative Holter tracing showed signs of ischemia, and controlling the heart rate 20% below the ischemia threshold or approximately 60 beats per minute with esmolol during vascular surgeries could reduce the risk of perioperative myocardial ischemia.

Recently, Feringa et al. demonstrated that tight heart rate control instead of just the use of β-blockers reduced perioperative myocardial ischemia and improved long-term outcome in vascular surgery patients.

Auerbach A, Goldman L. Assessing and reducing the cardiac risk of non-cardiac surgery. *Circulation* 2006;113:1361–1376.

Beattie WS. Evidence-based perioperative risk reduction. *Can J Anaesth* 2005; 52(Suppl 1):R3.

Feringa H, Bax J, Boersma E, et al. High dose beta-blockers and tight heart rate control reduce myocardial ischemia and troponin T release in vascular surgery patients. *Circulation* 2006;114:344–349.

Fleisher LA, Beckman JA, Freeman WK, et al. ACC/AHA guideline update for perioperative cardiovascular evaluation for noncardiac surgery: Focus update on perioperative Beta-blocker therapy. A report of the American College of Cardiology/American Heart Association Task Force on practice guidelines. *J Am Coll Cardiol* 2006;47:1–12.

Landesberg G. Pathophysiology of perioperative myocardial infarction: facts and perspectives. *J Cardiothorac Vasc Anesth* 2003;17:90–100.

Poldermans D, Boersma E, Bax J, et al. The effect of bisoprolol on perioperative mortality and myocardial infarction in high-risk patients undergoing vascular surgery. *N Engl J Med* 1999;341:1789–1794.

Priebe HJ. Perioperative myocardial infarction—aetiology and prevention. *Br J Anaesth* 2005;95:3–19.

Raby KE, Brull SJ, Timimi F, et al. The effect of heart rate control on myocardial ischemia among high-risk patients after vascular surgery. *Anesth Analg* 1999;88:477–482.

Slogoff S, Keats A. Myocardial ischemia revisited. *Anesthesiology* 2006;105:214–216.

C.14. When would you extubate the trachea? What could you do to prevent hypertension and tachycardia during extubation and emergence?

At the end of surgery, assuming no intraoperative complications, the trachea would be extubated when the patient is fully awake, breathing adequately, and neuromuscular blockade is fully reversed. To prevent tachycardia and hypertension associated with extubation and emergence, Low doses of medications such as 1 mg per kg of lidocaine, or esmolol or 0.015 to 0.03 mg per kg of nicardipine or 0.1 mg per kg of labetalol, diltiazem, or verapamil before emergence in order to reduce sympathetic response of emergence and extubation.

Atlee JL, Dhamee MS, Olund TL, et al. The use of esmolol, nicardipine, or their combination to blunt hemodynamic changes after laryngoscopy and tracheal intubation. *Anesth Analg* 2000;90:280.

Fujii Y, Kihara S, Takahashi S, et al. Calcium channel blockers attenuate cardiovascular responses to tracheal extubation in hypertensive patients. *Can J Anaesth* 1998;45: 655–659.

Mikawa K, Nishina K, Maekawa N, et al. Attenuation of cardiovascular responses to tracheal extubation: verapamil versus diltiazem. *Anesth Analg* 1996;82:1205–1210.

D. Postoperative Management

D.1. What are the postoperative predictors of perioperative cardiac morbidity (PCM)?

The postoperative period appears to present the highest risk for cardiac morbidity for the noncardiac surgical patient. It is during this period where 67% of the ischemic events occur.

This period is characterized by increase in heart rate, blood pressure, sympathetic discharge and hypercoagulability. Heart rate commonly increases postoperatively by 25% to 50% over intraoperative values, and tachycardia occurs in 10% to 25% of patients. Postoperative myocardial ischemia occurs in 27% to 41% of high-risk patients. Most of these events (50% or higher) are silent (without angina). Postoperative myocardial infarction (MI) is usually preceded by prolonged ST-segment depression. This change on ECG is easily missed if not continuously monitored because most of the changes will revert completely to baseline in almost all cases. Traditionally, ischemia monitoring has been of short duration following operation (24 to 72 hours), but data suggests that period should be increased to 7 days.

Perioperative myocardial infarction (PMI) may be associated with tachycardia and higher pain threshold. Studies involving large numbers of patients suggest that postoperative ischemia is the most important marker of immediate and long-term adverse cardiovascular events. It is associated with a 2.8-fold increase in the odds of all adverse cardiac outcomes.

Earlier observations suggested that most MIs would occur in the third postoperative day. However, this belief has changed. Many authors have found the highest incidence of troponins elevation, a biochemical marker of ischemia, frequently 8 to 24 hours after the surgical procedure; even mild elevations are associated with postoperative cardiac ischemia and they could help to categorize the short- and long-term risk of the surgical patient as they are independent predictors of mortality. The discrepancy of studies could be related to the different biochemical markers used in previous studies (CK/CK-MB vs. troponins).

Postoperative MI has also been associated with other clinical conditions as postoperative hypothermia, hypercoagulability, postoperative pain, and anemia.

Akhtar S, Silverman D. Assessment and management of patients with ischemic heart disease. *Crit Care Med* 2004;32(suppl):S126–S136.

Landesberg G. Pathophysiology of perioperative myocardial infarction: facts and perspectives. *J Cardiothorac Vasc Anesth* 2003;17:90–100.

Landesberg G, Mosseri M, Shatz V, et al. Cardiac troponin after major vascular surgery. The role of perioperative ischemia, preoperative thallium scanning, and coronary revascularization. *J Am Coll Cardiol* 2004;44:569–575.

Lee TH, Marcantonio ER, Mangione RC, et al. Derivation and prospective validation of a simple index for prediction of cardiac risk of major noncardiac surgery. *Circulation* 1999;100:1043–1049.

Priebe HJ. Perioperative myocardial infarction—aetiology and prevention. *Br J Anaesth* 2005;95:3–19.

D.2. How would you control postoperative pain?

The postoperative period can be stressful due to the onset of pain during emergence from anesthesia, fluid shifts, temperature changes, and alteration of respiratory function. Marked changes occur in plasma catecholamine concentration, hemodynamics, ventricular function, and coagulation following noncardiac surgery, particularly in patients with preexisting cardiac disease. These stresses place the patient at increased risk for development of adverse cardiac outcome. Effective pain management is essential to prevent adverse outcome. Patient-controlled intravenous analgesia (PCA) and/or patient-controlled epidural analgesia (PCEA) are popular methods for reducing postoperative pain. Several studies suggest that effective pain management leads to a reduction in postoperative catecholamine surges and hypercoagulability. Norris et al. found that using PCA or PCEA, the incidence of myocardial ischemia/infarction were comparable in patients undergoing abdominal aneurysm repair as long as the pain control and hemodynamics of the patients were similar.

Eagle KA, Berger PB, Calkins H, et al. ACC/AHA guideline update for perioperative cardiovascular evaluation for noncardiac surgery—executive summary. A report of the American College of Cardiology/American Heart Association Task Force on practice guidelines. *Anesth Analg* 2002;94:1052–1064.

Mangano DT, Siliciano D, Hollenberg M, et al. Postoperative myocardial ischemia. Therapeutic trials using intensive analgesia following surgery. *Anesthesiology* 1992;76:342–353.

Matot I, Oppenheim-Eden A, Ratro R, et al. Preoperative cardiac events in elderly patients with hip fracture randomized to epidural or conventional analgesia. *Anesthesiology* 2003;98:156–163.

Norris EJ, Beattie C, Perler BA, et al. Double-masked randomized trial comparing alternate combinations of intraoperative anesthesia and postoperative analgesia in abdominal aortic surgery. *Anesthesiology* 2001;95:1054–1067.

D.3. Is postoperative anemia associated with adverse cardiac outcome?

Patients with ischemic heart disease may be adversely affected by anemia. Based on existing literature the evidence is sufficient to state that transfusions are rarely beneficial if the hemoglobin level exceeds 10 g per dL (Hct >30%) in the absence of acute blood loss. It is also reasonable to state that the patient will benefit from a transfusion if the hemoglobin level falls below 7 g per dL. The controversy remains between Hg concentrations of 8.0 to 10.0 g per dL.

Two groups of investigators have now documented adverse clinical consequences of postoperative, iatrogenic acute anemia. Nelson et al. have identified a hematocrit of 28% as being the threshold associated with increased incidence of morbid cardiac events in postoperative vascular surgical patients. Wu et al. also demonstrated the benefit of higher hemoglobin levels in patients with acute myocardial infarction (MI). Since then two controversial publications: The TRICC trial (Transfusion Requirement in Critical Care) was not able to demonstrate a significant difference in 30-day mortality between patients who were "liberally" transfused (average hemoglobin, 10.7 g/dL) versus the restrictive group (no transfusion unless Hb <7g/dL). Rao et al., published the data from the combination of three large randomized trial stating the risk of death is 3.9 times greater in patients who were transfused compared with those who did not. The controversy remains, however, when confronted with high-risk patients or those who demonstrate myocardial ischemia, we are more likely to transfuse packed cells to raise the hematocrit to 30%.

Hebert PC, Wells G Blaichman MA, et al. Transfusion requirement in critical care investigators, Canadian Critical Care Trial Group. *N Engl J Med* 1999;340:409–417.

Nelson AH, Fleisher LA, Rosenbaum SH. Relationship between postoperative anemia and cardiac morbidity in high-risk vascular patients in the intensive care unit. *Crit Care Med* 1993;21:860.

Rao SV, Jolllis JG, Harrington RA, et al. Relationship of blood transfusion and clinical outcomes in patients with acute coronary syndromes. *JAMA* 2004;292:1555–1562.

Wu WC, Rathore SS, Wang Y, et al. Blood transfusion in elderly patients with acute myocardial infarction. *N Engl J Med* 2001;345:1230–1236.

D.4. Is postoperative hypothermia associated with postoperative myocardial ischemia?

Hypothermia is common during anesthesia and surgery owing to anesthetic-induced inhibition of thermoregulatory control. The principal initial cause of hypothermia is core-to-peripheral redistribution of body heat.

Perioperative hypothermia is associated with numerous complications: it triples the incidence of adverse myocardial outcomes in high-risk patients, increases blood loss. Even mild hypothermia has been associated with an increased incidence of wound infection following colon resection, Also it adversely affects oxygen availability in tissues, changes the kinetics and action of some anesthetic agents and muscle relaxants and is associated with delayed postanesthetic recovery.

Core hypothermia may increase circulating catecolamines levels, leading to tachycardia, hypertension, systemic vasoconstriction, and an imbalance between oxygen demand and supply. Frank et al. studied 100 patients undergoing lower extremity vascular surgery. They found that unintentional hypothermia (sublingual temperature less than 35°C (95°F) on arrival to postoperative intensive care unit [ICU]) is associated with a significantly higher incidence of myocardial ischemia (36% vs. 13%), angina (18% vs. 15%), and PaO_2 less than 80 mm Hg (52% vs. 30%) during the early postoperative period. Therefore, aggressive warming and heat conservation are mandatory during and after surgery. It is recommended to continue forced-air warming for the first several hours after surgery in hypothermic patients.

Auerbach A, Goldman L. Assessing and reducing the cardiac risk of noncardiac surgery. *Circulation* 2006;113(10):1361–1376.

Frank SM, Beattie C, Christopherson R, et al. The Perioperative Ischemia Randomized Anesthesia Trial Study Group. Unintentional hypothermia is associated with postoperative myocardial ischemia. *Anesthesiology* 1993;78:468–476.

Frank SM, Fleisher LA, Breslow MJ, et al. Perioperative maintenance of normothermia reduces the incidence of morbid cardiac events. A randomized clinical trial. *JAMA* 1997; 277:1127–1134.

Leslie K, Sessler D. Perioperative hypothermia in the high-risk surgical patient. *Best Pract Res Clin Anesthesiol* 2003;17:485–498.

Priebe HJ. Perioperative myocardial infarction—aetiology and prevention. *Br J Anaesth* 2005;95:3–19.

D.5. How would you make a diagnosis of perioperative myocardial infarction (PMI)?

The definition of myocardial infarction (MI), according to the World Health Organization, is based on cardiac symptoms, ECG changes and/or elevation in biomarkers.

Most ischemic episodes occur after and not during the operation: This is probably because of the high postoperative stresses related to anesthesia and surgery. Several studies have examined the optimal method for diagnosing a PMI. Clinical symptoms (mostly asymptomatic), postoperative ECG changes (even analysis of serial basal ECGs is limited in its sensitivity to new PMI, because most infarctions are non–Q wave in nature), and elevation of the MB fraction of creatine kinase (CK-MB) have been most extensively studied. Cardiac-specific enzyme elevations such as troponin I (cTn I), troponin T (cTn T) are currently the standard of care for biochemical diagnosis of a PMI.

In the purest physiologic sense, any detectable necrosis is an acute myocardial infarction (AMI). Consequently, even small elevations of specific markers of myocardial damage, such as cardiac troponins, should be acknowledged as indicative of significant injury. From a clinical perspective, there is clear evidence that any amount of detectable cardiac troponin release is associated with an increased risk of new adverse cardiac events

The literature has shown the increased sensitivity of troponins to myocardial injury that is not normally sufficient to cause CK-MB elevation, chest pain, or electrocardiographic abnormalities. The association between perioperative ischemia and the rise in cardiac troponin levels is still questioned by some. Landesberg et al. reported a good correlation between duration of ischemia and the rise in cardiac-specific troponin I. It should also be noted that the implications and clinical relevance of increases in troponins below the established cutoffs are still under investigation. Many investigators would agree that the increase in cardiac troponins postoperatively, even if no cardiovascular signs and symptoms are present, carries poor long-term outcome.

However, an important question is the meaning of abnormally elevated troponin and its diagnostic value in patients with chronic renal insufficiency. This patient population is among the highest-risk group. Nevertheless, the cut off for enzyme elevation is not clear.

Clinicians need to be sensitive to redundancy in testing. Some authors have demonstrated that routine cardiac troponin monitoring is an easy, effective, and inexpensive way to detect postoperative myocardial injury. However, the American College of Cardiology/American Heart Association (ACC/AHA) guidelines reserves the use of this biomarkers for patients at high risk and those with clinical, ECG or hemodynamic evidence of cardiovascular dysfunction. At best there is still lack of agreement regarding who should be tested.

Akhtar S, Silverman D. Assessment and management of patients with ischemic heart disease. *Crit Care Med* 2004;32(suppl):S126–S136.

Barash PG. Sequential monitoring myocardial ischemia in the perioperative period. *ASA annual refresher course lectures*. Park Ridge: American Society of Anesthesiologists, 2006:213.

Eagle KA, Berger PB, Calkins H, et al. ACC/AHA guideline update for perioperative cardiovascular evaluation for noncardiac surgery—executive summary. A report of the American College of Cardiology/American Heart Association Task Force on practice guidelines. *Anesth Analg* 2002;94:1052–1064.

Horvath KA, Parker MA, Frederiksen JW, et al. Postoperative troponin I values: insult or injury? *Clin Cardiol* 2000;23:731–733.

Jimenez F, Goldman L, Sacks DB, et al. Prognostic value of cardiac troponin T after noncardiac surgery: 6-month follow-up data. *J Am Coll Cardiol* 1997;29:1241–1245.

Landesberg G, Shatz V, Akopnik I, et al. Association of cardiac troponin, CK-MB, and post-operative myocardial ischemia with long-term survival after major vascular surgery. *J Am Coll Cardiol* 2003;42:1547–1554.

Lucrezzioti S, Foroni I, Fiorentini C. Perioperative myocardial infarction in noncardiac surgery: the diagnostic and prognostic role of cardiac troponins. *J Intern Med* 2002; 252:11–20.

Luepker RV, Apple FS, Christenson RH, et al. Case definition for acute coronary heart disease in epidemiology and clinical research studies: a statement from the AHA council on epidemiology and prevention; AHA statistics committee; world heart federation council on epidemiology and prevention; the European Society of Cardiology Working Group in epidemiology and prevention; Centers for Disease Control and Prevention and the National Heart Lung and Blood Institute. *Circulation* 2003;108:2543–2549.

D.6. How would you manage the patient with a suspected perioperative myocardial infarction (PMI)?

There is lack of control-evidence regarding management of PMI in the postsurgical patient. PMI could include three different clinical scenarios/diagnosis: unstable angina (UA), non-ST-elevation myocardial infarction non–ST-elevation myocardial infarction (NSTEMI), and ST-elevation myocardial infarction (STEMI).

The initial management should focus on the following diagnosis:

• Evaluation of chest pain if present.
• 12-Lead ECG and determination of changes if present.

- Measurement of biomarkers of cardiac injury. A cardiac-specific troponin is the preferred marker.
- Immediate consultation of a cardiologist and risk stratification to determine high-risk patients.

It is important to consider the recent surgical procedure and consultation with the surgical team regarding impact of aspirin and antithrombin therapy.

Unless a contraindication exists, patients with an acute coronary syndrome of the type UA or NSTEMI should be treated with oxygen, aspirin (ASA), sublingual/intravenous nitroglycerin (NTG) for chest pain relief, as long as blood pressure is adequate, a β-blocker, antithrombin therapy (unfractionated heparin or low molecular weight heparin), and/or a GP IIb/IIIa inhibitor.

The cardiology consultant should guide further management:

1. Option one is a routine angiographic approach in which coronary angiography and revascularization are performed unless a contraindication exists. Within this approach, the most common strategy advocates for a period of medical stabilization. A more aggressive approach calls for coronary angiography and revascularization performed within 24 hours of the onset of symptoms or diagnosis; the rationale for the more aggressive approach is the protective effect of carefully administered antithrombin and antiplatelet therapy on reperfusion procedures outcome.

2. The alternative approach, commonly referred to as the initially conservative strategy, is guided by ischemia, with angiography reserved for patients with recurrent ischemia or a "high-risk" stress test despite medical therapy.

Regardless of the angiographic strategy, an assessment of left ventricular (LV) function (echocardiography, ventriculogram or nuclear ventriculography) should be strongly considered because of the importance of treating patients who have impaired LV function with angiotensin-converting enzyme inhibitors, β-blockers and, surgical revascularization (CABG) when appropriate (e.g., three-vessel disease).

If the patient presents with a STEMI, recognized on the basis of the 12-lead ECG, the management will be initially similar to UA/NSTEMI (oxygen, ASA, NTG, β-blockers), then one should attempt to complete restoration of flow in the infarct artery by pharmacologic means (fibrinolysis: usually contraindicated after a surgical procedure due to the great increase in bleeding), percutaneous coronary intervention (PCI) (balloon angioplasty with or without deployment of an intracoronary stent under the support of pharmacologic measures to prevent thrombosis), or surgical measures (coronary artery bypass grafting [CABG]).

Evidence supports expeditious restoration of flow in the obstructed infarct artery after the onset of symptoms in patients with STEMI as a key determinant of short- and long-term outcomes regardless of whether reperfusion is accomplished by fibrinolysis or PCI. Early reperfusion of ischemic myocardium within the risk region of an occluded infarct-related artery interrupts the occurring necrosis, reduces ultimate infarct size, preserves regional and global ventricular function, and improves survival. A subset of patients will have severe three-vessel or left main disease or anatomic features unfavorable for PCI and may be candidates for urgent or emergency CABG.

Antman EM, Anbe DT, Kushner FG, et al. *ACC/AHA guidelines for the management of patients with ST-elevation myocardial infarction. A report of the American College of Cardiology/American Heart Association Task Force on practice guidelines (Committee to revise the 1999 Guidelines for the management of patients with acute myocardial infarction)*. American College of Cardiology Foundation and the American Heart Association, Inc, 2004.

Braunwald E, Antman EM, Beasley JW, et al. ACC/AHA guidelines for the management of patients with unstable angina and non–ST segment elevation myocardial infarction: a report of the American College of Cardiology/American Heart Association Task Force on practice guidelines (Committee on the Management of Patients with Unstable Angina). *J Am Coll Cardiol* 2000;36:970–1062.

Berger PB, Bellot V, Bell MR, et al. An immediate invasive strategy for the treatment of acute myocardial infarction early after non-cardiac surgery. *Am J Cardiol* 2001;87:1100–1102.

Eagle KA, Berger PB, Calkins H, et al. ACC/AHA guideline update for perioperative cardiovascular evaluation for noncardiac surgery—executive summary. A report of the American College of Cardiology/American Heart Association Task Force on practice guidelines. *Anesth Analg* 2002;94:1052–1064.

CHAPTER 16

Tetralogy of Fallot

James A. DiNardo

> ### A 5-MONTH-OLD INFANT
>
> recently adopted from South America is being evaluated for stable persistent cyanosis with arterial oxygen saturation (SaO_2) of 70% to 80% since birth. She feeds well and is in the 70th percentile for weight (6.5 kg). An echo done before her arrival at your institution suggests that she has tetralogy of Fallot (TOF). Although she has never been noted to have a "Tet spell," her SaO_2 was noted to decrease to 60% during a recent febrile episode. Repeat echocardiogram reveals TOF with severe valvular pulmonary stenosis (PS) and mild subvalvular PS secondary to anterior deviation of the conal septum into the right ventricle outflow tract (RVOT). There is a peak instantaneous gradient of 70 mm Hg across the RVOT as determined by continuous wave (CW) Doppler.

A. Medical Disease and Differential Diagnosis

1. What is tetralogy of Fallot (TOF)?
2. What is the pathophysiology of TOF with pulmonary stenosis (PS)?
3. What is shunting and how is $Q_P : Q_S$ calculated?
4. What is the pathophysiology of TOF with pulmonary artery (PA)?
5. How is the arterial saturation determined in single ventricle physiology?
6. What is a "pink Tet"?
7. What are hypercyanotic spells? How are they treated?
8. What palliative surgical procedures are available for treating this patient with **TOF/PS**?
9. What definite surgical procedures are available for treating this patient with **TOF/PS**?
10. What palliative and definite surgical procedures are available for treating a patient with **TOF/PA**?

B. Preoperative Evaluation and Preparation

1. What preoperative history and physical examination information do you want?
2. Which other abnormalities need to be considered in this patient?
3. In general, what nothing by mouth (NPO) guidelines will you follow and what premedication will you give to a child with congenital heart disease?

C. Intraoperative Management

1. How will you induce anesthesia in this patient if intravenous (IV) access cannot be obtained?

2. Why would end-tidal carbon dioxide ($ETCO_2$) monitoring be of particular use in a patient with TOF/PS?

3. What is near-infrared spectroscopy (NIRS) and what does it measure?

4. What are the important management issues during creation of a palliative shunt?

5. What is the effect of inhalation anesthetics on airway reflexes, myocardial contractility, systemic vascular resistance (SVR), and pulmonary vascular resistance (PVR) in children?

6. What are the pre–cardiopulmonary bypass (CPB) anesthetic goals for a patient undergoing definitive surgical correction of TOF/PS?

7. What interventions will reliably reduce PVR?

8. How does heparin administration and activated coagulation time (ACT) monitoring differ in children as compared to adults?

9. How is heparin reversed?

10. What is the incidence of protamine reactions in children?

11. What is the role of transesophageal echocardiography (TEE) in this patient?

12. What effect would a residual ventricular septal defect (VSD) have in this patient following separation from CPB?

D. Postoperative Management

1. How should postoperative ventilation be managed in this patient following placement of a transannular patch for TOF/PS?

2. Following complete repair of TOF/PS in an infant, what arterial oxygen saturation (SaO_2) is acceptable?

3. Following placement of a modified Blalock-Taussig shunt (MBTS) for TOF/PS in an infant what SaO_2 is acceptable?

4. What is junctional ectopic tachycardia (JET)?

A. Medical Disease and Differential Diagnosis

A.1. What is tetralogy of Fallot (TOF)?

In 1888, Fallot described a congenital heart defect composed of four characteristics (a) large ventricular septal defect (VSD), (b) right ventricular (RV) outflow obstruction, (c) overriding aorta, and (d) right ventricle hypertrophy (RVH). Broadly defined, TOF is a complex of anatomic malformations consisting of a large malalignment conoventricular VSD, a rightward and anterior displacement of the aorta such that it overrides the VSD, and a variable degree of subvalvular right ventricle outflow tract (RVOT) obstruction due to anterior, superior, and leftward deviation of the conal (infundibular) ventricular septum. In addition, abnormalities in the septal and parietal bands of the crista supraventricularis further exacerbate infundibular obstruction. RVH is the result of chronic RVOT obstruction. The most common associated lesion is a right aortic arch with mirror image arch vessel branching (innominate artery gives rise to left carotid and left subclavian, right carotid and right subclavian arise separately) present in 25% of patients. Two broad subsets of TOF exist: TOF with pulmonary stenosis (TOF/PS) and TOF with pulmonary artery (TOF/PA). A third much less common type of TOF known as *TOF with absent pulmonary valve* (*TOF/APV*) will not be considered here.

Tetralogy of fallot with pulmonary stenosis

TOF/PS involves the features of TOF in conjunction with varying degrees of valvular PS. At one end of the spectrum of TOF/PS the pulmonary valve may be mildly hypoplastic (reduced annulus size)

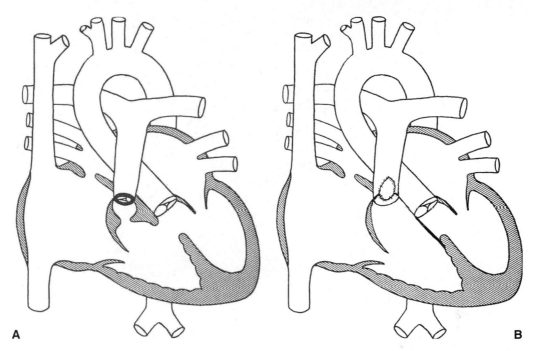

Figure 16.1 **A:** Uncorrected TOF/PS demonstrating malalignment VSD with aortic override, valvar and subvalvar (dynamic) PS. There is a left aortic arch. **B:** Definitively repaired tetralogy of Fallot with pulmonary stenosis (TOF/PS) with ventricular septal defect (VSD) closure creating left ventricle (LV) to aortic continuity, resection of subvalvar muscle bundles and deviated conal septum, and creation of a transannular patch (with pulmonary valvectomy) creating pulmonary insufficiency. A small atrial level communication has been left.

with minimal fusion of the pulmonary valve leaflets (Fig. 16.1). The pulmonary valve is almost always bileaflet. At the other end of the spectrum the pulmonary annulus may be very small with near fusion of the valve leaflets. It is important to point out that the valvular obstruction is a *fixed* obstruction while the subvalvular obstruction is *dynamic*. Left uncorrected, RVOT obstruction from both valvular and subvalvular obstruction begets progression of subvalvular obstruction as compensatory RVH increases the mass of the RV and infundibulum. The anatomy of TOF/PS can almost always be definitively delineated (including coronary anatomy) by two-dimensional echocardiography. Cardiac catheterization is rarely necessary or indicated.

Tetralogy of fallot with pulmonary artery

TOF with pulmonary artery involves the features of TOF and infundibular and pulmonary valvular atresia in conjunction with varying degrees of pulmonary arterial atresia. Four groups are said to exist. Group 1 patients have isolated infundibular and pulmonary valve atresia with a main pulmonary artery and distal pulmonary arteries of near normal size and architecture. In some of these patients the main pulmonary artery (PA) may extend to the atretic infundibulum. In others, there is short segment atresia of the main PA (Fig. 16.2). Patients in this group have pulmonary blood flow supplied from a patent ductus arteriosus (PDA). Group 2 patients have absence of the main PA but the PAs are in continuity and supplied by a PDA. Group 3 patients have severely hypoplastic native PAs; the left and right PA may not be in continuity. There are major aortopulmonary collateral arteries (vessels from the aorta to the PA) known as *MAPCAs*.

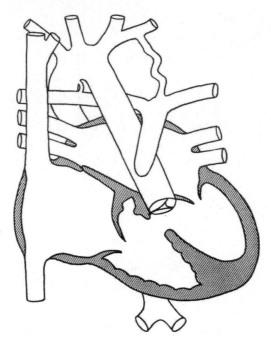

Figure 16.2 Illustration of tetralogy of Fallot with pulmonary artery group 1 with short segment pulmonary artery, good-sized PAs in continuity supplied by a right sided patent ductus arteriosus (PDA) and one large aortopulmonary collaterals (APC) from the left subclavian artery. There is a right aortic arch with mirror image arch vessel branching.

A PDA may be present as well. Some segments of lung may be supplied only by blood from MAPCAs, some only by the native PAs, and others by both sources (Fig. 16.3). Group 4 patients have no native PAs and all pulmonary blood flow is derived from MAPCAs.

The anatomy of MAPCAs in TOF/pulmonary artery can almost never be clearly delineated by two-dimensional echocardiography alone. Cardiac catheterization and/or magnetic resonance imaging (MRI)/magnetic resonance angiography (MRA) are necessary to delineate collateral anatomy and to determine $Q_P : Q_S$.

DiNardo JA. Anesthesia for congenital heart disease. In: DiNardo JA, ed. *Anesthesia for cardiac surgery*. Stamford: Appleton & Lange, 1998:141–200.

Jonas RA, ed. Tetralogy of Fallot with pulmonary atresia. *Comprehensive surgical management of congenital heart disease*. London: Arnold, 2004:440–456.

A.2. What is the pathophysiology of tetralogy of Fallot (TOF)/pulmonary stenosis (PS)?

TOF/PS is a complex shunt in which a communication (ventricular septal defect [VSD]) and a partial obstruction to right ventricle (RV) outflow (RV infundibular and valvular stenosis) are

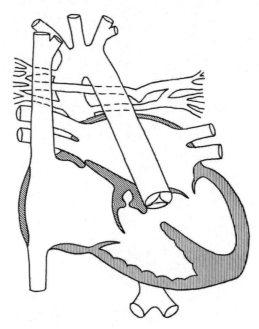

Figure 16.3 Illustration of tetralogy of Fallot with pulmonary artery (TOF/PA) group 3 with no main PA, small branch PAs in continuity supplied by major aortopulmonary collateral arteries (MAPCAs). Some lung segments are supplied by the native PAs while others are supplied directly by MAPCAs. There is a right aortic arch with mirror image arch vessel branching.

present. In complex shunts, the resistance to outflow is a combination of the resistance from the obstructive lesions and the vascular resistance. If the resistance from the RV obstructive lesions is high, changes in pulmonary vascular resistance (PVR) will have little effect on shunt magnitude and direction. In most patients with TOF/PS, there is a fixed and a dynamic component to RV outflow obstruction. The fixed component is produced by the valvular stenosis. The dynamic component is produced by variations in the caliber of the RV infundibulum. The pathophysiology present in TOF/PS is physiologic right-to-left (R-L) shunting induced by the presence of a VSD and right ventricle outflow tract (RVOT) obstruction. In addition, because the aorta overrides the VSD and the RV desaturated systemic venous blood tends to stream out the aorta even in the presence of mild RVOT obstruction.

The arterial oxygen saturation (SaO_2) is determined by the relative volumes and saturations of recirculated systemic venous blood and effective systemic blood flows that have mixed and reach the aorta. This is summarized in the following equation:

$$\text{Aortic } SaO_2 = \frac{\begin{array}{c}(\text{[pulmonary venous } O_2 \text{ saturation] [effective systemic blood flow]}\\ + \text{[systemic venous } O_2 \text{ saturation][recirculated systemic venous blood flow])}\end{array}}{(\text{total systemic blood flow})}.$$

This is demonstrated in Fig. 16.4 where the arterial oxygen saturation, $SaO_2 = [(98)(0.5) + (65)(0.5)]/1 = 81$.

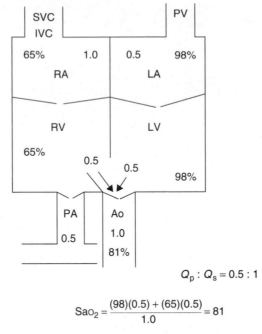

$$Q_p : Q_s = 0.5 : 1$$

$$Sao_2 = \frac{(98)(0.5) + (65)(0.5)}{1.0} = 81$$

Figure 16.4 Chamber oxygen saturations and relative flows for a patient with uncorrected tetralogy of Fallot with pulmonary stenosis (TOF/PS). Arterial, oxygen saturation (Sao_2) and $Q_P : Q_S$ are illustrated. Ao, aorta; IVC, inferior vena cava; LA, left atrium; LV, left ventricle; PA, pulmonary artery; PV, pulmonary vein; RA, right atrium; RV, right ventricle; SVC, superior vena cava.

A.3. What is shunting and how is $Q_P : Q_S$ calculated?

Shunting is the process whereby venous return into one circulatory system is recirculated through the arterial outflow of the same circulatory system. Flow of blood from the systemic venous atrium (right atrium [RA]) to the aorta produces recirculation of systemic venous blood. Flow of blood from the pulmonary venous atrium (left atrium [LA]) to the pulmonary artery (PA) produces recirculation of pulmonary venous blood. Recirculation of blood produces a physiologic shunt. Recirculation of pulmonary venous blood produces a physiologic left-to-right (L-R), whereas recirculation of systemic venous blood produces a physiologic right-to-left (R-L) shunt. A physiologic R-L or L-R shunt commonly is the result of an anatomic R-L or L-R shunt. In an anatomic shunt, blood moves from one circulatory system to the other through a communication (orifice) at the level of the cardiac chambers or great vessels. Physiologic shunts can exist in the absence of an anatomic shunt; transposition physiology is the best example.

Effective blood flow is the quantity of venous blood from one circulatory system reaching the arterial system of the other circulatory system. Effective pulmonary blood flow is the volume of systemic venous blood reaching the pulmonary circulation, whereas effective systemic blood flow is the volume of pulmonary venous blood reaching the systemic circulation. Effective pulmonary blood flow and effective systemic blood flows are the flows necessary to maintain life. Effective pulmonary blood flow and effective systemic blood flow are always equal, no matter how complex the lesions. Effective blood flow usually is the result of a normal pathway through the heart, but it may occur as the result of an anatomic R-L or L-R shunt.

Total pulmonary blood flow (Q_p) is the sum of effective pulmonary blood flow and recirculated pulmonary blood flow. Total systemic blood flow (Q_s) is the sum of effective systemic blood flow and recirculated systemic blood flow. Total pulmonary blood flow and total systemic blood flow do not have to be equal. Because Q_s (systemic cardiac output) tends to remain constant to supply end organs a physiologic L-R shunt (pulmonary recirculation) causes volume overload while a physiologic R-L shunt (systemic recirculation) allows Q_S to be maintained at the expense of arterial oxygen saturation (SaO₂).

Calculation of $Q_p : Q_s$ (the ratio of total pulmonary blood flow to systemic blood flow) is greatly simplified when the determination is made using low inspired concentrations of oxygen. This allows the contribution of oxygen carried in solution ($P_{O_2} \times 0.003$) to be ignored. Failure to account for this component when determination of $Q_p : Q_s$ is made using a fraction of inspired oxygen (F_{IO_2}) of 1.0 will introduce substantial (100%) error. If the F_{IO_2} is low the determination of $Q_p : Q_s$ can simplified to the following equation using just oxygen saturations:

$$(S_A O_2 - S_{SVC} O_2)/(S_{PV} O_2 - S_{PA} O_2)$$

where A = arterial, SVC = superior vena cava, PV = pulmonary vein that can be assumed to be 98% in the absence of significant pulmonary disease, PA = pulmonary artery.

DiNardo JA. Anesthesia for congenital heart surgery. In: Jonas RA, ed. *Comprehensive surgical management of congenital heart disease*. London: Arnold, 2004:45–65.

A.4. What is the pathophysiology of tetralogy of Fallot (TOF)/pulmonary artery?

The pathophysiology of TOF/pulmonary artery is single ventricle physiology. Single ventricle physiology describes the situation wherein complete mixing of pulmonary venous and systemic venous blood occurs at the atrial or ventricular level and the ventricle(s) then distributes output to both the systemic and pulmonary beds. As a result of this physiology the following are observed:

- Ventricular output is the sum of pulmonary blood flow (Q_p) and systemic blood flow (Q_s)
- Distribution of systemic and pulmonary blood flow is dependent on the relative resistances to flow (both intra and extracardiac) into the two parallel circuits
- Oxygen saturations are the same in the aorta and the pulmonary artery

This physiology can exist in patients with one well-developed ventricle and one hypoplastic ventricle as well as in patients with two well-formed ventricles. In the case of a single anatomic ventricle there is always obstruction to either pulmonary or systemic blood flow as the result of complete or near complete obstruction to inflow and/or outflow from the hypoplastic ventricle. In this circumstance there must be a source of both systemic and pulmonary blood flow to assure postnatal survival. In some instances of a single anatomic ventricle a direct connection between the aorta and the pulmonary artery through a patent ductus arteriosus (PDA) is the sole source of systemic blood flow (hypoplastic left heart syndrome or HLHS) or of pulmonary blood flow (pulmonary artery with intact ventricular septum). This is known as *ductal dependent circulation*. In other instances of a single anatomic ventricle intracardiac pathways provide both systemic and pulmonary blood flow without the necessity of a PDA. This is the case in tricuspid atresia with normally related great vessels, a nonrestrictive ventricular septal defect (VSD) and minimal or absent PS.

In certain circumstances single ventricle physiology can exist in the presence of two well-formed anatomic ventricles. This is generally the result of atresia or near atresia of outflow from one of the ventricles. Examples include:

- TOF/pulmonary artery where pulmonary blood flow is supplied through a large PDA or major aortopulmonary collateral arteries (MAPCAs)
- Truncus arteriosus
- Severe neonatal aortic stenosis and interrupted aortic arch; in both lesions a substantial portion of systemic blood flow is supplied through a PDA
- Heterotaxy syndrome

DiNardo JA. Anesthesia for congenital heart surgery. In: Jonas RA, ed. *Comprehensive surgical management of congenital heart disease*. London: Arnold, 2004:45–65.

A.5. How is arterial O_2 saturation determined in single ventricle physiology?

With single ventricle physiology, the arterial oxygen saturation (SaO_2) will be determined by the relative volumes and saturations of pulmonary venous and systemic venous blood flows that have mixed and reach the aorta. This is summarized in the following equation:

$$\text{Aortic } O_2 \text{ saturation} = \frac{\begin{array}{l}([\text{systemic venous saturation}]\,[\text{total systemic venous blood flow}] \\ + [\text{pulmonary venous saturation}]\,[\text{total pulmonary venous blood flow}])\end{array}}{(\text{total systemic venous blood flow} + \text{total pulmonary venous blood flow})}.$$

The primary goal in the management of patients with single ventricle physiology is optimization of systemic oxygen delivery and perfusion pressure. This is necessary if end-organ (myocardial, renal, hepatic, splanchnic) dysfunction and failure are to be prevented. This goal is achieved by balancing the systemic and pulmonary circulations. The term *balanced circulation* is used because both laboratory and clinical investigations have demonstrated that maximal systemic oxygen delivery (the product of systemic oxygen content and systemic blood flow) is achieved for single ventricle lesions when $Q_P : Q_S$ is at or just below 1:1. Increases in $Q_P : Q_S$ in excess of 1:1 are associated with a progressive decrease in systemic oxygen delivery because the subsequent increase in systemic oxygen content is more than offset by the progressive decrease in systemic blood flow and by diastolic hypotension due to run-off into the pulmonary circulation. Decreases in $Q_P : Q_S$ just below 1:1 are associated with a precipitous decrease in systemic oxygen delivery because the subsequent increase in systemic blood flow is more than offset by the dramatic decrease in systemic oxygen content.

DiNardo JA. Anesthesia for congenital heart surgery. In: Jonas RA, ed. *Comprehensive surgical management of congenital heart disease*. London: Arnold, 2004:45–65.

A.6. What is a "pink Tet"?

The term *pink Tet* refers to any noncyanotic patient with tetralogy of Fallot with pulmonary stenosis (TOF/PS) or TOF/pulmonary artery. In these patients $Q_P : Q_S$ is sufficiently high ($Q_P : Q_S$ generally greater than 0.8:1 in the presence of a normal mixed venous saturation and pulmonary vein saturation) to maintain a deoxyhemoglobin concentration less than 5 g per dL (arterial oxygen saturation [SaO_2] generally >80%). The designation of "pink Tet" would apply to TOF/PS patients with minimal valvular and subvalvular PS and to all patients with TOF/pulmonary atresia with pulmonary blood flow supplied from a large patent ductus arteriosus (PDA) and/or major aortopulmonary collateral arteries (MAPCAs).

DiNardo JA. Anesthesia for congenital heart disease. In: DiNardo JA, ed. *Anesthesia for cardiac surgery*. Stamford: Appleton & Lange, 1998:141–200.

A.7. What are hypercyanotic spells? How are they treated?

The occurrence of hypoxic spells in tetralogy of Fallot (TOF) patients may be life threatening and should be anticipated in every patient with TOF/pulmonary stenosis (PS) and any infundibular obstruction, even those who are not normally cyanotic. The peak frequency of spells is between 2 and 3 months of age; spells occur more frequently in severely cyanotic patients. The onset of spells usually prompts urgent surgical intervention, so it is not unusual for the anesthesiologist to care for an infant who is at great risk for spells during the preoperative period. The etiology of spells is not completely understood, but infundibular spasm or constriction plays a role. Crying, defecation, feeding, fever, and awakening all can be precipitating events. Paroxysmal hyperpnea is the initial finding. There is an increase in rate and depth of respiration, leading to increasing cyanosis and potential syncope, convulsions, or death. During a spell, the infant will appear pale and limp secondary to poor cardiac output. Hyperpnea has several deleterious effects in maintaining and worsening a hypoxic spell. Hyperpnea increases oxygen consumption through the increased work of breathing. Hypoxia induces a decrease in systemic vascular resistance (SVR), which further increases the right-to-left (R-L) shunt. Hyperpnea also lowers intrathoracic pressure and leads to an increase in systemic venous return. In the face of infundibular obstruction, this results in an increased right ventricle (RV) pressure and an increase in the R-L shunt. Treatment of a "Tet spell" includes the following:

- Administration of 100% oxygen.
- Compression of the femoral arteries or placing the patient in a knee-chest position transiently increases SVR and reduces the R-L shunt.
- Administration of morphine sulfate (0.05 to 0.1 mg/kg), which sedates the patient and may have a depressant effect on respiratory drive and hyperpnea.
- Administration of 15 to 30 mL per kg of a crystalloid solution. Enhancing preload will increase heart size, which may increase the diameter of the right ventricle outflow tract (RVOT).
- Administration of sodium bicarbonate to treat the severe metabolic acidosis that can be seen during a spell. Correction of the metabolic acidosis will help normalize SVR and reduce hyperpnea. Bicarbonate administration (1 to 2 mEq/kg) in the absence of a blood gas determination is warranted during a spell.
- Phenylephrine (dose 5 to 10 μg/kg IV or 2 to 5 μg/kg/minute as an infusion) can be used to increase SVR and reduce R-L shunting. In the presence of severe RV outflow obstruction, phenylephrine-induced increases of pulmonary vascular resistance (PVR) will have little or no effect in increasing RV outflow resistance. It is important to point out that treatment with α-adrenergic agents to increase SVR does nothing to treat the underlying cause of the spell although the decrease in unstressed venous volume induced by these agents may augment preload.
- β-Adrenergic agonists are absolutely contraindicated. By increasing contractility, they will cause further narrowing of the stenotic infundibulum.
- Administration of propranolol (0.1 mg/kg) or esmolol (0.5 mg/kg followed by an infusion of 50 to 300 μg/kg/minute) may reduce infundibular spasm by depressing contractility. In addition, slowing of heart rate (HR) may allow for improved diastolic filling (increased preload), increased heart size, and an increase in the diameter of the right ventricle outflow tract (RVOT).
- Manual compression of the abdominal aorta will increase SVR; this maneuver is particularly effective for the anesthetized patient. After the chest is open, the surgeon can manually

compress the ascending aorta to increase impedance to ejection through the LV. This can be effective in terminating a cyanotic episode.

- extracorporeal membrane oxygenation (ECMO) resuscitation is another alternative in refractory episodes when immediate operative intervention is not possible.

DiNardo JA. Anesthesia for congenital heart disease. In: DiNardo JA, ed. *Anesthesia for cardiac surgery*. Stamford: Appleton & Lange, 1998:141–200.

A.8. What palliative surgical procedures are available for treating this patient with tetralogy of Fallot with pulmonary stenosis (TOF/PS)?

Palliative shunt procedures to increase pulmonary blood flow can be used for patients with TOF/PS in whom complicated surgical anatomy precludes definitive repair at the time of presentation. In addition, some institutions delay elective complete repair until 12 to 18 months of age with placement of a palliative shunt if cyanosis occurs before that time interval. The palliative shunt procedures involve creation of a systemic-to-pulmonary arterial shunt analogous to a patent ductus arteriosus (PDA). Ideally, these surgical shunts should be mildly restrictive simple shunts. In the presence of a proximal obstruction to pulmonary blood flow, these shunts produce a left-to-right (L-R) shunt and an increase in pulmonary blood flow. The volume load imposed on the LV by these shunts parallels the increases in pulmonary flow that they produce. There will be progressive hypertrophy of the body and infundibulum of the right ventricle (RV) during the interval from shunt placement to definitive repair as right ventricle outflow tract (RVOT) obstruction will not be relieved. The shunts can be summarized as follows:

Waterston shunt—this shunt results from creation of a side-to-side anastomosis between the ascending aorta and the right pulmonary artery. This procedure is performed through a right thoracotomy without cardiopulmonary bypass (CPB).

Potts shunt—this shunt results from creation of a side-to-side anastomosis between the descending aorta and the left pulmonary artery. This procedure is performed through a left thoracotomy without CPB.

Waterston and Potts shunts are of historic interest only. It is difficult to size the orifice of this shunt correctly. Too small an orifice will limit pulmonary blood flow, whereas too large an orifice will create pulmonary overperfusion and congestion and predispose to development of unilateral pulmonary vascular obstructive disease (PVOD). These shunts may produce distortion of the pulmonary artery, making subsequent definitive repair difficult. In addition, they are difficult to take down at the time of the definitive procedure.

Central shunt—placing a synthetic tube graft between the ascending aorta and the main or branch pulmonary artery creates this shunt. This shunt can be performed with or without CPB through a thoracotomy or median sternotomy. It often is used when prior shunt procedures have failed.

Blalock-Taussig shunt (BTS)—as originally described this involved creation of an end-to-side anastomosis of the right or left subclavian artery to the ipsilateral branch pulmonary artery. Currently, a modification of this procedure known as the *modified Blalock-Taussig shunt* (*MBTS*) is used. It involves interposing a length of Gore-Tex tube graft (3.5 to 4.0 mm in infants) between the subclavian or innominate artery and the branch pulmonary artery. These shunts usually are performed on the side opposite the aortic arch through a thoracotomy without CPB (Fig. 16.5).

DiNardo JA. Anesthesia for congenital heart disease. In: DiNardo JA, ed. *Anesthesia for cardiac surgery*. Stamford: Appleton & Lange, 1998:141–200.

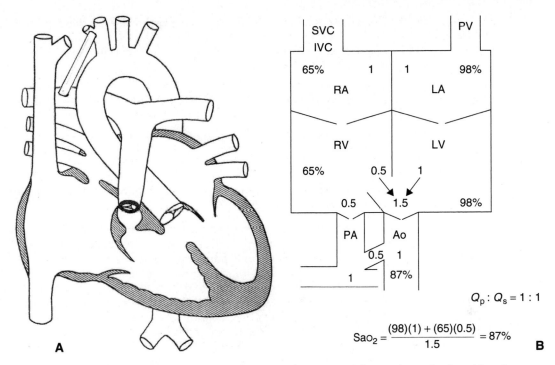

$$Q_p : Q_s = 1 : 1$$

$$Sao_2 = \frac{(98)(1) + (65)(0.5)}{1.5} = 87\%$$

Figure 16.5 A: Palliative modified Blalock-Taussig shunt (MBTS) for tetralogy of Fallot with pulmonary stenosis (TOF/PS). Shunt is seen to connect the innominate artery to the right pulmonary artery (PA). This patient has a left aortic arch. **B:** Chamber oxygen saturations and relative flows for a patient with MBTS and TOF/PS. Arterial oxygen saturation (Sao_2) and $Q_P : Q_S$ are illustrated. Ao, aorta; IVC, inferior vena cava; LA, left atrium; LV, left ventricle; PV, pulmonary vein; RA, right atrium; RV, right ventricle; SVC, superior vena cava.

A.9. What definite surgical procedures are available for treating this patient with tetralogy of Fallot with pulmonary stenosis (TOF/PS)?

Currently, most patients with TOF/PS have an elective full correction between the ages of 2 to 10 months of age. In some centers surgery is delayed as long as possible within this time interval with the precise timing of repair dictated by the onset of cyanotic episodes. Definitive repair for TOF/PS is being accomplished in neonates in some centers if favorable anatomy is present. Surgery is aimed at relieving the outflow obstruction by resection of hypertrophied, obstructing muscle bundles and augmentation and enlargement of the outflow tract with a pericardial patch. Unless the pulmonic annulus is near normal size and the pulmonary valve is only mildly stenotic enlargement of the outflow tract involves extension of the patch across the pulmonary valve annulus and into the main pulmonary artery. Because a transannular patch creates pulmonic insufficiency it is avoided when possible. If stenosis of the pulmonary artery extends to the bifurcation, the pericardial patch can be extended beyond the bifurcation of the pulmonary arteries. Finally, the ventricular septal defect (VSD) is closed. In neonates this is usually done through the right ventriculotomy created for resection of right ventricle outflow tract (RVOT) obstruction and placement of the transannular patch. In infants and older children the VSD can be closed through a transtricuspid valve approach.

An important surgical consideration for patients with TOF/PS is the occurrence of coronary artery abnormalities. Approximately 8% of patients have either the left main coronary artery or the left anterior descending artery as a branch of the right coronary artery. In these cases, a right ventriculotomy to enlarge the RVOT will endanger the left coronary artery. In such cases, an extracardiac conduit (right ventricle [RV] to main PA) may be necessary to bypass the outflow tract obstruction and avoid injury to the coronary artery.

DiNardo JA. Anesthesia for congenital heart disease. In: DiNardo JA, ed. *Anesthesia for cardiac surgery*. Stamford: Appleton & Lange, 1998:141–200.

Jonas RA, ed. Tetralogy of Fallot with pulmonary stenosis. *Comprehensive surgical management of congenital heart disease*. London: Arnold, 2004:279–300.

A.10. What palliative and definite surgical procedures are available for treating a patient with tetralogy of Fallot (TOF)/pulmonary artery?

Surgery in group 1 and 2 TOF/pulmonary artery patients is aimed at establishing a reliable source of pulmonary blood flow in the neonatal period, as these patients are dependent on PGE_1 to maintain a patent ductus arteriosus (PDA) and pulmonary blood flow. These patients may undergo a palliative shunt procedure or a definite procedure. The definite procedure would be creation of continuity between the right ventricle (RV) and the main PA through placement of a RV to PA conduit with ventricular septal defect (VSD) closure generally performed through the ventriculotomy used for the proximal end of the conduit. Patients in groups 3 and 4 present difficult management problems. As a rule these patients present with univentricular physiology with a tendency for pulmonary blood flow to become excessive ($Q_P : Q_S$ >2 to 3:1) as the pulmonary vascular resistance (PVR) drops following birth. In group 3 patients neonatal repair with placement of a RV to PA conduit is undertaken to place the PAs in continuity with the RV in an effort to promote native PA growth. In this circumstance the VSD is left open as a source of R to L shunting and delivery of desaturated blood to the systemic circulation as it would be impossible for the RV to deliver an adequate cardiac output to the left atrium (LA) across the hypoplastic pulmonary vascular bed. These infants then undergo multiple cardiac catheterization procedures in order to: (a) dilate and stent the hypoplastic native pulmonary arteries, and (b) to coil embolize major aortopulmonary collateral arteries (MAPCAs) which provide pulmonary blood flow which is competitive with blood flow supplied by native PAs. MAPCAs that provide pulmonary blood flow to segments of lung not supplied by native PAs must be unifocalized to the proximal pulmonary circulation.

Unifocalization may have to be performed and involves removal of the collateral vessel from the aorta with subsequent reanastomosis to the RV to PA conduit or a proximal PA branch. Although the traditional approach has been through a thoracotomy more recently most groups have favored a central approach working through a median sternotomy. It is only when 80% to 90% of the pulmonary vascular bed is direct continuity with the RV that closure or fenestrated closure of the VSD can be considered. Usually this will mean that at least 10 to 12 bronchopulmonary segments are now in direct continuity with the RV.

In group 4 patients it may be necessary to unifocalize several large collaterals to the distal end of conduit from the RV as the initial intervention. Alternatively several large collaterals could be unifocalized to a modified Blalock-Taussig shunt (MBTS) or central shunt. These procedures serve to promote pulmonary vascular growth, prevent the development of pulmonary vascular obstructive disease (PVOD), and control the $Q_P : Q_S$.

Jonas RA, ed. Tetralogy of Fallot with pulmonary atresia. *Comprehensive surgical management of congenital heart disease*. London: Arnold, 2004:440–456.

B. Preoperative Evaluation and Preparation

B.1. What preoperative history and physical examination information do you want?

Clinical history should include medications, allergies, past hospitalizations and operations (including prior anesthetic experiences), and a thorough review of systems. Performance of age-appropriate activities will aid in the evaluation of cardiac function and reserve. The neonate and infant in cardiac failure will manifest symptoms of low cardiac reserve during feeding, which is a strenuous activity, for even a normal newborn. A parent might report that sweating, tiring, dyspnea, and circumoral cyanosis occur during feeding. The observation by a parent that the patient cannot keep the same pace as siblings often is a reliable clinical sign that cyanosis or congestive heart failure is worsening.

Interpretation of vital signs must be age-specific. Growth curves also are useful. Congestive heart failure will inhibit, sequentially, age-appropriate gains in weight, height, and head circumference. It is not unusual for patients with severe congestive heart failure to weigh less at 3 or 4 months of age than at birth. Interestingly, cyanotic children often do not manifest this failure to thrive. Physical examination will reveal cyanosis, clubbing, or signs of congestive heart failure similar to those seen in adults, such as hepatomegaly, ascites, edema, or tachypnea. Rales may not be heard in infants and children with congestive heart failure, and the degree of heart failure may be determined more reliably by some of the signs and symptoms outlined in the preceding text. The degree of cyanosis is related to the percentage of desaturated hemoglobin. A markedly hypoxemic child with baseline arterial saturations in the 70% range may be anemic and clinically appear less cyanotic than another child with similar arterial saturation and a more appropriate hematocrit of 65%.

Physical examination should include an evaluation of the limitations to vascular access and monitoring sites imposed by previous surgery. A child who has undergone a palliative shunt procedure may have a diminished pulse or unobtainable blood pressure in the arm in which the subclavian artery has been incorporated into the shunt. This obviously has implications for arterial catheter placement, sphygmomanometric blood pressure monitoring, and use of pulse oximetry during surgery. Finally, the child who has undergone multiple palliative procedures may have poor venous access, which may influence the mode of induction.

It often is difficult to differentiate clearly between signs and symptoms of congestive heart failure and a mild upper respiratory tract infection. Because increased pulmonary blood flow seems to predispose multiple respiratory tract infections, the physical examination may show mild tachypnea, wheezing, or upper airway congestion and, in the absence of abnormal laboratory findings or fever, may be impossible to distinguish from congestive heart failure. The decision to proceed to surgery may be necessary even when the differentiation between worsening congestive heart failure and a respiratory tract infection cannot be made with certainty.

DiNardo JA. Anesthesia for congenital heart disease. In: DiNardo JA, ed. *Anesthesia for cardiac surgery*. Stamford: Appleton & Lange, 1998:141–200.

B.2. Which other abnormalities need to be considered in this patient?

Because approximately 8% of children with congenital heart disease have other congenital abnormalities, it is prudent to consider and define these defects. For example, patients with tetralogy of Fallot with pulmonary stenosis (TOF/PS) and TOF/pulmonary artery have a higher incidence of 22q11.2 deletion, a defect associated with DiGeorge syndrome, velocardiofacial syndrome, and conotruncal anomaly face syndromes leading to hypocalcemia, immunodeficiency, facial dysmorphia, palate anomalies, velopharyngeal dysfunction, renal anomalies, and speech and feeding disorders as well as neurocognitive, behavioral, and psychiatric disorders. Tracheal stenosis and bronchomalacia may be a serious problem for TOF/pulmonary artery patients who have undergone tracheoesophageal fistula repair. Needless to say many of these defects can seriously complicate airway management.

DiNardo JA. Anesthesia for congenital heart disease. In: DiNardo JA, ed. *Anesthesia for cardiac surgery*. Stamford: Appleton & Lange, 1998:141–200.

Goldmuntz E. DiGeorge syndrome: new insights. *Clin Perinatol* 2005;32:963–978.

B.3. In general, what NPO guidelines will you follow and what premedication will you give to a child with congenital heart disease?

Generally speaking the rule of 2, 4, 6, 8 can be used as the nothing by mouth (NPO) interval for neonates, infants and children with congenital heart disease:

- Two hours for clear liquids
- Four hours for breast milk
- Six hours for formula
- Eight hours for solid food

Premedication before induction can be used to facilitate a number of objectives. In older children it can be used to alleviate anxiety before an intravenous or inhalation induction. In younger children, premedication eases separation of the child from the parents. In infants judicious premedication alone or in combination with inhaled nitrous oxide can greatly simplify placement of an intravenous catheter in an otherwise struggling infant. Midazolam 1.0 mg per kg orally in infants and younger children who have not had prior cardiac surgery is useful. In children older than 1 year who have undergone prior operative procedures oral ketamine 7 to 10 mg per kg in combination with midazolam 1.0 mg per kg works well. These children are remarkably tolerant to midazolam as the result of either heightened anxiety or previous intra- and postoperative exposure to benzodiazepines. In circumstances where premedication is deemed important and the child will not take oral medication the intramuscular route can be used. Ketamine 2 to 3 mg per kg and glycopyrrolate (10 μg/kg) alone or in combination with midazolam 0.1 mg per kg works well.

DiNardo JA. Anesthesia for congenital heart surgery. In: Jonas RA, ed. *Comprehensive surgical management of congenital heart disease*. London: Arnold, 2004:45–65.

Ferrari LR, Rooney FM, Rockoff MA. Preoperative fasting practices in pediatrics. *Anesthesiology* 1999;90:978–980.

C. Intraoperative Management

C.1. How will you induce anesthesia in this patient if intravenous access cannot be obtained?

An alternative to intravenous induction in infants and neonates with difficult peripheral intravenous access is intramuscular induction with ketamine (3 to 5 mg/kg), succinylcholine (5 mg/kg), and glycopyrrolate (10 μg/kg). Glycopyrrolate is recommended to reduce the airway secretions associated with ketamine administration and to prevent the bradycardia, which may accompany succinylcholine administration. This technique provides prompt induction and immediate control of the airway with tracheal intubation and is useful in circumstances where it is anticipated that initial intravenous access will have to obtained through the external jugular vein, femoral vein, or internal jugular vein. This technique is hampered by the fact that the short duration of action of succinylcholine limits the period of patient immobility. An alternative technique combines intramuscular ketamine (4 to 5 mg/kg), glycopyrrolate (10 μg/kg) and rocuronium (1.0 mg/kg). This technique is hampered by the longer time interval until attainment of adequate intubating conditions and the longer duration of action of rocuronium as compared to succinylcholine.

DiNardo JA. Anesthesia for congenital heart surgery. In: Jonas RA, ed. *Comprehensive surgical management of congenital heart disease*. London: Arnold, 2004:45–65.

C.2. Why would end-tidal carbon dioxide (ETCO$_2$) monitoring be of particular use in a patient with tetralogy of Fallot with pulmonary stenosis (TOF/PS)?

ETCO$_2$ monitoring is routinely employed in patients with congenital heart disease with the caveat that the difference between PaCO$_2$ and ETCO$_2$ will vary as physiologic dead space varies and that in some circumstances the difference may be large (>10 to 15 mm Hg). Any acute reduction in pulmonary blood flow (decreased cardiac output, pulmonary embolus, increased intracardiac right-to-left shunting) will increase this gradient. In a patient with TOF/PS a gradual reduction in ETCO$_2$ will often precede a decrease in arterial oxygen saturation (SaO$_2$) as the first manifestation of the increased right-to-left intracardiac shunting associated with a "Tet spell."

DiNardo JA. Anesthesia for congenital heart surgery. In: Jonas RA, ed. *Comprehensive surgical management of congenital heart disease*. London: Arnold, 2004:45–65.

C.3. What is near-infrared spectroscopy (NIRS) and what does it measure?

NIRS is an evolving technology that holds promise as a real-time, on-line monitor of cerebral tissue oxygenation. This technology is based on the physical principle that light of an appropriate wavelength passing through a solution of a colored compound (chromophore) will be absorbed by the compound. As a result of this absorption the intensity of the light emerging from the solution will be lower than the intensity of the light projected into the solution. This principle through application of the Beer-Lambert equation "$\log [I_O/I] = c \; \alpha \; d$" allows quantification of the concentration (c) of a chromophore if the emergent light intensity (I) is measured and the following are known:

- Extinction coefficient (α), a constant that describes the absorption characteristics of a particular chromophore at a given wavelength of light.
- Thickness of the solution (d)
- Incident light intensity (I_O)

NIRS technology is particularly suited to use in neonates and infants because the thin skull and small head allow light to be transmitted through one side of the head and detected on the other side, a technique known as *transmission spectrometry*.

Cerebral oxygen saturation (ScO$_2$) as measured by all NIRS technology is the combined oxygen saturation of an uncertain mix of arterioles, capillaries, and venules. Traditional pulse oximetry differs in this respect from NIRS because it is capable of isolating and measuring the arteriole component by gating measurements to pulsatility. It has been previously assumed that ScO$_2$ represented contributions of cerebral arterial and venous blood in a ratio of 25:75 with the contribution of capillary blood felt to be negligible. More recent data suggests that in children the average ratio is 15:85. The issue is further complicated by the fact that there is significant variability in the ratio (from 0:100 to 40:60) between patients.

DiNardo JA. Anesthesia for congenital heart surgery. In: Jonas RA, ed. *Comprehensive surgical management of congenital heart disease*. London: Arnold, 2004:45–65.

C.4. What are the important management issues during creation of a palliative shunt?

- When a thoracotomy approach is used, unilateral lung retraction will be required for surgical exposure. The resulting atelectasis may severely compromise oxygenation and CO_2 removal. Intermittent reinflation of the lung may be necessary during the operative procedure. These reinflations should be coordinated with the surgeon. For all the shunts described, the main or branch pulmonary artery will have to be partially occluded by a clamp to allow creation of the distal anastomosis. The resulting increase in physiological dead space may compromise oxygenation and CO_2 removal and will increase the arterial-end-tidal carbon dioxide ($ETCO_2$) gradient.
- Efforts to increase pulmonary blood flow by reducing pulmonary vascular resistance (PVR) with ventilatory interventions and by increasing left-to-right (L-R) shunting should be initiated before pulmonary artery occlusion.
- Partial occlusion of the aorta with a clamp will be necessary during creation of Waterston, Potts, and central shunts. The resulting increase in LV afterload may compromise systolic function.
- All of the palliative shunts impose a volume load on the LV. Inotropic support may be necessary to ensure systemic and shunt perfusion after shunt creation.
- Palliative shunts are mildly restrictive simple shunts. It is important to maintain SVR and reduce PVR to maintain pulmonary blood flow in patients with surgical shunts.
- Be prepared to treat an episode of hypercyanosis.

DiNardo JA. Anesthesia for congenital heart disease. In: DiNardo JA, ed. *Anesthesia for cardiac surgery*. Stamford: Appleton & Lange, 1998:141–200.

C.5. What is the effect of inhalation anesthetics on airway reflexes, myocardial contractility, systemic vascular resistance (SVR), and pulmonary vascular resistance (PVR) in children?

Sevoflurane, isoflurane, and desflurane all induce dose related myocardial depression and SVR reduction with mild depression of contractility noted at 1 and 1.5 minimal alveolar concentration (MAC). Halothane induces a greater degree of myocardial depression at 1 and 1.5 MAC than sevoflurane, isoflurane, or desflurane. At these concentrations, neither sevoflurane, nor isoflurane or halothane alters the ratio of PVR to SVR substantially enough to induce any change in $Q_P : Q_S$.

Isoflurane and particularly desflurane are not good choices for inhalational induction because their pungency is responsible for a high incidence of airway complications in children. Desflurane has hemodynamic effects similar to isoflurane and may be useful as an adjuvant to narcotic anesthesia or as a primary maintenance agent after the airway has been secured. Sevoflurane has cardiovascular effects similar to isoflurane and is a good agent for inhalational induction in children; the incidence of airway complications is similar to that of halothane. Perhaps more important is the fact that inhalational induction with sevoflurane causes less myocardial depression than halothane in children.

DiNardo JA. Anesthesia for congenital heart disease. In: DiNardo JA, ed. *Anesthesia for cardiac surgery*. Stamford: Appleton & Lange, 1998:141–200.

Laird TH, Stayer SA, Rivenes SM, et al. Pulmonary-to-systemic blood flow ratio effects of sevoflurane, isoflurane, halothane, and fentanyl/midazolam with 100% oxygen in children with congenital heart disease. *Anesth Analg* 2002;95:1200–1206.

C.6. What are the pre–cardiopulmonary bypass (CPB) anesthetic goals for a patient undergoing definitive surgical correction of tetralogy of Fallot with pulmonary stenosis (TOF/PS)?

- Maintain heart rate (HR), contractility, and preload to maintain cardiac output. Euvolemia is important to prevent exacerbation of dynamic right ventricle outflow tract (RVOT) obstruction from hypovolemia and reflex increases in HR and contractility.
- Avoid increases in the pulmonary vascular resistance (PVR) : systemic vascular resistance (SVR) ratio. The less severe the right ventricle (RV) outflow obstructive lesions, the more important this becomes. Increases in PVR relative to SVR, and decreases in SVR relative to PVR, will increase right-to-left (R-L) shunting, reduce pulmonary blood flow, and produce or worsen cyanosis.
- Use ventilatory measures to reduce PVR.
- Maintain or increase SVR. This is particularly important when RV outflow obstruction is severe and changes in PVR will have little or no effect on shunt magnitude and direction.
- Aggressively treat episodes of hypercyanosis.
- Maintain contractility. Depression of contractility, particularly in the face of severe RV outflow obstruction, may produce RV afterload mismatch and drastically reduce pulmonary blood flow. The exception to this is patient in whom the dynamic component of infundibular obstruction is active. Reducing contractility in these patients may reduce RV outflow obstruction through relaxation of the infundibulum.

DiNardo JA. Anesthesia for congenital heart disease. In: DiNardo JA, ed. *Anesth Card Surg.* Stamford: Appleton & Lange, 1998:141–200.

C.7. What interventions will reliably reduce pulmonary vascular resistance (PVR)?

P_{O_2}. Both alveolar hypoxia and arterial hypoxemia induce pulmonary vasoconstriction. An arterial O_2 tension lower than 50 mm Hg increases pulmonary vascular resistance (PVR) over a wide range of arterial pH; however, this effect is enhanced when pH is lower than 7.40. Conversely, high levels of inspired O_2 can reduce an elevated PVR.

P_{CO_2}. Hypercarbia increases PVR, independent of changes in arterial pH. Hypocarbia, on the other hand, reduces PVR only through production of an alkalosis. In fact, reliable reductions in PVR and increases in pulmonary blood flow and P_{O_2} are seen in children with right-to-left (R-L) shunts when hyperventilation to a P_{CO_2} near 20 mm Hg and a pH near 7.60 is instituted. Similarly, postbypass hyperventilation to a P_{CO_2} of 20 to 33 mm Hg and a pH of 7.50 to 7.56 in patients with preoperative pulmonary hypertension results in a reduction in PVR when compared with ventilation that produces normocarbia or hypercarbia.

pH. Both respiratory and metabolic alkalosis reduce PVR, whereas both respiratory and metabolic acidosis increase PVR.

Variation in lung volumes. At small lung volumes, atelectasis results in compression of extraalveolar vessels, whereas at high lung volumes, hyperinflation of alveoli results in compression of intraalveolar vessels. Therefore, PVR is normally lowest at lung volumes at or near the functional residual capacity. Positive end-expiratory pressure (PEEP) may cause an increase in PVR by increasing alveolar pressure through hyperinflation. However, in situations in which PEEP works to recruit atelectatic alveoli and increase arterial P_{O_2}, a decrease in PVR generally is seen.

Vasodilator agents. There is no intravenous drug that selectively acts as a pulmonary vasodilator. In general, intravenous drugs intended to induce pulmonary vasodilation (PGE_1, PGI_2, nitroglycerin, sodium nitroprusside, and tolazoline) induce systemic vasodilation as well. Inhaled NO, PGE_1, and PGI_2 are the only specific pulmonary vasodilators available.

DiNardo JA. Anesthesia for congenital heart disease. In: DiNardo JA, ed. *Anesthesia for cardiac surgery*. Stamford: Appleton & Lange, 1998:141–200.

C.8. How does heparin administration and activated coagulation time (ACT) monitoring differ in children as compared to adults?

Before use of cardiotomy suction, cannulation, and commencing bypass, it is essential that adequate anticoagulation be obtained. Unfractionated heparin (UFH) is currently the anticoagulant used for cardiopulmonary bypass (CPB). It generally is acknowledged that an ACT in excess of 400 seconds is necessary to ensure adequate anticoagulation for the safe conduct of CPB.

While there is a large heparin anticoagulation monitoring literature in adults there is a very small literature in children. The ACT, commonly used to assess CPB anticoagulation is also prolonged by hypothermia, hemodilution, platelet dysfunction, and low coagulation factor levels. As a result, in children the ACT will overestimate the antifactor IIa and Xa effects of heparin.

Most institutions use an age or weight based protocol to administer the initial pre-CPB dose of heparin such as: patients less than 30 kg—200 IU per kg; patients greater than 30 kg—300 IU per kg. The large circuit prime volume to blood volume ratio would be expected to decrease plasma heparin levels with initiation of CPB unless an appropriate quantity of heparin is added to the CPB prime. Most institutions add heparin to the CPB prime as follows: patients less than 30 kg—2.5 IU per mL of CPB prime; patients greater than 30 kg—3.0 IU per mL of CPB prime.

Heparin should always be given into a central line through which venous return can be demonstrated easily or as is more common in infants/neonates directly into the heart (usually the right atrium) by the surgeon. This is necessary to ensure that the heparin dose has reached the central circulation. An ACT can be drawn within minutes of heparin administration as peak arterial ACT prolongation occurs within 30 seconds and peak venous ACT prolongation within 60 seconds.

DiNardo JA. Physiology and techniques of extracorporeal circulation in the pediatric patient. In: Lake CL, Booker, PD, eds. *Pediatric cardiac anesthesia*, 4th ed. Philadelphia: Lippincott Williams & Wilkins, 2005:228–252.

C.9. How is heparin reversed?

Protamine is a polyvalent cation derived from salmon sperm that is currently used to neutralize systemic heparinization. Protamine normally is given once stable hemodynamics are maintained after termination of cardiopulmonary bypass (CPB). It should not be administered until the likelihood that having to reinstitute CPB is small. After protamine neutralization of heparin begins, the cardiotomy suction should not be used and removal of the arterial and venous cannulas should proceed. This prevents contamination of the heparinized CPB circuit with protamine should prompt reinstitution of CPB be necessary and prevents thrombus formation on the cannulas.

There are several approaches to the neutralization of heparin with protamine, all with reportedly good clinical results. Some centers use 1.0 to 1.3 mg of protamine for each 100 units of heparin determined to exist at the termination of CPB. This ratio is based on the *in vitro* protamine-heparin neutralization ratio of 1.3:1.0. The amount of heparin present is determined by obtaining an activated coagulation time (ACT) when CPB terminates and using reverse extrapolation of the patient's heparin dose response curve to correlate ACT and heparin dose. This method has been criticized because the ACT obtained at the termination of CPB is prolonged by factors other than heparin, such as CPB-induced platelet dysfunction and hemodilution. This may result in an overestimation of the heparin present at the termination of CPB and a larger than necessary protamine dose.

Some centers simply administer a fixed dose of protamine based on the patient's weight (3 to 4 mg/kg) regardless of the heparin dose administered, whereas others administer 1.0 to 1.3 mg of protamine for each 100 units of heparin administered. Obviously, these methods do not rely on any post-CPB assessment of residual heparin effect (ACT) to determine the protamine dose. Nonetheless, these methods have been shown to result in adequate heparin reversal. In the case of the fixed dose regimen, heparin reversal is obtained at much lower protamine doses than predicted by the reverse extrapolation method.

The Hepcon automated heparin protamine titration method measures clotting times enhanced by addition of thromboplastin in several channels that contain varying quantities of protamine. The first channel to clot is the channel in which the protamine to heparin ratio is closest to neutralization. The absolute clotting time is not important; only the determination of the channel with the appropriate ratio. Therefore, the determination should be independent of nonheparin factors that prolong the ACT. In theory this method should allow determination of the appropriate dose of protamine independent of the nonheparin parameters that prolong ACT.

DiNardo JA. Physiology and techniques of extracorporeal circulation in the pediatric patient. In: Lake CL, Booker, PD, eds. *Pediatric cardiac anesthesia*, 4th ed. Philadelphia: Lippincott Williams & Wilkins, 2005:228–252.

C.10. What is the incidence of protamine reactions in children?

The incidence of protamine reactions in children following cardiac surgery is generally believed to be substantially lower than that in adults. A recent retrospective analysis of 1,249 children revealed the incidence of hypotension (at least 25% decrease in mean arterial pressure [MAP]) following protamine administration to be 1.76% to 2.88% depending on the stringency of criteria linking the episode to protamine administration. In this series no episodes of pulmonary hypertension or RV dysfunction were noted. There is a report of pulmonary hypertension and cardiovascular collapse in 6-week-old infant following protamine administration. Clinical experience indicates that pulmonary hypertensive episodes in children following protamine administration are very rare.

DiNardo JA. Physiology and techniques of extracorporeal circulation in the pediatric patient. In: Lake CL, Booker, PD, eds. *Pediatric cardiac anesthesia*, 4th ed. Philadelphia: Lippincott Williams & Wilkins, 2005:228–252.

C.11. What is the role of transesophageal echocardiography (TEE) in this patient?

It has been demonstrated that intraoperative TEE has a major impact on post-CPB decision making (such as return to CPB to repair residual lesions) in approximately 15% of cases when it is used nonselectively. In the subset of patients undergoing valve repair and outflow tract reconstruction TEE provides the best immediate assessment of the adequacy of the operative procedure and if necessary directs its revision. While detection of retained intracardiac air is certainly facilitated by use of intraoperative TEE it remains to be determined what role the technology will play in improving cardiac de-airing algorithms particularly in neonates/infants.

The role of TEE in the detection of residual VSDs following repair of both simple and complex defects deserves some discussion. Residual defects less than 3 mm are detectable by TEE but generally do not require immediate reoperation as they are hemodynamically insignificant. The majority (75%) of these small defects are not present at the time of hospital discharge as determined by transthoracic echocardiography. Residual defects greater than 3 mm detected by TEE require immediate reoperation only if they are associated with intraoperative hemodynamic (elevated left atrial pressure [LAP] and/or pulmonary artery pressure [PAP] in the presence of good ventricular function) and oximetric ($Q_P : Q_S$ >1.5 : 1 or right atrium [RA] to PA oxygen saturation step-up with fraction of inspired oxygen (FIO_2) ≤ 0.50) evidence that they are significant.

DiNardo JA. Anesthesia for congenital heart surgery. In: Jonas RA, ed. *Comprehensive surgical management of congenital heart disease*. London: Arnold, 2004:45–65.

Yang SG, Novello R, Nicolson S, et al. Evaluation of ventricular septal defect repair using intraoperative transesophageal echocardiography: frequency and significance of residual defects in infants and children. *Echocardiography* 2000;17:681–684.

C.12. What effect would a residual ventricular septal defect (VSD) have in this patient following separation from cardiopulmonary bypass (CPB)?

A residual VSD is likely to be very poorly tolerated in the patient with tetralogy of Fallot with pulmonary stenosis (TOF/PS). The most likely manifestation is low cardiac output syndrome associated with elevated central venous pressure (CVP), left atrial pressure (LAP), and pulmonary artery pressure (PAP). Right ventricle outflow tract (RVOT) obstruction will be completely or near completely eliminated postrepair. PVR is likely to be low and the pulmonary vasculature very compliant. As a result there will be potential for a large left-to-right intracardiac shunt with a residual VSD. This will place a large volume load on the LV and right ventricle (RV). An acute volume load will not be well tolerated by the RV that is likely to be concentrically hypertrophied and poorly compliant in response to the chronic pressure overload that existed preoperatively. The presence of pulmonary insufficiency will further exacerbate RV dysfunction by imposing an additional volume load.

DiNardo JA. Anesthesia for congenital heart disease. In: DiNardo JA, ed. *Anesthesia for cardiac surgery*. Stamford: Appleton & Lange, 1998:141–200.

D. Postoperative Management

D.1. How should postoperative ventilation be managed in this patient following placement of a transannular patch for tetralogy of Fallot with pulmonary stenosis (TOF/PS)?

The inspiratory phase of mechanical positive pressure ventilation increases impedance to right ventricle (RV) ejection by increasing RV afterload by elevating alveolar pressure and creating more West Zone I and II lung segments. As a result, the extent of this afterload elevation is directly related to the duration of inspiration (respiratory rate and I : E ratio) and to mean airway pressure. Increasing RV afterload will impede antegrade pulmonary blood flow and exacerbate the extent of pulmonary insufficiency induced by the transannular patch. RV afterload will also be increased by elevations in pulmonary vascular resistance (PVR).

As discussed in Question C.7, ventilation and gas mixture should be adjusted to minimize PVR. This should be accomplished with a tidal volume of 10 to 15 mL per kg, 3 to 5 mm Hg of positive end-expiratory pressure (PEEP), and a respiratory rate and I : E ratio adjusted to minimize mean airway pressure.

DiNardo JA. Anesthesia for congenital heart disease. In: DiNardo JA, ed. *Anesthesia for cardiac surgery*. Stamford: Appleton & Lange, 1998:141–200.

D.2. Following complete repair of tetralogy of Fallot with pulmonary stenosis (TOF/PS) in an infant what SaO₂ is acceptable?

Following complete repair of TOF/PS with no residual lesions and minimal intrapulmonary shunt the arterial oxygen saturation (SaO_2) should be 100%. In infants and small children, particularly those left with pulmonary insufficiency as the result of a transannular patch and those expected to have restrictive right ventricle (RV) function as a result of a ventriculotomy and/or extensive RV hypertrophy the surgeon may choose to leave a small (3 to 4 mm) atrial level communication or patent foramen ovale (PFO). This will allow intracardiac right-to-left shunting with the ability to augment systemic cardiac output at the expense of systemic oxygen saturation in the setting of RV dysfunction by allowing direct delivery of desaturated venous blood to the left atrium (LA). In these patients a PaO_2 of 40 to 50 mm Hg and a SaO_2 of 70% to 80% is acceptable until RV function improves over the course of days.

DiNardo JA. Anesthesia for congenital heart disease. In: DiNardo JA, ed. *Anesthesia for cardiac surgery*. Stamford: Appleton & Lange, 1998:141–200.

D.3. Following placement of a modified Blalock-Taussig shunt (MBTS) for tetralogy of Fallot with pulmonary stenosis (TOF/PS) in an infant what arterial oxygen saturation (SaO₂) is acceptable?

As illustrated in Fig. 16.5B in the presence of some antegrade pulmonary blood flow an appropriate SaO_2 would be 80% to 90%. In the absence of any antegrade pulmonary blood flow single ventricle physiology would exist and a SaO_2 of 70% to 80% would be more appropriate. SaO_2 is determined by the relative volumes and saturations of recirculated systemic venous blood and effective systemic blood flows that have mixed and reach the aorta. This is summarized in the following equation:

$$\text{Aortic } SaO_2 = \frac{([\text{pulmonary venous saturation}] [\text{effective systemic blood flow}] + [\text{systemic venous saturation}] [\text{recirculated systemic venous blood flow}])}{(\text{total systemic blood flow})}.$$

This is demonstrated in Fig. 16.5B where the $SaO_2 = [(98)(1) + (65)(0.5)]/1 = 87$
Three variables will ultimately affect SaO_2:

1. The ratio of total pulmonary to total systemic blood flow ($Q_p : Q_s$). A greater proportion of the arterial blood will consist of saturated blood (pulmonary venous blood) than of desaturated blood (systemic venous blood) when $Q_p : Q_s \geq 1 : 1$. $Q_p : Q_s$ will be increased when systemic arterial blood pressure is high and pulmonary vascular resistance (PVR) is low.

2. Systemic venous saturation. For a given $Q_P : Q_S$ and pulmonary venous saturation, a decrease in systemic venous saturation will result in a decreased arterial saturation. Decreases in systemic venous saturation occur as the result of decreases in systemic oxygen delivery or increases in systemic oxygen consumption. Recall that systemic oxygen delivery is the product of systemic blood flow and arterial oxygen content. Arterial oxygen content, in turn, is dependent on the hemoglobin concentration and the arterial saturation. Efforts should be made to increase hematocrit into the range of 35% to 45%, cardiac output should be enhanced with inotropes (dopamine 5 to 10 g/kg/minute), and systemic O_2 consumption reduced by appropriate levels of sedation/anesthesia and muscle relaxation if necessary.

3. Pulmonary venous saturation. In the absence of large intrapulmonary shunts and/or $\dot{V}/\dot{Q}$ mismatch pulmonary venous saturation should be close to 100% breathing room air. In the presence of pulmonary parenchymal disease, pulmonary venous saturation may be reduced. The $\dot{V}/\dot{Q}$ mismatch component of pulmonary venous desaturation will be largely eliminated with a fraction of inspired oxygen (F_{IO_2}) of 1.0 while the intrapulmonary shunt contribution will not be eliminated. For any given systemic venous saturation and $Q_P : Q_S$ a reduction in pulmonary venous saturation will result in a decreased arterial saturation.

DiNardo JA. Anesthesia for congenital heart disease. In: DiNardo JA, ed. *Anesthesia for cardiac surgery*. Stamford: Appleton & Lange, 1998:141–200.

D.4. What is junctional ectopic tachycardia (JET)?

Postoperative JET is a transient tachyarrhythmia that occurs immediately following congenital heart surgery. A much rarer form of congenital JET exists as well. JET is due to enhanced automaticity in the area of the atrioventricular (AV) node or proximal His Bundle. Associated with JET is a higher than average incidence of AV block. The incidence of JET following tetralogy of Fallot with pulmonary stenosis (TOF/PS) repair may be as high as 20% and is felt to be secondary to surgical trauma in the area of the AV node secondary to the retraction necessary to expose the ventricular septal defect (VSD) and right ventricle outflow tract (RVOT) from across the tricuspid valve.

JET typically manifests with a junctional rate only slightly faster than the sinus node rate and is the only narrow complex tachycardia in which the atrial rate is less than the ventricular rate (A : V ratio <1:1). Much less commonly (10%), there may be retrograde activation of the atrium with inverted p waves noted and A : V ratio = 1:1. In either case, there is loss of AV synchrony (loss of atrial kick). In many instances this arrhythmia is well tolerated. However, JET with heart rate (HR) greater than 170 bpm is associated with hemodynamic instability and increased postoperative mortality.

Cardioversion is ineffective as is adenosine. The most effective therapy for treatment of JET is atrial pacing at a rate slightly faster than the junctional rate such that A-V synchrony is reinitiated. This therapy is effective unless the junctional rate is very fast (>160 to 170 bpm) at which point atrial pacing at a faster rate is unlikely to improve hemodynamics because the reinitiation of A-V synchrony is offset by the dramatic reduction in diastolic filling time present at these rates. In this circumstance the most effective therapy is multimodal. JET requiring aggressive treatment prolongs postoperative ventilation times and intensive care unit (ICU) stay. The goal of aggressive therapy is to terminate JET or reduce the rate to point where atrial pacing can be reinitiated. In order, the following modalities are applied:

- Fever is aggressively treated with antipyretics.
- Sedation and hemodynamics are optimized.
- Reduction of inotrope doses is useful as most agents have chronotrophic activity. This may be difficult in the setting of hemodynamic instability and low cardiac out syndrome.

- Mild systemic hypothermia is introduced. A cooling blanket and icepacks are used to reduce patient temperature to 32°C (89.6°F) to 35°C (95°F). This usually requires sedation and paralysis to prevent shivering.
- Procainamide or amiodarone therapy is initiated.

Walsh EP. Automatic atrial and junctional tachycardias. In: Walsh EP, Saul JP, Triedman JK, eds. *Cardiac arrhythmias in children and young adults with congenital heart disease*. Philadelphia: Lippincott Williams & Wilkins, 2001:115–135.

CHAPTER 17

Transposition of the Great Arteries

JAMES A. DINARDO

A 3-DAY-OLD, FULL-TERM, 3.4-KG NEWBORN

is scheduled for an arterial switch operation (ASO). Shortly after birth, he demonstrated reverse differential cyanosis with a right arm arterial saturation of 40% and a lower extremity saturation of 60% despite prostaglandin E_1. A bedside balloon atrial septostomy was performed with resolution of reverse differential cyanosis and improvement of arterial saturation to 75%. Prostaglandin E_1 was discontinued 4 hours after the septostomy. He is extubated receiving 0.5 L per minute supplemental O_2 through nasal cannula. His arterial oxygen saturation is 75%; blood pressure 63/37 mm Hg, pulse 145 beats per minute, respiration 46 breaths per minute.

A. Medical Disease and Differential Diagnosis

1. What is transposition of the great arteries (D-TGA)?
2. What additional cardiac lesions are associated with D-TGA?
3. What is the natural history of D-TGA?
4. What is the pathophysiology of D-TGA?
5. What determines the oxygen saturation in patients with D-TGA?
6. Why did this infant have reverse differential cyanosis?
7. What are the preoperative issues pertaining to the coronary arteries in D-TGA?
8. What are the clinical subsets of D-TGA?
9. What is the differential diagnosis of D-TGA and how is the diagnosis made?
10. What preoperative interventions can help stabilize a patient with D-TGA?
11. What are the surgical options for repair? Why is one chosen over the others?

B. Preoperative Evaluation and Preparation

1. What information is important to prepare for this case?
2. What are the anesthetic goals before cardiopulmonary bypass (CPB)?
3. What is the plan for glucose management in this patient?

C. Intraoperative Management

1. How would you monitor this infant?
2. What would be the best method of induction?

3. Is CPB in infants and children different from adults?
4. What is modified ultrafiltration (MUF)?
5. Briefly describe the surgical techniques of the Mustard/Senning, arterial switch operation (ASO), and Rastelli procedures.
6. What is hypothermia and how is it classified? What is low-flow cardiopulmonary bypass (CPB)? What is deep hypothermic circulatory arrest (DHCA)?
7. Why is hypothermia beneficial to the brain during low flow CPB and DHCA?
8. Explain the difference between α-stat and pH-stat blood gas management.
9. What are the immediate post-CPB issues following ASO?

D. Postoperative Management

1. How is myocardial ischemia addressed in the intensive care unit (ICU) following the ASO?
2. What immediate postoperative problems would be anticipated following the Rastelli procedure?
3. What intermediate and long-term surgical problems are seen after ASO?
4. What are the long-term outcomes after ASO?
5. What are the long-term outcomes after Rastelli repair for D-TGA with left ventricular outflow tract (LVOT) obstruction?
6. What is long-term neurologic outcome like after ASO?

A. Medical Disease and Differential Diagnosis

A.1. What is transposition of the great arteries (D-TGA)?

D-TGA refers specifically to the anatomic circumstance wherein there is concordance of the atrioventricular (AV) connections associated with discordance of the ventriculoarterial connections. By far the most common manifestation of this anatomy occurs in patients with [S,D,D] segmental anatomy, also known as D-TGA. There is atrial situs solitus, D loop ventricles, and D-loop great arteries. A right-sided right atrium (RA) connects through a right-sided tricuspid valve and right ventricle (RV) to a right-sided and anterior aorta. A left-sided left atrium (LA) connects through a left-sided mitral valve and left ventricle (LV) to a left-sided and posterior pulmonary artery (PA). As a result, there is fibrous continuity between the mitral and pulmonic valves with a lack of fibrous continuity between the tricuspid and aortic valves (conus). In D-TGA, the combination of AV concordance (RA to RV; LA to LV) and ventriculoarterial discordance (RV to aorta; LV to PA) produces a parallel rather than a normal series circulation.

DiNardo JA. Anesthesia for congenital heart surgery. In: Jonas RA, ed. *Comprehensive surgical management of congenital heart disease*. London: Arnold, 2004:45–65.

DiNardo JA. Transposition of the great vessels. In: Lake CL, Booker PD, eds. *Pediatric cardiac anesthesia*, 4th ed. Philadelphia: Lippincott Williams & Wilkins, 2005:357–380.

A.2. What additional cardiac lesions are associated with transposition of the great arteries (D-TGA)?

The most commonly associated cardiac anomalies are a persistent patent foramen ovale (PFO), patent ductus arteriosus (PDA), ventricular septal defect (VSD), and subpulmonic stenosis or left ventricular outflow tract (LVOT) obstruction. Approximately 50% of patients with D-TGA will present with a PDA before prostaglandin E_1 administration. The foramen ovale is almost always patent, but a true secundum atrial septal defect (ASD) exists in only approximately 5% of patients. Although angiographically detectable VSDs may occur in 30% to 40% of patients, only approximately one third of these defects are hemodynamically significant. Therefore, for practical purposes, 75% of patients have an intact ventricular septum (IVS). LVOT obstruction is present in approximately 30% of patients with VSD and is most often due to an extensive subpulmonary fibromuscular ring or posterior malposition of the outlet portion of the ventricular septum.

Paul M. Complete transposition of the great arteries. In: Adams FH, Riemenschneider TA, eds. *Fetal and neonatal cardiology*. Philadelphia: WB Saunders, 1989:471–423.

A.3. What is the natural history of transposition of the great arteries (D-TGA)?

D-TGA is a common congenital heart lesion accounting for 5% to 7% of all congenital cardiac defects, second in frequency only to isolated VSDs. Without intervention, D-TGA has a high mortality rate: 45% will die within the first month and 90% will die within the first year of life. This is particularly unfortunate, because infants with D-TGA rarely have extracardiac defects. Advancements in medical and surgical therapy in the last 20 years have greatly improved the outlook for these infants. In fact, following stabilization with prostaglandin E_1 and the Rashkind-Miller balloon septostomy, many of these infants can be offered a definite surgical procedure (arterial switch) giving them a quality of life similar to that of normal children.

Hypoxia and intractable congestive heart failure (CHF) are the two primary causes of death. The early onset and progression of pulmonary vascular occlusive disease (PVOD) plays a major role in the dismal outlook in these patients. Compared to other forms of congenital heart disease, infants with transposition of great vessels (TGV) are at particular risk for accelerated development of PVOD. Systemic hypoxemia, the presence of bronchopulmonary collaterals (which deliver deoxygenated blood to the precapillary pulmonary arterioles), platelet aggregation in the lung, and polycythemia have all been implicated. Infants with TGV and large ventricular septal defect (VSD) without left ventricular outflow tract (LVOT) obstruction are at an even higher risk for the early development of PVOD due to exposure of the pulmonary vascular bed to high blood flow and systemic pressures. Advanced, nonreversible pulmonary hypertension reduces the corrective surgical options available to the patient.

DiNardo JA. Transposition of the great vessels. In: Lake CL, Booker, PD, eds. *Pediatric cardiac anesthesia*, 4th ed. Philadelphia: Lippincott Williams & Wilkins, 2005:357–380.

A.4. What is the pathophysiology of transposition of the great arteries (D-TGA)?

In the parallel arrangement of D-TGA, deoxygenated systemic venous blood recirculates through the systemic circulation without reaching the lungs to be oxygenated. This recirculated systemic venous blood represents a physiologic right-to-left shunt. Likewise oxygenated pulmonary venous blood recirculates uselessly through the pulmonary circulation. This recirculated pulmonary venous blood represents a physiologic left-to-right shunt. Therefore, in a parallel circulation, the physiologic shunt or the percentage of venous blood from one system that recirculates in the arterial outflow of the same system is 100% for both circuits. Unless there is one or more communications between the parallel circuits to allow intercirculatory mixing, this arrangement is not compatible with life.

The sites available for intercirculatory mixing in D-TGA can be intracardiac (patent foramen ovale [PFO], atrial septal defect [ASD], ventricular septal defect [VSD]) or extracardiac (patent ductus arteriosus [PDA], bronchopulmonary collaterals). Several factors affect the amount of intercirculatory mixing. The number, size, and position of anatomic communications are important. One large, nonrestrictive communication will provide better mixing than two or three restrictive communications. Reduced ventricular compliance and elevated systemic and pulmonary vascular resistance (PVR) tend to reduce intercirculatory mixing by impeding flow across the anatomic communications.

The position of the communication is also important. Poor mixing occurs even with large anterior muscular VSDs due to their unfavorable position. Finally, in the presence of adequate intercirculatory mixing sites, the extent of intercirculatory mixing is directly related to total pulmonary blood flow. Patients with reduced pulmonary blood flow secondary to subpulmonary stenosis or pulmonary vascular occlusive disease (PVOD) will have reduced intercirculatory mixing.

DiNardo JA. Anesthesia for congenital heart surgery. In: Jonas RA, ed. *Comprehensive surgical management of congenital heart disease*. London: Arnold, 2004:45–65.

DiNardo JA. Transposition of the great vessels. In: Lake CL, Booker PD, eds. *Pediatric cardiac anesthesia*, 4th ed. Philadelphia: Lippincott Williams & Wilkins, 2005:357–380.

A.5. What determines the oxygen saturation in patients with transposition of the great arteries (D-TGA)?

Intercirculatory mixing is the result of anatomic right-to-left and anatomic left-to-right shunts that are equal in magnitude. The anatomic right-to-left shunt produces effective pulmonary blood flow, which is the volume of systemic venous blood reaching the pulmonary circulation. The anatomic left-to-right shunt produces an effective systemic blood flow, which is the volume of pulmonary venous blood reaching the systemic circulation. Effective pulmonary blood flow, effective systemic blood flow, and the volume of intercirculatory mixing are always equal. The systemic blood flow is the sum of recirculated systemic venous blood plus effective systemic blood flow. Likewise, total pulmonary blood flow is the sum of recirculated pulmonary venous blood plus effective pulmonary blood flow. Recirculated blood makes up the largest portion of total pulmonary and systemic blood flow with effective blood flows contributing only a small portion of the total flows. This is particularly true in the pulmonary circuit where the total pulmonary blood flow (Q_P) and the volume of the pulmonary circuit (left atrium [LA]-left ventricle [LV]-pulmonary artery [PA]) is three to four times larger than the total systemic blood flow (Q_S) and the volume of the systemic circuit (right atrium [RA] right ventricle [RV]-aorta [Ao]). The net result is production of a transposition physiology, where the PA oxygen saturation is greater than the aortic oxygen saturation. Fig. 17.1 further elucidates these concepts.

Arterial saturation (Sao_2) is determined by the relative volumes and saturations of the recirculated systemic and effective systemic blood flows reaching the aorta. This is summarized in the following equation:

$$\text{Aortic saturation} = \frac{\begin{array}{c}([\text{systemic venous saturation}][\text{recirculated systemic blood flow}] \\ + [\text{pulmonary venous saturation}][\text{effective systemic blood flow}])\end{array}}{(\text{total systemic blood flow})}$$

This is illustrated in Fig. 17.1 where:

$$Sao_2 = ([50][1.2] + [99][1.1])/2.3 = 73\%$$

Obviously, the greater the effective systemic blood flow (intercirculatory mixing) relative to the recirculated systemic blood flow, the greater the aortic saturation. For a given amount of intercirculatory mixing and total systemic blood flow, a decrease in systemic venous or pulmonary venous saturation will result in a decrease in arterial saturation.

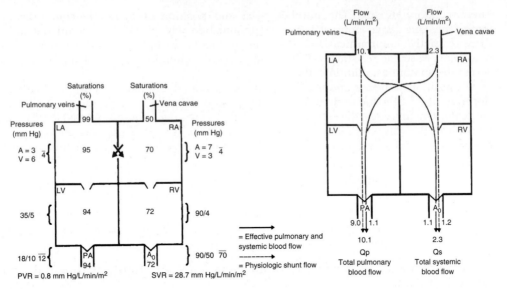

Figure 17.1 Depiction of saturations, pressures, and blood flows in complete transposition of the great vessels with intercirculatory mixing at the atrial level and a small left ventricular outflow tract gradient. It is apparent that total pulmonary blood flow (10.1 L/min/m^2) is almost five times total systemic blood flow (2.3 L/min/m^2). Effective (EFF) pulmonary and effective systemic blood flow are equal (1.1 L/min/m^2) and are the result of an anatomic shunt at the atrial level. The physiologic left-to-right shunt is 9 L/min/m^2; this represents blood recirculated from the pulmonary veins to the pulmonary artery. The physiologic right-to-left shunt is 1.2 L/min/m^2; this represents blood recirculated from the systemic veins to the aorta. In this depiction, pulmonary vascular resistance is low (approximately 1/35 of systemic vascular resistance) and there is a small (17 mm peak to peak) gradient from the left ventricle to the pulmonary artery. These findings are compatible with the high pulmonary blood flow depicted. (Modified from Freed MO, Keane JF. Profiles in congenital heart disease. In: Grossman W, ed. *Cardiac catheterization and angiography*. Philadelphia: Lea & Febiger, 1986:463, with permission.)

DiNardo JA. Anesthesia for congenital heart surgery. In: Jonas RA, ed. *Comprehensive surgical management of congenital heart disease*. London: Arnold, 2004:45–65.

DiNardo JA. Transposition of the great vessels. In: Lake CL, Booker PD, eds. *Pediatric cardiac anesthesia*, 4th ed. Philadelphia: Lippincott Williams & Wilkins, 2005:357–380.

A.6. Why did this infant have reverse differential cyanosis?

In transposition of the great arteries (D-TGA) with intact ventricular septum (IVS) the anatomic mixing sites are usually a patent ductus arteriosus (PDA) and a patent foramen ovale (PFO). The dynamics of intercirculatory mixing in D-TGA with IVS are complex. Anatomic shunting at the atrial level is ultimately determined by the size of the atrial communication and the cyclic pressure variations between the left and right atria. The volume and compliance of the atria, ventricles, and vascular beds in each circuit, as well as heart rate (HR) and phase of respiration all influence this relationship. Shunting is from the right atrium (RA) to the left atrium (LA) during diastole as the result of the reduced ventricular and vascular compliance of the systemic circuit (right ventricle [RV] and systemic arterial circuit). In systole, shunt is from the LA to the RA primarily because of the large volume of blood returning to the LA as a result of the high volume of recirculated pulmonary blood flow.

The direction of shunting across the PDA largely depends on the pulmonary vascular resistance (PVR) and the size of the intraatrial communication. When the PVR is low and the intraatrial communication is nonrestrictive, shunting is predominantly from the aorta to the PA through the PDA (effective pulmonary blood flow) and predominantly from the LA to RA across the atrial septum (effective systemic blood flow). When PVR is elevated, shunting across the PDA is likely to be bidirectional that in turn encourages bidirectional shunting across the atrial septum. When PVR is high and PA pressure exceeds aortic pressure shunting at the PDA will be predominantly from the PA to the aorta. This will create reverse differential cyanosis- physiology wherein the preductal arterial saturation (right arm) is lower than the postductal arterial saturation (legs). This physiology is usually the result of a restrictive atrial communication producing left atrial hypertension and is associated with low effective blood flows (poor mixing) and hypoxemia. A balloon atrial septostomy can be lifesaving in this setting. Decompression of the LA promotes mixing at the atrial level and also reduces PVR and PA pressure promoting mixing at the PDA. Other causes of reverse differential cyanosis to be considered in D-TGA are the presence of an interrupted aortic arch or severe aortic coarctation.

DiNardo JA. Anesthesia for congenital heart surgery. In: Jonas RA, ed. *Comprehensive surgical management of congenital heart disease.* London: Arnold, 2004:45–65.

DiNardo JA. Transposition of the great vessels. In: Lake CL, Booker PD, eds. *Pediatric cardiac anesthesia*, 4th ed. Philadelphia: Lippincott Williams & Wilkins, 2005:357–380.

A.7. What are the preoperative issues pertaining to the coronary arteries in transposition of the great arteries (D-TGA)?

As in normally related great vessels, the coronary arteries in D-TGA arise from the aortic sinuses that face the PA. In normally related vessels, these sinuses are located on the anterior portion of the aorta, whereas in D-TGA, they are located posteriorly. In most D-TGA patients (70%), the right sinus is the origin of the right coronary artery, whereas the left sinus is the origin of the left main coronary artery. In the remainder of cases, there is considerable variability, with the most common variations being shown in Fig. 17.2.

Most patients with D-TGA have a coronary anatomy that is suitable for the coronary reimplantation necessary in the arterial switch operation (ASO). Patients with certain types of coronary anatomy (intramural coronaries, single coronary artery) are at risk for postoperative myocardial ischemia and early mortality because reimplantation can result in the distortion of the coronary ostia or the narrowing of the artery itself. Patients with intramural coronaries generally require resuspension of the posterior leaflet of neopulmonary valve once the coronaries and a surrounding tissue cuff are excised.

The presence of a single coronary artery or intramural coronary arteries is a risk factor for mortality and this risk has persisted over the last two decades.

DiNardo JA. Transposition of the great vessels. In: Lake CL, Booker PD, eds. *Pediatric cardiac anesthesia*, 4th ed. Philadelphia: Lippincott Williams & Wilkins, 2005:357–380.

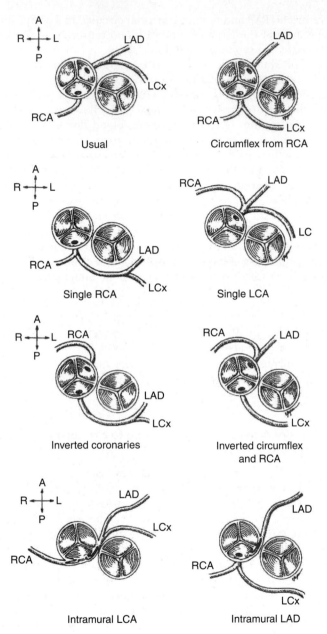

Figure 17.2 Depiction of the most common coronary artery patterns in transposition of the great vessels. The aorta is depicted anterior and to the right of the pulmonary artery. LAD, left anterior descending coronary artery; LCA, left coronary artery; LCx, left circumflex coronary artery; RCA, right coronary artery. (From Mayer JE, Sanders SP, Jonas RA, et al. Coronary artery pattern and outcome of arterial switch operation for transposition of the great arteries. *Circulation* 1990:82(Suppl III):144, with permission.)

Table 17.1 Clinical Subsets of Transposition of Great Arteries.

ANATOMY	PULMONARY BLOOD FLOW	INTERCIRCULATORY MIXING
D-TGA with IVS	Increased	Small
D-TGA with IVS; nonrestrictive atrial septum or PDA	Increased	Large
D-TGA with VSD	Increased	Large
D-TGA with VSD and LVOT obstruction	Reduced	Small
D-TGA with PVOD	Reduced	Small

D-TGA, transposition of great arteries; IVS, intact ventricular septum; PDA, patent ductus arteriosus; VSD, ventricular septal defect; LVOT, left ventricular outflow tract; PVOD, pulmonary vascular occlusive disease.
DiNardo JA. Transposition of the great vessels. In: Lake CL, Booker, PD, eds. *Pediatric cardiac anesthesia*, 4th ed. Philadelphia: Lippincott Williams & Wilkins, 2005:357–380.

A.8. What are the clinical subsets of transposition of the great arteries (D-TGA)?

Four clinical subsets based on anatomy, pulmonary blood flow, and intercirculatory mixing can be used to characterize patients with D-TGA. These are summarized in Table 17.1.

A.9. What is the differential diagnosis of transposition of the great arteries (D-TGA) and how is the diagnosis made?

Figure 17.3 delineates the differential diagnosis for D-TGA in the cyanotic newborn.

D-TGA may be associated with either cyanosis or congestive heart failure (CHF). In patients in whom intercirculatory mixing is limited, cyanosis is severe with little evidence of CHF. CHF is the more common finding in patients with increased pulmonary blood flow, a large quantity of intercirculatory mixing, and mild cyanosis.

Chest radiographs may appear normal in the first few weeks of life in infants with D-TGA and intact ventricular septum (IVS). Eventually, the triad of an enlarged egg-shaped heart (large right atrium [RA] and ventricle), narrow superior mediastinum, and increased pulmonary vascular markings evolve. In patients with D-TGA and ventricular septal defect (VSD) without left ventricular outflow tract (LVOT) obstruction, a large cardiac silhouette and prominent pulmonary vascular markings are seen at birth. Right axis deviation and right ventricular hypertrophy (RVH) are the electrocardiographic (ECG) findings in D-TGA with IVS, whereas right axis deviation, left ventricular hypertrophy (LVH), and RVH are seen with D-TGA and VSD.

Two-dimensional echocardiography is the diagnostic modality of choice in the diagnosis and assessment of infants with D-TGA. It accurately establishes the diagnosis of D-TGA and reliably, identifies associated abnormalities such as VSD, mitral and tricuspid valve abnormalities, and LVOT obstruction. It also reliably delineates coronary artery anatomy. Echocardiographic analysis of the ventricular septal position or left ventricle (LV) geometry is also used to noninvasively assess the LV to right ventricle (RV) pressure ratio and IV mass in neonates with D-TGA and IVS who are being evaluated as candidates for an arterial switch operation (ASO).

In institutions with high-level echocardiography, a comprehensive cardiac catheterization is no longer routinely performed in neonates with D-TGA. A limited catheterization may be performed in conjunction with a balloon atrial septostomy. In the rare instance where coronary anatomy cannot be clearly delineated by echocardiography, coronary angiography may be indicated. During catheterization of infants with pulmonary vascular occlusive disease (PVOD), a trial of ventilation at a FIO_2 of 1.0 may be used to determine whether pulmonary vascular resistance (PVR) is fixed or remains responsive to oxygen-induced pulmonary vasodilatation.

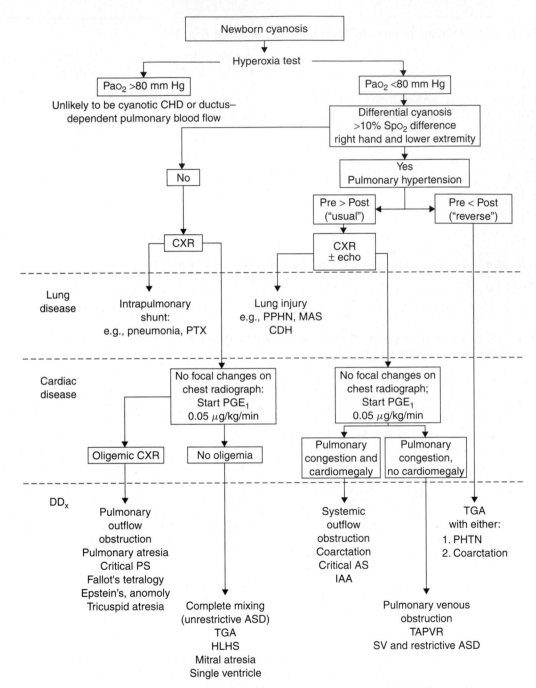

Figure 17.3 The differential diagnosis of transposition of the great arteries. AS, aortic stenosis; ASD, atrial septal defect; CHD, congenital heart disease; CXR, chest x-ray; HLHS, hypoplastic left heart syndrome; IAA, interrupted aortic arch; PHTN, pulmonary hypertension; PS, pulmonary stenosis; SA, single atrium; TAPVR, total anomalous pulmonary venous return; TGA, transposition of great arteries.

DiNardo JA. Anesthesia for congenital heart surgery. In: Jonas RA, ed. *Comprehensive surgical management of congenital heart disease*. London: Arnold, 2004:45–65.

DiNardo JA. Transposition of the great vessels. In: Lake CL, Booker PD, eds. *Pediatric cardiac anesthesia*, 4th ed. Philadelphia: Lippincott Williams & Wilkins, 2005:357–380.

A.10. What preoperative interventions can help stabilize a patient with transposition of the great arteries (D-TGA)?

Intact ventricular septum

Most neonates with D-TGA and intact ventricular septum (IVS) will be hypoxemic (arterial saturation $\leq 60\%$) within the first day of life. A proportion of these patients will have severely reduced effective pulmonary and systemic blood flow resulting in a PaO_2 less than 20 mm Hg, hypercarbia, and an evolving metabolic acidosis secondary to the poor tissue oxygen delivery. Prostaglandin E_1, (0.01 to 0.05 μg/kg/minute) is administered to dilate and maintain the patency of the ductus arteriosus. This will be effective in increasing effective pulmonary and systemic blood flow, and in improving PaO_2 and tissue oxygen delivery *if* (a) pulmonary vascular resistance (PVR) less than systemic vascular resistance (SVR) and (b) there is a nonrestrictive or minimally restrictive atrial septal communication. In some centers, all neonates stabilized on prostaglandin E_1 alone have a balloon atrial septostomy to enlarge the atrial septal communication so that prostaglandin E_1 can be stopped and surgery scheduled on a semielective basis. Prostaglandin E_1 infusion is associated with apnea, pyrexia, fluid retention, and platelet dysfunction.

If prostaglandin E_1 does not improve tissue oxygen delivery, then an emergent balloon atrial septostomy is performed in the catheterization laboratory utilizing angiography or in the intensive care unit (ICU) utilizing echocardiography. These patients also require tracheal intubation and mechanical ventilation. This allows reduction of PVR through induction of a respiratory alkalosis and elimination of pulmonary ventilation/pefusion ($\dot{V}/\dot{Q}$) mismatch. Sedation and muscle relaxation reduce oxygen consumption, thereby increasing mixed venous O_2 saturation. Recall that for a given amount of intercirculatory mixing and total systemic blood flow, an increase in systemic venous or pulmonary venous saturation will result in an increase in arterial saturation.

In rare instances, the combination of prostaglandin E_1, an atrial septostomy, and mechanical ventilation with sedation/muscle relaxation may be ineffective. In this circumstance, extracorporeal membrane oxygenation (ECMO) (either venoarterial [VA] or venovenous [VV]) support to improve tissue oxygenation and to reverse end-organ insult and lactic acidosis before surgery is an alternative approach to emergent surgery in a critically ill neonate.

Ventricular septal defect

Infants in this subset are mildly cyanotic with symptoms of congestive heart failure (CHF). Pulmonary blood flow is increased, and there is extensive intercirculatory mixing. Reducing PVR to further augment pulmonary blood flow and intercirculatory mixing will not greatly influence the systemic oxygenation. Reducing PVR in these patients may increase the recirculated volume in the pulmonary circuit by increasing circuit compliance. Maintaining systemic blood flow will then necessitate an increase in cardiac output from a failing heart. These patients are commonly stable enough not to require immediate surgical or catheterization laboratory intervention. They are, however, candidates for an arterial switch operation (ASO) before intractable CHF or advanced pulmonary vascular occlusive disease (PVOD) occur.

Ventricular septal defect and left ventricular outflow tract obstruction

The degree of cyanosis in these infants will depend on the extent of left ventricular outflow tract (LVOT) obstruction. LVOT obstruction reduces pulmonary blood flow and intercirculatory mixing, and it protects the pulmonary vasculature from the increased pressures and volumes that accelerate the development of PVOD. The more severe the LVOT obstruction, the less effective will be the efforts to increase pulmonary blood flow by decreasing PVR. When LVOT obstruction is severe, the infant is severely cyanotic and progressively develops polycythemia. These infants may require a palliative aortopulmonary shunt to increase pulmonary blood flow. Ideally, a definitive repair in the form of a Rastelli procedure is performed in the neonatal period.

Pulmonary vascular occlusive disease

The goal of diagnosis and treatment of infants with D-TGA is to intervene surgically before the development of PVOD. As PVOD advances, the child becomes progressively cyanotic and polycythemic. Efforts to reduce PVR will increase pulmonary blood flow and intercirculatory mixing in infants where PVR is not fixed. Infants with advanced PVOD (PVR >10 Wood units; histologic grade 4) are generally candidates only for palliative therapy. In particular, closure of a ventricular septal defect (VSD) in the presence of advanced pulmonary hypertension carries a high mortality rate owing to the afterload mismatch and the resultant pulmonary ventricular (left ventricle) dysfunction. These patients are candidates for a palliative intraatrial physiologic repair without closure or with fenestrated closure (4- to 5-mm hole in the center of the VSD patch) of the VSD.

DiNardo JA. Anesthesia for congenital heart surgery. In: Jonas RA, ed. *Comprehensive surgical management of congenital heart disease*. London: Arnold, 2004:45–65.

DiNardo JA. Transposition of the great vessels. In: Lake CL, Booker PD, eds. *Pediatric cardiac anesthesia*, 4th ed. Philadelphia: Lippincott Williams & Wilkins, 2005:357–380.

A.11. What are the surgical options for repair? Why is one chosen over the others?

Arterial anatomic repair: arterial switch (Jatene) operation

The arterial switch operation (ASO) anatomically corrects the discordant ventriculoarterial connections and is the procedure of choice for patients with transposition of great arteries (D-TGA). Following repair, the right ventricle (RV) is connected to the pulmonary artery (PA) and the left ventricle (LV) to the aorta. Clinical success with the ASO, summarized in Fig. 17.4, was achieved in 1975. In order for the ASO to be successful, the original pulmonary ventricle (LV) must have sufficient mass to be capable of functioning as the systemic ventricle following the switch. Patient selection and the timing of the surgical procedure are, therefore, important variables in determining the success of this procedure. The ASO was originally described in patients with D-TGA and a large ventricular septal defect (VSD) or a large patent ductus arteriosus (PDA). In these patients, the pulmonary ventricle (LV) remains exposed to systemic pressures, and the LV mass remains sufficient to support the systemic circulation. For this subset of patients, the ASO is generally performed within the first 2 to 3 months of life, before intractable congestive heart failure (CHF) or irreversible pulmonary vascular occlusive disease (PVOD) intervene.

In patients with D-TGA and intact ventricular septum (IVS), there is a progressive reduction in LV mass as the physiologic pulmonary hypertension present at birth resolves progressively over the first weeks following birth. Adequate LV mass to support the systemic circulation exists in these patients for only the first 2 or 3 weeks following birth. In patients with D-TGA and IVS, the ASO can be performed primarily or as the second phase of a staged procedure. A successful primary ASO must generally be performed within the first 3 weeks of life. Previously, favorable candidates for the procedure in the neonatal period were shown to have an LV to RV pressure ratio of at least 0.6 by catheterization. Currently, two-dimensional echocardiography is used to noninvasively assess the LV to RV pressure ratio. Three types of ventricular septal geometry have been described. Patients in whom the ventricular septum bulges to the left (type 3), indicating a

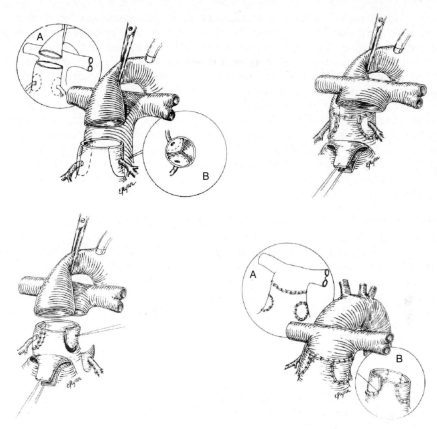

Figure 17.4 Details of the arterial switch procedure. **Upper left.** Aorta is transected and left and right main coronary arteries are excised using **(A)** either button of aortic wall or **(B)** segment of aortic wall extending from rim of aorta. **Lower left.** Equivalent segment of pulmonary arterial wall is excised, and coronary arteries are sutured to pulmonary artery. **Upper right.** Distal pulmonary artery is brought anterior to ascending aorta (LeCompte maneuver), and proximal pulmonary artery is anastomosed to distal aorta. **Lower right.** Sites of coronary explantation are repaired using either **(A)** patch of prosthetic material or **(B)** segment of pericardium. Finally, proximal aorta is sutured to distal pulmonary artery. (From: Castanda AR, Norwood WI, Jonas RA, et al. Transposition of the great arteries and intact ventricular septum: anatomical repair in the neonate. *Ann Thorac Surg* 1984;38:438–443. Reprinted with permission from the Society of Thoracic Surgeons.)

low pressure in the pulmonary ventricle (LV), are not candidates for a neonatal ASO. Patients with septal bulging to the right (type 1), indicating a high pressure in the pulmonary ventricle (LV), and those patients with an intermediate septal position (type 2) are considered good candidates. Most neonates with D-TGA and IVS who are suitable candidates for an ASO have type 2 septal geometry.

The staged ASO for D-TGA with IVS is used for those neonates in whom surgery cannot be performed in the first few weeks of life secondary to events such as prematurity, sepsis, low birth weight (<1.0 kg), or late referral. The LV is retrained to accept the systemic workload within the first 2 months of life. The preparatory surgery involves creation of a nonrestrictive atrial septum (if it does not already exist), placement of a PA band, and creation of an aortopulmonary shunt with entry to the PA distal to the band. The band must be tight enough to increase pressure in the pulmonary ventricle (LV) to approximately one half to two thirds of that in the systemic ventricle (RV). This will increase the afterload sufficiently to stimulate an increase in LV mass. Historically, after 3 to 6 months the PA was debanded, the shunt taken down, and an ASO performed. Currently a rapid two-stage repair is undertaken in which the ASO is performed as early as 1 week after preparatory PA banding, often during the same hospitalization. This approach is based on the fact that a doubling of LV mass is seen after 1 week of PA banding. The staged procedure is complicated by the fact that the adjustment of the PA band to the proper tightness is not an easy task and that the PA band and systemic to PA shunt may result in a distortion of the PA, making the definite ASO difficult. Intraoperative transesophageal echocardiography (TEE) is useful in guiding placement of the PA band. The band is tightened enough to flatten the intraventricular septum by shifting it toward the RV.

Intraatrial physiologic repairs: mustard and senning procedures

Both the Mustard and the Senning procedures are atrial switch procedures that surgically create discordant atrioventricular (AV) connections in D-TGA. Systemic venous blood is routed to the LV and the PA whereas pulmonary venous blood is routed to the RV and the aorta. This arrangement results in physiologic but not anatomic correction of D-TGA as the morphologic RV becomes the systemic ventricle. Given the current success with and the almost universal application of the more definitive ASO these intraatrial switch procedures are primarily of historic interest in patients with D-TGA.

Rastelli procedure

The Rastelli procedure was described in 1969 as a method of anatomically correcting D-TGA with VSD and left ventricular outflow tract (LVOT) obstruction. This surgery is used when LVOT obstruction in the form of subpulmonic and/or pulmonic stenosis is surgically uncorrectable. Performance of an ASO under these circumstances would leave the infant with residual LVOT obstruction (aortic or subaortic stenosis).

DiNardo JA. Transposition of the great arteries. In: Jonas RA, ed. *Comprehensive surgical management of congenital heart disease*. London: Arnold, 2004:256–278.

B. Preoperative Evaluation and Preparation

B.1. What information is important to prepare for this case?

The preoperative evaluation should begin with a careful history and physical examination. Gestational age, birth complications, family history, and any other medical problems should be noted. A comprehensive airway evaluation should be performed and the previous endotracheal tube size and leak pressure noted. Arterial and intravenous access should be assessed. A type and cross must be sent to the blood bank to ensure adequate red cells and blood component therapies are available in the operating room (OR).

The preoperative electrocardiography (ECG) and chest roentgenogram should be reviewed. The preoperative echocardiograms should be reviewed. Particular attention should be paid to septal geometry, biventricular function, coronary anatomy, and adequacy of mixing at the atrial septal and ductal levels. Prostaglandin E_1 was discontinued in the patient but the ductus arteriosus may remain patent.

Laboratory data should include a complete blood count, electrolytes, platelet count, arterial blood gas, calcium, blood urea nitrogen (BUN), creatinine, liver function tests (LFT)s and glucose.

Given that this infant presented with severe hypoxemia, end-organ dysfunction must be ruled out. The LFTs and creatinine should be normal; if they are elevated, consideration should be given to further medical optimization. A head ultrasonographic examination should be performed to rule out intraventricular hemorrhage (IVH).

DiNardo JA. Anesthesia for congenital heart surgery. In: Jonas RA, ed. *Comprehensive surgical management of congenital heart disease*. London: Arnold, 2004:45–65.

B.2. What are the anesthetic goals before cardiopulmonary bypass (CPB)?

- Maintain HR, contractility, and preload to maintain cardiac output; decreases in cardiac output decrease systemic venous saturation with a resultant fall in arterial saturation.
- Maintain ductal patency with prostaglandin E_1 (0.01 to 0.05 μg/kg/minute) in ductal-dependent patients.
- Avoid increases in pulmonary vascular resistance (PVR) relative to systemic vascular resistance (SVR); increases in PVR will decrease pulmonary blood flow and reduce intercirculatory mixing; in patients with pulmonary vascular occlusive disease (PVOD), ventilatory interventions should be used to reduce PVR; in patients with left ventricular outflow tract (LVOT) obstruction that is not severe, ventilatory interventions to reduce PVR increase pulmonary blood flow and intercirculatory mixing.
- Reductions in SVR relative to PVR should be avoided; decreased SVR increases recirculation of systemic venous blood and decreases arterial saturation.
- In patients with D-TGA and ventricular septal defect (VSD) with symptoms of congestive heart failure (CHF), ventilatory interventions to reduce PVR are not warranted as they will produce small improvements in arterial saturation at the expense of systemic perfusion.

DiNardo JA. Transposition of the great vessels. In: Lake CL, Booker PD, eds. *Pediatric cardiac anesthesia*, 4th ed. Philadelphia: Lippincott Williams & Wilkins, 2005:357–380.

B.3. What is the plan for glucose management in this patient?

Maintenance caloric requirements in the awake neonate/infant are 100 kcal/kg/day or 4 kcal/kg/hour. This caloric requirement can be met with glucose 25 g/kg/day or 1 g/kg/hour. From a practical point of view, this glucose requirement can be met with 10% dextrose (100 mg/mL) run at the maintenance volume replacement rate of 4 mL/kg/hour. Ten percent dextrose run at half this rate (2 mL/kg/hour) is usually sufficient to meet the caloric requirements of an anesthetized infant while avoiding both the hyper- and hypoglycemia that can be detrimental to neurologic outcome particularly following deep hypothermic circulatory arrest (DHCA). Dextrose infusions should be discontinued before commencement of cardiopulmonary bypass (CPB) as the associated neuroendocrine response to CPB generally produces mild hyperglycemia. Some infants receive nutritional support as part of medical stabilization before surgery. High-calorie total parenteral nutrition (TPN) and intralipid therapy should be discontinued and replaced with a 10% dextrose infusion several hours before transport to the OR. Continued administration of these high calorie infusions makes intraoperative serum glucose management problematic. In these patients, higher dextrose infusion rates may be necessary pre-CPB to avoid rebound hypoglycemia.

DiNardo JA. Anesthesia for congenital heart surgery. In: Jonas RA, ed. *Comprehensive surgical management of congenital heart disease*. London: Arnold, 2004:45–65.

C. Intraoperative Management

C.1. How would you monitor this infant?

Ideally, preinduction monitoring should include a blood pressure cuff, electrocardiography (ECG), pulse oximeter, and an end-tidal carbon dioxide monitor. In reality, a pulse oximeter and an ECG may be all that is practical in the early stages of induction. The other monitors are then quickly added as induction progresses. Pulse oximeter probes should be placed on an upper and lower extremity (pre- and postductal if relevant). An intraarterial catheter (radial or femoral) is placed just after induction. Many infants transferred from the intensive care unit (ICU) will have an umbilical artery or femoral artery catheter in place. A central venous pressure and drug infusion catheter is placed after intubation and stabilization. Double-lumen central venous catheters inserted through the femoral or internal jugular vein are preferred. Nasopharyngeal, tympanic, and rectal temperature probes are also placed following induction. A bladder catheter should be placed. A transesophageal echocardiography (TEE) probe can be inserted following induction and intubation.

DiNardo JA. Anesthesia for congenital heart surgery. In: Jonas RA, ed. *Comprehensive surgical management of congenital heart disease*. London: Arnold, 2004:45–65.

C.2. What would be the best method of induction?

This infant would have an IV catheter in place on transfer to the operating room (OR). Anesthesia is generally induced and maintained using a synthetic opioid-based (fentanyl or sufentanil) technique. These opioids may be used alone in high doses (25 to 100 μg/kg fentanyl or 2.5 to 10 μg/kg sufentanil) or in low to moderate doses (5 to 25 μg/kg fentanyl or 0.5 to 2.5 μg/kg sufentanil) in combination with an inhalation agent (generally isoflurane or sevoflurane) or a benzodiazepine (generally midazolam). The high-dose technique is particularly useful in neonates and infants. High-dose opioids provide hemodynamic stability, do not depress the myocardium, and blunt reactive pulmonary hypertension. In order to avoid bradycardia, pancuronium (0.1 mg/kg) is administered in conjunction with the opioid; its vagolytic activity offsets the vagotonic activity of the narcotics.

DiNardo JA. Anesthesia for congenital heart surgery. In: Jonas RA, ed. *Comprehensive surgical management of congenital heart disease*. London: Arnold, 2004:45–65.

DiNardo JA. Transposition of the great vessels. In: Lake CL, Booker PD, eds. *Pediatric cardiac anesthesia*, 4th ed. Philadelphia: Lippincott Williams & Wilkins, 2005:357–380.

C.3. Is cardiopulmonary bypass (CPB) in infants and children different from adults?

The major differences between adult and pediatric CPB are summarized in Table 17.2.

Flows of 2.0 to 2.5 L/minute/m^2 are commonly used for infants, children, and adults during mild to moderate systemic hypothermia. Owing to age-related differences in the relationship of surface area to weight, these flow rates expressed in mL/kg/minute will be substantially higher in the neonate than in the adult. The recommended full flow rates for pediatric CPB are summarized in Table 17.3.

The vast majority of operative procedures in children require the use of either total CPB or deep hypothermic circulatory arrest (DHCA). Venous cannulation for DHCA is usually accomplished with a single large venous cannula in the right atrium (RA). Once cooling is complete and circulatory arrest is established the cannula is removed to allow for maximum exposure. For

Table 17.2 Major Differences between Adult and Pediatric Cardiopulmonary Bypass.

PARAMETER	ADULT	PEDIATRICS
Hypothermic temperature	Rarely below 25°C–32°C	Commonly 15°C–20°C
Use of total circulatory arrest	Rare	Common
Pump prime		
Dilution effects on blood volume	25%–33%	200%–300%
Additional additives in ped primes		Blood, albumin
Perfusion pressures	50–80 mm Hg (some centers accept 30 mm Hg)	20–50 mm Hg
Influence of pH management strategy	Minimal at moderate hypothermia	Marked at deep hypothemia
Measured $Paco_2$ differences	30–45 mm Hg	20–80 mm Hg
Glucose regulation		
Hypoglycemia	Rare—requires significant hepatic injury	Common—reduced hepatic glycogen stores
Hyperglycemia	Frequent—generally easily controlled with insulin	Less common—rebound hypoglycemia may occur

total CPB once the cavae (and other sources of systemic venous return) are cannulated, surgical tourniquets or tapes are passed around the external circumference of the vessels. When these tapes are tightened around the cannulae, the right heart can be isolated completely and subsequently opened without entrainment of air into the venous circuit or obscuration of the surgical field by venous blood. During delivery of antegrade cardioplegia it is essential that at least one tape be left untightened to allow egress of cardioplegia solution from the coronary sinus without distention of the RA. A larger cannula is used in the inferior vena cava (IVC) as compared with the superior vena cava (SVC), because a larger portion of systemic venous return (two thirds) is from the IVC.

As with venous cannulation, arterial cannulation in children particularly infants/neonates can be technically challenging. It may be necessary in circumstances where the ascending aorta and aortic arch are hypoplastic and systemic blood flow is ductal dependant (as in hypoplastic left heart syndrome [HLHS]) to obtain systemic perfusion through the ductus arteriosus by cannulating the PA. When the aortic arch is interrupted, cannulation of the aorta both proximal and distal to the interruption is necessary. Because the arterial cannula is relatively large as compared to the aorta in infants/neonates complete or partial obstruction of the aorta by the cannula itself is possible. Constant vigilance is necessary to avoid this problem. If dampening of the arterial trace, distension of the systemic ventricle, or an increase in CPB line pressure occurs

Table 17.3 Recommended Full Flow Rates for Pediatric Cardiopulmonary Bypass.

PATIENT WEIGHT (kg)	FULL CPB FLOW RATES (mL/kg/min)
<3	150–200
3–10	125–175
10–15	120–150
15–30	100–120
30–50	75–100
>50	50–75

CPB, cardiopulmonary bypass.

with placement or manipulation of the arterial cannula, the surgeon should immediately be made aware of the situation so the cannula can be repositioned. Some centers utilize near-infrared spectroscopy (NIRS) and transcranial Doppler (TCD) ultrasonographic technology as adjunctive methods to assess cerebral blood flow during CPB.

Davies LK. Cardiopulmonary bypass in infants and children: how is it different? *J Cardiothorac Vasc Anesth* 1999;13(3):330–345.

DiNardo JA. Physiology and techniques of extracorporeal circulation in the pediatric patient. In: Lake CL, Booker PD, eds. *Pediatric cardiac anesthesia*, 4th ed. Philadelphia: Lippincott Williams & Wilkins, 2005:228–252.

DiNardo JA. Profound hypothermia and circulatory arrest. In: Lake CL, Booker PD, eds. *Pediatric cardiac anesthesia*, 4th ed. Philadelphia: Lippincott Williams & Wilkins, 2005: 253–265.

C.4. What is modified ultrafiltration (MUF)?

Ultrafiltrators are devices commonly added to the cardiopulmonary bypass (CPB) circuit to remove excess fluid and produce hemoconcentration. When used in conjunction with CPB, these devices produce an ultrafiltrate that occurs as the result of a hydrostatic pressure gradient across a semipermeable membrane. These are the same devices that can be used for hemodialysis when they are used in conjunction with a dialysate. When used in conjunction with CPB, they are commonly called *hemoconcentrators* as they produce an increase in hematocrit by removing excess fluid.

These devices consist of a core of microporous hollow fibers made of polysulfone, polyamide, or polyacrylonitrile material arranged in a bundle. The pore size is generally 0.30 to 0.40 μm. Owing to the pressure drop across the device, blood inflow must be obtained from the arterial side of the CPB circuit while blood outflow is diverted to the cardiotomy reservoir or venous reservoir. The ultrafiltrate is collected in a container connected to a vacuum source.

The ultrafiltrate is discarded and has the composition of glomerular filtrate. The rate at which ultrafiltrate is produced is dependent on the transmembrane pressure gradient (TMP). TMP is determined by the arterial inlet pressure (P_a), the venous outlet pressure (P_v), the absolute value of applied suction at the outlet (P_n), the oncotic pressure at the inlet (P_i), and the oncotic pressure at the outlet (P_o):

$$\text{TMP} = \frac{P_a + P_v}{2} + P_n - \frac{P_i + P_o}{2}$$

P_n is increased by using the regulated vacuum source connected to the outlet of the device. TMP should not exceed 500 mm Hg.

Continuous ultrafiltration (CUF) refers to ultrafiltration occurring throughout CPB or during those intervals when venous reservoir volume is sufficient to allow it. MUF is a technique that allows ultrafiltration to continue after weaning from CPB. MUF may be performed utilizing either an arteriovenous or venovenous system. In the arteriovenous system inflow to the ultrafiltrator during MUF is directly from the aortic cannula. Outflow from the ultrafiltrator is to the right atrium (RA). Blood volume is kept constant as ultrafiltrate is lost by replacing it with blood from the CPB circuit, which passes through the ultrafiltrator before being delivered to the RA. In this way, the CPB circuit can remain primed and the patient's blood, as well as the CPB blood, can be hemoconcentrated. In the venovenous system, the inferior vena cava (IVC) cannula provides inflow to the ultrafiltrator with the aid of a roller pump whereas outflow from the ultrafiltrator is returned to the superior vena cava (SVC) cannula. Blood volume is kept constant as ultrafiltrate is lost by replacing it with blood from the CPB circuit, which passes through the ultrafiltrator before being delivered to the SVC. The end point for termination of MUF following CPB varies from institution to institution with institutions terminating MUF after a set time interval (15 to 20 minutes), a set hematocrit (40%) or a set volume removed (750 mL/m^2). Heparin anticoagulation must be maintained during MUF with protamine reversal of heparin initiated after termination of MUF.

MUF may be an effective method of attenuating the deleterious consequences of a CPB strategy that involves large asanginous primes, particularly in neonates and infants. In the studies comparing MUF to no ultrafiltration, a CPB technique consisting of a very large asanginous pump prime (400 to 900 mL) with packed cells added to reach a hematocrit of 15% to 20% has generally been used. This is precisely the group of patients who would need and who would benefit from aggressive removal of excess fluid to reduce total body water and increase hematocrit and coagulation factors. Furthermore, it has been demonstrated that MUF and CUF during CPB are indistinguishable in their effect on hematocrit, mean arterial pressure (MAP), heart rate (HR), and LV shortening fraction when equal volumes of fluid are removed.

DiNardo JA. Physiology and techniques of extracorporeal circulation in the pediatric patient. In: Lake CL, Booker PD, eds. *Pediatric cardiac anesthesia*, 4th ed. Philadelphia: Lippincott Williams & Wilkins, 2005:228–252.

Thompson LD, McElhinney DB, Findlay P, et al. A prospective randomized study comparing volume-standardized modified and conventional ultrafiltration in pediatric cardiac surgery. *J Thorac Cardiovasc Surg* 2001;122:220–228.

C.5. Briefly describe the surgical techniques of the Mustard/Senning, arterial switch operation (ASO), and Rastelli procedures.

Intraatrial physiologic repairs: Mustard and Senning procedures

In both procedures the interatrial septum is excised, creating a large atrial septal defect (ASD). In the Mustard procedure, a baffle made of native pericardium or synthetic material is then used to redirect pulmonary and systemic venous blood. In the Senning procedure, autologous tissue from the right atrial wall and interatrial septum is used in place of the pericardium or synthetic material. In either case, pulmonary venous blood flows over the baffle and is directed across the tricuspid valve into the RV and out the aorta. Systemic venous blood flows on the underside of the baffle to be directed across the mitral valve into the left ventricle (LV) and out the PA. This arrangement results in physiologic but not anatomic correction of transposition of the great arteries (D-TGA), as the morphologic RV becomes the systemic ventricle. These procedures are performed with hypothermic cardiopulmonary bypass (CPB), bicaval cannulation, and aortic cross clamping during cardioplegic arrest. Intervals of low-flow CPB are customarily used.

Arterial anatomic repair: arterial switch (Jatene) operation

The PA and the aorta are transected distal to their respective valves. The coronary arteries are initially explanted from the ascending aorta with 3 to 4 mm of surrounding tissue. The explant sites are repaired either with pericardium or synthetic material. The coronary arteries are reimplanted into the proximal PA (neoaorta). The distal PA is brought anterior to the aorta (LeCompte maneuver) to be reanastomosed to the old proximal aorta (right ventricular outflow) and the distal aorta reanastomosed to the old proximal PA (left ventricular outflow). As a result the great arteries are switched to create ventriculoarterial concordance with both an anatomic and physiologic repair achieved. The ASO is done using hypothermic CPB with aortic cross clamping and cardioplegic arrest. Intervals of low-flow CPB are customarily used. A short interval of deep hypothermic circulatory arrest (DHCA) may be employed to close the atrial septum or ventricular septal defect (VSD) if a single venous cannula rather than bicaval venous cannulation is used. Closure of a VSD is preferentially done transatrially through the tricuspid valve. It is desirable to avoid approaching a VSD through the RV, because an incision in the RV may contribute substantially to postoperative RV dysfunction.

DiNardo JA. Transposition of the great arteries. In: Jonas RA, ed. *Comprehensive surgical management of congenital heart disease*. London: Arnold, 2004:256–278.

Jatene AD, Fontes VF, Paulista PP, et al. Anatomic correction of transposition of the great vessels. *J Thorac Cardiovasc Surg* 1976;72:364–370.

Rastelli procedure

The PA is transected and ligated just distal to or at the level of the pulmonary valve. A right ventriculotomy is performed, and the VSD is closed with a patch tunnel such that the LV is in continuity with the aorta. The VSD may have to be enlarged, in some cases, to prevent subaortic stenosis. Right ventricle (RV) to PA continuity is achieved by placement of valved conduit or valved homograft between the right ventriculotomy site and the proximal main PA. The result is LV to aortic continuity and RV to PA continuity with bypass of the subpulmonic and pulmonic stenosis. This procedure is performed with hypothermic CPB, bicaval cannulation, and aortic cross clamping during cardioplegic arrest. Intervals of low-flow CPB are customarily used.

Historically, most of these patients had a palliative systemic to PA shunt placed in the newborn period and then returned for the Rastelli procedure and takedown of the shunt at 2 to 3 years of age. The delay was felt necessary to avoid performing a right ventriculotomy in infants with immature myocardium and limited contractile elements and to allow adequate growth of the RV and pulmonary arteries to permit placement of an RV to pulmonary artery (PA) conduit. In the current era with improvements in myocardial protection, CPB technology, and surgical technique this procedure can be performed as a primary procedure in the neonatal period.

DiNardo JA. Transposition of the great arteries. In: Jonas RA, ed. *Comprehensive surgical management of congenital heart disease*. London: Arnold, 2004:256–278.

DiNardo JA. Transposition of the great vessels. In: Lake CL, Booker PD, eds. *Pediatric cardiac anesthesia*, 4th ed. Philadelphia: Lippincott Williams & Wilkins, 2005:357–380.

C.6. What is hypothermia and how is it classified? What is low-flow cardiopulmonary bypass (CPB)? What is deep hypothermic circulatory arrest (DHCA)?

The levels of systemic hypothermia employed during CPB are generally defined as follows: Mild (35°C [95°F] to 32°C [89.6°F]), moderate (31°C [87.8°F] to 26°C[78.8°F]), deep (25°C [77°F] to 20°C [68°F]), and profound (<20°C [68°F]). Unfortunately, it is not uncommon for temperatures less than 20°C (68°F) used in conjunction with pediatric cardiac surgery to be called *deep hypothermia*. Low-flow CPB in neonates/infants conducted in conjunction with temperatures of 18°C (64.4°F) to 25°C (77°F) is generally defined as 50 to 70 mL/kg/minute or approximately 1.0 to 1.5 L/minute/m^2.

Profound hypothermic circulatory arrest (PHCA) commonly referred to as *DHCA*, is a technique employed to improve exposure of intracardiac defects and to facilitate aortic arch reconstruction in infants and children. DHCA is conducted in conjunction with temperatures of 18°C (64.4°F) to 20°C (68°F) and allows cessation of CPB, venous and arterial cannula removal, and exsanguination of the patient into the venous reservoir of the CPB circuit. There has been substantial refinement of the technique of DHCA since its successful inception in the 1970s. In the current era, DHCA is used selectively and for short intervals. It is utilized primarily for the aortic arch reconstruction component of the Norwood procedure, repair of interrupted aortic arch, neonatal repair of total anomalous pulmonary venous connection, and complicated intracardiac repairs such as complete atrioventricular (AV) canal defects in small (<2.0 kg) neonates and infants.

Davies LK. Cardiopulmonary bypass in infants and children: how is it different? *J Cardiothorac Vasc Anesth* 1999;13(3):330–345.

DiNardo JA. Physiology and techniques of extracorporeal circulation in the pediatric patient. In: Lake CL, Booker PD, eds. *Pediatric cardiac anesthesia*, 4th ed. Philadelphia: Lippincott Williams & Wilkins, 2005:228–252.

DiNardo JA. Profound hypothermia and circulatory arrest. In: Lake CL, Booker PD, eds. *Pediatric cardiac anesthesia*, 4th ed. Philadelphia: Lippincott Williams & Wilkins, 2005: 253–265.

C.7. Why is hypothermia beneficial to the brain during low-flow cardiopulmonary bypass (LF CPB) and deep hypothermic circulatory arrest (DHCA)?

Hypothermia is arguably the most important component of low-flow CPB and DHCA. Hypothermia-induced reduction in cerebral metabolic rate for oxygen ($CMRO_2$) slows the rate of depletion of high-energy phosphates and the development of intracellular acidosis. This in turn delays or prevents the neuronal energy failure that leads to terminal membrane depolarization and subsequent neuronal injury or death during an ischemic episode. Q_{10} defines the ratio of organ O_2 consumption at a defined temperature to the O_2 consumption at a temperature 10°C (18°F) lower. The cerebral Q_{10} is approximately 3.65 in children [2] and 2.3 in adults. Despite this the cerebral metabolic rate will still be approximately 10% to 15% of its normothermic baseline at 15°C (59°F). If it is assumed that 3 to 5 minutes of cerebral ischemia can be tolerated at 37°C (98.6°F) and the Q_{10} is 3.0, 9 to 15 minutes of ischemia can be tolerated at 27°C (80.6°F) and 27 to 45 minutes can be tolerated at 17°C (62.6°F).

In addition to reducing $CMRO_2$, hypothermia also serves to ameliorate some of the sequalae of neuronal ischemia when instituted *before* the ischemia insult. Specifically, hypothermia markedly reduces release of the excitatory neurotransmitters glutamate, aspartate, and glycine that accompany cerebral ischemia and subsequent reperfusion. In energy-deprived cells, glutamate in particular is neurotoxic in part due to the role it plays in inducing massive calcium influx through NMDA receptors. Hypothermia also blunts the inhibitory effect of hypoxia on nitroxidergic (postganglionic parasympathetic nerve where NO is the neurotransmitter) induced cerebral vasodilatation. In addition, there is evidence that hypothermia may attenuate neutrophil migration into ischemic tissue.

DiNardo JA. Profound hypothermia and circulatory arrest. In: Lake CL, Booker PD, eds. *Pediatric cardiac anesthesia*, 4th ed. Philadelphia: Lippincott Williams & Wilkins, 2005: 253–265.

McCullough JN, Zhang N, Reich DL, et al. Cerebral metabolic suppression during hypothermic circulatory arrest in humans. *Ann Thorac Surg* 1999;67:1895–1899.

C.8. Explain the difference between α-stat and pH-stat blood gas management.

pH-stat and α-stat acid–base management are commonly discussed in association with management of CPB. pH-stat and α-stat regulation are acid–base management methods that directly influence blood flow to the brain and other organs. Although pH-stat and α-stat acid–base management are commonly mentioned in association with temperature–corrected and temperature–uncorrected blood gases, it must be emphasized that these are entirely different concepts. The method of blood gas interpretation (corrected or uncorrected) does not dictate the method of acid–base management (pH-stat or α-stat). α-Stat or pH-stat management is possible with use of both temperature–corrected and temperature–uncorrected blood gases. In addition, it is important to point out that at a patient temperature of 37°C (98.6°F) there is no difference between pH-stat and α-stat management. The difference between these two strategies becomes more marked as patient temperature progressively decreases below 37°C (98.6°F) and is not clinically relevant until patient temperature is less than 30°C (86°F).

When a blood gas sample is drawn from a patient at 25°C (77°F) and sent to the blood gas laboratory, the sample is warmed to 37°C (98.6°F) before measurement. The values obtained at 37°C (98.6°F) are called the *temperature-uncorrected values*. These values are converted to temperature-corrected values using a nomogram. The nomogram accounts for temperature-induced changes in pH, O_2 solubility, and CO_2 solubility in a closed-blood system. When pH and PCO_2 are measured at 37°C (98.6°F) and then corrected to a lower temperature, the electrochemically neutral pH will be higher and the corrected PCO_2 will be lower than the normal values at 37°C (98.6°F). Therefore, electrochemical neutrality is maintained by keeping pH alkalotic in temperature–corrected blood gases and normal in temperature-uncorrected gases. This is known as *α-stat regulation*. For practical purposes, it is easier to use uncorrected gases and keep pH and PCO_2 in the range considered normal at 37°C (98.6°F). It has been demonstrated clinically that cerebral blood flow and oxygen consumption are appropriately coupled when α-stat regulation is used. Deep hypothermia in the presence of α-stat regulation produces loss of cerebral autoregulation such that cerebral blood flow varies directly with arterial pressure.

pH-stat regulation refers to maintaining pH and PCO_2 at normal values for 37°C (98.6°F) when temperature-corrected gases are used and at acidotic values when temperature-uncorrected gases are used. For practical purposes, pH-stat is maintained by adding CO_2 to the ventilating gas during hypothermic CPB to increase PCO_2 and decrease the pH. In contrast to α-stat regulation, in which total CO_2 content is kept constant, pH-stat regulation results in an increase in total CO_2 content. The cerebral vasculature maintains vasomotor responses to varying PCO_2 during hypothermic CPB. This response is maintained during both moderate and deep hypothermia despite the fact that deep hypothermia induces loss of cerebral blood flow autoregulation. It has been demonstrated clinically that when pH-stat regulation is used with moderate hypothermic CPB there is uncoupling of cerebral blood flow and metabolism and loss of cerebral autoregulation. As a result, cerebral blood flow varies linearly with arterial blood pressure and cerebral hyperperfusion exists with cerebral blood flow far in excess of that dictated by cerebral metabolic rate. This hyperperfusion state is the result of: (a) reduced cerebral oxygen consumption induced by hypothermia and (b) cerebral vasodilation resulting from a disproportionately high PCO_2 for the degree of hypothermia present. The potential danger of the hyperperfused state is that it may result in increased delivery of microemboli into the cerebral circulation.

DiNardo JA. Physiology and techniques of extracorporeal circulation in the pediatric patient. In: Lake CL, Booker PD, eds. *Pediatric cardiac anesthesia*, 4th ed. Philadelphia: Lippincott Williams & Wilkins, 2005:228–252.

DiNardo JA. Profound hypothermia and circulatory arrest. In: Lake CL, Booker PD, eds. *Pediatric cardiac anesthesia*, 4th ed. Philadelphia: Lippincott Williams & Wilkins, 2005: 253–265.

C.9. What are the immediate post–cardiopulmonary bypass (CPB) issues following arterial switch operation (ASO)?

Bleeding from the extensive suture lines in the post-CPB period may be problematic. Efforts to reduce aortic blood pressure combined with aggressive blood component therapy are often required. In neonates it may require 1 to 2 units of platelets (0.25 to 0.5 units/kg) to obtain a therapeutic platelet count increase. Because platelets are suspended in fresh frozen plasma, a platelet transfusion of this size usually results in a fresh frozen plasma transfusion of 10 to 15 mL per kg.

Myocardial ischemia following reimplantation of the coronary arteries is a potential problem following the ASO. In some circumstances, the ischemia is transient secondary to coronary air emboli. TEE is very useful to assure adequate removal of air from the LA and ventricle before the termination of CPB. It is also useful in assessing the potency of the reimplanted coronary arteries. Maintenance of high perfusion pressures on CPB after aortic cross clamp removal will facilitate the distal migration of air emboli. In other instances, kinking of the reimplanted artery or compromise of the implanted coronary ostia may require immediate surgical intervention. Pharmacologic intervention with traditional therapies to improve the balance of myocardial oxygen demand and delivery such as nitroglycerin and β-blockade are never a long-term alternative to prompt surgical revision of the appropriate anastomosis.

Despite comprehensive preoperative evaluation, the LV of patients undergoing an ASO may be marginal in its ability to support the systemic circulation in the post-CPB period. This may occur as the result of myocardial ischemia, inadequate LV mass, poor protection of the LV during aortic cross clamping, or a combination of these variables. TEE is useful in identifying and continuously evaluating both global and regional LV systolic dysfunction. It also detects mitral regurgitation, which may occur secondary to papillary muscle dysfunction or to dilation of the mitral valve annulus. Inotropic support of the LV and afterload reduction may be necessary to terminate CPB.

DiNardo JA. Transposition of the great vessels. In: Lake CL, Booker PD, eds. *Pediatric cardiac anesthesia*, 4th ed. Philadelphia: Lippincott Williams & Wilkins, 2005:357–380.

D. Postoperative Management

D.1. How is myocardial ischemia addressed in the intensive care unit (ICU) following the arterial switch operation (ASO)?

Myocardial ischemia in the ICU following an ASO as heralded by ST-segment/T-wave changes or the development of atrial or ventricular arrhythmias requires immediate attention. Myocardial ischemia should be considered to be mechanical in nature until proved otherwise. Compression of the coronary ostia by swelling of thrombin gelform pads or thrombus formation around the coronary anastomoses must be considered. In this setting, surgical reexploration is likely to be immediately therapeutic.

Another source of mechanically induced myocardial ischemia in the ASO patient occurs as the result of left ventricle (LV) dilation. A unique cycle of LV dilation initiating and exacerbating myocardial ischemia exists in patients having undergone the ASO. Myocardial ischemia, afterload mismatch, or overzealous volume infusion can result in LV distension and left atrium (LA) hypertension. This will be particularly likely if there is mitral insufficiency from either papillary muscle dysfunction or dilation of the mitral valve annulus. LV distension may result in tension on and kinking of the coronary reanastomosis sites. LA hypertension produces elevations in PA pressure and distension of the PA. As the LeCompte maneuver brings the distal PA anterior to the ascending aorta, distension of the PA may actually compress or place tension on the coronary ostia. The resulting myocardial ischemia produces further LV dilation, progressive elevations in LA and PA pressures, and continuing compromise of coronary blood flow. Attempts to induce coronary vasodilatation with nitroglycerine are unlikely to be beneficial in this setting although its preload and afterload reducing may be beneficial. A more rational approach would be initiation of milrinone therapy.

DiNardo JA. Transposition of the great vessels. In: Lake CL, Booker PD, eds. *Pediatric cardiac anesthesia*, 4th ed. Philadelphia: Lippincott Williams & Wilkins, 2005:357–380.

DiNardo JA. Transposition of the great arteries. In: Jonas RA, ed. *Comprehensive surgical management of congenital heart disease*. London: Arnold, 2004:256–278.

D.2. What immediate postoperative problems would be anticipated following the Rastelli procedure?

Right (pulmonary) ventricular dysfunction may occur in the post–cardiopulmonary bypass (CPB) period. These patients are at risk because a right ventriculotomy is used to close the ventricular septal defect (VSD) and to create the new pulmonary outflow tract. Heart block may also occur given the proximity of the VSD to the intraventricular conduction pathways. A residual VSD may be present. Because the VSD closure to create left ventricle (LV) to aortic continuity is more of a tunnel than a patch closure LV outflow tract obstruction is also possible.

DiNardo JA. Transposition of the great vessels. In: Lake CL, Booker PD, eds. *Pediatric cardiac anesthesia*, 4th ed. Philadelphia: Lippincott Williams & Wilkins, 2005:357–380.

D.3. What intermediate and long-term surgical problems are seen after arterial switch operation (ASO)?

Supravalvular pulmonary stenosis is probably the most common complication of ASO. This stenosis is due to retraction of the tissue used to replace the tissue excised with the explanted coronaries and in most patients is not extensive enough to result in valvular pulmonary stenosis. Series with long-term follow-up (15 years) confirm that the incidence of supravalvular stenosis severe enough to require reoperation (generally a gradient >50 to 60 mm Hg) is approximately 4% to 8%. Aortic insufficiency occurs in approximately 10% to 15% of patients at long-term follow-up, with the majority (96%) graded as trivial or mild. Time has shown aortic insufficiency to be a rare source of morbidity or indication for reoperation following the ASO.

Early concerns existed regarding the long-term patency and growth potential of the reimplanted coronary arteries. Fortunately these problems have not materialized on a large scale.

DiNardo JA. Transposition of the great vessels. In: Lake CL, Booker PD, eds. *Pediatric cardiac anesthesia*, 4th ed. Philadelphia: Lippincott Williams & Wilkins, 2005:357–380.

Legendre A, Losay J, Touchot-Kone A, et al. Coronary events after arterial switch operation for transposition of the great arteries. *Circulation* 2003;108(Suppl 1):II186–II190.

Nogi S, McCrindle BW, Boutin C, et al. Fate of the neopulmonary valve after the arterial switch operation in neonates. *J Thorac Cardiovasc Surg* 1998;115:557–562.

D.4. What are the long-term outcomes after arterial switch operation (ASO)?

The initial result for the arterial switch in experienced institutions is excellent, with an actuarial survival at 1 year of 90% for patients with D-TGA and intact ventricular septum (IVS) and 83% for patients with D-TGA and ventricular septal defect (VSD). Other experienced groups have reported similar results. A recent review of 470 patients from one institution experienced in the ASO, however, revealed a 1-year survival rate of 92% and an 8-year survival rate of 91% for patients with both D-TGA and IVS and D-TGA and VSD. A similar review of 1,200 patients from another experienced institution revealed a 1- and 15-year survival rate of 92% for patients with D-TGA and IVS and 1- and 15-year survival respectively of 81% and 80% for D-TGA and VSD. A recent multiinstitution review of 631 patients with D-TGA and 167 patients with D-TGA and VSD reviewed similar initial and long-term (15 years) outcomes.

The overwhelming majority (90% to 97%) of patients have normal-sized, patent coronary arteries as assessed by coronary angiography. A recent study of a large cohort demonstrated that survival without coronary events (death from myocardial infarction [MI], sudden death, and reoperation for coronary stenoses) is 92.7% at 1 year and 88.2% at 15 years. The incidence of coronary events is bimodal with a high early and low late event rate. Eighty-nine percent of all coronary events occurred in the first 3 months after ASO. The event rate did not increase again until 6 years after ASO. Two types of coronary anatomy (a single coronary artery origin or two coronaries originating close to each other at a facing commissure) were risk factors for a coronary event.

One of the potential advantages of the ASO over the atrial switch procedure is the use of the native left ventricle (LV) as the systemic ventricle. Long-term follow-up indicates that patients who have undergone an ASO have higher systemic ventricular ejection fractions than do patients who have undergone atrial switch procedures. In fact, patients who had D-TGA and IVS repaired in infancy and patients who had D-TGA and VSD repaired later have LV end diastolic dimensions and contractile indices similar to normal patients. Myocardial contractility in patients having undergone a rapid or traditional two-stage arterial switch is mildly depressed as compared to patients having undergone a primary arterial switch. No progression of this ventricular dysfunction has been noted at either intermediate or long-term follow up.

DiNardo JA. Transposition of the great vessels. In: Lake CL, Booker PD, eds. *Pediatric cardiac anesthesia*, 4th ed. Philadelphia: Lippincott Williams & Wilkins, 2005:357–380.

Losay J, Touchota A, Serraf A, et al. Late outcome after arterial switch operation for transposition of the great arteries. *Circulation* 2001;104:I121–I126.

Pasquali SK, Hasselblad V, Li JS, et al. Coronary artery pattern and outcome of arterial switch operation for transposition of the great arteries: a meta-analysis. *Circulation* 2002;106:2575–2580.

Wernovsky G, Mayer JE Jr, Jonas RA, et al. Factors influencing early and late outcome of the arterial switch operation for transposition of the great arteries. *J Thorac Cardiovasc Surg* 1995;109:289–301; discussion 301–302.

Williams WG, McCrindle BW, Ashburn DA, et al. Outcomes of 829 neonates with complete transposition of the great arteries 12–17 years after repair. *Eur J Cardiothorac Surg* 2003;24:1–10.

D.5. What are the long-term outcomes after Rastelli repair for transposition of the great arteries (D-TGA) with left ventricular outflow tract (LVOT) obstruction?

Outcome following the Rastelli procedure for transposition of great vessels (TGV) with ventricular septal defect (VSD) and LVOT obstruction is good with a near 100% early survival rate. One large recent series reports freedom from death or transplantation to be 82% at 5 years with a progressive decrease to 52% by 20 years. Similar results are reported in another recent series[139]. The need for reintervention (either surgical or catheterization) increases over time. Intervention to relieve RVOT (right ventricle [RV] to pulmonary artery [PA] conduit) obstruction accounts for 75% of all interventions with pacemaker insertion and relief of LVOT obstruction (aortic outflow) accounting for most of the remaining interventions. Freedom from surgical or catheterization intervention for relief of conduit obstruction is 56% at 5 years, decreasing to 21% at 15 years.

Patients who had undergone the Rastelli procedure were reported to have increased left ventricle (LV) end-diastolic and end-systolic volumes and diminished LV contractile function compared with normal subjects. Despite this, the majority (98%) of these patients were found to be in New York Heart Association (NYHA) functional class 1 or 2 following the Rastelli procedure. It is unclear whether surgery at an earlier age and improvements in construction of the VSD tunnel patch has reduced the incidence of contractile dysfunction following the Rastelli procedure in the current era.

Dearani JA, Danielson DK, Puga FJ, et al. Late follow-up of 1095 patients undergoing operation for complex congenital heart disease utilizing pulmonary ventricle to pulmonary artery conduits. *Ann Thorac Surg* 2003;75:399–410.

D.6. What is long-term neurologic outcome like after arterial switch operation (ASO)?

The best assessment of neurologic outcome following ASO is data from the Boston Circulatory Arrest Trial. In this trial, infants undergoing ASO for transposition of the great arteries (D-TGA) with intact ventricular septum (IVS) or ventricular septal defect (VSD) randomized 171 infants to a strategy of either deep hypothermic circulatory arrest (DHCA) or low-flow cardiopulmonary bypass (CPB) using α-stat pH management. Infants in the DHCA group underwent an average of 52 minutes of DHCA whereas those in the low-flow CPB group underwent 14 minutes of DHCA.

At age 8 years, parents of children in the trial reported more problems with attention, learning, speech, and the frequency of developmental delay than parents of children in a normative sample. Despite this, children in the cohort had overall physical and psychosocial health status similar to the general population. Furthermore, there was no association between physical and psychosocial scores and the presence or absence of a VSD or the use of low-flow CPB versus DHCA. Neurodevelopmental outcome in this cohort was generally not adversely affected unless the duration of DHCA exceeded 41 minutes. Beyond 41 minutes, there was a nonlinear (steadily worsening) outcome with increasing duration of DHCA.

Eight-year data from the trial also demonstrated that neurologic status, intelligence quotient (IQ), academic achievement, memory, problem solving, and visual–motor integration did not differ between the DHCA and low-flow CPB groups. Nonetheless, DHCA was associated with greater functional deficiencies (motor function, speech apraxia, visual–motor tracking, phonic awareness) than LF CPB (impulsive behavior, worse behavior as rated by teachers).

Bellinger DC, Wypij D, duPlessis AJ, et al. Neurodevelopmental status at eight years in children with dextro-transposition of the great arteries: the Boston Circulatory Arrest Trial. *J Thorac Cardiovasc Surg* 2003;126:1385–1396.

DiNardo JA. Transposition of the great vessels. In: Lake CL, Booker PD, eds. *Pediatric cardiac anesthesia*, 4th ed. Philadelphia: Lippincott Williams & Wilkins, 2005:357–380.

Dunbar-Masterson C,Wypij D, Bellinger DC, et al. General health status of children with D-transposition of the great arteries after the arterial switch operation. *Circulation* 2001;104:I138–I142.

Wypij D, Newburger JW, Rappaport LA, et al. The effect of duration of deep hypothermic circulatory arrest in infant heart surgery on late neurodevelopment: the Boston Circulatory Arrest Trial. *J Thorac Cardiovasc Surg* 2003;126:1397–1403.

CHAPTER 18

Patent Ductus Arteriosus and Prematurity

RAJESH BHAT • ISOBEL RUSSELL • FUN-SUN F. YAO

A 7-DAY-OLD MALE INFANT

weighing 900 g was scheduled for ligation of patent ductus arteriosus (PDA). He was born at 30 weeks gestation and was intubated immediately after delivery because of respiratory distress. His condition improved over the next 4 days. However, on the fifth day of his life the respiratory distress worsened and a murmur was heard over his chest. Medical treatment for PDA was attempted unsuccessfully. His blood pressure was 56/32 mm Hg; heart rate, 160 beats per minute. The laboratory data were as follows: WBC, 17,000 per mm^3; hemoglobin, 11 g per dL; hematocrit, 34%; urine specific gravity 1.005; protein 1+; sugar 1+; serum calcium, 6.0 mg per dL; blood glucose, 60 mg per dL; arterial blood gases: pH 7.30; PaCO$_2$, 45 mm Hg; PaO$_2$, 60 mm Hg on FIO$_2$ 50%, inspiratory pressure, 30/4 cm H$_2$O; and ventilation rate, 25 per minute.

A. Medical Disease and Differential Diagnosis

1. How would you classify prematurity? What are the common problems associated with prematurity?
2. What are the survival rates of preterm infants?
3. What are the incidence and survival rates of respiratory distress syndrome (RDS)? Discuss its pathophysiology.
4. What is bronchopulmonary dysplasia? How would you treat it?
5. What are apnea spells? What are the possible causes of apneic spells?
6. Discuss the incidence and pathophysiology of patent ductus arteriosus (PDA) in preterm infants.
7. How would you make a diagnosis of PDA? Describe its treatment.
8. Would you give digitalis to treat congestive heart failure in preterm infants? Why?
9. How does indomethacin close the ductus? What are the adverse effects of indomethacin?
10. What is retinopathy of prematurity (ROP) (retrolental fibroplasia [RLF])? Discuss its etiology, pathophysiology, prognosis, and prevention.

11. Define neutral and critical temperatures. What are these values in the preterm neonate, in the term neonate, and in the adult? Discuss temperature regulation in the neonate.

B. Preoperative Evaluation and Preparation

1. How would you evaluate this patient preoperatively?
2. What are the normal values of arterial blood gases and pH in preterm and term pediatric patients?
3. Interpret the arterial blood gases: pH, 7.30; $Paco_2$, 45 mm Hg; Pao_2, 60 mm Hg; HCO_3^-, 20 mEq per L on 60% oxygen; and 5 cm H_2O of positive end-expiratory pressure (PEEP). How would you improve them?
4. What are the normal values of arterial blood pressure, heart rate, and respiratory rate for preterm infants?
5. What are the normal values of WBC, red blood cells (RBC), hemoglobin, glucose, electrolytes, calcium, blood urea nitrogen (BUN), and creatinine for preterm infants?
6. Would you transfuse blood to this patient preoperatively?
7. How would you interpret the urinalysis: specific gravity 1.005, sugar 1+, protein 1+?
8. Would you correct a serum calcium level of 6.0 mg per dL? What other information would you like to have? Which contains more calcium, 10 mL of 10% calcium chloride or 10 mL of 10% calcium gluconate? Could you hyperventilate this child safely?
9. How would you premedicate this patient?

C. Intraoperative Management

1. What monitors would you use for this child during surgery?
2. How does the oxygen analyzer work?
3. What is the Doppler effect? How does the Doppler transducer measure blood pressure?
4. What is the mechanism of pulse oximetry? Why is it important to monitor arterial oxygen saturation? What levels of arterial oxygen saturation would you like to keep during surgery?
5. How would you maintain the patient's body temperature?
6. How do the anesthetic requirements of the preterm infant differ from those of the adult?
7. What size endotracheal tube would you have used if the patient had not been intubated?
8. How would you have induced anesthesia if the patient had not been intubated?
9. How would you maintain anesthesia?
10. How would you ventilate the patient? What tidal volume, respiratory rates, and FIO_2 would you set for the infant?
11. Discuss blood and fluid therapy in this preterm infant.
12. During dissection of the ductus arteriosus, the arterial oxygen saturation dropped from 92% to 80% and the heart rate decreased from 140 beats per minute to 80 beats per minute. What were the causes? How would you correct this situation?

D. Postoperative Management

1. Would you reverse the muscle relaxants and extubate the patient at the end of surgery?
2. How can one minimize the risk of transporting the patient to the neonatal intensive care unit (ICU) after surgery?
3. The patient's condition deteriorated postoperatively in the ICU. Physical examination revealed persistent cardiac murmur. What was the possible diagnosis?

A. Medical Disease and Differential Diagnosis

A.1. How would you classify prematurity? What are the common problems associated with prematurity?

Preterm infants can be classified into three groups, as shown in Table 18.1. Infants of borderline prematurity usually require no special care, but, because of their susceptibility to respiratory distress syndrome (RDS), they should be observed closely for 24 to 48 hours in the newborn nursery. Further, those with a poor suck reflex may require gavage feedings. Infants classified as moderately premature require intense neonatal care, and neonatal mortality correlates inversely with gestational age. Neonates of extreme prematurity constitute only 1% of all preterm infants; however, mortality in this group is extremely high, accounting for greater than 70% of all neonatal deaths. Furthermore, morbidity in surviving infants is substantial, often secondary to irreversible neurologic or respiratory insult.

Behrman RE, Kliegman RM, Jenson HB, eds. *Nelson textbook of pediatrics*, 17th ed. Philadelphia: WB Saunders, 2004:550–558.

Gregory GA, ed. *Pediatric anesthesia*, 4th ed. New York: Churchill Livingstone, 2002:369.

Usher RH, Allen AC, McLean RH. Risk of respiratory distress syndrome related to gestational age, route of delivery and maternal diabetes. *Am J Obstet Gynecol* 1971;111: 826.

A.2. What are the survival rates of preterm infants?

The survival rates of preterm infants depend mainly on their maturity or birth weights. Because of the advancement in neonatal care, survival rates have increased twofold in the last two decades. Recently, the survival rates for infants with birth weights 500 to 750 g, 750 to 1,000 g, 1,000 to 1,250 g, 1,250 to 1,500 g, and 1,500 to 2,000 g have been approximately 53.9%, 86.3%, 94%,

Table 18.1 Classification of Prematurity.

	BORDERLINE PREMATURITY	MODERATE PREMATURITY	EXTREME PREMATURITY
Gestational age (wk)	37–38	31–36	24–30
Percentage live births	16%	6%–7%	<1%
Weight (g)	2,500–3,200	1,500–2,500	500–1,500
Associated problems	Poor suck	Poor suck	Poor suck
	RDS	RDS	RDS
	Temperature regulation	Temperature regulation	Temperature regulation
		Sepsis	Sepsis
		Intracranial hemorrhage	Intracranial hemorrhage
			Necrotizing enterocolitis
			Congestive heart failure
			Birth asphyxia
Level of care	Careful observation in newborn nursery	Neonatal ICU	Neonatal ICU

RDS, respiratory distress syndrome.

96.8%, and 97%, respectively. Recent reports showed the survival rates for premature infants born at 24, 25, and 26 weeks gestation to be 43%, 74%, and 83%, respectively.

Behrman RE, Kliegman RM, Jenson HB, eds. *Nelson textbook of pediatrics*, 17th ed. Philadelphia: WB Saunders, 2004:550–558.

Gregory GA, ed. *Pediatric anesthesia*, 4th ed. New York: Churchill Livingstone, 2002:370.

NICHD Neonatal Research Network. *Very low birth weight outcomes of the National Institute of Child Health and Human Development Neonatal Research Network*, Jan 1995 through Dec. 1996.

A.3. What are the incidence and survival rates of respiratory distress syndrome (RDS)? Discuss its pathophysiology.

RDS, formerly called hyaline membrane disease, is common in preterm infants. RDS is a life-threatening condition associated with 50% to 75% of all deaths of premature infants. It occurs three times more often in those born by cesarean section than in those born vaginally. The incidence of RDS depends on the birth weight. It happens in 86% of preterm infants weighing 501 to 750 g, 79% of preterm infants weighing 751to 1,000 g, 48% of preterm infants weighing 1,001 to 1,250 and 27% of preterm infants weighing 1,251 to1,500 g.

The survival rate has increased dramatically over the last 50 years. Survival depends on the infant's size. Ninety percent of those weighing 900 to 1,000 g survive, whereas approximately 70% of those weighing 500 to 700 g survive. Recently, an increase in survival and a decrease in severity of RDS have been associated with maternal steroid administration and routine administration of exogenous surfactant into the lungs of neonates of less than 28 weeks' gestation at birth. This may pose a problem for the anesthesiologist if these patients require surgery. Ventilation with high positive pressures and large volumes increases the likelihood of pulmonary gas leaks, pneumothorax and lung injury.

Physical examination of the infant with RDS will likely reveal cyanosis, tachypnea, intercostal retractions, and bilateral rales that fail to clear with suctioning. An arterial blood gas sample will demonstrate hypoxemia, metabolic acidosis, and respiratory alkalosis; a chest radiograph will show diffuse, hazy ("ground glass") infiltrates.

Deficiency of the alveolar phospholipid surfactant is thought to be the cause of RDS. The surfactant is produced by the type II alveolar cells and is necessary for the maintenance of alveolar stability. Surfactant production is usually inadequate before 35 weeks of gestational age. In its absence, alveolar collapse and a decrease in functional residual capacity (FRC) occur, with consequent right-to-left shunting, arterial hypoxemia, and metabolic acidosis.

Gregory GA, ed. *Pediatric anesthesia*, 4th ed. New York: Churchill Livingstone, 2002: 370.

Motoyama EK, Davis PJ, eds. *Smith's anesthesia for infants and children*, 7th ed. Philadelphia: Mosby, 2006:559.

Stoelting RK, Dierdorf SF, eds. *Anesthesia and coexisting disease*, 4th ed. New York: Churchill Livingstone, 2002:269.

A.4. What is bronchopulmonary dysplasia (BPD)? How would you treat it?

BPD is commonly defined as the need for supplemental oxygen beyond 30 days of life. BPD is a chronic lung disease found in many small preterm infants weighing 1,500 g or less as a result of mechanical ventilation, oxygen toxicity, infection, or a combination of these factors.

It includes interstitial fibrosis, lobar emphysema, and components of reactive airway disease, and may render the baby oxygen, steroid or ventilator dependent. With progressive disease, it may lead to pulmonary hypertension and right heart failure. It usually progresses through four stages:

Stage I: At 2 to 3 days of age, the chest x-ray shows classic respiratory distress syndrome (RDS). There are atelectasis, hyaline membrane, hyperemia, lymphatic dilation, metaplasia, and necrosis of bronchiolar mucosa.

Stage II: At 4 to 10 days of age, the chest x-ray shows obscure cardiac borders and nearly complete opacification of lung fields. The pathology reveals necrosis and repair of epithelium, persisting hyaline membrane, emphysematous coalescence of alveoli, and thickening of alveolar and capillary membranes.

Stage III: At 10 to 20 days of age, the chest film shows small rounded areas of sponge-like radiolucency. There are few hyaline membranes, regeneration of clear cells, bronchiolar metaplasia, mucous secretion, emphysematous alveoli, and focal thickening of basement membrane.

Stage IV: After 30 days of age, the radiolucent areas seen in stage III enlarge and alternate with thin strands of radiodensity. The pathology reveals emphysematous alveoli and marked hypertrophy of epithelium.

BPD causes maldistribution of ventilation and perfusion, resulting in hypoxemia and hypercarbia. The treatment is supportive. The goals of treatment are to minimize the FIO_2 and mean airway pressure, reduce the amount of lung water with diuretics (furosemide 5 to 10 mg per kg every 6 hours), and to support cardiac contractility with inotropes (e.g., digoxin).

Behrman RE, Kliegman RM, Jenson HB, eds. *Nelson textbook of pediatrics*, 17th ed. Philadelphia: WB Saunders, 2004:580–582, 1466–1467.

Gregory GA, ed. *Pediatric anesthesia*, 4th ed. New York: Churchill Livingstone, 2002:370.

Motoyama EK, Davis PJ, eds. *Smith's anesthesia for infants and children*, 7th ed. Philadelphia: Mosby, 2006:559–561.

Stoelting RK, Dierdorf SF, eds. *Anesthesia and coexisting disease*, 4th ed. New York: Churchill Livingstone, 2002:692–693.

A.5. What are apnea spells? What are the possible causes of apneic spells?

Apnea spells are defined as cessation of breathing lasting more than 20 seconds or more than 10 seconds and produces oxygen desaturatuion and bradycardia. Apneic spells are common in preterm infants, especially after the first week of life and almost universal in infants who are less than 1,000 g at birth. The causes are multiple and include the following:

- Hypothermia or hyperthermia
- Hypoglycemia or hyperglycemia
- Hypocalcemia or hypercalcemia
- Hypovolemia or hypervolemia
- Anemia
- Decreased functional residual capacity (FRC)
- Patent ductus arteriosus (PDA)
- Constipation
- Hypothyroidism
- Immature brain stem function

- Lack of type I muscle fibers in diaphragm
- Excessive handling
- Sepsis
- Gastroesophageal reflux disease.

Repeated apnea increases the likelihood of central nervous system damage because of repeated episodes of hypoxemia. Infants who have apneic spells do not breathe during anesthesia; therefore, they should be ventilated throughout anesthesia, including the induction phase. Inhaled and intravenous anesthetics affect the control of breathing and contribute to upper airway obstruction, thereby increasing the likelihood of apnea during the postoperative period, especially in preterm infants less than 60 weeks postconception age.

Behrman RE, Kliegman RM, Jenson HB, eds. *Nelson textbook of pediatrics*, 17th ed. Philadelphia: WB Saunders, 2004:561, 573–574.

Gregory GA, ed. *Pediatric anesthesia*, 4th ed. New York: Churchill Livingstone, 2002:370–371.

Neil NF, Rosemary H, John K, et al. Summary proceedings from the Apnea-of-Prematurity Group. *Pediatrics* 2006;117:47–51.

Rigatto H, Brady JP. Periodic breathing and apnea in preterm infants. I. Evidence of hypoventilation possibly due to central respiratory depression. *Pediatrics* 1972;50:202.

Stoelting RK, Dierdorf SF, eds. *Anesthesia and coexisting disease*, 4th ed. New York: Churchill Livingstone, 2002:694.

A.6. Discuss the incidence and pathophysiology of patent ductus arteriosus (PDA) in preterm infants.

Fifty percent of infants weighing less than 1,000 g and 20.2% of infants under 1,750 g have hemodynamically significant PDA. In term infants, the ductus arteriosus closes soon after birth in response to the increased arterial oxygen tension. However, in preterm infants, it has a thinner, poorly contractile muscular layer with diminished responsiveness to the increasing oxygen levels after birth. In addition, preterm infants often suffer from hypoxemia because of respiratory distress syndrome (RDS), so that there are both a reduced stimulus to and a reduced response to physiologic closure. As many as 20% of neonates with RDS have a PDA. However, on the third to fifth day of life, some resolution of the RDS usually occurs, with a concurrent decrease in pulmonary resistance. This allows blood shunting from the systemic to the pulmonary circulation by way of the PDA, resulting in pulmonary vascular overload and ultimately left heart failure. The pulmonary congestion worsens respiratory failure, resulting in further hypoxemia and CO_2 retention.

Emmanouilides GC, Riemenschneider TA, Allen HD, et al. eds. *Moss and Adams' heart disease in infants, children and adolescents, including the fetus and young adult*, 5th ed. Baltimore: Williams & Wilkins, 1995:746–761.

Lake CL, Booker PD, eds. *Pediatric cardiac anesthesia*, 4th ed. Philadelphia: Lippincott Williams & Wilkins, 2005:412–416.

Sethuraman G, Doty CI. *Patent ductus arteriosus*. eMedicine from WebMD, 2006.

Siassi B, Blanco C, Cabal LA, et al. Incidence and clinical features of patent ductus arteriosus in low birth weight infants: a perspective analysis of 150 consecutively born infants. *Pediatrics* 1976;57:347.

A.7. How would you make a diagnosis of patent ductus arteriosus (PDA)? Describe its treatment.

The diagnosis of PDA in preterm infants may be suspected when there is sudden increase in respiratory failure, tachycardia, tachypnea, and a widened pulse pressure. The typical continuous or machinery murmur of PDA is usually not present in this population, but a systolic murmur, sometimes extending into diastole, and a hyperdynamic precordium are nearly always present. The diagnosis is confirmed by echocardiography that demonstrates left atrial enlargement. Two-dimensional echocardiography can identify the aortic end of the ductus. Continuous-wave Doppler can detect abnormal flow in the pulmonary artery. Color Doppler can visualize the jet of abnormal flow.

The initial treatment of PDA is medical. It includes fluid restriction and administration of diuretics and indomethacin. Indomethacin, 0.1 to 0.2 mg per kg, three doses for every 12 hours, usually closes the ductus within 24 hours. If the ductus fails to close with medical treatment, surgical ligation is indicated. There is now the option of percutaneous closure of PDA with an Amplatzer Duct Occluder.

Gregory GA, ed. *Pediatric anesthesia*, 4th ed. New York: Churchill Livingstone, 2002:349–350.

Lake CL, Booker PD, eds. *Pediatric cardiac anesthesia*, 4th ed. Philadelphia: Lippincott Williams & Wilkins, 2005:412–416.

Pass RH, Hijazi Z, Hsu DT, et al. Multicenter USA amplatzer patent ductus arteriosus occlusion device trial: initial and one year results. *J Am Coll Cardiol* 2004;44:513–519.

A.8. Would you give digitalis to treat congestive heart failure in preterm infants? Why?

Digitalis should not be given to small preterm infants because it does not effectively improve stroke volume or ventricular emptying. However, it does decrease the heart rate, resulting in detrimental decrease in cardiac output. Meanwhile, digitalis toxicity increases mortality in preterm infants.

Berman W Jr, Dubynsky O, Whitman V, et al. Digoxin therapy in low birth weight infants with patent ductus arteriosus. *J Pediatr* 1978;93:652.

Emmanouilides GC, Riemenschneider TA, Allen HD, et al. eds. *Moss and Adams' heart disease in infants, children and adolescents, including the fetus and young adult*, 5th ed. Baltimore: Williams & Wilkins, 1995:746–761.

Gregory GA, ed. *Pediatric anesthesia*, 4th ed. New York: Churchill Livingstone, 2002:349.

A.9. How does indomethacin close the ductus? What are the adverse effects of indomethacin?

The ductus arteriosus functionally closes shortly after birth in term infants when the vascular smooth muscle contracts. The muscular contraction of the ductus is initiated by the increased oxygen content and is influenced by other factors, such as release of vasoactive substances, the relative resistances in the aorta and pulmonary artery, and the differences in sensitivity of the vessel to oxygen. The ductus arteriosus produces several prostaglandins, including PGI_2 and PGE_2; both prostaglandins relax the smooth muscle of the ductus and keep the ductus patent. Meanwhile, the ductus of preterm infants is far more sensitive to the vasodilating effects of prostaglandins than is the ductus of term infants. Indomethacin is one of the most potent inhibitors of the prostaglandin-forming cyclooxygenase. Therefore, indomethacin decreases the synthesis of prostaglandins, resulting in closure of the ductus. Adverse effects of indomethacin include decreased mesenteric, renal and cerebral blood flow. Ibuprofen is another nonselective cyclooxygenase inhibitor that can be used effectively to treat patent ductus arteriosus (PDA) and has less side effects on organ blood than indomethacin, although there is no clinical data to support its use in place of indomethacin.

Behrman RE, Kliegman RM, Jenson HB, eds. *Nelson textbook of pediatrics*, 17th ed. Philadelphia: WB Saunders, 2004:580.

Clyman RI. Ontogeny of the ductus arteriosus response to prostaglandins and inhibitors of their synthesis. *Semin Perinatol* 1980;4:115.

Emmanouilides GC, Riemenschneider TA, Allen HD, et al. eds. *Moss and Adams' heart disease in infants, children and adolescents, including the fetus and young adult*, 5th ed. Baltimore: Williams & Wilkins, 1995:747.

Stoelting RK, Dierdorf SF, eds. *Anesthesia and coexisting disease*, 4th ed. New York: Churchill Livingstone, 2002:50.

Wyllie J. Treatment of patent ductus arteriosus. *Semin Neonatol* 2003;8:425–432.

A.10. What is retinopathy of prematurity (ROP) (retrolental fibroplasia [RLF])? Discuss its etiology, pathophysiology, prognosis, and prevention.

Some degree of ROP occurs in approximately 50% of infants weighing 1,000 to 1,500 g at birth, 78% of those weighing 750 to 999 g and more than 90% of those weighing less than 750 g. At stage 3 ROP was not noted in infants with birth weight more than 1,500 g. No ROP was noted in infants born more than 32 weeks gestational age. ROP begins with retinal vascular obliteration, which is followed by increased vascularity, hemorrhage, cicatrization, and finally retinal detachment. ROP refers to all stages of the disease and its sequelae. RLF, the term previously used for this disease, described only the cicatricial stages.

The factors that cause ROP and determine its outcome are not fully known, but prematurity, the degree of retinal immaturity at birth, and days on supplemental oxygen therapy are major factors. Other contributing factors include respiratory distress, apnea, bradycardia, heart disease, infection, hypoxia, hypercarbia, acidosis, anemia, and the need for transfusion. The presence of fetal hemoglobin (HbF) may protect against ROP, and patients transfused with adult blood may be at great risk for developing ROP. Generally, the lower the birth weight and the sicker the infant, the greater the risk for ROP.

The retinal vasculature in the developing fetus spreads outward from the optic disc, reaching the nasal side of the retinal periphery by 36 weeks gestational age and the temporal side at 40 weeks. Classically, it was postulated that hyperoxia constricts the retinal arterioles, resulting in swelling and degeneration of the endothelium. This causes paradoxical retinal ischemia in spite of systemic hyperoxia. When normoxic conditions are restored, vascularization resumes in an aberrant manner, leading to retinal detachment and blindness. ROP is divided into five stages:

Stage 1: A thin white line separates the posterior vascularized portion of the retina from the anterior avascular retina.

Stage 2: The demarcation line increases in volume and elevates. At this point, it is known as the "ridge". The changes in stage 1 and 2 regress in 80% of patients. Between 5% and 10% of premature infants with stage 1 and 2 disease progress to stage 3.

Stage 3: Tissue proliferation develops from the ridge, usually posteriorly. Stage 3 can be mild, moderate, or severe, depending on the volume of the extraretinal tissue.

Stage 4: Partial retinal detachment occurs with the macula still attached (stage 4a). The macula is detached in stage 4b.

Stage 5: Total retinal detachment occurs.

Eighty-five percent of ROP cases undergo spontaneous recovery. Mild ROP regresses in 2 to 3 months, and moderate ROP in 6 months. The most severe ROP usually results in blindness or limited vision.

It is unclear what level of PaO_2 causes ROP, but a PaO_2 of 150 mm Hg for as short a time as 1 to 2 hours can do so. Furthermore, the retinal vessels of these neonates certainly constrict maximally with a PaO_2 of 100 mm Hg. In addition, it is also possible that ROP might develop at lower PaO_2 levels because infants of this age are normally exposed to a much lower PaO_2 (30 to 40 mm Hg) *in utero* than the levels found during the neonatal period. Therefore, in order to reduce the possibility of ROP, it is wise to maintain the PaO_2 levels between 50 and 70 mm Hg or the SaO_2 between 87% and 92% for infants <44 to 50 weeks gestation. However, prevention of ROP ultimately depends on the prevention of premature birth and its attendant problems. Oxygen alone is neither sufficient nor necessary to produce ROP, and no safe level of oxygen has yet been determined. Each infant must be treated with whatsoever is necessary to sustain life and neurologic function. Some investigations have suggested the use of vitamin E for its antioxidant effects in infants at risk for ROP. However, its efficacy has not been proved.

Behrman RE, Kliegman RM, Jenson HB, eds. *Nelson textbook of pediatrics*, 17th ed. Philadelphia: WB Saunders, 2004:2113–2114.

Betts EK, Downes JJ, Schaffer DB, et al. Retrolental fibroplasia and oxygen administration during general anesthesia. *Anesthesiology* 1977;47:518.

Gregory GA, ed. *Pediatric anesthesia*, 4th ed. New York: Churchill Livingstone, 2002:352–353.

Hussain N, Clive J, Bhandari V. Current incidence of retinopathy of prematurity, 1989–1997. *Pediatrics* 1999;104(3):e26.

Lucey JF, Dongman B. A reexamination of the role of oxygen in retrolental fibroplasia. *Pediatrics* 1984;73:82.

Motoyama EK, Davis PJ, eds. *Smith's anesthesia for infants and children*, 7th ed. Philadelphia: Mosby, 2006:781–782.

Stark DJ, Manning LM, Lenton L. Retrolental fibroplasia today. *Med J Aust* 1981;1:275.

Stoelting RK, Dierdorf SF, eds. *Anesthesia and coexisting disease*, 4th ed. New York: Churchill Livingstone, 2002:269.

A.11. Define neutral and critical temperatures. What are these values in the preterm neonate, in the term neonate, and in the adult? Discuss temperature regulation in the neonate.

Neutral temperature is the ambient temperature that results in minimal oxygen consumption. Critical temperature is the ambient temperature below which an unclothed, unanesthetized individual cannot maintain a normal core temperature (see Table 18.2).

Table 18.2 Neutral and Critical Temperature.

	NEUTRAL TEMPERATURE (°C)	CRITICAL TEMPERATURE (°C)
Preterm neonate	34	28
Term neonate	32	23
Adults	28	1

Normally, body heat is lost by conduction, convection, radiation, and evaporation. The neonate is particularly susceptible to heat loss owing to a large surface: volume ratio, lack of insulating fat, and naturally flaccid and open posture. When stressed by a cold environment, vasoconstriction occurs, but the neonate is unable to shiver. Further cold stress stimulates norepinephrine release, promoting the exothermic metabolism of brown fat deposits in an attempt to maintain core temperature. Continued cold stress often results in episodes of bradycardia, apnea, hypoglycemia, and metabolic acidosis.

When the infant's rectal temperature reaches 36.6°C to 37.3°C (97.88°F to 99.14°F), dilation of peripheral vessels occurs. The term neonate will perspire at 37.2°C (98.96°F) in an attempt to maintain a normal core temperature, whereas those infants born before 37 weeks gestation are unable to sweat.

Gregory GA, ed. *Pediatric anesthesia*, 4th ed. New York: Churchill Livingstone, 2002:347.

Silverman WA, Sinclair JC. Temperature regulation in the newborn infant. *N Engl J Med* 1966;279:146.

Stoelting RK, Dierdorf SF, eds. *Anesthesia and coexisting disease*, 4th ed. New York: Churchill Livingstone, 2002:689.

B. Preoperative Evaluation and Preparation

B.1. How would you evaluate this patient preoperatively?

The preoperative evaluation of preterm infants should be based on a clear understanding of the pathophysiology of prematurity. The preoperative evaluation of this patient should begin with a careful review of the medical record, followed by a systemic physical examination and laboratory evaluation, specifically:

- *History.* Birth trauma, asphyxia, maternal drug history, respiratory, cardiovascular, and fluid status
- *Physical examination.* Evaluation of the airway, cardiopulmonary system, fluid status (skin texture, turgor, mucous membranes, and fontanelles), and abdominal examination
- *Laboratory data.* White blood count; hemoglobin and hematocrit; serum electrolytes; serum coagulation profile, including prothrombin time (PT), partial thromboplastin time (PTT), and platelet count; serum calcium and serum protein; arterial blood gases; urinalysis and urine-specific gravity; chest and abdominal radiographs

B.2. What are the normal values of arterial blood gases and pH in preterm and term pediatric patients?

The normal blood gas and pH values for pediatric patients are shown in Table 18.3. The normal pH and $PaCO_2$ values for pediatric patients are similar to those for adults, whereas the normal PaO_2 values are lower in pediatric patients than in adult patients.

Table 18.3 Normal Values of Arterial Blood Gases and pH in Pediatric Patients.

AGE	PRETERM	TERM	1 MONTH	1 YEAR
pH	7.37 ± 0.03	7.40 ± 0.02	7.41 ± 0.04	7.39 ± 0.02
PaO_2 (mm Hg)	60 ± 8	70 ± 11	95 ± 8	93 ± 10
$PaCO_2$ (mm Hg)	37 ± 6	39 ± 7	40 ± 6	41 ± 7

Behrman RE, Kliegman RM, Jenson HB, eds. *Nelson textbook of pediatrics*, 17th ed. Philadelphia: WB Saunders, 2004:2410.

Gregory GA, ed. *Pediatric anesthesia*, 4th ed. New York: Churchill Livingstone, 2002:257, 355.

B.3. Interpret the arterial blood gases: pH, 7.30; $PaCO_2$, 45 mm Hg; PaO_2, 60 mm Hg; HCO_3^-, 20 mEq per L on 60% oxygen; and 5 cm H_2O of positive end-expiratory pressure (PEEP). How would you improve them?

The blood gases show mild respiratory and metabolic acidosis. The PaO_2 of 60 mm Hg is within normal range of preterm infants, although it is lower than normal values for adult patients. In order to prevent retinopathy of prematurity (ROP), it is wise to keep PaO_2 between 50 and 70 mm Hg. $PaCO_2$ of 45 mm Hg indicates hypoventilation, which can be corrected by increasing respiratory rate or tidal volume. In order to avoid the pulmonary oxygen toxicity, FIO_2 should be lowered to less than 40% by increasing levels of PEEP. Mild acidosis may be corrected by hyperventilation and by improving fluid balance and circulation.

B.4. What are the normal values of arterial blood pressure, heart rate, and respiratory rate for preterm infants?

The blood pressure is related to the size of infants, as shown in Table 18.4. The heavier the birth weight, the higher the blood pressure is. The normal heart rate is 120 to 160 beats per minute. The respiratory rate is normally between 30 and 60 breaths per minute. However, it can increase to 100 to 150 breaths per minute depending on how severely the lung compliance is decreased.

Gregory GA, ed. *Pediatric anesthesia*, 4th ed. New York: Churchill Livingstone, 2002:251.

B.5. What are the normal values of white blood cells (WBC), red blood cells (RBC), hemoglobin, glucose, electrolytes, calcium, blood urea nitrogen (BUN), and creatinine for preterm infants?

The WBC count usually ranges from 9,000 to 30,000 per mm^3 at birth and decreases to 5,000 to 20,000 per mm^3 during the 5th week of life.

The normal RBC and hemoglobin are $5.1 \pm 1.0 \times 10^6$ per mm^3 and 19.5 ± 5.0 g per dL, respectively, at birth and decrease to $4.5 \pm 0.7 \times 10^6$ per mm^3 and 12.2 ± 2.3 g per dL at 3 months of age. At birth, most of the hemoglobin is fetal hemoglobin (HbF), which has a greater affinity for oxygen. Therefore, the oxygen saturation (and content) of blood for a given PaO_2 is higher. By 7 months of age, the circulating hemoglobin is of the adult type.

Table 18.4 Normal Blood Pressure of Infants Weighing between 1,000 and 4,000 g.

	BIRTH WEIGHT (g)			
	1,000	**2,000**	**3,000**	**4,000**
Systolic BP (mm Hg)	50 ± 10	55 ± 10	60 ± 10	70 ± 10
Diastolic BP (mm Hg)	25 ± 10	30 ± 10	35 ± 10	40 ± 10
Mean BP (mm Hg)	35 ± 10	40 ± 10	45 ± 10	50 ± 10

BP, blood pressure.

The normal blood glucose level is between 45 and 90 mg per dL. A glucose level below 40 mg per dL is common in preterm infants. It should be corrected with a bolus of 10% to 20% glucose (2 to 5 g/kg) given over 5 minutes, followed by a continuous infusion of glucose. Severe hypoglycemia (<10 mg/dL) may cause brain damage.

The serum calcium concentration of preterm infants is normally lower than that of term infants because preterm infants have decreased serum proteins. Normal calcium level is over 8.0 mg per dL.

The normal values of sodium, potassium, and chloride are 135 to 145, 3.0 to 5.0, and 105 to 115 mEq per L, respectively.

The creatinine levels of term infants at birth are 0.6 to 1.2 mg per dL, but, within 1 month, fall to levels of 0.1 to 0.2 mg per dL. Preterm infants have relatively high serum creatinine levels compared with term infants. They are 0.8 to 1.8 mg per dL at birth and fall to 0.2 to 0.8 mg per dL in 1 month.

The normal BUN level is 10 to 20 mg per dL in term infants, whereas it is 16 to 28 mg per dL in preterm infants.

Behrman RE, Kliegman RM, Jenson HB, eds. *Nelson textbook of pediatrics*, 17th ed. Philadelphia: WB Saunders, 2004:2398–2409.

Gregory GA, ed. *Pediatric anesthesia*, 4th ed. New York: Churchill Livingstone, 2002:350–357.

B.6. Would you transfuse blood to this patient preoperatively?

The patient had a hemoglobin of 11 g per dL; we would not transfuse this patient. To ensure oxygen-carrying capacity, most clinicians agree that a hemoglobin of 10 g per dL is the lowest acceptable level if cardiorespiratory disease exists. If infants are well, a hemoglobin level of above 7.0 g per dL is usually tolerable.

Gregory GA, ed. *Pediatric anesthesia*, 4th ed. New York: Churchill Livingstone, 2002:357.

B.7. How would you interpret the urinalysis: specific gravity 1.005, sugar 1+, protein 1+?

In infants weighing 1,000 to 3,300 g, the normal urine-specific gravity is 1.005 to 1.010. A urine specific gravity of greater than 1.020 suggests dehydration.

Glucosuria 1+ normally presents in 13% of preterm infants who are less than 34 weeks gestational age because the preterm infant has a decreased renal tubular reabsorption for glucose. After 34 weeks of gestational age, glucosuria is usually associated with serum hyperglycemia.

Albumin is normally filtered by the glomerulus and is completely reabsorbed. However, because of tubular immaturity, 16% to 21% of preterm infants have proteinuria.

Grant BS Jr. Developmental patterns of renal functional maturation compared in the human neonate. *J Pediatr* 1978;92:705.

Jones MD, Gersham EL, Battaglia FC. Urinary flow rates and urea excretion rates in newborn infants. *Biol Neonate* 1972;21:321.

Rhodes PG, Hammel CL, Berman LB. Urinary constituents of the newborn infant. *J Pediatr* 1962;60:18.

B.8. Would you correct a serum calcium level of 6.0 mg per dL? What other information would you like to have? Which contains more calcium, 10 mL of 10% calcium chloride or 10 mL of 10% calcium gluconate? Could you hyperventilate this child safely?

Normally, the serum calcium is maintained at 8.0 mg per dL; however, in the preterm infant a level of 7.0 mg per dL is acceptable. This child's serum calcium is 6.0 mg per dL. Therefore, supplementation with 30 to 100 mg per kg of calcium gluconate or 10 to 20 mg per kg of calcium chloride is appropriate.

Hypocalcemia in neonate is defined as serum calcium less than 3.5 mEq per L or serum ionized calcium less than 1.5 mEq per L. When evaluating the serum calcium levels, it is important to know the serum protein concentration; neonatal hypocalcemia is usually due to hypoproteinemia. It is also important to determine the ionized calcium concentration (usually 45% of the total calcium concentration), because this is the calcium immediately available at the cellular level. The chloride molecule is approximately one-third the weight of the gluconate molecule. For this reason, approximately three times more calcium is given when an equivalent volume of calcium chloride is administered instead of 10% calcium gluconate. Respiratory alkalosis following hyperventilation will reduce serum ionized calcium levels and for this reason should be avoided in this infant.

Gregory GA, ed. *Pediatric anesthesia*, 4th ed. New York: Churchill Livingstone, 2002: 159,351–357.

Stoelting RK, Dierdorf SF, eds. *Anesthesia and coexisting disease*, 4th ed. New York: Churchill Livingstone, 2002:695.

B.9. How would you premedicate this patient?

Children under 1 year of age do not usually need sedation. However, atropine, 0.01 to 0.02 mg per kg, may be given to attenuate the vagal response to a host of different stimuli.

Lake CL, Booker PD, eds. *Pediatric cardiac anesthesia*, 4th ed. Philadelphia: Lippincott Williams & Wilkins, 2005:412–416.

C. Intraoperative Management

C.1. What monitors would you use for this child during surgery?

Proper monitoring of this child for safe administration of anesthesia includes the following:

- *Respiratory.* Precordial or esophageal stethoscope, end-tidal CO_2, inspiratory oxygen monitor, pulse oximeter, arterial blood gases, inspiratory pressure gauge
- *Cardiovascular.* Precordial or esophageal stethoscope, electrocardiogram, blood pressure cuff and Doppler transducer, and urinary bag
- *Thermoregulatory.* Esophageal or axillary temperature probe with servoloop overhead heater, and thermal blanket

If the patient has an umbilical artery catheter in place, it is useful for the measurement of blood pressure and arterial blood gases. However, it is probably unnecessary to establish an arterial line for the surgery alone because invasive monitoring in this age group is not without risk.

C.2. How does the oxygen analyzer work?

Oxygen analysis can be done by either parametric or ampometric analysis. Parametric analysis is based on the fact that oxygen is a dipole molecule. When a gas containing oxygen is passed through a magnetic field, the gas is deflected in proportion to the concentration of oxygen. Sensors can detect this deflection and give a readout of oxygen concentration. Ampometric analysis can be done with one of the two devices: the galvanic cell analyzer and the polarographic cell analyzer. In the galvanic or fuel cell analyzer, oxygen diffuses through a membrane of the sensor into an electrolyte solution from which the oxygen absorbs electrons and forms hydroxide ions. The hydroxide ions then diffuse to a lead anode where oxidation to lead oxide and water occurs with the resultant liberation of free electrons. An electron flow (current) is thereby generated between the anode and the cathode, which is proportional to the oxygen level at the sensor. This current is directly displayed by a meter that indicates oxygen percentage. These devices are relatively inexpensive to purchase but carry a high operating cost because the sensor is eventually exhausted and must be replaced.

The polarographic cell, or Clark electrode, uses a battery to induce a negative potential of 0.75 V between the anode and the cathode. As oxygen diffuses across a membrane and into the electrolyte solution separating the anode and cathode, the polarizing voltage at the cathode causes electrons to combine with oxygen molecules, reducing them to hydroxide ions. The hydroxide ions then move to the anode, causing electron flow (current) that is proportional to the initial oxygen concentration. This flow is read by a meter that translates to oxygen percentages. These monitors are initially more expensive than galvanic cell monitors, but they are less expensive to maintain, requiring only inexpensive electrolyte solution and battery replacement.

Saidman LJ, Smith NT, eds. *Monitoring in anesthesia*, 3rd ed. Boston: Butterworth-Heinemann, 1993:384.

C.3. What is the Doppler effect? How does the Doppler transducer measure blood pressure?

In 1841 Christian Doppler noted the change in observed frequency from a constant frequency sound generator when the source moved with respect to the observer. Ballot confirmed this "Doppler effect" in 1845 with the simple example of the frequency increase in a train's steam whistle as the train approached an observer. In the 1960s Ware described a practical ultrasonic system for transducing arterial wall motion to obtain blood pressure. The ultrasonic system consists of an occlusive cuff and a dual-crystal ultrasonic transducer placed over the artery distal to the occlusion. One crystal transmits the ultrasonic signal, whereas the other receives the signal reflected from the artery. Although the cuff occludes the artery, there is no arterial wall movement and the crystal receives a signal with an unchanged frequency. When the cuff pressure falls below systolic pressure, arterial wall motion occurs, causing a Doppler frequency shift, indicating systolic blood pressure. When the cuff pressure falls to diastolic pressure, the artery is open throughout the cycle: rhythmic arterial opening and closing does not occur and there is a loss of Doppler frequency shift. Therefore, one can easily and accurately obtain systolic and diastolic blood pressure.

Saidman LJ, Smith NT, eds. *Monitoring in anesthesia*, 3rd ed. Boston: Butterworth-Heinemann, 1993:121.

C.4. What is the mechanism of pulse oximetry? Why is it important to monitor arterial oxygen saturation? What levels of arterial oxygen saturation would you like to keep during surgery?

The mechanism of pulse oximetry is described in Chapter 58, question A.5.

Safe anesthesia practice requires the monitoring of arterial oxygen saturation in all patients to prevent hypoxia. However, in infants of less than 44 to 50 weeks gestation, it is also vital to guard against hyperoxia, which may cause retinopathy of prematurity (ROP).

The arterial oxygen saturation should be kept between 86% and 92% (some say 85% to 95%).

Lake CL, Booker PD, eds. *Pediatric cardiac anesthesia*, 4th ed. Philadelphia: Lippincott Williams & Wilkins, 2005:412–416.

Purohit DM, Ellison RC, Fierler S, et al. Risks of retrolental fibroplasia: experience with 3025 premature infants. *Pediatrics* 1985;76:339.

Wasunna A, Whitlaw AGL. Pulse oximetry in preterm infants. *Arch Dis Child* 1987;62:957.

C.5. How would you maintain the patient's body temperature?

Hypothermia greatly increases the metabolic rate and oxygen consumption of preterm infants. The preterm infant is particularly susceptible to heat loss because of a large surface-to-volume ratio, lack of insulating fat, and a naturally flaccid and open posture. In addition, the preterm infant often has impaired thermal regulatory ability; therefore, all precautions must be taken to ensure normothermia. The patient may be transported to the operating room in a battery-operated transport incubator if available. Otherwise, the infant should be covered with Saran Wrap and a warm blanket, and a cap should be put on his or her head to prevent heat loss. The operating room should be warmed to 35°C to 37°C (95°F to 98.6°F) and a servo-controlled infrared heater placed over the operating table. A water-circulating heating blanket should be put under the table sheet and kept at 37°C to 38°C (98.6°F to 100.4°F). All extremities should be wrapped in sheet wadding. All intravenous fluids and inspired gases should be warmed and humidified to help maintain the patient's body temperature. If the facility is available then in the very low birth weight infants the procedure can be done at the bedside with the appropriate equipment and using the intensive care unit (ICU) ventilator for airway management. This helps minimize the risks associated with transportation and also minimize the incidence of hypothermia.

Gregory GA, ed. *Pediatric anesthesia*, 4th ed. New York: Churchill Livingstone, 2002:358, 360.

C.6. How do the anesthetic requirements of the preterm infant differ from those of the adult?

Achieving proper anesthetic depth in the preterm infant presents a unique challenge to the anesthesiologist. Whereas anesthetic requirements (as determined by MAC) are decreased in the preterm infant as compared with the adult possibly due to immaturity of the central nervous system and to increase circulating concentrations of progesterone and β-endorphins. Cardiovascular sensitivity is greatly pronounced because of greater myocardial depression and a reduced peripheral response to catecholamines. Further, the baroreceptor reflex, often poorly developed in the preterm infant, is totally ablated by even light levels of inhalation anesthesia. Therefore, the preterm infant is extremely susceptible to anesthetic overdose, which produces cardiovascular depression leading to hypotension or cardiovascular collapse.

Unfortunately, an inadequate depth of anesthesia is also uniquely hazardous in the neonate. Because there is a lack of cerebral autoregulation, any systemic hypertension from inadequate depth of anesthesia may be transmitted directly to the cerebral circulation, resulting in intraventricular hemorrhage.

For these reasons, it is essential to carefully tailor anesthetic depth to surgical conditions, because the therapeutic margin between underdose and overdose is extremely narrow.

Gregory GA. The baroresponses of preterm infants during halothane anesthesia. *Can Anaesth Soc J* 1982;29:105.

Lou HC, Lassen PH, Fris-Hansen B. Impaired autoregulation of cerebral blood flow in the distressed newborn infant. *J Pediatr* 1979;94:118.

Stoelting RK, Dierdorf SF, eds. *Anesthesia and coexisting disease*, 4th ed. New York: Churchill Livingstone, 2002:690.

C.7. What size endotracheal tube would you have used if the patient had not been intubated?

The larynx of a full-term neonate usually accommodates a 3.0-mm or 3.5-mm endotracheal tube, whereas infants weighing less than 3,500 g tolerate a 3.0-mm tube. In infants weighing less than 1,500 g, a 2.5-mm (ID) tube is usually recommended. The endotracheal tube should be large enough to allow easy ventilation but small enough to permit leaking of gas between the tube and trachea when the lung is ventilated with 15 to 20 cm H_2O pressure. However, a higher leak pressure of 25 to 35 cm H_2O may be aimed for when high peak inspiratory pressures may be required during anesthesia, for example, during a thoracotomy or an upper laparotomy, or if the patient has decreased pulmonary compliance.

Gregory GA, ed. *Pediatric anesthesia*, 4th ed. New York: Churchill Livingstone, 2002:218.

Motoyama EK, Davis PJ, eds. *Smith's anesthesia for infants and children*, 7th ed. Philadelphia: Mosby, 2006:337.

C.8. How would you have induced anesthesia if the patient had not been intubated?

Preterm infants do need anesthesia for surgery. The patient should be preoxygenated with 100% oxygen, and ventilation should be controlled; otherwise, the preterm infant develops apnea and bradycardia. Anesthesia in the intensive care unit (ICU) is induced with fentanyl, 1 to 3 μg per kg. When the lid reflexes are lost, the infant is intubated after 0.05–0.1 mg per kg of pancuronium. After intubation, breath sounds should be checked bilaterally to ensure that the tube is properly positioned.

Alternatively, anesthesia may be induced in the operating room with an inhalation anesthetic such as sevoflurane followed by muscle relaxation with pancuronium before intubation.

Robinson SR, Gregory GA. Fentanyl-air oxygen anesthesia for ligation of patent ductus arteriosus in preterm infants. *Anesth Analg* 1981;60:504.

C.9. How would you maintain anesthesia?

Because preterm infants are extremely sensitive to cardiovascular depression from inhalation anesthetics, we prefer to use fentanyl with or without nitrous oxide for maintenance of anesthesia.

Increments of fentanyl, 3 to 5 μg per kg, are titrated to maintain hemodynamic stability. A bolus injection of high-dose fentanyl, 30 to 50 μg per kg, often causes hypotension because the infant is usually dehydrated as a result of fluid restriction and diuretic therapy for congestive heart failure from patent ductus arteriosus (PDA). Ketamine may be used alone or as a supplement to fentanyl-air-oxygen anesthesia.

Pancuronium, 0.1 mg per kg, is an attractive choice for muscle relaxation because it causes mild tachycardia and the infant's blood pressure is dependent on heart rate.

Lake CL, Booker PD, eds. *Pediatric cardiac anesthesia*, 4th ed. Philadelphia: Lippincott Williams & Wilkins, 2005:412–416.

Robinson SR, Gregory GA. Fentanyl-air-oxygen anesthesia for ligation of patent ductus arteriosus in preterm infants. *Anesth Analg* 1981;60:504.

C.10. How would you ventilate the patient? What tidal volume, respiratory rates, and FIO$_2$ would you set for the infant?

Controlled ventilation should be employed because preterm infants do not breathe well under anesthesia. The patient may be ventilated by hand with a Jackson-Reese device. The technique allows instantaneous compensation for changes in pulmonary compliance and resistance, especially during thoracotomy. It also permits the use of positive end-expiratory pressure (PEEP). If extra hands are not available, mechanical ventilation, preferably with a pediatric bellows, may be used to ventilate the infant.

During spontaneous respiration, normal tidal volume is 7 mL per kg for all ages. However, the ventilator tidal volumes calculated on the basis of body weight for adult patients, such as 10 mL per kg, are not applicable for pediatric patients, especially small infants. A large amount of ventilator-delivered tidal volume is lost through the large compression volume of the anesthesia breathing circuit and the leak around the uncuffed endotracheal tube. For example, if the compression volume of the anesthesia ventilator is 4.5 mL per cm H_2O (a value typical for adult ventilators) and the ventilator is set to deliver a 100 mL tidal volume to a patient at 20 cm H_2O peak inspiratory pressure, 90 mL is lost to compression volume: only 10 mL is delivered to the patient. In addition, if pulmonary and chest wall compliances change during anesthesia and surgery, the delivered tidal volume to the patient will also be changed. Therefore, it is wise to set tidal volume whatever necessary to achieve the desired inspiratory pressures, such as those used in the neonatal intensive care unit (ICU) before surgery. Usually the peak inspiratory pressures are set between 15 and 25 cm H_2O, depending on the patient's respiratory condition, to ensure adequate chest expansion.

The respiratory rates and inspiratory pressures are adjusted as needed to maintain the Paco$_2$ between 35 and 40 mm Hg or the end-tidal CO_2 between 30 and 35 mm Hg. The FIO$_2$ is adjusted to keep the Pao$_2$ between 50 and 70 mm Hg or the arterial oxygen saturation between 87% and 92% (practically 90% to 95%).

Gregory GA, ed. *Pediatric anesthesia*, 4th ed. New York: Churchill Livingstone, 2002:359.

Robins L, Crooker D, Smith RM. Tidal volume losses of volume limited ventilators. *Anesth Analg* 1967;46:428.

C.11. Discuss blood and fluid therapy in this preterm infant.

Fluid therapy should be aimed at correcting the preoperative deficit, providing maintenance fluid, and replacing intraoperative evaporative, third-space, and blood loss.

Intraoperative blood loss must be carefully estimated by weighing the sponges and using small-calibrated suction bottles in plain view of the anesthesiologist. The preterm infant's blood volume is only 80 to 95 mL (85 to 100 mL per kg); therefore, even a 10 mL blood loss can be critical. Despite these precautions, estimation of blood loss is inevitably inaccurate because of the unmeasured loss in the drapes and tissues. For this reason, it is recommended that 125% to 150% of measured blood loss be replaced. Each milliliter of estimated blood loss is replaced with 3 mL of Ringer's lactate or 1 mL of 5% albumin in saline. If the hematocrit is low (<30%) to begin with, blood losses are replaced with packed RBC.

Maintenance fluids consisting of 5% dextrose in one-fourth strength normal saline are given at 4 mL per kg per hour, whereas evaporative and third-space losses are replaced with Ringer's lactate at 8 to 12 mL per kg per hour for abdominal or thoracic procedures. The adequacy of blood and fluid therapy may be ensured by stable blood pressure, normal central venous pressure (over 3 cm H_2O), and an adequate urine output of >0.75 mL per kg per hour and specific gravity of less than 1.010. In addition, the infant's fontanelle should be above the inner table of the skull if there is no volume depletion.

Dierdorf SF, Krishna G. Anesthetic management of neonatal surgical emergencies. *Anesth Analg* 1981;60:204–214.

Gregory GA, ed. *Pediatric anesthesia*, 4th ed. New York: Churchill Livingstone, 2002:360.

C.12. During dissection of the ductus arteriosus, the arterial oxygen saturation dropped from 92% to 80% and the heart rate decreased from 140 beats per minute to 80 beats per minute. What were the causes? How would you correct this situation?

Pediatric patients, especially preterm infants, develop hypoxemia quickly after hypoventilation because they have high metabolism (increased oxygen demand) and low functional residual capacity (FRC) (decreased oxygen reserve). During dissection of the ductus arteriosus, the ipsilateral lung is retracted and compressed by the surgeon. Therefore, the pulmonary resistance increases and pulmonary compliance decreases. Consequently, the delivered tidal volume to the patient decreases and the gas leak around the endotracheal tube increases if the inspiratory pressures remain unchanged. Decreasing tidal volume causes hypoventilation, resulting in hypoxemia and CO_2 retention. In addition, compressing the lung tissue increases intrapulmonary shunt, which causes further hypoxemia. In pediatric patients, bradycardia is most commonly caused by hypoxemia. During dissection of the ductus arteriosus, surgical manipulation of the vagus nerve and lung tissue may initiate vagal reflex, with resultant bradycardia.

The infant should be manually ventilated with 100% oxygen to correct hypoxemia and bradycardia. If bradycardia persists, atropine, 0.01 to 0.02 mg per kg, should be given. The surgical manipulation should be stopped and the collapsed lung reexpanded. Blood loss or hypovolemia should also be corrected.

When the hemodynamic status and oxygenation are stabilized, the F_{IO_2} and respiratory pressures should be adjusted to ensure adequate ventilation and oxygenation.

D. Postoperative Management

D.1. Would you reverse the muscle relaxants and extubate the patient at the end of surgery?

No. Postoperative ventilatory support would be necessary for this preterm infant with respiratory distress syndrome (RDS); therefore, reversal of muscle relaxation and extubation are not indicated.

D.2. How can one minimize the risk of transporting the patient to the neonatal intensive care unit (ICU) after surgery?

The anesthesiologist's responsibilities do not end with the successful completion of the operative procedure. Removal of the surgical drapes must be done with caution to prevent inadvertent extubation or removal of the arterial or venous cannula. Transportation of the infant to the neonatal ICU is an extremely hazardous transition and requires watchful vigilance. Arrangements must be made in advance so that elevators are waiting and the nursery is ready to accept the patient. The anesthesiologist must accompany the child until satisfied that care has been appropriately transferred to the neonatal nursery staff.

The same monitors that were employed for surgery must be used in transport, including electrocardiogram ECG and monitors for arterial blood pressure and oxygen saturation. Ventilation should be maintained by hand with a Jackson-Reese device or by a battery-operated transport ventilator, and the child should not be transported with 100% oxygen unless it was used for the operative procedure. A precordial stethoscope is especially helpful to monitor the adequacy of respiration and heart sounds. Finally, every effort to ensure thermal stability must be made, including the use of a heated isolette (if possible), Saran Wrap, warm blankets, and a cap on the infant's head.

D.3. The patient's condition deteriorated postoperatively in the intensive care unit (ICU). Physical examination revealed persistent cardiac murmur. What was the possible diagnosis?

It has been reported that a large ductus arteriosus arising from the aortic arch proximal to the subclavian artery creates the illusion of the arch, leading to surgical closure of the distal left pulmonary artery instead of ductus arteriosus (Fig. 18.1). The ductus arteriosus was not

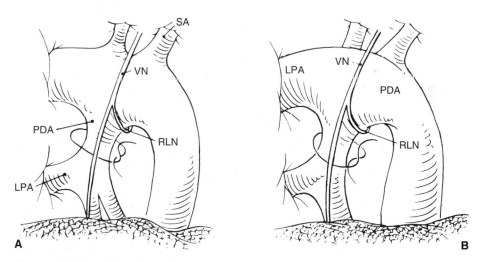

Figure 18.1   A: Anatomically atypical patent ductus arteriosus arising proximal to the left subclavian artery. **B:** Large patent ductus arteriosus sweeping into the descending aorta and appearing to be the arch. The ductus overlies the arch and hides it from view. A large distal left pulmonary artery is misinterpreted as the patent ductus (encircled by ligature). LPA, left pulmonary artery; PDA, patent ductus arteriosus; RLN, recurrent laryngeal nerve; SA, subclavian artery; VN, vagus nerve. (Reprinted with permission from Pontius RG, Danielson GK, Noonan JA, et al. Illusions leading to surgical closure to the distal left pulmonary artery instead of the ductus arteriosus. *J Thorac Cardiovasc Surg* 1981;82:103–107.)

ligated; therefore, the ductus murmur persisted. Inadvertent ligation of the distal left pulmonary artery resulted in pulmonary ischemia distal to the ligation. Meanwhile, the right lung was further flooded with the shunted blood through the unligated patent ductus arteriosus (PDA). The resultant ventilation/perfusion maldistribution ($\dot{V}/\dot{Q}$ abnormalities) caused further hypoxemia and CO_2 retention in this infant. The patient should be brought to the operating room for repair of the left pulmonary artery and ligation of the ductus arteriosus.

Pontius RG, Danielson GK, Noonan JA, et al. Illusions leading to surgical closure to the distal left pulmonary artery instead of the ductus arteriosus. *J Thorac Cardiovasc Surg* 1981;82:103–107.

The Gastrointestinal System

CHAPTER 19

Intestinal Obstruction

JOSEPH TJAN

A 73-YEAR-OLD WOMAN

with an acute abdomen was scheduled to undergo an emergency exploratory laparotomy. She complained of severe abdominal pain with periodic bouts of bilious vomiting. Past surgical history included a right hemicolectomy for colon cancer. Blood pressure 85/60 mm Hg, pulse 115 beats per minute, and hematocrit 45%.

A. Medical Disease and Differential Diagnosis

1. What is the differential diagnosis of the acute abdomen?
2. What are the causes of intestinal obstruction of the small bowel and of the large bowel?
3. Differentiate between simple and strangulated bowel obstruction.
4. Is it important to differentiate whether the bowel obstruction is located in the small bowel or large bowel? Why?
5. What are the signs and symptoms of intestinal obstruction?
6. What are the causes and effects of bowel distension?
7. Describe the fluid shifts during small bowel intestinal obstruction.
8. Discuss the systemic derangements that occur with intestinal obstruction.
9. Can there be actual losses of red cell mass?
10. What is an ileus? Discuss its causes and treatment.
11. What are the systemic effects from the absorption of bacteria and bacterial products?

B. Preoperative Evaluation and Preparation

1. Is it important to decompress the abdomen before surgical intervention? Why?
2. Describe the respiratory implications.
3. What are the implications of the tense abdominal wall?
4. Outline the methods of abdominal decompression.
5. Discuss the goals of fluid management.
6. What would you use as a guide to fluid volume replacement?
7. Would you premedicate this patient?

C. Intraoperative Management

1. What dangers are present during induction? How are they planned for?
2. Does the administration of antacids and/or H_2 blockers before the induction of anesthesia have a significant value in patients with small bowel obstruction?
3. In what position would you intubate this patient? Would you use Sellick's maneuver?
4. Is succinylcholine the best muscle relaxant to use for the rapid-sequence induction?
5. Would you remove or leave the nasogastric tube in place before inducing anesthesia?
6. Would you use nitrous oxide in this patient?
7. Are there any benefits to use a high concentration of inspired oxygen?

D. Postoperative Management

1. What are the principles of postoperative care in this patient?
2. Are there any postoperative respiratory problems associated with factors other than aspiration?
3. If the patient did aspirate gastric contents, what are the possible sequelae of this event? What is the treatment?
4. What is gram-negative sepsis? Describe the clinical picture and treatment.

A. Medical Disease and Differential Diagnosis

A.1. What is the differential diagnosis of the acute abdomen?

Intestinal obstruction accounts for approximately 15% to 20% of hospitalized patients with an acute abdomen. Abdominal pain can be divided into three categories: visceral, somatic, and referred. Visceral pain is transmitted through the autonomic nervous system through C fibers located intramurally in hollow viscera and in the capsule of abdominal organs. Visceral pain is dull, crampy, or aching in nature, and the factors that produce it include stretching and distension that result in increased wall tension, inflammation, ischemia, torsion, compression, and certain chemicals. Transmission of somatic pain occurs through A-δ fibers of spinal nerves to produce pain that is characteristically sharp, severe, and persistent. Somatic pain is caused by irritation of the parietal peritoneum and arises as a response to acute changes in pH or temperature, as seen with bacterial or chemical inflammation. Referred pain is that which is felt in a region of the body different from the point of its origin because of the sharing of common pathways for afferent neurons arising from different sites. A proper history and physical examination with early diagnosis is of utmost importance in the management of the patient with an acute abdomen. In a recent review of over 1,100 patients with abdominal pain who presented to the emergency room, the most common diagnosis overall was nonspecific abdominal pain. Appendicitis, intestinal obstruction, urologic disorders, and gallstones were the most common surgical causes in order of decreasing frequency. In 47% of the patients, surgical intervention was required. The gastrointestinal and intraperitoneal causes of abdominal pain are listed in Table 19.1. There are many extraperitoneal causes of abdominal pain, and these include pulmonary, cardiac, neurologic, metabolic, toxic, infectious, vascular, and hematologic conditions.

Table 19.1 Gastrointestinal and Intraperitoneal Causes of Abdominal Pain.

I. Inflammation/infection
  A. Peritoneum
    1. Chemical and nonbacterial peritonitis—perforated peptic ulcer, gallbladder, ruptured ovarian cyst, mittelschmerz
    2. Bacterial peritonitis
      a. Primary peritonitis—pneumococcal, streptococcal tuberculous
      b. Perforated hollow viscus—stomach, intestine, biliary tract
  B. Hollow intestinal organs
    1. Appendicitis
    2. Cholecystitis
    3. Peptic ulceration
    4. Gastroenteritis
    5. Regional enteritis
    6. Meckel's diverticulitis
    7. Colitis—ulcerative, bacterial, amebic
    8. Diverticulitis
  C. Solid viscera
    1. Pancreatitis
    2. Hepatitis
    3. Hepatic abscess
    4. Splenic abscess
  D. Mesentery
    1. Lymphadenitis
  E. Pelvic organs
    1. Pelvic inflammatory disease
    2. Tuboovarian abscess
    3. Endometritis

II. Mechanical (obstruction, acute distention)
  A. Hollow intestinal organs
    1. Intestinal obstruction—adhesions, hernia, tumor, volvulus, intussusception
    2. Biliary obstruction—calculi, tumor, choledochal cyst, hematobilia
  B. Solid viscera
    1. Acute splenomegaly
    2. Acute hepatomegaly—cardiac failure, Budd-Chiari syndrome
  C. Mesentery
    1. Omental torsion
  D. Pelvic organs
    1. Ovarian cyst
    2. Torsion or degeneration of fibroid
    3. Ectopic pregnancy

III. Vascular
  A. Intraperitoneal bleeding
    1. Ruptured liver
    2. Ruptured spleen
    3. Ruptured mesentery
    4. Ruptured ectopic pregnancy
    5. Ruptured aortic, splenic, or hepatic aneurysm
  B. Ischemia
    1. Mesenteric thrombosis
    2. Hepatic infarction—toxemia, purpura
    3. Splenic infarction
    4. Omental ischemia

IV. Miscellaneous
  A. Endometriosis

From Schwartz SI, Shires GT, Spencer FC, et al. eds. *Principles of surgery*, 7th ed. New York: McGraw-Hill, 1999:1036 with permission.

Brunicardi FC, ed. *Scchwartz's principles of surgery*, 8th ed. New York: McGraw-Hill, 2005:1017–1032.

A.2. What are the causes of intestinal obstruction of the small bowel and of the large bowel?

Intestinal obstruction can be of extraluminal (e.g., adhesions, hernias, or carcinomatosis), intraluminal (e.g., gallstones or foreign bodies), or intramural (e.g., Crohn's disease or tumors) origin. The term *mechanical bowel obstruction* denotes an actual physical barrier that interferes with the normal progression of intestinal contents. The most common cause of small bowel obstruction is postoperative adhesions, followed by incarcerated hernias and malignant tumors. Postoperative adhesions make up approximately 75% of cases of small bowel obstruction.

Alternatively, neoplasms account for most large bowel obstruction. Other causes of large bowel obstruction include diverticulitis and volvulus.

Brunicardi FC, ed. *Scchwartz's principles of surgery*, 8th ed. New York: McGraw-Hill, 2005: 1017–1032.

A.3. Differentiate between simple and strangulated bowel obstruction.

Simple obstruction occurs when the lumen is obstructed and the blood supply remains normal. Occlusion of the blood supply to the obstructed bowel results in a strangulated obstruction. Toxic fluid is discharged into the bowel lumen, bowel wall, and peritoneal cavity when venous outflow obstruction occurs. It is important to recognize strangulation preoperatively because the implications are more serious and the mortality rate is high at between 20% and 40%. However, the overall mortality rate for intestinal obstruction is under 10%. A closed-loop obstruction is present when both limbs of the loop are obstructed. This leads rapidly to strangulation, occasionally even before clinical evidence of intestinal obstruction exists.

Brunicardi FC, ed. *Scchwartz's principles of surgery*, 8th ed. New York: McGraw-Hill, 2005: 1017–1032.

A.4. Is it important to differentiate whether the bowel obstruction is located in the small bowel or large bowel? Why?

Yes. Simple mechanical obstruction of the small bowel results in altered bowel motility, bowel distension with progressive accumulation of fluid and gas, and systemic derangements. If the obstruction is not relieved promptly, strangulation ensues leading to bowel necrosis and the leakage of blood, fluid, and toxic substances into the bowel and peritoneal cavity. Approximately 60% to 80% of intestinal obstructions occur in the small bowel.

Although the signs and symptoms may be similar, large bowel obstruction is usually more insidious than small bowel obstruction. Except for a volvulus, large bowel obstruction has less of a propensity to strangulate. The colon is essentially a storage organ and has little secretory and absorptive functions. Therefore, systemic derangements are less severe with large bowel obstruction. The most important complication is progressive distension and rupture of the colon, especially in the presence of a competent ileocecal valve. The cecum is the usual site of rupture.

Brunicardi FC, ed. *Scchwartz's principles of surgery*, 8th ed. New York: McGraw-Hill, 2005: 1017–1032.

A.5. What are the signs and symptoms of intestinal obstruction?

The four cardinal signs and symptoms of intestinal obstruction are crampy abdominal pain, vomiting, obstipation, and abdominal distension. The colicky pain is often diffuse and alternates with quiescent periods. The duration of the quiescent period depends on the site of intestinal obstruction. With a high obstruction, the duration is approximately 4 to 5 minutes, and with lower ileal obstruction the duration is 15 to 20 minutes. Steady severe abdominal pain usually indicates strangulation.

Vomiting commonly occurs immediately after the onset of bowel obstruction, followed by a variable quiescent period before recurrence. Vomiting becomes more frequent and bilious the higher the level of obstruction, and, with the exception of a volvulus, it is uncommon in colonic obstruction. Abdominal distension is a late finding that may be absent in high small bowel obstruction that is associated with frequent bouts of emesis. Other signs of intestinal

Table 19.2   Radiologic Signs in Intestinal Obstruction.

SIGN	SIMPLE MECHANICAL OBSTRUCTION	ADYNAMIC ILEUS
Gas in intestine	Large bow-shaped loops in ladder pattern	Copious gas diffusely through intestine
Gas in colon	Less than normal	Increased, scattered through colon
Fluid levels in intestine	Definite	Often very large throughout
Tumor	None	None
Peritoneal exudate	None	Present with peritonitis; otherwise absent
Diaphragm	Somewhat elevated; free motion	Elevated: diminished motion

From Schwartz SI, Shires GT, Spencer FC, et al. eds. *Principles of surgery*, 7th ed. New York: McGraw-Hill, 1999:1061, with permission.

obstruction include localized tenderness, fever, tachycardia, and leukocytosis. White blood cell counts of 15,000 to 25,000 per μL is strongly suggestive of strangulation, but this is not a sensitive test because 40% of patients with strangulation have normal white blood cell counts. With the development of dehydration serum chemistries will change, hemoconcentration occurs, and urine output will diminish and become concentrated.

The most important initial diagnostic procedures are plain x-ray films of the abdomen in the supine and upright positions with upright and lateral chest x-ray films. In intestinal obstruction, gas-fluid levels are seen on the radiographs. Although normal within the stomach and colon, intestinal gas is usually minimal and infrequent in the small bowel. Therefore, gas-fluid levels are indicative of obstruction but may also be seen in gastroenteritis, severe constipation, sprue, and severe aerophagia. The radiologic findings and those features that differentiate simple mechanical obstruction from an ileus are summarized in Table 19.2.

Brunicardi FC, ed. *Scchwartz's principles of surgery*, 8th ed. New York: McGraw-Hill, 2005: 1017–1032.

A.6.   What are the causes and effects of bowel distension?

Intestinal obstruction results in the sequestration of fluid and gas within the lumen. Accumulation of fluid accounts for most of the bowel distension. As intraluminal pressure increases, the secretory function of the bowel increases progressively. Prostaglandin release seems to mediate this hypersecretion of fluid. In addition, reabsorption is impaired once intraluminal pressure exceeds 20 cm H_2O. The basic composition of the intestinal gas is that of swallowed air. As bowel distension continues from the ongoing gas and fluid accumulation, intraluminal and intramural pressures rise. The increased intramural pressures lead to progressive interference with the mesenteric blood supply, resulting in a strangulated obstruction with its associated morbidity and mortality.

Brunicardi FC, ed. *Scchwartz's principles of surgery*, 8th ed. New York: McGraw-Hill, 2005: 1017–1032.

A.7.   Describe the fluid shifts during small bowel intestinal obstruction.

Normally, approximately 7 to 9 L of fluid are secreted daily into the upper gastrointestinal tract. The secretions include saliva (500 to 2,000 mL), gastric juice (1,000 to 2,000 mL), bile (300 to 600 mL), pancreatic juice (300 to 800 mL), and succus entericus (2,000 to 4,000 mL) (Table 19.3). Because of small intestinal reabsorption only 400 mL passes the ileocecal valve.

Table 19.3 Volume and Composition of Gastrointestinal Fluids.

	24-HOUR VOLUME (mL)	NA+ (mEq/L)	K+ (mEq/L)	CL− (mEq/L)	HCO$_3^-$ (mEq/L)
Saliva	500–2,000	2–10	20–30	8–18	30
Stomach	1,000–2,000	60–100	10–20	100–130	0
Pancreas	300–800	135–145	5–10	70–90	95–120
Bile	300–600	135–145	5–10	90–130	30–40
Jejunum	2,000–4,000	120–140	5–10	90–140	30–40
Ileum	1,000–2,000	80–150	2–8	45–140	30
Colon	—	60	30	40	—

From Miller RD, ed. *Miller's anesthesia*, 6th ed. New York: Churchill Livingstone, 2005:1788, with permission.

In small bowel obstruction, several mechanisms contribute to fluid and electrolyte loss. The most important is the accumulation of fluid in the bowel lumen because the obstructed bowel becomes overly secretory instead of absorptive. Sequestration of fluid within the bowel wall accounts for the edematous appearance of the bowel. This in turn results in free peritoneal fluid because of transudation of fluid across the serosal surface of the bowel. Fluid accumulation above the obstruction can be remarkable. In early small bowel obstruction, 1,500 mL of fluid accumulates in the bowel. Once intestinal obstruction is well established and vomiting occurs, 3,000 mL of fluid may be present. When the patient exhibits hypotension and tachycardia, indicating circulatory instability, as much as 6,000 mL of fluid is in the gut. Lastly, vomiting and/or nasogastric suctioning further increase fluid losses.

Brunicardi FC, ed. *Scchwartz's principles of surgery*, 8th ed. New York: McGraw-Hill, 2005: 1017–1032.

Miller RD, ed. *Miller's anesthesia*, 6th ed. Philadelphia: Churchill Livingstone, 2005:1783–1798.

A.8. Discuss the systemic derangements that occur with intestinal obstruction.

The systemic derangements that occur can be categorized as follows: hemodynamic changes, electrolyte abnormalities, and disturbances in acid-base balance.

Hemodynamically, if fluid and electrolyte losses are not corrected, central venous pressure will fall. Hypotension and tachycardia will follow as the vascular volume decreases in relation to the size of the vascular bed. The shock state develops as the body calls forth sympathomimetic amines to increase cardiac output and decrease the size of the vascular bed.

Small bowel obstruction results in the loss of vast quantities of isotonic extracellular fluid. The extent of extracellular fluid loss may be monitored by serial hematocrit determinations. A rise in the hematocrit is proportionate to the amount of fluid loss. For example, if the hematocrit has risen to 55%, approximately 40% of plasma and extracellular fluid volume has been lost.

As the obstruction continues, there is a gradual decrease in the plasma sodium and chloride concentrations. Hyponatremia will aggravate hypovolemic hypotension, and confusion and somnolence will ensue. Hypokalemia will be manifested in delayed ventricular conduction, ST-T segment changes, and ventricular arrhythmias. With respect to acid-base balance, the most common occurrence is metabolic acidosis because of the effects of dehydration, starvation, ketosis, and loss of alkaline secretions. Metabolic alkalosis is rare and is the result of marked loss of acidic gastric fluid. Monitoring includes serial determinations of sodium, potassium, chloride, and CO_2.

Brunicardi FC, ed. *Scchwartz's principles of surgery*, 8th ed. New York: McGraw-Hill, 2005: 1017–1032.

Miller RD, ed. *Miller's anesthesia*, 6th ed. New York: Churchill Livingstone, 2005:1783–1798.

A.9. Can there be actual losses of red cell mass?

Yes. In longstanding intestinal obstruction, especially when it is associated with strangulation, increased permeability of the bowel wall occurs with loss of red cells into the bowel and peritoneal cavity. Whole blood or packed cells may be needed to restore circulating red blood cells.

Brunicardi FC, ed. *Scchwartz's principles of surgery*, 8th ed. New York: McGraw-Hill, 2005: 1017–1032.

A.10. What is an ileus? Discuss its causes and treatment.

An ileus is a functional failure of normal aboral intestinal transit. Except for the discomfort of abdominal distension, it is usually not painful. The pathogenesis of ileus is poorly understood, but stimulation of the inhibitory adrenergic neurons may play an important role. Classification of ileus is as follows:

- *Adynamic or inhibition ileus*—diminished or absent motility from neuromuscular inhibition
- *Spastic ileus*—contracted bowel musculature with resultant uncoordinated motility
- *Ileus of vascular occlusion*—disordered motility secondary to ischemia

Adynamic ileus is the most common form because it is present following every intraabdominal operation. Postoperative ileus affects different parts of the gastrointestinal tract differently. Small bowel function recovers within 24 hours, whereas gastric motility may take 24 to 48 hours to return. The colon is the most severely affected; ileus may persist for as long as 3 to 5 days.

If postoperative ileus is prolonged, other contributing causes should be sought that include:

- *Metabolic*—hypokalemia, hyponatremia, hypomagnesemia
- *Drugs*—narcotics, antacids, anticoagulants, phenothiazines, ganglionic blockers
- *Other*—intraperitoneal inflammation (e.g., acute appendicitis or acute pancreatitis), sepsis, hematoma, wound infection, ureteral colic, spine or rib fractures, basal pneumonia

Spastic ileus is rare and occurs with heavy metal poisoning, porphyria, and uremia. Management of ileus involves treatment of the underlying cause, nasogastric decompression, intravenous hydration, correction of metabolic abnormalities, and nutritional support if needed. No specific drug therapy has been shown to be effective.

Brunicardi FC, ed. *Scchwartz's principles of surgery*, 8th ed. New York: McGraw-Hill, 2005: 1017–1032.

A.11. What are the systemic effects from the absorption of bacteria and bacterial products?

The normal mucosa is impermeable to bacteria and toxins produced by bacterial degradation, but permeability is affected when there is impairment of the blood supply in a strangulated segment of bowel. Therefore, transperitoneal absorption of bacteria and toxins can result in bacteremia and septic shock.

Brunicardi FC, ed. *Scchwartz's principles of surgery*, 8th ed. New York: McGraw-Hill, 2005: 1017–1032.

B. Preoperative Evaluation and Preparation

B.1. Is it important to decompress the abdomen before surgical intervention? Why?

Yes, because of the respiratory and circulatory complications that ensue.

Brunicardi FC, ed. *Scchwartz's principles of surgery*, 8th ed. New York: McGraw-Hill, 2005: 1017–1032.

B.2. Describe the respiratory implications.

The distended bowel produces pressure on the diaphragm, limiting its downward movement, and resulting in inadequate ventilation and an increased work of breathing in a patient who may already be malnourished. The decrease in tidal volume and the reduction in functional residual capacity (FRC) result in a low PaO_2 and an elevated $PaCO_2$. It is especially true if the stomach is also distended. An additional reason for gastric decompression is to remove fluid and air from the stomach to lessen the likelihood of aspiration of gastric contents into the tracheobronchial tree during the induction of anesthesia. A longstanding obstruction and its associated respiratory compromise will result in a gasping, dusky, cyanotic, semicomatose patient.

Brunicardi FC, ed. *Scchwartz's principles of surgery*, 8th ed. New York: McGraw-Hill, 2005: 1017–1032.

B.3. What are the implications of the tense abdominal wall?

The first is related to the higher incidence of reverse peristalsis. Second, the stretched abdominal wall requires deeper anesthesia and more muscle relaxant to provide adequate operating conditions. These implications may increase morbidity. The distended abdomen significantly affects venous return by two mechanisms. First, distension decreases negative intrathoracic pressure and thereby decreases venous return. The second is due to direct vena caval compression from intraperitoneal tension. In longstanding intestinal obstruction, a large volume of intraperitoneal fluid may be present in the abdominal cavity. At the time of surgical incision, care must be taken to prevent the fluid from escaping rapidly from the abdomen to minimize severe hypotension. As fluid is slowly released from the abdominal cavity, the blood pressure should be checked frequently and the rate of fluid release adjusted to minimize a fall in blood pressure.

Benumof JL, ed. *Anesthesia and uncommon diseases*, 4th ed. Philadelphia: WB Saunders, 1998:205.

Brunicardi FC, ed. *Scchwartz's principles of surgery*, 8th ed. New York: McGraw-Hill, 2005: 1017–1032.

B.4. Outline the methods of abdominal decompression.

There are two types of tubes available for abdominal decompression: short tubes placed in the stomach and long tubes placed in the small intestine. To reduce the likelihood of regurgitation of gastric contents, it is important that the stomach be empty before induction of anesthesia. This is best done by the sump tube, which is more efficient than the simple Levin tube. The sump tube is composed of a double lumen, one for aspiration and the other to allow air into the stomach. The Miller-Abbott tube is a long intestinal tube that is initially passed into the stomach, and an incorporated balloon containing mercury at its tip aids in its passage through the pylorus into the small bowel.

Although gastric and intestinal tubes are employed to relieve abdominal distension, they do not function solely as definitive therapy for bowel obstruction except in postoperative ileus, partial small bowel obstruction, and intestinal obstruction resulting from inflammation that is expected to subside with conservative therapy. For all other bowel obstructions, the mainstay of therapy remains surgical intervention.

Brunicardi FC, ed. *Scchwartz's principles of surgery*, 8th ed. New York: McGraw-Hill, 2005: 1017–1032.

B.5. Discuss the goals of fluid management.

Estimating the degree of fluid deficit in intestinal obstruction is extremely difficult and often underestimated. There is significant sequestration of fluid within the bowel lumen, bowel wall, and transudation into the peritoneal cavity. Poor preoperative nutrition and protein loss into the bowel may lead to hypoalbuminemia and further fluid losses. The primary goal of fluid management is the initial restoration of intravascular volume to a state of normovolemia. This will lead to the optimization of oxygen delivery to the tissues and organs. The second goal is the correction of electrolyte disturbances, including acid-base derangements, which may exist. Because the fluid lost to an obstructed segment of bowel is similar to plasma in composition, a balanced salt solution such as lactated Ringer's solution is appropriate to use for fluid resuscitation.

Brunicardi FC, ed. *Scchwartz's principles of surgery*, 8th ed. New York: McGraw-Hill, 2005: 1017–1032.
Miller RD, ed. *Miller's anesthesia*, 6th ed. New York: Churchill Livingstone, 2005:1783–1798.

B.6. What would you use as a guide to fluid volume replacement?

Fluid losses can be calculated knowing that the body turns over 17 to 18 L of fluid a day, made up of intestinal secretions, urine excreted by the kidneys, fluid loss through the feces, and insensible losses from the lungs and skin. As mentioned previously, there is tremendous fluid loss into the gut, which may amount to 4,500 to 9,000 mL of functional fluid loss, including loss resulting from vomiting and nasogastric suctioning. If there is significant bowel wall edema and leakage of fluid into the peritoneal cavity because of peritonitis, an additional 7 L of fluid may be sequestered in the peritoneal space. Measurement of central venous pressure, hourly urine output, arterial blood pressure, heart rate, and skin turgor can be used to guide fluid replacement. In addition, there must be ongoing modifications in the management of fluid and electrolytes to achieve the desired physiologic goals.

Brunicardi FC, ed. *Scchwartz's principles of surgery*, 8th ed. New York: McGraw-Hill, 2005: 1017–1032.
Miller RD, ed. *Miller's anesthesia*, 6th ed. New York: Churchill Livingstone, 2005:1783–1798.

B.7. Would you premedicate this patient?

Because these individuals may have a diminished respiratory reserve because of the distended abdomen, any premedication that depresses respiratory drive will diminish the ability of the patient to ventilate. This will exaggerate any preexisting hypoxia and hypercarbia. Although the patient may be in considerable pain from the abdominal distension, narcotic analgesics should be avoided. The use of anticholinergic drugs has some value in protecting the heart from potent vagal stimulation associated with the use of vagomimetic drugs and endotracheal intubation. In those patients with preexisting tachycardia or hyperthermia, atropine or glycopyrrolate is omitted. Some physicians have advocated the use of antacids to increase the pH of gastric contents before induction of anesthesia, but this may actually stimulate vomiting in the bowel-obstructed patient. Antacids, especially particulate antacids, can produce serious pulmonary insufficiency if aspirated. In general, oral premedication should not be given to patients with intestinal obstruction.

Brunicardi FC, ed. *Scchwartz's principles of surgery*, 8th ed. New York: McGraw-Hill, 2005: 1017–1032.

C. Intraoperative Management

C.1. What dangers are present during induction? How are they planned for?

Regurgitation of stomach contents and subsequent aspiration into the tracheobronchial tree is the principal danger during induction of anesthesia for the patient with intestinal obstruction.

Mortality associated with aspiration of gastric contents ranges widely from 3% to 70%. Abdominal surgery in particular has been associated with up to 75% of the perioperative mortality resulting from aspiration pneumonitis. The incidence of aspiration for all anesthetics is almost 5 per 10,000 anesthetics. A rapid-sequence induction-intubation should be planned. An awake intubation, might be preferred if a difficult intubation is anticipated.

If the awake intubation route is chosen, the patient's lips, tongue, and upper oral pharynx should be sprayed with a topical anesthetic. When this is accomplished, additional spray further down into the pharynx can be done, but care must be taken to avoid anesthetizing the larynx because the defense mechanism for laryngeal closure will be lost in the event that regurgitation or vomiting should occur. Therefore, the performance of a superior laryngeal nerve block or a transtracheal injection is not warranted in these patients. Sedation should be limited or avoided altogether. A rapid-sequence induction allows the completion of tracheal intubation with a cuffed endotracheal tube to occur in the shortest possible time (from the period of loss of consciousness). The sequence consists of denitrogenation with 100% oxygen for approximately 3 to 4 minutes; precurarization with 1 mg of pancuronium to prevent vigorous fasciculations produced by succinylcholine, which may increase intragastric pressure; administration of thiopental sodium; application of cricoid pressure; rapid paralysis with succinylcholine; and endotracheal intubation with immediate cuff inflation. Cricoid pressure should not be released until the cuff is inflated and correct placement of the endotracheal tube has been verified by measures including auscultation and capnometry. Should the patient remain hemodynamically unstable following fluid and electrolyte resuscitation, ketamine or etomidate is preferable for induction of anesthesia.

Miller RD, ed. *Miller's anesthesia*, 6th ed. New York: Churchill Livingstone, 2005:1632–1636, 2456.

C.2. Does the administration of antacids and/or H_2 blockers before the induction of anesthesia have a significant value in patients with small bowel obstruction?

The volume and pH of gastric contents and the presence or absence of particulate matter appear to be the three most important factors determining the degree of pulmonary injury following aspiration. The classical term *at risk* is thought to imply a gastric volume greater than 25 mL with a pH less than 2.5. Approximately 40% of emergency surgical patients have a gastric pH below 2.5.

The more critical factor involved in determining the degree of lung injury appears to be the pH of gastric contents. Therefore, outcomes are better with aspirations of large volumes of nonacidic material compared with that of small volumes of acidic material. Normally, clear, nonparticulate antacids (0.3 M sodium citrate) are effective in raising gastric pH and likewise, histamine-2 (H_2) blocking agents are effective in reducing gastric volume and acidity. However, because of the large volumes of fluid sequestered in the bowel, antacids and/or H_2 blockers have little or no value in high mechanical intestinal obstruction. When there is time to prepare the patient, these agents may be of some value in partial small bowel obstruction to reduce both gastric volume and acidity.

Miller RD, ed. *Miller's anesthesia*, 6th ed. New York: Churchill Livingstone, 2005:2599–2601.

C.3. In what position would you intubate this patient? Would you use Sellick's maneuver?

Because gravity will aid in keeping gastrointestinal contents within the stomach, the sitting or semisitting position decreases the incidence of regurgitation and thereby lessens the risk of pulmonary aspiration. Some clinicians advise that the patient be intubated in the supine position for fear that if the patient did vomit and was in the sitting or semisitting position, there would be a greater tendency to aspirate. However, we believe the head-up position is preferable. Should massive reverse peristalsis and regurgitation occur, vigorous suctioning and the head-down position are the best methods of preventing soilage of the tracheobronchial tree. The head-down position must be at least 10 degrees to prevent aspiration into the lungs. Sellick's maneuver will aid in preventing refluxed material from reaching the pharynx by compression of the cricoid cartilage against the esophagus. When properly done, cricoid pressure will provide a barrier for at least 100 cm H_2O of esophageal pressure. Although some clinicians caution against using Sellick's maneuver in the vomiting patient for fear of rupture of the esophagus, this is mostly a theoretical concern. In fact, Sellick recently recommended that cricoid pressure should not be released in these situations.

Barash PG, Cullen BF, Stoelting RK, eds. *Clinical anesthesia*, 5th ed. Philadelphia: Lippincott Williams & Wilkins, 2006:613–615, 1053–1056.

Miller RD, ed. *Miller's anesthesia*, 6th ed. New York: Churchill Livingstone, 2005:1632–1636, 2456.

C.4. Is succinylcholine the best muscle relaxant to use for the rapid-sequence induction?

Yes. Succinylcholine is still the best muscle relaxant for use in the rapid-sequence induction technique despite the known complications associated with the use of this drug. More recently, however, several studies have appeared advocating the use of large doses of nondepolarizing muscle relaxants for rapid-sequence induction of anesthesia using the priming principle. The technique recommends the use of a small dose of a nondepolarizing muscle relaxant, followed 3 to 6 minutes later by a second intubating dose. These authors claim that patients can be intubated significantly earlier, by approximately 30 to 60 seconds, than if they are given a single intubating dose of a nondepolarizing muscle relaxant. With use of the priming principle, tracheal intubation can be achieved approximately 90 seconds following the second intubating dose of muscle relaxant. However, some argue that 90 seconds is not fast enough for a rapid-sequence induction technique and furthermore intubating conditions at 90 seconds may not be as ideal as that achieved at 60 seconds following succinylcholine administration. In addition one should keep in mind that large doses of nondepolarizing muscle relaxants will result in a longer duration of neuromuscular blockade. See Table 19.4 for the priming dose and intubating dose of various muscle relaxants.

Table 19.4   Rapid Tracheal Intubation[a] with Succinylcholine or Nondepolarizing Relaxants[b].

DRUG	PRIMING DOSE[c] (mg/kg)	INTUBATING DOSE[d] (mg/kg)	CLINICAL DURATION[e]	FULL RECOVERY[f]
Succinylcholine	None	1.0	5–10	12–15
Succinylcholine	Nondepolarizer pretreatment	1.5	5–10	12.15
Rapacuronium (ORG 9487)	None	1.5–2.0	15–30	35–55
Rocuronium	None	0.6–1.0	30–60	60–120
Mivacurium	0.02	0.25–0.3	15–20	25–35
Vecuronium	0.01	0.2	60–75	90–120
Vecuronium	None	0.3–0.4	90–150	120–180
Cisatracurium	0.01	0.25	55–75	75–100
Cisatracurium	None	0.4	75–100	100–120

[a]Intubation within 60 to 90 seconds following injection of the intubating dose of the relaxant.
[b]The administration of adequate dosage of intravenous anesthetic is assumed.
[c]This dose is given as preoxygenation is begun.
[d]This dose is given 2 to 4 minutes following the priming dose. For atracurium and mivacurium, slower injection (30 seconds) is recommended to minimize circulatory effects.
[e]Minutes from injection of the intubating dose to recovery of twitch to 25% of control.
[f]Minutes from injection of the intubating dose to recovery of twitch to 95% of control and train-of-four of 0.70.
From Miller RD, ed. *Anesthesia*, 5th ed. New York: Churchill Livingstone, 2000:427, with permission.

Miller RD, ed. *Miller's anesthesia*, 6th ed. New York: Churchill Livingstone, 2005:486–511.

C.5.   Would you remove or leave the nasogastric tube in place before inducing anesthesia?

The decision whether to remove or leave the nasogastric tube in place before induction of general anesthesia is somewhat controversial. Those clinicians who leave the nasogastric tube in place during induction and attach it to wall suction believe that the nasogastric tube allows for gastric decompression and reduces the chances of regurgitation and aspiration. In addition, the removal of the nasogastric tube may actually induce active vomiting and increase the likelihood of aspiration of gastric contents. However, the presence of a nasogastric tube for gastric decompression during induction does not reliably ensure an empty stomach and renders the lower esophageal sphincter (LES) incompetent by preventing complete closure of the LES. The LES is usually 2 to 3 cm long and functions as the major impediment to reflux of gastric contents into the esophagus. An incompetent LES will increase the likelihood of regurgitation and aspiration of gastric contents into the tracheobronchial tree. If left in place, the nasogastric tube may also interfere with visualization during laryngoscopy and endotracheal intubation.

Atlee JL, ed. *Complications in anesthesia*, 2nd ed. Philadelphia: WB Saunders, 2007.

Barash PG, Cullen BF, Stoelting RK, eds. *Clinical anesthesia*, 5th ed. Philadelphia: Lippincott Williams & Wilkins, 2006:1053–1056, 1393–1395.

C.6.   Would you use nitrous oxide in this patient?

Nitrous oxide should be avoided because its administration is associated with an undesirable increase in intraluminal gas volume and pressure that may lead to detrimental consequences. The blood-to-gas partition coefficient of nitrous oxide is 34 times that of nitrogen. Therefore, nitrous oxide in the blood can enter gas-filled cavities 34 times more rapidly than nitrogen can leave those cavities to enter the blood. When this happens during abdominal surgery, bowel distension will occur. The amount of distension will depend on the amount of gas already within the bowel and the duration of nitrous oxide administration. Normally, the bowel contains approximately 100 mL of gas that is mostly swallowed air, and nitrous oxide use results in a slow increase in bowel distension and intraluminal pressure. However, with bowel obstruction, the volume of gas within the bowel is greatly increased. Under these conditions, the increased intraluminal pressure associated with nitrous oxide administration may lead to bowel ischemia and necrosis. More commonly, it will cause difficulties with abdominal closure at the conclusion of surgery. Therefore, anesthesia should be maintained with oxygen, air and a volatile agent and increments of opioids and muscle relaxants as needed.

Barash PG, Cullen BF, Stoelting RK, eds. *Clinical anesthesia*, 5th ed. Philadelphia: Lippincott Williams & Wilkins, 2006:1058, 1065–1066.

C.7. Are there any benefits to use a high concentration of inspired oxygen?

Administration of a high concentration of inspired oxygen may lead to a reduction in the incidence of surgical wound infections. Wound infections are serious complications of surgery that can prolong hospitalization, thereby increasing morbidity and medical costs. The factors that may play a role in producing surgical wound infections include the site and complexity of surgery, the tissue oxygen tension, the presence of any underlying illness, prophylactic antibiotic use, the intravascular volume status, the patient's body temperature, and postoperative pain control. Compared with the administration of 30% inspired oxygen, those patients receiving 80% inspired oxygen had approximately half the number of postoperative surgical wound infections. The increased resistance to wound infections with administration of supplemental oxygen presumably reflects enhanced oxidative killing of bacteria by neutrophils in the now oxygen enriched environment of the surgical wound, which had been hypoxic because of the loss of the vascular supply.

Greif R, Akca O, Horn EP, et al. Supplemental perioperative oxygen to reduce the incidence of surgical wound infection. *N Engl J Med* 2000;342:161–167.

D. Postoperative Management

D.1. What are the principles of postoperative care in this patient?

The principles of postoperative management are the same as those in the preoperative care of the patient, namely fluids and electrolytes, antibiotics, and gastrointestinal decompression. In the immediate postoperative period, there continues to be significant ongoing fluid loss, mostly secondary to "third spacing." However, this fluid loss gradually diminishes over time and usually by about the third postoperative day reverses in direction as fluid is transferred back into the vascular compartment. The significant autoinfusion that ensues must, therefore, be accounted for in the computations of the daily fluid requirements of the patient. Otherwise, congestive failure may follow, especially because patients with intestinal obstruction are often older adults with limited reserves in several organ systems. As electrolyte loss continues postoperatively, serial determinations of serum sodium and potassium levels may be necessary. Hyponatremia and hypokalemia are factors that contribute to prolonged postoperative ileus. Because return of normal intestinal motility is usually prolonged after surgical relief of bowel obstruction, abdominal decompression often must be continued for 5 or 6 days postoperatively, whereas bowel function returns on about the third postoperative day after a routine abdominal operation. Finally, postoperative management may also include frequent monitoring of hemodynamic parameters, hemoglobin concentration, and urine output.

Brunicardi FC, ed. *Scchwartz's principles of surgery*, 8th ed. New York: McGraw-Hill, 2005: 1017–1032.

Miller RD, ed. *Miller's anesthesia*, 6th ed. New York: Churchill Livingstone, 2005:1783–1798.

D.2. Are there any postoperative respiratory problems associated with factors other than aspiration?

Yes. The postoperative respiratory problems are those related to hypoventilation. Although the intestinal obstruction has been relieved, there may still be significant abdominal distension that will inhibit diaphragmatic motion, and the patient may develop hypoxia and hypercarbia. In addition, abdominal pain and the residual effects of inhaled anesthetics, intravenous anesthetics, and neuromuscular blockers may contribute to respiratory inadequacy. The 15% to 20% reduction in functional residual capacity (FRC) associated with general anesthesia continues into the postoperative period and following upper abdominal surgery; vital capacity remains abnormal for more than a week. In summary, several pulmonary changes occur, including reductions in the following parameters: tidal volume, vital capacity, FRC, residual volume, and forced expiratory volume in 1 second (FEV_1). For these reasons, the endotracheal tube may be left in place to decrease anatomic dead space and make it possible to ventilate the patient during the immediate postanesthesia period. Leaving the endotracheal tube in place is also desirable for those patients with previous respiratory disease or in the morbidly obese individual. In both of these situations, the respiratory support will decrease residual atelectasis in the basilar portions of the lung. This will decrease any pulmonary shunt and lessen the need for a high inspired oxygen concentration (FIO_2). For those patients not requiring ventilatory support, a T-piece attached to the endotracheal tube will increase the FIO_2 to maintain the PaO_2 at an acceptable level. As the patient gradually regains respiratory adequacy (as shown by measuring inspiratory force and vital capacity), ventilation returns to normal and the patient can be safely extubated.

Longnecker DE, Tinker JH, Morgan GE, eds. *Principles and practice of anesthesiology*, 2nd ed. St. Louis: Mosby-Year Book, 1998:1881–1903.

D.3. If the patient did aspirate gastric contents, what are the possible sequelae of this event? What is the treatment?

Aspiration of gastric contents produces a chemical pneumonitis characterized initially by hypoxemia, bronchospasm, and atelectasis. In addition, the patient may exhibit signs of tachypnea, tachycardia, coughing, cyanosis, and shock. Arterial hypoxemia is the earliest and most reliable sign of aspiration. Even saline, when aspirated, causes significant hypoxemia.

Destruction of pneumocytes, lung parenchyma, and pulmonary microvasculature ensues, resulting in decreased surfactant activity, interstitial and alveolar edema, alveolar hemorrhage, and pulmonary hypertension (which results from hypoxic pulmonary vasoconstriction). The clinical picture may resemble that of the adult respiratory distress syndrome. Radiographic findings are variable and may not appear for several hours. In at least 10% of cases, the radiographic films are normal. Positive findings usually consist of diffuse infiltrates bilaterally located in either the perihilar or basal regions.

Once vomiting or regurgitation occurs, immediate lateral head positioning, vigorous suctioning, and the head-down position should be instituted. To avoid disseminating the aspirated material further distally, the trachea is suctioned before beginning positive pressure ventilation. Bronchoscopy is indicated only for those patients who have aspirated solid material resulting in significant airway obstruction. Use of bronchial irrigation with saline or sodium bicarbonate solution is of little value and may actually be more detrimental than beneficial. Management includes keeping the patient intubated and well ventilated, following arterial blood gases, and obtaining serial chest x-ray films. Depending on the arterial blood gases, regulation of the inspired oxygen concentration and the amount of ventilation to maintain PaO_2 and $PaCO_2$ within normal limits will be necessary. If the fraction of inspired oxygen (FIO_2) has to be maintained above 60%, the use of positive end-expiratory pressure (PEEP) may be necessary to recruit additional alveoli and improve oxygenation. The best PEEP will have the least effect on venous return and at the same time allow FIO_2 to be reduced to a safe level (40% or lower), thereby decreasing the likelihood of oxygen toxicity. It is important to realize that, although a patient may look well and have a clear chest without rhonchi or wheezes in the immediate postanesthetic period following aspiration, respiratory distress may still develop. It may take as long as 6 to 12 hours before the syndrome becomes manifest. The patient should be observed closely over 24 to 48 hours for the development of aspiration pneumonitis. Corticosteroid therapy remains controversial and the routine use of prophylactic antibiotics is not recommended because it may alter the normal flora of the respiratory tract and promote colonization by resistant organisms. However, antibiotics should be administered to those patients who show clinical signs of a secondary bacterial pulmonary infection with positive Gram stain and cultures or to those patients known to have aspirated gross fecal material, as with lower intestinal obstruction.

Barash PG, Cullen BF, Stoelting RK, eds. *Clinical anesthesia*, 5th ed. Philadelphia: Lippincott Williams & Wilkins, 2006:1393–1395.

D.4.   What is gram-negative sepsis? Describe the clinical picture and treatment.

Gram-negative sepsis frequently leads to a shock state caused by endotoxins from the cell walls of gram-negative bacteria circulating in the blood. The earliest signs of a gram-negative infection include an elevated temperature above 101°F (38.33°C), the development of shaking chills, mild hyperventilation, respiratory alkalosis, and an altered sensorium. The hemodynamic abnormalities of gram-negative sepsis are not clearly understood but seem to follow two distinct hemodynamic patterns, depending on the patient's volume status.

The first is a hyperdynamic circulatory pattern associated with early septic shock that occurs in patients who are normovolemic before the onset of sepsis. These patients present with hypotension, high cardiac output, normal or increased blood volume, normal or high central venous pressure, decreased peripheral resistance, warm and dry extremities, hyperventilation, and respiratory alkalosis. However, in a patient who is hypovolemic before the onset of sepsis as with a strangulated obstruction of the small bowel, a hypodynamic pattern is seen characterized by hypotension; low cardiac output; high peripheral resistance; low central venous pressure; and cold, clammy extremities. Both types of patterns will have a better outcome if early treatment is begun, but if therapy is delayed or unsuccessful, cardiac and circulatory failure ensues associated with a low, fixed cardiac output and a resistant metabolic acidosis.

Definitive therapy of gram-negative sepsis includes the administration of appropriate antibiotics and early surgical debridement or drainage of the source of infection when indicated. Supportive measures are provided by fluid replacement and the use of vasoactive drugs. Corticosteroid administration as part of the treatment regimen for sepsis is still a controversial issue. Direct arterial blood pressure monitoring and insertion of a pulmonary artery catheter may be necessary for proper management.

Brunicardi FC, ed. *Scchwartz's principles of surgery*, 8th ed. New York: McGraw-Hill, 2005:1017–1032.

Goldman L, Ausiello D, eds. *Cecil textbook of medicine*, 22nd ed. Philadelphia: WB Saunders, 2004:620–626.

CHAPTER 20

Liver Transplantation

WILTON C. LEVINE • ROBERT A. PETERFREUND • RAE M. ALLAIN

A 61-YEAR-OLD MAN

with a history of long standing hepatitis C complicated by cirrhosis and portal hypertension is scheduled for orthotopic liver transplantation. The history is remarkable for ascites, spontaneous bacterial peritonitis, upper gastrointestinal (GI) bleeding resulting from esophageal varices, and intermittent mild encephalopathy. He has previously undergone a transjugular intrahepatic portosystemic shunt (TIPS) procedure and multiple endoscopic variceal banding procedures. He has no history of significant alcohol use.

A. Medical Disease and Differential Diagnosis

1. What is the meaning of the term *orthotopic liver transplant* (OLT)? What are the potential graft options for liver transplantation?
2. What are the common causes of chronic liver disease resulting in referral for liver transplantation?
3. What are the common causes of fulminant hepatic failure?
4. What are the common problems related to chronic liver disease?
5. What medical criteria are used to determine a patient's status on the liver transplantation waiting list?
6. What types of electrolyte and acid–base abnormalities are present in patients with end-stage liver disease (ESLD)? Discuss Na, K, Mg, pH, and $PaCO_2$.
7. Is there a danger to treating hyponatremia?
8. What levels of albumin would you expect to find in this patient? How might this affect your anesthetic management?
9. What are the sequelae of portal hypertension? Does this affect the operative procedure?
10. What is a TIPS procedure? What is its role in the management of patients with ESLD?
11. What coagulation defects would you expect in this patient? How would you manage them preoperatively?
12. Why might this patient be hypoxemic preoperatively?
13. What are the expected hemodynamic changes encountered in ESLD?
14. What is the hepatorenal syndrome (HRS)? How would you differentiate this from prerenal azotemia or acute tubular necrosis (ATN)?
15. Discuss the neurologic manifestations of chronic liver disease and fulminant hepatic failure and their management.
16. What are the contraindications to liver transplantation?

B. Preoperative Evaluation and Preparation

1. What medications might this patient be receiving preoperatively?
2. What preoperative workup is desirable?
3. What immunosuppressive agents will be given perioperatively? What are the major side effects?
4. What risks associated with the anesthetic will you include in the informed consent?
5. What premedication would you choose for this patient?

C. Intraoperative Management

1. What are the three stages of the liver transplant operation?
2. What happens in the first stage of the liver transplant operation?
3. What monitors would you use? Why?
4. When would you place invasive monitors? Why?
5. What is the utility of intraoperative transesophageal echocardiography (TEE)?
6. When is intraoperative renal replacement therapy indicated?
7. What initial hemodynamic findings might be anticipated in this case?
8. What are the considerations for the induction of anesthesia?
9. Which anesthetic agents would be useful for maintenance?
10. Are there any drugs that should be avoided?
11. Is there a role for a combined anesthetic technique (regional/epidural plus general anesthesia) in liver transplantation?
12. What happens in the second stage of the liver transplant operation?
13. Which blood vessels are isolated and ligated?
14. What are the surgical options for completing the vascular anastomoses?
15. What is the order of reconstruction of the vascular anastomoses?
16. What is the "test clamp" maneuver?
17. What is venovenous bypass? What are potential advantages and disadvantages of this procedure?
18. What are the potential advantages of the "piggyback" (vena cava preservation) technique?
19. What physiologic disturbances should be anticipated during the second stage (anhepatic phase) of the liver transplant operation?
20. How would you treat hyperkalemia?
21. Why should you anticipate hypocalcemia?
22. What is the postreperfusion syndrome? What should you be prepared to do?
23. What happens during the third stage of the liver transplant operation?
24. What intraoperative findings suggest that the hepatic graft is functioning?
25. What disorders of coagulation should be anticipated? How can they be monitored and treated? What is thromboelastography (TEG)?
26. How would you treat a hyperfibrinolytic state?

D. Early Postoperative Management

1. What are the possible postoperative vascular catastrophes that should be kept in mind?
2. What coagulation disturbances should be anticipated in the postoperative period?
3. List the complications of massive transfusion.

4. How might renal function change?

5. What other early postoperative complications should be anticipated?

A. Medical Disease and Differential Diagnosis

A.1. What is the meaning of the term orthotopic liver transplant (OLT)? What are the potential graft options for liver transplantation?

The term *OLT* refers to the surgical procedure of removing the patient's diseased native liver and replacing it in the same location with a new organ. The procedure is accepted treatment for a number of irreversible liver diseases. Since the advent of the procedure in 1963, the number of patients awaiting liver transplantation has grown exponentially. In June 2006 over 17,000 patients in the United States were on the waiting list. A total of 6,444 liver transplants were performed in the United States in the year 2005 with 323 living donations. Traditionally, grafts for transplantation have been procured from brain-dead donors. However, due to an increasing gap between the number of patients awaiting transplant and the number of organs available from brain-dead donors, there has been a recent renewal of interest in DCD (donation after cardiac death) procurement. This type of procurement occurs when a specified amount of time has passed (usually 5 minutes) after asystolic death in a critically ill, but not brain dead, patient who has been withdrawn from life support after consent from family and/or health care proxy. The clinical significance of a liver from a DCD donor is that it has been exposed to a longer warm ischemic time than a graft from a brain-dead donor and, therefore, may be of inferior initial functional quality. Once procured, the liver may be placed into one recipient or may be "split" to provide grafts for two recipients (usually one adult and one pediatric).

An alternate source for a liver graft is living donor transplantation, either from related or unrelated individuals. This procedure usually involves removal of the right hepatic lobe from a healthy individual and transplantation into an adult recipient. Pediatric or very small adult patients may be transplanted with the smaller left hepatic lobe, which usually confers less risk of complication to the donor. This chapter focuses mainly on cadaveric liver transplantation into adult recipients.

Cronin DC, Millis JM, Siegler M. Transplantation of liver grafts from living donors into adults—too much, too soon. *N Engl J Med* 2001;344:1633–1637.

Marcos A, Fisher RA, Haon JM, et al. Selection and outcome of living donors for adult to adult right lobe transplantation. *Transplantation* 2000;69:2410–2415.

Organ Procurement and Transplantation. Website: www.optn.org, accessed June 19, 2006.

A.2. What are the common causes of chronic liver disease resulting in referral for liver transplantation?

Chronic liver diseases may be divided into two general categories: hepatocellular diseases and cholestatic diseases. Hepatocellular diseases include hepatitis (infectious, toxic, or auto immune), alcoholic liver disease, and hemochromatosis. Cholestatic liver diseases include primary biliary cirrhosis and primary sclerosing cholangitis. Uncommon liver diseases that may be treated with transplant include α_1-antitrypsin deficiency, cystic fibrosis, Wilson's disease, Budd-Chiari syndrome, amyloidosis, and various inborn errors of metabolism. Finally, if certain criteria are met, hepatic malignancy may be a reason for liver transplantation. For hepatocellular carcinoma, there must be only a single tumor smaller than 5 cm in diameter, or three or fewer tumors, the largest of which is smaller than 3 cm in diameter.

Alcoholic liver disease is the most common cause of end-stage liver disease (ESLD) in the United States, but cirrhosis resulting from hepatitis C is the most common indication for orthotopic liver transplant (OLT). Most patients infected with Hepatitis C Virus develop chronic infection; approximately 20% to 30% of these progress to cirrhosis. Hepatitis B, which infects approximately 5% of the world's population, is the most important global cause of chronic liver disease. This virus causes chronic infection in 5% to 10% of individuals affected. The development of cirrhosis is closely correlated to the degree of active replication of the virus, detectable by serum antigenic markers. Cirrhotic liver disease secondary to hepatitis B or C infection places patients at high risk for hepatocellular carcinoma, which may be detected by serial serum screening for α-fetoprotein elevation.

Biliary atresia, which may have been treated initially by Kasai portoenterostomy, is the most common indication for pediatric liver transplantation.

Haydon GH, Neuberger J. Liver transplantation of patients in end-stage cirrhosis. *Ballieres Best Pract Res Clin Gastroenterol* 2000;14:1049–1073.

Ramrakhiani S, Bacon BR. Hepatology in the new millennium: advances in viral hepatitis, hepatic disorders, and liver transplantation. *Med Clin North Am* 2000;84:1085–1105.

Rosen HR, Shackleton CR, Martin P. Indications for and timing of liver transplantation. *Med Clin North Am* 1996;80:1069–1102.

A.3. What are the common causes of fulminant hepatic failure?

The most common causes of fulminant hepatic failure are acetaminophen toxicity (39%), idiosyncratic (13%) and acute viral hepatitis (12%, with hepatitis B the culprit in most cases). Other etiologies include drugs (phenytoin and halothane), autoimmune, Wilson's Disease, Budd-Chiari Syndrome, and toxins (e.g., trichloroethylene and tetrachloroethane found in cleaning solvents and sniffed glue), and *Amanita phalloides*, the "death-cap" mushroom that grows wild in parts of the United States.

Larson A, Polson J, Fontana RJ, et al. Acetaminophen-Induced Acute Liver Failure : Results of a United States Multicenter, Prospective study, *Hepatology* 2005;42:1364–1372.

Ostapowicz G, Fontana RJ, Schiodt FV, et al. Results of a prospective study of acute liver failure at 17 tertiary care centers in the United States. *Ann Int Med* 2002;137:947–954.

A.4. What are the common problems related to chronic liver disease?

Chronic hepatic disease leads to a myriad of medical problems for the patient, involving virtually all other organ systems. General complaints include fatigue, poor appetite, and pruritus. Dyspnea related to ascites-induced abdominal distention or pleural effusions is common. Ascites predisposes to spontaneous bacterial peritonitis (SBP). Portal hypertension often results in upper gastrointestinal (GI) bleeding from gastroesophageal varices. Neurologic signs of hepatic encephalopathy range from mild forgetfulness (stage 1) to deep coma (stage 4) in decompensated liver disease. Renal dysfunction, manifested as elevated creatinine or oliguria, may be the result of prerenal azotemia (e.g., hypovolemia resulting from over aggressive diuretic or lactulose use), acute tubular necrosis (ATN) (e.g., infection resulting from SBP with sepsis), or hepatorenal syndrome (HRS). The coagulopathy associated with chronic liver disease results in easy skin bruising and mucosal bleeding. Enhanced sodium retention, plasma expansion, and low serum oncotic pressure may cause peripheral edema. Malnourishment leads to muscle wasting, weakened integument, and osteoporosis.

Baker J, Yost CS, Niemann CU. Organ transplantation. In: Miller RD, ed. *Miller's anesthesia*, 6th ed. Philadelphia: Churchill Livingstone, 2005:2231–2284.

Haydon GH, Neuberger J. Liver transplantation of patients in end-stage cirrhosis. *Ballieres Best Pract Res Clin Gastroenterol* 2000;14:1049–1073.

Wiklund RA. Preoperative preparation of patients with advanced liver disease. *Crit Care Med* 2004;32:S106–S115.

A.5. What medical criteria are used to determine a patient's status on the liver transplantation waiting list?

In 2002, the United network for organ sharing (UNOS) implemented a major change in the policy for matching donated livers to patients awaiting transplants. Except for the most severe and acute cases of liver failure, an adult (>12 years old) patient's status on the waiting list is now determined by the model for end-stage liver disease (MELD) (Equation 20.1). The MELD score is mathematically calculated from the patient's serum creatinine, bilirubin, and international normalized ratio (INR). It ranges in value from 6 to 40. Patients with a higher score have a greater short-term risk of dying from liver disease and are ranked higher on the liver transplant waiting list. The MELD score replaces the Child-Turcotte-Pugh (CTP) score (Table 20.1) which was previously used by UNOS. The CTP score is still commonly used clinically to determine a patient's severity of disease. For the CTP score, points are assigned based on severity of encephalopathy and ascites and on measurements of serum albumin, serum bilirubin, and INR. Total points equal the CTP score. Ascites and encephalopathy are not included in the MELD score as they are not predictors of death in patients with end-stage liver disease (ESLD). Relation between MELD score and 3 month survival can be seen in Figure 20.1.

Exceptions to the MELD classification exist for patients with fulminant hepatic failure and life expectancy of less than 7 days without a liver transplant. These patients are termed *Status 1* and are ranked highest on the waiting list. This group includes patients without a prior history

Table 20.1 Child-Turcotte-Pugh Scoring System to Assess Severity of Liver Disease.

POINTS	1	2	3
Encephalopathy	None	Grade 1–2	Grade 3–4
Ascites	Absent	Slight (or controlled by diuretics)	At least moderate despite diuretics
Bilirubin (mg/dL)	<2	2–3	>3
Albumin (g/dL)	>3.5	2.8–3.5	<2.8
INR	<1.7	1.7–2.3	>2.3
For PBC, PSC, or other cholestatic liver disease, substitute following values of bilirubin (mg/dL)[a]	<4	4–10	>10

[a]United Network for Organ Sharing. website: www.unos.org, accessed August 5, 2001, with permission.
INR, international normalized ratio; PBC, primary biliary cirrhosis; PSC, primary sclerosing cholangitis.

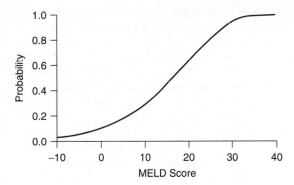

Figure 20.1 Relation between MELD score and 3-month mortality in patients with cirrhotic liver disease. MELD, model for end-stage liver disease. (Wiesner RH, McDiarmid SV, Kamath PS, et al. MELD and PELD: Application of Survival Models to Liver Allocation. *Liver Transplant* 2001;7(7):567–580.)

of liver disease who develop acute fulminant hepatic failure, patients who suffer primary graft nonfunction or hepatic artery thrombosis within 7 days of a liver transplant, and patients with acutely decompensated Wilson's disease. Additionally, special case exceptions are in place for patients with diagnoses such as hepatocellular carcinoma.

Pediatric patients under 12 years of age are ranked on the transplant waiting list according to the Pediatric End-Stage Liver Disease model (PELD). The PELD score is similar in derivation to the MELD, but uses bilirubin, INR, and albumin, and incorporates the child's age and growth failure into the formula.

Equation 20.1 MELD Formula

$$\begin{aligned} \text{MELD score} &= 0.957 \times \text{Log}_e(\text{creatinine mg/dL}) \\ &+ 0.378 \times \text{Log}_e(\text{bilirubin mg/dL}) \\ &+ 1.120 \times \text{Log}_e(\text{INR}) \\ &+ 0.643 \end{aligned}$$

Multiply the score by 10 and round to the nearest whole number

Laboratory values less than 1.0 are set to 1.0 for the purposes of the MELD calculation. The maximum serum creatinine considered within the MELD score equation is 4.0 g per dL. For patients receiving dialysis, creatinine is set to 4.0 mg per dL.

Organ Procurement and Transplantation Network. Website: www.optn.org, accessed April 5, 2006.

A.6. What types of electrolyte and acid–base abnormalities are present in patients with end-stage liver disease (ESLD)? Discuss Na, K, Mg, pH, and $PaCO_2$.

Patients with chronic liver disease commonly are hyponatremic because of low sodium diets, impaired renal handling of free water, and elevated levels of antidiuretic hormone (ADH). Hyponatremia may be exacerbated by overaggressive diuretic use. It is best treated by discontinuation of diuretics combined with free water restriction, not by infusion of hypertonic saline. When severe (sodium <120 mEq/L), hyponatremia is an indication to postpone liver transplantation because of the risk of central pontine myelinolysis (CPM). Serum potassium levels may be either high or low in patients awaiting liver transplant. Hypokalemia may occur from diminished intake, diuretic treatment, or intestinal losses. Alternatively, hyperkalemia may be seen with potassium-sparing diuretics, renal failure, and metabolic acidemia. Preoperative hyperkalemia may significantly complicate the intraoperative management of patients for liver transplantation. Hypomagnesemia is a common finding in patients with cirrhosis. The mechanisms include poor dietary intake, intestinal malabsorption, hypophosphatemia, hyperaldosteronism, and diuretic therapy.

The most common acid–base disturbance in ESLD is a compensated respiratory alkalosis. The pH is usually normal, but $Paco_2$ is low (mean value 32 mm Hg in one prospective study). The mechanism is hyperventilation triggered by unknown combinations of centrally acting hormones and/or metabolic changes. The degree of hyperventilation is not directly related to the level of hypoxemia. Sometimes metabolic alkalosis may be seen secondary to loop diuretics, hyperaldosteronism, vomiting, or diarrhea. In critically ill patients (especially those with renal failure), a metabolic acidosis is common.

Haydon GH, Neuberger J. Liver transplantation of patients in end-stage cirrhosis. *Ballieres Best Pract Res Clin Gastroenterol* 2000;14:1049–1073.

Krowka MJ, Dickson ER, Wiesner RH, et al. A prospective study of pulmonary function and gas exchange following liver transplantation. *Chest* 1992;102:1161–1166.

Merritt WT. Metabolism and liver transplantation: review of perioperative issues. *Liver Transpl Surg* 2000;6(4 Suppl 1):S76–S84.

A.7. Is there a danger to treating hyponatremia?

Patients undergoing orthotopic liver transplantation are at increased risk for development of perioperative central pontine myelinolysis (CPM). CPM is a neurologic condition characterized by symmetric noninflammatory demyelinating lesions in the basis pontis. Clinical signs include altered level of consciousness progressing to inability to speak or swallow (pseudobulbar palsy) and then the classic "locked-in" syndrome with quadriplegia. CPM is a very serious condition that causes permanent structural changes in the brain and often is associated with death. The etiology of CPM is uncertain, but osmotic stress on central nervous system (CNS) cells is theorized and a correlation with rapid correction of hyponatremia has been noted. Many patients awaiting liver transplantation suffer from electrolyte disturbances, including hyponatremia related to renal dysfunction or medication effect (e.g., overaggressive diuretic therapy). Because patients with ESLD are at risk for CPM and these patients commonly present for transplant surgery with hyponatremia, the anesthesiologist must be cognizant of the risks of rapid changes in serum sodium concentration. Intraoperative fluid replacement should avoid delivering high sodium loads that may cause rapid swings in serum sodium, or even hypernatremia, by the end of the case. For example, if sodium bicarbonate is to be used, it must be done with extreme caution given its high sodium concentration. Rapid change in serum sodium concentration is certainly not the only risk factor for CPM, and a "safe" rate of correction of hyponatremia has not been definitively established; some experts recommend sodium correction at a rate no greater than 12 mEq/L/day. Physicians must have a high index of suspicion for CPM in postoperative liver transplant patients with neurologic dysfunction.

Estol CJ, Faris AA, Martinez AJ, et al. Central pontine myelinolysis after liver transplantation. *Neurology* 1989;39:493–498.

Fryer JP, Fortier MV, Metrakos P, et al. Central pontine myelinolysis and cyclosporine neurotoxicity following liver transplantation. *Transplantation* 1996;61:658–661.

Wszolek ZK, McComb RD, Pfeiffer RF, et al. Pontine and extrapontine myelinolysis following liver transplantation: relationship to serum sodium. *Transplantation* 1989; 48:1006–1012.

A.8. What levels of albumin would you expect to find in this patient? How might this affect your anesthetic management?

Hypoalbuminemia from impaired hepatic synthesis of albumin is characteristic of liver disease. Low serum albumin levels contribute to ascites formation. Because many anesthetic drugs (e.g., opioids, barbiturates) are bound to albumin in the circulation, a low albumin level can increase the free fraction of drug administered, theoretically resulting in an exaggerated clinical effect. ESLD alters many aspects of normal pharmacokinetics, however, including drug volume of distribution, hepatic extraction and metabolism, renal excretion, and levels of serum proteins other than albumin. The net effect of these changes is unpredictable, making general recommendations for drug administration ill-advised. A safe approach in these patients is to titrate the drug to the desired effect.

Baker J, Yost CS, Niemann CU. Organ transplantation. In: Miller RD, ed. *Anesthesia*, 6th ed. Philadelphia: Churchill Livingstone, 2005:2231–2284.

Sandberg WS, Raines D. Anesthesia for liver surgery. In: Longnecker DE, Tinker JH, Morgan GE, eds. *Principles and practice of anesthesiology*, 3rd ed. St. Louis: Mosby, 2007.

Wiklund RA. Preoperative preparation of patients with advanced liver disease. *Crit Care Med* 2004;32:S106–S115.

A.9. What are the sequelae of portal hypertension? Does this affect the operative procedure?

The normal gradient between portal vein and inferior vena cava (IVC) pressures is 2 to 6 mm Hg. Portal hypertension, defined as a gradient greater than 10 mm Hg, is caused both by increased resistance to portal vein flow and by splanchnic hyperemia. A pressure gradient of 8 to 10 mm Hg results in engorgement of alternate vascular channels to restore portal-systemic flow. Bleeding often occurs once the gradient increases above 12 mm Hg. Gastroesophageal collaterals produce esophageal varices, a cause for upper gastrointestinal (GI) bleeding. Lower abdominal collaterals in the hemorrhoidal plexus predispose to lower GI bleeding. Finally, intraabdominal collaterals may significantly complicate liver dissection during the transplant operation because they cause bleeding; they are also difficult to control.

Nietsch HH. Management of portal hypertension. *J Clin Gastroenterol* 2005;39:232–236.

Wright AS, Rikkers LF. Current management of portal hypertension. *J Gastrointest Surg* 2005;9:992–1005.

A.10. What is a transjugular intrahepatic portosystemic shunt (TIPS) procedure? What is its role in the management of patients with end-stage liver disease (ESLD)?

TIPS stands for transjugular intrahepatic portosystemic shunt. An expandable stent is placed into the liver parenchyma to provide a portosystemic communication for treatment of portal hypertension. This decreases the risk of recurrent variceal bleeding and helps with the treatment of refractory ascites. The procedure may be performed under local or general anesthesia and is often used as a "bridge" to liver transplantation in patients with severe liver disease. Unlike older, surgically created portosystemic (e.g., splenorenal) and peritoneovenous (e.g., LeVeen shunt) shunts, a TIPS does not require abdominal operation or vascular diversion, both of which impose technical hazards to future liver transplantation.

Complications associated with the TIPS procedure include bleeding, infection, hemobilia, stent migration, and worsened encephalopathy resulting from enhanced systemic delivery of biogenic amines normally cleared by the liver. The long-term patency of TIPS procedures is poor, with many patients requiring revisions before liver transplantation.

Boyer TD, Haskal ZJ. The role of transjugular intrahepatic portosystemic shunt in the management of portal hypertension (American Association for the study of liver disease practice guideline). *Hepatology* 2005;41:386–400.

Ochs A, Rossle M, Haag K, et al. The transjugular intrahepatic portosystemic stent-shunt procedure for refractory ascites. *N Engl J Med* 1994;332:1192–1197.

Rossle M, Haag K, Ochs A, et al. The transjugular intrahepatic portosystemic stent-shunt procedure for variceal bleeding. *N Engl J Med* 1994;330:165–171.

Yonker-Sell AE, Connolly LA. Mortality during transjugular intrahepatic portosystemic shunt placement. *Anesthesiology* 1996;84:231–233.

A.11. What coagulation defects would you expect in this patient? How would you manage them preoperatively?

The coagulopathy associated with most cases of end-stage liver disease (ESLD) may be the anesthesiologist's most challenging aspect of care. The liver is the primary site of synthesis for enzymes involved in the coagulation cascade (except Factor VIII and von Willebrand's factor). Therefore, diminished synthesis of clotting factors results in a coagulopathy. The vitamin K-dependent factors (II, VII, IX, X, protein C, and protein S) are depressed earlier and more significantly than others. This is usually manifested as a prolonged prothrombin time (PT) and international normalized ratio (INR) on laboratory testing and a clinical tendency to bleed. Some patients may improve with preoperative vitamin K treatment, but impaired hepatic carboxylation of the clotting factors, which is not correctable with vitamin K, is usually the rule in severe liver disease. Levels of fibrinogen, an acute phase reactant, may be normal or increased in ESLD; fibrinogen levels often drop precipitously in patients who are critically ill. ESLD may also cause a dysfibrinogenemic state, measurable by a prolonged thrombin time. Thrombocytopenia is characteristic of ESLD with portal hypertension resulting from sequestration of platelets in the enlarged spleen. Because the liver not only synthesizes clotting factors but also clears activated clotting factors, ESLD may be accompanied by low-grade disseminated intravascular coagulation (DIC) when the normal balance between endogenous procoagulants and anticoagulants is disturbed. Rarely, the coagulation abnormalities of ESLD may produce a hypercoagulable state, but clinical experience indicates that a hypocoagulable state with high risk for hemorrhage exists in most patients.

In summary, patients presenting for orthotopic liver transplant (OLT) usually have severe perturbations in coagulation parameters, but it is neither necessary nor possible to correct them preoperatively. Certainly, patients with active sites of bleeding should be transfused with fresh frozen plasma (FFP), packed red blood cells (PRBCs), cryoprecipitate, and platelets as dictated by clinical assessment and laboratory parameters. In addition, desmopressin (DDAVP) may be considered for patients with concomitant renal dysfunction and uremic bleeding (Chapter 36, section A.3). Some transplant anesthesiologists will transfuse FFP or platelets preoperatively in patients with severely abnormal coagulation profiles to diminish bleeding risks associated with central venous and arterial line placements. However, potentially curative transplant surgery ought not be postponed by efforts to correct coagulation defects.

Kang Y. Blood coagulation during liver, kidney, and pancreas transplantation. In: Lake CL, Moore RA, eds. *Blood: hemostasis, transfusion, and alternatives in the perioperative period.* New York: Raven Press, 1995:529–537.

Sandberg WS, Raines D. Anesthesia for liver surgery. In: Longnecker DE, Tinker JH, Morgan GE, eds. *Principles and practice of anesthesiology*, 3rd ed. St. Louis: Mosby, 2007.

Wiklund RA. Preoperative preparation of patients with advanced liver disease. *Crit Care Med* 2004;32:S106–S115.

A.12. Why might this patient be hypoxemic preoperatively?

Hypoxemia, defined as arterial PaO_2 less than 70 mm Hg when breathing room air, is a common finding in ESLD, occurring in about one third of patients. The etiology is multifactorial. Ventilation/perfusion ($\dot{V}/\dot{Q}$) mismatch may occur because of compressive effects of ascites and pleural effusions ("hepatic hydrothorax") on basilar lung tissue. The normal pulmonary vasoconstrictive response to hypoxemia is often blunted in cirrhosis, causing worsened $\dot{V}/\dot{Q}$ mismatch. Patients' prior smoking histories or underlying reasons for liver failure (e.g., α_1-antitrypsin deficiency, cystic fibrosis) may result in $\dot{V}/\dot{Q}$ mismatch with hypoxemia.

Some patients with ESLD may be hypoxemic because of hepatopulmonary syndrome (HPS). The triad of liver disease, arterial hypoxemia, and intrapulmonary vascular dilatations defines HPS, which exists in approximately 5% to 15% of patients with liver disease. Patients with HPS often complain of dyspnea and fatigue; they may have clubbing and spider angiomata on physical examination. Platypnea (shortness of breath occurring in the upright position) and orthodeoxia (arterial deoxygenation occurring in the upright position) are characteristic. Resting upright room air arterial PaO_2 is low (<80 mm Hg) and the alveolar-arterial oxygen gradient is high (>20 mm Hg). Contrast enhanced echocardiography demonstrates abnormal pulmonary vasodilation. These vascular anomalies contribute to hypoxemia through $\dot{V}/\dot{Q}$ mismatch, frank shunt, or diffusion limitation. Depending on the predominant mechanism of hypoxemia, some patients with HPS may respond to 100% oxygen administration with improved PaO_2, whereas others with true shunts do not improve. HPS is not a contraindication to liver transplantation, and, in fact, resolution of the syndrome posttransplant is reported. The exact cause for HPS remains unknown, but enhanced production or impaired hepatic clearance of endogenous vasodilators (possibly nitric oxide) is theorized.

Fallon MB, Abrams GA. Hepatopulmonary syndrome. *Curr Gastroenterol Rep* 2000;2: 40–45.

Krowka MJ. Pathophysiology of arterial hypoxemia in advanced liver disease. *Liver Transpl Surg* 1996;2:308–312.

Krowka MJ, Porayko MK, Plevak DJ, et al. Hepatopulmonary syndrome with progressive hypoxemia as an indication for liver transplantation: case reports and literature review. *Mayo Clin Proc* 1997;72:44–53.

Lange PA, Stoller JK. The hepatopulmonary syndrome. *Ann Intern Med* 1995;122:521–529.

A.13. What are the expected hemodynamic changes encountered in end-stage liver disease (ESLD)?

Patients with ESLD usually demonstrate a hyperdynamic circulation with tachycardia, elevated cardiac output, low arterial blood pressure, and low systemic vascular resistance. The pathophysiology is thought to involve arterial vasodilation because of enhanced endogenous production, or diminished hepatic clearance, of various vasodilating substances. Definitive identification of these substances remains elusive, but nitric oxide and glucagon have been implicated. Recent experimental evidence supports nitric oxide's role. Increased venous capacitance resulting from formation of portosystemic shunts from portal hypertension also contributes to the genesis of the hyperdynamic circulation. Despite the frequent finding of a high cardiac output in cirrhotics, echocardiography may reveal myocardial contractile impairment similar to that seen in sepsis. In fact, all the hemodynamic changes seen in the patient with ESLD may mimic those of sepsis.

Mandell MS, Katz JJ, Wachs M, et al. Circulatory pathophysiology and options in hemodynamic management during adult liver transplantation. *Liver Transpl Surg* 1997; 3:379–387.

Steadman RH. Anesthesia for liver transplant surgery. *Anesthesiol Clin North America* 2004; 22:687–711.

A.14. What is the hepatorenal syndrome (HRS)? How would you differentiate this from prerenal azotemia or acute tubular necrosis (ATN)?

HRS is a functional renal failure seen in patients with advanced liver disease without specific clinical findings. Two types exist: Type I involves rapid and progressive impairment of renal function with a doubling of the initial serum creatinine to a level greater than 2.5 mg per dL or a 50% reduction in the 24 hour creatinine clearance to lower than 20 mL per minute in less than 2 weeks. Type II involves impairment in renal function with a serum creatinine greater than 1.5 mg per dL not meeting the criteria for type I. HRS is often associated with severe oliguria (<500 mL/24 hours), low urine sodium (<10 mEq/L), and spontaneous dilutional hyponatremia (serum sodium <130 mEq/L). HRS is a diagnosis of exclusion. HRS may be differentiated from prerenal failure by a lack of response to a 1.5 L volume challenge. ATN, on the other hand, is differentiated by a urine sodium greater than 10 mEq per L and the presence of granular casts in the urine sediment.

The pathogenesis of HRS involves severe vasoconstriction of the renal circulation in conjunction with splanchnic arterial vasodilation. The vasodilation of the splanchnic system leads to compensatory activation of the renin-angiotensin-aldosterone system and the sympathetic nervous system. These systems cause renal retention of sodium and water in addition to renal vasoconstriction. When the tenuous local balance between vasoconstrictors and vasodilators is destroyed, however, profound intrarenal arterial vasoconstriction ensues, causing HRS. Medical management of HRS is marginally effective, but liver transplantation usually reverses the process. Interestingly, kidneys transplanted from patients with HRS function normally in new hosts, pointing out the essential role of hepatic disease in the pathogenesis.

Arroyo V, Gines P, Gerbes AL, et al. Definition and diagnostic criteria of refractory ascites and hepatorenal syncrome in cirrhosis. *Hepatology* 1996;23:164–176.

Bataller R, Gines P, Arroyo V, et al. Hepatorenal syndrome. *Clin Liver Dis* 2000;4:487–507.

Cardenas A. Hepatorenal syndrome: a dreaded complication of end-stage liver disease. *Am J Gastroenterol* 2005;100:460–467.

Gines P, Guevara M, Arroyo V, et al. Hepatorenal syndrome. *J Lancet* 2003;362:1819–1827.

A.15. Discuss the neurologic manifestations of chronic liver disease and fulminant hepatic failure and their management.

Hepatic encephalopathy occurs in 50% to 70% of patients with chronic liver disease. The pathogenesis is incompletely understood but is likely multifactorial. Etiologic theories include cerebral circulation of toxins incompletely cleared by the diseased liver, production of false neurotransmitters resulting from increased concentrations of aromatic amino acids, the existence of abnormal endogenous agonists binding to the central nervous system (CNS) γ-amino butyric acid (GABA) receptor, and manganese deposition in the basal ganglia. High serum ammonia levels are characteristic of patients with hepatic encephalopathy, although the degree of elevation does not correlate with neurologic severity. Encephalopathy is classified in grades one through four, with grade one being mild confusion and grade four indicating coma. Therapy for hepatic encephalopathy involves identifying and treating any reversible causes (e.g., gastrointestinal (GI) bleeding, infection), using cathartics (lactulose), and administering short courses of antibiotics (neomycin or metronidazole) to diminish intestinal ammonia production. The benzodiazepine antagonist flumazenil has been reported to temporarily improve hepatic encephalopathy and may be helpful as a diagnostic tool, but its use is not routinely recommended.

As in chronic liver disease, patients who develop fulminant hepatic failure are at risk for hepatic encephalopathy, but the consequences are more serious because of accompanying cerebral edema with resultant increased intracranial pressure (ICP) and a threat of herniation. For this reason, ICP monitoring should be seriously considered for patients with fulminant hepatic failure and encephalopathy, even given the bleeding risks associated with invasive monitors. It is this risk that seems to be the greatest deterrent against ICP monitoring. A review of recent data indicates a risk of approximately 10% for intracranial hemorrhage with insertion of ICP monitoring. To minimize the risk, it has been recommended that epidural transducers be utilized rather than intradural monitors. With or without ICP monitoring, 30-day outcomes are similar.

ICP elevations to greater than 25 mm Hg should be treated with mannitol to achieve hyperosmolarity. Preoperative hyperventilation has not been shown to improve outcome and corticosteroids are not indicated. Pentobarbital coma may be indicated for patients unresponsive to mannitol, but it may worsen cerebral hypoperfusion by causing systemic hypotension. Many centers consider sustained cerebral hypoperfusion (cerebral perfusion pressure <40 mm Hg) a contraindication to transplant because of the high risk for brain death as an outcome. In the future, transcranial Doppler ultrasonography (TCD) may offer a noninvasive means of monitoring for elevated ICP in these patients. The anesthetic plan must include careful attention to avoiding drugs or conditions that may exacerbate elevations in ICP.

Cordoba J, Blei AT. Cerebral edema and intracranial pressure monitoring. *Liver Transpl Surg* 1995;1:225–228.

Jalan R, Hayes PC. Hepatic encephalopathy and ascites. *Lancet* 1997;350:1309–1315.

Riordan SM, Williams R. Treatment of hepatic encephalopathy. *N Engl J Med* 1997;337:473–479.

Saab S, Han SH, Martin P. Liver transplantation: selection, listing criteria, and preoperative management. *Clin Liver Dis* 2000;4:513–532.

Vaquero J, Fontana RJ, Larson AM, et al. Complications and use of intracranial pressure monitoring in patients with acute liver failure and severe encephalopathy. *Liver Transpl* 2005;11:1581–1589.

A.16. What are the contraindications to liver transplantation?

As the outcome of liver transplantation has improved, the list of absolute contraindications diminishes. At present, the list includes:

- Sepsis
- Advanced cardiopulmonary disease
- Extra hepatic malignancy
- AIDS (but not necessarily HIV infection)
- Alcohol or illicit drug use in the previous 6 months by a patient with a known substance abuse history
- Unfavorable psychosocial circumstance (e.g., psychiatric illness precluding medication compliance)

Whereas old age was previously thought to be a contraindication, recent survival data suggest that elderly patients suffer no greater mortality in the first years posttransplant than do younger recipients. Important to good outcomes in this population is a careful preoperative evaluation for comorbid disease and referral for transplantation in the early stages of liver disease. In April 2006, more than 11% of patients on the liver transplant waiting list in the United States were older than 65 years whereas approximately 60% were 50 to 64 years old.

Baker J, Yost CS, Niemann CU. Organ transplantation. In: Miller RD, ed. *Anesthesia*, 6th ed. Philadelphia: Churchill Livingstone, 2005:2231–2284.

Rosen HR, Shackleton CR, Martin P. Indications for and timing of liver transplantation. *Med Clin North Am* 1996;80:1069–1102.

Saab S, Han SH, Martin P. Liver transplantation: selection, listing criteria, and preoperative management. *Clin Liver Dis* 2000;4:513–532.

Sandberg WS, Raines D. Anesthesia for liver surgery. In: Longnecker DE, Tinker JH, Morgan GE, eds. *Principles and practice of anesthesiology*, 3rd ed. St. Louis: Mosby, 2007.

United Network for Organ Sharing. Website: www.unos.org, accessed April 4, 2006.

B. Preoperative Evaluation and Preparation

B.1. What medications might this patient be receiving preoperatively?

Typical medications for a patient with end-stage liver disease (ESLD) include diuretics (e.g., spironolactone, furosemide) to control ascites, β-blockers (e.g., propranolol) to treat portal hypertension, cathartics (e.g., lactulose) to control encephalopathy, antibiotic prophylaxis (e.g., levofloxacin) for spontaneous bacterial peritonitis (SBP), and vitamins (including vitamin K) to counter dietary or absorptive deficiencies.

Sandberg WS, Raines D. Anesthesia for liver surgery. In: Longnecker DE, Tinker JH, Morgan GE, eds. *Principles and practice of anesthesiology*, 3rd ed. St. Louis: Mosby, 2007.

B.2. What preoperative workup is desirable?

Ideally, the preoperative evaluation of a patient scheduled for orthotopic liver transplant (OLT) is a deliberate, multidisciplinary process in all cases except the most urgent (e.g., fulminant hepatic failure). Evaluation by a dedicated team of hepatologists, transplant surgeons, social workers, and psychologists is usual before listing the patient for transplant. Cardiology, pulmonary, infectious disease and nephrology consultation may be requested in specific cases in which comorbid illness exists. Patients who may have received multiple previous transfusions, such as patients with a history of gastrointestinal (GI) bleeding, should be evaluated in advance for problems with crossmatching large quantities of blood products for a transplant operation. Consultation by a blood bank physician may be advisable. An evaluation by the transplant anesthesiologist may occur at the time of listing for the procedure. Patients of advanced age or those with particular risk factors may undergo cardiopulmonary testing to evaluate for myocardial ischemia (e.g., dobutamine stress echocardiography), cardiac dysfunction (e.g., transthoracic echocardiography), or lung disease (e.g., pulmonary function tests). The anesthesiologist should be familiar with these common tests and their interpretations to formulate an anesthetic plan.

Preoperative myocardial evaluation is recommended, typically with a functional stress echo using dobutamine. It is critical to ensure that the heart rate reaches 85% of the maximum predicted heart rate for the stress test to be considered adequate. A vasodilatory (e.g., adenosine, persantine) myocardial stress is less optimal because in patients with end-stage liver disease (ESLD), the resting vascular tone is so low as to render provocation of further pharmacologic vasodilation impossible. Transthoracic echo in this setting is also useful to estimate right ventricular systolic pressure as an estimate of pulmonary artery pressure. If elevated, pre-transplant right heart catheterization may be warranted.

In cases of altered mental status, a head CT is often indicated to evaluate intracranial bleeding, herniation and/or the extent of cerebral edema.

Immediately before the transplant, laboratory determination of complete blood count (CBC), coagulation parameters, electrolytes, blood urea nitrogen (BUN), creatinine, bilirubin, and albumin should be obtained. A recent electrocardiogram (ECG) and chest radiograph are also helpful. Large quantities of blood products should be typed, crossmatched and readily available. If intraoperative renal replacement (continuous venovenous hemofiltration [CVVH]) therapy is a consideration, consultation with a nephrologist should be sought.

Sandberg WS, Raines D. Anesthesia for liver surgery. In: Longnecker DE, Tinker JH, Morgan GE, eds. *Principles and practice of anesthesiology*, 3rd ed. St. Louis: Mosby, 2007.

Sharma P, Rakela J. Management of pre-liver transplant patients—part 1. *Liver Transpl* 2005;11:124–133.

Sharma P, Rakela J. Management of pre-liver transplant patients—part 2. *Liver Transpl* 2005;11:249–260.

Wiklund RA. Preoperative preparation of patients with advanced liver disease. *Crit Care Med* 2004;32:S106–S115.

B.3. What immunosuppressive agents will be given perioperatively? What are the major side effects?

A combination of immunosuppressant medications is key to successful transplantation and organ viability. Particular protocols vary significantly from center to center. A usual regimen includes cyclosporine or FK-506 (tacrolimus), azathioprine or mycophenolate mofetil (MMF), and prednisone. Antibodies directed against T-cell lymphocytes (e.g., OKT3 or antithymocyte globulin) may be substituted for cyclosporine or tacrolimus in patients with renal dysfunction, or they may be used in short courses to treat rejection. New drugs being used for immunosuppression in liver transplantation include monoclonal antibodies to IL-2 receptors (CD25) of T lymphocytes

Table 20.2 Major Side Effects of Immunosuppressant Medications.

MEDICATION	SIDE EFFECTS
Cyclosporine	Nephrotoxicity
	Hypertension
FK-506 (tacrolimus)	Nephrotoxicity
	Hypertension
Mycophenolate mofetil	Hypertension
	Leukopenia
	Abdominal pain
	Diarrhea
	Vomiting
Azathioprine	Leukopenia
	Anemia
	Thrombocytopenia
Prednisone	Glucose intolerance
	Osteoporosis
	Peptic ulcer disease
	Adrenal suppression
OKT3	Symptoms of cytokine release (fever, chills, dyspnea, wheezing, chest pain)
	Leukopenia
Antithymocyte globulin	Fever
	Chills
	Leukopenia
	Thrombocytopenia
Basiliximab	GI upset
Daclizumab	GI upset

GI, gastrointestinal.

(basiliximab and daclizumab). Major side effects of the immunosuppressants are listed in Table 20.2.

Baker J, Yost CS, Niemann CU. Organ transplantation. In: Miller RD, ed. *Anesthesia*, 6th ed. Philadelphia: Churchill Livingstone, 2005:2231–2284.

Feng SF, Ko DSC, Cosimi AB. Liver transplantation. In: Morris PJ, Wood WC, eds. *Oxford textbook of surgery*, 2nd ed. New York: Oxford University Press, 2000:685–707.

Moser MAJ. Options for induction immunosuppression in liver transplant recipients. *Drugs* 2002;62:995–1011.

B.4. What risks associated with the anesthetic will you include in the informed consent?

Potential risks associated with anesthesia for liver transplantation, which should be discussed with the patient preoperatively, include massive blood product transfusion, respiratory failure and prolonged mechanical ventilation, cardiac dysfunction and vasopressor support, renal failure and dialysis, stroke, and death. The patient should be informed that initial postoperative care is provided in the critical care unit. The known risks of central venous cannulation (e.g., bleeding, stroke, pneumothorax) may also be discussed, especially if the patient is severely coagulopathic or has a history of previous cannulations.

Carton EG, Plevak DJ, Kranner PW, et al. Perioperative care of the liver transplant patient: part 2. *Anesth Analg* 1994;78:382–399.

Sandberg WS, Raines D. Anesthesia for liver surgery. In: Longnecker DE, Tinker JH, Morgan GE, eds. *Principles and practice of anesthesiology*, 3rd ed. St. Louis: Mosby, 2007.

B.5. What premedication would you choose for this patient?

The decision to premedicate this patient should be based on an assessment of the severity of his end-stage liver disease (ESLD) and the need for anxiolysis. Patients with ESLD are exceptionally sensitive to medications with central nervous system (CNS) effects. Benzodiazepines have been noted to have an exaggerated effect thought to be due to the presence of endogenous substances with γ-aminobutyric acid (GABA) receptor agonist activity in the brain and up regulation of GABA receptors. Prudence dictates the avoidance of CNS depressants for patients with obvious signs of encephalopathy. For patients without CNS impairment, incremental, low doses of the usual premedications (e.g., midazolam, fentanyl, morphine) may be safely titrated to effect. Because "full stomach" concerns apply to the induction of anesthesia for many of these patients, pretreatment with antacid medications (e.g., ranitidine, sodium bicitrate) may be considered.

Riordan SM, Williams R. Treatment of hepatic encephalopathy. *N Engl J Med* 1997;337: 473–479.

Sandberg WS, Raines D. Anesthesia for liver surgery. In: Longnecker DE, Tinker JH, Morgan GE, eds. *Principles and practice of anesthesiology*, 3rd ed. St. Louis: Mosby, 2007.

C. Intraoperative Management

C.1. What are the three stages of the liver transplant operation?

The three stages of the liver transplant operation are (a) the preanhepatic phase from the start of surgery to clamping of the hepatic artery, (b) the anhepatic phase from clamping of the hepatic artery to reperfusion of the new liver, and (c) the postanhepatic phase from reperfusion of the liver to the end of the case.

Steadman RH. Anesthesia for liver transplant surgery. *Anesthesiol Clin North America* 2004;22:687–711.

C.2. What happens in the first stage of the liver transplant operation?

During the preanhepatic phase, the anesthesia team completes the induction of the anesthetic and the placement of lines and monitors. A maintenance anesthetic is established. The anesthesia team also addresses physiologic abnormalities such as acid-base or electrolyte disturbances, fluid imbalances, disorders of coagulation, or unstable hemodynamics, and may elect to intervene and treat some or all of the concerns.

The principle surgical team prepares the patient for a large subcostal incision. In addition, one of the axillae and a groin area may be prepared for the possible institution of venovenous bypass (see Question C.17). After incision, the abdomen is evaluated for previously unsuspected pathologic conditions. Ascites, which is often present in liver disease complicated by portal hypertension, will be drained. The anesthesia team must be aware of, and vigilant for, hemodynamic effects related to drainage of large volumes of ascites. The liver is dissected from its ligamentous attachments and the vascular structures are exposed.

A second team of surgeons will simultaneously prepare the graft liver for implantation. This is carried out on a separate table and does not involve the anesthesia team.

C.3. What monitors would you use? Why?

In addition to routine basic monitors (electrocardiogram [ECG], pulse oximetry, capnography, temperature, and noninvasive blood pressure), an arterial line is placed for close systemic pressure monitoring and to facilitate frequent sampling for blood tests. Central venous pressure monitoring is established to help assess the volume status and provide a route for central drug administration. The use of a pulmonary artery catheter depends on local practice and the physiologic state of the patient. The pulmonary artery catheter may be particularly useful when the patient has renal insufficiency (e.g., acute tubular necrosis [ATN], hepatorenal syndrome [HRS]), respiratory compromise (pulmonary edema, hepatopulmonary syndrome [HPS]), mild to moderate pulmonary hypertension, or unstable hemodynamics before surgery. Transesophageal echocardiography (TEE) and intracranial pressure (ICP) monitoring (either directly or with noninvasive methods) may be indicated in particular cases for which concerns exist for cardiac dysfunction or cerebral edema. All patients receive nasogastric tubes and bladder catheters.

Cordoba J, Blei AT. Cerebral edema and intracranial pressure monitoring. *Liver Transpl Surg* 1995;1:187–194.

Lidofsky SD, Bass NM, Prager MC, et al. Intracranial pressure monitoring and liver transplantation for fulminant hepatic failure. *Hepatology* 1992;16:1–7.

Philips BJ, Armstrong IR, Pollock A, et al. Cerebral blood flow and metabolism in patients with chronic liver disease undergoing orthotopic liver transplantation. *Hepatology* 1998;27:369–376.

Pregler J, Csete M. Anesthesia for liver transplantation. *Curr Opin Anesth* 1996;9:263–266.

Suriani RJ. Transesophageal echocardiography during organ transplantation. *J Cardiothorac Vasc Anesth* 1998;12:686–694.

Suriani RJ, Cutrone A, Feierman D, et al. Intraoperative transesophageal echocardiography during liver transplantation. *J Cardiothorac Vasc Anesth* 1996;10:699–707.

C.4. When would you place invasive monitors? Why?

Invasive monitors may be placed before or after the induction of the anesthetic and endotracheal intubation. An advantage of placing the monitors before induction is that the information will be available for induction. Also, an assessment can be made of the patient's baseline hemodynamic state before any anesthesia-associated perturbations. However, patients with encephalopathy, tense ascites, or respiratory compromise (atelectasis, pleural effusions) may be poor candidates for the Trendelenburg position and the draping of the face associated with central vein cannulation. Therefore, it may be advantageous to place major monitoring and access lines after induction of anesthesia and endotracheal intubation. Because massive hemorrhage sometimes complicates the procedure, large-bore intravenous access is critical.

C.5. What is the utility of intraoperative transesophageal echocardiography (TEE)?

TEE may be useful during liver transplantation to help provide clinical information regarding left and right heart filling and function, detection of myocardial ischemia and monitoring of emboli.

TEE is not without risk in liver transplant patients especially given the significant prevalence of esophageal varices and risk for variceal hemorrhage. In fact, esophageal varices are considered to be relative contraindications to TEE in most circumstances. As always, a risk-benefit analysis must be done before performing a TEE in these patients. TEE is not used routinely for patients undergoing liver transplantation in many institutions.

Suriani RJ. Transesophageal echocardiography during organ transplantation. *J Cardiothorac Vasc Anesth* 1998;12:686–694.

C.6. When is intraoperative renal replacement therapy indicated?

Renal replacement therapy or continuous venovenous hemofiltration (CVVH) may be used intraoperatively to help manage a transplant patient's fluid and electrolyte status. The literature and experience on this topic is just emerging. In the Massachusetts General Hospital, indications for intraoperative CVVH include patients on CVVH preoperatively, patients with preoperative glomerular filtration rates (GFRs) less than 30 mL per minute, and severe hyponatremia with or without renal failure.

C.7. What initial hemodynamic findings might be anticipated in this case?

Patients with cirrhosis and end-stage liver disease (ESLD) often exhibit tachycardia (pulse rates 90 to 110 beats/minute) and low-normal blood pressures (systolic blood pressure 90 to 110 mm Hg). In addition, a high cardiac output (6 to 20 L/minute, even in a normal-sized adult), elevated stroke volume (80 to >120 mL), and reduced systemic vascular resistance are commonly encountered. Central venous and pulmonary artery pressures may be low, normal, or high. Drainage of ascites often rapidly and significantly alters hemodynamics. The anesthesiologist should anticipate hypotension following ascites drainage.

Sandberg WS, Raines D. Anesthesia for liver surgery. In: Longnecker DE, Tinker JH, Morgan GE, eds. *Principles and practice of anesthesiology*, 3rd ed. St. Louis: Mosby, 2007.

C.8. What are the considerations for the induction of anesthesia?

Because of tense ascites, recent food ingestion, or a propensity for delayed gastric emptying, it is often appropriate to consider a liver transplant patient as having a full stomach, thereby a candidate for the rapid-sequence induction of general endotracheal anesthesia. However, renal dysfunction with elevated potassium levels or recent debilitation with prolonged immobilization may preclude the use of succinylcholine. Intravascular volume depletion (diuresis, diarrhea, dialysis, etc.) should be considered when choosing drugs and drug dosages for induction. Liver disease, perhaps in conjunction with renal dysfunction, may result in altered volumes of distribution, alterations in plasma protein binding, and reduced metabolism and clearance of induction drugs. For the induction of anesthesia in a setting of a lengthy procedure, termination of the effects of induction drugs assumes less importance.

Sandberg WS, Raines D. Anesthesia for liver surgery. In: Longnecker DE, Tinker JH, Morgan GE, eds. *Principles and practice of anesthesiology*, 3rd ed. St. Louis: Mosby, 2007.

C.9. Which anesthetic agents would be useful for maintenance?

In principle, any maintenance regimen can be used for patients undergoing liver transplantation. Because it is unusual to emerge and extubate the patients in the operating room, titration of long acting intravenous agents such as benzodiazepines, opioids, and muscle relaxants to allow for extubation is generally unnecessary. Some practitioners avoid nitrous oxide because of the propensity to distend the bowel and because intravenous air embolism is sometimes encountered during the operation. Hemodynamic fluctuations are often encountered during the liver transplant procedure; it may be advisable to avoid high concentrations of inhalation agents such as isoflurane.

Steadman RH. Anesthesia for liver transplant surgery. *Anesthesiol Clin North America* 2004;22:687–711.

Wiklund RA. Preoperative preparation of patients with advanced liver disease. *Crit Care Med* 2004;32:S106–S115.

C.10. Are there any drugs that should be avoided?

Although halothane has been nearly removed from clinical practice, it is still used in the care of many pediatric patients. Halothane metabolism by the liver can produce metabolites including free radicals. There is less evidence for hepatotoxicity from exposure to the other potent inhalation agents. Isoflurane is a recommended agent for use during the liver transplant anesthetic. The newer gases desflurane and sevoflurane may better preserve hepatic oxygen supply and demand balances compared with the older anesthetics. Nitrous oxide appears to possess little direct hepatotoxicity.

Baden JM, Rice SA. Metabolism and toxicity of inhaled anesthetics. In: Miller RD, ed. *Anesthesia*, 5th ed. Philadelphia: Churchill Livingstone, 2000:158–160.

Merritt WT. Metabolism and liver transplantation: review of perioperative issues. *Liver Transpl* 2000;6(4 Suppl 1):S76–S84.

Sandberg WS, Raines D. Anesthesia for liver surgery. In: Longnecker DE, Tinker JH, Morgan GE, eds. *Principles and practice of anesthesiology*, 3rd ed. St. Louis: Mosby, 2007.

C.11. Is there a role for a combined anesthetic technique (regional/epidural plus general anesthesia) in liver transplantation?

Patients with end-stage liver disease (ESLD) often exhibit coagulation disorders. The presence of a coagulopathy is a contraindication to regional anesthesia, particularly epidural anesthesia. Patients without an initial disorder of coagulation may develop a coagulopathy intraoperatively or postoperatively. This should be considered in planning the anesthetic.

C.12. What happens in the second stage of the liver transplant operation?

The second stage of the liver transplant operation, known as the anhepatic phase, begins when the native liver is devascularized by ligation of the inflow vessels (portal vein, hepatic artery). The surgical team will then complete the dissection of the diseased liver and evaluate the site for bleeding, particularly from retroperitoneal areas. The graft is brought to the surgical field to begin the vascular anastomoses. The anhepatic phase terminates when the graft is reperfused. Unclamping of the vena cava and portal vein usually precedes restoration of the arterial supply.

Evidence of hepatocyte metabolic function may be seen when the graft receives blood flow from the portal system. However, the graft only receives oxygen-rich blood at systemic perfusion pressures when the hepatic artery inflow is reconstituted. This may be delayed minutes to hours, depending on the complexity of the arterial vascular anatomy. Some centers reperfuse with portal vein and hepatic arterial supplies simultaneously. Some centers use an infusion of prostaglandin E_1 because evidence suggests a role for this drug in improvement of hepatic blood flow, suppression of the immune system, and general cytoprotection.

Pregler J, Csete M. Anesthesia for liver transplantation. *Curr Opin Anesth* 1996;9:263–266.

C.13. Which blood vessels are isolated and ligated?

The liver receives inflow from the portal vein as well as from the hepatic artery. Both vessels must be identified, dissected free, and ultimately clamped and divided. The hepatic veins drain the liver, feeding into the inferior vena cava (IVC). The suprahepatic and infrahepatic portions of the IVC must be identified and isolated. In addition, the native liver's biliary drainage is interrupted.

C.14. What are the surgical options for completing the vascular anastomoses?

In the standard method of reconstructing the vascular connections, the suprahepatic vena cava and the infrahepatic vena cava are clamped and divided. Blood flow through the inferior vena cava (IVC) is completely interrupted. A cylinder of the recipient's IVC, the segment receiving the hepatic veins, is removed *en bloc* with the diseased liver, often with venovenous bypass to support the circulation. The graft supplies a cylinder of IVC to reconstruct the IVC (Fig. 20.2A). In the piggyback method, the diseased liver is dissected off the IVC. The recipient's IVC is thereby preserved and blood flow is not completely interrupted, usually preventing the need for venovenous bypass. One end of the graft's segment of IVC is oversewn, and the open end is anastomosed to the preserved recipient IVC. The anastomosis may be constructed with the stump of the recipient's hepatic veins (Fig. 20.2B). Rarely, a side-to-side cavo-caval anastomosis is created (Fig. 20.2C).

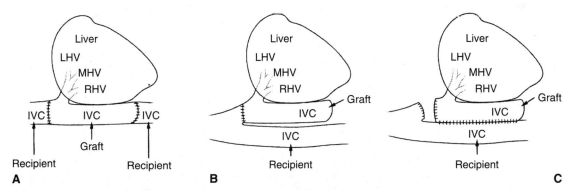

Figure 20.2 Three different techniques to reconstruct the hepatovenous outflow. **A:** End-to-end interposition of the donor vena cava to the recipient vena cava. **B:** End-to-end anastomosis of the vena cava to the hepatic veins. **C:** Side-to-side cavo-cavostomy. IVC, inferior vena cava; LHV, left hepatic veins; MHV, middle hepatic veins; RHV, right hepatic veins. (Reproduced and modified with permission from Hesse UJ, Berrevoet F, Troisi R, et al. Hepato-venous reconstruction in orthotopic liver transplantation with preservation of the recipients' inferior vena cava and veno-venous bypass. *Langenbecks Arch Surg* 2000;385:350–356.)

Reconstruction of the arterial supply may be a direct connection of the donor and recipient hepatic arteries. Unfavorable arterial anatomy may mandate more complex reconstructions.

Busque S, Esquivel CO, Concepcion W, et al. Experience with the piggyback technique without caval occlusion in adult orthotopic liver transplantation. *Transplantation* 1998;65:77–82.

Hesse UJ, Berrevoet F, Troisi R, et al. Hepato-venous reconstruction in orthotopic liver transplantation with preservation of the recipients' inferior vena cava and veno-venous bypass. *Langenbecks Arch Surg* 2000;385:350–356.

Reddy KS, Johnston TD, Putnam L, et al. Piggyback technique and selective use of veno-venous bypass in adult orthotopic liver transplantation. *Clin Transplant* 2000;14: 370–374.

C.15. What is the order of reconstruction of the vascular anastomoses?

In the standard method, the suprahepatic inferior vena cava (IVC) anastomosis is completed, followed by the infrahepatic IVC anastomosis, the portal vein anastomosis, and the arterial reconstruction. The biliary drainage is reconstituted last. In the piggyback method, which preserves the recipient's IVC, there is only one IVC anastomosis. This connection is accomplished first, followed by the portal vein, arterial, and biliary anastomoses.

C.16. What is the "test clamp" maneuver?

In the standard method of reconstruction, the recipient's inferior vena cava (IVC) is divided. This completely interrupts blood return to the heart from below the diaphragm. Recipients' circulatory systems vary in their tolerance of this loss of preload. In preparation for clamping and dividing the IVC, a test clamp maneuver is performed to assess the resilience of the circulatory system. This may be accomplished by occlusion of the suprahepatic IVC. Arterial pressure and cardiac output will fall with the loss of venous return. Excessive circulatory depression during the test clamp warrants a delay in proceeding with the surgery and a reassessment of volume status, cardiac performance, metabolic state (particularly ionized calcium levels), and other possible depressant factors such as the effects of anesthetics. Venovenous bypass may be instituted if, after optimizing these variables, there is excessive circulatory depression following a second test clamp maneuver.

C.17. What is venovenous bypass? What are potential advantages and disadvantages of this procedure?

Venovenous bypass is a method to provide temporary rerouting of blood flow from below the diaphragm to the heart when the inferior vena cava (IVC) is interrupted. Some centers routinely use this procedure, some never do. Other centers reserve venovenous bypass for situations when excessive depression of the recipient's circulatory system follows the interruption of venous return through the IVC. A Y-shaped tubing is used. One limb of the tubing is inserted into the recipient's portal vein to drain the splanchnic beds. Another limb of the tubing is placed through a groin cut down into an iliac vein or the distal IVC. The outflow tubing passes through a pump. Blood returns to the patient through a cutdown access to an axillary vein or through percutaneous access to an internal jugular or subclavian vein (Fig. 20.3).

Proposed advantages of venovenous bypass include a decompression of the splanchnic circulation (thereby promoting an earlier return of gut motility), preserved drainage of the renal veins (potentially reducing acute renal dysfunction), and improved filling of the heart when the IVC is interrupted. Disadvantages include the need for additional surgical incisions, heat loss

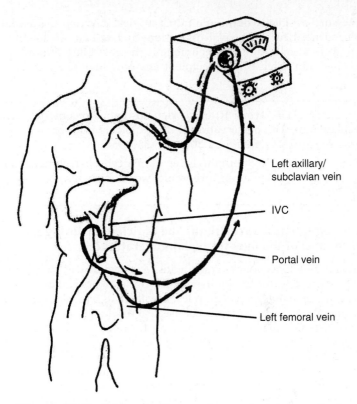

Left axillary/
subclavian vein

IVC

Portal vein

Left femoral vein

Figure 20.3 Schematic diagram of venovenous bypass circuit during liver transplantation. Venous return comes from drainage of the femoral and portal veins connected together into a single venous return line. The centrifugal pump returns the blood into the axillary or subclavian vein. IVC, inferior vena cava.

with exteriorization of blood flow, and risks of air and thromboembolism. The efficacy and benefits of routine use of venovenous bypass remain controversial. However, portal decompression clearly improves surgical visualization in certain circumstances, such as in Budd-Chiari syndrome.

Kaufman RD, Khoury GF. Hemodynamic changes with initiation of veno-venous bypass in orthotopic liver transplant patients. *Am J Anesthesiol* 1995;22:184–188.

Paulsen AW, Whitten CW, Ramsey MAE, et al. Considerations for anesthetic management during veno-venous bypass in adult hepatic transplantation. *Anesth Analg* 1989; 68:489–496.

Steadman RH. Anesthesia for liver transplant surgery. *Anesthesiol Clin North America* 2004;22:687–711.

C.18. What are the potential advantages of the "piggyback" (vena cava preservation) technique?

Advantages of the piggyback technique for vascular reconstruction potentially include hemodynamic stability resulting from preservation of cardiac filling, preservation of renal perfusion pressure, avoidance of the additional surgical interventions associated with venovenous bypass, reduced need for retrocaval dissection, and a lessened likelihood of damage to the adrenal vein. A disadvantage of the technique is the possibility of outflow obstruction resulting in hepatic congestion. Unfavorable recipient anatomy may preclude the use of the piggyback technique.

Hesse UJ, Berrevoet F, Troisi R, et al. Hepato-venous reconstruction in orthotopic liver transplantation with preservation of the recipients' inferior vena cava and veno-venous bypass. *Langenbecks Arch Surg* 2000;385:350–356.

Reddy KS, Johnston TD, Putnam L, et al. Piggyback technique and selective use of veno-venous bypass in adult orthotopic liver transplantation. *Clin Transplant* 2000;14: 370–374.

C.19. What physiologic disturbances should be anticipated during the second stage (anhepatic phase) of the liver transplant operation?

An accumulation of endogenous organic acids (e.g., lactic acid) that are ordinarily metabolized to carbon dioxide and water by the liver leads to metabolic acidosis. If citrate is infused (such as during transfusions), ionized calcium levels will fall as a result of chelation. Magnesium levels will also decline. Plasma potassium levels rise as a result of acidemia, reduced urine output, and the absence of hepatic uptake of this ion. Transfusions of packed red blood cells (PRBCs) also deliver a potassium load to the recipient. The liver is a major organ for the regulation of glucose levels. In the anhepatic phase, there is no gluconeogenesis, but glucose is often delivered to the patient during transfusions. Blood glucose levels should be monitored, both for hyperglycemia and hypoglycemia.

Merritt WT. Metabolism and liver transplantation: review of perioperative issues. *Liver Transpl* 2000;6(4 Suppl 1):S76–S84.

C.20. How would you treat hyperkalemia?

Hyperkalemia may be treated by forcing diuresis, infusing β-adrenergic agonists, or by administering insulin in combination with glucose. However, these approaches may be slow to achieve reductions in plasma potassium. Alkalinization, achieved by hyperventilation or with sodium bicarbonate, will reduce potassium levels more rapidly. The dysrhythmic effects of elevated potassium may be countered with calcium. Rarely, when hyperkalemia is refractory to the preceding treatments, continuous venovenous hemofiltration (CVVH) may be utilized to reduce the elevated serum potassium level.

De Wolf A, Frenette L, Kang Y, et al. Insulin decreases the serum potassium concentration during the anhepatic stage of liver transplantation. *Anesthesiology* 1993;78:677–682.

Merrit WT. Metabolism and liver transplantation: review of perioperative issues. *Liver Transpl* 2000;6(4 Suppl 1):S76–S84.

C.21. Why should you anticipate hypocalcemia?

The principal reason to anticipate hypocalcemia is the failure to clear the citrate that is normally metabolized by the liver. This calcium chelating agent accumulates in patients who receive transfusions of citrated blood products.

C.22. What is the postreperfusion syndrome? What should you be prepared to do?

With the completion of the venous anastomoses, the graft is perfused by the portal vein with drainage into the vena cava. At this juncture, acute systemic hypotension, bradycardia, elevated pulmonary artery pressures, and supraventricular or ventricular dysrhythmias may be encountered. Right heart failure or ventricular tachycardia or fibrillation occur in extreme situations. Potential etiologies include (a) an acute acid or potassium load released into the systemic circulation from the graft, the splanchnic bed, or the lower extremities; (b) the effects of cold blood from the graft on the heart; (c) the release of cytokines; or (d) the release of unidentified vasoactive substances. Bleeding and pulmonary embolization of air or thrombus may complicate the situation. Preexisting hypovolemia, acidemia, hyperkalemia, hypocalcemia, and hypothermia are likely to exacerbate the acute changes. Careful flushing of the graft just before completion of the anastomoses may attenuate the reperfusion disturbances by removing the preservative solution. Before reperfusing the new graft, the following measures should be considered: (a) preemptive administration of calcium to correct hypocalcemia; (b) sodium bicarbonate, dichloroacetate, or tris-hydroxymethyl aminomethane (THAM) to adjust pH; and (c) inotropes or vasopressors for circulatory support. The surgical and anesthesia teams must be prepared to diagnose and treat dysrhythmias or cardiac arrest.

Steadman RH. Anesthesia for liver transplant surgery. *Anesthesiol Clin North America* 2004;22:687–711.

Merritt WT. Metabolism and liver transplantation: review of perioperative issues. *Liver Transpl* 2000;6(4 Suppl 1):S76–S84.

Nahas GG, Sutin KM, Fermon C, et al. Guidelines for the treatment of acidaemia with THAM. *Drugs* 1998;55:191–224.

C.23. What happens during the third stage of the liver transplant operation?

The third stage of the liver transplant operation, the neohepatic phase, follows reperfusion of the new liver. In the neohepatic phase, surgical efforts are directed toward construction of a biliary drainage system. This may be straightforward, with an anastomosis between the graft's common bile duct and the biliary stump of the recipient. More complex reconstructions are sometimes required, such as the creation of a choledochojejunostomy. A donor cholecystectomy is generally performed. A T-tube is often placed in the reconstructed biliary outflow system, with external drainage. An intraoperative cholangiogram, with contrast dye instilled through the T-tube, is often used to assess the patency and integrity of the biliary reconstruction. The third stage ends with closure of all wounds and transport to the intensive care unit.

During the third stage of the procedure, the anesthesia team focuses on monitoring for evidence of graft function, assessing the coagulation state of the patient and initiating treatment as needed, and optimizing hemodynamics.

Kang Y. Liver transplantation. *Int Anesthesiol Clin* 1991;29(3):59–86.

Steadman RH. Anesthesia for liver transplant surgery. *Anesthesiol Clin North America* 2004;22:687–711.

C.24. What intraoperative findings suggest that the hepatic graft is functioning?

An early indication of graft function is enhanced production of carbon dioxide attributable to metabolism of organic acids by the new liver. This may first be detected by observing a rise in end-tidal carbon dioxide ($ETCO_2$). Hypocalcemia often resolves quickly as the graft metabolizes citrate during the final phases of the procedure. Metabolic alkalemia can develop as a result of citrate metabolism. Potassium levels tend to normalize with the onset of hepatocyte function. A number of recipients exhibit hyperglycemia resistant to insulin. Clotting disorders resulting from factor depletion will not be corrected by new synthesis of coagulation factors for hours to days after the transplant.

C.25. What disorders of coagulation should be anticipated? How can they be monitored and treated? What is thromboelastography (TEG)?

The patient's coagulation status at the start of the operation depends on the nature of the hepatic disease. Conditions in which the hepatocytes are uniformly affected, such as hepatitis C (HCV), often present with biosynthetic failure leading to reduced levels of clotting factors. Portal hypertension can produce hypersplenism resulting in thrombocytopenia. In contrast, in conditions in which normal hepatic parenchyma is preserved, such as isolated hepatoma, or in which hepatocyte function is nearly normal, such as in an isolated genetic deficiency, there may be little or no evidence of deranged coagulation. Factor deficiency leads to elevated prothrombin time (PT) or activated partial thromboplastin time (aPTT). Fibrinogen, which is synthesized in the liver, may be depleted. Some patients have disseminated intravascular coagulation (DIC) or primary fibrinolysis. Uremia, commonly associated with liver disease, will lead to platelet dysfunction.

During the preanhepatic phase of the liver transplant procedure, platelet and clotting factor depletion from consumption, or dilutional coagulopathy, may be encountered. During the anhepatic phase and the postanhepatic phase, dilutional coagulopathy may continue. A hyperfibrinolytic state sometimes develops during the anhepatic phase, with clinical evidence of severe nonsurgical bleeding after graft reperfusion. Heparin or heparin-like substances may be released into the circulation with reperfusion of the graft. Finally, DIC occasionally results from reperfusion and massive transfusion.

The coagulation status should always be monitored clinically, by inspection of the surgical field. Routine laboratory tests (PT, aPTT, platelet count, fibrinogen levels) are used in some centers for evaluating the coagulation status and directing treatment. Other centers use TEG, a test of whole blood clotting function, to diagnose disorders of coagulation. TEG assesses the viscoelastic properties of a whole blood sample as a function of time (see Chapter 13; Question A.22). Potential advantages of TEG include the ability to detect a hypercoagulable state, and the ability to distinguish hyperfibrinolysis from other causes of clinical coagulopathy such as factor depletion or thrombocytopenia. Heparinase may be used to help diagnose coagulopathy resulting from the presence of heparinoids.

Dzik WH. Massive transfusion in the adult patient: lessons from liver transplantation. In: Jeffries LC, Brecher ME, eds. *Massive transfusion*. Bethesda, MD: American Association of Blood Banks, 1994:65–93.

Dzik WH, Arkin CF, Jenkins RL. Fibrinolysis during liver transplantation in humans: role of tissue-type plasminogen activator. *Blood* 1990;71:1090–1095.

Harding SA, Mallett SV, Peachey TD. Use of heparinase modified thromboelastography in liver transplantation. *Br J Anaesth* 1997;78:175–179.

Hickman R, Bracher M, Pienaar BH. Heparin as the cause of coagulopathy which may complicate grafting of the liver. *Surg Gynecol Obstet* 1991;172:197–206.

Kang Y. Thromboelastography in liver transplantation. *Semin Thromb Hemost* 1995;21(Suppl 4):34–44.

McCormick PA, Murphy KM. Splenomegaly, hypersplenism and coagulation abnormalities in liver disease. *Baillieres Best Pract Res Clin Gastroenterol* 2000;14:1009–1031.

Srinivasa V, Gilbertson LI, Bhavani-Shankar K. Thromboelastography: where is it and where is it heading. *Int Anesthesiol Clin* 2001;39:35–49.

C.26. How would you treat a hyperfibrinolytic state?

One option for the management of a presumed or diagnosed hyperfibrinolytic state is to wait for the hepatic graft to clear the causative substances. Tissue plasminogen activator (TPA) has been implicated as a causal agent in hyperfibrinolysis. A functioning graft liver should eventually clear excess TPA from the circulation. A second option is pharmacologic therapy with antifibrinolytic agents (tranexamic acid, ε-aminocaproic acid [Amicar]), or aprotinin [Trasylol]). These substances block fibrin degradation by plasmin, but the full spectrum of their actions remains incompletely defined. The use of prophylactic antifibrinolytic agents in liver transplant surgery has been advocated, but this is controversial. Potential disadvantages of antifibrinolytic agents include the development of thromboses that may be catastrophic.

Dzik WH. Massive transfusion in the adult patient: lessons from liver transplantation. In: Jeffries LC, Brecher ME, eds. *Massive transfusion*. Bethesda, MD: American Association of Blood Banks, 1994:65–93.

Fitzsimons MG, Peterfreund RA, Raines DE. Aprotinin administration and pulmonary thromboembolism during orthotopic liver transplantation: report of two cases. *Anesth Analg* 2001;92:1418–1421.

Mannucci PM. Hemostatic drugs. *N Engl J Med* 1998;339:245–253.

Porte RJ, Molenaar IQ, Begliomini B, et al. Aprotinin and transfusion requirements in orthotopic liver transplantation: a multicentre randomised double-blind study. *Lancet* 2000;355:1303–1309.

Xia VW, Steadman RH. Antifibrinolytics in orthotopic liver transplantation: current status and controversies. *Liver Transpl* 2005;11:10–18.

D. Early Postoperative Management

D.1. What are the possible postoperative vascular catastrophes that should be kept in mind?

Failure or leakage of a vascular anastomosis can lead to rapid intravascular volume loss. Thrombosis of the portal vein or hepatic artery will compromise viability of the graft. Persistent portal hypertension can lead to variceal bleeding or intraabdominal bleeding.

Haydon GH, Neuberger J. Liver transplantation of patients in end-stage cirrhosis. *Baillieres Best Pract Res Clin Gastroenterol* 2000;14:1049–1073.

D.2. What coagulation disturbances should be anticipated in the postoperative period?

Typically, heparin effects, disseminated intravascular coagulation (DIC), or hyperfibrinolysis have been resolved in the operating room. However, dilutional coagulopathy, along with ongoing platelet and factor consumption in the early postoperative phase, and poor graft function, may contribute to clinical bleeding. Postoperative uremia compromises platelet function as well. Even the best functioning graft liver may not produce substantial levels of clotting factors for several days. Therefore, there may be a requirement for plasma, cryoprecipitate, and/or platelets in the early postoperative period.

D.3. List the complications of massive transfusion.

Massive transfusion, usually defined as transfusion of volumes greater than one blood volume, is associated with several metabolic and cardiopulmonary consequences. The incidence and/or severity of these consequences may depend on the function of the recipient's organs. For example, patients with renal insufficiency will be less likely to tolerate the acid–base and electrolyte disturbances associated with massive transfusion.

Complications of massive transfusion include (a) hyperkalemia, (b) hypocalcemia, (c) hypomagnesemia, (d) acidemia, (e) rebound alkalemia (after citrate anticoagulant is metabolized), (f) volume overload and pulmonary edema, (g) transfusion-related acute lung injury (TRALI), (h) hypothermia, (i) dilutional coagulopathy, (j) disseminated intravascular coagulation (DIC), and (k) myocardial dysfunction (also see Chapter 56, Questions C.11 and C.13).

Cobas M. Preoperative assessment of coagulation disorders. *Int Anesthesiol Clin* 2001; 39(1):1–15.

Dzik WH. Massive transfusion in the adult patient: lessons from liver transplantation. In: Jeffries LC, Brecher ME, eds. *Massive transfusion*. Bethesda, MD: American Association of Blood Banks, 1994:65–93.

Merrit WT. Metabolism and liver transplantation: review of perioperative issues. *Liver Transpl* 2000;6(4 Suppl 1):S76–S84.

D.4. How might renal function change?

Renal function may deteriorate as a result of intraoperative hypoperfusion. Inferior vena cava (IVC) preservation techniques or venovenous bypass are believed to preserve renal perfusion and reduce the likelihood of dysfunction. Postoperatively, sepsis and the nephrotoxic calcineurin inhibitors (CNI) such as cyclosporin A and FK506 (tacrolimus) may contribute to renal dysfunction. Balanced immunosuppression with steroids, mycophenolate mofetil (MMF), anti-CD25 (basilximab/daclizumab) and antithymoglobulin (ATG) can help minimize posttransplant renal dysfunction.

Distant DA, Gonwa TA. The kidney in liver transplantation. *J Am Soc Nephrol* 1993;4: 129–136.

Varo E, Lopez A, Rivero C. Initial immunosuppression in liver transplant recipients with impaired renal function. *Transplant Proc* 2005;37:3309–3312.

D.5. What other early postoperative complications should be anticipated?

Neurologic complications including peripheral nerve injury related to positioning and central nervous system (CNS) damage from drugs, hypoperfusion, bleeding, or central pontine myelinolysis (CPM) have been described. Appropriate evaluation may include CNS imaging studies, electroencephalography, and monitoring of drug levels and metabolic parameters. Infection, especially pulmonary infection, is a particular risk in the immunosuppressed patient. Other pulmonary complications include pulmonary edema, atelectasis, injury to the diaphragm, and lung injury from massive transfusion. Monitoring of metabolic parameters, and liver function tests and liver biopsies, contribute to an assessment for possible acute graft failure or acute rejection of the graft. Biliary complications include leakage at the anastomosis site, stricture with obstruction, and ischemic necrosis.

Other complications include graft reinfection (with hepatitis B or C), portal vein or hepatic artery thrombosis, biliary complications, chronic rejection of the graft, and viral, bacterial, or fungal infections.

Afessa B, Gay PC, Plevak DJ, et al. Pulmonary complications of orthotopic liver transplantation. *Mayo Clin Proc* 1993;68(5):427–434.

Baker J, Yost CS, Niemann CU. Organ transplantation. In: Miller RD, ed. *Anesthesia*, 6th ed. Philadelphia: Churchill Livingstone, 2005:2231–2284.

Golfieri R, Gianpalma E, Morselli Labate AM, et al. Pulmonary complications of liver transplantation: radiological appearance and statistical evaluation of risk factors in 300 cases. *Eur Radiol* 2000;10:1169–1183.

Haydon GH, Neuberger J. Liver transplantation of patients in end-stage cirrhosis. *Baillieres Best Pract Res Clin Gastroenterol* 2000;14:1049–1073.

Moreno E, Gomez SR, Gonzalez I, et al. Neurologic complications in liver transplantation. *Acta Neurol Scand* 1993;87:25–31.

CHAPTER 21

Pyloric Stenosis

Vinod Malhotra • Aarti Sharma

A 3-WEEK-OLD FIRST-BORN MALE INFANT

had projectile vomiting, which contained the ingested formula but no bile. His body weight was 2.5 kg. Serum electrolytes: K^+ 2.2 mEq per L, Cl^- 86 mEq per L. Blood pH 7.68. This infant was also noted to have a systolic murmur heard best at the second intercostal space along the left sternal border, which was assessed by a cardiologist and diagnosed as a ventricular septal defect (VSD).

A. Medical Disease and Differential Diagnosis

1. What is the diagnosis in this patient?
2. What is the differential diagnosis of pyloric stenosis?
3. What are the metabolic problems in this newborn secondary to his disease?
4. What are the adverse effects of metabolic alkalosis?
5. How would you treat this infant?
6. How would you determine fluid replacement in a newborn and what fluids would you use?
7. How would you correct the metabolic alkalosis in this patient?
8. What causes a cardiac murmur?

B. Preoperative Evaluation and Preparation

1. How would you evaluate this patient preoperatively?
2. How would you evaluate a heart murmur?
3. How would you differentiate between functional versus organic murmur?
4. What are the types of ventricular septal defect (VSD)? What type of shunt do they cause?
5. What are the risks of surgery and anesthesia in a patient with VSD?
6. How would you prepare this patient rapidly for emergency surgery? Is surgical intervention an acute emergency in this case?
7. How would you prepare this patient for anesthesia?

C. Intraoperative Management

1. What anesthetic techniques or agents would you use?
2. What induction–intubation sequence would you use?
3. What are the anatomic characteristics of the airway in the newborn and how do they differ from those in the adult?
4. How do you determine the size of the endotracheal tube in a pediatric patient?
5. What anesthesia system would you use and why?

6. What are the advantages and disadvantages of commonly employed nonrebreathing systems?
7. How would you monitor this patient intraoperatively?
8. How does the pulse oximeter function?
9. What factors affect the measurement of oxygen saturation by the pulse oximeter?

D. Postoperative Management

1. What are the complications that can occur in the postanesthesia recovery period?
2. How would you treat postextubation "croup" in this infant?

A. Medical Disease and Differential Diagnosis

A.1. What is the diagnosis in this patient?

The most likely diagnosis in this patient is pyloric stenosis. The factors that favor the diagnosis are as follows:

- Age—3 weeks (average age at onset; range 5 days to 5 months)
- Boy child (boy to girl ratio = 4:1)
- Projectile vomiting (characteristic)
- Contents—ingested formula, no bile

The resultant biochemical abnormality in this patient is a hypokalemic, hypochloremic, metabolic alkalosis.

Pyloric stenosis occurs in 3 of 1,000 infants born in the United States; its incidence may be increasing. It is more common in whites of Northern European ancestry, less common in blacks, and rare in Asians.

Behrman RE, Kleigman RM, Jenson HB, et al eds. *Nelson textbook of pediatrics*, 17th ed. Philadelphia: WB Saunders, 2004:1229.

A.2. What is the differential diagnosis of pyloric stenosis?

Pyloric stenosis is distinguished from other congenital anomalies that cause obstruction of the alimentary tract in the newborn. These other anomalies include chalasia of the esophagus, hiatus hernia, duodenal atresia, jejunal atresia, ileal atresia, pancreatic annulus, malrotation of the gut, intraabdominal hernias, and Meckel's diverticulum. Pathognomonic features of pyloric stenosis include absence of bile staining of the vomitus and visible gastric peristaltic waves on abdominal examination along with the palpable pyloric mass. The diagnosis is commonly made clinically. An "olive" is sometimes palpated in the epigastrium just to the right of the midline. Diagnosis can be confirmed by abdominal ultrasound. Occasionally, an upper gastrointestinal (GI) series with barium may be necessary.

Behrman RE, Kleigman RM, Jenson HB, et al eds. *Nelson textbook of pediatrics*, 17th ed. Philadelphia: WB Saunders, 2004:1230.

A.3. What are the metabolic problems in this newborn, secondary to his disease?

Metabolic changes occur secondary to protracted vomiting and comprise the characteristic hypokalemic, hypochloremic alkalosis, as evident in this infant. Hyponatremia, although present, may not be manifested in serum value determinations because of severe dehydration.

Table 21.1 Metabolic Findings in the Newborn Secondary to Pyloric Stenosis.

SEVERITY OF DEHYDRATION	ARTERIAL BLOOD GASES				SERUM ELECTROLYTES			
	PH	P_{CO_2}	CO_2	PO_2	NA	K	CL	HCO_3
Mild	↑	↑	↑	↔	↓↔	↓	↓↓	↑
Moderate	↑↑	↑↑	↑↑	↔	↓	↓↓	↓↓↓	↑↑
Severe	↓↓	↓	↓↓	↓	↓	↓↓	↓↓↓	↓↓

(↔), no change; ↑/↓, slight change; ↑↑/↓↓, moderate change; ↑↑↑/↓↓↓, marked change.

Compensatory respiratory acidosis is a frequent finding; it results from hypoventilation that may be marked and associated with periods of apnea. In severe dehydration leading to circulatory shock, the lack of adequate perfusion coupled with impaired renal and hepatic function may produce an entirely different picture of metabolic acidosis with hyperventilation, resulting in respiratory alkalosis. Therefore, depending on the severity and duration of vomiting and the type of fluid replenishment, one can encounter wide variation in findings on arterial blood gas and electrolyte determinations. However, most frequent findings are hypokalemia, hyponatremia, hypochloremia, and primary metabolic alkalosis with secondary respiratory acidosis. The renal response to vomiting is twofold: serum pH initially is maintained by excretion of alkaline urine with sodium and potassium loss; with depletion of these electrolytes, the kidneys secrete acidic urine (paradoxic acidosis), further increasing the metabolic alkalosis. These findings are summarized in Table 21.1.

Behrman RE, Kleigman RM, Jenson HB, et al. eds. *Nelson textbook of pediatrics*, 16th ed. Philadelphia: WB Saunders, 2004:1229.

Cote' CJ, Todres ID, Goudsouzian NG, et al. eds. *A practice of anesthesia for infants and children*, 3rd ed. WB Saunders, 2001:306–307.

A.4. What are the adverse effects of metabolic alkalosis?

- An increase in pH results in shifting of the oxygen-dissociation curve to the left, thereby binding more oxygen to the hemoglobin and unloading less oxygen at the tissue level. This phenomenon assumes even more importance in newborns because at 3 weeks they still have up to 70% fetal hemoglobin with an already low value of P50 (i.e., 20 to 22 mm Hg).
- Respiratory compensation is affected by hypoventilation with increased potential for atelectasis, as well as periods of apnea.
- Decrease in ionized calcium.
- Increased potential for seizures.

Behrman RE, Kleigman RM, Jenson HB, et al. eds. *Nelson textbook of pediatrics*, 16th ed. Philadelphia: WB Saunders, 2004:1229–1230.

A.5. How would you treat this infant?

Medical management of infant with pyloric stenosis is of acute urgency and should be taken early and vigorously. The principles of management can be grouped under the following three categories: supportive therapy, to stabilize the patient; diagnostic tests, to confirm the diagnosis and to monitor therapy; and surgery as the corrective therapy.

Supportive therapy

- Circulatory support
- Correction of electrolyte imbalance
- Prevention of aspiration

Fluids

The infant with pyloric stenosis is hypovolemic and dehydrated secondary to persistent vomiting. Dehydration severity can vary from mild hypovolemia to circulatory shock. The following parameters are good indicators of dehydration severity:

- Physical appearance—skin turgor, parched mucous membranes, sunken fontanels, sunken eyeballs
- Blood pressure—decreased
- Pulse—increased
- Urine output—decreased
- Weight (birth and present) and weight loss

Quantitative assessment of these parameters gives a fair estimate of the amount of total body fluid depletion. A wide bore intravenous cannula should be placed and an infusion started immediately to correct the deficits and provide maintenance fluids.

Electrolytes

The patient is alkalotic, hypokalemic, hypochloremic, and hyponatremic and must be provided with necessary ions to replenish the deficit. Albumin or Ringer's lactate may be used to treat the shock first. Next, the deficit should be corrected; 0.45% to 0.9% saline is adequate for this purpose. Potassium (usually 40 mEq/L) must be added to this to correct hypokalemia and aid in the correction of alkalosis. However, potassium infusion should be withheld until satisfactory renal function is established. Maintenance fluid should be added to this regimen, and for this purpose 5% dextrose in 0.225% saline is usually adequate.

Prevention of aspiration

A nasogastric tube should be inserted to thoroughly empty the stomach, and the upper airway reflexes should be preserved.

Diagnostic tests

- To assess the severity of fluid and electrolyte derangement and to monitor therapy, the following should be evaluated: complete blood count, serum electrolytes, blood gases, blood urea nitrogen (BUN), electrocardiogram (ECG) (for marked hypokalemia)
- To confirm the diagnosis—barium swallow, ultrasound imaging

Surgery

Pyloromyotomy is the definitive treatment for these infants. Ramstedt pyloromyotomy through a right upper quadrant transverse incision has been the traditional treatment for hypertrophic pyloric stenosis. Recently, laparoscopic and circumumbilical approaches have been introduced as alternative methods to improve cosmesis, but concerns about greater operative times, costs, and complications remain. Surgery should be carried out early, but only after the patient has been stabilized satisfactorily.

Behrman RE, Kleigman RM, Jenson HB, et al. eds. *Nelson textbook of pediatrics*, 17th ed. Philadelphia: WB Saunders, 2004:1230–1231.

Gregory GA, ed. *Pediatric anesthesia*. 4th ed. Churchill Livingstone, 2002:579–580.

Table 21.2 **Estimation of the Degree of Dehydration in a Newborn.**

	MILD	**MODERATE**	**SEVERE**
Percent fluid loss	5	10	15–20
Skin turgor	Poor	Very poor	Parched
Mucous membrane and tongue	Dry	Dry	Parched
Fontanelle and eyes	normal	Sunken fontanelle	Sunken eyes
Urine	Concentrated oliguria	Oliguria	Oliguria, anuria
Pulse	Normal	Tachycardia	Marked tachycardia
Blood pressure	Normal	Hypotension	Marked hypotension, shock

A.6. **How would you determine fluid replacement in a newborn and what fluids would you use?**

The general principles of fluid therapy are based on fluid maintenance, correction of deficits, and replacement of losses.

Maintenance fluids

In the newborn maintenance fluids are as follows:

- First 48 hours of life—75 mL/kg/day or 3 mL/kg/hour
- 2 days to 1 month—150 mL/kg/day or 6 mL/kg/hour
- 1 month onward (up to 10 kg)—100 mL/kg/day or 4 mL/kg/hour

Estimation of the degree of dehydration in a newborn is shown in Table 21.2.

The maintenance fluids take into account the fluid losses occurring normally through the kidney, bowel, skin, and lungs. At birth, the kidney is still undergoing maturation and what may be called "a glomerular imbalance" exists. What it implies is that some mature glomeruli may be connected to the immature tubules and vice versa. Hence, the kidney is functionally limited at birth but undergoes rapid maturation during the first week of life.

Electrolytes

The newborn is an obligate sodium loser as well as a poor tolerator of excessive sodium overload. The maintenance electrolytes are as follows:

- Sodium—3 to 5 mEq/kg/day
- Potassium—2 to 3 mEq/kg/day
- Chloride—1 to 3 mEq/kg/day

Correction of deficits

Deficits take into account the previous unreplaced losses because of a period of no intake by mouth and dehydration resulting from increased losses (e.g., from vomiting, diarrhea, and increased body temperature). The amount of deficit can be assessed by physical examination (see Table 21.2), body weight loss, and hematocrit.

Replacement of losses

Replacing losses covers ongoing abnormal losses not covered by maintenance fluids. Intraoperatively, it covers evaporative losses from the operative site, third spacing, and losses from the lungs if dry gases are used in nonrebreathing circuits (Table 21.3).

The younger and more physically immature the patient, the higher skin permeability, the ratio of body surface area to weight and the metabolic demand. In addition the use of radiant warmers and phototherapy increases insensible water loss.

Table 21.3   Fluid Requirement to Replace Intraoperative Fluid Losses (Except Blood Loss) in the Newborn.

	FLUID REPLACEMENT (mL/kg/hr)
Minor surgery (e.g., herniorrhaphy)	1–3
Moderate surgery (e.g., pyloromyotomy)	3–5
Major surgery (e.g., intestinal)	5–7
Respiratory water loss due to dry gases	2

Miller RD, ed. *Anesthesia*, 6th ed. New York: Churchill Livingstone, 2005:2388–2389.

A.7.   How would you correct the metabolic alkalosis in this patient?

To correct the metabolic alkalosis in this patient the underlying electrolyte derangements (hyponatremia, hypokalemia, and hypochloremia) must be corrected. We correct the deficits by using calculated volumes of 5% dextrose in normal saline or Ringer's lactate solution, which helps to restore sodium and chloride mainly. Dextrose, 5% with one-fourth strength normal saline, may be used to provide maintenance fluids. Once renal function is established, potassium supplements are added to the infusion. Depending on the deficit, this therapy can require anywhere from 12 to 72 hours. In severely alkalotic patients, HCl and NH_4Cl have been used to correct the derangement. However, we have rarely found it necessary.

Barash PG, Cullen BF, Stoelting RK, eds. *Clinical anesthesia*, 5th ed. Philadelphia: Lippincott Williams & Wilkins, 2006:1201–1202.

A.8.   What causes a cardiac murmur?

Cardiac murmurs are caused by turbulent blood flow across cardiac valves or septal defects and are audible sound waves in the range of 20 to 2,000 Hz. Most murmurs in pediatric patients are normal or innocent, occurring in almost 50% of all school-aged children but must be distinguished from those murmurs associated with significant structural heart disease. Auscultation is critically important in diagnosing these murmurs; however, echocardiography remains the gold-standard.

Pelech AN. The cardiac murmur. When to refer? *Pediatr Clin North Am* 1998;45:107–122.

B.   Preoperative Evaluation and Preparation

B.1.   How would you evaluate this patient preoperatively?

The following information is necessary in evaluating this patient:

History

Onset of illness, frequency and amount of vomiting, last feeding, diarrhea, urine output, activity of the newborn (active or lethargic), and birth weight.

Physical examination

Present body weight (to determine the weight loss), temperature, signs of dehydration (skin turgor, mucous membranes, fontanels, eyeballs, blood pressure, pulse, color, and volume of urine), muscle tone, and level of consciousness.

Laboratory findings

Complete blood count, electrolytes, blood urea nitrogen (BUN) and blood sugar, urinalysis, and arterial blood gases.

Based on the data available, we can determine the fluid and electrolyte status of the patient and correct these accordingly to stabilize for surgery and anesthesia.

B.2. How would you evaluate a heart murmur?

Heart murmurs can be innocent or organic. By definition, innocent murmurs occur in the absence of structural or physiologic cardiac disease. The clinical diagnosis of a normal or innocent murmur should occur in the setting of an otherwise normal history, physical examination, and appearance. The presence of a family history of hypertrophic cardiomyopathy; congenital cardiac disease; or unexplained infant, childhood, or early adult death is particularly worrisome. Perinatal history of prematurity, maternal diabetes, drug or toxin ingestion, fetal distress, and clearly definable chromosomal disorders have particular cardiorespiratory relevance. The initial approach to the evaluation of the cardiovascular system should include an assessment of the cardiorespiratory system functionality as a pump and delivery system. An index of exercise or play capacity should be sought as a component of assessing growth and development. I would ask about exercise tolerance, shortness of breath, cyanotic episodes, growth (because congestive heart failure may manifest as failure to thrive), and symptoms of congestive heart failure.

Park MK, ed. *Pediatric cardiology for practitioners*, 4th ed. Mosby, 2002:23–33.

B.3. How would you differentiate between functional versus organic murmur?

Normal murmurs of childhood are comprised of five systolic and two continuous types but never solely diastolic (Table 21.4). A functional murmur is usually soft, 1/6 or 2/6 and never associated with palpable thrill. Pathologic murmurs are usually louder, 3/6 or greater and are associated with other cardiovascular pathologic features.

Park MK, ed. *Pediatric cardiology for practitioners*, 4th ed. Mosby, 2002:23–33.

Table 21.4   Innocent Murmurs of Childhood.

Systolic murmurs	*Continuous murmurs*
Vibratory Still's murmur	Venous hum
Pulmonary flow murmur	Mammary arterial souffle
Peripheral pulmonary artery stenosis murmur	
Supraclavicular systolic murmur	
Aortic systolic murmur	

B.4. What are the types of ventricular septal defect (VSD)? What type of shunt do they cause?

One common classification of VSD is based on anatomic location.

- Type I defects, or supracristal defects (5% of all VSDs), are outflow defects located above the crista supraventricularis just under the annulus of aorta.
- Type II defects, or infracristal defects (80% of all VSDs), are lower in membranous septum beneath the crista supraventricularis.
- Type III defects, or canal type (11% incidence), are inlet VSDs that accompany complete atrioventricular (AV) canal. They result from partial failure of the endocardial cushions to fuse.
- Type IV, or muscular, defects (2% to 7% incidence), probably results from excessive resorption of septal tissue during the muscular septal formation. They may be located anywhere in the muscular septum and may be multiple (also known as the Swiss cheese defect).

VSD is left-to-right shunt. Pathophysiologic effects of VSD include left-to-right shunting, pulmonary hypertension, and heart failure resulting from volume overload.

Park MK, ed. *Pediatric cardiology for practitioners*, 4th ed. Mosby, 2002:133–134.

B.5. What are the risks of surgery and anesthesia in a patient with ventricular septal defect (VSD)?

Infective endocarditis is a complication of most congenital cardiac anomalies, so the patient requires antibiotic prophylaxis. There is also risk of increasing the flow in the shunt or reversing the flow in the shunt, resulting from acute and persistent increases in systemic vascular resistance or decreases in pulmonary vascular resistance causing hypoxemia and congestive heart failure. Right ventricular infundibular hypertrophy may be present in the patients with a VSD. Normally, this is a beneficial change, because it increases the resistance to right ventricular ejection, leading to decrease in magnitude of the left-to-right shunt. Nevertheless, perioperative events that exaggerate this obstruction to right ventricular outflow, such as increased myocardial contractility or hypovolemia, must be minimized. Therefore, these patients are often anesthetized with a volatile anesthetic. In addition, intravascular fluid volume should be maintained by prompt replacement of blood loss. During the anesthetic, a normal end-tidal carbon dioxide should be maintained and routine air bubble precautions should be taken.

Stoelting RK, Dierdorf SF. *Anesthesia and co-existing disease*, 4th ed. New York: Churchill Livingstone, 2002:37–41.

B.6. How would you prepare this patient rapidly for emergency surgery? Is surgical intervention an acute emergency in this case?

Hypertrophic pyloric stenosis is a medical emergency and not a surgical emergency. Therefore, no newborn should be subjected to the additional hazards of anesthesia and surgery until stabilized medically.

Barash PG, Cullen BF, Stoelting RK, eds. *Clinical anesthesia*, 5th ed. Philadelphia: Lippincott Williams & Wilkins, 2006:1201–1202.

B.7. How would you prepare this patient for anesthesia?

Fluid and electrolyte replacement should be accomplished satisfactorily- this may take anywhere from 12 to 72 hours depending on the patient's status. The next step is to empty the stomach through a wide bore nasogastric tube, lavaging out the gastric contents and any leftover barium. Alternatively, an oral-gastric approach allows for passage of a tube with wider lumen that ensures better stomach emptying. Premedication is usually atropine (0.01 to 0.02 mg/kg) intravenous or intramuscular if the patient does not have intravenous line.

Barash PG, Cullen BF, Stoelting RK, eds. *Clinical anesthesia*, 5th ed. Philadelphia: Lippincott Williams & Wilkins, 2006:1201–1202.

Gregory GA, ed. *Pediatric anesthesia*, 4th ed. New York: Churchill Livingstone, 2002:101, 579–580.

C. Intraoperative Management

C.1. Which anesthetic techniques or agents would you use?

These children should arrive to the operating room with an intravenous access. Standard monitors are placed. The stomach is emptied by inserting an orogastric tube after (atropine may be used as premedication). Because the stomach may not be completely emptied, a rapid-sequence induction and intubation with cricoid pressure is highly recommended. Nevertheless, a recent survey of anesthetists in the United Kingdom revealed that 66% of all inductions were performed intravenously with only 56% of cases applying cricoid pressure. There is also some controversy regarding the appropriateness of awake intubations in this situation. A recent study comparing awake, rapid-sequence, or modified rapid-sequence induction demonstrated faster and more successful tracheal intubations in babies whose vocal cords were paralyzed using cis-atracurium (0.4 to 0.5 mg/kg), vecuronium (0.1 to 0.2 mg/kg), or rocuronium (0.6 to 1 mg/kg).

Cook-Sather SD, Tulloch HV, Cnaan A, et al. A comparison of awake versus paralyzed tracheal intubation for infants with pyloric stenosis. *Anesth Analg* 1998;86:945–951.

C.2. What induction–intubation sequence would you use?

The patient can be induced with a mixture of 50% O_2 and 50% N_2O and sevoflurane or halothane, with spontaneous ventilation and gentle assist through the cricoid pressure as respiration is depressed. The trachea is intubated with muscle relaxant but can be intubated without muscle relaxant if sufficient deeper planes of anesthesia are achieved. Awake intubation may be accomplished in skillful hands in a lethargic neonate or in a critically sick infant. In most cases, however, neonates presenting for this procedure are fit and do not require awake intubation, which can be more traumatic.

Barash PG, Cullen BF, Stoelting RK, eds. *Clinical anesthesia*. 5th ed. Philadelphia: Lippincott Williams & Wilkins, 2006:1201–1202.

C.3. What are the anatomic characteristics of the airway in the newborn and how do they differ from those in the adult?

The special characteristics of the upper airway in the newborn are as follows:

Table 21.5 Comparative Anatomy of the Larynx and Trachea in the Newborn and the Adult.

ANATOMIC FEATURES	NEWBORN	ADULT
Size	4 cm	10–13 cm
Shape	Funnel	Cylindrical
Position of the glottis	C3–4	C6
Narrowest point	1 cm below vocal cords	At vocal cords
Vocal cords	Slanting anteriorly	Transverse or slightly Slanting posteriorly
Mucous membrane	Loose (swells easily)	More firmly bound

- Nasopharynx—narrow nasal passages, obligate nasal breathers
- Oropharynx—large tongue, long and pendulous epiglottis
- Larynx—the distinctive features shown in Table 21.5

It is apparent, therefore, that the newborn who has low respiratory reserve can develop airway obstruction easily. The infant may present problems during intubation and tolerate airway trauma poorly.

Comparative anatomy of the larynx and trachea in the newborn and the adult is shown in Table 21.5.

Gregory GA, ed. *Pediatric anesthesia*, 4th ed. New York: Churchill Livingstone, 2002:224–225.

C.4. How do you determine the size of an endotracheal tube in a pediatric patient?

The two parameters of endotracheal tube sizes are the tube length and diameter, depending on the age of the child, as shown in Table 21.6. However, these are approximate sizes and one must have one size bigger and one size smaller tube available when selecting any size tube. A simple way to remember these numbers is to know the sizes at newborn, 6 months, and 1 year. Between 2 and 12 years the following guide may be used:

- Tube length from tip to incisor teeth (cm) = 11+ age in years
- Tube internal diameter (mm) = 4+ age/4
  French size (French) = 18 + age

Table 21.6 Endotracheal Tube Size for Pediatric Patient.

AGE	LENGTH	INTERNAL DIAMETER (mm)	FRENCH SIZES
Newborn	10	3.0	14
6 mo	12	3.5	16
1 y	14	4.0	18
2 y	15	4.5	20
4 y	16	5.0	22
6 y	17	5.5	24
8 y	18	6.0	26
10 y	19	6.5	28
12 y	20	7.0	30

External circumference (French) = ID (mm) × 4 + 2
(French size means external circumference in millimeters, which equals π times external diameter; π = 3.1416)

Barash PG, Cullen BF, Stoelting RK, eds. *Clinical anesthesia*, 5th ed. Philadelphia: Lippincott Williams & Wilkins, 2006:1214–1215.

Gregory GA, ed. *Pediatric anesthesia*, 4th ed. New York: Churchill Livingstone, 2002:206–208.

C.5. What anesthesia system would you use and why?

We employ the circle system with alight circuit. The circle system is more advantageous because it maintains heat and humidification better and offers the freedom of choosing varying gas flows. The controversy about the increased resistance in adult system is discounted by the fact that the respiration is assisted or controlled intraoperatively. Newer anesthesia machines use valves with much less resistance than older models. Dead space in these systems is no more than that of the Mapleson circuits.

Barash PG, Cullen BF, Stoelting RK, eds. *Clinical anesthesia*, 5th ed. Philadelphia: Lippincott Williams & Wilkins, 2006:1215.

C.6. What are the advantages and the disadvantages of commonly employed nonrebreathing systems?

Commonly used nonrebreathing systems include Bain Breathing circuit (Mapleson D system) and Jackson-Rees modification of Ayre's T-piece. They offer the following advantages and disadvantages.

Advantages
- Minimal dead space
- No valves, low resistance
- Lightweight
- Reservoir bag to assist ventilation
- Good appreciation of patient's respiratory exchange

Disadvantages
- High flow of fresh gases required
- Low flows may allow rebreathing of gases without CO_2 absorption
- Loss of heat and humidity because of high flow of cold, dry gases (Bain's circuit allows some heating of inspired gases by surrounding fresh gas flow tubing with expired gas tubing)
- Scavenging problems of waste gases

Barash PG, Cullen BF, Stoelting RK, eds. *Clinical anesthesia*, 5th ed. Philadelphia: Lippincott Williams & Wilkins, 2006:578–585.

Gregory GA, ed. *Pediatric anesthesia*, 4th ed. New York: Churchill Livingstone, 2002:196–206.

C.7. How would you monitor this patient intraoperatively?

Monitoring should include blood pressure, electrocardiogram (ECG), rectal temperature, precordial stethoscope, pulse oximeter, and an end-tidal CO_2 monitor.

C.8. How does the pulse oximeter function?

The commonly used pulse oximeter (Nellcor pulse oximeter Model 100) combines the scientific principles of spectrophotometric oximetry and plethysmography. Light of two wavelengths, 660 nm (red) and 925 nm (infrared), is emitted by a pair of light-emitting diodes (LED) and is passed through the tissue being measured to a photodetector. Because the saturated hemoglobin absorbs more blue light than unsaturated hemoglobin, the absorption of light for each color is an indication of the ratio of oxygen saturated blood to unsaturated blood. The pulsating vascular bed, by expanding and relaxing, creates a change in light-path length that modifies the amount of light detected. The microprocessor-controlled circuitry in the unit senses the pulsatile waveform, which is solely produced by the arterial blood, thereby allowing measurement of pulse rate and arterial saturation. The oximeter is reliably accurate in 50% to 100% saturation range.

Instruction manual. *Nellcor pulse oximeter model N-100, instruction manual.* Hayward: Nellcor Inc, 1984.

Tremper KK, Barker SJ. Pulse oximetry. *Anesthesiology* 1989;70:98–108.

C.9. What factors affect the measurement of oxygen saturation by the pulse oximeter?

Dysfunctional hemoglobin, as with carboxyhemoglobin and methoxyhemoglobin, can affect the accuracy of the oximeter. Intravascular dyes such as cardiogreen can also interfere with the accuracy of the instrument. Skin color, tissue thickness, venous blood, light intensity, and ambient light do not affect the accuracy of the instrument because they do not pulse.

Instruction manual. *Nellcor pulse oximeter model N-100, instruction manual.* Hayward: Nellcor Inc, 1984.

Tremper KK, Barker SJ. Pulse oximetry. *Anesthesiology* 1989;70:98–108.

D. Postoperative Management

D.1. What are the complications that can occur in the postanesthesia recovery period?

The patient should be carefully observed for signs of respiratory depression and periods of apnea secondary to combination of metabolic alkalosis, general anesthesia, and decreased body temperature. However, these infants do not appear to be at increased risk of postoperative apnea. Hypoventilation predisposes to atelectasis. Patient should be awake and responsive to avoid aspiration. Severe hypoglycemia resulting from depletion of liver glycogen stores has been reported 2 to 3 hours after surgery. Postextubation "croup" is a potentially dangerous complication in this age group.

Barash PG, Cullen BF, Stoelting RK, eds. *Clinical anesthesia*, 5th ed. Philadelphia: Lippincott Williams & Wilkins, 2006:1201–1202.

Chipps BE, Moynihan R, Schieble T, et al. Infants undergoing pyloromyotomy are not at risk for postoperative apnea. *Pediatr Pulmonol* 1999;27:278.

D.2. How would you treat postextubation "croup" in this infant?

Treatment of the potentially catastrophic postextubation laryngeal edema should be immediate, vigorous, and carried out under direct observation of the anesthesiologists. It consists of the following:

- Increasing inspired oxygen concentration (50% to 60%)
- Humidification of inspired gases
- Adequate hydration using parenteral fluids
- Light sedation to calm the patient and allow for cooperation in therapy
- Avoidance of any significant respiratory depression
- Epinephrine through hand-held nebulizer and mask, 50 μg/kg/minute of active isomer
  - Racemic epinephrine (2.25%) 0.05 mL per kg diluted in 5-mL saline solution delivered in 10 minutes

Treatment should be given over 10 minutes and may be repeated every 30 minutes, as necessary. Rebound phenomenon may be expected approximately 2 hours after cessation of this therapy.

- Steroids—dexamethasone, 0.5 to 1 mg per kg intravenously
- Reintubation—if signs of deterioration or hypoxia appear
- Tracheostomy, if necessary—rarely, subglottic edema may be so rapid and so severe that tracheostomy is the only choice

The age group most likely to manifest this complication is 1 to 4 years. Infants younger than 1 year are at most risk, mainly because of the size of the airway. Fortunately, an infant of this age is most amenable to early and vigorous intervention and should always be treated as an emergency requiring the continued presence of and evaluation by a physician who is adept at securing an airway for the child.

Hall S. The child with a difficult airway: recognition and management. *ASA annual meeting refresher course lectures*. Park Ridge: American Society of Anesthesiologists, 2006:412.

SECTION IV

The Nervous System

CHAPTER 22

Brain Tumor and Craniotomy

KANE O. PRYOR • HUGH C. HEMMINGS, JR.

A PREVIOUSLY HEALTHY 47-YEAR-OLD WOMAN

presents with a 4-month history of headache, with intermittent diplopia and limb ataxia developing over the last month. She is admitted following an episode of vomiting and lethargy. Physical examination reveals bilateral papilledema, nystagmus, and subtle cranial nerve V, VII, and VIII signs on the right. Magnetic resonance imaging (MRI) shows a large, right posterior fossa mass consistent with a petroclival meningioma, exerting mass effect on the pons and fourth ventricle. Computed tomography angiogram shows a highly vascular tumor with the principal blood supply arising from the ascending pharyngeal branch of the external carotid artery. The patient is scheduled for craniotomy and resection of the tumor. Two days before the surgery, the patient underwent cerebral angiography and embolization of the tumor. The anesthetic course during that case was uneventful. The operative report states that there are "substantial residual feeding arteries."

A. Medical Disease and Differential Diagnosis

1. What are the determinants of intracranial pressure (ICP)?
2. How does the presence of a mass alter the ICP in this patient?
3. What are the determinants of cerebral blood flow (CBF), and how are they altered by the presence of an intracranial tumor?
4. Are there any issues specific to posterior cranial fossa pathology?

5. What are the cerebral steal syndromes?
6. What is the role of preoperative embolization therapy?

B. Preoperative Evaluation and Preparation

1. What is the approach to the preoperative evaluation of the posterior fossa craniotomy patient?
2. If the patient had presented with intracranial hypertension, what management may have already been initiated preoperatively, and what are the implications for anesthetic management?
3. How will intraoperative electromyogram (EMG), sensory evoked potential (SEP) or brainstem auditory evoked response (BAER) monitoring affect the anesthetic management plan?
4. What are the options for patient positioning during posterior fossa surgery?
5. What are the principal disadvantages associated with the common posterior fossa craniotomy positions?
6. How should the patient position ultimately be determined?
7. If the surgeon insists that the surgery should be performed in the sitting position, how will this affect your preoperative assessment and planning?
8. Should this patient receive premedication?

C. Intraoperative Management

1. What are the anesthetic goals for craniotomy?
2. What monitors should be used during craniotomy?
3. What specific risks are associated with induction?
4. How would you induce anesthesia?
5. What are the effects of anesthetics on cerebral metabolic rate of oxygen ($CMRo_2$), cerebral blood flow (CBF), and intracranial pressure (ICP)? With this in mind, how would you maintain anesthesia?
6. How would you approach the management of CO_2?
7. How would you approach diuretic therapy?
8. How would you manage serum glucose?
9. How will you approach maintenance fluid management?
10. Once the bone plate is removed and the dura retracted, the surgeon reports that the brain is still "tight." In consideration of the issues discussed above, what would be your response?
11. If deliberate hypotension is indicated, how would you achieve it?
12. While the surgeon is resecting tumor from near the brainstem, the patient's heart rate suddenly drops to 20. What is your assessment and management?
13. Would you monitor for venous air embolism (VAE)? What are the monitoring options?
14. Are there any measures you can take to prevent VAE?
15. During the procedure, the precordial Doppler becomes loud and turbulent. The end-tidal carbon dioxide ($ETCO_2$) drops from 31 mm Hg to 13 mm Hg, and the systemic pressure from 121/63 mm Hg to 64/32 mm Hg. What is your assessment and management?
16. What is your approach to emergence? What if the patient does not wake up?

D. Postoperative Management

1. What postoperative complications are of greatest concern? What level of monitoring is required?

A. Medical Disease and Differential Diagnosis

A.1. What are the determinants of intracranial pressure (ICP)?

The intracranial cavity is a rigid structure with minimal compliance. The structures within this cavity can be conceived of as belonging to one of three compartments:

- The *parenchymal compartment*, which is made up of two subcompartments—the cellular compartment, consisting of the neuronal, glial, and tumor cells, and the fluid compartment, consisting of intracellular and extracellular fluid;
- The *cerebrospinal fluid (CSF) compartment*; and
- The *blood compartment*, consisting of the arterial and venous subcompartments.

If the volume of any one of these compartments increases, there is limited compensatory potential. Initially, CSF can drain to the spinal CSF reservoir, and venous blood to the extracranial veins. Therefore, during the early phase of intracranial volume expansion, only a minimal increase in ICP may occur. However, at a critical point these compensatory mechanisms are exhausted, and even small increases in intracranial volumes will result in significant increases in ICP. As ICP increases, the pressure gradient may eventually lead to herniation of brain tissue through a noncompliant space—rapidly resulting in often irreversible injury.

Normal ICP is 5 to 15 mm Hg. Normal adult brain tissue volume is approximately 1,400 mL, intracranial CSF volume is 75 to 100 mL, and cerebral vascular volume is approximately 150 mL.

Bergsneider M, Becker D. Intracranial pressure monitoring. In: Cottrell J, Smith D, eds. *Anesthesia and neurosurgery*, 4th ed. St. Louis: Mosby, 2001:101–113.

A.2. How does the presence of a mass alter the intracranial pressure (ICP) in this patient?

As the intracranial cavity is essentially of fixed volume, the volume of any intracranial mass must be accommodated by reduction in the volume of other intracranial contents. The neurological sequelae of the mass will be determined largely by its anatomic location and the rapidity of growth. Elevated ICP in the presence of supratentorial masses is usually the result of their direct space occupying effects. This may also be true of masses in the posterior fossa, but in addition, these masses may obstruct cerebrospinal fluid (CSF) outflow at the fourth ventricle, resulting in a noncommunicating hydrocephalus and elevated ICP. Slow-growing tumors, such as meningiomas, can become astoundingly large without causing substantial increases in ICP as volume remodeling occurs; this is especially true of supratentorial hemispheric tumors. Conversely, even small fast-growing tumors in critical neuroanatomic locations in the posterior fossa may rapidly lead to symptoms of elevated ICP, especially if CSF outflow is obstructed. It is important to remember that while compensatory mechanisms may be able to maintain a normal or near-normal ICP, the patient with an intracranial mass will always have diminished reserve to accommodate increases in the volume of other intracranial contents.

In this patient, a slow-growing meningioma has been able to attain a large size before becoming symptomatic. The patient is demonstrating early signs and symptoms of elevated ICP, which most likely results from the combination of mass effect and obstruction of CSF outflow at the fourth ventricle. This patient would have very little volume reserve; even small further increases in volume—such as an increase in cerebral blood volume (CBV)—would likely cause a precipitous spike in ICP.

Langfitt TW. Increased intracranial pressure. *Clin Neurosurg* 1969;16:436–471.

Ropper AH. Lateral displacement of the brain and level of consciousness in patients with an acute hemispheral mass. *N Engl J Med* 1986;314:953–958.

A.3. What are the determinants of cerebral blood flow (CBF), and how are they altered by the presence of an intracranial tumor?

The brain receives a disproportionate percentage of cardiac output, due to its high metabolic requirement ($\sim$3.5 mL O_2/minute/100 g brain tissue). CBF is coupled to cerebral metabolic rate (CMR). At a wide range of mean arterial pressures (MAPs), the cerebral circulation alters its resistance to maintain a constant CBF—this is termed *autoregulation*. When intracranial pressure (ICP) is normal, autoregulation maintains constant CBF between MAPs of approximately 50 to 150 mm Hg. Above and below these values, CBF will be pressure-dependent. In the presence of chronic hypertension, autoregulation will be shifted to occur at higher values.

CBF also varies with changes in $Paco_2$ between values of approximately 25 and 100 mm Hg. Increasing the $Paco_2$ from 40 to 80 mm Hg will roughly double CBF, and decreasing from 40 to 20 mm Hg will halve the CBF.

The presence of an intracranial mass may cause localized regions of high tissue pressure gradients, inflammation, and ischemia. These may all contribute to a dysfunction of normal autoregulation; therefore, in the brain regions surrounding the mass, regional cerebral blood flow (rCBF) may be pressure-dependent over a greater range of pressures than in normal tissue. Further, if ICP become elevated above the level of the central venous pressure (CVP), the cerebral perfusion pressure (CPP = MAP − ICP) decreases. The ability of autoregulation to compensate for decreases in CPP is limited, and therefore in the presence of elevated ICP, CBF may be low even in the presence of normally adequate MAPs.

Giulioni M, Ursino M. Impact of cerebral perfusion pressure and autoregulation on intracranial dynamics: a modeling study. *Neurosurgery* 1996;39:1005–1014.

Schaller B, Graf R. Different compartments of intracranial pressure and its relationship to cerebral blood flow. *J Trauma* 2005;59:1521–1531.

A.4. Are there any issues specific to posterior cranial fossa pathology?

Surgery for tumors in the posterior fossa presents several challenges not seen with supratentorial surgery. The posterior fossa is a tightly enclosed space in which tumors are often in direct contact with highly critical structures, such as cranial nerves or the brainstem. The margin for error when operating near these structures is extremely small, as can be the spatial reserve for postoperative inflammation. Indeed, the patient with a posterior fossa tumor may worsen neurologically in the hours following surgery due to edema or hematoma formation, and this possibility must be considered when determining the appropriateness of extubation and postoperative management.

In addition to the risk for neuronal damage, surgery in the proximity of the brainstem nuclei can trigger significant intraoperative autonomic and collateral hemodynamic instability, which can be extremely challenging to manage. The risk to cranial nerves and other structures often demands intraoperative neurophysiologic monitoring—such as sensory evoked potentials (SEPs), brainstem auditory evoked potentials (BAEPs), or electromyography (EMG)—all of which can substantially restrict and dictate anesthetic management.

Finally, the posterior fossa cannot be accessed with the patient in the conventional supine position. The positions that do permit access to the posterior fossa all present unique difficulties (see subsequent text), most notably the risk of venous air embolism (VAE) and jugular venous outflow obstruction.

Drummond JC, Todd MM. Acute sinus arrhythmia during surgery in the fourth ventricle: an indicator of brainstem irritation. *Anesthesiology* 1984;60:232–235.

Little KM, Friedman AH, Sampson JH, et al. Surgical management of petroclival meningiomas: defining resection goals based on risk of neurological morbidity and tumor recurrence rates in 137 patients. *Neurosurgery* 2005;56:546–559.

Patel S, Wen D, Haines S. Posterior fossa: surgical considerations. In: Cottrell J, Smith D, eds. *Anesthesia and neurosurgery*, 4th ed. St. Louis: Mosby, 2001:319–334.

A.5. What are the cerebral steal syndromes?

Any intracranial pathology, including marginal ischemia and inflammation surrounding a mass lesion, may cause a localized dysfunction of normal cerebral autoregulation and response to vasoactive agents. Therefore, the microvasculature in the pathologic region may have an essentially fixed resistance. In this case, if vasodilation occurs in other normal regions of the brain, the decreased vascular resistance in the normal tissue will theoretically shunt blood flow away from the pathologic regions, which are already most vulnerable. This phenomenon is known as *"cerebral steal."* In anesthesia management, cerebral steal is most relevant in the context of hypercapnia and the use of high concentrations (>1 MAC) of volatile anesthetics. Both of these will cause vasodilation of normal vasculature and potentially cause decreased regional cerebral blood flow (CBF) in pathological areas. During hypocapnia, when there is vasoconstriction in normal tissue, the opposite may occur. In this case, blood flow to pathologic regions may actually increase. This phenomenon is known as *"inverse steal"* or the *"Robin Hood Effect."* The clinical relevance of steal and inverse steal phenomena has never been established.

Artru AA, Merriman HG. Hypocapnia added to hypertension to reverse EEG changes during carotid endarterectomy. *Anesthesiology* 1989;70:1016–1018.

Darby JM, Yonas H, Marion DW, et al. Local "inverse steal" induced by hyperventilation in head injury. *Neurosurgery* 1988;23:84–88.

Sato K, Shirane R, Kato M, et al. Effect of inhalational anesthesia on cerebral circulation in Moyamoya disease. *J Neurosurg Anesthesiol* 1999;11:25 30.

A.6. What is the role of preoperative embolization therapy?

Highly vascular tumors, especially those that are anatomically difficult to access, present a high risk of substantial intraoperative bleeding. In addition to the systemic risks associated with gross blood loss, surgical exposure may be severely compromised, and neuronal and neurovascular inflammation and irritation exacerbated by excessive tracking of blood into brain tissue.

To reduce this risk, patients will often undergo embolization of the feeding vessels in the days immediately before the surgery. An arterial catheter is inserted, usually in the femoral artery, and guided under fluoroscopy to vessels that are supplying only the tumor. A viscous "glue" (usually polyvinyl chloride [PVC] based) is delivered, which occludes the vessel, thereby reducing the vascularity of the tumor. Vascular anatomy may not always permit embolization, and embolization itself may precipitate swelling and hyperemic changes in blood flow dynamics, which must be considered.

Dowd CF, Halbach VV, Higashida RT. Meningiomas: the role of preoperative angiography and embolization. *Neurosurg Focus* 2003;15:E10.

Engelhard HH. Progress in the diagnosis and treatment of patients with meningiomas. Part I: diagnostic imaging, preoperative embolization. *Surg Neurol* 2001;55:89–101.

B. Preoperative Evaluation and Preparation

B.1. What is the approach to the preoperative evaluation of the posterior fossa craniotomy patient?

In addition to the thorough preoperative evaluation required for all anesthetic patients, the evaluation of the craniotomy patient should answer several questions that critically affect anesthesia management:

- What is the patient's intracranial pressure (ICP) and its relation to the intracranial compliance curve?
- How is autoregulation likely to be affected by the pathology and chronic changes in blood pressure?
- Does the patient have any of the electrolyte and endocrine abnormalities associated with intracranial pathology?
- Is the lesion highly vascular, or difficult to access?
- What is the likely positioning, and does it incur a risk of venous air embolism (VAE) or obstruction of jugular venous outflow?
- Will the neurological status affect the ability to extubate or to establish an early neurological assessment after general anesthesia?
- Will the anesthetic technique need to accommodate specific monitoring requirements, such as electroencephalography (EEG), electrocorticography, brainstem auditory evoked responses (BAERs), or sensory evoked potentials (SEPs)?

Fischer SP. Preoperative evaluation of the adult neurosurgical patient. *Int Anesthesiol Clin* 1996;34:21–32.

Jellish WS, Murdoch J, Leonetti JP. Perioperative management of complex skull base surgery: the anesthesiologist's point of view. *Neurosurg Focus* 2002;12:e5.

Smith D, Osborn I. Posterior fossa: anesthetic considerations. In: Cottrell J, Smith D, eds. *Anesthesia and neurosurgery*, 4th ed. St. Louis: Mosby, 2001:335–352.

B.2. If the patient had presented with intracranial hypertension, what management may have already been initiated preoperatively, and what are the implications for anesthetic management?

A patient with evidence of intracranial hypertension will be aggressively monitored and treated preoperatively; it is likely that your preoperative assessment will occur in an intensive care setting. The anesthesiologist should be aware of the implications of preoperative management of intracranial hypertension.

A likely hierarchy of management, and some common implications for anesthetic management, is as follows:

- *Corticosteriods.* May have resulted in hyperglycemia, which should be aggressively treated.
- *Head elevation.* Care should be taken to avoid rapidly lowering the head during transport.
- *Diuretics (mannitol, furosemide).* May result in electrolyte or acid-base abnormalities. Decreased preload may increase the risk of hypotension in the peri-induction period.
- *Iso- or hypertonic saline therapy.* May have resulted in hypernatremia, or a hyperchloremic, non-anion gap metabolic acidosis.
- *Intubation and institution of hyperventilation.* If prolonged, cerebral blood flow (CBF) response may be diminished or absent, with risk of increase in CBF and intracranial pressure (ICP) if hyperventilation is rapidly ceased. Can lead to underlying compensatory metabolic acidosis. Care should be taken to avoid hypoventilation during transport.

- *Ventriculostomy.* Should be clamped during transport, because of difficulty in maintaining appropriate level. Should be attended to on arrival to operating room, as even relatively short periods of clamping can result in elevations of ICP.
- *Manipulation of systemic pressures to optimize cerebral perfusion pressure (CPP).* Care should be taken to ensure drug infusions are maintained during transport to avoid rebound hypertension or hypotension.
- *Drug-induced cerebral vasoconstriction and/or coma.* Thiopental is usually used. This signifies a critical neurological status. The therapy is often continued as the primary anesthetic.
- *Deliberate hypothermia.* Signifies a critical neurological status. Requires discussion of intraoperative temperature management goals with the neurosurgeon, as the neuroprotective benefits may be countered by hypothermia-induced coagulopathy.

Stevens RD, Bhardwaj A. Evolving paradigms in the management of severe traumatic brain injury. *Crit Care Med* 2005;33:2415–2417.

Vincent JL, Berre J. Primer on medical management of severe brain injury. *Crit Care Med* 2005;33:1392–1399.

B.3. How will intraoperative electromyography (EMG), sensory evoked potential (SEP) or brainstem auditory evoked response (BAER) monitoring affect the anesthetic management plan?

The most common EMG monitoring during posterior fossa surgery is for cranial nerve VII, although monitoring of V, IX, X, and XI is frequently encountered. Usually, the surgeon will deliver a very low current to a structure they believe could be the cranial nerve of interest, and muscular activity is monitored in the distribution of the nerve; mechanical manipulation of a nerve will often also cause muscular activity. Therefore, during EMG monitoring, muscle relaxants should not be used.

The most common evoked potential monitoring encountered during resection of posterior fossa tumors is the BAER, which monitors cranial nerve VIII. Somatosensory evoked potentials (SSEPs) can also be used to monitor cortical integrity. Many common anesthetic drugs cause decreases in amplitude and increases in latency of the responses, thereby mimicking neuronal ischemia or trauma. Volatile agents should be kept at less than 0.5 MAC, and nitrous oxide should not be used. The anesthetic plan will often rely heavily on opioids; low-dose propofol infusions are also often incorporated. Importantly, the anesthetic should be kept constant throughout the monitoring phase—an infusion pump device greatly facilitates this goal.

Fisher RS, Raudzens P, Nunemacher M. Efficacy of intraoperative neurophysiological monitoring. *J Clin Neurophysiol* 1995;12:97–109.

Harper CM. Intraoperative cranial nerve monitoring. *Muscle Nerve* 2004;29:339–351.

Peterson DO, Drummond JC, Todd MM. Effects of halothane, enflurane, isoflurane, and nitrous oxide on somatosensory evoked potentials in humans. *Anesthesiology* 1986;65:35–40.

B.4. What are the options for patient positioning during posterior fossa surgery?

- *Sitting position.* Although this has fallen out of favor, it is important for the anesthesiologist to understand. The patient is in a reclined sitting posture, such that the feet are at or near the level of the heart. The head is held in a flexed position with a skull fixation device, and the arms crossed over the chest.
- *Prone position.* This is especially suitable for lesions in the midline. Depending upon body habitus, supporting rolls may be placed horizontally across the chest and hips, or in parallel

along the longitudinal axis of the body. The head is held with a skull fixation device with the neck in a flexed position.

- *Lateral decubitus position.* This is suited to cerebellopontine angle tumors and cerebellar hemispheric lesions.
- *Park bench (semiprone) position.* The patient is turned toward a more prone position, moving the upper shoulder out of the surgeon's view, and permitting better access to midline lesions.
- *Supine position.* This can sometimes be used with the patient's head rotated. To reduce the amount of rotation of the neck, which may obstruct venous outflow, a supporting roll may be placed under the ipsilateral shoulder, and the whole bed rotated away from the surgeon.

Black S, Ockert DB, Oliver WC Jr, et al. Outcome following posterior fossa craniectomy in patients in the sitting or horizontal positions. *Anesthesiology* 1988;69:49–56.

Kikuta KI, Miyamoto S, Kataoka H, et al. Use of the prone oblique position in surgery for posterior fossa lesions. *Acta Neurochir (Wien)* 2004;146:1119–1124.

Orliaguet GA, Hanafi M, Meyer PG, et al. Is the sitting or the prone position best for surgery for posterior fossa tumours in children. *Paediatr Anaesth* 2001;11:541–547. ?

Porter JM, Pidgeon C, Cunningham AJ. The sitting position in neurosurgery: a critical appraisal. *Br J Anaesth* 1999;82:117–128.

B.5. What are the principal disadvantages associated with the common posterior fossa craniotomy positions?

In the sitting position, the head is elevated well above the right atrium, and usually greater than the height of the central venous fluid column. This will reduce venous bleeding; however, it will also make it much easier for large volumes of air to be entrained into the central venous circulation, especially through the large dural sinuses, which are tented open. When propagated through the right heart to the pulmonary circulation, this will cause a venous air embolism (VAE), which can range in severity from the subclinical to precipitating acute hemodynamic collapse and death. In a patient with a patent foramen ovale (PFO), air can traverse to the arterial circulation, causing embolic strokes. Although VAE can occur with the other positions, the risk and severity is substantially higher in the sitting position. The risk is such that a right heart catheter is almost obligatory, the placement of which incurs associated risks of pneumothorax, infection, bleeding, and arrhythmias. Further, the treatment of VAE is complicated by the sitting position, as it is difficult to rapidly move the patient's head below the level of the heart. The sitting position is also associated with increased hypotension. As neurosurgeons have gained experience in accessing the posterior fossa from other positions, the risks associated with the sitting position have caused its popularity to dramatically decrease.

In the prone position, the head is usually slightly elevated above the heart; therefore there is a risk of VAE, although it is much less than in the sitting position. Prone positioning can cause a significant decrease in pulmonary compliance, and will increase ventilation-perfusion mismatch, leading to atelectasis, venous admixture, and shunting. There is virtually no access to the airway, chest, or limbs, and therefore in the event of an airway, pulmonary, or cardiovascular emergency, the prone position places the anesthesiologist in a substantially compromised position.

The supine position alleviates many of the issues described preceding text. However, to access even the lateral posterior fossa from the supine position usually requires substantial rotation of the neck. This can cause obstruction of jugular venous outflow, leading to cerebral venous engorgement, with potentially undesirable effects on intracranial pressure (ICP), cerebral perfusion pressure (CPP), surgical exposure, and bleeding. The neck rotation can also cause brachial plexus injury as well as significant pressure on laryngeal structures with potential vocal cord injury.

Black S, Ockert DB, Oliver WC Jr, et al. Outcome following posterior fossa craniectomy in patients in the sitting or horizontal positions. *Anesthesiology* 1988;69:49–56.

Porter JM, Pidgeon C, Cunningham AJ. The sitting position in neurosurgery: a critical appraisal. *Br J Anaesth* 1999;82:117–128.

B.6. How should the patient position ultimately be determined?

Surgical exposure will be the principal determinant of patient position. However, because interruption of a posterior fossa craniotomy for anesthesia crisis management is highly undesirable, the anesthesiologist and neurosurgeon should discuss alternate positioning if there are significant anesthetic concerns. For example, alternatives to the prone position should be sought for patients with minimal pulmonary reserve and/or very large body habitus. The risk of venous air embolism (VAE) is such that we are very reluctant to use the sitting position except where the surgical exposure considerations are overwhelming.

B.7. If the surgeon insists that the surgery should be performed in the sitting position, how will this affect your preoperative assessment and planning?

The first step is to establish whether the patient has any contraindications to the sitting position that might have been overlooked. The presence of any intracardiac defects, pulmonary arteriovenous malformations, or carotid artery stenosis should be sought. The presence of a patent foramen ovale (PFO) can lead to a catastrophic paradoxical air embolus if air is entrained; this has led to some advocacy for routine preoperative echocardiography, although it is not commonly performed. The presence of any of these comorbidities argues against use of the sitting position, and must be discussed with the surgeon. Severe hypovolemia, cachexia, and extremes of age may diminish the ability of autonomic reflexes to maintain adequate cerebral and upper lung perfusion in the upright position, leading to extremely difficult intraoperative cardiopulmonary management. It must always be remembered that the critical pressure is the cerebral perfusion pressure (CPP), and not the mean arterial pressure (MAP), and that pressure must therefore be evaluated at the level of the head.

Anesthesia planning must recognize the physiological implications of the sitting position. Venous pooling will result in lower left atrial filling pressures, leading to reduced stroke volume and cardiac output. Although there will be an increase in both systemic and pulmonary vascular resistance, the net effect is a tendency to arterial hypotension, leading to decreased CPP. The temptation to counter reduced preload with intraoperative fluid administration may run counter to attempts to diurese, and may result in an exaggerated increase in filling when the patient in repositioned supine at the conclusion of surgery. Conversely, it must be understood that because the hypotension is not the result of afterload reduction, the use of vasopressors, while increasing arterial pressures, may have the effect of reducing organ blood flow. Due to the beneficial effects of gravity, pulmonary compliance and functional residual capacity (FRC) are greater in the sitting position than in the horizontal positions; however, the simultaneous cardiovascular effects may lead to increased ventilation–perfusion mismatch, countering any significant benefit.

Finally, if the sitting position is to be adopted, there must be a preoperative plan for the detection and management of venous air embolism (VAE), should it occur. The patient's neck must be evaluated to assess for any difficulties in the placement of a right atrial catheter. In some patients, such as those who have previously had chemotherapy or dialysis through central catheters, those who have had prior neck irradiation, and those who are morbidly obese, placement of a right atrial catheter may be extremely difficult or impossible, and necessitates the consideration of alternate positions, or radiologically-guided placement preoperatively.

Dalrymple DG, MacGowan SW, MacLeod GF. Cardiorespiratory effects of the sitting position in neurosurgery. *Br J Anaesth* 1979;51:1079–1082.

Guggiari M, Lechat P, Garen-Colonne C, et al. Early detection of patent foramen ovale by two-dimensional contrast echocardiography for prevention of paradoxical air embolism during sitting position. *Anesth Analg* 1988;67:192–194.

Kwapisz MM, Deinsberger W, Muller M, et al. Transesophageal echocardiography as a guide for patient positioning before neurosurgical procedures in semi-sitting position. *J Neurosurg Anesthesiol* 2004;16:277–281.

Perkins-Pearson NA, Marshall WK, Bedford RF. Atrial pressures in the seated position: implication for paradoxical air embolism. *Anesthesiology* 1982;57:493–497.

Stendel R, Gramm HJ, Schroder K, et al. Transcranial Doppler ultrasonography as a screening technique for detection of a patent foramen ovale before surgery in the sitting position. *Anesthesiology* 2000;93:971–975.

Tindall GT, Craddock A, Greenfield JC Jr. Effects of the sitting position on blood flow in the internal carotid artery of man during general anesthesia. *J Neurosurg* 1967;26:383–389.

B.8. Should this patient receive premedication?

With rare exceptions, standard pharmacologic approaches to premedication should be avoided in patients with intracranial pathology. Benzodiazepenes and other psychoactive drugs may confound the ability to accurately assess changes in neurological function. Opioids may precipitate hypoventilation, leading to hypercapnia and increased cerebral blood flow (CBF); in a patient with minimal compliance reserve, such as this patient, even a small increase in CBF may precipitate a dangerous increase in intracranial pressure (ICP). A professional and unrushed visit by the anesthesiologist remains the optimal approach to preoperative anxiolysis.

Costello TG, Cormack JR. Clonidine premedication decreases hemodynamic responses to pin head-holder application during craniotomy. *Anesth Analg* 1998;86:1001–1004.

Tohmo H, Karanko M, Scheinin M, et al. Enalapril premedication attenuates the blood pressure response to tracheal intubation and stabilizes postoperative blood pressure after controlled hypotension with sodium nitroprusside in neurovascular patients. *J Neurosurg Anesthesiol* 1993;5:13–21.

C. Intraoperative Management

C.1. What are the anesthetic goals for craniotomy?

The anesthetic goals specific to craniotomy aim to directly or indirectly protect the brain from further injury due to mechanical or physiologic insult during the perioperative period. The principal elements are as follows:

- Management of intracranial pressure (ICP), especially before the removal of the bone plate
- Management of cerebral blood flow (CBF) and cerebral perfusion pressure (CPP)
- Provide a "relaxed" brain. This will optimize surgical exposure (critically important as the field of view may be extremely narrow), and will reduce the pressure exerted by the retraction devices on underlying brain tissue (which may lead to ischemia)
- Implement any pharmacological measures that may help directly protect brain tissue, such as inducing burst-suppression

- Minimize the anesthetic interference with neuronal monitoring modalities, such as electroencephalography (EEG), brainstem auditory evoked responses (BAERs), or somatosensory evoked potentials (SSEPs)
- Facilitate an early neurologic assessment

Bekker AY, Mistry A, Ritter AA, et al. Computer simulation of intracranial pressure changes during induction of anesthesia: comparison of thiopental, propofol, and etomidate. *J Neurosurg Anesthesiol* 1999;11:69–80.

Jellish WS, Murdoch J, Leonetti JP. Perioperative management of complex skull base surgery: the anesthesiologist's point of view. *Neurosurg Focus* 2002;12:e5.

Leslie K, Troedel S. Does anaesthesia care affect the outcome following craniotomy? *J Clin Neurosci* 2002;9:231–236.

Peterson DO, Drummond JC, Todd MM. Effects of halothane, enflurane, isoflurane, and nitrous oxide on somatosensory evoked potentials in humans. *Anesthesiology* 1986; 65:35–40.

C.2. What monitors should be used during craniotomy?

As with all patients undergoing general anesthesia, monitoring must include electrocardiography (ECG), blood pressure, pulse oximetry temperature, and capnography. Placement of an arterial line is routine for tumor craniotomies, and should be regarded as mandatory for everything except the most superficial and nonvascular supratentorial tumors. Arterial lines can often be placed following induction, but should be placed before induction in patients with significantly deranged autoregulation or minimal intracranial compliance reserve, as cerebral blood flow (CBF) and perfusion will be highly pressure dependent in such situations. The arterial line transducer should be zeroed at the level of the Circle of Willis. The decision on whether to place a central venous line for central venous pressure (CVP) or right heart monitoring is generally determined by the patient's overall physiological state, and usually offers very little, if any, benefit in a generally healthy patient. One exception is during posterior fossa procedures in the sitting position, in which case a right heart catheter should be placed.

In any case where there is a risk of venous air embolism (VAE), precordial Doppler monitoring (or some other detection method such as transesophageal echocardiography [TEE] or end-tidal N_2) should be used. The use of neurophysiology monitoring, such as electroencephalography (EEG), electromyography (EMG), brainstem auditory evoked responses (BAERs), or somatosensory evoked potentials (SSEPs) will be determined by the location of the tumor; although often performed by neurophysiologists, the anesthesiologist should understand the principles of these methods and be able to interpret basic elements.

C.3. What specific risks are associated with induction?

An unstable induction is, of course, not desirable for any general anesthetic. However, the patient with intracranial pathology will have dramatically diminished ability to compensate for the hemodynamic changes occurring during induction. Hypotension may result in inadequate cerebral perfusion pressure (CPP) and cerebral ischemia, whereas hypertension and sympathetic activation may lead to hyperemia, increased cerebral blood flow (CBF) and volume, and increased intracranial pressure (ICP). The implication of rapid changes in $Paco_2$ are often underappreciated—hypoventilation as the patient is sedated will increase cerebral blood volume (CBV), and may be sufficient to lead to decompensation in a patient with minimal ICP reserve. Episodes of coughing, especially relevant if the airway has to be secured by an awake fiberoptic technique, will precipitate short but dramatic increases in ICP. Finally, hypoxia will be very poorly tolerated by brain tissue with marginal reserve.

Bozeman WP, Idris AH. Intracranial pressure changes during rapid sequence intubation: a swine model. *J Trauma* 2005;58:278–283.

Lanier WL, Albrecht RF 2nd, Laizzo PA. Divergence of intracranial and central venous pressures in lightly anesthetized, tracheally intubated dogs that move in response to a noxious stimulus. *Anesthesiology* 1996;84:605–613.

Petersen KD, Landsfeldt U, Cold GE, et al. Intracranial pressure and cerebral hemodynamic in patients with cerebral tumors: a randomized prospective study of patients subjected to craniotomy in propofol-fentanyl, isoflurane-fentanyl, or sevoflurane-fentanyl anesthesia. *Anesthesiology* 2003;98:329–336.

Pinaud M, Lelausque JN, Chetanneau A, et al. Effects of propofol on cerebral hemodynamics and metabolism in patients with brain trauma. *Anesthesiology* 1990;73:404–409.

C.4. How would you induce anesthesia?

The specific drug combinations used during induction are less important than the ultimate goal of maintaining tight hemodynamic stability during the periinduction period. We favor an opioid-based intravenous or mixed intravenous-inhalational induction. After thorough preoxygenation and the administration of midazolam as an amnestic, fentanyl is slowly titrated to a total dose of 5 to 10 μg per kg. The airway can then usually be taken over by the addition of a small dose of propofol or thiopental, after which an inhalational agent is added. Alternatively, the final phase of the induction can often be achieved with only the addition of sevoflurane, with a careful transition from spontaneous breathing to assisted ventilation; although this mixed technique takes an extra minute or two, we have found the tremendous hemodynamic stability to be worthwhile. A nondepolarizing muscle relaxant should be used for intubation; succinylcholine is not absolutely contraindicated, but because it can cause a transient increase in intracranial pressure (ICP), its use should be reserved for situations in which it is strongly indicated. Although hypoventilation is obviously undesirable, care should also be taken to avoid excessive hyperventilation.

One benefit of an opioid-based induction is the attenuation of tachycardia and hypertension during direct laryngoscopy, and during the placement of the head fixation pins that usually occurs approximately 5 minutes following intubation. Alternatively, lidocaine 1.5 mg per kg can be given 1 to 2 minutes before laryngoscopy.

Bekker AY, Mistry A, Ritter AA, et al. Computer simulation of intracranial pressure changes during induction of anesthesia: comparison of thiopental, propofol, and etomidate. *J Neurosurg Anesthesiol* 1999;11:69–80.

Bozeman WP, Idris AH. Intracranial pressure changes during rapid sequence intubation: a swine model. *J Trauma* 2005;58:278–283.

Todd MM, Warner DS, Sokoll MD, et al. A prospective, comparative trial of three anesthetics for elective supratentorial craniotomy. Propofol/fentanyl, isoflurane/nitrous oxide, and fentanyl/nitrous oxide. *Anesthesiology* 1993;78:1005–1020.

C.5. What are the effects of anesthetics on CMRO$_2$, cerebral blood flow (CBF), and intracranial pressure (ICP)? With this in mind, how would you maintain anesthesia?

Volatile anesthetics

All volatile anesthetics reduce CMRO$_2$, with isoflurane having the most substantial effect at normal clinical doses. At concentrations less than 1 MAC, some degree of autoregulation is maintained, which will tend to decrease CBF; however, volatile agents also have a direct vasodilatory effect. The net result may be an overall increase in CBF, greater in deeper structures than in cerebral cortex. This increase in CBF may potentially lead to elevation in ICP, although the effect is generally weak except when there is minimal compliance reserve. A more likely consequence is that the increased CBF will be an impediment to optimal surgical exposure once the bone plate is removed. Lastly, $PaCO_2$ reactivity is preserved in healthy brain at concentrations less than 1 MAC, but pathologic brain may have diminished or absent CO_2 responsiveness.

Nitrous oxide

Studies to date have shown substantial variation in the effects of N_2O, which probably relates to the heterogeneity of the anesthetic combinations in which it has been studied. The balance of evidence suggests that N_2O increases $CMRO_2$, CBF, and ICP. ICP increases can be marked, especially if used in combination with a volatile agent; the effect can be attenuated by the addition of an intravenous anesthetic. At best, N_2O offers no neuroprotection, and at worst, its effects may be neurotoxic and counter productive to surgical exposure. Because alternative approaches to maintenance are readily available, we regard N_2O as relatively contraindicated in craniotomy for intracranial pathology, although this view is by no means universal.

Intravenous anesthetics

The intravenous anesthetics that act through GABAergic mechanisms (e.g., barbiturates, propofol, and etomidate) cause a dose-dependent reduction in $CMRO_2$, CBF, cerebral blood volume (CBV), and ICP. In contrast to volatile anesthetics, CBF remains coupled to $CMRO_2$, with no direct vasodilatory effect. In other words, the direct drug effect is a reduction in $CMRO_2$, and the decreases in CBF, CBV, and ICP result from intact normal physiological responses. CO_2 reactivity is preserved. $CMRO_2$ can be reduced to as low as 40% of resting values in the presence of an isoelectric electroencephalogram (EEG). The NMDA-antagonist ketamine may increase $CMRO_2$, CBF and ICP. Although traditionally thought of as relatively neurotoxic, recent studies suggest a predominantly neuroprotective effect of ketamine, especially when combined with GABAergic agents.

Opioids

The effects of the opioid drugs on $CMRO_2$, CBF, and ICP are generally far less significant than the effect of the other intravenous or gaseous anesthetics. Most evidence suggests that opioids have no effect or slightly reduce $CMRO_2$, CBF, and ICP. In the awake patient, opioids will cause hypoventilation, elevated $PaCO_2$, and a consequent increase in CBF and potentially in ICP. Vigilance must be maintained during preinduction sedation and in the immediate postextubation period.

Theoretically, the optimal maintenance anesthetic technique is probably total intravenous anesthesia (TIVA) in an oxygen/air mixture, provided hyperventilation is not excessive. We favor the use of propofol 100 to 200 μg/kg/minute, titrated to EEG, with the addition of sufficient remifentanil or other opioid to blunt hemodynamic responses. Unless precluded by monitoring, a nondepolarizing muscle relaxant should be added to ensure that the patient does not move while the head is fixed. A TIVA approach maximizes the ability to reduce $CMRO_2$ without impairing surgical exposure through increased CBF, or causing cerebral steal. If a TIVA is impractical or not possible, an alternative approach is to use a low concentration of a volatile anesthetic in conjunction with high-dose opioid infusion. There will be a reduction in $CMRO_2$, but the impairment of surgical exposure will be minimal.

Fraga M, Rama-Maceiras P, Rodino S, et al. The effects of isoflurane and desflurane on intracranial pressure, cerebral perfusion pressure, and cerebral arteriovenous oxygen content difference in normocapnic patients with supratentorial brain tumors. *Anesthesiology* 2003;98:1085–1090.

Guy J, Hindman BJ, Baker KZ, et al. Comparison of remifentanil and fentanyl in patients undergoing craniotomy for supratentorial space–occupying lesions. *Anesthesiology* 1997;86:514–524.

Todd MM, Drummond JC. A comparison of the cerebrovascular and metabolic effects of halothane and isoflurane in the cat. *Anesthesiology* 1984;60:276–282.

Todd MM, Warner DS, Sokoll MD, et al. A prospective, comparative trial of three anesthetics for elective supratentorial craniotomy. Propofol/fentanyl, isoflurane/nitrous oxide, and fentanyl/nitrous oxide. *Anesthesiology* 1993;78:1005–1020.

Warner DS, Hindman BJ, Todd MM, et al. Intracranial pressure and hemodynamic effects of remifentanil versus alfentanil in patients undergoing supratentorial craniotomy. *Anesth Analg* 1996;83:348–353.

C.6. How would you approach the management of CO_2?

A reduction of $PaCO_2$ results in decreased cerebral blood flow (CBF) and cerebral blood volume (CBV) within minutes. Therefore, hyperventilation is a rapidly effective measure that can be instituted to decrease intracranial pressure (ICP) or to improve surgical exposure. However, hyperventilation has substantial limitations. At $PaCO_2$ values less than 25 mm Hg cerebral ischemia may result from a critical reduction in CBF combined with a large left shift of oxyhemoglobin dissociation, preventing oxygen unloading. Prolonged hyperventilation may result in the development of an underlying metabolic acidosis through normal compensatory mechanisms, which may result in a decrease in pH if hyperventilation is rapidly terminated. Further, prolonged hyperventilation may result in a decrease in ionized Ca^{2+}, leading to hemodynamic difficulties and prolonged emergence from effects on synaptic function.

It is important to remember that the difference between $PaCO_2$ and end-tidal carbon dioxide ($ETCO_2$) can vary greatly. Therefore, an arterial blood gas should be taken as soon as possible after induction to establish the arterial-end tidal gradient in CO_2 partial pressure. We initially aim for a $PaCO_2$ of approximately 35 mm Hg unless there is elevated ICP. If, once the bone plate is removed, the surgeons determine that their exposure is suboptimal, we hyperventilate to a $PaCO_2$ of 30 mm Hg. Further hyperventilation is reserved for situations in which establishing adequate exposure is extremely difficult. To avoid postoperative acid-base instability, hyperventilation can be gradually reduced throughout the closure, permitting a steady reestablishment of bicarbonate and Ca^{2+} equilibrium.

Brian JE Jr. Carbon dioxide and the cerebral circulation. *Anesthesiology* 1998;88:1365–1386.

Muizelaar JP, Marmarou A, Ward JD, et al. Adverse effects of prolonged hyperventilation in patients with severe head injury: a randomized clinical trial. *J Neurosurg* 1991; 75:731–739.

Rowney DA, Fairgrieve R, Bissonnette B. Cerebrovascular carbon dioxide reactivity in children anaesthetized with sevoflurane. *Br J Anaesth* 2002;88:357–361.

C.7. How would you approach diuretic therapy?

The purpose of diuretic therapy in intracranial procedures is to dehydrate the brain, thereby leading to a reduction in the volume of the fluid compartment. This facilitates surgical exposure and reduces the requirement for brain retraction. Through the same principal, mannitol is used as therapy for elevated intracranial pressure (ICP) states when the cranium is closed.

Mannitol is an osmotic diuretic that is usually prepared in a 20% solution (20 g/100 mL), and should initially be given in a dose of 0.5 to 1.0 g per kg; the total dose can be increased to 1.5 g per kg if initial efforts are ineffective. Higher doses have been reported to lead to cardiac arrest from disruption of cardiac cellular function. Because mannitol initially draws water into the vascular space before it is excreted, rapid dosing can cause a transient increase in ICP, and so it should be infused over 20 to 30 minutes. If there is very little intracranial compliance reserve, aggressive dosing should be synchronized with the removal of the bone plate.

If mannitol does not provide adequate surgical conditions, the loop diuretic furosemide can be used. In a naïve adult patient, a dose as low as 5 mg may be adequate. Furosemide does not have the problem of an initial increase in vascular volume, and so may preferred in patients with marginal cardiac function who can develop congestive heart failure with a large mannitol load. However, the combination of mannitol and furosemide can cause electrolyte abnormalities and severe systemic dehydration, necessitating fluid resuscitation. Because mannitol therapy alone is often adequate, we do not administer furosemide routinely, and instead reserve its use for situations when surgical exposure is suboptimal.

In cases of extreme cerebral edema, hypertonic saline, in concentrations up to 7.5%, can be used. This can be effective in refractory intracranial hypertension, but is limited by the development of severe hypernatremia.

Gemma M, Cozzi S, Tommasino C, et al. 7.5% hypertonic saline versus 20% mannitol during elective neurosurgical supratentorial procedures. *J Neurosurg Anesthesiol* 1997;9: 329–334.

Schettini A, Stahurski B, Young HF. Osmotic and osmotic-loop diuresis in brain surgery. Effects on plasma and CSF electrolytes and ion excretion. *J Neurosurg* 1982;56:679–684.

Suarez JI, Qureshi AI, Bhardwaj A, et al. Treatment of refractory intracranial hypertension with 23.4% saline. *Crit Care Med* 1998;26:1118–1122.

Thenuwara K, Todd MM, Brian JE Jr. Effect of mannitol and furosemide on plasma osmolality and brain water. *Anesthesiology* 2002;96:416–421.

C.8. How would you manage serum glucose?

For reasons that are incompletely understood, hyperglycemia worsens neurologic injury. At the same time, even nondiabetic patients undergoing craniotomy are at risk of hyperglycemia secondary to steroid therapy. There is no study that has clearly identified the level of serum glucose that requires intraoperative treatment; however, its intraoperative management is too often overlooked. Serum glucose should be checked intraoperatively, and hyperglycemia treated by reducing glucose to the normal range with intravenous insulin.

Lukins MB, Manninen PH. Hyperglycemia in patients administered dexamethasone for craniotomy. *Anesth Analg* 2005;100:1129–1133.

Rovlias A, Kotsou S. The influence of hyperglycemia on neurological outcome in patients with severe head injury. *Neurosurgery* 2000;46:335–342.

C.9. How will you approach maintenance fluid management?

If the blood–brain barrier (BBB) is intact, the principal determinant of brain tissue water is the osmotic gradient across the BBB. It is this principal that guides the use of hypertonic solutions such as mannitol or hypertonic saline to reduce interstitial water and reduce intracranial pressure (ICP) or optimize surgical exposure. Under the same principal, the use of hypotonic solutions, such as Lactated Ringer's solution, favor the transport of water into the brain interstitium, and thereby the development of edema.

In regions where the BBB is not intact, due to pathology and surgical tissue injury, osmotic particles will be able to cross from the capillaries into the interstitial tissue. Therefore, the benefits of hypertonic solutions are lost in these areas. It follows that the benefit obtained from the use of hypertonic solutions is because of an *overall* effect on the brain, and not from a *specific* effect in localized regions of brain injury.

The above considerations favor the use of isotonic normal (0.9%) saline as maintenance fluid in craniotomies. More controversial is the approach to volume. Historically, craniotomy patients have been kept deliberately hypovolemic in the belief that this will increase the passage of free water from the brain in situations involving a disrupted BBB. However, recent evidence suggests that there is in fact very little reduction in interstitial water, and that it comes at the price of significant systemic hypoperfusion and hypotension. Therefore, the favored approach to fluid management is now maintenance of isovolemia with normal saline. In prolonged cases, the chloride loading may result in a mild hyperchloremic non-anion gap metabolic acidosis. Dextrose-containing solutions should never be used unless for specifically treating hypoglycemia. 5% albumin can be used when volume expansion is a requirement. Albumin has a plasma half-life of 16 hours, and little is known about how the passage of albumin molecules across a damaged BBB influences interstitial water movements over these time periods. Therefore, its routine use is not recommended.

Drummond JC, Moore SS. The influence of dextrose administration on neurologic outcome after temporary spinal cord ischemia in the rabbit. *Anesthesiology* 1989;70:64–70.

Jelsma LF, McQueen JD. Effect of experimental water restriction on brain water. *J Neurosurg* 1967;26:35–40.

Lanier WL, Stangland KJ, Scheithauer BW, et al. The effects of dextrose infusion and head position on neurologic outcome after complete cerebral ischemia in primates: examination of a model. *Anesthesiology* 1987;66:39–48.

Prough DS, Bidani A. Hyperchloremic metabolic acidosis is a predictable consequence of intraoperative infusion of 0.9% saline. *Anesthesiology* 1999;90:1247–1249.

C.10. Once the bone plate is removed and the dura retracted, the surgeon reports that the brain is still "tight." In consideration of the issues discussed in the preceding text, what would be your response?

In almost all cases, the most effective initial response is to increase hyperventilation to a $Paco_2$ of approximately 27 to 30 mm Hg. If mannitol 1 g per kg has already been administered, furosemide should be given until a diuresis is established. If the patient has a cerebrospinal fluid (CSF) drain, this should be opened and CSF removed in no greater than 10 to 20 mL aliquots, with reassessment in between. Hypertension should be addressed and treated, and the patient well anesthetized to attenuate cerebral blood flow (CBF) responses to surgical stimulation. Positioning should be reassessed to eliminate any obstruction to jugular venous outflow. A change in anesthetic maintenance strategy to reduce or eliminate volatile agents may occasionally be helpful. Finally, deliberate hypotension can be instituted.

Brian JE Jr. Carbon dioxide and the cerebral circulation. *Anesthesiology* 1998;88:1365–1386.

Thenuwara K, Todd MM, Brian JE Jr. Effect of mannitol and furosemide on plasma osmolality and brain water. *Anesthesiology* 2002;96:416–421.

C.11. If deliberate hypotension is indicated, how would you achieve it?

Although sodium nitroprusside (SNP) and volatile anesthetics (especially isoflurane) are historically the most commonly used drugs to achieve hypotension, both are very far from ideal. SNP is very effective and is titratable over very short time periods, but because it causes cerebral vasodilation it may actually increase vascular engorgement. Nitroglycerin (NTG) is also a potent cerebral vasodilator and has the same limitation. Similarly, high levels of volatile anesthetic will have direct cerebral vasodilatory effects. Further, the uncoupled cerebral vasodilation caused by nitrates and volatiles can theoretically cause a cerebral steal phenomenon.

In most cases, the required level of hypotension can be achieved with the use of high-dose remifentanil and propofol, possibly with the addition of a β-adrenergic blocker. Remifentanil enables a profound but rapidly reversible opioid level to be achieved without unfavorable effects on cerebral blood flow (CBF) or dilation. Similarly, propofol can cause hypotension through systemic vasodilation, but does not cause cerebral vasodilation and is rapidly reversible. The β-blocker labetalol is often highly effective as an adjunctive "background." The calcium channel blocker nicardipine is titratable over relatively short time periods, and is an excellent choice if hypotension is required in a non-anesthetized patient (such as during an awake procedure, during emergence, or in the intensive care unit (ICU)), although it may impair autoregulation. Esmolol infusions can be utilized for a more titratable β-blocker therapy. With the advent of newer drugs, the ganglionic blocker trimethaphan is now rarely used.

Degoute CS, Ray MJ, Manchon M, et al. Remifentanil and controlled hypotension; comparison with nitroprusside or esmolol during tympanoplasty. *Can J Anaesth* 2001; 48:20–27.

Endoh H, Honda T, Ohashi S, et al. The influence of nicardipine-, nitroglycerin-, and prostaglandin E(1)-induced hypotension on cerebral pressure autoregulation in adult patients during propofol-fentanyl anesthesia. *Anesth Analg* 2002;94:169–173.

Hoffman WE, Edelman G, Ripper R, et al. Sodium nitroprusside compared with isoflurane-induced hypotension: the effects on brain oxygenation and arteriovenous shunting. *Anesth Analg* 2001;93:166–170.

Jordan D, Shulman SM, Miller ED Jr. Esmolol hydrochloride, sodium nitroprusside, and isoflurane differ in their ability to alter peripheral sympathetic responses. *Anesth Analg* 1993;77:281–290.

Michenfelder JD, Milde JH. The interaction of sodium nitroprusside, hypotension, and isoflurane in determining cerebral vasculature effects. *Anesthesiology* 1988;69:870–875.

Ornstein E, Young WL, Ostapkovich N, et al. Deliberate hypotension in patients with intracranial arteriovenous malformations: esmolol compared with isoflurane and sodium nitroprusside. *Anesth Analg* 1991;72:639–644.

Thomsen LJ, Riisager S, Jensen KA, et al. Cerebral blood flow and metabolism during hypotension induced with sodium nitroprusside and captopril. *Can J Anaesth* 1989; 36:392–396.

C.12. While the surgeon is resecting tumor from near the brainstem, the patient's heart rate suddenly drops to 20. What is your assessment and management?

Surgery near the brainstem nuclei can result in dramatic autonomic disturbances. Profound vagal reflexes can be alarming, sometimes resulting in complete asystole. These can often be followed by a sympathetic reflex, and under such circumstances the hemodynamics can shift from extreme bradycardia and hypotension to tachycardia and hypertension in a matter of seconds.

The first step is to alert the surgeon to stop operating, which almost always alleviates the problem. Once the hemodynamic status has stabilized, an "autonomic blunting" prophylactic regimen can be given. Glycopyrrolate should be titrated until a 15% to 20% increase in heart rate is observed; if sympathetic reflexes are also involved, β-adrenergic blockade can be added. This approach is usually highly effective in attenuating the reflexes.

The sudden development of bradycardia should always alert the anesthesiologist to the possibility of a sudden increase in intracranial pressure (ICP), leading to the Cushing reflex. In this case, hypertension will be seen, and the surgeon should be immediately notified.

Koerbel A, Gharabaghi A, Samii A, et al. Trigeminocardiac reflex during skull base surgery: mechanism and management. *Acta Neurochir (Wien)* 2005;147:727–733.

Schaller B, Probst R, Strebel S, et al. Trigeminocardiac reflex during surgery in the cerebellopontine angle. *J Neurosurg* 1999;90:215–220.

C.13. Would you monitor for venous air embolism (VAE)? What are the monitoring options?

Although the risk for VAE is most marked when the sitting position is used, it can occur whenever the height of the surgical site is further above the heart than the venous column. As this applies in many approaches to the posterior fossa, some form of monitoring for VAE is recommended, with the *caveat* that invasiveness should be proportionate to risk.

A precordial Doppler ultrasound transducer is highly sensitive and non-invasive- we use it routinely for posterior fossa procedures. Positioning over the right heart can be difficult, and its ability to detect turbulence cause by VAE should be assessed by rapidly injecting 5 to 10 mL of saline peripherally and listening for the characteristic change in sound quality. The combination of precordial Doppler and end-tidal carbon dioxide ($ETco_2$) monitoring is extremely effective at detecting clinically significant VAE. Transesophageal echocardiography (TEE) is extremely sensitive, and can detect air bubbles in the left heart, but it requires operator expertise and is often impossible in the horizontal operating positions. End-tidal nitrogen (ETN_2) is specific for air, and non-invasive, but can be difficult to interpret if an air–oxygen mix is being used in the anesthetic. A pulmonary artery catheter can detect pulmonary hypertension resulting from reflex vasoconstriction and direct obstruction in the presence of VAE, but because of its invasiveness, it should only be used when another indication is present.

The use of a right atrial catheter should be strongly considered in any situation when the risk of VAE is high, and many regard it as mandatory when the sitting position is used. The tip of the catheter is placed near the sino-atrial node by electrocardiograph (ECG) guidance. The catheter is flushed with $NaHCO_3$ and the right arm lead attached to a conductive connector placed on the line. The catheter should then be advanced into the right ventricle, which can be detected by transducing the pressure waveform. It should then be drawn back until the P wave on the catheter lead is biphasic (mid-atrium), and then back further to the point at which the P wave and QRS complex are of equal amplitude. The catheter is then pulled back another centimeter and secured. The right atrial catheter can confirm the presence of VAE through the aspiration of air, but its principal utility is therapeutic.

Cucchiara RF, Nugent M, Seward JB, et al. Air embolism in upright neurosurgical patients: detection and localization by two-dimensional transesophageal echocardiography. *Anesthesiology* 1984;60:353–355.

Gildenberg PL, O'Brien RP, Britt WJ, et al. The efficacy of Doppler monitoring for the detection of venous air embolism. *J Neurosurg* 1981;54:75–78.

Martin RW, Colley PS. Evaluation of transesophageal Doppler detection of air embolism in dogs. *Anesthesiology* 1983;58:117–123.

Matjasko J, Petrozza P, Mackenzie CF. Sensitivity of end-tidal nitrogen in venous air embolism detection in dogs. *Anesthesiology* 1985;63:418–423.

Schubert A, Deogaonkar A, Drummond JC. Precordial Doppler probe placement for optimal detection of venous air embolism during craniotomy. *Anesth Analg* 2006;102:1543–1547.

C.14. Are there any measures you can take to prevent venous air embolism (VAE)?

The most effective prevention of VAE derives from the surgical technique, and the surgeon's tolerance of lower head positions. The anesthesiologist can contribute by ensuring adequate hydration (increasing the height of the venous column), and by avoiding drugs that dilate the venous capacitance vessels, such as nitroglycerin (NTG). Positive end-expiratory pressure (PEEP) does not reduce the incidence of VAE, but it does impair surgical conditions through reducing venous return, and increases the chance of a paradoxical air embolus in a patient with a patent foramen ovale (PFO); therefore, it should not be used in craniotomies unless there is a strong rationale based on respiratory pathology.

Considerable controversy remains over the use of N_2O in the sitting position and other circumstances in which there is a high risk of VAE. No study has demonstrated an effect of N_2O on VAE. The controversy extends to the effect of N_2O on pneumocephalus, because some studies suggest that it increases the size of the gas collection, risking the development of tension, but other studies suggest that it may promote the resorption of the gas. When combined with the possible deleterious effects of N_2O on neuroprotection outlined in Question C.5, we see no role for N_2O in posterior fossa craniotomy, given that viable alternatives in anesthetic management are readily available.

Giebler R, Kollenberg B, Pohlen G, et al. Effect of positive end-expiratory pressure on the incidence of venous air embolism and on the cardiovascular response to the sitting position during neurosurgery. *Br J Anaesth* 1998;80:30–35.

Kytta J, Tanskanen P, Randell T. Comparison of the effects of controlled ventilation with 100% oxygen, 50% oxygen in nitrogen, and 50% oxygen in nitrous oxide on responses to venous air embolism in pigs. *Br J Anaesth* 1996;77:658–661.

Losasso TJ, Muzzi DA, Dietz NM, et al. Fifty percent nitrous oxide does not increase the risk of venous air embolism in neurosurgical patients operated upon in the sitting position. *Anesthesiology* 1992;77:21–30.

C.15. During the procedure, the precordial Doppler becomes loud and turbulent. The end-tidal carbon dioxide ($ETCO_2$) drops from 31 to 13 mm Hg, and the systemic pressure from 121/63 to 64/32. What is your assessment and management?

This is a classic presentation of venous air embolism (VAE). Immediately inform the surgeon, institute 100% oxygen, and request assistance. The surgeon should flood the field with fluid, and urgently prepare the field for lowering the head (e.g., placement of a protective drape). An assistant should reach under the drapes and apply pressure to the jugular veins to prevent further entrainment (but not enough to occlude carotid flow), although this should only be a transient measure. Intravenous fluids should be opened to full flow. The head should then be lowered to a level below the heart, or at least as much as is possible. The left lateral decubitus position has been advocated, but is probably of little benefit. If a right atrial catheter is in place, air should be aspirated; if not, then placement should be considered, depending on the ability of the above measures to alleviate the instability. Other management will be supportive.

If the VAE is detected early, the episode will usually resolve, and it is almost always appropriate to resume and complete the surgery, although the placement of additional monitors before resumption may be warranted. However, an undetected, rapid, or prolonged entrainment of air can lead to cardiac arrest. If cardiac arrest is present or imminent, and the patient is in a prone or semiprone position, the anesthesiologist must prepare the surgeon and others in the room for an emergent move to the supine position to enable resuscitation. For this reason, a stretcher must always be available outside the operating room when patients are in the prone position.

Archer DP, Pash MP, MacRae ME. Successful management of venous air embolism with inotropic support. *Can J Anaesth* 2001;48:204–208.

Bunegin L, Albin MS, Helsel PE, et al. Positioning the right atrial catheter: a model for reappraisal. *Anesthesiology* 1981;55:343–348.

Palmon SC, Moore LE, Lundberg J, et al. Venous air embolism: a review. *J Clin Anesth* 1997;9:251–257.

C.16. What is your approach to emergence? What if the patient does not wake up?

Providing an early neurological assessment is one of the most valuable contributions of the anesthesiologist to outcome. Therefore, there is an imperative to have patients emerge quickly, even when surgery has been prolonged. At the same time, the emergence from anesthesia may incur substantial changes in pressure, $PaCO_2$, cerebral blood flow (CBF), and autonomic activity, and therefore must be carefully planned. Transitioning from hyperventilation should be gradual, to prevent a precipitous acidosis. Adrenergic blocking agents may be administered to attenuate the sympathetic effects often seen during and following emergence in these patients. Reversal of neuromuscular block should be carefully titrated to avoid autonomic instability, with care taken to ensure that the patient does not move while the head is fixed in pins. Antiemetic therapy should be aggressive, as the elevation in intracranial pressure (ICP) caused by retching and vomiting are particularly undesirable in craniotomy patients.

Coughing or "bucking" during emergence causes dramatic spikes in ICP, and must be avoided. There are several approaches to avoiding this, including the use of intravenous lidocaine, an opioid-based anesthetic, or a deep extubation. In the case of a deep extubation, there is always a risk that a neurological event may prevent the patient from waking up, in which case reintubation may be required. Although an opioid-based anesthetic often results in a smooth emergence, excessive hypoventilation in the immediate postoperative period may cause an elevation in ICP in patients with no compliance reserve.

A failure to emerge may represent a neurologic event resulting from the surgery, such as an intracranial bleed, vessel occlusion, embolic event, or seizure. In such cases, the time to diagnosis is a critical determinant of outcome. The anesthesiologist must be able to state with confidence that the delayed emergence is unlikely to be the secondary to the anesthetic. The usual approach is to immediately obtain a computed tomography (CT) scan; the operating room should be left available in the event that an emergent return is required.

In some posterior fossa surgery, especially that near the brainstem, postoperative edema can lead to an anticipated worsening of neurological status before an improvement on the first or second postoperative day, thereby necessitating prolonged intubation. In these cases, the patient can be awoken, and once an original neurological assessment is obtained, sedated for transport to the intensive care unit (ICU).

Diachun CA, Tunink BP, Brock-Utne JG. Suppression of cough during emergence from general anesthesia: laryngotracheal lidocaine through a modified endotracheal tube. *J Clin Anesth* 2001;13:447–451.

Fagan C, Frizelle HP, Laffey J, et al. The effects of intracuff lidocaine on endotracheal-tube-induced emergence phenomena after general anesthesia. *Anesth Analg* 2000;91:201–205.

Gonzalez RM, Bjerke RJ, Drobycki T, et al. Prevention of endotracheal tube-induced coughing during emergence from general anesthesia. *Anesth Analg* 1994;79:792–795.

Kim ES, Bishop MJ. Cough during emergence from isoflurane anesthesia. *Anesth Analg* 1998;87:1170–1174.

Leech P, Barker J, Fitch W. Proceedings: changes in intracranial pressure and systemic arterial pressure during the termination of anaesthesia. *Br J Anaesth* 1974;46:315–316.

Mendel P, Fredman B, White PF. Alfentanil suppresses coughing and agitation during emergence from isoflurane anesthesia. *J Clin Anesth* 1995;7:114–118.

Todd MM, Warner DS, Sokoll MD, et al. A prospective, comparative trial of three anesthetics for elective supratentorial craniotomy. Propofol/fentanyl, isoflurane/nitrous oxide, and fentanyl/nitrous oxide. *Anesthesiology* 1993;78:1005–1020.

D. Postoperative Management

D.1. What postoperative complications are of greatest concern? What level of monitoring is required?

Part of the neurological assessment conducted immediately on emergence should be an evaluation of the lower cranial nerves. Damage to the nerves or to nuclei can result in difficulty swallowing and protecting the airway. The principal concern, however, is the development of edema or hematoma causing compression of the brainstem or midbrain structures. The brainstem sits in an anatomic location with very little compliance; therefore, even small degrees of edema that would be well tolerated following supratentorial procedures may lead to catastrophic neurological compromise. It is critical to appreciate that edema and hematoma can develop over the course of several hours following the procedure; a patient that had a satisfactory emergence may deteriorate neurologically in the middle of the night. In certain circumstances, the risk for postoperative edema is so high that the patient is left intubated prophylactically, as discussed in Question C.16. However, deterioration cannot always be anticipated, and therefore these patients should be initially monitored in an intensive care setting in all cases.

Bucciero A, Quaglietta P, Vizioli L. Supratentorial intracerebral hemorrhage after posterior fossa surgery. Case report. *J Neurosurg Sci* 1991;35:221–224.

Pollack IF, Polinko P, Albright AL, et al. Mutism and pseudobulbar symptoms after resection of posterior fossa tumors in children: incidence and pathophysiology. *Neurosurgery* 1995;37:885–893.

Porter JM, Pidgeon C, Cunningham AJ. The sitting position in neurosurgery: a critical appraisal. *Br J Anaesth* 1999;82:117–128.

Suri A, Mahapatra AK, Bithal P. Seizures following posterior fossa surgery. *Br J Neurosurg* 1998;12:41–44.

Wilder BL. Hypothesis: the etiology of midcervical quadriplegia after operation with the patient in the sitting position. *Neurosurgery* 1982;11:530–531.

CHAPTER 23

Carotid Endarterectomy

MARIA BUSTILLO • CYNTHIA A. LIEN

A 71-YEAR-OLD WOMAN

is scheduled for a left carotid endarterectomy (CEA) for asymptomatic left carotid stenosis. She has 90% occlusion of her left carotid artery. Her past medical history is positive for hypertension, insulin dependent diabetes mellitus, and coronary artery disease with angioplasty 2 years ago. Her blood pressure is 180/75 mm Hg and her pulse is 65 beats per minute and regular.

A. Medical Disease and Differential Diagnosis

1. What are the presenting symptoms of carotid stenosis?
2. What is the prevalence of carotid artery disease?
3. What is the natural course of carotid artery disease?
4. Discuss diabetes mellitus as a risk factor for CEA.
5. What are the indications for surgical intervention in the management of carotid atherosclerotic disease?
6. Discuss the anatomy of the cerebral vasculature, including the carotid artery and the circle of Willis.
7. Discuss cerebral perfusion in the presence of carotid artery disease.
8. Discuss the different surgical approaches to carotid revascularization.
9. What is normal cerebral blood flow (CBF)?
10. What is critically low CBF as measured by the electroencephalogram (EEG)?
11. What is cerebral autoregulation?
12. How does $Paco_2$ affect CBF?
13. What are the principal determinants of CBF?
14. What is meant by the term "luxury perfusion"?
15. What is meant by the term "intracerebral steal"?
16. What is "inverse steal" or the "Robin Hood" syndrome?

B. Preoperative Evaluation and Preparation

1. What would you be looking for in your preoperative evaluation?
2. Is this patient's blood pressure too high for elective surgery?
3. What laboratory data would be required preoperatively?
4. Would you premedicate this patient?

C. Intraoperative Management

1. How would you monitor this patient?
2. How would you know that the patient's cerebral perfusion is adequate during surgery?

3. Discuss the differences and relative advantages and disadvantages of the unprocessed EEG and the processed EEG.
4. How would you measure CBF intraoperatively? What are the relative advantages and disadvantages of each technique? How much CBF is considered adequate?
5. Does internal carotid stump pressure accurately reflect cerebral perfusion?
6. Discuss somatosensory evoked potentials (SSEPs) as a monitor of CBF during CEA.
7. Describe the role of the transcranial Doppler as a monitor of cerebral perfusion during CEA.
8. What type of anesthesia would you choose for this patient? Why?
9. How would you induce and maintain general anesthesia in this patient?
10. How would you proceed if the patient were to receive regional anesthesia?
11. Discuss the effects of anesthetics on CBF.
12. Discuss the protective effects of anesthetic agents on cerebral function.
13. How would you manage this patient's ventilation under general anesthesia?
14. How would you manage this patient's blood pressure intraoperatively?
15. Discuss reperfusion injury following CEA.
16. What intravenous fluids would you give this patient intraoperatively?

D. Postoperative Management

1. The patient does not "wake up" from general anesthesia. Why?
2. Postoperatively the patient's blood pressure is 170/96 mm Hg. Would you treat this? If so, why and how?
3. What immediate postoperative complications might you expect?
4. Discuss postoperative neurocognitive dysfunction following uncomplicated CEA.

A. Medical Disease and Differential Diagnosis

A.1. What are the presenting symptoms of carotid stenosis?

Carotid stenosis is commonly asymptomatic. It can, although, present with amaurosis fugax, a transient ischemic attack or a cerebrovascular accident. Amaurosis fugax is a temporary monocular blindness caused by a transient ischemia attack (TIA) of the retina. It is an indication of an evolving arterial thrombus in the internal carotid artery, which is the main blood supply to the optic nerve and retina through the ophthalmic artery. The symptoms of amaurosis fugax, which have been described as a shade descending over one eye, often last less than 10 minutes, and are ipsilateral to the evolving and symptomatic vascular disease.

Brunicardi FC, Andersen DK, Billian TR, et al. eds. *Schwartz's principles of surgery*, 8th ed. New York: McGraw-Hill, 2005:780–788.

Kasper DL, Braunwald E, Fauci AS, et al. eds. *Harrison's principle of internal medicine*, 16th ed. New York: McGraw-Hill, 2005:2377–2381.

A.2. What is the prevalence of carotid artery disease?

Carotid artery disease is a manifestation of generalized arteriosclerosis. A review of data contained in the medical records of Mayo Medical Center shows the incidence of transient ischemia attacks (TIAs) to be 31 per 100,000 people in Rochester, Minnesota. The incidence increases with age: 1 per 100,000 in people less than 45 years old increasing to 293 per 100,000 in people 75 years and older. In patients with an asymptomatic carotid stenosis of less than 75%, the risk of developing a TIA is 1% to 2% per year.

Similar rates have been reported in the former Union of Soviet Socialist Republics. Stroke remains the third most common cause of death in the United States. Death from heart disease and cancer are the first and second leading causes of death.

Meyer FB, ed.*Sundt's occlusive cerebrovascular disease*. 2nd ed. Philadelphia: WB Saunders, 1994:60.

Minino AM, Smith BL. *Deaths: preliminary data from 2000. National vital statistics reports*. Hyattsville: National Center for Health Statistics, 2000;49(12):1–40.

Wilke HJ, Ellis JE, McKinsey JF. Carotid endarterectomy: perioperative and anesthetic considerations. *J Cardiothorac Vasc Anesth* 1996;10:928–949.

A.3. What is the natural course of carotid artery disease?

In carotid artery disease, atherosclerotic plaques develop at the lateral aspect of the bifurcation of the carotid artery. The severity of the process parallels that in other major vessels. Thrombosis is most likely to occur where the plaque narrows the lumen to the greatest degree. Thromboembolic stroke accounts for the greatest percentage of cerebral vascular accidents (CVAs).

Sixty percent of thrombotic strokes are preceded by one or more transient ischemia attacks (TIAs). Most frequently one or two TIAs will occur before the final stroke, and each will last less than 10 minutes. In greater than 25% of cases, a complete stroke will follow a TIA within 1 month. In approximately 30% of cases, TIAs do not precede a stroke. Embolic and hemorrhagic strokes are rarely preceded by TIAs.

In a patient population in Rochester, Minnesota, the 50% survival time after the first TIA was 7 to 8 years. The highest mortality rate was in the first 2 years following a TIA. However, 2 years following a TIA, the mortality rate stabilized at one and one-half times that of the general population.

Barash PG, Cullen BF, Stoelting RK, eds. *Clinical anesthesia*, 5th ed. Philadelphia: Lippincott Williams & Wilkins, 2006:946–954.

Fields WS, Maslenikov V, Meyer JS, et al. Joint study of extracranial arterial occlusion. V. Progress report of prognosis following surgery or nonsurgical treatment for cerebral ischemic attacks and cervical carotid artery lesions. *JAMA* 1970;211:1993.

Matsumoto N, Whisnant JP, Kurland LT, et al. Natural history of stroke in Rochester Minnesota, 1955 through 1969: an extension of a previous study, 1945 through 1954. *Stroke* 1973;4:20.

Meyer FB, ed. *Sundt's occlusive cerebrovascular disease*, 2nd ed. Philadelphia: WB Saunders, 1994:60.

A.4. Discuss diabetes mellitus as a risk factor for carotid endarterectomy (CEA).

Diabetes is a major risk factor for stroke. When matched for associated risk factors, symptomatic cerebrovascular disease is more common in patients who have diabetes mellitus than in the nondiabetic population. The risk of stroke is at least 2.5 fold greater in diabetic than in nondiabetic patients. Additionally, mortality and the severity of stroke are greater in patients with diabetes.

In a study from 1992 to 1995, 732 carotid endarterectomies were performed in diabetic and nondiabetic patients. A greater percentage of patients with diabetes who underwent CEA were woman than nondiabetic patients. Patients with diabetes were younger at presentation than nondiabetic patients and were more likely to have history of coronary artery disease. This may contribute to the higher incidence of postoperative cardiac morbidity in diabetic patients. By itself diabetes mellitus is not a risk factor for postoperative cardiac morbidity in patients who undergo carotid surgery.

Diabetes mellitus and obesity are considered independent risk factors for neurocognitive decline after CEA.

Akabari CM, Pomposelli FB, Gibbons GW, et al. Diabetes mellitus: a risk factor for carotid endarterectomy? *J Vasc Surg* 1997;24(6):1070–1074.

Heyer EJ, Wilson DA, Sahlein DH, et al. APOE-ε 4 predisposes to cognitive dysfunction following uncomplicated carotid endarterectomy. *Neurology* 2005;65:1–5.

Kannel WB, McGee DL. Diabetes and cardiovascular disease the Framinghan study. *JAMA* 1979;241:235–238.

Stokes J, Kannel WB, Wolf PA, et al. The relative importance of selected risk factors for various manifestations of cardiovascular disease among men and women from 35 to 64 years old: 30 years of follow-up in the Framingham study. *Circulation* 1987;75:65–73.

A.5. What are the indications for surgical intervention in the management of carotid atherosclerotic disease?

Currently in the United States there are more than 700,000 new strokes per year and it is estimated that 20% to 30% are due to carotid atherosclerotic disease.

Accepted indications for surgery currently include the following:

- Transient ischemic attacks with angiographic evidence of stenosis.
- Reversible ischemic neurologic deficits with greater than 70% stenosis of the vessel wall or an ulcerated plaque, with or without stenosis.
- An unstable neurologic status that persists despite anticoagulation.

In the North American Symptomatic Endarterectomy Trial (NASCET), carotid endarterectomy (CEA) decreased the risk of an ipsilateral stroke from 26% to 9%, yielding an absolute risk reduction of 65%. Similar results were obtained in the European Carotid Surgery Trial (ESCT), which demonstrated a 39% risk reduction, and the Veterans Affairs Cooperative Trial which demonstrated a 60% risk reduction from a severe stroke with surgical versus medical therapy.

A multicenter study of 1,662 asymptomatic patients (asymptomatic carotid atherosclerosis study [ACAS]) with carotid stenosis of 60% or more determined by Doppler studies, demonstrated that patients undergoing CEA in addition to medical therapy had a 53% reduction in aggregate risk for stroke or death compared to patients receiving only medical therapy. Additional outcome studies are warranted before CEA is recommended as a routine therapy for asymptomatic carotid artery disease.

Barash PG, Cullen BF, Stoelting RK, eds. *Clinical anesthesia*, 5th ed. Philadelphia: Lippincott, Williams & Wilkins, 2006:946–954.

Barnett HJM, Meldrum HE, Eliasziw M. The dilemma of surgical treatment for patients with asymptomatic carotid disease. *Ann Intern Med* 1995;123:723–725.

Brunicardi FC, Andersen DK, Billian TR, et al. eds. *Schwartz's principles of surgery*, 8th ed. New York: McGraw-Hill, 2005:780–788.

European Carotid Surgery Trialists Collaborative Group. MRC European Carotid Surgery Trial: interim results for symptomatic patients with severe (70–90%) or with mild (0–29%) carotid stenosis. *Lancet* 1991;337:1235–1243.

Asymptomatic Carotid Atherosclerosis Study Group. Executive committee for the Asymptomatic Carotid Atherosclerosis Study: endarterectomy for asymptomatic carotid artery stenosis. *JAMA* 1995;273:1421–1428.

Hobson RW, Weiss DG, Fields WS, et al. Efficacy of carotid endarterectomy for asymptomatic carotid stenosis. The Veterans Affairs Cooperative Study Group. *N Engl J Med* 1993;328:221–227.

Mayberg MR, Wilson SE, Yatsu F, et al. The Veterans Affair Cooperative Studies Program 309 Trialist Group. Carotid endarterectomy and prevention of cerebral ischemia is symptomatic carotid stenosis. *JAMA* 1991;226:3289–3294.

Mayo Asymptomatic Carotid Endarterectomy Study Group. Results of a randomized controlled trial of carotid endarterectomy of asymptomatic carotid stenosis. *Mayo Clin Proc* 1992;67:513–518.

North American Symptomatic Carotid Endarterectomy Trial Collaborators. Beneficial effect of carotid endarterectomy in symptomatic patients with high-grade carotid stenosis. *N Engl J Med* 1991;325:445–453.

The CASANOVA Study Group. Carotid surgery versus medical therapy in asymptomatic carotid stenosis. *Stroke* 1991;22:1229–1235.

A.6. Discuss the anatomy of the cerebral vasculature, including the carotid artery and the circle of Willis.

The common carotid arteries originate in the thorax. The right common carotid artery originates at the bifurcation of the brachiocephalic trunk, and the left originates from the aortic arch. In the neck, the common carotid arteries travel within the carotid sheath. At the level of the thyroid cartilage each common carotid artery bifurcates into internal and external carotid arteries.

Branches of the external carotid artery include the superior thyroid, lingual, facial, ascending pharyngeal, occipital, and posterior auricular arteries.

The internal carotid artery passes through the neck without branching to enter the middle cranial fossa through the carotid canal of the temporal bone, adjacent to the sphenoid bone. It supplies the hypophysis cerebri, the orbit, and the major portion of the supratentorial region of the brain. Cerebral arteries are derived from the internal carotid and vertebral arteries. The anastomosis they form at the base of the brain is known as the *Circle of Willis*. The two anterior cerebral arteries form the circle anteriorly. They are connected through the anterior communicating artery. The two posterior cerebral arteries form the circle posteriorly, which then ends at the junction of the basilar artery. The posterior cerebral arteries are connected to the internal carotid arteries by the two posterior communicating arteries (Fig. 23.1). The middle cerebral artery primarily supplies the lateral surface of each cerebral hemisphere. The anterior cerebral and posterior cerebral arteries supply the medial and inferior surfaces of the cerebral hemisphere.

Hemmings HC, Hopkins PM, eds. *Foundations of anesthesia basic science for clinical practice*, 2nd ed. Elsevier 2006;245.

Moore KL. *Clinically oriented anatomy*, 5th ed. Baltimore: Lippincott Williams & Wilkins, 2006;930–931.

A.7. Discuss cerebral perfusion in the presence of carotid artery disease.

Autoregulation is assumed to be lost in areas of threatened ischemia. Vascular regions subjected to chronic hypoperfusion and relative ischemia are maximally vasodilated and unresponsive to

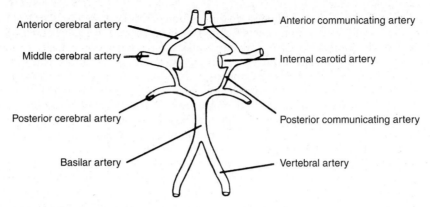

Figure 23.1 Arterial circle of Willis.

factors that induce vasoconstriction in normally reactive vascular beds. Therefore, in patients with carotid artery disease, blood flow through ischemic regions is passive and dependent on systemic blood pressure. For this reason, hypotension is best avoided in the period before restoration of unobstructed cerebral blood flow (CBF).

Barash PG, Cullen BF, Stoelting RK, eds. *Clinical anesthesia*, 5th ed. Philadelphia: Lippincott Williams s& Wilkins, 2006:946–954.

Ehrenfeld WK, Hamilton FN, Larson CP, et al. Effect of CO2 and systemic hypertension on downstream cerebral arterial pressure during carotid endarterectomy. *Surgery* 1970;67:87.

Fourcade HE, Larson CP, Ehrenfeld WK, et al. The effects of CO2 and systemic hypertension on cerebral perfusion pressure during carotid endarterectomy. *Anesthesiology* 1970; 33:383.

A.8. Discuss the different surgical approaches to carotid revascularization.

Carotid endarterectomy (CEA) involves the removal of atheromatous plaque from the vessel lumen through a fairly standardized surgical procedure. This involves occluding the common, external, and internal carotid arteries, isolating the diseased segment, opening the vessel wall, and removing the plaque. The vessel is then closed. If the remaining intima is too thin, the vessel is closed with a vein graft or a synthetic (Dacron) patch. The use of a shunt during the period of carotid cross clamping depends on whether evidence of cerebral ischemia becomes apparent with cross clamping of the carotid artery. Variations in shunt usage exist because there is little evidence that one therapy is superior to the others. Placement of a shunt allows hemispheric cerebral blood flow (CBF) to be maintained during cross clamping and may be especially advantageous when the endarterectomy is expected to be complex and require a long period of time.

On the other hand, shunt usage is not without its problems. It may make the surgery technically more difficult. Technical problems with shunts include plaque or air embolism, kinking of the shunt, shunt occlusion on the side of the vessel wall, and injury to the distal internal carotid artery. The use of a shunt does not guarantee adequate CBF nor prevent thromboembolic strokes.

Another intervention to treat carotid stenosis is percutaneous transluminal angioplasty and stenting by interventional radiologists. Advantages to endovascular techniques include: avoidance of surgical incision, minimal anesthetic requirements, avoidance of minor complications associated with endarterectomy including cranial nerve injury and wound infections, shorter duration of induced carotid occlusion by the balloon catheter than with surgical clamping of the carotid artery and lower hospital costs for shorter hospital and intensive care unit (ICU) stays.

Clinical trials comparing CEA with angioplasty have been done. Early trials were stopped prematurely because of significantly worse outcomes among patients treated with angioplasty. In the carotid and vertebral artery transluminal angioplasty study (CAVATAS), comparison of endovascular treatment and CEA for severe carotid stenosis found that at 1 year after treatment, the endovascular treatment group had more severe (70% to 99%) ipsilateral carotid stenosis. Although there was no difference in outcome based on the treatment, the perioperative rate of disabling stroke or death of 5.9% from endovascular treatment was double the average perioperative rate of 2.3% from previous larger clinical trials of CEA.

The Carotid revascularization using endarterectomy or stenting systems (CaRESS) phase I study was a multicenter, prospective, non-randomized trial designed to address the question of whether carotid artery stenting (CAS) with cerebral protection was comparable to CEA in patients with symptomatic and asymptomatic carotid stenosis. A total of 397 patients (254 CEA and 143 CAS) were enrolled in the study: 32% were symptomatic and 68% were asymptomatic. There were no significant differences in patient demographics, symptoms, or surgical risk profiles between groups at baseline. There were no significant differences in combined death/stroke rates at 30 days or at 1 year after treatment. Similarly, there was no significant difference in the combined end point of death, stroke or myocardial infarction (MI) at 30 days or 1 year between the two groups. There were also no significant differences between CEA and CAS in the secondary end points or residual stenosis, restenosis, repeat angiography, carotid revascularization, or change in quality of life. The CaRESS phase I study suggests that the 30-day and 1-year risk of death, stroke, or MI with CAS is equivalent to that with CEA in symptomatic and asymptomatic patients with carotid stenosis.

Sundt TM, Houser OW, Sharbrough FW, et al. Carotid endarterectomy: results, complications and monitoring techniques. *Adv Neurol* 1977;16:97–119.

The CaRESS Investigators. Carotid Revascularization using Endarterectomy or Stenting Systems (CaRESS) phase I clinical trial: 1-year results. *J Vasc Surg* 2005;42:213–219.

The CAVATAS Investigators. Endovascular versus surgical treatment in patients with carotid stenosis in the Carotid and Vertebral Artery Transluminal Angioplasty Study (CAVATAS): a randomized trial. *Lancet* 2001;357:1729–1737.

Thompson JE, Talkington CM. Carotid endarterectomy. *Ann Surg* 1978;184:1–15.

Wylie EJ, Stoney RJ, Ehrenfeld WK, eds. *Manual of vascular surgery*, Vol. I. *Comprehensive manuals of surgical specialties series*. New York: Springer-Verlag, 1980:49–84.

Wilke HJ, Ellis JE, McKinsey JF. Carotid endarterectomy: perioperative and anesthetic considerations. *J Cardiothorac Vasc Anesth* 1996;10:928–949.

A.9. What is normal cerebral blood flow (CBF)?

Normal CBF is approximately 50 mL/100 g/minute for the entire brain. However, blood flow is about four times higher in gray matter than it is in white matter, with the flows being 80 and 20 mL/100 g/minute, respectively.

Hemmings HC, Hopkins PM, eds. *Foundations of anesthesia basic science for clinical practice*, 2nd ed. Philadelphia: Elsevier Science, 2006:248–249.

Kety SS, Schmidt CF. The nitrous oxide method for the quantitative determination of cerebral blood flow in man: theory, procedure and normal values. *J Clin Invest* 1948;27:476.

Lassen NA, Munch O. The cerebral blood flow in man determined by the use of radioactive krypton. *Acta Physiol Scand* 1955;33:30.

A.10. What is critically low cerebral flow as measured by the electroencephalogram (EEG)?

Assuming a normal temperature and hematocrit, 100 mL of blood contains approximately 20 mL of oxygen. A normal global cerebral blood flow (CBF) of 50 mL/100 g/minute delivers oxygen to the brain at a rate of 10 mL/100 g/min. This is in excess of the high metabolic requirements of the brain for oxygen (3 to 5 mL/100 g/minute), which affords a relative margin of safety. The CBF at which ischemia becomes apparent on the EEG is approximately 20 mL/100 g/minute. EEG changes may be delayed for up to 150 seconds following the onset of ischemia. It is impossible to define the specific changes that represent irreversible ischemia. In the setting of an isoelectric EEG, oxygen delivery to the brain may be adequate to keep the neurons alive but may provide insufficient energy for them to function.

The development of cerebral infarction depends on both the degree and duration of ischemia. Jones showed in an animal model of reversible ischemia, that with CBF of 18 to 23 mL/100 g/minute animals would recover from impaired neurologic function when blood flow was returned to normal levels, regardless of the duration of the ischemic period. Infarction development at lower flows depends on both the degree of regional cerebral blood flow (rCBF) reduction and the duration of ischemia. Neurons that are nonfunctional but that will recover fully with restoration of adequate flow are said to be in an ischemic penumbra. Neuronal destruction occurs with CBF less than 10 mL/100 g/minute.

Barash PG, Cullen BF, Stoelting RK, eds. *Clinical anesthesia*, 5th ed. Philadelphia: Lippincott Williams & Wilkins, 2006:946–954.

Boysen G, Engell HC, Pitolese GR, et al. On the critical level of cerebral blood flow in man with particular reference to carotid surgery. *Circulation* 1974;49:1023.

Jones TH, Morawetz RB, Crowell RM, et al. Threshold of focal cerebral ischemia in awake monkeys. *J Neurosurg* 1981;54:773.

Levy WJ. Intraoperative EEG patterns: Implications for EEG monitoring. *Anesthesiology* 1984;60:430.

Trojaborg W, Boysen G. Relation between EEG, regional cerebral blood flow and internal carotid artery pressure during carotid endarterectomy. *Electroencephalogr Clin Neurophysiol* 1973;34:61.

A.11. What is cerebral autoregulation?

Cerebral autoregulation is the tendency of the tissue to maintain normal blood flow despite variations in blood pressure. In normotensive individuals, cerebral blood flow (CBF) is constant between mean arterial pressures of 50 and 150 mm Hg. What this means is that cerebrovascular resistance increases, through vasoconstriction, as mean arterial pressure increases from 50 to 150 mm Hg. At pressures greater than 150 mm Hg, the cerebral vasculature is maximally vasoconstricted and CBF increases with increasing pressure. At pressures less than 50 mm Hg, cerebral vessels are maximally vasodilated, so that as mean arterial pressure falls CBF decreases.

In hypertensive patients, autoregulation still exists. The upper and lower limits of the autoregulatory curve, however, have been shifted to the right in these individuals, to higher pressures (Fig. 23.2). What this means is that a mean arterial pressure of 60 mm Hg, which would be well tolerated in a normotensive individual, may actually be below the lower limit of autoregulation in the hypertensive individual, resulting in cerebral hypoperfusion. Conversely,

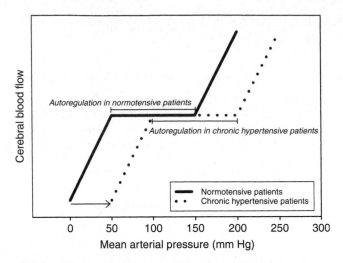

Figure 23.2 Cerebral autoregulatory curves in normotensive and chronic hypertensive patients. New autoregulation curve is achieved with chronic hypertension. The curve shifts back to normotensive range once hypertension is well controlled.

hypertensive patients tolerate marked increases in mean arterial pressure much better than their normotensive counterparts. In treated hypertensive patients, the limits of autoregulation are shifted with time toward normal.

Haggendal E, Lofgren J, Nilsson NJ, et al. Effects of varied cerebrospinal fluid pressure on cerebral blood flow in dogs. *Acta Physiol Scand* 1970;79:262.

Hemmings HC, Hopkins PM, eds. *Foundations of anesthesia basic science for clinical practice*, 2nd ed. Philadelphia: Elsevier Science, 2006:249–250.

Symon L, Pasztor E, Dorsch NWC, et al. Physiological responses of local areas of the cerebral circulation in experimental primates determined by the method of hydrogen clearance. *Stroke* 1973;4:632.

A.12. How does PCO_2 affect cerebral blood flow (CBF)?

Hypercarbia results in cerebral vasodilation and hypocarbia in cerebral vasoconstriction. CBF changes approximately 4% for each mm Hg increase or decrease in arterial PCO_2 for partial pressures of arterial carbon dioxide between 20 and 80 mm Hg.

Hemmings HC, Hopkins PM, eds. *Foundations of anesthesia basic science for clinical practice*, 2nd ed. Philadelphia: Elsevier Science, 2006:249–250.

Skinhoj E, Paulson OB. Carbon dioxide and cerebral circulatory control: evidence of a nonfocal site of action of carbon dioxide on the cerebral circulation. *Arch Neurol* 1969; 20:249.

A.13. What are the principal determinants of cerebral blood flow (CBF)?

The principal determinants of CBF are nerve cell activity, cerebral perfusion pressure, $PaCO_2$, the pH of the extracellular fluid in the brain, PaO_2, and neurogenic influences.

Cottrell JE, Smith DS. *Anesthesia and neurosurgery*, 4th ed. St. Louis: CV Mosby, 2001:19–32.

Hemmings HC, Hopkins PM, eds. *Foundations of anesthesia basic science for clinical practice*, 2nd ed. Philadelphia: Elsevier Science, 2006:247–250.

A.14. What is meant by the term "luxury perfusion"?

Luxury perfusion is blood flow that is in excess of metabolic need (increased cerebral blood flow [CBF] relative to cerebral metabolic rate for O_2). It is most frequently observed in tissues surrounding tumors or areas of infarction. It has also been described in tissues that have been manipulated during surgery.

Paulson OB. Cerebral apoplexy (stroke): pathogenesis, pathophysiology and therapy as illustrated by regional blood flow measurements in the brain. *Stroke* 1971;2:327–360.

A.15. What is meant by the term intracerebral steal?

Intracerebral steal is a paradoxical response to carbon dioxide in which hypercapnea decreases the blood flow in an ischemic area. It is the consequence of the vasodilatory effect of carbon dioxide on the normally perfused arterioles at the periphery of an ischemic lesion. Because chronically ischemic vascular beds are maximally vasodilated, they cannot dilate further in response to hypercapnea.

Paulson OB. Cerebral apoplexy (stroke): pathogenesis, pathophysiology and their therapy as illustrated by regional blood flow measurements in the brain. *Stroke* 1971;2:327–360.

A.16. What is "inverse steal" or the "Robin Hood" syndrome?

Inverse steal is the effect of hypocapnea producing increased blood flow to ischemic regions of the brain. Vasoconstriction occurs in adjacent, normal arterioles, thereby causing a local increase in perfusion pressure and augmenting collateral flow to the ischemic, unreactive, maximally vasodilated area of the brain.

Betz E. Cerebral blood flow: its measurement and regulation. *Physiol Rev* 1972;52:595–630.

B. Preoperative Evaluation and Preparation

B.1. What would you be looking for in your preoperative evaluation?

Once the presence of a carotid lesion amenable to surgical treatment has been documented through Doppler, angiographic, or oculoplethysmographic studies, the anesthesiologist will be asked to evaluate the patient regarding her readiness for surgery. The anesthesiologist should determine whether or not other manifestations of generalized arteriosclerosis, such as coronary artery disease, hypertension, and renal disease, are present. Medical conditions associated with arteriosclerosis, such as obesity, diabetes mellitus, and pulmonary disease secondary to cigarette smoking, should be sought. The patient's neurologic status and airway will need to be evaluated.

Because 30% to 50% of patients undergoing carotid endarterectomy (CEA) have coronary artery disease, evidence of heart disease should be sought in the patient's history. Patients should be specifically asked whether they have angina, or have had a myocardial infarction (MI) or congestive heart failure. An indication of daily activity level should be obtained. A patient unable to ambulate for distances because of claudication may never develop angina or left ventricular failure; henceforth, more invasive evaluation of the patient's cardiac function may be required. Evidence of cardiac disease should also be sought on physical examination. This would include heart rate and rhythm, and presence of jugular venous distention, basilar rales on auscultation of the chest, cardiac enlargement as determined by lateral displacement of the point of maximal impulse, and an S3 gallop.

Based on the Cardiac Risk Stratification for noncardiac surgical procedures by the American Heart Association/American College of Cardiology Task force on assessment of therapeutic cardiovascular procedures, CEA is classified as an intermediate risk procedure with a reported cardiac risk generally less than 5%.

Whether or not the patient has hypertension should be determined. Hypertension is present in 55% to 80% of patients with carotid artery disease, and its presence would alter intraoperative blood pressure management. Blood pressure should be measured in both arms with the patient in both the supine and the upright positions. A range of acceptable blood pressures, where the patient is free of symptoms of both cardiac and cerebral ischemia, should be determined. This is done, in part, by reviewing the patient's chart and making note of the highest and the lowest blood pressures that were measured. Knowing this range allows the anesthesiologist to determine the range of blood pressures, which are likely to be tolerated without treatment in the operating room. Raising the blood pressure excessively to improve cerebral perfusion may exacerbate myocardial ischemia, and lowering the blood pressure to reduce the work of the heart may compromise cerebral perfusion, exacerbating cerebral ischemia.

The presence of other disorders associated with vascular disease, such as obesity, diabetes, and cigarette smoking with their sequelae, should be determined. Evidence of other end-organ effects of vascular disease, such as renal dysfunction, should also be sought.

The patient's neurologic status also needs to be evaluated preoperatively. Although it would be preferable to medically optimize the patient with uncontrolled hypertension or untreated metabolic disease, or if possible, delay surgery in the patient with a recent MI, the presence of crescendo transient ischemia attacks (TIAs) may not allow that option.

The patient's airway needs to be assessed for ease of ventilation and intubation. A patient in whom it is difficult to establish ventilation may become hypercarbic during induction, and the increase in $PaCO_2$ may have adverse effects on regional cerebral blood flow (CBF). As part of this evaluation, the range of motion of the patient's neck that is tolerated without evidence of cerebral ischemia needs to be determined so that relative extremes of extension and lateral rotation of the neck during ventilation, intubation, and finally patient positioning can be avoided. Extreme extension and rotation of the neck may occlude the patient's vertebral artery and contribute to postoperative neurologic deficits.

Asiddao CB, Donegan JH, Whitesell RC, et al. Factors associated with perioperative complications during carotid endarterectomy. *Anesth Analg* 1982;61:631.

Barash PG, Cullen BF, Stoelting RK, eds. *Clinical anesthesia*, 5th ed. Philadelphia: Lippincott Williams & Wilkins, 2006:946–954.

Eagle K, Brundage B, Chaitman B, et al. Guidelines for perioperative cardiac evaluation of the noncardiac surgery. A report of the American Heart Association/American College of Cardiology Task Force on assessment of diagnostic and therapeutic cardiovascular procedures. *Circulation* 1996;93:1278.

B.2. Is this patient's blood pressure too high for elective surgery?

Although hypertension is present in most patients presenting for carotid endarterectomy (CEA), its rapid correction is not recommended because this may exacerbate cerebral ischemia. If this patient had evidence of myocardial ischemia at this blood pressure and was stable from a neurologic standpoint, blood pressure could be gradually decreased with antihypertensive medications.

Normal myocardial and cerebral function need to be preserved. These goals are not necessarily at odds with each other. To decrease myocardial oxygen consumption, one would want to decrease heart rate, blood pressure, and myocardial contractility. In this patient population, decreasing heart rate can decrease myocardial work; whereas cerebral perfusion pressure is maintained with an adequate mean arterial pressure. If a hypertensive patient presents with an unstable neurologic status, it may be necessary to control blood pressure only once the obstruction to cerebral blood flow (CBF) has been relieved.

A single blood pressure measurement is of little use in the preoperative assessment of the patient. It is the range of the blood pressures normally tolerated by the patient that will guide perioperative blood pressure management. For example, if a patient's blood pressure is measured at 80/50 mm Hg and at 170/100 mm Hg preoperatively and at these blood pressures, she does not develop any new neurologic deficits or myocardial ischemia, the clinician will be inclined to treat blood pressures only beyond these two extremes.

Because this patient is hypertensive, one can expect that wide swings in her blood pressure will occur under anesthesia. The anesthesiologist must be prepared for these fluctuations by having both vasopressors and vasodilators readily available. Variations in blood pressure should be minimized because these have been related to increased cardiac and neurologic morbidity.

Barash PG, Cullen BF, Stoelting RK, eds. *Clinical anesthesia*, 5th ed. Philadelphia: Lippincott Williams & Wilkins, 2006:946–954.

Hamilton WP. Do let the blood pressure drop and do use myocardial depressants? *Anesthesiology* 1976;45:273–274.

Smith JS, Roizen MF, Cahalan MK, et al. Does anesthetic technique make a difference? Augmentation of systolic blood pressure during carotid endarterectomy: effects of phenylephrine versus light anesthesia and of isoflurane versus halothane on the incidence of myocardial ischemia. *Anesthesiology* 1988;69:846–853.

B.3. What laboratory data would be required preoperatively?

Laboratory tests should be ordered to determine the patient's baseline cardiac, respiratory, and metabolic status.

Hemoglobin and hematocrit should be obtained preoperatively because values may be abnormal in a patient with advanced age, renal, or pulmonary disease and because significant blood loss may occur intraoperatively.

A urine analysis and data on blood urea nitrogen and creatinine should be obtained to determine the patient's baseline renal status.

An electrocardiogram (ECG) should be examined preoperatively to look for arrhythmias, evidence of ischemia, previous myocardial infarctions (MIs), or left ventricular hypertrophy. Where appropriate, the preoperative ECG should be compared with earlier studies to determine whether interval changes have occurred.

A chest x-ray should be examined to look for cardiomegaly, evidence of pulmonary edema or chronic obstructive pulmonary disease (COPD), or pneumonia. If the patient has a history of COPD, a preoperative arterial blood gas should be obtained to identify the patient's baseline $PaCO_2$. In patients who are chronically hypercarbic, rapid adjustment to normocarbia intraoperatively will be interpreted by the body as relative hypocarbia. Cerebral blood flow (CBF) will be reduced accordingly. Management of intraoperative ventilation should be aimed at maintaining the patient's normal arterial carbon dioxide level.

Further preoperative evaluation would be based on the presence of concurrent disease.

Barash PG, Cullen BF, Stoelting RK, eds. *Clinical anesthesia*, 5th ed. Philadelphia: Lippincott Williams & Wilkins, 2006:946–954.

B.4. Would you premedicate this patient?

Some disagreement exists as to whether patients should be premedicated before a carotid endarterectomy (CEA). Ideally the patient should present to the operating room calm and awake. Preoperative anxiety should be alleviated in these patients because anxiety can lead to preoperative hypertension, which has been associated with adverse neurologic outcome. Increases in heart rate in the anxious patient lead to increased myocardial oxygen consumption and, potentially, ischemia, ventricular dysfunction, and arrhythmias.

Premedication may lead to ventilatory depression, with resultant hypercarbia and alterations in cerebral blood flow (CBF) that can exacerbate cerebral ischemia. Sedation can also interfere with the immediate postoperative neurologic assessment of the patient because it may cause delayed awakening from anesthesia. One of the anesthetic goals for CEA under general anesthesia is to have a patient who promptly emerges from anesthesia and is able to cooperate with a basic neurologic evaluation. A patient who is too sedated at the end of surgery is problematic.

To achieve these goals, a thorough and reassuring preoperative visit alone may provide sufficient anxiolysis. The anesthesiologist should explain the preoperative procedure and what can be expected in the postoperative period, answering any questions that the patient has. If a pharmacologic premedication is required, a benzodiazepine (e.g., diazepam 5 mg orally, 1 hour preoperatively or midazolam 1 to 2 mg intravenously) will provide anxiolysis and minimal respiratory depression.

Bailey PL, Andriano KP, Goldman M, et al. Variability of the respiratory response to diazepam. *Anesthesiology* 1986;64:460.

Barash PG, Cullen BF, Stoelting RK, eds. *Clinical anesthesia*, 5th ed. Philadelphia: Lippincott Williams & Wilkins, 2006:946–954.

Freeman LJ, Nixon PGF, Sallabank P, et al. Psychological stress and silent myocardial ischemia. *Am Heart J* 1987;114:477.

Leigh JM, Walker J, Janaganathan P. Effect of preoperative anaesthetic visit on anxiety. *Br Med J* 1977;2:987.

C. Intraoperative Management

C.1. How would you monitor this patient?

Patients who are about to undergo carotid endarterectomy (CEA) are monitored with routine monitors of cardiovascular, pulmonary, and metabolic function, which include electrocardiogram (ECG) leads II and V_5; noninvasive blood pressure monitor; pulse oximetry; end-tidal capnometry; and esophageal temperature.

An intraarterial catheter should be used to monitor the patient's blood pressure closely. Its presence will permit immediate identification of blood pressure changes and allow for repetitive sampling of arterial blood gases.

Whether a pulmonary artery catheter is required to monitor the patient's cardiac function would be dictated solely by the patient's preoperative cardiac status. CEA is not an operation in which large fluid shifts are anticipated. A pulmonary artery catheter should not be required in the patient with normal left ventricular function.

Barash PG, Cullen BF, Stoelting RK, eds. *Clinical anesthesia*, 5th ed. Philadelphia: Lippincott Williams & Wilkins, 2006; 951–952.

C.2. How would you know that the patient's cerebral perfusion is adequate during surgery?

In the awake patient undergoing carotid endarterectomy (CEA) under local anesthesia, repeated neurologic examinations can be done to assess the adequacy of cerebral perfusion.

If the patient receives general anesthesia, cerebral perfusion or function should be monitored. No currently available clinical monitor is as sensitive and specific for cerebral dysfunction as repeated neurologic examinations, and no one monitor is used routinely in all operating rooms. A number of monitors have been used to monitor cerebral perfusion or function. These include the electroencephalograph (EEG), somatosensory evoked potentials (SSEP), transcranial Doppler, internal carotid stump pressure, and jugular venous oxygen saturation.

There has been recent interest in cerebral oximetry as a monitor as it is noninvasive, continuous, and easy to use. In recent studies, a relative decrease of 20% or greater in regional cerebral oxygen saturation (rSO_2) suggested cerebral ischemia. The monitor, though, had a low positive predictive value and low specificity. If used exclusively, it would suggest the need for unnecessary shunting and lead to over-shunting of patients.

Barash PG, Cullen BF, Stoelting RK, eds. *Clinical anesthesia*, 5th ed. Philadelphia: Lippincott Williams & Wilkins, 2006:950–951.

Evans WE, Hayes JP, Waltke EA, et al. Optimal cerebral monitoring during carotid endarterectomy: neurologic response under local anesthesia. *J Vasc Surg* 1985;2:775.

Grubhofer G, Plochl W, Skolka M, et al. Comparing doppler ultrasonography and cerebral oximetry as indicators for shunting in carotid endarterectomy. *Anesth Analg* 2000; 91:1339–1344.

Grundy BL, Sanderson AC, Webster MW, et al. Hemiparesis following carotid endarterectomy: comparison of monitoring methods. *Anesthesiology* 1981;55:462.

Rosenthal D, Stanton PE Jr, Lamis PA. Carotid endarterectomy: the unreliability of intraoperative monitoring having had stroke or reversible ischemic neurological deficit. *Arch Surg* 1981;116:1569.

Samra SK, Dy EA, Welch K, et al. Evaluation of a cerebral oximeter as a monitor of cerebral ischemia during carotid endarterectomy. *Anesthesiology* 2000;93:964–970.

C.3. Discuss the differences and relative advantages and disadvantages of the unprocessed electroencephalogram (EEG) and the processed EEG.

The EEG is neither a measure of cerebral blood flow (CBF) nor a way to determine whether irreversible neuronal damage has occurred. Rather, it is an indicator that areas of the brain may be at risk for infarction. EEG changes that occur with hypothermia, hypocarbia, hypoxemia, and deep anesthesia mimic electroencephalographic signs of ischemia. In patients who have had a cerebral vascular accident (CVA), the processed EEG does not predict cerebral ischemia.

A number of problems associated with monitoring the 16-lead EEG intraoperatively have detracted from its popularity. These include difficulty in obtaining a meaningful recording in the electrically noisy environment of the operating room, the bulk of the equipment required, and the need for specially trained personnel for interpretation. The 16-channel EEG is, however, a sensitive indicator of ischemia.

The processed EEG has eliminated many of the problems associated with the 16-channel EEG. The equipment is generally compact and the data display allows for ease of interpretation. The most commonly used processed EEG is the power spectrum analysis. For this analysis the EEG is studied in short time intervals of 2 to 16 minutes, called *epochs*. Each epoch then is subjected to a fast Fourier transform analysis during which the complex waveform of the unprocessed EEG is broken down into its component sine waves of varying amplitudes and frequencies. The power spectrum is calculated by squaring the amplitude of the individual frequency components. The power spectrum can then be displayed in a number of graphic forms, two of which are the compressed spectral array and the density modulated spectral array. Data are displayed in these two forms as relative power versus frequency (Fig. 23.3).

It must be remembered that the processed EEG is only as good as the original from which it was obtained. Therefore, meticulous recording techniques are required even when monitoring a processed EEG. During carotid endarterectomy (CEA) generally two or four EEG channels are monitored in order to determine right and left symmetry in neuronal activity during interruption of CBF.

Barash PG, Cullen BF, Stoelting RK, eds. *Clinical anesthesia*, 5th ed. Philadelphia: Lippincott Williams & Wilkins, 2006:758–760.

Harris EJ, Brown WH, Pavy RN, et al. Continuous electroencephalographic monitoring during carotid artery endarterectomy. *Surgery* 1978;83:306.

Kearse LA, Lopez-Bresnahan M, McPeck K, et al. Preoperative cerebrovascular symptoms and electroencephalographic abnormalities do not predict cerebral ischemia during carotid endarterectomy. *Stroke* 1995;26:1210.

Levy W, Shapiro HM, Maruchak G, et al. Automated EEG processing for intraoperative monitoring. *Anesthesiology* 1980;53:223.

Rampil IJ, Holzer JA, Quest DO, et al. Prognostic value of computerized EEG analysis during carotid endarterectomy. *Anesth Analg* 1983;62:186.

Sundt TM, Sharbrough FW, Peipgras DG, et al. Correlation of cerebral blood flow and electroencephalographic changes during carotid endarterectomy. *Mayo Clin Proc* 1981;56:533.

C.4. How would you measure cerebral blood flow (CBF) intraoperatively? What are the relative advantages and disadvantages of each technique? How much CBF is considered adequate?

Measurement of regional CBF is the single best method for detecting decreases in CBF during general anesthesia. A number of different ways are used to measure CBF. These include the Kety-Schmidt method, later modifications on this, the intracarotid injection method, and the inhalation and intravenous techniques.

The Kety-Schmidt method, as originally described, involved 10 to 16 minutes of inhalation of 15% nitrous oxide. During this period of time equilibration would occur between arterial, venous, and tissue concentrations of nitrous oxide. Blood samples would intermittently be taken from a peripheral artery and the jugular bulb to determine tracer concentration. The amount of tracer taken up by the brain in a certain period of time is equivalent to the amount delivered to the brain in the arterial blood supply minus that recovered in the cerebral venous blood in the same period of time. If it is assumed that the brain concentration of the tracer is proportional to the tracer

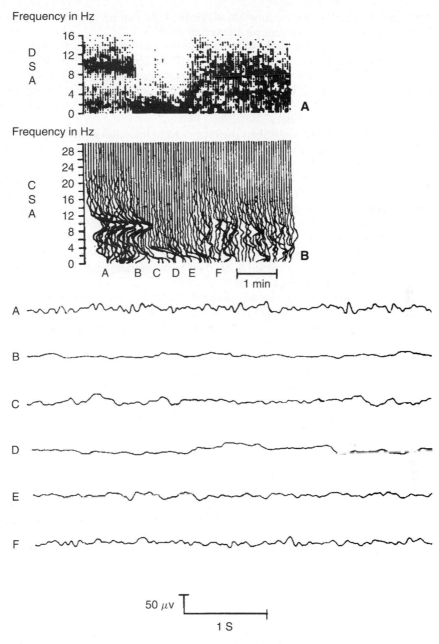

Figure 23.3 An example of density spectral analysis (**A**) and the unprocessed EEG (**B**) compressed during a period of marked hypotension during initiation of bypass. Slowing wave form activity in the unprocessed EEG (*B to E*) is also evident in the density modulated spectral array (DSA) and compressed spectral array (CSA). (Reprinted with permission from Levy W, Shapiro HM, Maruchak G, et al. Automated EEG processing for intraoperative monitoring. *Anesthesiol* 1980;53:223.)

concentrations in the cerebral venous blood, global CBF can be determined with knowledge of the blood brain partition coefficient for the tracer used.

Later modifications of this technique employ the radioactive tracers krypton 85 (^{85}Kr) or xenon 133 (^{133}Xe). CBF, as measured using the Kety-Schmidt method and its modifications, may overestimate CBF in the case of low perfusion states in which brain and venous blood may not equilibrate. One cannot measure regional cerebral blood flow (rCBF) using these techniques because jugular venous blood is a mixed venous sample with varying amounts of contamination from the contralateral hemisphere.

In 1961, Lassen and Ingva described the intracarotid injection method of CBF determination. The technique involves injecting a radioactive tracer, ^{85}Kr or ^{133}Xe, as a bolus into the cerebral arterial supply and following the cerebral washout with external scintillation counting. Use of external scintillation counters makes it possible to determine rCBF, and the sensitivity of the technique is improved by increasing the number of detectors. The tracer is injected directly into either an internal carotid or a vertebral artery, minimizing the number of counts obtained from the extracranial circulatory distribution. This method assumes that the tracer mixes completely with brain. Because the tracer is almost completely exhaled on passage through the lungs, it has essentially no recirculation. A typical tracer washout curve in normal brain is the summation of two exponential curves. Two separate flows, fast (gray matter) and slow (white matter), can be calculated using compartmental analysis.

The more noninvasive techniques to determine CBF are the inhalation and the intravenous techniques. The inhalation method involves a 1-minute period of inhalation of ^{133}Xe followed by a 10-minute period of washout with external detection. The washout of tracer from the brain is similar to that obtained with intraarterial injection except that, because of mixing in the heart and the lungs, the input of tracer is not instantaneous. Because the slow component of CBF is contaminated by extracranial clearance of the tracer, the noninvasive methods are suited primarily for determination of gray matter flow. The inhalation and intravenous methods may be less reliable in the presence of pulmonary disease because the end-tidal concentration of tracer may not adequately reflect arterial concentration. With these techniques, extracranial contamination can result in an underestimation of CBF results, and under extremely low flow states, they may not give reliable quantitative information.

One thing to bear in mind with all tracer washout techniques is that, in general, they only provide flow information about cortical CBF and not about deeper structures. Furthermore, with any of these techniques, CBF is a calculated number, and it will vary depending on the specific technique used to measure it. Average global CBF is 50 mL/100 g/minute, gray matter flow is 80 mL/100 g/minute, and white matter flow is 20 mL/100 g/minute. A measured flow intraoperatively of greater than 24 mL/100 g/minute is considered to be sufficient and that of less than 18 mL/100 g/minute is inadequate. The specific flow differences compatible with ischemia depend on the anesthetic agents used. The expense and expertise required to collect and interpret CBF data have limited its use to only a few centers.

Barash PG, Cullen BF, Stoelting RK, eds. *Clinical anesthesia*, 5th ed. Philadelphia: Lippincott Williams & Wilkins, 2006:946–954.

Bell BA. A history of the study of the cerebral circulation and the measurement of cerebral blood flow. *Neurosurgery* 1984;14:238.

C.5. Does internal carotid stump pressure accurately reflect cerebral perfusion?

The internal carotid stump pressure, the pressure in the portion of the internal carotid artery cephalad to the carotid cross-clamp, has been used to determine whether cerebral blood flow (CBF) during cross clamping was adequate to avoid neuronal damage. The stump pressure presumably reflects pressure transmitted through collateral vessels. Maintaining stump pressures from 25 to 70 mm Hg has been described as necessary to avoid neurologic injury. However, this range of stump pressures may not reliably represent the adequacy of collateral CBF, as it does not correlate consistently with changes in the electroencephalogram (EEG), regional cerebral blood flow (rCBF), or changes in the neurologic status of the awake patient. Furthermore, anesthetic agents can alter carotid stump pressure without changing regional CBF. Inadequate stump pressures have been demonstrated when measured rCBF was adequate. Therefore, if shunting during carotid endarterectomy (CEA) were to be done only on the basis of stump pressures, some patients would unnecessarily receive shunts.

Barash PG, Cullen BF, Stoelting RK, eds. *Clinical anesthesia*, 5th ed. Philadelphia: Lippincott Williams & Wilkins, 2006:946–954.

Harada RN, Comerota AJ, Good GM, et al. Stump pressure, electroencephalographic changes, and the contralateral carotid artery: another look at selective shunting. *Am J Surg* 1995;170:148.

Kelly JJ, Callow AD, O'Donnell TF, et al. Failure of carotid stump pressure: its incidence as a predictor for a temporary shunt during carotid endarterectomy. *Arch Surg* 1979; 114:1361.

C.6. Discuss somatosensory evoked potentials (SSEPs) as a monitor of cerebral blood flow (CBF) during carotid endarterectomy (CEA).

SSEPs are a specialized form of electrophysiologic monitoring that reflects the presence of intact sensory pathways from a stimulated peripheral nerve to the cortex where electrical activity is monitored. Evidence exists that distortion of certain waveforms is associated with ischemia. These SSEP changes, however, are not consistently associated with changes in the electroencephalogram (EEG). Questions have been raised regarding whether SSEPs can over predict the presence of ischemia and the need for shunting. Further work in this area is warranted because, if SSEPs are a useful indicator of ischemia, they may be used when ischemia cannot be detected on an EEG tracing, such as during barbiturate anesthesia. During barbiturate anesthesia the isoelectric EEG can only indicate that neurons are quiet. It cannot indicate whether these same neurons are ischemic. The SSEP tracing would remain intact with barbiturate anesthesia and, therefore, would potentially be more useful as a clinical monitor. In patients who have had prior strokes, there is some asymmetry to their baseline SSEP waveforms. This asymmetry does not appear to affect the SSEP as an effective clinical monitor, which may also be a relative advantage over the EEG in patients with prior cerebral vascular accidents (CVAs).

Lam AM, Teturswamy G. Monitoring of evoked responses during carotid endarterectomy and extracranial-intracranial anastomosis. *Int Anesthesiol Clin* 1984;22:107.

Manninen PH, Tan TK, Sarjeant RM. Somatosensory evoked potential monitoring during carotid endarterectomy in patients with a stroke. *Anesth Analg* 2001;93:39.

Moorthy SS, Markand ON, Dilley RS, et al. Somatosensory-evoked responses during carotid endarterectomy. *Anesth Analg* 1982;61:879.

C.7. Describe the role of the transcranial Doppler as a monitor of cerebral perfusion during carotid endarterectomy (CEA).

By allowing for continuous assessment of the velocity of the blood flow in the ipsilateral middle cerebral artery, the transcranial Doppler may be useful throughout CEA. It can aid in determining the need for a shunt by detecting a decrease in the middle cerebral artery blood flow velocity with placement of the carotid cross-clamp. It allows for continuous assessment of shunt function. It can be used to assess the adequacy of pharmacologically induced intraoperative hypertensive therapy. The transcranial Doppler also allows for the detection of air or particulate embolization. The disadvantage of the transcranial Doppler is that it is technically demanding and not obtainable in approximately 20% of patients.

A good correlation has been shown between intraoperative electroencephalography (EEGs) and transcranial Doppler. Patients who have unchanged EEGs have a middle cerebral artery velocity of 24.1 cm per second during cross clamping, whereas those with a middle cerebral artery velocity of 14.7 cm per second develop EEG changes. The ratio of the mean velocity while the cross-clamp is in place compared with the mean velocity before placement of the clamp may also be used to predict alteration in neurologic function. A ratio below 0.4 detects 97% of patients with EEG evidence of cerebral ischemia.

Barash PG, Cullen BF, Stoelting RK, eds. *Clinical anesthesia*, 5th ed. Philadelphia: Lippincott Williams & Wilkins, 2006:951.

Grubhofer G, Plochl W, Skolka M, et al. Comparing Doppler ultrasonography and cerebral oximetry as indicators for shunting in carotid endarterectomy. *Anesth Analg* 2000; 91:1339.

Jansen C, Vriens EM, Eikelboom BC, et al. Carotid endarterectomy with transcranial Doppler and electroencephalographic monitoring: a prospective study in 130 operations. *Stroke* 1993;24:665.

Jorgensen LG, Schroeder TV. Transcranial Doppler for detection of cerebral ischaemia during carotid endarterectomy. *Eur J Vasc Surg* 1992;6:142.

Schneider PA, Rossman ME, Torem S, et al. Transcranial Doppler in the management of extracranial cerebrovascular disease: implications in diagnosis and monitoring. *J Vasc Surg* 1988;7:223.

C.8. What type of anesthesia would you choose for this patient? Why?

Patients undergoing carotid endarterectomy (CEA) may have either regional or general anesthesia. Each type of anesthesia has its own advantages and disadvantages, which must be considered when choosing the optimal anesthetic for a patient. Benefits of general anesthesia include a still patient and a quiet operative field, early control of the airway and ventilation, and the ability to "protect" the brain should ischemia, which cannot be eliminated, develop. A disadvantage of general anesthesia is the inability to perform repeated neurologic evaluations during surgery. Therefore, patients receiving general anesthesia should have their cerebral blood flow (CBF) or function monitored as previously discussed.

The primary advantage of a regional anesthetic is that the patient remains awake allowing for repeated neurologic evaluations. Although anecdotal reports support that regional anesthesia allows for greater stability of blood pressure, decreased requirement for vasoactive medications to support blood pressure, and decreased incidence of perioperative myocardial infarction (MI), further outcome studies are warranted. Potential complications associated with regional anesthesia include the following:

- Seizures
- Alteration of mental status with cerebral ischemia
- Loss of patient cooperation associated with cerebral hypoperfusion, inadequate ventilation, and sedation

A metaanalysis of 3 randomized studies of 143 patients and 17 nonrandomized retrospective studies demonstrated that within 30 days of operation, there was a 50% reduction in the relative odds of death, stroke, MI and pulmonary complications with regional anesthesia. However, there are still no large randomized prospective studies to draw definitive conclusions in terms of which type of anesthesia is optimal.

Allen BT, Anderson CB, Rubin BG, et al. The influence of anesthetic technique on perioperative complications after carotid endarterectomy. *J Vasc Surg* 1994;19:834.

Barash PG, Cullen BF, Stoelting RK, eds. *Clinical anesthesia*, 5th ed. Philadelphia: Lippincott Williams & Wilkins, 2006:946–954.

Corson JD, Chang BB, Shah DM, et al. The influence of anesthetic choice on carotid endarterectomy outcome. *Arch Surg* 1987;122:807.

Ombrellaro MP, Freeman MB, Stevens SL, et al. Effect of anesthetic technique on cardiac morbidity following carotid artery surgery. *Am J Surg* 1996;171:387.

Stoneham MD, Knighton JD. Regional anaesthesia for carotid endarterectomy. *Br J Anaesth* 1999;82:910.

C.9. How would you induce and maintain general anesthesia in this patient?

Following preoxygenation, all anesthetics should be titrated slowly with special attention to their effect on the patient's blood pressure. Control of the airway should be taken as soon as the patient is no longer able to breathe adequately to maintain normocarbia. While breathing oxygen, the patient is given small doses of fentanyl and reminded to breathe to maintain normocapnea. Opioids are administered until the patient is comfortably sedated. This may be accomplished with a dose of 3 μg per kg of fentanyl. Lidocaine (0.5 to 1 mg/kg) is administered intravenously with at least 2 minutes before laryngoscopy and intubation to blunt the hyperdynamic response to airway manipulation. Following administration of 2 to 3 mg per kg of thiopental, controlled ventilation is instituted with 100% oxygen to avoid hypoxia and hypercarbia. A muscle relaxant is administered to facilitate endotracheal intubation. Succinylcholine should be avoided in hemiparetic patients because of the possibility of a hyperkalemic response to its administration. Nondepolarizing muscle relaxants with significant hemodynamic effects such as sympathomimetic activity, vagolysis, or histamine release should be avoided. Once the patient is relaxed, an expeditious laryngoscopy and intubation are performed. The time spent intubating the patient's trachea is minimized to decrease the hemodynamic response to airway manipulation.

During the induction and intubation sequence, the patient's blood pressure is kept in his normal range by the use of vasopressors such as phenylephrine and vasodilators such as nitroglycerin or sodium nitroprusside as indicated.

Anesthesia can be maintained with a combination of volatile anesthetics and opioids. The addition of opioids to an isoflurane anesthetic will decrease heart rate, reduce the requirements for volatile anesthetics and, when properly dosed, allow for a prompt, smooth emergence from general anesthesia. Their use should not be avoided because of anecdotal reports of adverse neurologic outcome after focal ischemia in rodents. Any anesthetic regimen is suitable if it provides hemodynamic stability, does not exacerbate cerebral ischemia, and allows for a prompt emergence from anesthesia at the conclusion of surgery.

Maintenance of a light anesthetic appears to have several advantages over deep anesthesia. It allows ischemic patterns on the electroencephalogram (EEG) to be recognized easily. It also facilitates maintenance of the patient's blood pressure. In addition, administration of a light anesthetic, compared to a deep anesthetic using phenylephrine to maintain blood pressure, results in a lower incidence of perioperative myocardial infarction (MI).

Barash PG, Cullen BF, Stoelting RK, eds. *Clinical anesthesia*, 5th ed. Philadelphia: Lippincott Williams & Wilkins, 2006:948–949.

Barone FC, Feuerstein GZ, White RF. Brain cooling during transient focal ischemia provides complete neuroprotection. *Neurosci Biobehav Rev* 1997;21:31.

Schmid-Elsaesser R, Hungerguber E, Zausinger S, et al. Combination drug therapy and mild hypothermia: a promising treatment strategy for reversible, focal cerebral ischemia. *Stroke* 1999;30:1891.

Smith JS, Roizen MF, Cahalan MK, et al. Does anesthetic technique make a difference? Augmentation of systolic blood pressure during carotid endarterectomy: effects of phenylephrine versus light anesthesia and of isoflurane versus halothane on the incidence of myocardial ischemia. *Anesthesiology* 1988;69:836.

C.10. How would you proceed if the patient were to receive regional anesthesia?

Patient cooperation is essential for a regional anesthetic to proceed successfully. For a patient to be adequately anesthetized, a sensory blockade is required in the C2 to C4 dermatomes. This can be accomplished with either deep or superficial cervical plexus blocks. In doing the blocks, care must be taken not to excessively palpate the neck, because part of the plaque in the carotid artery may dislodge and embolize.

Superficial cervical plexus blocks are performed by infiltrating along with middle third of the posterior border of the sternocleidomastoid muscle with local anesthesia. Deep cervical plexus blocks are performed with three injections along a line drawn from Chassaignac's tubercle (C6) to the mastoid process. The C4 nerve root is located at the intersection of that line with one drawn horizontally from the lower border of the mandible. C2 and C3 are located by dividing the distance between the mastoid process and the horizontal line into thirds. Alternatively, a single injection of local anesthetic can be made on the line between the mastoid process and Chassaignac's tubercle at the level of C4 with the needle directed medially and slightly caudad.

Patients receiving regional anesthesia must be both cooperative and not oversedated with intravenous medications. If they are unable to cooperate and become obtunded, the primary advantage of regional anesthesia (which is continuous neurologic evaluation) is lost. Intravenous sedation therefore must be given judiciously, if at all, to these patients.

Bosilejevac JE, Farha SJ. Carotid endarterectomy: results using regional anesthesia. *Am J Surg* 1980;46:403.

Brown DL. *Atlas of regional anesthesia*, 2nd ed. Philadelphia: WB Saunders, 1999:181–183.

Cousins MJ, Bridenbaugh PO, eds. *Neural blockade in clinical anesthesia and management of pain*, 3rd ed. Philadelphia: Lippincott-Raven, 1997:507–513.

Peitzman AB, Webster MW, Loubeau J, et al. Carotid endarterectomy under regional (conductive) anesthesia. *Ann Surg* 1982;196:59.

C.11. Discuss the effects of anesthetics on cerebral blood flow (CBF).

It is important to remember that all general anesthetics affect CBF and cerebral metabolic oxygen consumption. This can be used to the anesthesiologist's advantage when the decrease in oxygen consumption is greater than the decrease in CBF.

In general, volatile anesthetics are considered to be vasodilators and intravenous anesthetics to be vasoconstrictors. Ketamine is an exception, as it will cause increases in both CBF and cerebral metabolic rate. Volatile anesthetics, as vasodilators produce a dose-dependent increase in CBF.

The magnitude of vasodilation is dependent on the balance between the anesthetic's intrinsic vasodilatory property and vasoconstriction secondary to its decrease in cerebral metabolic rate.

It has been suggested that anesthetic agents only affect the blood flow in normally perfused areas of the brain. If this is the case, volatile anesthetics would cause a steal phenomenon, where the blood vessels in normal brain dilate and steal blood flow away from ischemic areas of the brain that are both already maximally vasodilated and unresponsive to the vasodilating effects of the anesthetics.

Barash PG, Cullen BF, Stoelting RK, eds. *Clinical anesthesia*, 5th ed. Philadelphia: Lippincott Williams & Wilkins, 2006:752–754.

Matta BF, Heath KJ, Tipping K, et al. Direct cerebral vasodilatory effects of sevoflurane and isoflurane. *Anesthesiology* 1999;91:677.

C.12. Discuss the protective effects of anesthetic agents on cerebral function.

Although it has not been proved that general anesthetics afford brain protection, agents that cause the greatest decrease in cerebral metabolic oxygen consumption should lessen the risk of cerebral ischemia. Whether or not a particular anesthetic is optimal for these patients is an area of debate. Obviously, avoiding or eliminating ischemia is preferable to protecting against it.

Messick looked at the effects of volatile anesthetics on critical regional cerebral blood flow (CBF), that is, the regional CBF at which electroencephalogram (EEG) evidence of cerebral ischemia became apparent. He found that critical regional CBF in patients receiving isoflurane was less than 10 mL/100 g/minute and in patients receiving halothane was 18 to 20 mL/100 g/minute. This decrease in critical CBF suggests that isoflurane may offer some protective effect and may be the best of the volatile anesthetics for use during this operation. Because of its potential to cause a decrease in blood pressure and reflex increase in heart rate, however, it probably should not be used at high concentrations as the sole anesthetic. A significant proportion of patients with carotid artery disease also have coronary artery disease, and they may not tolerate the hypotension and tachycardia associated with the use of high-dose isoflurane. By using this anesthetic in low concentrations in combination with other anesthetic agents, one can better maintain hemodynamic stability while perhaps providing for an increased tolerance of cerebral hypoperfusion. Other evidence, however, suggests that isoflurane may not offer protection during regional cerebral ischemia.

The newer agents, sevoflurane and desflurane, have been investigated for their possible role in neuroanesthesia. Compared to isoflurane, desflurane has no significant difference in its effects on decreasing cerebral glucose utilization, increasing blood flow, and maintaining coupling between local CBF and local cerebral glucose utilization. Although sevoflurane showed no significant difference in its effects on decreasing cerebral glucose utilization, and coupling between local CBF and local cerebral glucose utilization at 1 MAC, it did show less of an increase in CBF. This difference between isoflurane and sevoflurane was independent of their effects on systemic blood flow and cardiac output. Hence, desflurane and sevoflurane may have similar neuroprotective effects as isoflurane and, with their lower blood gas solubility coefficients, they may promote a more rapid recovery from anesthesia allowing faster evaluation of neurologic status.

Thiopental affords cerebral protection against focal or incomplete global cerebral ischemia. It is a cerebral vasoconstrictor, as are most other intravenous anesthetics. It will also transiently decrease cerebral metabolism to 40% to 50% of baseline. The combined effect is that cerebral metabolic oxygen consumption is decreased more than oxygen delivery. The reduction in oxygen demand is the result of inhibition of functioning neurons, which can be seen as a quiet or isoelectric EEG. When dosing barbiturates for cerebral protection, the EEG should be monitored and repeated doses given to achieve and then maintain a bust suppression pattern on the EEG. Once the EEG is isoelectric, indicating lack of neuronal function, further doses of thiopental do not provide additional protection. It is generally not recommended that thiopental be used for cerebral protection during carotid endarterectomy (CEA). As mentioned previously, avoidance of ischemia is preferable to its treatment. If thiopental is used, the EEG, because of its isoelectricity, becomes useless as a monitor of cerebral ischemia. This is especially problematic if selective shunting is to be done. Furthermore, the doses of thiopental required to suppress the EEG may cause hypotension and a delayed emergence from anesthesia.

Barbiturate use to minimize the possibility of cerebral ischemia has been advocated for the patient undergoing carotid bypass procedures where temporary occlusion of the recipient vessel is required. Whether treatment of patients with a 3 to 5 mg per kg dose of thiopental affects their outcome in terms of neurologic deficit is not known. It has, however, been shown to be efficacious in animal models.

Dexmedetomidine is a selective α_2-adrenergic agonist with sedative, analgesic, and anxiolytic properties without respiratory depression. In animal studies, dexmedetomidine reduces ischemic damage after transient and permanent ischemia. Its mechanism of neuroprotection is still unclear. One hypothesis suggests that with the onset of cerebral ischemia, one of the initial responses in the central nervous system is the excessive release of norepinephrine and glutamate during energy failure. If the increase in norepinephrine release is a causative component of injury, an α_2-adrenergic agonist may decrease the damage afforded by cerebral ischemia. Dexmedetomidine has been shown to reduce arousal and decrease CBF in volunteers.

Barash PG, Cullen BF, Stoelting RK, eds. *Clinical anesthesia*, 5th ed. Philadelphia: Lippincott Williams & Wilkins, 2006:946–954.

Hicks RG, Kerr DR, Horton DA. Thiopentone cerebral protection under EEG control during carotid endarterectomy. *Anaesth Intensive Care* 1988;14:22.

Holzer A, Greher M, Hetz H, et al. Influence of aortic blood flow velocity on changes of middle cerebral artery blood flow velocity during isoflurane and sevoflurane anaesthesia. *Eur J Anaesthesiol* 2001;18:238.

Jolkkonen J, Puurunen K, Koistinaho J, et al. Neuroprotection by the α2-adrenoceptor agonist, dexmedetomidine, in rat focal cerebral ischemia. *Eur J Clin Pharmacol* 1999; 372:31.

Kuhmonen J, Haapalinna A, Sivenius J. Effects of dexmedetomidine after transient and permanent occlusion of the middle cerebral artery in the rat. *J Neural Transm* 2001; 108:261.

Kuhmonen J, Pokorny J, Miettinen R, et al. Neuroprotective effects of dexmedetomidine in the gerbil hippocampus after transient global ischemia. *Anesthesiology* 1997;87:371.

Lenz C, Rebel A, van Ackern K, et al. Local cerebral blood flow, local cerebral glucose utilization, and flow-metabolism coupling during sevoflurane versus isoflurane anesthesia in rats. *Anesthesiology* 1998;89:1480.

Lenz C, Frietsch T, Futterer C, et al. Local coupling of cerebral blood flow to cerebral glucose metabolism during inhalational anesthesia in rats. *Anesthesiology* 1999;91:1720.

Matta BF, Heath KJ, Tipping K, et al. Direct cerebral vasodilatory effects of sevoflurane and isoflurane. *Anesthesiology* 1999;91:677.

Messick JM Jr, Casement B, Sharbrough FW, et al. Correlation of regional cerebral blood flow (rCBF) with EEG changes during isoflurane anesthesia for carotid endarterectomy: critical rCBF. *Anesthesiology* 1987;66:344.

Michenfelder JD, Sundt TM, Fode N, et al. Isoflurane when compared to enflurane and halothane decreases the frequency of cerebral ischemia during carotid endarterectomy. *Anesthesiology* 1987;67:336.

Moffat JA, McDougall MJ, Brunet D, et al. Thiopental bolus during carotid endarterectomy–rational drug therapy? *Can Anaesth Soc J* 1983;30:615.

Nehls DG, Todd MM, Spetzler RF, et al. A comparison of the cerebral protective effects of isoflurane and barbiturates during temporary focal ischemia in primates. *Anesthesiology* 1987;66:453.

Nussmeier NA, Arlund C, Slogoff S. Neuropsychiatric complications after cardiopulmonary bypass: cerebral protection by a barbiturate. *Anesthesiology* 1986;64:165.

Shapiro HM. Barbiturates in brain ischaemia. *Br J Anaesth* 1985;57:82.

Prielipp RC, Wall MH, Tobin JR, et al. Dexmedetomidine-induced sedation in volunteers decreases regional and global cerebral blood flow. *Anesth Analg* 2002;95:1052.

C.13. How would you manage this patient's ventilation under general anesthesia?

Because carbon dioxide is a potent cerebral vasodilator, it was initially recommended that patients undergoing carotid endarterectomy (CEA) be hypoventilated intraoperatively to achieve hypercarbia. It is now well accepted that hypercapnea should be avoided in patients with carotid artery disease. Carbon dioxide causes vasodilation in normally reactive, nonischemic, vascular beds. In patients with carotid artery disease this means that blood flow is diverted away from the already maximally dilated vessels in the territory of the occluded carotid and toward normal areas of the brain. This decrease in regional cerebral blood flow (rCBF) in ischemic areas of the brain with increased cerebral blood flow (CBF) in normal areas of the brain is known as *intracerebral steal*.

Other authors have recommended extreme hypocapnea during CEA, reasoning that this would result in an "inverse steal" or "Robin Hood" phenomenon. Hypocapnea would cause constriction of cerebral vessels in normally perfused areas of the brain, diverting blood flow into the maximally vasodilated, unreactive, hypoperfused regions of the brain. Clinical trials have been unable to demonstrate any benefit from hypocapnea, and animal studies have shown that it may, in fact, exacerbate ischemia. This most likely happens not only because of intense vasoconstriction, but also because of a leftward shift of the oxyhemoglobin dissociation curve so that hemoglobin is less able to give its oxygen to tissues.

The general recommendation for patients with cerebrovascular disease is that normocarbia or mild hypocarbia be maintained. After repair of their carotid stenosis, some patients will have a marked hyperemia with CBFs of 100 mL/100 g/minute. In these patients decreasing both blood pressure and arterial carbon dioxide tension to decrease their CBF is indicated. Without a decrease in CBF, these patients are at risk for postoperative intracerebral hemorrhage.

Baker WH, Rodman JA, Barnes RW, et al. An evaluation of hypocarbia and hypercarbia during carotid endarterectomy. *Stroke* 1976;7:451.

Barash PG, Cullen BF, Stoelting RK, eds. *Clinical anesthesia*, 5th ed. Philadelphia: Lippincott Williams & Wilkins, 2006:946–954.

Roizen MF, ed. *Anesthesia for vascular surgery*. New York: Churchill Livingstone, 1990: 128–129.

C.14. How would you manage this patient's blood pressure intraoperatively?

A number of factors need to be considered in blood pressure management of patients undergoing carotid endarterectomy (CEA). In the patient with carotid artery disease, a loss of autoregulation occurs in ischemic areas of the brain. In areas of chronic hypoperfusion, vessels are maximally vasodilated and unresponsive to vasomotor stimuli. Perfusion in these ischemic areas is pressure dependent.

During cerebral arterial occlusion, systemic blood pressure may need to be increased to augment collateral blood flow. The primary collateral pathways include the Willisian channels. If Willisian channels are not available, either because of the patient's anatomy or a therapeutic intervention, there are also secondary collateral channels that bridge adjacent major vascular territories. These pathways are known as the *pial-to-pial collateral* or *leptomeningeal* pathways.

Because of the adjustment of the autoregulatory limits in hypertensive patients and because of a lack of autoregulation in ischemic areas of the brain, hypotension should be avoided. The patient's blood pressure should be maintained in its high normal range. During arterial occlusion or vasospasm the only practical way to increase collateral blood flow may be by increasing the collateral perfusion pressure by raising the systemic blood pressure. The extent to which the blood pressure should be raised depends on the nature of the disease. During deliberate hypertension the systemic blood pressure is raised by 30% to 40% above the baseline or until ischemic symptoms resolve. Both maintenance of and increases in blood pressure can be accomplished with light anesthesia and, when necessary, infusion of the α agonist phenylephrine. Phenylephrine has no direct effect on the cerebral vasculature; so cerebral perfusion is increased by an elevation in the cerebral perfusion pressure. Phenylephrine increases blood pressure, cerebral perfusion pressure, stump pressure, and regional cerebral blood flow (CBF). It also increases myocardial oxygen consumption. Because it increases afterload, care must be taken when it is used in patients with coronary artery disease because it can exacerbate ischemia and failure. In patients with coronary artery disease, blood pressure should not be increased above baseline unless evidence of cerebral ischemia develops. Extreme increases in blood pressure can, and should be managed with easily titratable intravenous vasodilators such as sodium nitroprusside or nitroglycerin.

After the bifurcation of the carotid artery is exposed, the surgeon often infiltrates the carotid sinus with lidocaine to eliminate the unpredictable hemodynamic response to manipulation of the carotid artery.

Once the stenosis has been relieved and the carotid cross-clamp removed, the patient's blood pressure should be maintained in its low normal range. This lowering of blood pressure offers several advantages. It decreases myocardial oxygen consumption by decreasing the work of the heart, it decreases the amount of stress on the suture line in the carotid artery, and finally, it minimizes the possibility of reperfusion hemorrhage.

Aaslid R, Lindegaard KF, Sorteberg W, et al. Cerebral autoregulation dynamics in humans. *Stroke* 1989;20:45.

Barash PG, Cullen BF, Stoelting RK, eds. *Clinical anesthesia*, 5th ed. Philadelphia: Lippincott Williams & Wilkins, 2006:951–952.

Boysen G, Engell HC, Henrickson H. The effect of induced hypertension on internal carotid artery pressure and regional cerebral blood flow during temporary carotid clamping for endarterectomy. *Neurology* 1986;17:891.

Smith JS, Roizen MF, Cahalan MK, et al. Does anesthetic technique make a difference? Augmentation of systolic blood pressure during carotid endarterectomy: effects of phenylephrine versus light anesthesia and of isoflurane versus halothane on the incidence of myocardial ischemia. *Anesthesiology* 1988;69:846.

Young WL, Pile-Spelman J. Anesthetic considerations for interventional neuroradiology (Review). *Anesthesiology* 1994;80:427–456.

C.15. Discuss reperfusion injury following carotid endarterectomy (CEA).

Reperfusion injury involves cerebral hemorrhage or the development of cerebral edema after obstruction to flow through the carotid artery has been relieved. Although rare, it is an often-fatal complication of CEA. Patients with a previous stroke are most likely to suffer reperfusion hemorrhage, but it can occur in otherwise normal brain tissue. Poorly controlled blood pressure after the carotid cross-clamp has been removed, contributes to this complication. One proposed mechanism for this injury is that once flow is returned to normal, vascular beds in previously hypoperfused areas of the brain are unable to respond properly with vasoconstriction, to maintain normal flow with increased perfusion. Because hypoperfusion distal to the carotid stenosis has been long-standing, these vessels have lost their ability to autoregulate. Once the carotid stenosis is eliminated, the perfusion pressure distal to the former site of the stenosis is markedly increased. Because of the lack of autoregulation in this area, cerebral blood flow (CBF) increases with increasing perfusion. The patients at highest risk for reperfusion injury have the greatest degree of stenosis and the greatest pressure drop across the carotid lesion. Again, maintaining good blood pressure control with antihypertensive medications once the carotid obstruction is eliminated decreases the incidence of reperfusion injury.

Barash PG, Cullen BF, Stoelting RK, eds. *Clinical anesthesia*, 5th ed. Philadelphia: Lippincott Williams & Wilkins, 2006:953.

Breen JC, Caplan LF, DeWitt LD, et al. Brain edema after carotid surgery. *Neurology* 1996;46:175.

Peipgras D, Morgan M, Sundt T, et al. Intracerebral hemorrhage after carotid endarterectomy. *J Neurosurg* 1988;68:532.

Schroeder T, Sillisen H, Sorensen O, et al. Cerebral hyperperfusion following carotid endarterectomy. *J Neurosurg* 1987;66:824.

Solomon R, Loftus C, Quest DQ, et al. Incidence and etiology of intracerebral hemorrhage following carotid endarterectomy. *J Neurosurg* 1986;64:29.

C.16. What intravenous fluids would you give this patient intraoperatively?

Because moderate hyperglycemia has been shown to worsen neurologic outcome after ischemia, care must be taken to avoid increasing the patient's glucose with exogenously administered dextrose. Intravenous fluids such as Normosol R, Lactated Ringer's, or normal saline would be appropriate choices for patients undergoing carotid endarterectomy (CEA).

These patients should not be vigorously hydrated intraoperatively. It is best to limit their intraoperative fluids to that required for maintenance, with additional colloid and blood replacement being given as needed. Intraoperative overhydration may lead to some of the frequently observed postoperative hypertension and in patients with myocardial disease, may exacerbate congestive heart failure.

Barash PG, Cullen BF, Stoelting RK, eds. *Clinical anesthesia*, 5th ed. Philadelphia: Lippincott Williams & Wilkins, 2006:946–954.

Li PA, Siesjo BK. Role of hyperglycaemia-related acidosis in ischaemic brain damage. *Acta Physiol Scand* 1997;161(4):567–580.

Pulsinelli WA, Levy DE, Sigsbee B, et al. Increased damage after ischemic stroke in patients with hyperglycemia with or without established diabetes mellitus. *Am J Med* 1983;74:540.

Pulsinelli WA, Waldman S, Rawlingson D, et al. Moderate hyperglycemia augments ischemic brain damage: a neuropathologic study in the rat. *Neurology* 1983;33:222.

D. Postoperative Management

D.1. The patient does not "wake up" from general anesthesia. Why?

Once other causes of slow emergence from general anesthesia (such as hyperglycemia or hypoglycemia, hypothermia, anesthetic overdose, hypercarbia, and hypoxemia) have been ruled out, the possibility of an adverse intraoperative event having occurred needs to be considered. Patency of the carotid artery on which the surgery was done should be evaluated. This can be done by means of Doppler studies although the patient is still in the operating room. If no blood flow is seen in the carotid artery, the incision can be immediately reexplored. If Doppler studies are normal, the possibility of a cerebral infarction from prolonged hypoperfusion or from emboli must be considered. The patient should remain intubated while further studies, including a computed tomography scan and cerebral angiography, are done as expeditiously as possible. The incidence of new perioperative neurologic deficits is 3% in centers where the operation is done commonly.

Graber JN, Vollman RW, Johnson WC, et al. Stroke after carotid endarterectomy: risk as predicted by preoperative computerized tomography. *Am J Surg* 1984;147:492.

Paciaroni M, Eliasziw M, Kappelle LJ, et al. Medical complications associated with carotid endarterectomy. *Stroke* 1999;30:1759.

D.2. Postoperatively the patient's blood pressure was 170/96 mm Hg. Would you treat this? If so, why and how?

This patient's blood pressure needs to be carefully controlled because postoperative hypertension is associated with bleeding at the operative site, myocardial ischemia, arrhythmias, and intracerebral hemorrhage and cerebral edema.

Hypertension is observed more commonly than hypotension after carotid endarterectomy (CEA). Causes of hypertension include hypoxemia, hypercarbia, pain, and a full bladder. Obviously, if any or all of these causes are present, they need to be dealt with promptly and appropriately. Another common cause of postoperative hypertension and tachycardia has been attributed to blunting of the carotid baroreceptor mechanism secondary to carotid sinus dysfunction caused by surgical trauma. If this is the cause of hypertension, therapy with antihypertensive agents should be started.

The patient's blood pressure should be maintained in her low normal range postoperatively. Elevated blood pressure can be treated with hydralazine in 5-mg increments or if the patient is not bradycardic, labetalol may be used in 10-mg increments. Alternatively, infusions of sodium nitroprusside or nitroglycerin may be used. β-Blockade with 1-mg increments of propranolol or an infusion of esmolol may be added to this regimen.

Barash PG, Cullen BF, Stoelting RK, eds. *Clinical anesthesia*, 5th ed. Philadelphia: Lippincott Williams & Wilkins, 2006:946–954.

Wong JH, Findlay JM, et al. Hemodynamic instability after carotid endarterectomy: risk factors and associations with operative complications. *Neurosurgery* 1997;41(1): 1992–1998.

D.3. What immediate postoperative complications might you expect?

Immediate postoperative complications include neurologic deficits, hemodynamic instability, and respiratory insufficiency. Evaluation of the North American symptomatic carotid endarterectomy trial (NASCET) showed that 8.1% of patients had medical complications: 1% with myocardial infarctions (MIs), 7.1% with other cardiovascular disorders such as arrhythmias and congestive heart failure, 0.8% with respiratory complications, 0.4% with transient confusion, and 0.7% with other complications. Carotid endarterectomy (CEA) was 1.5 times more likely to have medical complications in patients with a history of cardiac disease or hypertension.

Postoperative neurologic complications are usually embolic in nature, occurring during surgery whereas the remainder is from reperfusion injury, intracranial hemorrhage, and anesthetic effects.

Circulatory instability is common after CEA, with either hypotension or hypertension being observed. Hypotension may have any of several causes, as does hypertension as noted previously. These include hypovolemia, depression of the circulation by residual anesthetics, prolonged effect of intraoperatively administered antihypertensives, dysrhythmias, and myocardial ischemia. Each of these causes needs to be sought and, if present, treated appropriately. Another possible cause of hypotension is an excessive reflex response because of increased sensitivity of the carotid sinus after exposure of the baroreceptor mechanism to a higher pressure with removal of the plaque. If this is the cause, therapy needs to be instituted with fluids and vasopressors.

Postoperative respiratory insufficiency is a rare but potentially life-threatening complication. This can be due to vocal cord paralysis from intraoperative traction on the laryngeal nerves. Should this present with inability to protect the airway, the patient should be immediately reintubated.

A prospective study found that 12.5% of patients had nerve injuries after CEA, but all were transient, lasting from 1 week to 37 months. No patient had life-threatening respiratory insufficiency from the nerve injuries. The most commonly injured nerves were the hypoglossal, recurrent laryngeal, superior laryngeal, and greater auricular nerves.

Airway obstruction can also occur from hematoma formation at the operative site, from either arterial or venous bleeding. The hematoma needs to be evacuated as quickly as possible and, depending on ventilatory status, the patient may need to be intubated. This is most easily done after evacuation of the hematoma, if the clinical condition allows.

Supraglottic edema may also be a rare cause of postoperative upper airway obstruction after CEA. Computed tomographic analysis of airways postoperatively showed reduction in the volume of the airway in all patients, with a greater reduction seen in intubated patients (63% ± 9%) than in nonintubated patients (32% ± 7%).

Tension pneumothorax can result from air dissecting through the wound and the mediastinum to the pleura. This diagnosis should be considered in all patients after CEA, who seem to have respiratory distress and no evidence of upper airway obstruction. Absence of breath sounds over half of the chest and hemodynamic instability would support this diagnosis.

Chemoreceptor function is irreversibly suspended in most patients after CEA for up to 10 months. Lack of chemoreceptor function means that there is a loss of circulatory response to hypoxia and an increase in resting $PaCO_2$ of approximately 6 mm Hg. This complication is potentially very serious, and one needs to be most concerned about its development in patients who have had a previous contralateral CEA, where function may be lost bilaterally. In all patients after CEA supplemental oxygen should be provided and opioids administered cautiously.

Ballotta E, Da Giau G, Renon L, et al. Cranial and cervical nerve injuries after carotid endarterectomy: a prospective study. *Surgery* 1999;125:85.

Barash PG, Cullen BF, Stoelting RK, eds. *Clinical anesthesia*, 5th ed. Philadelphia: Lippincott Williams & Wilkins, 2006:953–954.

Carmichael FJ, McGuire GP, Wong DT, et al. Computed tomographic analysis of airway dimensions after carotid endarterectomy. *Anesth Analg* 1996;83:12.

Paciaroni M, Eliasziw M, Kappelle LJ, et al. Medical complications associated with carotid endarterectomy. *Stroke* 1999;30:1759.

Wade JC, Larson CP Jr, Hickey RF, et al. Effects of carotid endarterectomy on carotid chemoreceptor and baroreceptor function in man. *N Engl J Med* 1970;282:823.

D.4. Discuss postoperative neurocognitive dysfunction following uncomplicated carotid endarterectomy (CEA).

CEA will reduce the incidence of stroke in patients with high-grade carotid artery stenosis. There is, however, increasing evidence that as many as to 28% of surgical patients have significant neuropsychological dysfunction 1 day after CEA. Between 9% and 23% of these patients continue to exhibit cognitive decline 1 month after surgery.

The APOE-ε4 allele has been associated with worse outcome following stroke. In a prospective trial, 75 patients undergoing CEA were studied. Twelve of 75 (16%) patients possessed the APOE-ε4 allele. Eight of the 75 patients (11%) experienced cognitive dysfunction on postoperative day 30. One month after CEA, APOE-ε4-positive patients were more likely to have suffered a neurocognitive injury (42%) than APOE-ε4-negative patients (5%).

The presence of APOE-ε4 allele increase the risk of neurocognitive dysfunction 62-fold 1 month after surgery. Diabetes and obesity also predisposed to injury.

Heyer EJ, Wilson DA, Sahlein DH, et al. APOE-ε4 predisposes to cognitive dysfunction following uncomplicated carotid endarterectomy. *Neurology* 2005;65:1–5.

CHAPTER 24

Awake Craniotomy for Deep Brain Stimulation

Elizabeth A.M. Frost • J. Lance LaFleur

A 79-YEAR-OLD MAN

with Parkinson's disease was scheduled for insertion of electrodes for deep brain stimulation (DBS). He was right handed, English speaking and of normal intelligence. He had good memory function but a marked tremor. His current medications, levodopa (Sinemet), bromocriptine (Parlodel), selegiline (Eldepryl), pramipexole (Mirapex), and amantadine (Symmetrel), afforded only fair movement control. He had recently become very depressed and sertraline hydrochloride (Zoloft) had been prescribed. He also had a history of hypertension, treated with hydrochlorothiazide

---

A. Medical Disease and Differential Diagnosis

1. What is Parkinson's disease (PD)?
2. What is the underlying pathology of PD?
3. What constitutes current drug therapy?
4. What are the criteria for surgical treatment of PD and what types of surgery are available?

B. Preoperative Evaluation and Preparation

1. What are the anesthetic implications of the patient's medication?
2. What laboratory evaluations should be made?
3. How should the anesthesiologist explain the anesthetic plan for the procedure to the patient?
4. Is premedication indicated?
5. What precautions should be taken for airway management?

C. Intraoperative Management

1. What are the anesthetic considerations in a magnetic resonance imaging (MRI) unit?
2. The surgeon wants to implant electrodes. What are the anesthetic implications?
3. How can the airway best be maintained?
4. Which and how much fluids should be given?
5. What constitutes required monitoring?
6. Is invasive monitoring advisable?

7. How should the brain be monitored?
8. Which anesthetic agents should be used?
9. How is blood pressure controlled?
10. The case lasts longer than anticipated: what could be the complications?
11. The patient begins to cough. What is the differential diagnosis? Treatment?
12. The surgeon asks that the patient become more responsive. What would you do?
13. The patient is complaining of pain. How would you manage it?

D. Postoperative Management

1. The patient became hemiplegic postoperatively. What is the differential diagnosis?
2. How would you manage postoperative pain?
3. About 1 hour into the postoperative period, the patient became comatose. What should be done?
4. If there are no complications, is this patient suitable for same day discharge?
5. How would you manage the second stage of the procedure? When? Are the requirements different from those for electrode insertion?
6. Are results successful on a long-term basis

A. Medical Disease and Differential Diagnosis

A.1. What is Parkinson's disease (PD)?

James Parkinson (1755 to 1824), an English surgeon, political radical, and paleontologist established the disease as an entity with "An Essay on the Shaking Palsy" in 1817. Sorting through several palsied conditions which he had observed, Parkinson gave the classic clinical description of the disease: *"Involuntary, tremulous motion with lessened muscular power, in parts not in action and even when supported; with a propensity to bend the trunk forewards, and to pass from a walking to a running pace: the sense and intellect being uninjured."* Four decades later, Jean-Martin Charcot added rigidity to Parkinson's excellent description and attached the name Parkinson's disease to the syndrome. Parkinson is also noted for the earliest description in English of a case of perforated and gangrenous appendix (1812).

Parkinson's disease (PD) is a neurodegenerative condition resulting from neuronal loss in the dopaminergic substantia nigra pars compacta (SNc) (Fig 24.1). Projections from the SNc to the striatum normally allow for refined movements. Initially, the dopamine receptors in the striatum of PD patients are upregulated in response to a reduction in dopaminergic input. As increasing populations of somata are lost in the SNc, clinical symptoms begin to appear (Fig. 24.2). Dysfunction initially occurs unilaterally in the form of micrographia, hand tremor, decreased arm swing, and foot dragging. Eventually, bilateral symptoms appear as bradykinesia, resting tremor, postural instability. A therapeutic response to levodopa (L-dopa) occurs. Almost 90% of patients with PD have significant vocal fold bowing and adduction and pharyngeal residues of solids can be found on evaluation of swallowing.

Blumin JH, Pcolinsky DE, Atkins JP. Laryngeal findings in advanced Parkinson's disease. *Ann Otol Rhinol Laryngol* 2004;113(4):253–258.

Carpenter CCJ, Griggs RC, Loscalzo J. *Cecil essentials of medicine*, 6th ed. Philadelphia: WB Saunders, 2004:1020–1024.

Parkinson J. *An essay on the shaking palsy*. London: Whittingham & Rowland, 1817.

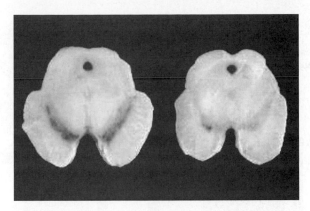

Figure 24.1 Midbrain comparison. Normally, neurons in the substantia nigra pars compacta (SNc) release dopamine. A by-product of dopamine synthesis is neuromelanin, which is easily visualized on midbrain section (*left*). In the Parkinson disease patient, a loss of neurons in the SNc leads to midbrain pallor (*right*). (Adapted from Kumar V, Abbas A, Fausto N. *Pathologic basis of disease*, 7th ed. Philadelphia: WB Saunders, 2005:1391–1393.)

A.2. What is the underlying pathology of Parkinson's disease (PD)?

PD is a clinical diagnosis (Table 24.1), confirmed in postmortem analysis by demonstration of Lewy bodies and the loss of dopaminergic neurons in the substantia nigra pars compacta (SNc). The degeneration of SNc dopaminergic neurons, which project to the striatum as the nigrostriatal pathway, leads to a reduction in striatal dopamine content and eventually to the clinical phenotype.

The genetics of PD suggest a mechanism for the presence of diagnostic Lewy bodies: oxidative stress, mitochondrial dysfunction, decreased adenosine triphosphate (ATP) production, diminished degradative action of highly energy dependent ubiquitin proteosome system (UPS), protein aggregation, and eventual disease. Administration of synthetic and endogenous proteasome inhibitors disrupts the UPS in rats causes both the clinical signs of PD (bradykinesia, rigidity, and tremor) and the pathologic findings (neuronal degeneration and Lewy body-like inclusions in the SNc and other areas similarly affected in PD patients) within 2 weeks.

Environmental factors may be involved in the pathogenesis of PD. An acute form of PD can be caused by exposure to MPTP (1-methyl-4-phenyl-1,2,3,6-tetrahydropyridine), which is a neurotoxic by-product of the illicit synthesis of meperidine analogues. Once administered parentally, MPTP readily enters the brain and is metabolized by astrocytic monoamine oxidase B to MPP$^+$ (1-methyl-4-phenylpyridinium). MPP$^+$ concentrates in dopaminergic SNc neurons where it inhibits the mitochondrial electron transport chain resulting in ATP depletion and selective cell death. Exposure to pesticides or other toxins may increase the risk of development of PD.

Many studies have attempted to link PD with family history. Rocca et al. performed a historical cohort study at the Mayo Clinic on 162 PD patients and more than 1,000 first-degree relatives. In patients with early onset of PD, there was a small relative risk for first-degree relatives in developing the disorder. However, there was no increased risk for relatives of patients that had late onset PD.

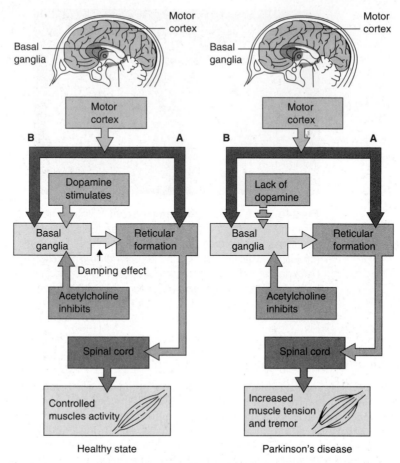

Figure 24.2 Pathways involved in Parkinson's disease. During movement, fibers from the primary motor cortex in the precentral gyrus project to the reticular formation and spinal cord (pathway A), then to the muscles. Modulatory fibers through pathway B project to the basal ganglia. These signals dampen and refine the signals in pathway A, allowing for smooth, controlled movement. If there is a lack of dopamine, as in Parkinson's disease, inhibitory acetylcholine (ACh) predominates in the basal ganglia. The damping effect on the reticular formation is diminished, and movement symptoms result.

Table 24.1 Clinical Features of Parkinson's Disease.

PRIMARY FEATURES	SECONDARY FEATURES
Bradykinesia	Dysphagia
Resting tremor	Masked facies
Muscular rigidity	Autonomic dysfunction (constipation, urinary retention, orthostatic hypotension)
Therapeutic response to L-dopa treatment	Depression, dementia,
Postural and gait abnormalities; cog wheel movements	Sleep disorder
Difficulty with voice, speech, swallowing	

Approximately 20% of elderly PD patients develop a dementia similar to Alzheimer's disease, which may coexist. Also, depression occurs in approximately 40% of all patients with PD. Although this widespread comorbidity is often untreated, therapy is appropriate and must be approached cautiously because of the risks of drug interactions.

Du Y, Ma Z, Lin S, et al. Minocycline prevents nigrostriatal dopaminergic neurodegeneration in the MPTP model of Parkinson's disease. *Proc Natl Acad Sci USA* 2001;98:14669–14674.

Eriksen J, Wszolek Z, Petrucelli L. Molecular pathogenesis of parkinson disease. *Arch Neurol* 2005;62:349–350.

Kumar V, Abbas A, Fausto N. *Robbins and Cotran pathologic basis of disease*, 7th ed. Philadelphia: WB Saunders, 2005:1391–1393.

McNaught KS, Perl DP, Brownell AL, et al. Systemic exposure to proteasome inhibitors causes a progressive model of Parkinson's disease. *Ann Neurol* 2004;56:149–162.

Rocca WA, McDonnell SK, Strain KJ, et al. Familial aggregation of Parkinson's disease: The Mayo Clinic family study. *Ann Neurol* 2004;56(4):495–502.

A.3. What constitutes current drug therapy?

Treatment of Parkinson's disease (PD) aims to enhance the effects of dopamine and/or reduce the effects of acetylcholine (ACh) by the administration of centrally acting drugs. Agents that combine actions on dopaminergic and cholinergic components of the extrapyramidal system are used. L-dopa and α-methylhydrazine (carbidopa) in combination (Sinemet), bromocriptine and lergotrile in combination with Sinemet, amantadine, and anticholinergics (e.g., benztropine) are most commonly used. Dopamine levels are increased in the brain, whereas peripheral effects are decreased.

Many side effects occur: nausea, orthostatic hypotension, hallucinations, psychosis, and dyskinesia. Long-term administration (>5 years) of anti-Parkinson medication is associated with a pattern of motor fluctuations. The progression to motor complications from these drugs affects nearly half of all patients and is often debilitating

Several different classes of drugs and combinations have been prescribed:

Levodopa/Carbidopa

L-dopa, a metabolic precursor to dopamine, was among the first drugs used to treat PD. Taken orally, L-dopa crosses the blood–brain barrier unlike dopamine. Remaining dopaminergic neurons take up L-dopa in the SNc and metabolize it to produce more dopamine neurotransmitter. Administered alone, it is rapidly decarboxylated to dopamine in the body outside of the central nervous system (CNS) by the dopamine decarboxylase enzyme. Consequently, this enhanced dopamine concentration in the periphery causes many side effects: nausea, vomiting, hypotension. Moreover, as much of the original dose is metabolized before reaching the CNS, large doses of L-dopa must be administered to achieve the desired effects. To combat the issues of monotherapy with L-dopa, dual therapy of L-dopa and carbidopa is recommended. Carbidopa blocks the peripheral conversion of L-dopa to dopamine and increases the bioavailability of L-dopa. Peripheral effects are decreased.

Problems associated with L-dopa therapy usually center on a "wearing off" effect of the drug over time. As L-dopa treatment requires viable neurons in the substantia nigra pars compacta (SNc), progressive loss of these neurons reduces the efficacy of the drug. Also, an "on/off" motor effect has been described, primarily due to the fact that L-dopa has an extremely short half-life

(1 to 2 hours). Therefore, concentrations in the CNS can vary greatly and lead to fluctuations in symptomatic relief. Other studies have shown that L-dopa therapy can eventually lead to dyskinesia due to fluctuating dopamine concentrations, prompting some physicians to save L-dopa therapy for more advanced cases.

L-dopa exhibits several drug interactions. Pyridoxine, or B_6 increases the peripheral breakdown of L-dopa, effectively reducing the bioavailability. L-dopa should not be administered simultaneously with monoamine oxidase (MAO) inhibitors as the enhanced catecholamine production can cause a hypertensive crisis. MAO inhibitors increase peripheral dopamine and other catecholamines and inhibit the breakdown of L-dopa, further increasing peripheral dopamine and blood pressure. Patients medicated with antipsychotic medications such as phenothiazines, butyrophenones, and thioxanthines should also be wary of taking L-dopa as it may exacerbate psychotic symptoms by increasing CNS dopamine concentrations. These drugs block dopamine receptors and can cause PD symptoms themselves. Cardiac patients are advised to take L-dopa cautiously due to an increased susceptibility to arrhythmias.

Dopamine agonists

Dopamine agonists, mainly bromocriptine, pergolide (Permax), pramipexole, and ropinirole, are coadministered with L-dopa to reduce the effective dose of L-dopa. These drugs rapidly cross the blood–brain barrier and require no metabolism or conversion once in the brain. Dopamine agonists directly bind to dopamine receptors in the striatum. Similar side effects occur (nausea, hypotension, and vomiting due to increased peripheral dopamine) and may be more intense than with L-dopa alone. Dopamine agonists do not produce dyskinesia.

Dopamine agonists are primarily used as first line drugs or for patients with severe dyskinesias associated with L-dopa therapy. Also, younger patients may respond better. But this class may be contraindicated for patients with a history of myocardial infarction or peripheral vascular disease, as peripheral dopamine worsens arterial spasm. Much like L-dopa, dopamine agonists have been shown to increase symptoms in patients with psychiatric disorders.

Monoamine oxidase inhibitors

Selegiline, similar to dopamine agonists, is typically used for treatment of early PD as a means of delaying the onset of L-dopa administration. Selegiline acts by selectively inhibiting monoamine oxidase (MAO) B, the enzyme that breaks down dopamine in the brain. Some forms of PD have been linked to too much dopamine metabolism directly increasing the concentration of toxic free radicals that destroy dopamine neurons. Selegiline, by blocking the breakdown of dopamine and subsequent free radical production, may have a neuroprotective effect. Early administration of selegiline can delay the onset of severe symptoms of PD by as much as 50%. Side effects of this drug are generally mild, but high doses can cause hypertensive crisis.

Catechol-O-methyltransferase inhibitors

Catechol-O-methyltransferase (COMT) inhibitors, mainly tolcapone (Tasmar) and entacapone, are relatively new drugs in the treatment of PD. The mechanism of action is similar to that of carbidopa; inhibition of the breakdown of L-dopa. The enzyme COMT selectively metabolizes L-dopa in the CNS and the periphery, decreasing bioavailability. The COMT inhibitors block this enzyme, effectively increasing central uptake of L-dopa. Simultaneous administration of COMT inhibitors with L-dopa reduces some of the negative motor side effects of L-dopa therapy. In a study of the "on/off" motor effect of L-dopa, COMT inhibitors increased the duration of the "on" time and decreased the duration of the "off" time. As COMT inhibitors increase effective concentrations of L-dopa, side effects are similar to those of L-dopa, mainly orthostatic hypotension, nausea, and vomiting. Tolcapone has been shown to cause frequent diarrhea and has been linked to liver failure through fulminant hepatitis. Liver function should be closely monitored. The drug is only used as an adjunct to L-dopa/carbidopa in patients with severe symptom fluctuations.

AntiViral agents

Amantadine, the popular antiviral drug, has anti-Parkinson effects. The mechanism is not entirely clear, but it is believed that amantadine enhances synthesis, release, or reuptake of dopamine in remaining neurons of the SNc. Side effects of amantadine—orthostatic hypotension, urinary retention, peripheral edema, dry mouth, restlessness, agitation—are less frequent and less severe as compared to L-dopa therapy. Amantadine has not been shown to have any effect on tremor, but it decreases rigidity and bradykinesia.

Anticholinergic agents

The anticholinergic agents—trihexyphenidyl (Artane), benztropine (Cogentin), biperiden (Akineton)—are adjuncts in treating PD. These drugs block ACh-dominated cholinergic transmission and restore the ACh/dopamine balance in the striatum. Side effects result from blocking of parasympathetic stimulation of various organs and include mood changes, dry mouth, dilated pupils, constipation, urinary retention, and visual problems. Anticholinergic drugs are contraindicated in patients with glaucoma, prostatic hypertrophy, or pyloric stenosis.

Borges N. Tolcapone in Parkinson's disease: liver toxicity and clinical efficacy. *Expert Opin Drug Saf* 2005;4(1):69–73.

Kondo T. Comment on guidelines for treatment of Parkinson's disease. *Rinsho Shinkeigaku* 2004;44(11):830–832.

A.4. What are the criteria for surgical treatment of Parkinson's disease (PD) and what types of surgery are available?

Medical therapy is palliative because drug therapy does not halt the progression of neuronal degeneration. Also, drug therapy loses its efficacy in many patients and therefore surgical strategies have been developed. Although bradykinesis may continue to respond to drug therapy, symptoms such as dysarthria, gait disorders, and postural instability emerge, progress and respond poorly to treatment. Stereotactic surgery employs precise lesioning with the basal ganglia to dampen pathologic neuronal discharge. Procedures such as pallidotomy and thalamotomy were initially performed but are now less frequently utilized. Lesions are permanent and there is risk of severe side effects such as stroke or neurologic injury. Some years ago, experimentation with implantation of fetal neural tissue showed early promise in improving the clinical symptoms of patients with PD or MPTP (1-methyl-4-phenyl-1,2,3,6-tetrahydropyridine)-induced PD. This technique stereotactically implants fetal mesencephalic neurons or adrenal chromaffin cells into the striatum. However, any benefit from neural transplantation may be due to associated acute and reactive host brain injury. Also, the process is politically charged as it involves fetal tissue, usually collected during abortions. Recently other studies indicate that stem cells are more suitable as cellular replacements.

The procedure of choice now is deep brain stimulation (DBS), which involves first the implantation of stimulatory electrodes and later placement of a generator that allows control. of the electrodes. Deep brain stimulating devices are implanted in two stages: the first stage is performed with the patient awake or with minimal sedation. The second stage is performed under general anesthesia. Patients chosen for surgical implantation must be carefully evaluated for comorbidities. They should have a documented preoperative improvement from dopaminergic medication of at least 30% in the patient's Unified Parkinson's Disease Rating Scale motor disability scores. A L-dopa challenge may be needed to document the best "on" state. They should be able to lie still for several hours. Communication is essential during the procedure. Therefore they should have little or no dementia and active psychiatric disease should be treated preoperatively. Cardiorespiratory stability is also important. Hypertension should be well controlled. Patients with obstructive pulmonary disease and those who smoke must be able to lie not only supine with minimal head up position but should not have a chronic cough. Patients must be motivated with good support systems and committed to the postoperative management of DBS.

As DBS techniques have also been shown to improve intractable epilepsy, cephalgias, restless legs syndrome, and other movement disorders; anesthesiologists may soon be called on to assist in many different situations and in patients with a host of pathologies.

Bronte-Stewart H. Parkinson's disease: surgical options. *Curr Treat Options Neurol* 2003; 5(2):131–147.

Driver-Dunckley E, Evidente VG, Adler CH, et al. Restless legs syndrome in Parkinson's disease patients may improve with subthalamic stimulation. *Mov Disord* 2006;21:1287–1289.

Green A, Owen S, Davies P, et al. Deep brain stimulation for neuropathic cephalgia. *Cephalgia* 2006;26(5):561–567.

Landau WM. Positive potential of fetal nigral implants for Parkinson's disease. *Arch Neurol* 2004;61:1808–1809.

Perlmutter JS, Mink JW. Deep brain stimulation. *Annu Rev Neurosci* 2006;29:229–257.

Shingo T. Cell therapy in Parkinson's disease. *Rinsho Shinkeigaku* 2004;44(11):951–953.

Takagi Y, Takahashi J, Saiki H, et al. Dopaminergic neurons generated from monkey embryonic stem cells function in a Parkinson's primate model. *J Clin Invest* 2005; 115(1):102–109.

B. Preoperative Evaluation and Preparation

B.1. What are the anesthetic implications of the patient's medications?

As noted in the preceding text there are many side effects associated with Parkinson's disease (PD) medications including dry mouth, orthostatic hypotension, nausea, visual disturbances, and urinary retention. Typically, in order to produce maximum effect during stimulation, the surgeon requires that no PD medications be given for several hours before surgery. Thus patients may present to the operating room with significant movement disorders. Also, if the indication for deep brain stimulation (DBS) is epilepsy, side effects of the many agents used for this disease must also be considered including hepatic enzyme induction, competitive metabolic inhibition, plasma protein level, and binding, all of which may cause drug interactions and change doses and duration of effect of other agents. Gum hypertrophy may add to the difficulties of securing an airway emergently (Table 24.2). In addition, the anesthesiologist should not fail to inquire as to any herbal preparations that the patient may have taken as interference with clotting has been reported with gingko, ginger, garlic, and gengsing among others.

Many antiepileptic drugs induce hepatic enzyme activities. If two drugs share a similar pathway for metabolism, the second drug is cleared at a faster rate due to increased hepatic enzyme activity. Phenytoin, barbiturates, and carbamazepine are potent hepatic enzyme inducers causing faster elimination of other drugs. Because antiseizure drugs increase the activity of the nonspecific drug metabolizing enzyme system, cytochrome P-450, the duration of action of muscle relaxants, narcotics or other anesthetic agents may decrease. Chronic alcoholic

Table 24.2   Commonly Used Drugs in Seizure Control.

TYPE OF SEIZURE	FIRST LINE DRUG	SECOND LINE DRUG
Generalized tonic-clonic	Carbamazepine Phenytoin Valproate	Clobazam Clonazepam Lamotrigine Phenobarbital Vigabatrin Felbamate Acetazolamide
Generalized absence	Valproate Ethosuximide	Clonazepam Lamotrigine Acetazolamide
Tonic, atonic, atypical absences	Valproate Clobazam Clonazepam Lamotrigine Phenytoin	Carbamazepine Phenobarbital Felbamate Acetazolamide
Myoclonic seizures	Valproate Clonazepam	Phenobarbital Acetazolamide
Simple partial, complex partial, secondarily generalized	Carbamazepine Valproate Phenytoin	Clobazam Lamotrigine Gabapentin Vigabatrin Phenobarbital Felbamate Acetazolamide

patients who take phenytoin can have even higher hepatic enzyme activity, which decreases the serum concentration of anesthetic agents and increases the elimination rate. The dosage of benzodiazepines or barbiturates for premedication may need to be increased. Also, induction doses of thiopental or propofol may also have to be greater. Frequent administration of muscle relaxants may be required due to increased hepatic drug metabolism.

Chang VC, Chou KL. Deep brain stimulation for Parkinson's disease: patient selection and motor outcomes. *Med Health R I* 2006;89(4):142–144.

Levy RH, Mattson RH, Meldrum BS. *Antiepileptic drugs*, 4th ed. New York: Raven Press, 1994.

Shorvon SD. Medical assessment and treatment of chronic epilepsy. *Brit Med J* 1991; 302:363–366.

B.2. What laboratory evaluations should be made?

Routine evaluations include complete blood count, electrolyte screening panel including blood sugar level (which should be controlled at or below 120 mg/dL), urinalysis to exclude urinary tract infection, and assessment of renal and liver function. A chest x-ray will help to exclude evidence of aspiration, which is a common occurrence in Parkinson's disease (PD) patients. Depending on other comorbidities and the clinical situation, an electrocardiogram should also be available. It is advisable to secure a blood specimen for type and screening of blood before surgery. Although blood transfusion is rarely necessary, should it be required it will be an emergent situation. One of the serious complications of deep brain stimulation (DBS) is intracerebral hemorrhage. Antiseizure medications such as carbamazepine or valproate may cause thrombocytopenia although leukopenia is more common. Therefore, the type of antiseizure drugs used and any history of bleeding should be carefully evaluated preoperatively and platelet and white blood cell counts measured.

B.3. How should the anesthesiologist explain the anesthetic plan for the procedure to the patient?

Cooperation from the patient is essential. The anesthesiologist must explain that the patient will be awake during part if not all of the procedure and that this is required so that the healthy part of the brain can be identified and not injured. It is important to review with the patient what will be required of him/her such as the questions that may be asked to assess the speech center and tasks he/she may be expected to perform such as "move your toes." The patient may be asked to read from a paper. In such circumstances the anesthesiologist should ensure that the patient can read without glasses or that the print is large enough that enhanced vision is not necessary. Clearly, the anesthesiologist must ascertain the language and competency of the patient. The patient must be reassured that the anesthesiologist will be close by to monitor and to give pain medications if necessary. The anesthesiologist should also be aware of any aura that the patient may experience before a seizure so that appropriate medications may be promptly given to avert a major attack. Although urinary catheters are not usually placed in awake patients, especially men, the patient should be told that if there is a need to urinate, a bottle will be made available. The procedure usually requires 2 to 4 hours. If arthritis prevents the patient from lying comfortably, pillows and appropriate padding must be available.

Usually, a frame is attached to the patient's head after infiltration with local anesthesia. In the holding area, a circumferential or ring block around the head may be applied by the anesthesiologist or surgeon. The patient is then taken to radiology where images are obtained. In the operating room, the procedure is started under local anesthesia and sedation, if necessary, until the optimal positions for the electrodes are identified. Following placement of the stimulators and testing, the patient returns to magnetic resonance imaging (MRI) or computed tomography (CT) for a scan to confirm placement and to rule out hematoma formation. Parkinson's medications are given as soon as possible, which usually relieves patient discomfort. Patients are observed carefully overnight for any neurologic changes and are generally ready for discharge the following day. Discussion between all the specialties (neurology, neurosurgery, neurophysiology, and anesthesiology) involved is necessary to ensure that each is aware of the requirements and concerns of the others.

B.4. Is premedication indicated?

If the patient is to undergo radiologic procedures in which seizure activity is not to be provoked (e.g., if DBS is performed to ablate epileptic foci, the seizure threshold should not be increased) a benzodiazepine is a suitable agent. Also, intravenous diazepam given before contrast injection may reduce the incidence of contrast, associated seizures. The exception is the amytal test, which is preceded by cerebral angiography (amobarbital 30 mg is injected into an artery supplying eloquent cerebral areas to determine neurologic function before devascularization). Under these circumstances, no sedative drugs are given. For patients scheduled for definitive mapping and resection, no sedative drugs should be given and premedication should consist of antiemetics and antacids. Thereby the importance of the preanesthetic visit is underscored. Anticonvulsants are usually given preoperatively but in reduced doses at the discretion of the neurosurgeon. Most antiepileptic drugs are not available in intravenous form. Some evidence suggests that hemodynamic stability may be increased during pinhead holder insertion if clonidine is given orally 90 minutes before placement.

Costello TG, Cormack JR. Clonidine premedication decreases responses to pin head holder application during craniotomy. *Anesth Analg* 1998;86:1001–1004.

Optiz A, Marschall R, Degan R, et al. General anesthesia in patients with epilepsy and status epilepticus. *Adv Neurol* 1983;34:531–535.

Pagani JJ, Hayman LA, Bigelow RH, et al. Prophylactic diazepam in prevention of contrast media associated seizures in glioma patients undergoing cerebral computed tomography. *Cancer* 1984;54:2200–2204.

B.5. What precautions should be made for airway management?

Airway evaluation is especially important in these patients. As the effects of the maintenance drugs wear off, the patient may become rigid and mouth opening may be very difficult. Primary laryngospasm is a known complication of Parkinson's disease (PD) and acute withdrawal of treatment can cause airway obstruction. Dentition is often impaired in the ill, geriatric population. Patients who have been receiving Dilantin for many years may have gum hypertrophy and loosening of teeth that may hamper placement of an airway. The head is encased in a frame and a bar crosses in front of the mouth. Also, the frame is attached to the bed making it impossible to extend the head. Not infrequently, if the procedure becomes prolonged, the degree of sedation must be increased, occasionally to general anesthesia, especially if there are intraoperative complications. Should aspiration, vomiting, or respiratory depression occur, a means to support oxygenation must be immediately available. Therefore, as well as careful preoperative assessment of the airway, the difficult airway cart should be available. Laryngeal mask and cuffed oropharyngeal airways are particularly valuable as they can be placed with little or no head movement and minimal opening of the mouth. A tracheostomy kit should also be available. It is essential that the anesthesiologist be aware preoperatively of the location of the key to the frame and know how the face piece can be immediately released should a problem occur.

Fikkers BF, Zandstra DF. Primary laryngospasm in a patient with Parkinson's disease: treatment with CPAP via a minitracheostomy following extubation. *Intensive Care Med* 1995;21:863–864.

Santos P, Valero R, Arguis MJ, et al. Preoperative adverse events during stereotactic microelectrode-guided deep brain surgery in Parkinson's disease. *Rev Esp Anestesiol Reanim* 2004;51(9):523–530.

C. Intraoperative management

C.1. What are the anesthetic considerations in an magnetic resonance imaging (MRI) unit.

Three types of energy in the MRI suite affect monitors and equipment and thus anesthetic delivery: a powerful static magnetic field of 1.5 Tesla (15,000 times greater than the magnetic field of the earth's surface), radiofrequency (RF) pulses that cause magnetic resonance by superenergizing cells which then emit RF signals, and time-varied magnetic field (TVMF) gradients that encode the emitted RF to produce two-dimensional and three-dimensional images.

Equipment and monitors must be adaptable to the MRI suite. All devices must meet three criteria: they must function normally at the site, they must present no danger to the patient or personnel, and they must not affect successful completion of the procedure or imaging. For most locations, these goals can be met by selecting commercially available portable monitoring devices. In general, nonferromagnetic equipment must be used. Only certain metals, iron, nickel, and cobalt to name a few, are magnetic. Items made of nonmagnetic aluminum, titanium, copper, silver, and gold are safe as far as missile dangers are concerned and are among the materials used to make MR-compatible intravenous (IV) poles, fixation devices, and nonmagnetic anesthesia machines. Often one must bring into the MRI magnet room susceptible metal items such as infusion pumps for IV lines. In such cases, it is safer to position those objects securely in the magnet room before the patient enters the magnet bore. Biomedical engineers with expertise in magnetic imaging should be consulted before installation or use of any electronic devices.

Implanted metals such as hip prostheses and Harrington rods are made of stainless steel, a metal usually only weakly magnetic. Information about the presence of such devices should be obtained and appropriate consultation sought from radiologists as to safety. Issues with large, weakly magnetic metal objects usually center on image degradation rather than the danger of the patient experiencing an uncontrollable magnetic force. Metals do not need to be missiles to be dangerous to the patient. Dangers from wires in epidural or pulmonary artery catheters relate to radiofrequency (RF) and the risk of burns.

Systems for central wall gases (oxygen, nitrous oxide, and air) are commercially available for MRI centers and should be installed during construction. Electrical power sources for monitoring systems are usually available in the magnet room itself and consist of isolated duplex power circuits with filtered 120 V (alternating current) to prevent electrical noise artifacts from interfering with the images. Monitors plugged into these outlets should be located as far from the core of the magnet as possible, beyond the gauss line. Also, they should be free of ferromagnetic material, and RF shielded. If possible, monitors should be outside the magnet room, and an external power source used. Then cables should be passed through wave guides (used to prevent leakage of RF pulses from the magnet and interference from outside sources) in the wall to limit the effects of magnetization, RF, and TVMF on the equipment.

Electrocardiography (ECG) is difficult within a static magnetic field. Maximum voltage charges are induced in any column of conducting fluid. The superimposed potentials are greatest in ST segments and T waves of leads I, II, V_1, V_2 and increase with field strength. Spike artifacts that mimic R waves are often produced due to the changing magnetic fields of the imaging gradients. Changes in the ECG wave form are present even in filtered systems designed for MRI use and make it impossible to reliably monitor for ischemia or to interpret arrhythmias. Plethysmography can be used as cardiac monitor, but is not useful for ischemia detection. Telemetry units have been used with low magnetic fields (0.6T), but their use may interfere with the RF needed for imaging. In patients highly susceptible to ischemia, a 12-lead ECG pre- and post-MRI is recommended.

Several MRI compatible ECG systems are currently available, and use ECG electrodes made of carbon graphite to lower resistance, eliminate ferromagnetism and minimize RF interference. The skin must be adequately prepared (dried or abraded). ECG cables are coaxialized to avoid any coils and subsequent burning of the skin. A small towel is folded and placed on the patient's chest, to avoid contact with the skin as an extra precaution.

Automated oscillometric blood pressure monitoring, based on pneumatic principles, eliminates the problems of electromagnetic interference. Units should be placed away from the magnet's core, and the tubing extended to accommodate this distance using plastic connectors as necessary. A conventional noninvasive blood pressure unit is not shielded from either RF or the magnetic field and uses a 120 V electrical outlet. Consequently, there is usually some interference with RF during scanning. Manual mercury sphygmomanometers have been adapted in for use in MRI by replacing all ferromagnetic hardware with brass or aluminum pieces.

Invasive blood pressure monitoring in the MRI center has certain practical limitations. Conventional disposable transducers may function adequately outside of the gauss line, although their accuracy should be determined by a biomedical engineer. Because disposable transducers have a predictably high natural frequency, a modest addition of tubing to move the transducers away from the patient is unlikely to cause damping. Self-contained multiple-monitor systems designed for MRI suites are now built with modes for invasive monitoring (Magnetic Resonance Equipment, Bay Shore, NY).

Because of the length of the tube, it is usually impossible to visualize the patient's face and chest for adequacy of ventilation during scanning. Alternative techniques include respiratory capnography, available in both conventional systems placed beyond the gauss line and MR-compatible systems. Should general anesthesia be required and in deeply sedated, spontaneously breathing patients the Jackson Rees circuit can be attached to either the endotracheal tube or a tight-fitting mask (using a mask strap). When the circuit is placed on the chest, visualization of bag movement outside of the magnet indicates adequacy of ventilation. Direct visualization of the airway by observing the scan image is also useful to confirm airway patency. Acoustic noise produced by the rapidly changing electric current pulsing through a static magnetic field makes useful auscultation during scanning impossible. Alternative monitoring techniques for confirmation of heart rate and ventilation include a system for remote auscultatory monitoring using microphones. The sounds are transmitted to a remote receiver and headphone set as infrared light, which does not interfere with imaging.

Many commercially available pulse oximeters function well in the magnet but burns to extremities have been caused by the induction of current within a loop of wire in the presence of magnetic flux with resultant heating of the wires. MR-specific pulse oximeters use heavy fiberoptic cables, which do not overheat and cannot be looped. These cables are expensive and easily damaged. If conventional oximeters are used, burns can usually be avoided by placing the sensor on the extremity distal to the magnet, keeping the sensor wires free of coils and protecting the digits with clear plastic wrap.

Quench monitors are usually present within each MRI suite. The magnet superconductors are kept cool in liquid nitrogen. Should this coolant evaporate due to leaky housing ("quench") the ambient oxygen supply of the room can drop precipitously causing hypoxia and the potential for cryo injury.

By replacing the machine's ferromagnetic components of the anesthetic machine with brass, aluminum, and plastic, the ferromagnetic content can be reduced to less than 2% of the total weight. One such machine, the Excel-210 MRI (Ohmeda, Madison, WI) is 99.8% stainless steel, brass, aluminum, and plastic. A similar model has recently been marketed by Drager (Doylestown, PA). The position of the machine in the scanner suite should be determined by a biomedical engineer. Medical gas cylinders constructed from aluminum should be used exclusively. Vaporizers, however, are affected little by the powerful magnetic field, and function accurately.

Plastic battery-operated laryngoscopes should be available. Batteries last longer if shielded with a paper casing or if plastic coated. If MRI compatible laryngoscopes are not available, the airway must be secured outside the magnet room using conventional ferromagnetic laryngoscopes.

Both circle and rebreathing anesthesia systems can be used for ventilation but may require additional lengths of tubing. Nonferromagnetic ventilators powered by compressed oxygen are commercially available for use with MRI (Omnivent, Topeka, KS). Standard ventilators on anesthesia machines can be modified by reducing the ferromagnetic content. A standard Air Shields Ventimeter Controller II (Hatboro, PA) has been used successfully at a distance of 12 ft from the core of the magnet at the 70 gauss line.

The difficulties of administering general anesthesia with an anesthesia machine can be avoided by using total intravenous anesthesia with a continuous infusion of propofol. However, all commercially available infusion pumps contain ferromagnetic circuitry which can be damaged and malfunction in the presence of a high magnetic field. Several pumps are accurate in the MR environment outside the gauss line including the IVAC 530 33(R), the IMED 960/960A 35, and the Medfusion 2010 (also see Chapter 61 Questions C.4, C.5, and C.6).

American Society of Anesthesiologists. *Anesthesia in remote locations safety [videotape]. Patient safety videotape series: videotape no. 26.* American Society of Anesthesiologists, www.asahq.org/NEWSLETTERS/1997/12_97/Anesthesia_1297.html, 1997.

Litt L, Cauldwell CB. Being extra safe when providing anesthesia for MRI examinations. *Anesth Saf Newsl* 2002;66:6.

Rezai AR, Phillips M, Baker KB, et al. Neurostimulation system used for deep brain stimulation (DBS) MR safety issues and implications of failing to follow safety recommendations. *Invest Radiol* 2004;39(5):300–303.

C.2. The surgeon wants to implant electrodes. What are the anesthetic implications?

A surgical team consisting of a neurosurgeon, an electrophysiologist, and a neurologist adjust measurements such as pulse, amplitude, and electrical port to optimally inhibit subthalamic nuclei (STN) output to the thalamus. After the experience in the magnetic resonance imaging (MRI) unit, the patient usually does not experience pain as much anxiety. With the return to the operating room, the anesthesiologist can now utilize all familiar equipment. Essential monitors are applied. Before further injection by the surgeon around the operative site, a small dose of midazolam (1 to 1.5 mg) and/or fentanyl (25 to 50 μg) is appropriate. If necessary, a bolus injection of propofol (20 to 30 mg) may be used. Thereafter, a propofol infusion of 10 to 20 μg/kg/minute allows sedation with consciousness.

As the surgeon places the electrodes, communication is essential both with the operator and the patient. Movement by the latter may seriously compromise precise placement. Until cooperation has been achieved, a patient attitude must be maintained.

C.3. How can the airway best be maintained?

Hopefully spontaneous ventilation with adequate oxygen saturation is maintained. Supplemental humidified oxygen should be provided with side stream capnography. A jaw thrust maneuver by the anesthesiologist, although improving oxygenation, might well alter the position and distort the electrode placement. Therefore sedation must be extremely well balanced to ensure that the patient continues to breathe nasally but does not experience pain. In the event of ventilatory compromise, an laryngeal mask airway (LMA), and nasal and oral airways of all sizes must be immediately available. The key is preparedness. As long as the patient is awake, he/she can maintain his/her own airway. Should circumstances change, the anesthesiologist must be able to secure the airway rapidly by fiberoptic means or through an intubating laryngeal mask if necessary. In some instances, it suffices to pass a LMA and allow continued spontaneous ventilation. Controlled ventilation may also be possible through an LMA if there is no leak. Communication with the surgeon is essential.

Watson NC, Hokanson M, Maltby JR, et al. The intubating laryngeal mask in failed fiberoptic intubation. *Can J Anaesth* 1999;46(4):376–378.

C.4. Which and how much fluids should be given?

Sugar containing solutions should be avoided in all situations where there is risk of cerebral damage. Some practitioners prefer to limit fluid intake if a urinary catheter has not been placed. Others place a condom catheter preoperatively. Patients with chronic hypertension may be hypovolemic and become hypotensive after administration of sedatives. Appropriate care requires replacement of fluids.

Many patients with Parkinson's disease (PD) have problems with urinary retention and urgency. Communication with the patient is essential to ensure him/her that a bottle or bedpan is available. Blood replacement is seldom required except in emergent situations.

Zornow M. Crystalloids, colloids and the brain. Intraoperative fluid therapy for the neurosurgical patient. *ASA Ann Refresher Course Lect.* Park Ridge,IL. American Society of Anesthesiologists, 2000;311.

C.5.   What constitutes required monitoring?

Monitoring as required by the guidelines of the ASA should be instituted. Monitors include, pulse oximetry, electrocardiography (ECG), capnography, noninvasive blood pressure monitoring and the availability of temperature measurement.

American Society of Anesthesiologists. *Directory of members. Standards for basic anesthetic monitoring.* Obtained on the web at: www.asa.org, 2006.

C.6.   Is invasive monitoring advisable?

If the patient is awake, I prefer not to insert an arterial cannula, although such a monitor additionally allows for blood gases analysis and for assessment of electrolytes and blood sugar levels. Use of a noninvasive blood pressure monitor set at 5-minute intervals is generally adequate (shorter duration is often uncomfortable for the patient). Also, during conscious sedation, placement of a central venous cannula probably is not warranted as the complication rate is significant and the information gained is scant. Should the requirements change to the need for general anesthesia, invasive blood pressure monitoring is recommended..

C.7.   How should the brain be monitored?

The neurosurgeon is monitoring electrical activity. The best monitor for the anesthesiologist in the awake patient is the response, either verbal or movement. Use of the BIS monitor (Aspect, Natick, MA) may add useful information in determining wakefulness if more sedation becomes necessary. Such a monitor may also help in determining sudden deterioration if the activity decreases although no medication has been given.

If the indication for deep brain stimulation (DBS) is location and control of epilepsy, then identification of speech or motor areas may be indicated to avoid accidental damage. Preservation of speech and motor function is essential. Mapping processes should be planned well in advance with involved personnel including the neurosurgeon, neurologist, and anesthesiologist. Speech mapping is performed under local anesthesia with monitored anesthesia care (MAC), while the patient is awake, because full cooperation is an essential aspect of the process. On the other hand, motor mapping is usually done under general anesthesia. The usual process is direct cortical stimulation on the suspected brain surface to elicit movements in various parts of the face, eyelids, tongue, neck, shoulders, and upper and lower extremities. Emesis should be prevented and ondansetron, dexamethasone and/or metoclopramide added to the preoperative medication schedule. An H_2-histamine blocker may help to reduce gastric acidity and volume.

C.8.   Which anesthetic agents should be used?

Anesthetic concerns for Parkinson's disease (PD) patients include an increased sensitivity to anesthetic agents, increased risk of laryngospasm and diaphragmatic spasm, increased risk of aspiration, hallucinations (visual and tactile), decreased vital capacity which may lead to pulmonary complications, violent tremors, postoperative delirium, muscle tremors that produce

ECG changes mimicking ventricular fibrillation, and extrapyramidal symptoms (EPS). Possible side effects of L-dopa consist of depletion of myocardial norepinephrine stores, peripheral vasoconstriction, hypovolemia, and orthostatic hypotension. Glycopyrrolate offers protection against neostigmine-induced bronchoconstriction in healthy subjects. However, in patients with PD, obstructive dysfunction is probably caused by parasympathetic hyperactivity and susceptibility to the muscarinic effects of neostigmine and bronchospasm is increased. Therefore, glycopyrrolate in usual doses may be inadequate. It is probably best to avoid the use of neostigmine.

The patient who undergoes deep brain stimulation (DBS) insertion should understand the sequence throughout this prolonged procedure. Preoperative cessation of anti-Parkinson therapy begins the evening before surgery to allow the symptoms to be observed during the procedure and demonstrate accurate placement of stimulating electrodes. Unfortunately, skeletal muscle rigidity, cramping, and other side effects ensue.

In some centers, no sedation is used. At others, a combination of midazolam, fentanyl in small divided doses, and a propofol infusion (acts at the γ-aminobutyric acid [GABA] receptors) has been used to allow adequate sedation for many hours. Remifentanil 0.1 μg/kg/minute may also be used. An agent that has been shown to mimic natural sleep is dexmedetomidine. It is a potent and highly selective α_2-adrenoreceptor agonist that provides dose dependent sedation, analgesia, sympatholysis, and anxiolysis without respiratory depression. Dose is approximately 0.1 to 0.2 μg/kg/minute without the need for bolus injection. At this level, the patient is sedated and comfortable but able to answer questions. Generally, sedation is discontinued before stimulation to allow the patient to be awake and cooperative. Spasticity may dictate that deeper sedation is essential.

Herrick IA, Craen RA, Gelb AW, et al. Propofol sedation during awake craniotomy for seizures: electrocorticography and epileptogenic effects. *Anesth Analg* 1997;84:1280–1284.

Manninen PH, Burke SJ, Wennberg R, et al. Intraoperative localization of an epileptogenic focus with alfentanil and fentanyl. *Anesth Analg* 1999;88:1101–1106.

Moore TA, Markert JM, Knowlton RC. Dexmedetomidine as rescue drug during awake craniotomy for cortical mapping and tumor resection. *Anesth Analg* 2006;102:1556–1558.

Schulz U, Keh D, Fritz G, et al. "Asleep-awake-asleep" anaesthetic technique for awake craniotomy. *Anaesthetist* 2006;55(5):585–598.

Sehgal A, Panchal I. Postoperative bronchospasm in a patient with Parkinson's disease. *Can J Anaesth* 2001;48(2):214–215.

C.9. How is blood pressure controlled?

As noted in the preceding text, hemodynamic stability can best be achieved with small doses of narcotics such as fentanyl, remifentanil or alfentanil. Labetalol, 5 to 10 mg may be used in a patient with a history of hypertension. Hydralazine is another choice in low dose. Least perturbations of blood pressure on incision can be achieved by scalp infiltration with bupivacaine. Hypertension has been associated with an increased risk of intracerebral hemorrhages. Dexmedetomidine offers better control and less need for antihypertensive medications.

Bloomfield EL, Schubert A, Secic M, et al. The influence of scalp infiltration on hemodynamics and postoperative pain in adult patients undergoing craniotomy. *Anesth Analg* 1998;87:579–582.

Rozet I, Muangman S, Vavialala MS, et al. Clinical experience with dexmedetomidine for functional neurosurgical procedures. *J Neurosurg Anesthesiol* 2004;16:362.

C.10. The case lasts longer than anticipated: what could be the complications?

Over time the patient is likely to become restless and less cooperative. He may wish to urinate and may complain of cold, hunger, or thirst. Everything possible should be done to ensure the patient's comfort, including a warming blanket and moistening of the lips. Small doses of benzodiazepines may be indicated with the understanding that the effect can be reversed. As the patient's head is secured to the table, even small movements should be avoided as the scalp may be torn. Dexmedetomidine may have remarkably beneficial effects. Additionally, dexmedetomidine has been shown to be both preventive and therapeutic for delirium, which is common in such elderly population, in particular, following administration of benzodiazepines. Again, communication with the surgeon is essential to understand all the options.

Difficulties can include technical problems in isolating the appropriate area or achieving appropriate readings and movement by the patient. Should there be sudden bleeding, then the patient should be released from the frame, general anesthesia induced and the airway secured immediately by endotracheal intubation. Blood should be obtained and preparation made for transfusion. Open craniotomy may be required to identify and secure the bleeding point.

C.11. The patient begins to cough. What is the differential diagnosis? Treatment?

The differential diagnosis rests between a dry mouth, "smoker's cough," and an embolic event. The patient is positioned in a slightly head up position. The negative pressure gradient between the surgical field and the right atrium allows entrainment of air into the venous circulation from the epidural veins, opened either at the incision or at any of the pin head holder sites. Occurrence in awake and spontaneously breathing patients may be increased over the frequency seen in ventilated and paralyzed patients because of the transfer of negative intrathoracic pressure to the central venous system with the initiation of each breath. Coughing is the first symptom, followed by chest pain, dyspnea, and tachypnea. While side stream capnography will detect decrease in end-tidal carbon dioxide ($ETCO_2$) very quickly and should be standard equipment, continuous Doppler monitoring interferes with neural recording. Decreases in $ETCO_2$ (usually dramatic) and SpO_2 (4 to 5 points) are also early changes and allow for prompt therapy. The surgeon must be informed immediately; the field flooded with saline and wax applied to the bone edges. The head should be lowered and the legs elevated. Lidocaine 50 mg may help to decrease coughing. Arterial blood gas analyses confirm the diagnosis with high $PaCO_2$ and low PaO_2. It is rarely necessary to abandon the procedure. Hemodynamic parameters are often stable throughout although some amount of tachycardia is common.

Suarez S, Ornaque I, Fabregas N, et al. Venous air embolism during Parkinson surgery in patients with spontaneous ventilation. *Anesth Analg* 1999;88(4):793–794.

C.12. The surgeon asks that the patient become more responsive. What would you do?

Depending on the medications that have been used for sedation, naloxone or flumazenil may be given to reverse narcotic and benzodiazepine effects. Naloxone should be given in increments of 0.1 mg as sudden reversal of analgesia may cause the patient to move unduly and cause scalp tearing. Even if it has been necessary to place a laryngeal mask airway (LMA), patients can still be awakened and tolerate the airway, especially if lidocaine 50 mg has been given intravenously. Intelligible sounds can be appreciated through an LMA.

C.13. The patient is complaining of pain. What would you do?

Small doses of remifentanil 0.01 to 0.05 μg/kg/minute for 3 to 5 minutes combined with propofol 15 μg/kg/minute have been shown to be effective in relieving pain during conscious sedation.

Onset of action of fentanyl is longer than that of remifentanil, making it less useful. Fentanyl is also cumulative. However, in doses of 25 μg the drug may be beneficial. Alfentanil offers no particular advantage.

Berkenstadt H, Perel A, Hadani M, et al. Monitored anesthesia care using remifentanil and propofol for awake craniotomy. *J Neurosurg Anesthesiol* 2001;13(3):246–249.

D. Postoperative Management

D.1. The patient became hemiplegic postoperatively. What is the differential diagnosis?

Surgical results are generally favorable with combined morbidity and mortality rates below 5% for epileptogenic foci resection and approximately 4% for deep brain stimulation (DBS) for Parkinson's disease (PD). However, hematoma formation related to surgery or decreased clotting due to a drug effect or herbal ingestion may occur. The patient requires an immediate computed tomography (CT) scan and preparations should be made for reexploration. Other causes include vasospasm, which may be managed by increased fluid administration and slight elevation of the blood pressure. Central pressure monitoring should be instituted.

National Institute of Health. *Surgery for epilepsy. National Institute of Health consensus statement*, Vol. 8. Bethesda: National Institute of Health, 1990:1–20.

D.2. How would you manage postoperative pain?

Postoperative pain is generally not severe as the brain itself has no pain endings. Morphine may be administered in small increments (2 to 4 mg), intravenously or acetaminophen (Tylenol) with or without codeine may be ordered.

D.3. About 1 hour into the postoperative period, the patient becomes comatose. What should be done?

The patient has most likely sustained a seizure. During a convulsion, the patient must be protected from injuring him/herself. If vital signs, especially oxygen saturation, are stable and if the seizure stops within seconds spontaneously, it may not be necessary to intubate. Rather, close observation is indicated. The dosing schedule of the patient's anticonvulsant drugs should be reviewed, serum levels obtained and a dose of Dilantin given. Should the patient not recover promptly, computed tomography (CT) scan is indicated. Intracranial hemorrhage and cerebral edema are included in the differential diagnosis. Serum electrolytes should be evaluated as hyponatremia is associated with diminished consciousness. The anesthetic agents given should also be reviewed, especially as to the use of reversal agents during periods of stimulation. Flumazenil, a benzodiazepines antagonist that involves the receptor site on the GABAa receptor–chloride channel complex has been implicated in neuroexcitatory phenomena, especially seizures. Also, the duration of action of flumazenil is shorter than that of midazolam or diazepam. Therefore, the sedative effects of these latter drugs may resurface in the postoperative period, especially in older patients in whom the half-life of the benzodiazepines is extended.

Spivey WH. Flumazenil and seizures: analysis of 43 cases. *Clin Ther* 1992;14:292–305.

D.4. If there are no complications, is this patient suitable for same day discharge?

A review of 154 patients showed that it is feasible to perform awake craniotomies, discharging patients on the same or next day. Patient selection must be stringent with respect to several factors. A shorter operating time requires less sedation and less blood loss and fluid shift. Although some neurosurgeons prefer monitored care for their patients for at least 24 hours postoperatively, such a routine may not always be necessary. In the study of Blanshard, cited in the preceding text, 29% patients were discharged on the same day. Only one case was readmitted because of a seizure at home, which was found to be related to mild cerebral edema that responded to steroids. One patient, scheduled as an ambulatory case was admitted overnight for treatment of headache and nausea.

Another study (1996 to 2003) of 262 patients indicated a frequency of minor complications of 4.2%. Transient and permanent neurologic deficits occurred in 0.2% and 0.4%, respectively. Intracranial hemorrhage was reported in 0.2%. Skin infection rate was 3% initially and increased to 6%, requiring removal of the stimulation system in 4.6%. Hardware related problems occurred in 13.9% and was the main reason for extended hospital stay. Analyzing data from 109 patients (1998 to 2002) indicated 16 serious adverse events in 14 patients including 2 perioperative deaths from pulmonary embolism, 4 intracranial hemorrhages, 4 infections, 1 cerebrospinal leak, 1 venous infarction, 1 seizure and 1 skin erosion. Authors emphasize the importance of extending informed consent to include all potential complications

Berie A, Kelly PJ, Rezai A, et al. Complications of deep brain stimulation surgery. *Stereotact Funct Neurosurg* 2001;77(1–4):73–78.

Blanshard HJ, Chung F, Manninen PH, et al. Awake craniotomy for removal of intracranial tumour a feasible technique for ambulatory patients. *Br J Anaesth* 1999;82:8–9.

Umemura A, Jaggi JL, Hurtig HI, et al. Deep brain stimulation for movement disorders: morbidity and mortality in 109 patients. *J Neurosurg* 2003;9894:779–784.

Venkatraghavan L, Manninen P, Mak P, et al. Anesthesia for functional neurosurgery: review of complications. *J Neurosurg Anesthesiol* 2006;18:64–67.

Voges J, Waerzeggers Y, Maarouf M, et al. Deep brain stimulation; long term analysis of complications caused by hardware and surgery a single centre experience. *J Neurop Neurosurg psychiatry* 2006;77:868–872.

D.5. How would you manage the second stage of the procedure? When? Are the requirements different from those for electrode insertion?

Patients who present for insertion of generators (usually 2 weeks later) may be relieved to undergo general anesthesia for the procedure. Generally Parkinson's disease (PD) patients are sensitive to hypnotic agents unless they frequently medicate with benzodiazepines for anxiety. Induction of anesthesia may produce fluctuations in blood pressure and heart rate caused by intravascular volume depletion and an inadequate response to hypotension (due to decreased renin release and depletion of noradrenergic stores secondary to L-dopa therapy). The use of ketamine has been known to cause an exaggerated sympathetic response, and there is a potential hyperkalemic response to succinylcholine.

During maintenance of anesthesia, there is a normal response to nondepolarizing muscle relaxants. It is suggested that the choice of agents used are those that provide for a rapid recovery, avoiding neostigmine as noted in the preceding text. Sensitivity to anesthetic agents is increased. Intraoperative monitoring should include standard monitors, including temperature. The ECG should be closely monitored in the presence of arrhythmogenic anti-Parkinson agents (e.g., L-dopa). The patient's airway is of concern due to possible muscle rigidity, which may impede airway manipulation and impair ventilation. The risk of aspiration is increased. The avoidance of phenothiazines, butyrophenones, and metoclopramide which may exacerbate extrapyramidal symptoms (EPS), the avoidance of meperidine if the patient is on selegiline combination therapy, assessment of the status of the intravascular volume, and instruction on the importance of deep breathing are all important considerations. Common manifestations of autonomic disturbances include esophageal dysfunction that puts the PD patient at risk for aspiration. Also, orthostatic hypotension may result in exaggerated decreases in blood pressure in response to volatile anesthetics. Additional anesthetic considerations include the avoidance of indirect-acting sympathomimetic amines if the patient is on selegiline.

Before extubation, a full recovery from neuromuscular blockade should be ensured and the anesthesia provider should be prepared for laryngospasm and impaired ventilation secondary to muscle rigidity and a hyperparasympathetic response. Also, emergence from anesthesia may produce tremors and hallucinations. The postoperative course may see these patients develop transient mental confusion. Their respiratory status must be observed closely, and the use of incentive spirometry is often indicated.

D.6. Are results successful on a long-term basis?

Deep brain stimulation (DBS) can be performed bilaterally, and improves symptoms of bradykinesia, rigidity, and tremor (gait and postural instability are often refractory to treatment). Postoperative dyskinesias are observed which often resolve with subsequent reductions in doses of pharmacologic agents. Eventually, a net reduction in dyskinesia results in most patients. Stimulation produces significant improvement in all "off" medication conditions, resulting in close to 50% improvement in Unified Parkinson's Disease Rating Scales but no improvement in conjunction with medication. The duration of "off" periods is significantly reduced. While young, dementia-free Parkinson's disease (PD) patients who respond well to drug therapy are ideal DBS candidates, patients who fail to respond favorably to L-dopa are unlikely to benefit from DBS.

Jaggi JL, Umemura A, Hurtig HI, et al. Bilateral stimulation of the subthalamic nucleus in Parkinson's disease: surgical efficacy and prediction of outcome. *Stereotact Funct Neurosurg* 2004;82(2):104–114.

CHAPTER 25

Management of Head Injury

EUGENE S. FU • JONATHAN JAGID • LEO T. HARRIS

A 37-YEAR-OLD MAN

with a history of atrial fibrillation, receiving Coumadin therapy, was struck by a motor vehicle. On admission, the patient had a Glasgow Coma Scale (GCS) of five and vital signs were blood pressure 112/63 mmHg, heart rate 60 beats per minute, respiratory rate 18, breaths per minute. The patient received fresh frozen plasma for a prothrombin time (PT) of 36.5 seconds and an activated partial thromboplastin time (aPTT) of 35 seconds. Head computed tomography (CT) scan showed bifrontal contusions and an expanding intracerebral hematoma in the right frontal region (Fig. 25.1). The patient was taken to the operating room (OR) for a bifrontal craniectomy for evacuation of the anterior frontal lobe and a frontal intracerebral hematoma.

A. Pathophysiology and Differential Diagnosis

1. What types of intracranial injuries are most likely to have occurred in this patient?
2. What is the difference between primary and secondary injury? What factors contribute to secondary injury?
3. What are the risks and benefits of administering mannitol?
4. What is the effect of hyperglycemia on neurologic outcome following head trauma?
5. What alterations in sodium and potassium balance can occur in head injury patients?
6. In addition to sodium and potassium, what other electrolyte abnormalities can be present after head trauma?
7. What are the neuroprotective effects of administering magnesium?
8. What role does gender and female sex hormones have in the pathophysiology of traumatic brain injury?

B. Preoperative Evaluation and Preparation

1. What is the GCS? What is the significance of a GCS of five in this patient?
2. In addition to the GCS, what other assessments can be done to evaluate neurologic function?
3. What is the role of CT scanning in the initial evaluation of the head-injured patient? What management options can be done in patients whose neurologic condition is deteriorating before obtaining a CT scan?
4. What is the role of intracranial pressure (ICP) monitoring in the management of head injury?
5. How can you clear this patient's cervical spine?

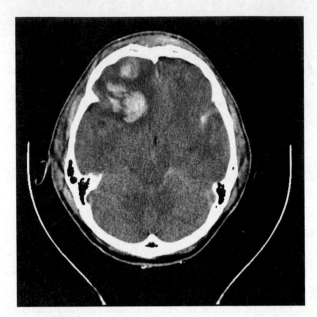

Figure 25.1 Head computed tomography (CT) scan showing bifrontal contusions and intracerebral hematoma expansion of the right frontal contusion.

6. What are the benefits of early endotracheal intubation in this patient?

7. What is your plan for airway management in this patient? How would it change if the patient were combative? How would it change if the patient had facial fractures with significant swelling of the head and neck?

8. What are the effects of succinylcholine on ICP? What is the significance of the effect, if any?

9. What coagulation abnormalities are present after traumatic brain injury? What treatment modalities can be used to provide hemostasis and reduce intracranial hematoma expansion?

C. Intraoperative Management

1. What is appropriate hemodynamic monitoring during CT scanning and during craniotomy for evacuation of a subdural hematoma?

2. Should hyperventilation be used in this patient?

3. What are the implications of arterial hypertension in head-injured patients? How should blood pressure be managed?

4. What should be done about intravenous fluid replacement? Should corticosteroids be given empirically?

5. Should hypertonic saline be administered to this patient? How is hypertonic saline administered?

6. The patient underwent a craniotomy for a bifrontal craniectomy for evacuation of the anterior frontal lobe and a frontal intracerebral hematoma. Are there anesthetic agents that should be avoided in this situation? Which ones? What agents might be preferred in this situation?

7. Should hypothermia be employed in this patient?

D. Postoperative Neurointensive Care Management

1. What are the postoperative ventilation considerations in this patient?
2. What specific measures should be used to control the patient's intracranial pressure (ICP)? What type of monitoring devices can be used to monitor ICP?
3. What is neurogenic pulmonary edema? Would you avoid positive end-expiratory pressure (PEEP) in a patient with increased ICP?
4. What is the role of antiseizure prophylaxis in the perioperative management of head trauma?
5. How can cerebral oxygenation monitoring be used in the clinical management of traumatic brain injury?
6. What methods can be used in the neurointensive care unit to prevent hyperthermia?

A. Pathophysiology and Differential Diagnosis

A.1. What types of intracranial injuries are most likely to have occurred in this patient?

In a patient without obvious signs of localizing neurologic deficits, the most probable intracranial injury is cerebral contusion. This is usually a diffuse or multifocal process that results in disruption of the blood–brain barrier, causing widespread brain swelling due to edema. The diagnosis can be made with certainty only after ruling out other focal injuries, such as intracranial hematoma. Traumatic intracranial hematomas include epidural hematoma, subdural hematoma, and cerebral hematoma. The clinical hallmark signifying a mass lesion is the presence of generalized elevated intracranial pressure (ICP) in conjunction with focal deficits. Interestingly, most patients who were able to talk and then deteriorate into coma had a mass lesion requiring surgery, indicating the importance of quickly diagnosing mass lesions with computed tomography (CT) scanning.

Epidural hematomas, located between the skull and dura, are almost always caused by skull fractures. Most epidural hematomas occur in the temporoparietal region as skull fractures in this area cross the path of the middle meningeal artery. Consequently, epidural hematomas can rapidly expand in the presence of a lacerated meningeal artery. The classic presentation of an epidural hematoma is a patient who appears lucid but then deteriorates into a comatose state, with a fixed dilated pupil ipsilateral to the skull fracture and contralateral hemiparesis. Subdural hematomas are located between the inner surface of the dura mater and the pial surface of the brain. In contrast to epidural hematomas, subdural hematomas are caused by lacerations of the venous sinuses (e.g., lateral sinus or sagittal sinus) and tend to develop more insidiously.

Intracerebral hematomas are collections of blood ranging from petechial hemorrhages to large collections usually in the temporal or frontal lobes. Some lesions are pure hematomas or hemorrhagic contusions. Often, these hemorrhagic areas can be managed medically with follow-up CT scans. Indications for surgical evacuation of intracerebral hematomas include rapid mental deterioration, mass effect, and marked elevations in ICP.

Eisenberg HM, Gary HE Jr, Aldrich EF, et al. Initial CT Findings in 753 patients with severe head injury. A report from the NIH Traumatic Coma Bank. *J Neurosurg* 1990;73: 688–698.

Lobato RD, Rivas JJ, Gomez PA, et al. Head-injured patients who talk and deteriorate into coma. Analysis of 211 cases studied with computerized tomography. *J Neurosurg* 1991;75:256–261.

Schmidek HH, ed. *Operative neurosurgical techniques*, 4th ed. Philadelphia: WB Saunders, 2000:83–85.

A.2. What is the difference between primary and secondary injury? What factors contribute to secondary injury?

Primary injury represents neurologic damage that occurs at the time of impact. Secondary injury is the consequence of ischemic insults to the brain that occur subsequent to the primary injury. Prevention of further hypoxemia and hypotension are the mainstay of managing head-injury patients. Pathophysiological processes contributing to secondary injury include (a) alterations in the balance between cerebral blood flow and metabolism, (b) disruption of cerebral autoregulation, (c) loss of cerebral vascular reactivity to carbon dioxide, and (d) vasogenic fluid accumulation leading to brain swelling.

Unfortunately, many patients with severe head trauma arrive to the hospital after having episodes of hypotension and hypoxemia. Improvement in outcomes depends on trauma centers having emergency teams that provide rapid treatment in the field and direct transport to the hospital. Initial management entails oxygenation by early intubation and maintenance of cerebral perfusion pressure (CPP) with rapid resuscitation to treat hemorrhagic or hypovolemic shock. However, the difficulty with fluid administration is that brain swelling increases intracranial pressure (ICP) and lowers the threshold of the systemic blood pressure for cerebral ischemia. Elevation in ICP, which heralds cerebral herniation, leads to further brain damage and increased morbidity. The use of ICP monitoring has been important in decreasing secondary injury as a means to quantify and treat cerebral hypoperfusion. Improved outcome in patients with severe head trauma has been attributed to the approach of "squeezing oxygenated blood through a swollen brain."

Chestnut RM, Marshall LF, Klauber MR, et al. The role of secondary brain injury in determining outcome from severe head injury. *J Trauma* 1993;34:216–222.

Ghajar J. Traumatic brain injury. *Lancet* 2000;356:923–929.

Young A, Willats S. Controversies in management of acute brain trauma. *Lancet* 1998; 352:164–165.

A.3. What are the risks and benefits of administering mannitol?

Mannitol is an osmotic diuretic that has been a mainstay in decreasing intracranial pressure (ICP). Traditionally, it was thought that mannitol could aggravate elevated ICP by crossing a disrupted blood–brain barrier and inducing additional edema. Following mannitol administration, cerebrospinal fluid (CSF) pressure transiently increases in normal patients but immediately decreases in the presence of intracranial hypertension. Mannitol is effective in reversing brain swelling and is recommended for the treatment of traumatic intracranial hypertension. Indications for administering mannitol before ICP monitoring include transtentorial herniation and progressive neurologic deterioration. The standard adult dose has been 1 g per kg as a rapid intravenous infusion. However, in one study involving patients with severe traumatic brain injury, patients receiving high-dose mannitol ($\sim$1.4 g/kg) had improved recovery of pupillary responses and 6-month outcome parameters compared to patients receiving 0.7 g per kg.

Cruz J, Minoja G, Okuchi K, et al. Successful use of the new high-dose mannitol treatment in patients with Glasgow Coma Scale scores of 3 and bilateral abnormal pupillary widening: a randomized trial. *J Neurosurg* 2004;100:376–383.

Eckstein M. The prehospital and emergency department management of penetrating head injuries. *Neurosurg Clin N Am* 1995;6:741–751.

Hartwell RC, Sutton LN. Mannitol, intracranial pressure, and vasogenic edema. *Neurosurgery* 1993;32:444–450.

Nortje J, Menon DK. Traumatic brain injury: physiology, mechanisms, and outcome. *Curr Opin Neurol* 2004;17:711–718.

Ravussin P, Abou-Madi M, Archer D, et al. Changes in CSF pressure after mannitol in patients with and without elevated CSF pressure. *J Neurosurg* 1988;69:869–876.

A.4. What is the effect of hyperglycemia on neurologic outcome following head trauma?

The release of catecholamines and hyperglycemia are manifestations of the stress response to severe head injury. Patients with severe head injury have higher blood glucose levels compared to patients with moderate and minor injury. Postoperative glucose levels above 200 mg per dL have been associated with a worse neurologic outcome. Early hyperglycemia is a significant indicator of severity of injury and a predictor of outcome. Nevertheless, hyperglycemia should be treated aggressively, especially when the risk of cerebral ischemia is present. Elevated plasma glucose levels provide a substrate for anaerobic metabolism, allowing increased production of lactate during ischemia. The approach to glucose control in traumatic brain injury patients is a subject to debate as the downside of aggressive therapy is hypoglycemia and cerebral glucopenia. In one study, intense insulin therapy, with the goal of maintaining blood glucose levels at 80 to 100 mg per dL, was associated with increased microdialysis levels of glutamate, which is a marker for cellular distress.

Diringer MN. Is aggressive treatment of hyperglycemia for everyone? *Crit Care Med* 2006;34:930–931.

Rovlias A, Kotsou S. The influence of hyperglycemia on neurological outcome in patients with severe head injury. *Neurosurgery* 2000;46:335–342.

Vespa P, Boonyaputthikul R, McArthur DL, et al. Intensive insulin therapy reduces microdialysis glucose values without altering glucose utilization or improving the lactate/pyruvate ratio after traumatic brain injury. *Crit Care Med* 2006;34:850–856.

Yang SY, Zhang S, Wang ML. Clinical significance of admission hyperglycemia and factors related to its patients with acute severe head injury. *Surg Neurol* 1995;44:373–377.

A.5. What alterations in sodium and potassium balance can occur in head injury patients?

Neurologically injured patients are at risk for electrolyte imbalance. Perioperative fluid administration, mannitol administration, syndrome of inappropriate antidiuretic hormone secretion (SIADH), and cerebral salt wasting syndromes are potential causes of hyponatremia. Severe hyponatremia (Na <120 mEq/L) may be associated with cerebral edema and seizures. The correction of hyponatremia must be gradual to avoid precipitating central pontine myelinolysis. Hypernatremia can occur as a result of enteral tube feedings, diuresis with mannitol, and diabetes insipidus (DI). Basilar skull fractures may predispose to the development of DI as a consequence of shearing of the pituitary stalk. Treatment of DI entails administration of 1-desamino-8-D-arginine-vasopressin (DDAVP) in conjunction with hypoosmolar fluids.

Hypokalemia may result from potassium loss secondary to polyuresis in association with diuretic administration and high urine output states such as SIADH and cerebral salt wasting syndrome. Concurrent hypomagnesemia, as seen with alcoholic and diabetic patients, can aggravate hypokalemia. The loss of cellular magnesium depletes intracellular potassium, making hypokalemia more difficult to treat if magnesium supplementation is not given. In addition, serum potassium levels may decrease despite normal total body stores. Common causes of intracellular shifts of potassium include hyperventilation and insulin administration.

Cucchiara RF, Black S, Michenfelder JD, eds. *Clinical neuroanesthesia*, 2nd ed. New York: Churchill Livingstone, 1998:241–242.

Polderman KH, Bloemers FW, Peerdeman SM, et al. Hypomagnesemia and hypophosphatemia at admission in patients with severe head injury. *Crit Care Med* 2000;28: 2022–2025.

A.6. In addition to sodium and potassium, what other electrolyte abnormalities can be present after head trauma?

Potassium and sodium levels are routinely checked perioperatively. However, magnesium and phosphate levels are not routinely ordered so low levels of these electrolytes are more likely to remain undetected. Hypomagnesemia has been associated with cardiac arrhythmia such as torsades de pointes, sudden death, seizures, and neuromuscular irritability. Hypophosphatemia has been associated with weakness of the respiratory muscles and respiratory infections.

Polderman KH, Bloemers FW, Peerdeman SM, et al. Hypomagnesemia and hypophosphatemia at admission in patients with severe head injury. *Crit Care Med* 2000;28: 2022–2025.

A.7. What are the neuroprotective effects of administering magnesium?

Magnesium homeostasis is altered after traumatic brain injury because magnesium falls on the order of 50%. In addition to treating hypomagnesemia, administration of magnesium affords neuroprotection. Magnesium is an *N*-methyl-D-aspartate (NMDA) antagonist that suppresses excitotoxic mechanisms. Excitatory amino acids such as glutamate and aspartate are released after traumatic injury, which initiates a cascade of events leading to secondary injury. Glutamate-induced ionic depolarization leads to calcium influx and cell death. Magnesium works at the postsynaptic receptor to reduce the neurotoxic effect of glutamate. In animal models, traumatic brain injury decreases intracellular free concentrations of magnesium. Magnesium crosses the blood–brain barrier. Repeated administration of magnesium attenuates brain edema and improves neurologic recovery. Although prophylactic magnesium administration has received some enthusiasm in the management of stroke, its clinical use in the treatment of head injury remains to be seen.

Cottrell JE. Brain protection in neurosurgery. *ASA annual refresher course lectures*, Park Ridge: American Society of Anesthesiologists, 2004;145.

Feldman Z, Gurevitch B, Artru AA, et al. Effect of magnesium given 1 hour after head trauma on brain edema and neurological outcome. *J Neurosurg* 1996;85:131–137.

Fu ES, Tummala RP. Neuroprotection in brain and spinal cord trauma. *Curr Opin Anaesth* 2005;18:181–187.

Heath DL, Vink R. Traumatic brain axonal injury produces sustained decline in intracellular free magnesium concentration. *Brain Res* 1996;738:150–153.

A.8. What role does gender and female sex hormones have in the pathophysiology of traumatic brain injury?

Women account for approximately 20% to 30% of the head injury population. Laboratory evidence indicates that estrogen and progesterone mediate neuroprotection by decreasing lipid peroxidation and reducing production of inflammatory cytokines. Compared to women, increases in cerebrospinal fluid (CSF) levels of glutamate, lactate, and F_2-isoprostane (marker for lipid peroxidation) are observed in men after traumatic brain injury. However, there appears to be a paradox between the acute neuroprotective properties of female sex hormones and actual recovery for women as functional outcome has been worse for women. It has been suggested that female sex hormones may be detrimental to neuroplasticity and recovery. In addition to gender differences, the effect of hormonal status in females in the pathophysiology of head injury remains unclear. Consequently, gender selection and the relation of hormonal status at time of injury become important in the design of clinical trials involving therapeutic interventions in brain trauma patients.

> Fu ES, Tummala RP. Neuroprotection in brain and spinal cord trauma. *Curr Opin Anaesth* 2005;18:181–187.
>
> Wagner AK, Fabio A, Puccio AM, et al. Gender associations with cerebrospinal fluid glutamate and lactate/pyruvate levels after severe traumatic brain injury. *Crit Care Med* 2005;33:407–413.

B. Preoperative Evaluation and Preparation

B.1. What is the Glasgow Coma Scale (GCS)? What is the significance of a GCS of 5 in this patient?

The GCS is the most widely used method to assess neurologic status and severity of brain dysfunction following head trauma. The scale, which ranges from 3 to 15 points, is based on evaluating the best motor response, the best verbal response, and eye opening (Table 25.1). Of the patients who

Table 25.1 Glasgow Coma Scale.

Eye Opening:	None	1
	To pain	2
	To verbal command	3
Best verbal response:	No verbal response	4
	Incomprehensible sounds	1
	Inappropirate words	2
	Disoriented, conversing	3
	Oriented, conversing	4
Best motor response:	No response (flaccid)	1
	Extension (decerebrate)	2
	Abnormal flexion (decorticate)	3
	Flexion/withdrawal	4
	Localizes to pain	5
	Obeys verbal commands	6

initially survive traumatic brain injury, 80% have minor injury (GCS 13 to 15), 10% have moderate injury (GCS 9 to 12), and 10% have severe injury (GCS <9). Serial determination of GCS is essential to monitor the patient's condition as patients GCS can change in a rapid or delayed manner. Decreases in the GCS of three or more points are indicative of catastrophic neurologic deterioration.

Alvarez M, Narva JM, Rue M, et al. Mortality prediction in head trauma patients: performance of Glasgow Coma Score and general severity systems. *Crit Care Med* 1998;26:142–148.

Longnecker DE, Tinker JH, Morgan GE Jr, eds. *Principles and practice of anesthesiology*, 2nd ed. St. Louis: Mosby, 1998:581–582.

Schmidek HH, ed. *Operative neurosurgical techniques*, 4th ed. Philadelphia: WB Saunders, 2000:83–85.

B.2. In addition to the Glasgow Coma Scale (GCS), what other assessments can be done to evaluate neurologic function?

The Glasgow Coma Score assesses spontaneous activity. Further neurologic evaluation includes pupillary examination, checking for brainstem reflexes in unconscious patients, and looking for lateralizing signs. Fixed bilateral enlarged pupils may signify an ominous prognosis whereas unilateral papillary enlargement occurs in the presence of an expanding hematoma. Deeply comatose patients lacking spontaneous eye opening should have evaluation of the brainstem reflexes. The oculocephalic reflex or doll's eye maneuver is elicited by rotating the head horizontally to one side. In the intact brainstem, the eyes deviate conjugately to the other side. This maneuver should be performed only when the cervical spine has been cleared. If the doll's eye response is abnormal, then testing of the oculovestibular reflex (cold caloric test) is another method to evaluate brainstem function. The cold caloric test entails irrigation of the external auditory canal with ice water. In the intact brainstem, the eyes should deviate to the side of cold stimulation. Abnormal oculocephalic and oculovestibular signify severe brainstem dysfunction extending to the pons. However, other causes for abnormal responses need to be ruled out, which include drugs (e.g., phenytoin), nerve injuries (e.g., oculomotor, abducens, vestibular), and labyrinthine disease. Additional lateralizing signs include asymmetric posturing, hemiparesis, and facial weakness. The presence of these findings could indicate the possibility of a mass lesion.

Cucchiara RF, Black S, Michenfelder JD, eds. *Clinical neuroanesthesia*, 2nd ed. New York, Churchill Livingstone, 1998:241–242.

Ivatury RR, Cayten CG, eds. *The textbook of penetrating trauma*. Baltimore: Williams & Wilkins, 1996:251–253.

B.3. What is the role of computed tomography (CT) scanning in the initial evaluation of the head-injured patient? What management options can be done in patients whose neurologic condition is deteriorating before obtaining a CT scan?

If there has been a loss of consciousness or if the Glasgow Coma Scale (GCS) is less than 15, a head CT scan should be obtained. Evidence of an intracranial hematoma that causes compression of the ventricles or a midline shift of greater than 5 mm is an indication for surgical intervention. Conversely, absence of a mass lesion or compression of the ventricles is an indication for conservative management.

In a patient whose neurologic condition is deteriorating, prompt intubation, ventilation, and mannitol administration usually provides sufficient time to obtain a preoperative CT scan.

In rare circumstances, the surgeon may need to initiate emergency surgical exploration of an expanding intracranial hematoma without CT scanning. In acute situations, urgent partial surgical decompression through a burr hole close to the fracture may be required.

Miller RD, ed. *Miller's anesthesia*, 6th ed. New York: Churchill Livingstone, 2005:2152.

Prough DS. Perioperative management of traumatic brain injury. *ASA annual refresher course lectures*. Park Ridge: American Society of Anesthesiologists, 2004:221.

Schmidek HH, ed. *Operative neurosurgical techniques*, 4th ed. Philadelphia: WB Saunders, 2000:83–85.

B.4. What is the role of intracranial pressure (ICP) monitoring in the management of head injury?

Life-threatening emergencies such as impending herniation or hemorrhagic wounds in the abdomen/thorax require rapid surgical intervention. Definitive surgery for non–life-threatening injuries should be delayed until the patient is hemodynamically stable to minimize hypotension, hypovolemia, and cerebral hypoxemia. If the patient is not emergently taken to the OR, ICP monitoring becomes helpful in optimizing blood pressure management because cerebral perfusion pressure (CPP) can be calculated by measuring mean arterial pressure (MAP) and ICP. Patients with head trauma often sustain other injuries requiring nonneurologic surgery. The decision to have an ICP monitor placed before nonneurologic surgery includes neurologic status in conjunction with computed tomography (CT) findings, the nature and duration of the surgical procedure, and surgical procedures requiring occlusion of the aorta.

Although there have been no prospective, randomized, clinical trials to establish the clinical efficacy of ICP monitoring, ICP monitoring has become widely used for the management of intracranial hypertension. ICP monitoring helps in the early detection of expanding hematomas and can be useful in reducing ICP by cerebrospinal fluid (CSF) drainage.

In this patient, ICP monitoring is appropriate because this patient has severe brain injury and an abnormal CT scan. In patients with severe head injury but a normal CT scan, ICP monitoring is indicated when systolic blood pressure is less than 90 mm Hg and there is motor posturing. ICP monitoring is rarely indicated in patients with mild to moderate injury.

Marion DW, Spiegel TP. Changes in the management of severe traumatic brain injury. 1991–1997. *Crit Care Med* 2000;28:16–18.

Marshall LF. Head Injury: recent past, present and future. *Neurosurgery* 2000;47:546–561.

Prough DS. Perioperative management of traumatic brain injury. *ASA annual refresher course lectures*. Park Ridge: American Society of Anesthesiologists, 2004:221.

Schmidek HH, ed. *Operative neurosurgical techniques*, 4th ed. Philadelphia: WB Saunders, 2000:83–85.

B.5. How can you clear this patient's cervical spine?

Two percent of patients presenting to trauma units following closed head injury have a concomitant cervical spine fracture. Adequate cervical spine x-rays, especially in the uncooperative patient, are very difficult to obtain following many traumas. Furthermore, injuries in the atlantooccipital region are especially difficult to identify radiographically, and up to 26% of lateral radiographs failed to show fractures. Even in the face of normal radiographic studies, patients may still have significant ligamentous injuries with cervical instability necessitating particular care during airway management. Typically, patients are examined carefully, their cervical spine is palpated, and tenderness or weakness is identified. In the uncooperative or unconscious patient, the cervical spine should be considered not cleared, even in light of normal x-rays. On the other hand, if the cervical spine is cleared radiographically, the mental status is normal, and the patient is asymptomatic, then the examination can be considered cleared.

Brooks RA, Willett KM. Evaluation of the Oxford protocol for total spinal clearance in the unconscious trauma patient. *J Trauma* 2001;50:862–867.

Kirshenbaum KJ, Nadimpalli SR, Fantus R, et al. Unsuspected upper cervical spine fractures associated with significant head trauma: role of CT. *J Emerg Med* 1990;8:183–198.

Miller RD, ed. *Miller's anesthesia*, 6th ed. New York: Churchill Livingstone, 2005:2152–2153.

O'Malley KF, Ross SE. The incidence of injury to the cervical spine in patients with craniocerebral injury. *J Trauma* 1988;28:1476–1478.

Stiell IG, Wells GA, Clement C, et al. The role of clinical assessment in the evaluation of patients with potential cervical spine injury. *Acad Emerg Med* 2001;8:457.

B.6. What are the benefits of early endotracheal intubation in this patient?

Endotracheal intubation not only provides a secure airway in a patient with an altered ability to protect his airway, but also allows for the ability to hyperventilate the patient, providing a rapid tool for lowering intracranial pressure (ICP) if necessary. Also, patients with facial trauma can often have progressive swelling and anatomic distortion, making subsequent intubation attempts more difficult.

Miller RD, ed. *Miller's anesthesia*, 6th ed. New York: Churchill Livingstone, 2005:2152–2153.

Prough DS. Perioperative management of traumatic brain injury. *ASA annual refresher course lectures*. Park Ridge: American Society of Anesthesiologists, 2004:221.

B.7. What is your plan for airway management in this patient? How would it change if the patient were combative? How would it change if the patient had facial fractures with significant swelling of the head and neck?

Patients with a Glasgow Coma Scale (GCS) of less than 8 often require intubation and controlled ventilation to lower the intracranial pressure (ICP) and protect the airway. Direct laryngoscopy following induction and muscle relaxation should be accompanied by in-line stabilization by an assistant, with many authors recommending leaving the posterior portion of the rigid collar in place, so that it can act as a stabilizer to prevent further movement. Earlier recommendations for in-line traction are no longer popular due to concerns for spinal cord damage in patients with gross instability. Emergency airway equipment should always be available in case of the inability to intubate with direct laryngoscopy. Another option is awake fiberoptic intubation, however, a compliant patient is a necessity, as thrashing and fighting can cause more harm to the unstable spine than laryngoscopy itself. A combative patient would make one lean more towards rapid sequence induction and intubation with in-line stabilization, whereas a patient with facial fractures and facial swelling would lead one to fiberoptic intubation. Mid-face and basilar skull fractures should preclude attempts at nasal intubation due to concerns for entering the cranial vault inadvertently. Blood in the airway can complicate fiberoptic intubation in these patients, and alternate intubation devices and plans should be readily available. In any event, the goals of preoxygenation and securing an airway with a minimum of cervical spine motion should be observed, while being cognizant of the risk of regurgitation and aspiration in a patient with a full stomach.

Criswell JC, Parr MJ, Nolan JP. Emergency airway management in patients with cervical spine injuries. *Anaesthesia* 1994;49:900.

Miller RD, ed. *Miller's anesthesia*, 6th ed. New York: Churchill Livingstone 2005:2152–2153.

Prough DS. Perioperative management of traumatic brain injury. *ASA annual refresher course lectures*. Park Ridge: American Society of Anesthesiologists, 2004:221.

B.8. What are the effects of succinylcholine on intracranial pressure (ICP)? What is the significance of the effect, if any?

Succinylcholine has been shown in animal and human studies to increase ICP through increased muscle spindle activation with depolarization. The effect, however, can be avoided by using a defasciculating dose of a nondepolarizing drug before succinylcholine administration. It is important to remember that the elevation in ICP from succinylcholine will be much less than the elevation during intubation attempts in awake struggling patients.

Lanier WL, Milde JH, Michenfelder JD. Cerebral stimulation following succinylcholine in dogs. *Anesthesiology* 1986;64:551–559.

Miller RD, ed. *Miller's anesthesia*, 6th ed. New York: Churchill Livingstone, 2005:2153.

Stirt JA, Grosslight KR, Bedford RF, et al. "Defasciculation" with metocurine prevents succinylcholine-induced increases in intracranial pressure. *Anesthesiology* 1987;67: 50–53.

B.9. What coagulation abnormalities are present after traumatic brain injury? What treatment modalities can be used to provide hemostasis and reduce intracranial hematoma expansion?

Abnormalities in blood clotting occur in the setting of traumatic brain injury, which is further aggravated in patients taking anticoagulant medication. The presentation of coagulopathy is diverse, ranging from abnormalities in clotting studies to clinically significant bleeding diathesis. Disseminated intravascular coagulation (DIC) is a consequence of traumatic brain injury, presumably related to release of tissue thromboplastins. One explanation for secondary brain injury after intracranial bleeding is ischemia secondary to cerebral herniation, increased intracranial pressure (ICP), and direct blood vessel occlusion by the hematoma. An alternative explanation is intravascular microthrombosis secondary to DIC.

Traditionally, the administration of fresh frozen plasma and clotting factors has been used in correcting coagulation abnormalities after head injury. Early hemostatic therapy for acute hemorrhage has been proposed to reduce the growth of hematoma expansion. Recombinant activated factor VII has been administered to promote hemostasis in patients with acute intracerebral hemorrhage. One randomized trial showed that factor VIIa given within 4 hours after onset of intracerebral hemorrhage limited the growth of hematoma and improved functional outcome. However, in this trial, only patients with spontaneous intracerebral hemorrhage were studied whereas traumatic brain injury patients were excluded. Moreover, the exclusion criteria also included: (a) patients with Glasgow Coma Scale (GCS) less than 5, (b) patients that underwent surgical evacuation within 24 hours after admission, and (c) patients taking oral anticoagulants or with known coagulopathy. Given these study limitation, further research is needed to evaluate the role of factor VIIa in traumatic brain injury patients that undergo surgical intervention and may have concomitant abnormalities in coagulation.

Mayer SA, Brun NC, Begtrup K, et al. Recombinant activated factor VII for acute intracerebral hemorrhage. *N Engl J Med* 2005;352:777–785.

Mayer SA. Ultra-early hemostatic therapy for primary intracerebral hemorrhage: a review. *Can J Neurol Sci* 2005;2(Suppl):S31–S37.

Stein S, Smith DH. Coagulopathy in traumatic brain injury. *Neurocrit Care* 2004;1:479–488.

C. Intraoperative Management

C.1. What is appropriate hemodynamic monitoring during computed tomography (CT) scanning and during craniotomy for evacuation of a subdural hematoma?

It is axiomatic that hemodynamic monitoring should be commensurate with the anticipated changes in cardiovascular status during the planned procedure. Assuming there is no evidence of occult blood loss or major intrathoracic injury, the most aggressive monitoring during CT scanning should consist of direct arterial pressure assessment. This is based on the requirement for arterial blood gas analysis and the possible need to administer vasoactive drugs to control blood pressure. Conversely, if there is evidence of occult bleeding or a major thoracic injury, placement of a central venous pressure (CVP) or pulmonary arterial (PA) catheter may be required in guiding fluid management before CT scanning.

If no invasive monitors were placed during CT scanning, an arterial line is needed before craniotomy surgery. Placement of a CVP or PA catheter in the OR is helpful in managing blood pressure in conjunction with fluid administration. If cardiac contusion is a consideration, placement of a PA catheter would be more preferable than placement of a CVP catheter, because both cardiac output and right ventricular pressures can be measured. Cardiac contusion is most often associated with right ventricular dysfunction.

C.2. Should hyperventilation be used in this patient?

The theoretical advantages of hyperventilation are control of intracranial pressure (ICP) and reversal of acidosis in brain tissue. However, cerebral blood flow in head-injured tissue is low and vasoconstriction can result in ischemia. In areas of severe injury (e.g., subdural hematomas, diffuse contusions), there is local variability in perfusion as well as loss of autoregulation and CO_2 reactivity. A randomized, clinical trial has shown hyperventilation is potentially deleterious, suggesting that prophylactic hyperventilation ($PaCO_2 \leq 35$ mm Hg) should be avoided. It has been suggested that the use of monitors such as jugular venous hemoglobin oxygen saturation monitoring and cerebral oximeters may help determine the effects of hyperventilation on cerebral oxygenation. Measures of cerebral metabolism may predict which patients benefit from hyperventilation.

Currently, it has been recommended that hyperventilation be used on a selective rather than on a routine basis. Hyperventilation may be necessary to lower ICP for brief periods in which there is acute neurologic deterioration or intracranial hypertension that is refractory to other treatment modalities such as mannitol and cerebrospinal fluid (CSF) drainage. If ICP monitoring is present in the OR, hyperventilation could be used to lower ICP to less than 20 mm Hg. Other goals such as facilitating surgical access and minimizing surgical retraction are still important considerations in the intraoperative management of head injury.

Marshall LF. Head injury: recent past, present and future. *Neurosurgery* 2000;47:546–561.

Miller RD, ed. *Miller's anesthesia*, 6th ed. New York: Churchill Livingstone, 2005:2155.

Muizelaar JP, Maramarou A, Ward JD. Adverse effects of prolonged hyperventilation in patients with severe head injury: a randomized clinical trial. *J Neurosurg* 1991; 75:731–739.

C.3. What are the implications of arterial hypertension in head-injured patients? How should blood pressure be managed?

Hypertension is a common feature of head injury in patients who do not have massive blood loss associated with their injuries. The etiology of hypertension appears to be catecholamine related. Some experts believe that cerebral perfusion is optimized when there is a high arterial pressure opposing the effects of elevated intracranial pressure (ICP). Others feel that in the presence of a disrupted blood–brain barrier, arterial hypertension contributes to extravasation of edema fluid and aggravation of brain swelling.

Although some experts advocate maintaining cerebral perfusion pressure (CPP) above 60 mm Hg, proponents of high CPP recommend maintaining CPP greater than 70 mm Hg with the use of volume expansion and vasoactive drugs. Several clinical studies have suggested improved outcomes when systemic arterial pressure is raised to keep CPP at 70 to 90 mm Hg, but they were not controlled, blinded, or randomized. Other studies have questioned the necessity of vasopressors to maintain cerebral perfusion above 70 mm Hg and the role of CPP as a determinant of cerebral blood flow. The majority impression at this time is to maintain arterial pressure at normal to slightly elevated levels. Above all, arterial hypotension is to be avoided, because it profoundly increases neuronal damage in the presence of elevated ICP.

Cruz J, Jaggi JL, Hoffstad OJ. Cerebral blood flow, vascular resistance, and oxygen metabolism in acute brain trauma: redefining the role of cerebral perfusion. *Crit Care Med* 1995;23:1412–1417.

Marshall LF. Head injury: recent past, present and future. *Neurosurgery* 2000;47:546–561.

Miller RD, ed. *Miller's Anesthesia*, 6th ed. New York: Churchill Livingstone, 2005:2154–2155.

Rosner MJ, Daughton S. Cerebral perfusion management in head injury. *J Trauma* 1990; 30:933–940.

Rosner MJ, Rosner SD, Johnson AH. Cerebral perfusion pressure: management protocol and clinical results. *J Neurosurg* 1995;83:949–962.

Talmor D, Roytblat L, Artru AA, et al. Phenylephrine-induced hypertension does not improve outcome after closed head trauma in rats. *Anesth Analg* 1998;87:574–578.

C.4. What should be done about intravenous fluid replacement? Should corticosteroids be given empirically?

Often, many head-injured patients sustain multiple injuries, which require aggressive resuscitation with crystalloids, plasma expanders, and blood. Once the patient arrives to the operating room (OR), packed red blood cells should be administered to maintain normal central venous pressure (CVP) along with crystalloid or colloid solutions in quantities sufficient to replace blood loss. The problem with aggressive resuscitation is that excessive crystalloid administration may exacerbate brain edema.

Rapid formation of brain edema is a common reaction associated with most neuropathological processes, including intracranial hematomas. Although crystalloid administration decreases colloid oncotic pressure (COP), the reduction of COP does not cause edema in normal or injured brain tissue. It is the administration of free water and the decrease in osmolality that appears to be important in edema formation. In experimental studies, $D_5 W$ solutions increase edema, increase blood glucose, and worsen neurologic outcome. Isotonic solutions such as Ringer's lactate and 0.9% saline have no adverse effect on edema formation, blood glucose, and neurologic outcome. The worsening of neurologic outcome with $D_5 W$ has been attributed to edema formation rather than hyperglycemia.

Corticosteroids have been shown to be effective in reducing cortical edema associated with brain tumors and abscesses, but prospective studies evaluating their efficacy in head trauma have failed to demonstrate any benefit and are occasionally associated with iatrogenic complications such as sepsis. Glucocorticoids do not lower intracranial pressure (ICP) and its routine use in not recommended for head injury. Moreover, their potential for raising plasma glucose make their use less desirable in the setting of traumatic brain injury.

Feldman Z, Zachari S, Reichenthal E, et al. Brain edema and neurological status with rapid infusion of lactated Ringer's or 5% dextrose solution following head trauma. *J Neurosurg* 1995;83:1060–1066.

Kaieda R, Todd MM, Warner DS. Prolonged reduction in colloid osmotic pressure does not increase brain edema following cryogenic injury in rabbits. *Anesthesiology* 1989; 71:554–560.

Marshall LF. Head injury: recent past, present and future. *Neurosurgery* 2000;47:546–561.

Talmor D, Shapira Y, Artru AA, et al. 0.45% saline and 5% dextrose in water, but not 0.9% or 5% dextrose in 0.9% saline, worsen brain edema two hours after closed head trauma in rats. *Anesth Analg* 1998;86:1225–1229.

C.5. Should hypertonic saline be administered to this patient? How is hypertonic saline administered?

The rationale for hyperosmolar therapy is to decrease cerebral edema by creating an osmolar gradient between the intravascular space and cerebral tissue. Water moves from the cells and interstitial spaces into the capillaries, to decrease cerebral water content and intracranial pressure (ICP). Hypertonic saline and mannitol are the modalities for hyperosmolar therapy. Hypertonic saline has been shown to decrease ICP even when other conventional measures such as barbiturates and mannitol have been exhausted. Hypertonic saline is a volume expander in the systemic circulation and does not impair renal function as seen with mannitol administration. Often, with hypertonic saline administration, the goal is to maintain normovolemia with the help of central venous pressure (CVP) or pulmonary arterial catheter monitoring.

Typically, a 3% saline solution is administered at a rate of 75 to 150 mL per hour whereas a bolus of 250 mL may be given for aggressive therapy. Of further note, the use of 7.5% hypertonic saline has been reported. Preliminary evidence supports the use of hypertonic saline in reducing ICP, suggesting that controlled clinical trials should be performed to determine if hypertonic saline improves outcome. Currently, the human data is still inconclusive to recommend the use of hypertonic saline as a standard of management. In one study, patients receiving 2 mL per kg of 7.5% saline had better control of ICP compared to patients receiving mannitol, but no changes in mortality and neurologic outcome were observed. In another study involving the prehospital administration of hypertonic saline for resuscitation in hypotensive traumatic brain injury patients, ICP control was better in the hypertonic saline patients, but again no differences in outcome were demonstrated.

Cooper DJ, Myles PS, McDermott FT, et al. Prehospital hypertonic saline resuscitation of patients with hypotension and severe traumatic brain injury: a randomized controlled trial. *JAMA* 2004;291:1350–1357.

Horn P, Munch E, Vajkoczy P, et al. Hypertonic saline solution for control of elevated intracranial pressure in patients with exhausted response to mannitol and barbiturates. *Neurol Res* 1999;21:758–764.

Qureshi AI, Suarez JI. Use of hypertonic saline solutions in treatment of cerebral edema and intracranial hypertension. *Crit Care Med* 2000;28:3301–3313.

Qureshi AI, Suarez JI, Bhardwaj A, et al. Use of hypertonic (3%) saline/acetate infusion in the treatment of cerebral edema: effect on intracranial pressure and lateral displacement of the brain. *Crit Care Med* 1998;26:440–446.

Vialet R, Albanese J, Thomachot L. Isovolume hypertonic solutes (sodium chloride or mannitol) in the treatment of refractory posttraumatic intracranial hypertension: 2 ml/kg 7.5% saline is more effective that 2 ml/kg 20% mannitol. *Crit Care Med* 2003;31:1683–1687.

C.6. **The patient under went a craniotomy for a bifrontal craniectomy for evacuation of the anterior frontal lobe and a frontal intracerebral hematoma. Are there anesthetic agents that should be avoided in this situation? Which ones? What agents might be preferred in this situation?**

The principles of anesthetic management for patients with rapidly expanding intracranial mass lesions are based on the ideal of maximizing intracranial compliance by minimizing the volume within the intracranial compartment. This means that any maneuver that increases cerebral blood volume should be avoided. All intravenous induction agents (e.g., thiopental, etomidate, and propofol) except for ketamine are known for their vasoconstrictive effects and are reasonable choices provided that the hemodynamic stability is maintained. Ketamine has been out of favor in the neurosurgical setting because early studies showed that it increases cerebral metabolic rate, cerebral blood flow, and intracranial pressure (ICP). However, a more recent study showed that in ventilated patients receiving propofol sedation, ketamine actually decreased ICP and did not adversely alter cerebral hemodynamics. These authors surmised that when ketamine is added to a background anesthetic, the central nervous excitation effects of ketamine are blunted and increases the depth of anesthesia. Because ketamine is an NMDA antagonist, with possible neuroprotective effects, it has been suggested that the use of ketamine in head injury warrants reevaluation.

All the volatile inhalation agents and nitrous oxide have some cerebral vasodilatory effects. Caution must be exercised in using inhalation agents in patients with rapidly expanding intracranial mass lesions. When the surgical field is "tight", eliminating inhalation agents and going with a total intravenous anesthetic (TIVA) technique may be appropriate. For example, a propofol or thiopental infusion may render the patient sufficiently anesthetized for a craniotomy. Finally, there is concern that opioids may act as cerebral vasodilators and raise ICP. Several studies have shown that sufentanil increases ICP in head-injured patients possibly secondary to indirect cerebral vasodilatation caused by autoregulatory compensation when mean arterial pressure (MAP) decreases. Direct cerebral vasodilatation has been implicated in the increase in ICP seen after morphine and fentanyl administration.

Albanèse J, Arnaud S, Rey M, et al. Ketamine decreases intracranial pressure and electroencephalographic activity in traumatic brain injury patients during propofol sedation. *Anesthesiology* 1997;87:1328–1334.

Albanèse J, Durbec O, Viviand X, et al. Sufentanil increases intracranial pressure in patients with head trauma. *Anesthesiology* 1993;79:493–497.

de Nadal M, Munar F, Poca MA, et al. Cerebral hemodynamic effects of morphine and fentanyl in patients with severe head injury: absence of correlation to cerebral autoregulation. *Anesthesiology* 2000;92:11–19.

Werner C, Kochs E, Bause H, et al. Effects of sufentanil on cerebral hemodynamics and intracranial pressure in patients with brain injury. *Anesthesiology* 1995;83:721–726.

C.7. Should hypothermia be employed in this patient?

In experimental models, hypothermia has been shown to decrease the amount of edema and necrosis volume after cerebral damage. A temperature of 32°C (89.6°F) has been considered to be the safe limit for patients with head injury. Several clinical trials, involving less than 100 patients, have shown that inducing moderate (32°C to 33°C [89.6°F to 91.4°F]) or mild hypothermia (33°C to 35°C [91.4°F to 95°F]) in patients with severe head trauma (GCS <8), improves neurologic outcome. However, a multicenter phase III head injury trial, involving almost 400 patients, showed that inducing hypothermia in patients who already arrived to the hospital normothermic did not improve outcome. In general, enthusiasm for the application of hypothermia in neurosurgical patients has faded as another multicenter trial of hypothermia involving cerebral aneurysm patients also demonstrated negative findings in improving neurologic outcome. Despite, negative findings from the most recent comprehensive trials on hypothermia, various researchers contend that the complete abandonment of hypothermia is premature and that newer technologies which induce hypothermia (e.g., intravascular cooling) should be further investigated.

Clifton GL, Miller ER, Choi SC, et al. Lack of effect of induction of hypothermia after acute brain injury. *N Engl J Med* 2001;344:556–563.

Jiang J, Yu M, Zhu C. Effect of long-term mild hypothermia therapy in patients with severe traumatic brain injury: 1-year follow-up review of 87 cases. *J Neurosurg* 2000; 93:718–719.

Marion DW, Penrod LE, Kelsey SF, et al. Treatment of traumatic brain injury with moderate hypothermia. *N Engl J Med* 1997;336:540–546.

Pomeranz S, Safar P, Radovsky A, et al. The effect of resuscitative moderate hypothermia following epidural brain compression injury cerebral damage in a canine outcome model. *J Neurosurg* 1993;79:241–251.

Sahuquillo J, Mena MP, Vilalta A, et al. Moderate hypothermia in the management of severe traumatic brain injury: a good idea proved ineffective? *Curr Pharm Des* 2004; 10:2193–2204.

Todd MM, Hindman BJ, Clarke WR, et al. Mild intraoperative hypothermia during surgery for intracranial aneurysm. *N Engl J Med* 2005;352:135–145.

D. Postoperative Neurointensive Care Management

D.1. What are the postoperative ventilation considerations in this patient?

If the patient had normal consciousness preoperatively, early extubation would be preferable once it is confirmed that the patient is able to follow commands and move extremities. Efforts should be made to avoid bucking and coughing on the endotracheal tube and to treat hypertension that occurs on emergence. Intravenous lidocaine is a useful drug to smooth the coughing associated with emergence. Short acting opiates, particularly remifentanil, can provide a patient that is hemodynamically stable, tolerating the endotracheal tube, and following commands. However, many traumatic brain injury patients undergoing emergency surgery remain intubated postoperatively due to severity of the brain injury. In that case, blood pressure control to prevent hypertension is needed to prevent further hemorrhage. In some patients, sedatives and muscle relaxants may be administered on transport to prevent changes in intracranial pressure (ICP) associated with stimulation and agitation. In ventilated patients, the use of a cerebral oxygen monitor may be useful in optimizing brain O_2 delivery in relation to arterial carbon dioxide ($Paco_2$).

Guy J, Hindman BJ, Baker KZ, et al. Comparison of remifentanil and fentanyl in patients undergoing craniotomy for supratentorial space-occupying lesions. *Anesthesiology* 1997;86:514–524.

Miller RD, ed. *Miller's anesthesia*, 6th ed. New York: Churchill Livingstone, 2005:2152–2157.

Prough DS. Perioperative management of traumatic brain injury. *ASA annual refresher course lectures*. Park Ridge: American Society of Anesthesiologists, 2004:221.

D.2. What specific measures should be used to control the patient's intracranial pressure (ICP)? What type of monitoring devices can be used to monitor ICP?

After removal of an intracranial hematoma, control of ICP is of paramount importance in the patient's recovery. Briefly, those patients whose ICP can be maintained below 20 to 25 mm Hg tend to have significantly better outcomes than do patients whose ICP remain elevated. It has become common practice, therefore, to monitor ICP in the postoperative period in these patients. This enables the intensivist to adjust treatment with hyperventilation, mannitol, cerebrospinal fluid (CSF) drainage, and head-up tilt, to the desired ICP response. If these maneuvers fail, the next intervention is to maintain barbiturate coma to a level where the electroencephalogram (EEG) shows burst suppression. This is continued until it is no longer required to control intracranial hypertension. After weaning, from barbiturate therapy, the patient can be weaned from diuretics and/or hyperventilation, as appropriate. As aforementioned, the use of hyperventilation in head-injury patients must be used on a selective basis because hyperventilation has potentially deleterious effects on cerebral perfusion.

The classic intraventricular catheter or ventriculostomy was introduced by Lundberg in 1960 and has been the gold standard for ICP monitoring and CSF drainage. Placement of an intraventricular catheter has been associated with the potential for infection and brain parenchyma injury. Placement of a subarachnoid bolt used to be a less invasive modality but limitations included accuracy and stability. Subarachnoid bolts have been supplanted by a variety of implantable pressure transducer devices. Current ICP monitoring systems utilize a twist drill for bolt placement in the skull to allow a catheter to be rapidly placed in the parenchyma or subarachnoid space. Some systems allow CSF drainage in which a catheter containing a transducer at the tip is placed into the ventricles.

Cucchiara RF, Black S, Michenfelder JD, eds. *Clinical neuroanesthesia*, 2nd ed. New York, Churchill Livingstone, 1998:83–84.

Marshall LF. Head injury: recent past, present and future. *Neurosurgery* 2000;47:546–561.

D.3. What is neurogenic pulmonary edema? Would you avoid positive end-expiratory pressure (PEEP) in a patient with increased intracranial pressure (ICP)?

Neurogenic pulmonary edema is a commonly seen disorder following head injury or intracranial bleed. The mechanisms are unclear, but are thought to be due to a combination of increased pulmonary pressures due to massive catecholamine release with increased ICP (Cushing's response) and altered pulmonary capillary permeability from as-yet undescribed neurogenic factors. The onset can be immediate or delayed, and treatment consists of supportive care as with other cases of pulmonary edema, including PEEP.

Positive pressure ventilation, PEEP, and increased ICP have been studied in animal and human models, and although there is a slight increase in ICP with higher levels of PEEP (10 to 12 cm H_2O) in patients with normal ICP, patients with elevated ICP do not seem to demonstrate a clinically significant change in ICP with even high levels of PEEP. On the other hand, avoidance of PEEP, in such setting, may lead to hypoxemia that, in turn, can exacerbate cerebral ischemia.

McGuire G, Crossley D, Richards J, et al. Effects of varying levels of positive end-expiratory pressure on intracranial pressure and cerebral perfusion pressure. *Crit Care Med* 1997;25:1059–1062.

Rosen P, ed. *Emergency medicine: concepts and clinical practice*, 4th ed. St. Louis: Mosby, 1998:436.

D.4. What is the role of antiseizure prophylaxis in the perioperative management of head trauma?

Seizures may cause secondary injury as a result of increases in intracranial pressure (ICP), changes in oxygen supply and demand, and increases in neurotransmitter release. Early posttraumatic seizures (PTS) occur in the first week after injury, mostly within the first 24 hours. Late PTS occurs after the first week. Often early PTS occurs within hours after injury, especially in patients with depressed or open skull fractures and hemorrhagic brain contusions. Short-term prophylactic administration of anticonvulsant drugs (e.g., phenytoin, carbamazepine) for early PTS is recommended. Administration of anticonvulsant medicines, however, has not been shown to prevent late PTS. Therefore, routine antiseizure prophylaxis is not recommended later than 1 week following head injury.

Marshall LF. Head injury: recent past, present and future. *Neurosurgery* 2000;47:546–561.

Schmidek HH, ed. *Operative neurosurgical techniques*, 4th ed. Philadelphia: WB Saunders, 2000:54–56.

D.5. How can cerebral oxygenation monitoring be used in the clinical management of traumatic brain injury?

An indwelling parenchymal device that measures local oxygenation can be used to gain information regarding tissue oxygenation in real time at the bedside. In a severely injured brain autoregulatory mechanisms fail. As a result, various areas of the brain will be ischemic. Use of an oxygen sensor allows for more precise management to optimize oxygen delivery and eliminate progression of ischemia. A cerebral oxygen monitor is placed either intraoperatively or at the bedside, much like a ventriculostomy. Many studies have shown it to be equally as useful as a jugular bulb catheter. The device can either be placed in an ischemic penumbra of a lesion or in an uninjured area of the brain. In the first case, the monitor will yield information that can be used to prevent further ischemia and cell death. In the second case, the device is used as a global indicator of cerebral oxygenation and may be useful in guiding ventilatory management.

Cerebral oxygenation monitoring also offers the ability to measure parenchymal temperatures simultaneous to oxygen content. This is of critical importance when using hypothermia or maintaining normothermia. By definition, brain oxygen tension or partial pressure (P_bO_2) is not adequate if it drops below a value of 20 mm Hg. In recent studies, values of less than 20 mm Hg for short intervals of time have correlated with worse neurologic outcome. A value of greater than 30 mm Hg is optimal. Currently, there are several devices on the market that measure oxygen content.

Jaeger M, Soehle M, Meixensberger J. Brain tissue oxygen (PtiO₂): a clinical comparison of two monitoring devices. *Acta Neurochir (Wien)* 2005;95(Suppl):79–81.

Jaeger M, Soehle M, Schuhmann MU, et al. Correlation of continuously monitored regional cerebral blood flow and brain tissue oxygen. *Acta Neurochir (Wien)* 2005;147: 51–56.

Stiefel MF, Heuer GG, Smith MJ, et al. Cerebral oxygenation following decompressive hemicraniectomy for the treatment of refractory intracranial hypertension. *J Neurosurg* 2004;101:241–247.

D.6. What methods can be used in the neurointensive care unit to prevent hyperthermia?

Fever continues to be a problem in critically ill neurosurgical patients. One retrospective study noted that greater than 50% of closed head injury patients had one febrile episode in the neurointensive care unit. Fever and hyperthermia accentuate excitotoxic release of neurotransmitters, increases production of free radicals, and accelerates cytoskeletal protein degradation. Although the enthusiasm to induce perioperative hypothermia for neuroprotection has waned, interventions are needed to cool patients to prevent hyperthermia.

Conventional water circulating cooling blankets have been considered to be ineffective due to poor surface contact with the skin. A newer external cooling device has been developed which utilizes self-adhesive, hydrogel-coated pads that circulate temperature-controlled water under negative pressure. Intravascular central venous catheters have been developed for both placed for cooling and rewarming. These catheters contain special built-in balloons through which cooled or warmed saline is circulated in a closed loop design. The patient's temperature is continuously compared with a user-defined target temperature and the controller systems is equipped with a safety system that alarms when the temperature is above or below programmed levels or when there is a system malfunction. Fig. 25.2 shows a comparison of brain and rectal temperatures after intravascular cooling through a femoral catheter. Intracranial temperature measurements were obtained through an indwelling cerebral oxygen catheter placed into the brain parenchyma of the left frontal region.

In view of the recent advances in technologies to lower temperature, experts contend that it is premature to completely abandon the use of hypothermia. Future avenues of research include: (a) evaluating the impact of fever and hyperthermia on neurologic outcome, (b) treating refractory elevations in intracranial pressure (ICP) with hypothermia, and (c) exploring methods for intraventricular or lumbar irrigation for rapid brain cooling.

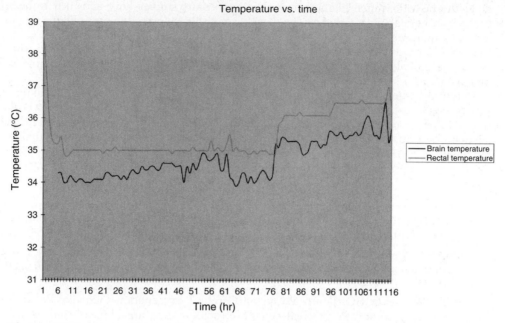

Figure 25.2 Comparison of brain and rectal temperatures following intravascular cooling. Intracranial temperatures were measured with a brain tissue oxygen catheter placed into the parenchyma of the left frontal region.

Kilpatrick MM, Lowry DW, Firlik AD, et al. Hyperthermia in the neurosurgical intensive care unit. *Neurosurgery* 2000;47:850–856.

Mayer SA, Kowalski RG, Presciutti M, et al. Clinical trial of a novel surface cooling system for fever control in neurocritical care patients. *Crit Care Med* 2004;32:2508–2515.

Sahuquillo J, Mena MP, Vilalta A, et al. Moderate hypothermia in the management of severe traumatic brain injury: a good idea proved ineffective? *Curr Pharm Des* 2004; 10:2193–2204.

CHAPTER 26

Cerebral Aneurysm

PATRICIA FOGARTY MACK

A 43-YEAR-OLD WHITE WOMAN

presented to the emergency room 2 days ago, complaining of severe headache, nausea, and vomiting, followed by a witnessed 3-minute loss of consciousness. On regaining consciousness, the patient was noted by her family to be confused. A computed tomography (CT) scan showed subarachnoid blood. You are called to the angiography suite because four-vessel angiography has revealed an 18-mm basilar tip aneurysm and a 10-mm right middle cerebral artery (MCA) aneurysm. The interventional neuroradiologist wishes to coil the basilar tip aneurysm but believes the MCA aneurysm will require craniotomy and clipping.

At present, she was oriented only to person. She had no previous medical history; however, she had smoked one pack of cigarettes per day for the last 20 years. Blood pressure was 130/80 mm Hg, pulse 90 beats per minute, and respiration 18 breaths per minute. She had no focal neurologic deficits. Laboratory examination revealed normal electrolytes and complete blood count (CBC). Electrocardiogram (ECG) demonstrated normal sinus rhythm (NSR) with flipped T waves throughout the precordium.

A. Medical Disease and Differential Diagnosis

1. What are the incidence, prevalence, and causes of subarachnoid hemorrhage (SAH) and what are the risk factors associated with rupture of intracranial aneurysms?
2. What are common sizes and locations of intracranial aneurysms?
3. What is the pathophysiology of aneurysmal rupture and SAH?
4. What are symptoms and signs of SAH?
5. How does one assess the severity of SAH?
6. What are the cardiovascular effects of SAH?
7. How is the diagnosis of SAH made?
8. What is the risk of rebleeding for a patient with SAH?

B. Preoperative Evaluation and Preparation

1. What are some concerns in going to the interventional neuroradiology (INR) suite in the midst of an angiogram to follow immediately with coiling of an aneurysm?
2. What type of anesthesia is required for coiling of an aneurysm?
3. Would you proceed with induction of general anesthesia under these circumstances?

4. What types of emergencies can occur during coiling of an aneurysm and how should they be managed?

5. A craniotomy is planned for the following day to clip the middle cerebral artery (MCA) aneurysm. Should surgery be postponed because of the patient's elevated creatinine phosphokinase (CPK) MB fractions?

6. Would you premedicate this patient before craniotomy?

C. Intraoperative Management

1. What are the goals of the induction and maintenance of anesthesia for this patient?

2. Is placement of an arterial line necessary for induction of anesthesia in this patient in the INR suite?

3. How would you assess fluid status in this patient?

4. Would a monitor of central venous pressure (CVP) be useful in this patient for craniotomy for clipping?

5. What other forms of monitoring would you consider?

6. What are your particular concerns during induction of anesthesia in this patient?

7. How would you accomplish a smooth and safe induction and intubation of this patient?

8. Would you perform a rapid-sequence induction and intubation on this patient?

9. What are the effects of hypoxemia and hypercapnia, such as would be seen with loss of the airway on induction, on cerebral blood flow (CBF)?

10. What is optimal fluid management for aneurysm clipping? Would you use a dextrose-containing solution?

11. After the bone plate was removed and as the dura was being opened the surgeon complained that the brain was "tight." What could you do to achieve better brain relaxations and facilitate surgical exposure?

12. How might transmural pressure be decreased to allow for aneurysm clip placement?

13. What is the purpose of controlled hypotension and how is it achieved?

14. What are some of the potential drawbacks of controlled hypotension?

15. What methods of cerebral protection might you employ during this operation?

16. Would you induce mild hypothermia as a means of cerebral protection?

17. What are the indications for deep hypothermic circulatory arrest?

18. What steps should be taken in the case of intraoperative rupture of an intracranial aneurysm?

19. How would you plan the emergence from an anesthetic for aneurysm clipping?

D. Postoperative Management

1. Would you extubate the patient postoperatively?

2. What would be the differential diagnosis if the patient did not return to her preoperative neurologic condition?

3. On postoperative day 2, the patient became disoriented and developed hemiplegia. A computed tomography (CT) scan was performed, which shows no new intracranial bleeding. What other diagnostic studies should be performed?

4. What is cerebral vasospasm and what causes it?

5. What are pathophysiologic changes seen in cerebral vasospasm?

6. How is the diagnosis of cerebral vasospasm made?

7. What steps can be taken to prevent cerebral vasospasm?

8. What treatments can be undertaken once a diagnosis of cerebral vasospasm is made?

9. What are other neurologic complications following SAH and aneurysm clipping?

10. What other organ systems may manifest problems postoperatively in aneurysm clipping patients?

A. Medical Disease and Differential Diagnosis

A.1. What are the incidence, prevalence, and causes of subarachnoid hemorrhage (SAH) and what are the risk factors associated with rupture of intracranial aneurysms?

The prevalence of SAH is 2% to 5% with an incidence of 10 to 28 per 100,000 people. There are 25,000 cases of SAH each year in the United States, comprising 10% of all cases of stroke. Sixty percent of the cases occur in young individuals between the ages of 40 and 60. Therefore, a poor neurologic outcome is a devastating condition to be endured over a potentially long period.

Approximately one third of patients die as a result of the acute bleed. Of the two thirds who survive the acute bleed, one half (one third of total) later die or are severely disabled and one half (one third of total) have an acceptable outcome.

Cerebral aneurysms account for 75% to 80% of SAH; arteriovenous malformations are the cause in 4% to 5%, whereas no specific cause can be found in 15% to 20% of SAH. Other causes of SAH include trauma, mycotic aneurysm, sickle cell disease, cocaine use, and coagulation disorders.

Risk factors for rupture of cerebral aneurysms include hypertension, pregnancy, and vascular abnormalities (e.g., type III collagen deficiency and elastase abnormalities). One third of patients with polycystic kidney disease have been found to have intracranial aneurysms at autopsy. Genetic predisposition plays a role: 7% of berry aneurysms are familial, and 5% to 10% of patients with ruptured aneurysm have a first-order relative with ruptured aneurysm. The rupture rate for aneurysm has been estimated at 0.14% per year for a 5-mm lesion to 1.1% per year for a 10-mm lesion.

Smoking and alcohol abuse also appear to predispose to aneurysm formation and rupture. Smoking at any time and female gender are related to the presence of multiple intracranial aneurysms, as well as for accelerated aneurysm growth. Cocaine abuse and resultant episodic hypertension may predispose to aneurysmal rupture at an early age.

Death and disability are primarily due to the initial bleed, vasospasm, and rebleeding. Other causes include surgical complications, parenchymal hemorrhage, hydrocephalus, and complications of medical therapy.

Albin MS, ed. *Textbook of neuroanesthesia: with neurosurgical and neuroscience perspectives*. New York: McGraw-Hill, 1997:846.

Chang HS. Simulation of the natural history of cerebral aneurysms based on data from the International Study of Unruptured Intracranial Aneurysms. *J Neurosurg* 2006;104:188–194.

Juvela S, Pooras M, Poussa K. Natural history of unruptured intracranial aneurysms: probability and risk factors for aneurysm rupture. *J Neurosurg* 2000;93:379–387.

Juvela S, Poussa K, Porras M. Factors affecting formation and growth of intracranial aneurysms: a long term follow-up study. *Stroke* 2001;32:485–491.

Krex D, Schackert HK, Schackert G. Genesis of cerebral aneurysms–an update. *Acta Neurochir (Wien)* 2001;143:429–448.

N Engl J Med. International Study of Unruptured Intracranial Aneurysms Investigators. Unruptured intracranial aneurysms–risk of rupture and risk of surgical intervention. 1998;339: 1725–1733.

Tsutsumi K, Ueki K, Morita A, et al. Risk of rupture from incidental cerebral aneurysms. *J Neurosurg* 2000;93:550–553.

Yoshimoto Y. A mathematical model of the natural history of intracranial aneurysm: quantification of the benefit of prophylactic treatment. *J Neurosurg* 2006;104:195–200.

A.2. What are common sizes and locations of intracranial aneurysms?

Small (<12 mm) aneurysms make up 78% of the total, whereas large (12 to 24 mm) are 20%, and giant (>24 mm) comprise 2%. Most aneurysms are located in the anterior circulation, with the junction of the anterior communicating and anterior cerebral arteries being the most common (39%). Thirty percent of aneurysms occur in the internal carotid artery, 22% in the middle cerebral artery (MCA), and 8% in the posterior circulation (posterior cerebral, basilar, and vertebral arteries).

Kasell NF, Torner JC, Haley C, et al. The international cooperative study on the timing of aneurysm surgery. Part 1. Overall management results. *J Neurosurg* 1990;73:18–32.

Kasell NF, Torner JC, Haley C, et al. The international cooperative study on the timing of aneurysm surgery. Part 2. Surgical results. *J Neurosurg* 1990;73:37–47.

A.3. What is the pathophysiology of aneurysmal rupture and subarachnoid hemorrhage (SAH)?

On the basis of experimental models, aneurysmal rupture leads to the leakage of arterial blood and a rapid increase in intracranial pressure (ICP), approaching diastolic blood pressure in the proximal intracerebral arteries. This increase in ICP causes a decrease in cerebral perfusion pressure (CPP) and a fall in cerebral blood flow (CBF), leading to a loss of consciousness. The decrease in CBF diminishes bleeding and stops the SAH. A gradual reduction in ICP and an increase in CBF indicates improved cerebral function and possibly a return to consciousness. A persistent increase in ICP (perhaps resulting from thrombi in the cranial cisterns), however, indicates a persistent no-flow pattern with acute vasospasm, cell swelling, and death.

A.4. What are symptoms and signs of subarachnoid hemorrhage (SAH)?

Headache occurs in 85% to 95% of patients. Often a brief loss of consciousness occurs, followed by diminished mentation; however, consciousness may be impaired to any degree or may be unaffected at the time of presentation. Symptoms may be similar to infectious meningitis (nausea, vomiting, and photophobia) secondary to subarachnoid blood. The patient may also experience motor and sensory deficits, visual field disturbances, and cranial nerve palsies. Finally, blood in the subarachnoid space may cause an elevated temperature.

Albin MS, ed. *Textbook of neuroanesthesia: with neurosurgical and neuroscience perspectives.* New York: McGraw-Hill, 1997:847.

Guy J, McGrath BJ, Borel CO, et al. Perioperative management of aneurysmal subarachnoid hemorrhage. Part 1. Operative management. *Anesth Analg* 1995;81:1060–1072.

A.5. How does one assess the severity of subarachnoid hemorrhage (SAH)?

Two grading scales are commonly used to assess neurologic status following SAH, the Hunt and Hess grade (Table 26.1) and the World Federation of Neurologic Surgeons' grade (Table 26.2), based on the Glasgow Coma Scale. The scales are useful in identifying a baseline neurologic status from which any acute changes should be assessed. In addition, the scales may correlate with

Table 26.1 Modified Hunt and Hess Clinical Grades.

GRADE[a]	CRITERIA
0	Unruptured aneurysm
I	Asymptomatic or minimal headache and slight nuchal rigidity
II	Moderate to severe headache, nuchal rigidity, but no neurologic deficit other than cranial nerve palsy
III	Drowsiness, confusion, or mild focal deficit
IV	Stupor, mild to severe hemiparesis, possible early decerebrate rigidity, vegetative disturbance
V	Deep coma, decerebrate rigidity, moribund appearance

[a]Serious systemic disease such as hypertension, diabetes, severe arteriosclerosis, chronic pulmonary disease, and severe vasospasm seen on arteriography result in placement of the patient in the next less favorable category.
From Hunt WE, Hess RM. Surgical risk as related to time of intervention in the repair of intracranial aneurysms. *J Neurosurg* 1968; 28:14–20, with permission.

physiologic status. Patients who are Hunt and Hess grades I and II have near-normal cerebral autoregulation and intracranial pressure (ICP).

Drake CG. Report of World Federation of Neurologic Surgeons Committee on a universal subarachnoid hemorrhage grading scale. *J Neurosurg* 1988;68:985–986.

Hunt WE, Hess RM. Surgical risk as related to time of intervention in the repair of intracranial aneurysms. *J Neurosurg* 1968;28:14–20.

A.6. What are the cardiovascular effects of subarachnoid hemorrhage (SAH)?

Injury to the posterior hypothalamus from SAH causes the release of norepinephrine from the adrenal medulla and cardiac sympathetic efferents. Norepinephrine can cause an increase in afterload and direct myocardial toxicity, leading to subendocardial ischemia. Pathologic analysis of myocardium of patients who have died of acute SAH has revealed microscopic subendocardial hemorrhage and myocytolysis.

Electrocardiographic abnormalities are present in 50% to 80% of patients with SAH. Most commonly these involve ST segment changes and T wave inversions; however, they also include prolonged QT interval, U waves, and P-wave changes. ST-T wave changes are usually scattered and not related to a particular distribution.

Dysrhythmias occur in 80% of patients, usually in the first 48 hours. Premature ventricular contractions are the most common abnormality. However, any type of dysrhythmia is possible.

Table 26.2 World Federation of Neurological Surgeons' (WFNS) Grading Scale.

WFNS GRADE	GLASGOW COMA SCALE	MOTOR DEFICIT
I	15	Absent
II	14–13	Absent
III	14–13	Present
IV	12–7	Present or absent
V	6–3	Present or absent

From Drake CG. Report of World Federation of Neurologic Surgeons Committee on a universal subarachnoid hemorrhage grading scale. *J Neurosurg* 1988; 68:985–986, with permission.

They include severely prolonged QT interval, torsades de pointes, and ventricular fibrillation. In one series, 66% of the arrhythmias were considered mild, 29% moderate, and 5% severe. In addition to increased catecholamine secretion, hypercortisolism and hypokalemia have been suggested as causes for the dysrhythmias seen with SAH.

Ventricular dysfunction, possibly leading to pulmonary edema, is present in approximately 30% of patients with SAH.

Cardiac troponin I predicts myocardial dysfunction in SAH with a sensitivity of 100% and a specificity of 91%. This compares with a sensitivity and specificity of 60% and 94% for CK-MB in predicting myocardial dysfunction. In order to plan optional anesthetic management, it would be important to determine if cardiac dysfunction is due to myocardiac infarction or reversible neurogenic left ventricular dysfunction. A retrospective study from Duke determined that reversible neurogenic cardiac dysfunction was associated with a troponin level 0.22 to 0.25 ng per mL and an ejection fraction of less than 40% by echocardiograms.

Albin MS, ed. *Textbook of neuroanesthesia: with neurosurgical and neuroscience perspectives.* New York: McGraw-Hill, 1997:862.

Bulsara KR, McGirt MJ, Liao L, et al. Use of peak troponin value to differentiate myocardial infarction from reversible neurogenic left ventricular dysfunction associated with aneurysmal subarachnoid hemorrhage. *J Neurosurg* 2003;98:524–528.

A.7. How is the diagnosis of subarachnoid hemorrhage (SAH) made?

Noncontrast computed tomography (CT) scan can determine the magnitude and location of the bleed. It may also be useful in assessing ventricular size and aneurysm location. High-resolution CT (CT angiogram) with contrast can more precisely determine the location of the aneurysm.

Lumbar puncture can be used to diagnose SAH if CT is negative, especially when the patient presents more than 1 week after an initial bleed. Xanthochromia, a yellow discoloration of the cerebrospinal fluid (CSF) after centrifugation, is present from 4 hours to 3 weeks after SAH. The lumbar puncture can cause herniation or rebleeding. Therefore, a CT scan should be performed first if the patient presents within 72 hours of suspected SAH, once subarachnoid blood is confirmed.

Four-vessel angiography (right and left carotid and vertebral arteries) is used to visualize all intracranial vessels, to localize the source of bleeding, and to rule out multiple aneurysms (5% to 33% of patients). Three-dimensional reconstructive angiograms and magnetic resonance angiography (MRA) also may be used.

Guy J, McGrath BJ, Borel CO, et al. Perioperative management of aneurysmal subarachnoid hemorrhage. Part 1. Operative management. *Anesth Analg* 1995;81:1060–1072.

Kasell NF, Torner JC, Haley EC, et al. The International Cooperative Study on the Timing of Aneurysm Surgery. Part 2. Surgical results. *J Neurosurg* 1990;73:37–47.

A.8. What is the risk of rebleeding for a patient with subarachnoid hemorrhage (SAH)?

The risk of rebleeding from a ruptured aneurysm is highest, 4%, in the first 24 hours after the initial bleed and 1.5% per day thereafter. Cumulative risk is 19% in 14 days and 50% at 6 months. After 6 months, the rebleeding risk is 3% per year.

Kasell NF, Torner JC. Aneurysmal rebleeding: a preliminary report from the Cooperative Aneurysm Study. *Neurosurgery* 1983;13:479–481.

B. Preoperative Evaluation and Preparation

B.1. What are some concerns in going to the interventional neuroradiology (INR) suite in the midst of an angiogram to follow immediately with coiling of an aneurysm?

Whenever an anesthesiologist assumes care of a patient when the patient is already sedated it may be more difficult to obtain an accurate medical history. In addition the physical examination will be limited by the patient's position for the diagnostic study. Finally, the patient's capacity to consent may also be impaired by previous sedation.

B.2. What type of anesthesia is required for coiling of an aneurysm?

In most institutions general anesthesia is required for coiling of an intracranial aneurysm. First, intraoperative neurologic testing is generally not required. Second, akinesis is very important not only when the coils are actually deployed but also while the interventionist is navigating the intracranial vessels to reach the aneurysm.

B.3. Would you proceed with induction of general anesthesia under these circumstances?

Yes, I would proceed. Obliteration of the aneurysm with coils has become the standard of care for basilar tip aneurysm and it would be best for the patient to have this done in the same setting as the angiography, provided there were no contradictions to induction of general anesthesia (e.g., hemodynamic instability).

Lee CZ, Young WL. Anesthetic considerations for interventional neuroradiology. *ASA Refresher Courses Anesthesiol* 2005;33(1):145–154.

B.4. What types of emergencies can occur during coiling of an aneurysm and how should they be managed?

Basically, intraoperative emergencies can be divided into two categories—hemorrhage and thrombotic. Appropriate management requires constant communication between the radiologist/surgeon and the anesthesiologist. If an intracranial hemorrhage occurs, the intervenionalist may try to glue the hole in the aneurysm or repair the vessel with N-butyl cyanoacrylate (NBCA). If this is not possible, heparin should be rapidly reversed with protamine and a ventriculostomy will generally be placed by the surgical team. Management of $Paco_2$ can then be guided by the intracranial pressure (ICP). In the case of catheter-induced thrombosis, induced hypertension is usually desirable while tissue plasminogen activator (TPA) or rheoprotherapy is considered.

If a coil is malpositioned, anticoagulation would be continued while the interventional radiologist attempts to snare the coil. As in a thrombosis it may be desirable to augment the blood pressure.

B.5. A craniotomy is planned for the following day to clip the middle cerebral artery (MCA) aneurysm, should surgery be postponed because of the patient's elevated creatinine phosphokinase (CPK) MB fractions?

Fifty percent of patients will have an increase in CPK-MB fraction; however, CPK-MB per total CPK fraction is usually not consistent with transmural myocardial infarction (MI). As discussed previously, troponin I levels are more sensitive. In addition, although some patients (0.7%) do sustain an MI in the setting of subarachnoid hemorrhage (SAH), little correlation is found between electrocardiographic abnormalities and ischemia in this population.

An echocardiogram may be useful in determining the severity of reversible neurogenic left ventricular dysfunction. If LV function is found to be depressed, a pulmonary artery (PA) catheter or intraoperative transesophageal echocardiography may be helpful for intraoperative management.

The desire to delay surgery because of cardiac abnormalities must be weighed against the risk of rebleeding and vasospasm. In most cases the risk of recurrent hemorrhage outweighs the risk of perioperative MI. Furthermore, even if coronary artery disease is present, these patients are not candidates for angioplasty or myocardial revascularization, which requires heparinization. If pulmonary edema or malignant dysrhythmias are present, it may be prudent to postpone surgery until such problems are controlled medically. However, if these problems are not present, then clipping of the aneurysm may be indicated. Bulsara, et al. found that 2.9% of patients had severe cardiac dysfunction. In this study, neurogenic LV dysfunction resolved over 4 to 5 days.

Bulsara KR, McGirt MJ, Liao L, et al. Use of peak troponin value to differentiate myocardial infarction from reversible neurogenic left ventricular dysfunction associated with aneurysmal subarachnoid hemorrhage. *J Neurosurg* 2003;98:524–528.

B.6. Would you premedicate this patient before craniotomy?

No. When the patient is in a Hunt and Hess grade III–V state, anxiety is unlikely. Furthermore, heavy sedation may decrease ventilation, raising $PaCO_2$ and increasing cerebral blood flow (CBF) and intracranial pressure (ICP), which, at the very least, may hinder preoperative and postoperative neurologic evaluation. If patients are Hunt and Hess grade I–II and it appears that preoperative anxiety might lead to hemodynamic instability, a small dose of benzodiazepine may be appropriate.

Medications such as calcium channel blockers (nimodipine), anticonvulsants, and steroids should be continued preoperatively on the day of surgery.

If the patient is at risk for aspiration, medications to decrease gastric acidity and volume are appropriate. Most patients will already be receiving an H_2-blocker if they are on dexamethasone.

Albin MS, ed. *Textbook of neuroanesthesia: with neurosurgical and neuroscience perspectives.* New York: McGraw-Hill, 1997:868.

C. Intraoperative Management

C.1. What are the goals of the induction and maintenance of anesthesia for this patient?

The primary goal is to prevent aneurysm rupture on induction or intraoperatively while maintaining adequate cerebral perfusion pressure (CPP). The goal of matching anesthetic depth to surgical stimulation is more important than which specific drugs are used. In general, the anesthesiologist should provide for rapid and reversible titration of blood pressure, maintain CPP, and protect against cerebral ischemia. An additional goal is to provide a relaxed brain for ease of surgical exposure with minimal brain retraction. Finally, the anesthetic should be planned to achieve a rapid, smooth emergence, allowing prompt neurologic assessment. This can be accomplished with a combination of balanced anesthesia, muscle relaxation, and sympathetic blockers.

Bendo AA. Intracranial vasculary surgery. *Anesthesiol Clin North America* 2002;20:377–388.

Cottrell JE, Smith DS, eds. *Anesthesia and neurosurgery*, 4th ed. St. Louis: Mosby, 2001:376–378.

Guy J, McGrath BJ, Borel CO, et al. Perioperative management of aneurysmal subarachnoid hemorrhage. Part 1. Operative management. *Anesth Analg* 1995;81:1060–1072.

C.2. Is placement of an arterial line necessary for induction of anesthesia in this patient in the interventional neuroradiology (INR) suite?

In this case, because a femoral sheath is in place at the time that anesthesia is being induced, one may transduce femoral arterial pressure during induction. However, because the patient has two aneurysms and because the sheath will be removed at the end of the procedure it would be prudent to place an additional arterial line at some point before removal of the sheath. When a large coaxial catheter is placed through the femoral sheath, systolic pressure is underestimated. The mean pressure, however, should be accurate. Recent studies have suggested that placement of an arterial line for induction is not essential when an unruptured aneurysm is to be coiled. At Cornell, we do not usually place an arterial line before induction for embolization of unruptured aneurysm.

Lai YC, Manninen PH. Anesthesia for cerebral aneurysms: a comparison between interventional neuroradiology and surgery. *Can J Anaesth* 2001;48:391–395.

Young WL, Pile-Spellman J. Anesthetic consideration for international neuroradiology. *Anesthesiology* 1994;80:427–455.

C.3. How would you assess fluid status in this patient?

Several issues in interventional radiology complicate fluid management. First, contrast material acts as an osmotic diuretic. Often these patients have had a computed tomography (CT) scan with contrast before the angiograms and may become intravascularly depleted. Second, the femoral sheath and other catheters are constantly flushed with a heparinized saline solution. It is not uncommon for a patient to receive 1,000 mL or more of flush fluid during the case. This must be taken into account when calculating fluid balance.

C.4. Would a monitor of central venous pressure (CVP) be useful in this patient for craniotomy for clipping?

At our institution we reserve placements of CVP catheter for those patients who have a history of cardiac disease, have documented cardiac dysfunction or if we are unable to secure large-bore peripheral IV access. Although not always directly monitored, advantages of CVP may be useful in assessing volume replacement needs, especially because urine output will be affected by osmotic or loop diuretics administered to facilitate surgical exposure. If vasoactive medication becomes necessary, it can be most effectively administered through a central venous catheter.

One disadvantage of CVP monitoring is catheter placement. Some clinicians are concerned that placement of an internal jugular venous CVP will compromise venous outflow of the head, thereby predisposing to bleeding or brain swelling; however, this remains controversial. A "long-arm" or antecubital CVP line may be more difficult to insert and have a higher incidence of thrombophlebitis.

Finally, a poor correlation between CVP and left ventricular end-diastolic pressure has been documented in subarachnoid hemorrhage (SAH), so a pulmonary artery (PA) catheter may be more useful in assessing volume status as well as providing a monitor of cardiac output in those patients who have had preoperative cardiac problems. Patients who are expected to be candidates for hypertensive hypervolemic hemodilution (HHH) therapy for vasospasm or for barbiturate coma may also benefit from placement of a PA catheter.

Central pressure monitoring is usually instituted after the patient is asleep to minimize stress to the patient. One should be careful to use the minimal degree of head-down tilt necessary to access the central circulation, because a severe Trendelenburg position may have deleterious effects on intracranial pressure (ICP) and cerebral perfusion pressure (CPP).

Lai YC, Manninen PH. Anesthesia for cerebral aneurysms: a comparison between interventional neuroradiology and surgery. *Can J Anaesth* 2001;48:391–395.

C.5. What other forms of monitoring would you consider?

Electroencephalography (EEG) and somatosensory evoked potentials (SSEPs) have been advocated by some authors; however, they are not standard monitoring in most hospitals. Although EEG has been used to monitor cerebral ischemia, scalp electrodes may not reflect activity of brain areas most at risk. Cortical electrodes, such as those used in epilepsy surgery, may avoid the problem of attenuation of the scalp electroencephalographic signal by CSF drainage and air between scalp electrodes and brain surface during surgery. EEG is useful in titrating barbiturate or propofol infusion if burst suppression is desired during temporary clipping.

SSEPs may detect reversible ischemia during temporary vessel occlusion; however, they may not detect ischemia in subcortical structures and motor cortex. Furthermore, SSEPs have relatively high false-positive (38% to 60%) and false-negative (5% to 34%) rates. Brainstem auditory evoked responses (BAERs) may be useful in monitoring during posterior circulation aneurysm clipping.

Monitoring of intracranial pressure (ICP) is common, with the probability of increased ICP greatest at 24 to 48 hours after subarachnoid hemorrhage (SAH). An intraventricular catheter not only allows for ICP monitoring but also allows for CSF drainage to improve operating conditions. If an intraventricular catheter is not present, lumbar spinal drain may be placed. One must be careful not to allow substantial CSF drainage before dural opening because this may decrease ICP allowing for an increase in transmural pressure and possible rupture.

Intraoperative angiography is one means by which to ensure complete obliteration of the aneurysm without clip occlusion of the parent artery or perforating branches.

Bekker AY, Baker KZ, Baker CJ, et al. Anesthetic considerations for cerebral aneurysm surgery. *Am J Anesthesiol* 1995;22:248–258.

Bendo AA. Intracranial vasculary surgery. *Anesthesiol Clin North America* 2002;20:377–388.

Manninen PH, Lam AM, Nantau WE. Monitoring of somatosensory evoked potentials during temporary arterial occlusion in cerebral aneurysm surgery. *J Neurosurg Anesthesiol* 1990;2:97–104.

Schramm J, Antou L, Gerhard S, et al. Surgical and electrophysiological observations during clipping of 134 aneurysms with evoked potential monitoring. *Neurosurgery* 1990;26:61–70.

Young WL, Solomon RA, Pedley TA, et al. Direct cortical EEG monitoring during temporary vascular occlusion for cerebral aneurysm surgery. *Anesthesiology* 1989;71:794–799.

C.6. What are your particular concerns during induction of anesthesia in this patient?

If an aneurysm ruptures during anesthetic induction, mortality is high ($\sim$75%). Therefore, precise control of transmural pressure is important in preventing aneurysm rupture.

$$\text{Transmural pressure} = \text{CPP} = \text{MAP–ICP or CVP (whichever is greater),}$$
$$\text{where MAP} = \text{mean arterial pressure}$$

On the other hand, one does not want CPP to be so low that ischemia develops, especially in areas of vasospasm.

Tsementzis SA, Hitchcock ER. Outcome from "rescue clipping" of ruptured intracranial aneurysms during induction of anesthesia and endotracheal intubation. *J Neurol Neurosurg Psychiatry* 1985;48:160–163.

C.7. How would you accomplish a smooth and safe induction and intubation of this patient?

Assuming that evaluation of the airway indicated that intubation would not be difficult, one would begin with preoxygenation. Thiopental (3 to 5 mg/kg), propofol (1.5 to 2.5 mg/kg), or etomidate (0.5 to 1.0 mg/kg) all have similar effects on cerebral blood flow (CBF) and cerebral metabolic rate. Given that this woman had no other medical problems, thiopental is a reasonable choice. One may want to avoid ketamine for induction because of its associated increase in CBF and intracranial pressure (ICP).

After loss of consciousness and apnea, care must be taken to maintain a normal $Paco_2$ and to avoid extreme hyperventilation. Vigorous hyperventilation will lower $Paco_2$, decreasing CBF. This may lower ICP to such a degree that if mean arterial pressure (MAP) is maintained or increased, transmural pressure may be increased, leading to rupture of the aneurysm.

A nondepolarizing muscle relaxant, which has no effect on ICP or CBF, should be added to facilitate intubation. The neuromuscular junction should be monitored to ensure that paralysis is adequate to avoid coughing with intubation.

Fentanyl (3 to 5 μg/kg), sufentanil (0.5 to 1.0 μg/kg), or remifentanil (0.25 to 1.0 μg/kg) can be added 3 to 5 minutes before laryngoscopy to blunt the hemodynamic response. Isoflurane/desflurane/sevoflurane is added to deepen the anesthetic. Finally, approximately 90 seconds before laryngoscopy, lidocaine (1.5 to 2.0 mg/kg) or esmolol (0.5 mg/kg) can be added to further blunt the hemodynamic response to intubation.

Lidocaine decreases both CBF and cerebral metabolic rate for oxygen, and at high concentrations it can cause seizures. Esmolol and labetalol have no effect on CBF and ICP, even in brain areas where autoregulation may not be intact. Extreme reductions in MAP (>35%) may compromise cerebral perfusion pressure (CPP) in patients with increased ICP.

Albin MS, ed. *Textbook of neuroanesthesia: with neurosurgical and neuroscience perspectives*. New York: McGraw-Hill, 1997:873.

Cottrell JE, Smith DS, eds. *Anesthesia and neurosurgery*, 4th ed. St. Louis: Mosby, 2001:376–379.

Guy J, McGrath BJ, Borel CO, et al. Perioperative management of aneurysmal subarachnoid hemorrhage. Part 1. Operative management. *Anesth Analg* 1995;81:1060–1072.

C.8. Would you perform a rapid-sequence induction and intubation on this patient?

No indication is seen for a rapid-sequence induction and intubation on this patient. Overall risk of aspiration during general anesthesia has been estimated at 0.05%; however, the risk of aneurysm rupture during induction is 1% to 2%. Therefore, unless a clear indication exists for rapid-sequence induction it is best avoided.

If rapid-sequence induction is indicated, one may consider using vecuronium (0.15 to 0.20 mg/kg) or rocuronium (0.9 mg/kg) rather than succinylcholine. Succinylcholine may cause an increase in intracranial pressure (ICP), although this increase can be attenuated or eliminated by deep anesthesia or prior defasciculation. Succinylcholine, more importantly, may lead to hyperkalemia and possibly ventricular fibrillation in those patients presenting with motor deficits following subarachnoid hemorrhage (SAH).

In the case of a full stomach or an anticipated difficult airway, careful awake fiberoptic intubation, with use of appropriate sedation and topical application of local anesthesia, is an appropriate alternative. Under such circumstances, it is useful to have an assistant so that while one person is securing the airway, the other is solely focused on controlling the hemodynamics with titration of β-blockers and sodium nitroprusside.

Cottrell JE, Smith DS, eds. *Anesthesia and neurosurgery*, 4th ed. St. Louis: Mosby, 2001: 377–378.

Guy J, McGrath BJ, Borel CO, et al. Perioperative management of aneurysmal subarachnoid hemorrhage. Part 1. Operative management. *Anesth Analg* 1995;81:1060–1072.

Iwasuta N, Kuroda N, Amaha K, et al. Succinylcholine induced hyperkalemia in patients with ruptured central aneurysms. *Anesthesiology* 1980;53:64–67.

Lanier WL, Milde JH, Michenfelder JD. Cerebral stimulation following succinylcholine in dogs. *Anesthesiology* 1986;64:551–559.

Olsson GL, Hullen B, Hambraeus-Johnzonk K. Aspiration during anesthesia: a computer-aided study of 185,838 anesthetics. *Acta Anesthesiol Scand* 1986;30:84–92.

Stirt JA, Grosslight KR, Bedford RF, et al. Defasciculation with metocurine prevents succinylcholine associated increases in intracranial pressure. *Anesthesiology* 1987;67:50–53.

Tsementzis SA, Hitchcock ER. Outcome from "rescue clipping" of ruptured intracranial aneurysms during induction of anesthesia and endotracheal intubation. *J Neurol Neurosurg Psychiatry* 1985;48:160–163.

C.9. What are the effects of hypoxemia and hypercapnia, such as would be seen with loss of the airway on induction, on cerebral blood flow (CBF)?

Each mm Hg increase in $PaCO_2$ increases CBF 3% to 4%, when $PaCO_2$ is in the range of 20 to 80 mm Hg. In addition, the hypoxia that will ensue if the airway is not secured in a timely manner will also cause an increase in CBF once PaO_2 is less than 60 mm Hg (Fig. 26.1).

C.10. What is optimal fluid management for aneurysm clipping? Would you use a dextrose-containing solution?

Maintenance fluid requirements and blood loss should be replaced. One wants to avoid profound hypovolemia not only for its detrimental cardiovascular effects but also because it is associated with cerebral ischemia and perioperative neurologic deficits resulting from vasospasm. Some authors advocate mild hypervolemia to maximize cerebral blood flow (CBF) and minimize vasospasm; however, one must keep in mind the possibility of cerebral edema.

In general, dextrose-containing solutions should be avoided because an increased incidence of neurologic deficits associated with glucose administration has been found in experimental models of focal cerebral ischemia. At Cornell, we try to maintain blood glucose less than 180 mg per dL.

Use of crystalloid versus colloid for fluid management and which type of crystalloid solution, lactated Ringer's versus normal saline or Normosol, has long been a matter of controversy. Although some authors advocate colloid solutions to diminish the risk of brain swelling, no evidence exists that colloid use improves outcome. However, giving large amounts of hyposmolar (lactated Ringer's) solution may predispose to brain edema and contribute to hyponatremia,

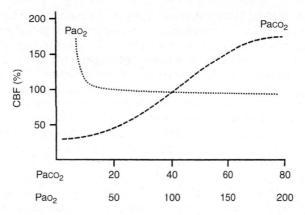

Figure 26.1 Change in cerebral blood flow as a function of arterial carbon dioxide ($Paco_2$) and oxygen (Pao_2) tension. CBF, cerebral blood flow. (From Albin MS, ed. *Textbook of neuroanesthesia: with neurosurgical and neuroscience perspectives.* New York: McGraw-Hill, 1997:30, with permission.)

which may increase the incidence of delayed ischemic neurologic deficits. Therefore, normal saline is the fluid of choice at Cornell.

A moderate degree of hemodilution to a hematocrit of 30% to 35% usually lowers blood viscosity, thereby increasing CBF. The goal is to increase oxygen delivery by increasing CBF, without allowing the hematocrit to decrease to the degree that reduction in oxygen content negates the increase in CBF. Hematocrit, serum sodium, and serum osmolality measurements may be followed to guide fluid therapy. Serum sodium should be maintained within normal limits, both to maintain serum oncotic pressure and to avoid the hyponatremia associated with cerebral salt wasting.

Guy J, McGrath BJ, Borel CO et al. Perioperative management of aneurysmal subarachnoid hemorrhage. Part 1. Operative management. *Anesth Analg* 1995;81:1060–1072.

Lanier WL, Stangland KJ, Scheithauer BW, et al. The effects of dextrose infusion and head position on neurologic outcome after complete cerebral ischemia in primates: examination of a model. *Anesthesiology* 1987;66:39–48.

Maroon JC, Nelson PB. Hypovolemia in patients with subarachnoid hemorrhage: therapeutic implications. *Neurosurgery* 1979;4:223–226.

McGirt MJ, Blessing R, Ninjee SM, et al. Correlation of serum brain natriuretic peptide with hyponatremia and delayed ischemic neurologic deficits after subarachnoid hemorrhage. *Neurosurgery* 2004;54:1369–1374.

C.11. After the bone plate was removed and as the dura was being opened the surgeon complained that the brain was "tight." What could you do to achieve better brain relaxations and facilitate surgical exposure?

Any method that rapidly decreases intracranial pressure (ICP) before dural opening may suddenly increase transmural pressure and lead to aneurysm rupture. After dural opening, one of the fastest ways to decrease cerebral blood volume and improve exposure is through hyperventilation. Mild hypocarbia ($PaCO_2$ = 30 to 35 mm Hg) can usually be established before dural opening, with moderate hypocarbia ($PaCO_2$ = 25 to 30 mm Hg) after dural opening. However, because of the risk of cerebral ischemia secondary to diminished cerebral blood flow (CBF), normocarbia should be maintained whenever possible in patients with vasospasm.

Mannitol is the most frequently used diuretic at our institution. It is given as an infusion for a total dose of 0.7 g per kg (0.25 to 1.0 g/kg). Its immediate effect is a transient rise in intravascular volume, which may pose problems in patients with impaired ventricular function. In addition, too rapid an infusion can lead to decreases in systemic vascular resistance. Its onset of diuretic action is in 10 to 15 minutes with peak effect occurring at 60 to 90 minutes. If mannitol does not produce the desired brain relaxation and the serum osmolality is greater than 320 mOsm, additional mannitol is unlikely to produce additional effect. In those patients who may not tolerate the initial effects of mannitol, intravenous furosemide (0.1 to 0.3 mg/kg) can be substituted. Both medications can cause derangements in fluid status and serum electrolytes that require close monitoring.

Drainage of CSF from either a lumbar drain or an intraventricular catheter is usually effective in optimizing surgical exposure. One must be careful to avoid significant CSF drainage before dural opening to prevent either brainstem herniation or a sudden decrease in transmural pressure. Similarly, hemodynamic instability can ensue if CSF is drained too rapidly at any point in the operation.

If tight brain remains a problem, one must ascertain that there is no hypoxemia or hypercarbia. In addition, one should consider eliminating N_2O, if it is in use and reducing the amount of volatile anesthetic, because all inhalational agents are cerebral vasodilators and may potentially increase ICP. Of course, if inhaled agents are reduced, appropriate intravenous agents should be substituted to ensure adequate anesthesia.

One may give a bolus of thiopental to decrease $CMRO_2$ and CBF; however, one must maintain mean arterial pressure (MAP) to maintain cerebral perfusion pressure (CPP). At the time of patient positioning, one must ensure that no impediment exists to venous outflow of the brain (i.e., that extreme flexion or rotation of the head is avoided and that no monitor cables [electrocardiogram (ECG) leads] are draped across the neck).

Albin MS, ed. *Textbook of neuroanesthesia: with neurosurgical and neuroscience perspectives*. New York: McGraw-Hill, 1997:869.

Bendo AA. Intracranial vasculary surgery. *Anesthesiol Clin North America* 2002;20:377–388.

Sullivan HG, Keenan RL, Isrow L. The critical importance of $PaCO_2$ during intracranial aneurysm surgery. *J Neurol Neurosurg* 1980;52:426–431.

C.12. How might transmural pressure be decreased to allow for aneurysm clip placement?

The most widely accepted method for producing a slack aneurysm to allow for clip placement is the use of temporary clip occlusion of one or more parent vessels. For example, to place a permanent clip on an anterior communicating artery aneurysm, a temporary clip can be placed on either the right or left anterior cerebral artery or both. Advantages of temporary clip use include a greater reduction in transmural pressure and greater ease in clipping, decreased incidence of intraoperative rupture, and avoidance of controlled hypotension.

The maximal duration of temporary clip application before a neurologic deficit occurs is unknown, but it is probably related to the location of the aneurysm and distribution of perforating vessels distal to the temporary clip. White matter and major deep nuclei are likely to be more susceptible than gray matter to temporary ischemia. Risk factors for neurologic deficit following temporary clip placement include poor preoperative neurologic condition, age older than 61 years, and distribution of perforating arteries in distal basilar and horizontal segments of middle cerebral artery (MCA).

Akyuz AA, Erylmaz M, Ozdemir C, et al. Effect of temporary clipping on frontal lobe functions in patients with ruptured aneurysm of the anterior communicating artery. *Acta Neurochir Scan* 2005;112 (5):293–297.

Kett-White R, Hutchinson PJ, Al-Ravie PG, et al. Cerebral oxygen and microdialysis monitoring during aneurysm surgery: effects of blood pressure, cerebral spinal fluid drainage and temporary clipping on infarction. *J Neurosurgery* 2002;96:1013–1019.

C.13. What is the purpose of controlled hypotension and how is it achieved?

In the past controlled hypotension was used to decrease transmural pressure, making the aneurysm neck slack enough to allow placement of a clip without vessel rupture. Various agents were used to achieve controlled hypotension, including volatile agent, nitroprusside, esmolol, labetalol, nitroglycerin, and trimethaphan. Specific agents were selected based on the patient's preexisting medical conditions, especially coronary ischemia or poor ventricular function. In an otherwise healthy patient, sodium nitroprusside infusion may be used for its rapid onset, easy titratability, and quick offset. An esmolol infusion can be added to augment hypotension and to counteract the reflex tachycardia and cyanide toxicity seen with nitroprusside. Side effects of nitroprusside include cyanide toxicity, rebound hypertension, and intrapulmonary shunting. Direct measurement of central venous pressure (CVP) is useful when planning to use controlled hypotension in these patients.

During controlled hypotension, mean arterial pressure (MAP) is usually maintained at a minimum of 50 mm Hg in previously normotensive individuals. Neurologic function monitors (electroencephalography [EEG], somatosensory evoked potential [SSEP], brainstem auditory evoked responses [BAER], cerebral oximetry) may be useful in guiding target level of MAP.

Albin MS, ed. *Textbook of neuroanesthesia: with neurosurgical and neuroscience perspectives.* New York: McGraw-Hill, 1997:877–878.

Ornstein E, Young WL, Ostapkovich N, et al. Deliberate hypotension in patients with intracranial arteriovenous malformations: esmolol compared with isoflurane and sodium nitroprusside. *Anesth Analg* 1991;72:639–644.

C.14. What are some of the drawbacks of controlled hypotension?

The main drawback of controlled hypotension is that it leads to a global decrease in cerebral perfusion pressure (CPP). CPP is then further diminished in the presence of vasospasm or in areas of brain retraction. In a retrospective study, multiple regression analysis indicated that patients who underwent even limited periods of controlled hypotension had a worse outcome, both in terms of Glasgow Outcome Scale (multiple regression) and higher incidence and severity of vasospasm. At Cornell we avoid controlled hypotension in neurosurgery.

Chang HS, Hongo K, Nakagawa H. Adverse effects of limited hypotensive anesthesia on the outcome of patients with subarachnoid hemorrhage. *J Neurosurg* 2000;92:971–975.

Ruta TS, Mutch WAC. Controlled hypotension for cerebral aneurysm surgery: are the risks worth the benefits? *J Neurosurg Anesthesiol* 1991;3:153–156.

C.15. What methods of cerebral protection might you use during this operation?

Cerebral protection has long been a matter of much investigation and controversy. Barbiturate loading has been shown in animals to be protective against focal ischemia; however, no controlled human studies have been performed. Barbiturates decrease both cerebral metabolic rate for glucose and oxygen and lower cerebral blood flow (CBF) and intracranial pressure (ICP). The dose is usually titrated to electroencephalographic silence or burst suppression. At doses used to suppress electroencephalographic activity, the patient may experience cardiovascular depression. The dose of barbiturate traditionally used for cerebral protection may also prolong emergence and hinder postoperative neurologic evaluation. Although barbiturates were originally thought to protect against ischemia through metabolic depression, other factors such as redistribution of blood flow to ischemic areas, blockade of the sodium channels and glutamate receptors, attenuation of *N*-methyl D-aspartate (NMDA) and α-amino-3-hydroxy-5-methyl-4-isoxazole propionic acid (AMPA)-mediated glutamate toxicity all play a role.

Propofol has also been used as an alternative to thiopental sodium. Cerebral protection due to propofol is thought to result from scavenging of free radicals, inhibition of glutamate release and prevention of lipid peroxidation. In studies involving both volatile anesthetics and propofol, apoptotic cell death is delayed, but not prevented, if the ischemic result is mild.

Etomidate decreases cerebral metabolic rate at electroencephalographic burst suppression and prevents an increase in excitatory neurotransmitters during cerebral ischemia in animal models; however, it has been associated with a greater volume of injured brain than thiopental and control groups in focal ischemia in hypertensive rats.

Deliberate mild hypothermia (32.5°C to 35.5°C) although promising in animal models, did not demonstrate efficacy with good grade aneurysm patients in the intraoperative hypothermia for aneurysm surgery trial (IHAST) 2. Magnesium has been proposed as a cerebroprotective agent during aneurysm clipping. Magnesium is a cerebral vasodilator which, in animal models, blocks voltage-dependent calcium channels and reverses experimental vasospasm. In humans, magnesium has been found to attenuate brain tissue hypoxia during temporary occlusion. Finally, erythropoietin is being investigated as a cerebroprotectant.

Chan MTV, Boet R, Ng SCP, et al. Magnesium sulfate for brain protection during temporary cerebral artery occlusion. *Acta Neurochir* 2005;95(suppl):107–111.

Drummond JC, Cole DJ, Patel PM, et al. Focal cerebral ischemia during anesthesia with etomidate, isoflurane, or thiopental: a comparison of the extent of cerebral injury. *Neurosurgery* 1995;37:742–748.

Engelhard K, Werner C, Eberspacher E, et al. Influence of propofol on neuronal damage and apoptotic factors after incomplete cerebral ischemia and reperfusion in rats: a long-term observation. *Anesthesiology* 2004;101:912–917.

Engelhard K, Werner C, Hoffman WE, et al. The effect of Sevoflurane and propofol on cerebral neurotransmitter concentrations during cerebral ischemia in rats. *Anesth Analg* 2003;97(4):1155–1161.

Guy J, McGrath BJ, Borel CO, et al. Perioperative management of aneurysmal subarachnoid hemorrhage. Part 1. Operative management. *Anesth Analg* 1995;81:1060–1072.

Kawaguchi M, Furuya H, Patel PM. Neuroprotective effects of anesthetic agents. *J Anesth* 2005;19:150–156.

Liu R, Suzuki A, Guo Z, et al. Intrinsic and extrinsic erythropoietin enhances neuroprotection against ischemia and reperfusion injury *in vitro*. *J Neurochem* 2006;96:1101–1110.

Ravussin P, Detribolet N. Total intravenous anesthesia with propofol for burst suppression in cerebral aneurysm surgery—a preliminary report of 42 patients. *Neurosurgery* 1990;32:236–240.

Warner DS, Takaoka S, Wu B, et al. Electroencephalographic burst suppression is not required to elicit maximal neuroprotection from pentobarbital in a rat model of focal cerebral ischemia. *Anesthesiology* 1996;84(6):1475–1484.

C.16. Would you induce mild hypothermia as a means of cerebral protection?

Hypothermia causes a greater reduction in cerebral metabolic rate for glucose and oxygen than the level attained at electroencephalographic silence because its reduction of metabolism is caused by a reduction both in neuronal electrical activity and in enzyme activity related to maintenance of cellular function. Hypothermia also reduces the release of excitatory neurotransmitters. Significant reduction in infarct size after global and focal ischemia has been demonstrated in several animal studies. Unfortunately, these advantages have not been documented in clinical trial. The intraoperative hypothermia for aneurysm surgery trial (IHAST) showed no differences in Glasgow Outcome Scale at 3 months in good grade patients.

Disadvantages of unintentional hypothermia documented in the literature include an increased incidence of myocardial ischemia in peripheral vascular surgery, increased incidence of postoperative wound infection in abdominal surgery, coagulopathy, prolonged drug clearance, and hyperglycemia. In the IHAST study, the hypothermic group had a small increase in infection rate. As a result of IHAST, we no longer deliberately induce hypothermia in good grade patients for aneurysm clippings.

Albin MS, ed. *Textbook of neuroanesthesia: with neurosurgical and neuroscience perspectives.* New York: McGraw-Hill, 1997:878.

Frank SM, Beattie C, Christopherson R, et al. Unintentional hypothermia is associated with postoperative myocardial ischemia. *Anesthesiology* 1993;78:468–476.

Kurz A, Sesler DI, Lenhardt R, et al. Perioperative normothermia to reduce the incidence of surgical wound infection and shorten hospitalization. *N Engl J Med* 1996;334: 1209–1215.

Todd MM, Handman BJ, Clarke WR, et al. Intraoperative hypothermia for aneurysm surgery trial. *N Engl J Med* 2005;352(2):135–145.

C.17. What are the indications for deep hypothermic circulatory arrest?

Hypothermic circulatory arrest at body temperature less than 22°C (71.6°F) is reserved for giant aneurysms, difficult basilar artery aneurysms, and anatomically complex aneurysms that are not clippable without complete cessation of blood flow and are not amenable to the use of temporary clips. Deep hypothermic circulatory arrest requires cooperation between several services including anesthesiology, neurosurgery, cardiac surgery, and perfusionists. In addition to all the concerns mentioned regarding anesthesia for the person with an intracranial aneurysm and the need for prompt awakening for ease of neurologic assessment, deep hypothermic circulatory arrest adds the concerns regarding institution of and separation from cardiopulmonary bypass, systemic heparinization and protamine reversal, and, of course, rewarming from profound hypothermia. This is rarely performed now that coil embolization is possible for many of these aneurysms.

Young WL, Lawtom MI, Gupta DK, et al. Anesthetic management of deep hypothermic circulatory arrest for cerbral aneurysm clipping. *J Neurosurg Anesthesiol* 2003;15(3): 274–277.

C.18. What steps should be taken in the case of intraoperative rupture of an intracranial aneurysm?

The incidence of intraoperative rupture is 2% to 19%. The stage of the operation at which rupture occurs affects outcome, with rupture at induction being the worst. After induction the most common times for rupture are when the dura matter or arachnoid matter are being opened, during intracranial hematoma removal, and of course during dissection exposure of the aneurysm. At any point in the operation, a sudden sustained increase in blood pressure with or without bradycardia is suggestive of rupture. If rupture is suspected on induction, one must institute measures to control intracranial pressure (ICP) while maintaining cerebral perfusion pressure (CPP).

If rupture occurs during surgical dissection, mortality is lower. The primary concern is to control bleeding while maintaining systemic perfusion. Bleeding is controlled by placement of temporary clips or by clamping or compression of the ipsilateral carotid artery in the neck if the aneurysm is too proximal. If bleeding is not controlled in a timely manner and a significant amount of blood accumulates in the subarachnoid space, severe brain swelling that is refractory to all treatment may develop. At Cornell, we do not use controlled hypotension at any point in the surgery even in the face of intraoperative rupture.

Bendo AA. Intracranial vasculary surgery. *Anesthesiol Clin North America* 2002;20:377–388.

Guy J, McGrath BJ, Borel CO, et al. Perioperative management of aneurysmal subarachnoid hemorrhage. Part 1. Operative management. *Anesth Analg* 1995;81:1060–1072.

Hawkin K, Kuroda S, Takahashi A, et al. Intraoperative premature rupture of the cerebral aneurysms. Analysis of the causes and management. *Acta Neurochir (Wien)* 1999;141: 1255–1263.

Sundt TM, Whisnant JP. Subarachnoid hemorrhage from intracranial aneurysm: surgical management and natural history of disease. *N Engl J Med* 1978;299:116–122.

C.19. How would you plan the emergence from an anesthetic for aneurysm clipping?

The goal is to have a patient comfortable and not coughing or straining or subject to hypercarbia or wide variations in blood pressure.

After discontinuing all anesthetic agents and reversing neuromuscular blockade, the use of a lidocaine (1.5 mg/kg) bolus may minimize bucking and reaction to the endotracheal tube. Strict control of blood pressure must be observed especially in the presence of ischemic heart disease or in patients suspected of having multiple aneurysms. One should keep the blood pressure within 20% of the patient's normal measurement.

D. Postoperative Management

D.1. Would you extubate the patient postoperatively?

Most patients who are in Hunt and Hess grades I and II can be extubated postoperatively with no need for airway support. Patients in grades IV and V usually require mechanical ventilation postoperatively, whereas grade III patients may or may not require intubation and mechanical ventilation. Patients with vertebral or basilar artery aneurysms may require airway protection secondary to cranial nerve damage and loss of protective reflexes.

If this patient was able to follow commands, was clinically recovered from the effects of muscle relaxants, and had established an adequate ventilatory pattern with return of protective airway reflexes, extubation would be appropriate.

Bendo AA. Intracranial vasculary surgery. *Anesthesiol Clin North America* 2002;20:377–388.

Guy J, McGrath BJ, Borel CO, et al. Perioperative management of aneurysmal subarachnoid hemorrhage. Part 1. Operative management. *Anesth Analg* 1995;81:1060–1072.

D.2. What would be the differential diagnosis if the patient did not return to her preoperative neurologic condition?

If the patient had a focal neurologic deficit on awakening in the operating room, the cause most likely would be a surgical one, although new-onset vasospasm is also a possibility.

If, however, the patient failed to awaken, the first step would be to ensure that all inhalational and infused anesthetics had been discontinued. Second, one should make sure that neuromuscular blockade was fully reversed. One should make sure that the patient had been appropriately rewarmed, because hypothermia would prolong the duration of action of most intravenous medications. While considering reversal of benzodiazepines and narcotics, one should rule out other causes such as hypoxia, hypercarbia, hyponatremia, and hypoglycemia. One should consider the possibility of intraoperative seizure, with delayed emergence resulting from a postictal state. If after reversal of all anesthetic agents, the patient had not awakened, a computed tomography (CT) scan should be obtained to rule out subdural hematoma, intracranial hemorrhage, hydrocephalus, and pneumocephalus. An angiogram may also be obtained to rule out vascular occlusion. An electroencephalogram might be appropriate to rule out subconvulsive status epilepticus.

Cottrell JE, Smith DS, eds. *Anesthesia and neurosurgery*, 4th ed. St. Louis: Mosby, 2001.385.

D.3. On postoperative day 2, the patient became disoriented and developed hemiplegia. A computed tomography (CT) scan was performed, which shows no new intracranial bleeding. What other diagnostic studies should be performed?

If transcranial Doppler (TCD) is available, an increased value for cerebral arterial flow velocity would be suggestive for vasospasm. Tissue oximetry may also be useful as a monitor for vasospasm. Angiography, however, is the gold standard for the diagnosis of cerebral vasospasm and this should be obtained to confirm the diagnosis and characterize the number and location of the vessels involved.

Cerebral vasospasm may be localized to the area of aneurysm rupture or in an area of the brain remote from the subarachnoid hemorrhage (SAH). The worst prognosis is in those patients in whom vasospasm is diffuse. Of course, as these studies are being obtained, laboratory values should be checked to make sure no new or worsening metabolic derangement is contributing to the neurologic deterioration.

D.4. What is cerebral vasospasm and what causes it?

Vasospasm, which occurs in 35% of patients with subarachnoid hemorrhage (SAH), is a segmental or diffuse narrowing of the lumen of one or more intracranial arteries. It is the most common cause of delayed cerebral ischemia and may be seen angiographically in 60% of patients, even if clinical manifestations are not apparent.

The severity of vasospasm is apparently related to the amount and location of subarachnoid blood. Injection of blood into the subarachnoid space causes vasospasm in experimental animals and antifibrinolytics apparently worsen the spasm. On a molecular level, one theory is that oxyhemoglobin causes the production of superoxide radicals that lead to a decrease in nitric oxide (NO) production in endothelial cells. This decrease in NO increases protein kinase C and intracellular calcium, resulting in myofilament activation and vasospasm. Other theories involve prostaglandins and lipid peroxidases. There may also be a genetic predisposition to development of vasopasm. Preliminary studies suggest that patients with a certain polymorphism of haptoglobin ($\alpha_1\alpha_1$) maybe protected against vasospasm as compared to patients with haptoglobin $\alpha_2\alpha_2$ which is less effective at neutralizing free radical formation by free hemoglobin.

Borosody M, Burke A, Caplin W, et al. Haptoglobin and the development of cerebral vasospasm after subarachnoid hemorrhage. *Neurology* 2006;66:634–640.

Vollrath AM, Weir BKA, Macdonald RL, et al. Intracellular mechanisms involved in the responses of cerebrovascular smooth-muscle cells to hemoglobin. *J Neurosurg* 1994; 80:261–268.

D.5. What are pathophysiologic changes seen in cerebral vasospasm?

Structurally, leukocytes, red blood cells, and macrophages are seen in arterial walls. Inflammatory mediators, such as eicosanoids, interleukin 1, and immune complexes, are increased. Eventually, the vessel wall thickens, and smooth muscle proliferation and collagen deposition accompany degenerative changes in the tunica intima and media.

Functionally CO_2 reactivity is impaired, and autoregulation is often impaired, perhaps correlating to the degree of vasospasm. Cerebral blood flow (CBF) in some areas appears to be pressure dependent, hence the reasoning behind hypertensive therapy.

D.6. How is the diagnosis of cerebral vasospasm made?

The clinical diagnosis of cerebral vasospasm is made when the patient experiences an altered level of consciousness (drowsiness, disorientation) or a new focal neurologic deficit. These may be accompanied by increasing headache, meningismus, and fever. Vasospasm is rare in the first 3 days following subarachnoid hemorrhage (SAH). It reaches peak incidence at 3 to 10 days and usually resolves by 10 to 14 days after SAH. In this patient, the new onset of hemiplegia suggests that the middle cerebral artery (MCA) is involved. If vessels in the posterior fossa are involved, respiratory and hemodynamic abnormalities may develop.

The differential diagnosis includes rebleeding, hydrocephalus, seizure, hyponatremia, and drug effects. Transcranial Doppler (TCD), cerebral blood flow (CBF), velocity greater than 120 cm per second in association with a new focal neurologic deficit are usually sufficient to make the diagnosis of cerebral vasospasm; however, a change in TCD values over time may be more useful than an absolute value. CBF velocity greater than 200 cm per second is associated with a high risk of cerebral infarct, whereas a velocity less than 100 cm per second indicates that cerebral vasospasm is unlikely.

Angiographic cerebral vasospasm can be found in 60% of patients following SAH but only 50% of these patients will develop clinical focal neurologic deficits.

Albin MS, ed. *Textbook of neuroanesthesia: with neurosurgical and neuroscience perspectives*. New York: McGraw-Hill, 1997:852.

McGrath BJ, Guy J, Borel CO, et al. Perioperative management of aneurysmal subarachnoid hemorrhage. Part 2. Postoperative management. *Anesth Analg* 1995;81:1295–1302.

D.7. What steps can be taken to prevent cerebral vasospasm?

Calcium channel blockers are standard prophylactic therapy to prevent vasospasm. The mechanism is unknown, but presumably calcium channel blockers aid in maintaining cellular integrity by preventing calcium entry into ischemic cells. Nimodipine, taken orally, improves neurologic outcome. Patients given nimodipine have no change in overall incidence of vasospasm, but they have a lower incidence of severe narrowing. In addition, although no improvement is found in mortality, there is improvement in outcome for survivors. Intravenous nimodipine is not available in the United States.

Nicardipine, an intravenous agent, showed a lower incidence of vasospasm but no improvement in outcome versus a placebo group; however, both groups received hypertensive hypervolemic hemodilution (HHH) therapy. The main complication of calcium channel blocker therapy is hypotension (0% to 8%), which may make it difficult to achieve HHH therapy.

Other steps to limit cerebral vasospasm include the removal of subarachnoid blood as quickly as possible, instillation of thrombolytic agents (e.g., urokinase), and use of pharmacologic agents to reduce inflammatory response (high-dose glucocorticoids, ibuprofen). In Europe and Japan, protease inhibitors have been used in the treatment of vasospasm.

Haley EC, Kassell NF, Torner JC, et al. A randomized, controlled trial of high-dose intravenous nicardipine in aneurysmal subarachnoid hemorrhage. *J Neurosurg* 1993;78: 537–547.

Weyer GW, Nolanc CP, Macdonald RL. Evidence-based cerebral vasospasm management. *Neurosurg Focus* 2006;21:E8.

D.8. What treatments can be undertaken once a diagnosis of cerebral vasospasm is made?

Treatment for cerebral vasospasm is multifactorial and includes continuation of prophylactic measures. Hypertensive hypervolemic hemodilution (HHH) therapy is a plan to augment cerebral blood flow (CBF) past the stenotic areas. It begins with hypervolemic hypertension, with intravascular volume expansion with crystalloid or colloid to increase cardiac output. Some recommended target values are central venous pressure (CVP) 10 to 12 mm Hg, pulmonary artery occlusion pressure (PAOP) 15 to 18 mm Hg, cardiac index 3.0 to 3.5 L/minute/m^2, and hematocrit 30% to 35%. Various blood pressure targets have been reported but a reasonable plan is systolic blood pressure 160 to 200 mm Hg if the aneurysm is clipped and 120 to 150 mm Hg if unclipped. Vasoactive infusions are added if hypervolemia alone is inadequate. Endpoints of therapy are resolution of neurologic deficits or occurrence of complications of therapy, such as pulmonary edema (26%), myocardial ischemia, and rebleeding or rupture of a secondary aneurysm. A pulmonary artery (PA) catheter is often indicated.

Fluid used for HHH should be isotonic and have enough sodium to avoid hyponatremia. Vasopressin, fludrocortisone, or hydrocortisone may be administered to counteract excessive sodium and fluid loss.

Other treatments for vasospasm, including intraarterial verapamil, papaverine or nitroprusside infusions, or angioplasty, are usually reserved for those cases that fail HHH therapy.

Hoh BH, Ogilvy CS. Endovascular treatment of cerebral vasospasm: transluminal balloon angioplasty, intra-arterial papaverine, and intra-arterial nicardipine. *Neurosurg Clin N Am* 2005;16:501–516

D.9. What are other neurologic complications following subarachnoid hemorrhage (SAH) and aneurysm clipping?

Hydrocephalus, manifesting with a gradual decrease in level of consciousness, occurs in 25% of patients surviving SAH. Diagnosis is confirmed by computed tomography (CT) scan. Treatment is by ventricular drainage.

Seizures, which occur in 13% of patients with SAH, may herald rebleeding or vasospasm. Seizures cause an increase in mean arterial pressure (MAP), cerebral blood flow (CBF), intracranial pressure (ICP), and lactate production, predisposing to rebleeding in those patients with unclipped aneurysms and cerebral ischemia in those patients with vasospasm. Most patients receive prophylactic anticonvulsants.

Hyponatremia occurs in 10% to 34% of patients with SAH in a time course that parallels that of vasospasm. It may be due to syndrome of inappropriate antidiuretic hormone secretion (SIADH), "cerebral salt wasting," or prolonged or excessive mannitol use. Cerebral salt wasting syndrome is thought to be mediated by release of atrial natriuretic factor by the hypothalamus secondary to distention of the cerebral ventricles from hydrocephalus. After SAH, patients also have elevated serum. In these patients, fluid restriction is not the treatment of choice, because hypovolemia may predispose to vasospasm. Brain nutriuretic peptide patients may be treated with an isotonic or hypertonic salt containing fluid. In addition, treatment with hydrocortisone may be considered.

Finally, patients may experience brain swelling or edema, which is treated with mannitol and/or dexamethasone.

Albin MS, ed. *Textbook of neuroanesthesia: with neurosurgical and neuroscience perspectives.* New York: McGraw-Hill, 1997:861.

Hart RG, Byer JA, Slaughter JR, et al. Occurrence and implications of seizures in subarachnoid hemorrhage due to ruptured intracranial aneurysms. *Neurosurgery* 1982; 8:417–421.

Heros RC. Acute hydrocephalus after subarachnoid hemorrhage. *Stroke* 1989;20:715–717.

McGirt MJ, Blessing R, Ninjee SM, et al. Correlation of serum brain natriuretic peptide with hyponatremia and delayed ischemic neurologic deficits after subarachnoid hemorrhage. *Neurosurgery* 2004;54:1369–1374.

Moro N, Katayam V, Kojima J, et al. Prophylactic management of excessive natriuresis with hydrocortisone for efficient hypervolemic therapy after subarachnoid hemorrhage. *Stroke* 2003;34:2807–2811.

Nelson PB, Seif SM, Maroon JC, et al. Hyponatremia in intracranial disease: perhaps not the syndrome in inappropriate secretion of antidiuretic hormone (SIADH). *J Neurosurg* 1981;55:938–941.

D.10. What other organ systems may manifest problems postoperatively in aneurysm clipping patients?

The lungs can be affected by pneumonia or neurogenic pulmonary edema, in which disruption of the pulmonary capillary membrane occurs secondary to increased sympathetic nervous system activity. Because of inactivity, patients may be predisposed to developing deep venous thrombosis and pulmonary embolism. Patients may have fever secondary to subarachnoid blood, which may make workup of postoperative infection more difficult. In addition, as in most patients with head injury, those with subarachnoid hemorrhage (SAH) may have increased metabolic rate.

McGrath BJ, Guy J, Borel CO, et al. Perioperative management of aneurysmal subarachnoid hemorrhage. Part 2. Postoperative management. *Anesth Analg* 1995;81:1295–1302.

SECTION V

Pain Management and Neuraxial Blocks

CHAPTER 27

Brachial Plexus Block

JOSEPH TJAN • VINOD MALHOTRA

A 46-YEAR-OLD MAN

suffered a severe crush injury to his left hand at the construction site where he worked. On arrival to the emergency room, he received 75 mg of meperidine intramuscularly. Past medical history included psychiatric treatment for depression.

A. Medical Disease and Differential Diagnosis
1. What were the presenting problems in this patient?
2. Do you have any concerns about the use of meperidine in the emergency room?
3. What are the possible drug interactions between meperidine and the commonly used psychotropic drugs?
4. What are the anesthetic implications of tricyclic antidepressants (TCAs) and monoamine oxidase inhibitors (MAOIs)?
5. In an elective case, would you discontinue the use of tricyclics or MAOIs preoperatively?
6. What precautions should be taken to anesthetize a patient receiving MAOIs?

B. Preoperative Evaluation and Preparation
1. What premedication would you order?

C. Intraoperative Management
1. What anesthetic technique would you employ?
2. Describe the formation and major branches of the brachial plexus.
3. What regional technique would you choose to block the brachial plexus in this patient?

641

4. What are the advantages and disadvantages of axillary, interscalene, subclavian, and supraclavicular nerve blocks?
5. Describe the landmarks and procedure of an axillary nerve block.
6. Describe the landmarks and procedure of an interscalene nerve block.
7. What is the incidence of hemidiaphragmatic paresis after an interscalene brachial plexus block?
8. Describe the pulmonary function changes that occur after an interscalene brachial plexus block.
9. What would you do if the patient complained of dyspnea after performing an interscalene block?
10. What are the most commonly missed nerves with an axillary nerve block and an interscalene nerve block? How can you circumvent this problem?
11. After an axillary block, the patient complained of tourniquet-related pain. How would you manage this problem?
12. What local anesthetic agent would you use and why?
13. What is the maximum safe dose of the local anesthetics?
14. What would be your choice of technique if a bilateral block were required?

D. Postoperative Management

1. In the recovery room, the patient complained of shortness of breath. How would you manage this problem?
2. How do you treat a systemic reaction to a local anesthetic?
3. On the second postoperative day, the patient complained of persistent numbness and paresthesia in the right forearm and the hand. How would you manage this neurologic dysfunction?

A. Medical Disease and Differential Diagnosis

A.1. What were the presenting problems in this patient?

This patient presented for emergency surgery for a crush injury to the hand. Blood loss, which might be significant, was unknown. He probably had a full stomach. A possibility of recent ingestion of alcohol or a central nervous system (CNS) depressant drug should be entertained. It is important to determine the type of drug therapy he received for his psychiatric illness.

A.2. Do you have any concerns about the use of meperidine in the emergency room?

In this patient, meperidine presents several potential problems. Meperidine would potentiate the effects of recently ingested alcohol or any central nervous system (CNS) depressant drug, which might lead to respiratory depression. If the patient has bled significantly, meperidine may induce hypotension. The emetic side effects of meperidine, along with its effect on gastroesophageal sphincter tone, may increase the likelihood of nausea and vomiting in this patient. It would be prudent to determine which psychotropic medication the patient was taking, because the potential for serious drug interaction exists.

Miller RD, ed. *Miller's anesthesia*, 6th ed. New York: Churchill Livingstone, 2005:379–437.

A.3. What are the possible drug interactions between meperidine and the commonly used psychotropic drugs?

The psychotropic agents commonly employed and of concern to the anesthesiologist include antidepressants, antipsychotic agents, and lithium. This patient is most likely taking antidepressants. Two types of antidepressants are available: tricyclics and monoamine oxidase inhibitors (MAOIs). The commonly used tricyclics include imipramine, amitriptyline, desipramine, nortriptyline, doxepin, and protriptyline. Tricyclics enhance the effects of meperidine, namely analgesia, respiratory depression, and cholinergic side effects. MAOIs are usually the second line of antidepressants. They include tranylcypromine, phenelzine, pargyline, nialamide, furazolidone, and isocarboxazid. In the presence of MAOIs, meperidine may cause profound respiratory depression, hypotension, agitation, excitement, restlessness, hypertension, headache, rigidity, convulsions, hyperpyrexia, and coma.

Miller RD, ed. *Miller's anesthesia*, 6th ed. New York: Churchill Livingstone, 2005:423, 658, 1122–1124.

Wells DG, Bjorksten AR. Monoamine oxidase inhibitors revisited. *Can J Anaesth* 1989; 36:64–74.

A.4. What are the anesthetic implications of tricyclic antidepressants (TCAs) and monoamine oxidase inhibitors (MAOIs)?

TCAs block the reuptake of norepinephrine and serotonin or dopamine at the presynaptic nerve endings. This predisposes the patients receiving chronic tricyclic therapy to perioperative hypotension. The response to pressor agents is exaggerated two to ten times. Therefore, a possibility of hypertensive crisis exists with the usual doses of sympathomimetic amines. Other interactions are summarized in Table 27.1. It is conceivable that additive toxicity exists when drugs with similar effects on presynaptic nerve endings (e.g., cocaine, pancuronium, and ketamine) are used concomitantly. Ventricular tachycardia and fibrillation have been described when halothane and pancuronium were used together in patients receiving TCAs.

MAOIs prevent deamination of serotonin, norepinephrine, and dopamine. This causes an exaggerated response with the likelihood of hypertensive crisis, particularly when indirect-acting pressors (e.g., ephedrine or metaraminol) are used. Potentially lethal interactions (although uncommon) occur with narcotics, especially meperidine. Other interactions with anesthetic drugs are summarized in Table 27.2.

Table 27.1 Some Interactions between Tricyclic Antidepressants and Drugs Used in Anesthesia.

DRUGS USED IN ANESTHESIA	INTERACTION
Narcotics	↑ Analgesia
	↑ Respiratory depression
Barbiturates	↑ Sleep time
Anticholinergics	↑ Central activity
	↑ Peripheral activity
Sympathomimetics	↑ Effect of direct-acting agents

↑, increase.
From Smith NT, Corbascio AN, eds. *Drug interactions in anesthesia,* 2nd ed. Philadelphia: Lea & Febiger, 1986:268, with permission.

Table 27.2 **Some Interactions between Monoamine Oxidase Inhibitors and Drugs Used in Anesthesia.**

DRUGS USED IN ANESTHESIA	INTERACTION
Inhalation drugs	Muscle stiffness, hyperpyrexia (halothane in animals)
Narcotics	Meperidine → excitatory syndrome → ↑ narcotic effect and coma
Barbiturates	↑ Sleep time
Anticholinergics	↑ Central activity
Sympathomimetics	↑↑ Effects of indirect-acting agents
	↑ Effects of direct-acting agents
	↑ Dopamine effects
Muscle relaxants	↑ Duration of block with succinylcholine (phenelzine decreases plasma cholinesterase)

↑, increase; ↑↑, much increase; →, cause.
From Smith NT, Corbascio AN, eds. *Drug interactions in anesthesia,* 2nd ed. Philadelphia: Lea & Febiger, 1986:270, with permission.

Ebrahim ZY, O'Hara JF, Borden L, et al. Monoamine oxidase inhibitors and elective surgery. *Cleve Clin J Med* 1993;60:129.

El-Ganzouri AR, Ivankovich AD, Braverman E, et al. Monoamine oxidase inhibitors: should they be discontinued preoperatively? *Anesth Analg* 1985;64:592.

Miller RD, ed. *Miller's anesthesia*, 6th ed. New York: Churchill Livingstone, 2005:1122–1124.

Stack CG, Rogers P, Linters PK. Monoamine oxidase inhibitors in anesthesia: a review. *Br J Anaesth* 1988;60:222.

Wells DG, Bjorksten AR. Monoamine oxidase inhibitors revisited. *Can J Anaesth* 1989; 36:64–74.

A.5. **In an elective case, would you discontinue the use of tricyclics or monoamine oxidase inhibitors (MAOIs) preoperatively?**

Until recently, the common belief has been that MAOIs should be discontinued for at least 2 weeks before surgery and that tricyclic antidepressants (TCAs) be substituted for therapy. A closer scrutiny of the literature reveals that the adverse drug reactions occur only in a few patients receiving MAOIs and that anesthesia can be safely administered in these patients. Therefore, a 2-week discontinuation is not necessary if MAOI therapy is appropriate and properly monitored. Moreover, patients receiving MAOIs often have severe depressive illness and run a major risk of suicide. Consequently, discontinuation of the drugs may be life threatening. Direct adrenergic agonists or antagonists should be used to treat hypotension, hypertension, or arrhythmias. TCAs, on the other hand, can be continued to the day of surgery. Again, only direct adrenergic agonists or antagonists should be used in smaller than usual doses to treat any cardiovascular instability.

Ebrahim ZY, O'Hara JF, Borden L, et al. Monoamine oxidase inhibitors and elective surgery. *Cleve Clin J Med* 1993;60:129.

El-Ganzouri AR, Ivankovich AD, Braverman E, et al. Monoamine oxidase inhibitors: should they be discontinued preoperatively? *Anesth Analg* 1985;64:592.

Smith NT, Corbascio AN, eds. *Drug interactions in anesthesia*, 2nd ed. Philadelphia: Lea & Febiger, 1986:261–281.

Stack CG, Rogers P, Linters PK. Monoamine oxidase inhibitors in anesthesia: a review. *Br J Anaesth* 1988;60:222.

Wells DG, Bjorksten AR. Monoamine oxidase inhibitors revisited. *Can J Anaesth* 1989; 36:64–74.

A.6. What precautions should be taken to anesthetize a patient receiving monoamine oxidase inhibitors (MAOIs)?

It is not possible to define those patients in whom adverse reactions are likely to occur. Therefore, all patients receiving MAOIs should be assumed at potential risk of adverse drug reactions. The following precautions should be taken:

- Preoperative liver function test should be done because of the possibility of drug-induced abnormalities.
- Premedication should be generous to prevent overreaction to anxiety.
- Close monitoring of heart rate and blood pressure through an arterial cannula is recommended.
- Avoid sympathetic stimulation.
- Avoid meperidine. If narcotics are required, morphine or preferably fentanyl may be used.
- Avoid indirect-acting sympathomimetic amines such as ephedrine, methamphetamine, and mephentermine, because they markedly increase the intraneuronal storage of norepinephrine. If needed, direct-acting sympathomimetics should be titrated carefully.
- Avoid cocaine because it inhibits reuptake of endogenous norepinephrine, resulting in a buildup of norepinephrine.

Ebrahim ZY, O'Hara JF, Borden L, et al. Monoamine oxidase inhibitors and elective surgery. *Cleve Clin J Med* 1993;60:129.

Mangano DT, ed. *Preoperative cardiac assessment*. Philadelphia: JB Lippincott, 1990:162.

Stack CG, Rogers P, Linters PK. Monoamine oxidase inhibitors in anesthesia: a review. *Br J Anaesth* 1988;60:222.

Wells DG, Bjorksten AR. Monoamine oxidase inhibitors revisited. *Can J Anaesth* 1989; 36:64–74.

B. Preoperative Evaluation and Preparation

B.1. What premedication would you order?

No single premedication regimen has been shown to be consistently better than others. This patient has already received meperidine. If careful history rules out any significant problems or other drug intake, intravenous midazolam that is carefully titrated in the operating room may be beneficial if a plexus block with local anesthetics is planned. Benzodiazepines have been shown to elevate the patient's convulsion threshold to local anesthetics.

Cousins MJ, Bridenbaugh PO, eds. Neural blockade. In: *Clinical anesthesia and management of pain*, 3rd ed. Philadelphia: Lippincott Williams & Wilkins, 1998:179–199.

C. Intraoperative Management

C.1. What anesthetic technique would you employ?

Left brachial plexus block is preferred to a general anesthetic in this patient because it provides adequate anesthesia with good operating conditions while decreasing the likelihood of aspiration.

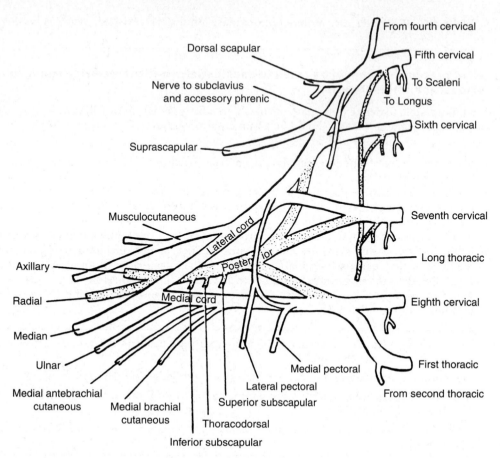

Figure 27.1 Plan of brachial plexus. (From Clemente CD, ed. *Gray's anatomy*, 30th ed. Philadelphia: Lea & Febiger, 1985:1205, with permission.)

C.2. Describe the formation and major branches of the brachial plexus.

The brachial plexus supplies the nerves to the upper limb. It is formed by the ventral primary divisions of the fifth to the eighth cervical and the first thoracic nerves, with contributions from the fourth cervical and the second thoracic roots. The roots join to form the superior, middle, and inferior trunks, which divide into anterior and posterior divisions (Fig. 27.1). The three posterior divisions form the posterior cord whose major branches are the radial and the axillary nerves. The upper two anterior divisions form the lateral cord whose major branches are the musculocutaneous nerve and the lateral root of the median nerve. The lowest anterior division forms the medial cord, which gives the medial root to the median nerve and terminates as the ulnar nerve. The sympathetic contributions to the brachial plexus are derived from the middle cervical ganglion and the stellate ganglion.

C.3. What regional technique would you choose to block the brachial plexus in this patient?

We would prefer an axillary perivascular technique of brachial plexus block. It is the easiest and the safest block to perform, and it provides adequate anesthesia for a surgical procedure on the hand.

C.4. What are the advantages and disadvantages of axillary, interscalene, subclavian, and supraclavicular nerve blocks?

Four classic routes were described for blocking the brachial plexus: paravertebral (Kappis); axillary (Hirschel); infraclavicular (Louis, Bazy); and supraclavicular (Kulenbampff). The first two techniques have been virtually abandoned, but the infraclavicular and supraclavicular techniques have seen a resurgence in their use with the aid of ultrasound imaging. The use of ultrasound imaging directs the anesthesiologist to the targeted nerve under live guidance, with concurrent visualization of important vascular and other adjacent structures. It is being used with increasing frequency in the performance of several peripheral nerve blocks (e.g., brachial plexus, femoral, and sciatic). However, there are only two controlled studies at present comparing ultrasound to conventional techniques, and these two studies involve a femoral nerve block. The study results showed a decreased onset time, greater block intensity, and the need for a smaller volume of local anesthetic. Further studies are needed comparing conventional and ultrasound-guided techniques for the brachial plexus, but the obvious advantages of a decreased onset time, greater block intensity, and smaller volume of local anesthetic requirement, if they are proved, are very encouraging. The perivascular techniques of brachial plexus block (Winnie, Collins) by axillary, interscalene, or subclavian approach are by far the most commonly employed techniques. The advantages and disadvantages of these techniques are described as follows:

Perivascular axillary block

Advantages:

- Excellent anesthesia for forearm and hand
- Easy technique
- Landmark (axillary artery) easy to identify
- Safest of all techniques
- Easiest of techniques to perform in children
- Paresthesias not necessary

Disadvantages:

- Insufficient anesthesia for shoulder and upper arm
- Abduction of the arm required to perform the technique (e.g., for painful shoulders or radius fractures)
- Intravascular injection (rare)
- Hematoma (extremely rare)

Perivascular interscalene block

Advantages:

- Ideal for shoulder surgery
- Cervical plexus can be blocked as well
- Can be performed if arm is immobilized
- Landmarks usually clear
- Lower volume of local anesthetic can be employed
- Much reduced likelihood of pneumothorax compared with supraclavicular block

Disadvantages:

- Lower trunk anesthesia may be missed
- May block phrenic, vagus, recurrent laryngeal, or cervical sympathetic nerves
- Inadvertent epidural, subdural, or spinal anesthesia reported
- Intravascular injection into vertebral artery possible

Perivascular subclavian block

Advantages:

- Landmarks (interscalene groove and subclavian artery) easy to identify
- Can be performed even if arm is immobilized
- Smaller volume of local anesthetic can be used compared with the axillary block
- Less likelihood of missing the lower trunk than with the interscalene block

Disadvantages:

- Paresthesias needed to ensure the success of the block (less pleasant for the patient)
- Pneumothorax (extremely rare)
- Block of phrenic, recurrent laryngeal, and cervical sympathetics possible, especially with large volumes of local anesthetic

Supraclavicular block

Advantages:

- Brachial plexus blocked where most compactly arranged
- Most intense block produced
- Smaller volume required
- Quick onset
- All of the nerves are reliably blocked
- Can be performed if arm is immobilized

Disadvantages:

- Paresthesias required (unpleasant for patient)
- Pneumothorax (0.5% to 6%)
- Phrenic nerve block (40% to 60%)
- Stellate ganglion block (70% to 90%)
- Possible neuritis

Adriani J, ed. *Labat's regional anesthesia techniques and clinical applications*, 4th ed. St. Louis: Warren H. Green, 1985:254–280.

Brown DL. Brachial plexus blocks: an update. *ASA annual meeting refresher course lectures*. Park Ridge: American Society of Anesthesiologists, 2005:245.

Miller RD, ed. *Miller's anesthesia*, 6th ed. New York: Churchill Livingstone, 2005:1685–1695.

Tetzlaff JE, Yoon HJ, Dilger J, et al. Subdural anesthesia as a complication of an interscalene brachial plexus block. *Reg Anesth* 1994;19:357–359.

Urmey WF, Talts KH, Sharrock NE. One hundred percent incidence of hemidiaphragmatic paresis associated with interscalene brachial plexus anesthesia as diagnosed by ultrasonography. *Anesth Analg* 1991;72:498–503.

Winnie AP. *Plexus anesthesia, Perivascular techniques of brachial plexus block*. Vol I. Denmark: Schultz, 1983:197–203.

Sites BD. Introduction to ultrasound-guided regional anesthesia: seeing is believing. *ASA annual meeting refresher course lectures*. Park Ridge: American Society of Anesthesiologists, 2005:319.

C.5. Describe the landmarks and procedure of an axillary nerve block.

The major landmark for the axillary perivascular technique is the axillary artery. The patient lies supine with the arm abducted 75 to 90 degrees and the forearm flexed at the elbow. The axillary artery is palpated and followed as far proximally as possible under the pectoralis major. At this point, with the index finger directly over the pulse, a 1.5-in., 21-gauge short-bevel needle is inserted just above the fingertip and advanced toward the apex of the axilla at a 10- to 20-degree angle to the artery. (For the beginner, an easy procedure is to aim for the artery when advancing the needle, as if attempting to place an intraarterial catheter.) When a "click" is felt, caused by penetration of the fascial sheath, 20 to 40 mL of the anesthetic solution is injected. The amount is determined by the patient's age. The finger over the pulse is pressed against the humerus to decrease the distal spread of the solution, thereby promoting the cephalad spread to anesthetize the entire brachial plexus. Repeated aspiration is a must during injection to prevent accidental injection of a large dose of a local anesthetic intravascularly.

Miller RD, ed. *Miller's anesthesia*, 6th ed. New York: Churchill Livingstone, 2005:1685–1695.

Winnie AP. *Plexus anesthesia, Perivascular techniques of brachial plexus block*. Vol I. Denmark: Schultz, 1983:197–203.

C.6. Describe the landmarks and procedure of an interscalene nerve block.

The landmarks for the interscalene block include the cricoid cartilage, the transverse process of C6 vertebra, the interscalene groove, and the external jugular vein.

The patient lies supine with the head turned slightly to the contralateral side. The posterior border of the sternocleidomastoid muscle is palpated, and the fingers are rolled back to the interscalene groove at the level of C6 vertebra (cricoid cartilage). The needle is inserted at this point and directed caudad, mesiad, and posteriorly. Once paresthesia is elicited, 10 to 40 mL of solution is injected. In an adult, 20 mL of solution should anesthetize the brachial plexus (the lower trunk may often be spared with this volume). Increasing the volume to 40 mL blocks the cervical and brachial plexuses effectively.

Miller RD, ed. *Miller's anesthesia*, 6th ed. New York: Churchill Livingstone, 2005: 1685–1695.

Winnie AP. *Plexus anesthesia, Perivascular techniques of brachial plexus block*. Vol I. Denmark: Schultz, 1983.

C.7. What is the incidence of hemidiaphragmatic paresis after an interscalene brachial plexus block?

Interscalene brachial plexus block with 40 to 50 mL of local anesthetic virtually ensures a 100% incidence of ipsilateral hemidiaphragmatic paresis. The fibrous sheath that encases the cervical and brachial plexuses allow for the spread of local anesthetic to occur.

Decreasing the injected volume of local anesthetic to 20 mL does not reduce the likelihood of diaphragmatic paresis or significantly lessen the pulmonary effects. The pulmonary changes and diaphragmatic paresis following interscalene brachial plexus block are completed within the first 15 minutes, making worsening of respiratory function unlikely postoperatively. Within 3 to 4 hours, most patients will exhibit the return of normal hemidiaphragmatic motion. Compared with an interscalene brachial plexus block, a supraclavicular block has a lower incidence of ipsilateral hemidiaphragmatic paresis, and an axillary block will usually have no effect on hemidiaphragmatic function.

Neal JM, Moore JM, Kopacz DJ, et al. Quantitative analysis of respiratory, motor, and sensory function after supraclavicular block. *Anesth Analg* 1998;86:1239–1244.

Urmey WF, Gloeggler PJ. Pulmonary function changes during interscalene brachial plexus block: effects of decreasing local anesthetic injection volume. *Reg Anesth* 1993;18:244–249.

Urmey WF, McDonald M. Hemidiaphragmatic paresis during interscalene brachial plexus block: effects on pulmonary function and chest wall mechanics. *Anesth Analg* 1992;74:352–357.

Urmey WF, Talts KH, Sharrock NE. One hundred percent incidence of hemidiaphragmatic paresis associated with interscalene brachial plexus anesthesia as diagnosed by ultrasonography. *Anesth Analg* 1991;72:498–503.

C.8. Describe the pulmonary function changes that occur after an interscalene brachial plexus block.

In addition to ipsilateral hemidiaphragmatic paresis, an interscalene brachial plexus block will also produce other changes in pulmonary function and chest wall mechanics. Measures of pulmonary function, such as forced vital capacity (FVC) and forced expiratory volume in 1 second are reduced by approximately 25% after an interscalene block. Similar to the onset of hemidiaphragmatic paresis, the degree of reduction of pulmonary function begins to plateau at 15 minutes. With regard to chest wall mechanics, an interscalene block will result in increased upper rib cage expansion and ipsilateral paradoxical inward motion of the hemiabdomen during inspiration (Fig. 27.2). Increased expansion of the rib cage presumably reflects increased activity of the intercostals and accessory muscles of inspiration.

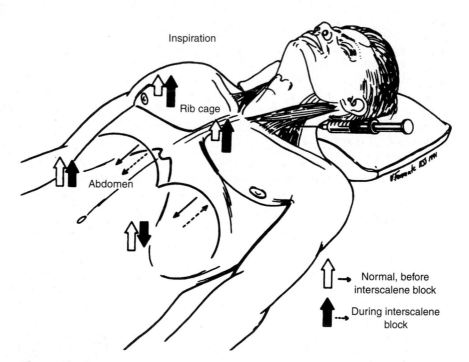

Figure 27.2 Illustration of typical changes in chest wall motion measured by magnetometry during interscalene anesthesia. The ipsilateral hemiabdomen no longer expanded, contracting instead with tidal inspiration 10 minutes after interscalene brachial plexus injection of mepivacaine. (From Urmey WF, McDonald M. Hemidiaphragmatic paresis during interscalene brachial plexus block: effects on pulmonary function and chest wall mechanics. *Anesth Analg* 1992;74:356, with permission.)

In summary, patients who receive an interscalene brachial plexus block can be expected to have decreased inspiratory strength secondary to hemidiaphragmatic paresis, as well as a reduced ability to cough and clear secretions. Given the undesirable changes in pulmonary function that would occur from an interscalene block, patients with preexisting pulmonary disease may require a different anesthetic technique if it is anticipated that they will not tolerate the reductions in pulmonary function. Absolute contraindications include patients with contralateral hemidiaphragmatic paresis, pneumothorax, or a history of contralateral pneumonectomy, as well as patient refusal.

Neal JM, Moore JM, Kopacz DJ, et al. Quantitative analysis of respiratory, motor, and sensory function after supraclavicular block. *Anesth Analg* 1998;86:1239–1244.

Urmey WF, Gloeggler PJ. Pulmonary function changes during interscalene brachial plexus block: effects of decreasing local anesthetic injection volume. *Reg Anesth* 1993;18:244–249.

Urmey WF, McDonald M. Hemidiaphragmatic paresis during interscalene brachial plexus block: effects on pulmonary function and chest wall mechanics. *Anesth Analg* 1992; 74:352–357.

Urmey WF, Talts KH, Sharrock NE. One hundred percent incidence of hemidiaphragmatic paresis associated with interscalene brachial plexus anesthesia as diagnosed by ultrasonography. *Anesth Analg* 1991;72:498–503.

C.9. What would you do if the patient complained of dyspnea after performing an interscalene block?

Respiratory symptoms can occur after an interscalene brachial plexus block, even in patients without evidence of preexisting pulmonary pathology. If symptoms are present, complaints are usually of mild dyspnea or altered respiratory sensation. For these reasons, pulse oximetry and supplemental oxygen should always be used on patients receiving an interscalene block. If the patient complains of dyspnea, all that is usually needed is reassurance and observation. To optimize diaphragmatic mechanics, one should place the patient in the sitting position if possible. The sitting position will result in an increased forced vital capacity (FVC) compared with the supine position. Because auscultation of the ipsilateral side will likely show diminished breath sounds, a chest radiograph is required if a pneumothorax is suspected. Positive pressure ventilation through a mask or endotracheal tube should be performed if clinically indicated.

Neal JM, Moore JM, Kopacz DJ, et al. Quantitative analysis of respiratory, motor, and sensory function after supraclavicular block. *Anesth Analg* 1998;86:1239–1244.

Urmey WF, Gloeggler PJ. Pulmonary function changes during interscalene brachial plexus block: effects of decreasing local anesthetic injection volume. *Reg Anesth* 1993;18:244–249.

Urmey WF, McDonald M. Hemidiaphragmatic paresis during interscalene brachial plexus block: effects on pulmonary function and chest wall mechanics. *Anesth Analg* 1992; 74:352–357.

Urmey WF, Talts KH, Sharrock NE. One hundred percent incidence of hemidiaphragmatic paresis associated with interscalene brachial plexus anesthesia as diagnosed by ultrasonography. *Anesth Analg* 1991;72:498–503.

C.10. What are the most commonly missed nerves with an axillary nerve block and an interscalene nerve block? How can you circumvent this problem?

In axillary block, the nerves missed most often are the musculocutaneous and circumflex nerves, because the exits from the sheath are higher up. Injecting a large volume (at least 40 mL in an adult man), keeping distal digital pressure to prevent distal spread of the solution, and avoiding abduction of the arm more than 90 degrees during and after the injection can promote the cephalad spread of the solution to block these nerves. In addition, the musculocutaneous nerve can be blocked in the substance of the coracobrachialis muscle by injecting 5 to 7 mL of the local anesthetic solution. The cutaneous branches can also be blocked at the lateral border of the biceps, just above the elbow crease. If a tourniquet is to be used, T2 must be blocked, which can be done easily by injecting 3 to 4 mL of local anesthetic subcutaneously as the needle is withdrawn after the axillary block.

In the interscalene approach, the most frequently missed nerves are the nerves derived from the lower trunk (C8, T1), namely, the ulnar, the medial brachial cutaneous, and the medial antebrachial cutaneous nerves. Use of a larger volume of anesthetic solution (40 mL in an adult man) and digital pressure proximal to the injection promotes distal spread of the solution, thereby producing complete block of the brachial plexus. For surgery of the hand, the ulnar nerve can be blocked behind the medial epicondyle at the elbow. If surgery involves the forearm, or if a tourniquet is to be used, the medial antebrachial nerve must be blocked in the arm subcutaneously and T2 must be blocked as described.

Winnie AP. *Plexus anesthesia, Perivascular techniques of brachial plexus block*. Vol I. Denmark: Schultz, 1983:197–203.

C.11. After an axillary block, the patient complained of tourniquet-related pain. How would you manage this problem?

Tourniquet-related pain seems to be mediated by the somatic and the sympathetic nerves. This entity is not completely understood and occasionally may be refractory to the usual means of management. Several steps can be taken to manage tourniquet-related pain: The intercostobrachial nerves can be blocked by injecting 3 to 5 mL of the local anesthetic subcutaneously in the axilla; the musculocutaneous nerve can be blocked in the substance of the coracobrachialis using 5 to 7 mL of the local anesthetic solution; a circumferential subcutaneous infiltration with local anesthetic may be used, although its use has been questioned by many; intravenous analgesic sedation may be added; nitrous oxide analgesia may be added to the regimen; and if conditions allow, the tourniquet can be released temporarily and reinflated after a rest period. Occasionally, the surgeon may be able to finish the rest of the procedure without the tourniquet. If none of these steps is helpful or practical, general anesthesia may have to be induced, with intubation of the trachea to protect the airway. Each of the aforementioned measures can be instituted separately or in combination with others, depending on the individual demands of each situation.

Miller RD, ed. *Miller's anesthesia*, 6th ed. New York: Churchill Livingstone, 2005:1685–1695, 2423–2425.

C.12. What local anesthetic agent would you use and why?

A wide spectrum of local anesthetics is available and the choice is dictated primarily by the duration of the procedure (Table 27.3).

Miller RD, ed. *Miller's anesthesia*, 6th ed. New York: Churchill Livingstone, 2005:573–603.

Table 27.3 Duration of Procedure and Selection of Local Anesthetics.

ANTICIPATED DURATION OF OPERATION	LOCAL ANESTHETIC RECOMMENDED
20–30 min	2% procaine
30–60 min	2% procaine with epinephrine or 2% chloroprocaine[a]
60–90 min	2% chloroprocaine with epinephrine or 1% lidocaine
2–3 hr	1% lidocaine with epinephrine or 1% mepivacaine
	1% mepivacaine with epinephrine or 1% prilocaine or mixture of mepivacaine and tetracaine with epinephrine
5–6 hr	0.15%–0.2% tetracaine with epinephrine
10–12 hr	0.5% bupivacaine or 0.5% ropivacaine

All durations are approximate guidelines at best, because fairly wide standard deviations exist when durations of local anesthetic actions are measured clinically.
[a]Epinephrine is recommended in 1:200,000 concentrations.

Rosenblatt MA. Practical regional anesthesia for outpatients. *ASA annual refresher course lectures*. Park Ridge: American Society of Anesthesiologists, 2005:137.

Winnie AP. *Plexus anesthesia, Perivascular techniques of brachial plexus block*. Vol I. Denmark: Schultz, 1983:197–203.

C.13. What is the maximum safe dose of the local anesthetics?

The maximum safe doses of the commonly used local anesthetics for infiltration and blocks are shown in Table 27.4.

Miller RD, ed. *Miller's anesthesia*, 6th ed. New York: Churchill Livingstone, 2005:573–603.

C.14. What would be your choice of technique if a bilateral block were required?

Bilateral blocks in the neck (i.e., interscalene, subclavian, and supraclavicular) should not be performed because of the potentially fatal complications of bilateral phrenic nerve block, recurrent laryngeal nerve block, and pneumothorax. Bilateral blocks in the axilla would require a total local anesthetic dose in excess of the maximum safe dose; hence, they should be avoided. To circumvent this problem, the anesthesiologist may perform one block in the axilla and the other in the neck, to reduce the total dose of local anesthetic used. Alternatively, the two blocks can

Table 27.4 Maximum Safe Doses of Local Anesthetics for Infiltration and Blocks.

LOCAL ANESTHETIC	DOSE PLAIN (mg)	DOSE WITH EPINEPHRINE (mg)
Lidocaine	400	500 (7 mg/kg)
Prilocaine	400	600
Mepivacaine	400	500
Etidocaine	300	400
Bupivacaine	175	250 (3 mg/kg)
Procaine	500	750–1,000
Chloroprocaine	600	800–1,000
Tetracaine	100	150–200

be spaced to allow for biodegradation of the drug. General anesthesia should also be considered, and its risks and benefits weighed against bilateral brachial plexus block.

D. Postoperative Management

D.1. In the recovery room, the patient complained of shortness of breath. How would you manage this problem?

Pneumothorax should always be ruled out if the patient has shortness of breath after receiving a brachial plexus block. The presence of subcutaneous emphysema is indicative of a pneumothorax. Supportive therapy, including oxygen, should be instituted immediately and a chest radiograph obtained to determine the extent of the pneumothorax. Pneumothorax resolves spontaneously in most cases. Patients with more than 50% pneumothorax invariably require treatment. Air can be aspirated by means of a wide-bore needle through the second intercostal space, or a chest tube may need to be inserted and connected to underwater drainage.

D.2. How do you treat a systemic reaction to a local anesthetic?

Refer to Chapter 29, Question C.3.

D.3. On the second postoperative day, the patient complained of persistent numbness and paresthesia in the right forearm and the hand. How would you manage this neurologic dysfunction?

Persistent neurologic dysfunction following brachial plexus block has been reported to be from 0.1% to 1.9%. However, before assuming anesthetic technique or neurotoxicity of local anesthetic to be the cause, other causes must be carefully ruled out. In this patient, they include the crush injury to the hand and lacerated nerves, tourniquet pressure, retractors used during surgery, a tight cast or dressing, positioning of the arm during surgery and in the immediate postoperative period although the neural block is still present, and any undiagnosed preexisting conditions such as previous injury, diabetes, or alcoholic neuropathy.

A detailed history for preexisting conditions must be sought. Assuming none exists, a careful history of current anesthetic technique including eliciting of paresthesia should be obtained. Anesthetic drugs, their concentration and dose, and any additives should be documented. A review of pattern of onset of regional block and its regression is necessary.

A detailed focused physical examination is helpful in localizing the nerve injury and therefore useful in differential diagnosis. For example, a glove and stocking type of distribution may suggest tourniquet-induced injury, whereas a neurologic injury in the dermatomal distribution where paresthesia was obtained might indicate a needle-induced nerve lesion.

Most nerve injuries resolve within days or weeks; however, some may persist and become permanent. Therefore, a neurologic consultation is recommended for initial evaluation and follow-up. Electromyograph and nerve conduction study results may or may not be abnormal initially but will become abnormal in subsequent weeks if symptoms persist. Reassuring the patient and effective communication between the anesthesiologist, the neurologist, and the surgeon are a must.

Cooper K, Kelley H, Carrithers J. Perception of side-effects following axillary block used for outpatient surgery. *Reg Anesth* 1995;20:212–216.

Kroll DA, Caplan RA, Posner K. Nerve injury associated with anesthesia. *Anesthesiology* 1990;73:202–207.

Selander D. Neurotoxicity of local anesthetics: animal data. *Reg Anesth* 1993;18:461–468.

Winchell SW, Wolfe R. The incidence of neuropathy following upper extremity blocks. *Reg Anesth* 1985;10:12–15.

CHAPTER 28

Nerve Blocks of the Lower Extremity

Jeffrey Y.F. Ngeow • Philip S.L. Chan • David Y. Wang

A 35-YEAR-OLD MAN

is scheduled for drainage of an abscess in his left great toe. He also has an effusion in his right knee that may need arthroscopy, pending the Gram stain result of intraoperative needle aspiration. His medical history is significant for heavy smoking (40 pack-years), severe aortoiliac occlusive disease, and recurrent attacks of lower extremity pain that are associated with sloughing of the pulp tissues of the digits. His anesthetic history is significant for a difficult intubation three years ago during laparoscopic cholecystectomy. His only regular medication is clopidogrel (Plavix), which he stopped 4 days ago. He has had a previous magnetic resonance angiogram, which was read as abnormal.

A. Medical Disease and Differential Diagnosis
  1. What are the possible causes of abscess in the digits?
  2. What is a Charcot joint?
  3. What is thromboangiitis obliterans?

B. Preoperative Evaluation and Preparation
  1. How is the status of the local perfusion in the foot assessed? Why is the abnormal magnetic resonance angiogram a concern?
  2. Will you be concerned with the status of neurologic function in this patient?
  3. What investigations should be reviewed in evaluating this patient?
  4. What anesthetic options should be discussed with the patient preoperatively?

C. Intraoperative Management
  1. What monitoring should be employed intraoperatively?
  2. What are the landmarks for an ankle block?
  3. What are the advantages and disadvantages of an ankle block?
  4. What other peripheral regional anesthetic techniques may be appropriate for incision and drainage of an abscess?
  5. What peripheral nerve blocks can be used for the arthroscopy?
  6. Why is ultrasound guidance potentially useful in performing peripheral nerve blocks?

D. Postoperative management

   1. How should the postoperative pain management of this patient be handled?

   2. Why should the neurovascular status of the patient subsequently be followed?

A. Medical Disease and Differential Diagnosis

A.1. What are the possible causes of abscess in the digits?

There are different types of bacterial infections of the digits—felon (infection of the pulp of the digit), paronychia (infection localized to the area around the nail root), suppurative flexor tenosynovitis, and pyogenic arthritis.

Acute infection may result from traumatic contamination (e.g., animal bites or puncture with a contaminated needle) or from foreign bodies such as splinters or inclusion cysts. Abscess may also be caused by chronic infections such as osteomyelitis with sequestrum.

A number of conditions may produce local neurovascular insufficiency, which predisposes the patient to localized infection. These include arterial insufficiency from atherosclerosis, venous stasis disease, previous surgery or trauma that resulted in denervation and fibrosis, Charcot joint (see question A.2), syringomyelia, Hansen's disease (leprosy), and tabes dorsalis (tertiary syphilis).

Various systemic diseases may also predispose a patient to abscesses. These include diabetes mellitus, generalized vascular insufficiency such as Buerger's disease (thromboangiitis obliterans; see question A.3), Reynaud's disease, disseminated lupus erythematosis, human immunodeficiency (HIV), sickle cell disease, gout, intravenous drug abuse, and neurologic deficiencies secondary to chemical or nutritional neuropathies, multiple sclerosis, and cerebral vascular accidents. Embolization from valvular vegetation in bacterial endocarditis is a rare cause of abscess in the digits.

Harris ED Jr ed. *Kelley's textbook of rheumatology*, 7th ed. Philadelphia: WB Saunders, 2005:633–634.

LeFrock JL, Joseph WS. Bone and soft tissue infections of the lower extremity in diabetics. *Clin Podiatr Med Surg* 1995;12:87–103.

A.2. What is a Charcot joint?

A Charcot joint is an arthropathy (bone and joint destruction) secondary to sensory neuropathy associated with a wide range of disorders. Although the pathogenesis is not fully understood, it is believed that a lack of protective sensations in the affected joint results in continuous microtrauma. A Charcot joint is often swollen, warm, and erythematous, making it difficult to distinguish initially from an infection; gout and rheumatoid arthritis should also be considered on the differential diagnosis. The underlying neurologic dysfunction may be the result of a wide range of diseases including metabolic disturbances such as diabetes mellitus (the most common cause), chronic uremia and chronic alcoholism. Conditions specifically resulting in destruction of dorsal column fibers such as in syringomyelia or tabes dorsalis can also result in Charcot joint formation. In children, one must consider spinal bifida with meningomyelocele as the underlying cause of the Charcot joint. In the elderly, spinal cord tumors and degenerative diseases with nerve root compression may be responsible in causing Charcot joints. There is also a sizeable group of hereditary neuropathic conditions that may cause a Charcot joint, including Charcot-Marie-Tooth disease. The incidence of osteomyelitis is increased in patients with neuropathic joints.

Trepman E, Nihal A, Pinzur MS. Current topics review: Charcot neuroarthropathy of the foot and ankle. *Foot Ankle Int* 2005;26:46–63.

A.3. What is thromboangiitis obliterans?

Also known as *Buerger's disease*, this is a condition in which there is an inflammatory, nonatherosclerotic obliteration of medium and small blood vessels in the extremities, resulting in distal extremity ischemia, ischemic ulcers, or gangrene. The sloughing of the pulp tissues of the digits seen in this patient is most likely due to thromboangiitis obliterans; the typical victim is a young adult male who is a heavy smoker (tobacco use is an absolute requirement for diagnosis). The presenting symptom is typically claudication of the foot or leg, progressing to ischemic ulcerations of the toes or fingers. The condition is reversible with smoking cessation as long as gangrene or tissue loss has not already occurred.

Olin JW, Shih A. Thromboangiitis obliterans (Buerger's disease). *Curr Opin Rheumatol* 2006;18:18–24.

B. Preoperative Evaluation and Preparation

B.1. How is the status of the local perfusion in the foot assessed? Why is the abnormal magnetic resonance angiogram a concern?

Local perfusion in an extremity can be evaluated at the bedside by palpating for arterial pulses, observing the skin temperature and color, and estimating the adequacy of capillary refill. If there is tissue edema due to inflammation, infection or gangrene, a zone of demarcation may be apparent. When arterial pulses cannot be palpated, the Doppler ultrasound flow detector may be used to locate the blood vessel. A low Ankle-Brachial Index (ABI) (ratio of blood pressure measured at the ankle over blood pressure measured over the brachial artery; normal 0.95 to 1.2) may further indicate the severity of the peripheral vascular disease.

In this patient, who has an abnormal magnetic resonance angiogram with a history of aortoiliac occlusive disease, there is a high likelihood that arterial blood flow to the foot is decreased. Therefore, any intervention that may further compromise the perfusion of the extremity, such as injection of solutions containing a vasoconstrictor, or prolonged use of a tourniquet, should be avoided.

B.2. Will you be concerned with the status of neurologic function in this patient?

In this patient with infections at multiple sites, one must consider possible systemic causes for his immunocompromise, such as diabetes mellitus. As part of the preoperative evaluation, any neurologic deficiencies associated with systemic conditions should be documented. As this patient suffers from thromboangiitis obliterans, any peripheral nerve damage, especially in the foot, should be documented prior to the conduct of regional anesthesia. Furthermore, given that the patient was on clopidogrel, and the risk of hematomas and subsequent nerve damage is unknown, it is advisable to thoroughly document any preexisting deficits.

B.3. What investigations should be reviewed in evaluating this patient?

Preoperative workup in this patient should include a review of the chest x-ray film, as well as the x-ray films of the foot, biochemistry, and the coagulation profile.

The chest x-ray may show unsuspected an immobile or elevated hemi-diaphragm in a demyelination condition. Pulmonary scarring, or even pericardial effusion, may suggest intravenous drug abuse. Such findings may have a bearing on postoperative analgesic requirements.

It may also be helpful to look at x-rays of the foot itself. If necrotic bone is present and sequestrum excision is part of the surgical plan, harvesting of bone graft either around the ankle or in the iliac crest may be required. This possibility will certainly need to be considered in the anesthetic plan.

Biochemistry test results will help to rule out systemic conditions that may be contributing to abscess formation. Analysis of blood glucose level will help rule out diabetes mellitus; blood urea nitrogen (BUN) and creatinine are useful indicators of renal function. If a history of alcohol abuse is suspected, liver enzymes and function studies (albumin, coagulation studies, etc.) should be reviewed. There is no reliable laboratory test to indicate the degree of platelet impairment for patients on clopidogrel.

B.4. What anesthetic options should be discussed with the patient preoperatively?

The simplest anesthetic method that is compatible with the requirements of the surgery, and is acceptable to the patient, should be used. In this case study, the history of difficult intubation makes general anesthesia a less desirable option for peripheral surgery. The use of neuraxial techniques is also not desirable given the recent use of clopidogrel. Although there are no studies documenting the actual risk of vertebral canal (spinal) hematoma in patients taking clopidogrel, surgical experience, as well as pharmacokinetic data, suggests discontinuation of the medication for a minimum of seven days to reduce this risk.

There is even less data on the safety of peripheral nerve blocks in the presence of clopidogrel. All the major bleeding complications associated with anticoagulation and nonneuraxial regional techniques that have been reported in the literature occurred after psoas compartment or lumbar sympathetic nerve blocks. Unlike neuraxial techniques, case reports suggest that the major risk related to nerve blocks in the presence of anticoagulation relates to blood loss, rather than neurologic complications. If surgery is deemed urgent by the surgeon, a reasonable anesthetic plan includes performing an ankle block for the left foot and peripheral nerve blocks for the right knee and iliac crest, in anticipation of the need for arthroscopy and/or bone graft harvesting.

At all times one should be cognizant that the mention of nerve blocks may evoke fear of painful needles, and anxiety at the possibility of intraoperative pain and/or awareness. A full discussion of the risks and benefits of any regional anesthetic techniques is an important part of the preoperative anesthetic consultation. Irrespective of the anesthetic techniques ultimately used, the patient must be assured of adequate relief from anxiety and pain during the induction of anesthesia, the operation itself, and the postoperative period.

There should also be a discussion of the nature and possible side effects of the drugs involved, including the medications used for intraoperative sedation, as well as the local anesthetic agents. The patient should be informed that regardless of the anesthetic technique employed, neither complete anesthesia, nor amnesia, can be assured at all stages of the operation.

Horlocker T, Wedel D, et al Regional anesthesia in the anticoagulated patient: defining the risks (the second ASRA consensus conference on neuraxial anesthesia and anticoagulation). *Reg Anesth Pain Med* 2003;28:172–197.

Shah S, Tsai T, Iwata T, et al. Outpatient regional anesthesia for foot and ankle surgery. *Int Anesthesiol Clin* 2005;43:143–151.

Spitellie PH, Holmes MA, Domino KB. Awareness during anesthesia. *Anesthesiol Clin North Am* 2002;20:555–570.

C. Intraoperative Management

C.1. What monitoring should be employed intraoperatively?

In addition to the routine vital signs monitors (electrocardiogram [ECG], blood pressure, pulse oximetry and body temperature), specific items for monitoring in this case may include Doppler ultrasonography flow detector probe on the operated limb before and after induction of anesthesia. In most cases, an increase in blood flow occurs after successful neural blockade. Any change, or lack of change, in the perfusion status of the foot should be documented. When continuous intraoperative blood flow monitoring is necessary, a sterile probe for a pulse oximeter with plethysmographic display may be attached to a nearby digit, if the operating condition permits. If a tourniquet is required, which is usually the case when blood flow is not severely compromised, the tourniquet pressure and acceptable ischemia time must be discussed with the surgeon beforehand and carefully followed. With noncritical cases of vascular insufficiency, a simple preoperative test noting the reperfusion time following a brief period of ischemia can be used as a guide for acceptability of the tourniquet.

Couse NF, Delaney CP, Horgan PG, et al. Pulse oximetry in the diagnosis of non-critical peripheral vascular insufficiency. *J R Soc Med* 1994;87:511–512.

C.2. What are the landmarks for an ankle block?

For complete anesthesia of the foot, each of the five nerves to the foot must be individually blocked. With the exception of the saphenous nerve (which is the extension of the femoral nerve), all the nerves are derived from the sciatic nerve. Various techniques and landmarks have been described by numerous authors, but essentially the two major nerves supplying motor function to the foot, the posterior tibial and the deep peroneal, require individual needle insertion whereas the sensory nerves to the foot (superficial peroneal, saphenous and sural) can be blocked by a common subcutaneous ring.

To approach the posterior tibial nerve, the foot is dorsiflexed to 90 degrees. The patient is placed either prone with the leg straight, or supine with the operated leg flexed and supported by the opposite leg. A fine gauge needle (25 to 27 G) is inserted along the medial border of the Achilles tendon at the level of the medial malleolus and advanced to contact the posterior tibia. One must be aware that the posterior tibial artery often lies between the nerve and the tibial periosteum. Three to 5 mL of the local anesthetic solution (without epinephrine) is injected if paresthesia is encountered during needle insertion; otherwise 5 to 7 mL is injected just superficial to the periosteum (Fig. 28.1).

The deep peroneal nerve at the ankle lies deep between the tendons of the tibialis anterior (TA) and the extensor hallucis longus (EHL). These tendons are identified by asking the patient to dorsiflex the big toe (EHL) and the ankle (TA). Traditionally, the nerve is blocked here. But since this nerve courses behind the EHL to emerge just lateral to the EHL tendon on the dorsum of the foot in close proximity to the anterior tibial artery, it can be more easily blocked by using the "midtarsal" approach as described by Sharrock et al. (Fig. 28.2). With this method, the dorsalis pedis pulsation is first located lateral to the EHL tendon at the midfoot, just distal to the extensor retinaculum. A fine gauge needle is inserted immediately lateral to the arterial pulse until contact is made with periosteum. After withdrawing the needle two to three mm off the periosteum, 2 to 3 mL of the local anesthetic solution (without epinephrine) should be injected.

From the same needle puncture site as the deep peroneal nerve block, the needle can be redirected to block both the branches of the superficial peroneal, saphenous, and sural nerves by making a subcutaneous ring across the dorsum of the foot using 3 to 5 mL of the anesthetic solution (without epinephrine). An alternative to blocking the sural nerve (which is not necessary

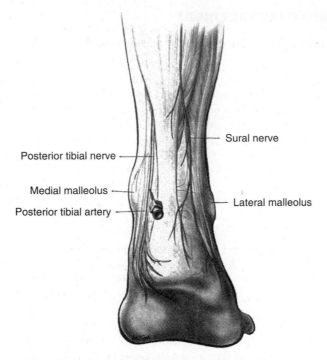

Figure 28.1 The posterior tibial nerve block.

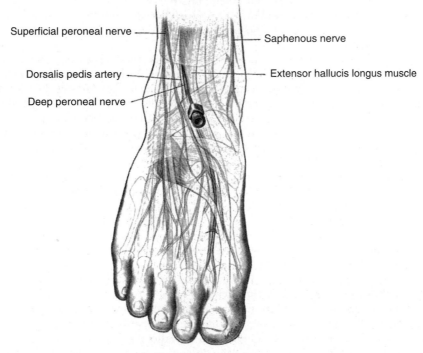

Figure 28.2 The deep peroneal nerve block.

for surgery on the great toe), the patient is positioned as for the posterior tibial nerve block, and the needle is inserted immediately lateral to the Achilles tendon at the level of the lateral malleolus in an anterolateral direction. The needle is advanced until contact is made with bone or paresthesia is elicited, and 3 to 5 mL of the local anesthetic is injected.

Brown DL. *Atlas of regional anesthesia*, 3rd ed. Philadelphia: WB Saunders, 2006:139–143.

Sharrock NE, Waller JF, Fierro LE. Midtarsal block for surgery of the forefoot. *Br J Anaesth* 1986;58:37–40.

C.3. What are the advantages and disadvantages of an ankle block?

The main advantages of an ankle block lies in its relative simplicity and safety compared to other regional methods. The landmarks used in performing this block are readily identified in most patients, and precise localization of each nerve is not necessary with this "field block" technique. Furthermore, because only a small part of the extremity is anesthetized, the major hemodynamic changes associated with neuraxial techniques will be avoided. The main complication of the ankle block is direct intraneural injection of the local anesthetic solution. Short of direct intravascular injections, systemic toxic effect from the usual volume (15 to 20 mL) of local anesthetic agents used rarely occurs. This may be due to slower uptake and distribution of the local anesthetic into the central compartment.

The two main disadvantages of this block are the discomfort associated with the performance of the block and the inability to use a pneumatic tourniquet, unless it is placed just supramalleolarly around the well-padded ankle. The ankle block is exceedingly uncomfortable for most patients because of the multiple needle insertions involved, as well as the abundance of nerve endings in the foot and ankle region, which makes it extremely sensitive to needle injections. Adequate sedation is recommended prior to carrying out the block. In addition, the long tendons of the foot continue to work, because the muscles have their nerve supply more proximally and so the patient must be reminded not to move the foot during surgery.

When prolonged numbness can be tolerated by the patient and is acceptable to the surgeon, the patient can be relieved of postsurgical pain for many hours with long acting local anesthetic agents such as bupivacaine. Both the patient and the surgical team must be forewarned of the anticipated delay in sensory and motor recovery to allay anxiety during the immediate postoperative period.

Hadzic A, Vloka J. New York school of regional anesthesia; Peripheral Nerve Blocks: "Principles and Practice". Available at: http://www.nysora.com/techniques/ankle_block/. Accessed August 20, 2006.

Lichtenfeld NS. The pneumatic ankle tourniquet with ankle block anesthesia for foot surgery. *Foot Ankle* 1992;13:344–349.

Mineo R, Sharrock NE. Venous levels of lidocaine and bupivacaine after midtarsal ankle block. *Reg Anesth* 1992;17:47–49.

C.4. What other peripheral regional anesthetic techniques may be appropriate for incision and drainage of an abscess?

There are several other ways to provide regional anesthesia for this patient. It is possible to use an intravenous regional block, when venous access is available. For tourniquets placed on the calf, 30 mL of a 0.5% lidocaine solution injected after exsanguination usually suffices. If the tourniquet is placed on the thigh, then 50 to 60 mL will be needed. The downside of this technique is that the exsanguination process may be painful for patients with an abscess.

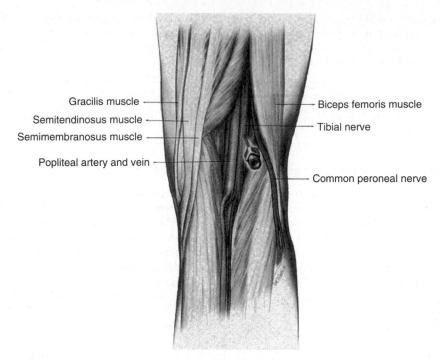

Gracilis muscle

Semitendinosus muscle

Semimembranosus muscle

Popliteal artery and vein

Biceps femoris muscle

Tibial nerve

Common peroneal nerve

Figure 28.3 Classic posterior approach of tibial nerve block.

Alternatively, the tibial, common peroneal, and saphenous nerve blocks can be done around the knee joint. At this level, the exact location of the saphenous nerve is variable. It may be blocked easily by a transverse skin wheal just inferior to the medial tibial condyle. The sciatic nerve can be consistently found at the top center of the popliteal fossa just lateral to the popliteal pulse, prior to its division into the tibial and common peroneal nerves (so-called popliteal block; see Fig. 28.3). The sciatic nerve can be blocked at this level with the patient in the prone, lateral, or supine positions (with the leg flexed at the hip and the knee).

The classic intertendinous technique involves the identification of the popliteal triangle, which is defined by the tendon of the biceps femoris laterally, the tendons of the semitendinosus and semimembranosus medially, and the popliteal fossa crease. The point of needle insertion varies among different authors, but generally the nerve can be identified 7 cm above the popliteal crease, at the midpoint between the tendons, or 9 cm above the popliteal crease, 1 cm lateral to the midline of the triangle. Localization of the nerve can be achieved using a paresthesia-seeking technique or a nerve stimulation technique. Ideally, the paresthesia elicited should be below the knee. Using a nerve stimulation technique, plantar flexion and inversion of the foot (ideally) or dorsiflexion and eversion of the foot, is sought at 0.2 to 0.5 mA current.

Using anesthetic solutions in higher concentrations (such as 2% lidocaine or 0.75% bupivacaine) with these nerve blocks, the motor nerves to the long tendons of the ankle, as well as the sensory supply to the lower leg and foot, are anesthetized. Patient movement during foot surgery is therefore minimized. Two major benefits of popliteal block are that analgesia lasts significantly longer than analgesia from an ankle block. It also allows the use of a calf tourniquet.

Enneking FK, Chan V, Greger J, et al. Lower-extremity peripheral nerve blockade: Essentials of our current understanding. *Reg Anesth Pain Med* 2005;30:4–35.

Rogers JN, Ramamurthy S. Lower extremity blocks. In: Brown DL, ed. *Regional anesthesia and analgesia*. Philadelphia: WB Saunders, 1996:279–291.

Shah S, Tsai T, Iwata T, et al. Outpatient regional anesthesia for foot and ankle surgery. *Int Anesthesiol Clin* 2005;43:143–151.

C.5. What peripheral nerve blocks can be used for the arthroscopy?

Combined femoral and sciatic nerve blocks provide an alternative to neuraxial techniques for achieving anesthesia of the knee. Although the obturator nerve also innervates the knee, its sensory terminals supply only a small area of skin just medial and superior to the knee joint. The area involved (usually just beyond the medial portal for the arthroscopy), can easily be anesthetized, if necessary, with local infiltration by the surgeon.

The femoral nerve provides sensory innervation to most of the anterior knee and can be blocked in the supine patient by injection at the femoral triangle (Fig. 28.4). The needle insertion site is immediately lateral to the femoral pulse at the level of the inguinal ligament (classical landmark) or at the level of the femoral crease. The further one moves from the inguinal canal, the more likely the nerve has divided into posterior and anterior divisions. If using a nerve stimulator, a patellar twitch (stimulation of quadriceps contraction) at 0.2 to 0.5 mA current is sought. Otherwise, the nerve can be localized by seeking paresthesia consistent with the distribution of the nerve. Injection of 10 to 25 mL of 0.5% bupivacaine here will usually provide adequate surgical anesthesia. Consideration should also be made for placement of an indwelling catheter for postoperative infusion.

A variation of the femoral nerve block is the fascia iliaca block, which was first described by Dalens. This technique does not require a nerve stimulator or the seeking of paresthesia. A line is

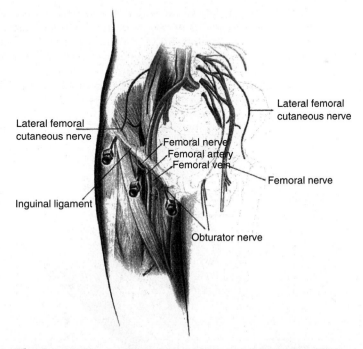

Figure 28.4 The femoral nerve block, lateral femoral cutaneous nerve block, and the obturator nerve block.

drawn between the anterior superior iliac spine (ASIS) and the pubic tubercle, and divided into thirds. The needle insertion point is made one cm caudad to this line, two thirds of the distance from the pubic tubercle. Two "pops" may be felt as the needle pierces the fascia lata, then the fascia iliaca; the use of a short bevel or pencil tipped needle may enhance the appreciation of the "pops". Twenty to 25 mL of the local anesthetic solution is then injected. Both the fascia iliaca and femoral nerve blocks are effective in providing postoperative analgesia, but the fascia iliaca block is more likely to block the lateral femoral cutaneous nerve as well.

The sciatic nerve can be blocked using a number of different approaches. The posterior approach (classically described by Labat, with modified approaches described by Winnie, Raj, DiBenedetto and others) requires placement of the patient on his/her side with the operative side up and the hip and knee flexed (Sims position). A description of all the posterior approaches to the sciatic nerve is beyond the scope of this chapter. In essence, these modified approaches utilize anatomic landmarks that are easier to locate in patients than with the Labat technique, and they block the sciatic nerve more distally in the leg, thereby avoiding painful needle insertion through the gluteal muscles.

The landmarks for the classical approach by Labat are determined by first drawing a line from the greater trochanter to the posterior superior iliac spine (PSIS) (Fig. 28.5). Winnie modified this approach by adding a second line, drawn from the greater trochanter to the sacral hiatus. From the midpoint of the PSIS line another line is drawn perpendicularly to meet the sacral hiatus line. The intersection of the perpendicular line and the sacral hiatus line is the needle insertion point. As with the popliteal block (which in essence is a distal sciatic nerve block; see C4), localization of the nerve can be achieved using a paresthesia-seeking technique or a nerve stimulation technique. Ideally, the paresthesia should be below the knee. Using a nerve stimulation technique, plantar flexion and inversion of the foot (ideally) or dorsiflexion and eversion of the foot is sought at 0.2 to 0.5 mA current. A volume of 20 to 25 mL of the anesthetic solution will be needed to cover the nerve adequately.

If the patient cannot be turned lateral, an anterior approach to the sciatic nerve may be employed. In the supine patient, a line is drawn along the inguinal ligament from the ASIS to the pubic tubercle and is trisected. Another line is drawn from the tip of the greater trochanter inferomedially parallel to the inguinal line. At the junction of the medial and second third of the trisected line a perpendicular line is drawn to meet the trochanteric line. The intersection is the point of needle entry. A needle inserted vertically here will contact the medial border of the femur

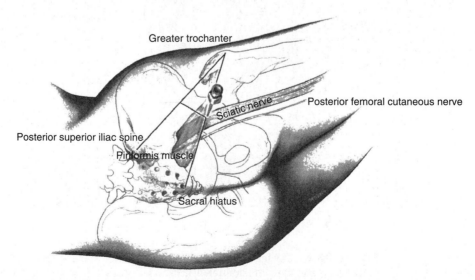

Figure 28.5 Sciatic nerve block, the Labat approach.

at the lesser trochanter. The needle is then directed slightly medially to pass the medial femoral surface. Either muscle stimulation (as described in the preceding text) or paresthesia should be sought about 5 cm deep to the femur. The posterior femoral cutaneous nerve, which leaves the main trunk early, may be missed by this approach.

Dalens B, Vanneuville G, Tanguy A. Comparison of the fascia iliaca compartment with "3-in-1" block in children. *Anesth Analg* 1989;69:705–713.

Enneking FK, Chan V, Greger J, et al. Lower-extremity peripheral nerve blockade: essentials of our current understanding. *Reg Anesth Pain Med* 2005;30:4–35.

Sharrock N, Pinchot H. Anesthetic considerations in arthroscopy. In: Scott WN, ed. *Arthroscopy of the knee, diagnosis and treatment*. Philadelphia: WB Saunders, 1990: 37–42.

C.6. Why is ultrasound guidance potentially useful in performing peripheral nerve blocks?

Most peripheral nerve blocks rely upon surface anatomic landmarks (bony, vascular, muscular, grooves) to guide initial needle placement. However, many studies have demonstrated the unreliability of these landmarks due to the wide inter-patient variability in nerve location. Furthermore, in patients with peripheral vascular disease, pulses that help in performing nerve blocks may be absent or severely diminished.

Anatomic landmarks only guide the initial needle placement; techniques such as electrical nerve stimulation or seeking of paresthesia are used to more precisely localize the nerve. Neither of these techniques are able to confirm whether the needle is intraneural, and once the local anesthetic injection has begun, it is impossible to know whether the needle position has changed.

Ultrasonography imaging offers several potential clinical benefits. Firstly, it allows visualization of nerves, which helps to define the best possible site for needle insertion. Secondly, it provides real-time guidance for the needle during its advancement toward the target nerve, thereby minimizing "hunting" for the nerve and potential complications such as vascular injury. Lastly, direct observation of local anesthetic spread at the time of injection helps ensure that the local anesthetic is deposited completely around the nerves (Figs. 28.6 to 28.8).

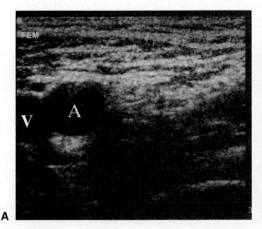
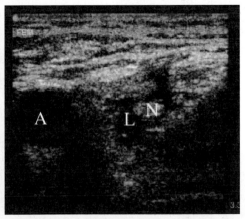

Figure 28.6 Femoral nerve block. **A:** The probe is at the top of the image. The neurovascular bundle is identified at the femoral crease. The femoral nerve (*N*) is lateral to the femoral artery (*A*). Blood vessels appear black; arteries are distinguishable from veins by its noncompressibility by the probe (*A*). **B:** The local anesthetic solution (*L*) is injected under ultrasound guidance. The appearance of a local anesthetic "doughnut" or ring around the nerve (*N*) indicates proper placement of the solution.

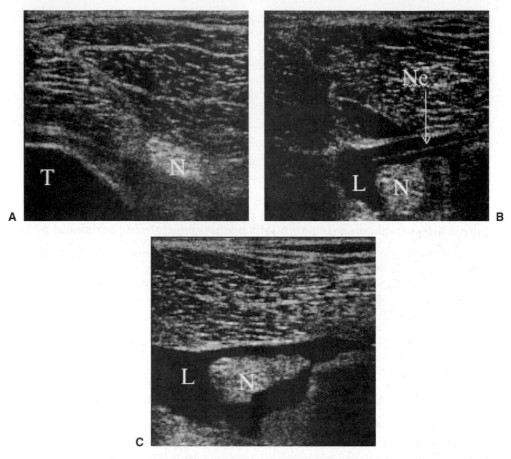

Figure 28.7 Popliteal nerve block. **A:** The nerve (*N*) is identified with the tibia (*T*) nearby. **B:** The block needle (*Ne*) is seen on the ultrasound image, and local anesthetic (*L*) is seen being deposited around the nerve. **C:** After the injection is completed, the local anesthetic is seen ringing the nerve.

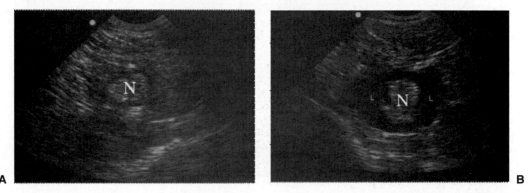

Figure 28.8 "Doughnut Sign." **A:** The nerve (*N*) is identified on ultrasound (probe on the skin is at the top of the image). **B:** A ring of local anesthetic (*L*) is seen around the nerve after injection, showing proper placement of the solution.

Despite the purported benefits, few studies exist demonstrating the superiority of ultrasound-guided blocks over nerve blocks done by traditional means; no studies have looked at whether it decreases the incidence of inadvertent intravascular injection or nerve injuries. Studies by Marhofer et al and Williams et al have shown shorter onset of sensory block time, improved block quality, and less arterial puncture (Marhofter's study only) in the performance of femoral nerve blocks and supraclavicular blocks, respectively. Nevertheless, in this clinical scenario, where performance of the nerve block may be difficult due to lack of pulses as landmarks, and the need for the block to be completely effective, ultrasound guidance may be indicated.

Awad IT, Chan V. Ultrasound imaging of peripheral nerves: a need for a new trend. *Reg Anesth Pain Med* 2005;30:321–323.

Marhofer P, Schrogendorfer K, Koining H, et al. Ultrasonographic guidance improves sensory block and onset time of three-in-one blocks. *Anesth Analg* 1997;85:854–857.

Williams SR, Chouinard P, Arcand G, et al. Ultrasound guidance speeds the execution and improves the quality of supraclavicular block. *Anesth Analg* 2003;97:1518–1523.

D. Postoperative Management

D.1. How should the postoperative pain management of this patient be handled?

The four cornerstones of postoperative pain management are the following: opioids, regional anesthesia, acetaminophen, and nonsteroidal antiinflammatory drugs (NSAIDs). Intraoperative ketorolac, or preoperative administration of a COX-II inhibitor may be useful in reducing opioid requirements. Opioids, whether given through patient-controlled systems or by nurses, should be given before sensations fully recover from the regional anesthetic technique and pain becomes severe.

Drainage of the abscess should not result in excessive postoperative pain. However, with knee arthroscopy, postoperative pain management requires preoperative planning. If the patient undergoes a synovectomy for inflammatory conditions during the knee arthroscopy, he is more likely to experience severe pain in the knee joint after the nerve block subsides. Options for postoperative pain control include preoperative insertion of a continuous femoral catheter, and/or intraoperative intraarticular injection of local anesthetic, morphine, clonidine, and/or ketorolac by the surgeon.

Brill S, Plaza M. Non-narcotic adjuvants may improve the duration and quality of analgesia after knee arthroscopy: a brief review. *Can J Anesth* 2004;51:975–978.

Macario A, Lipman A. Ketorolac in the era of cyclo-oxygenase-2 selective nonsteroidal anti-inflammatory drugs: a systematic review of efficacy, side effects, and regulatory issues. *Pain Med* 2001;2:336–351.

Straube S, Derry S, McQuay HJ, et al. Effect of preoperative Cox-II-selective NSAIDs (coxibs) on postoperative outcomes: a systematic review of randomized studies. *Acta Anaesthesiol Scand* 2005;49:601–613.

D.2. Why should the neurovascular status of the patient subsequently be followed?

It is important to follow the neurovascular function of the lower extremity for a period of 24 to 36 hours after any peripheral nerve block. In general, neurovascular dysfunction after foot and ankle surgery may arise as a result of: (a) unappreciated preexisting peripheral vascular disease; (b) accidental injury of the peripheral nerves during the surgery; (c) nerve damage during the performance of regional anesthesia; (d) tourniquet use; (f) complex regional pain syndrome; (g) deep vein thrombosis; (h) stretching of blood vessels after surgical correction of foot deformities.

The frequency of peripheral neurologic complications after single-shot peripheral nerve blocks is not well established. In their 1997 study, Auroy et al. reported nerve injury rates of 0.02% for lower extremity blocks. In their 2002 study, the incidence of neurologic complications after lower extremity blocks was 0.04%, ranging from 0.02% for sciatic nerve blocks, 0.03% for femoral blocks, and 0.31% for popliteal nerve blocks. Fanelli et al. noted a 2.1% incidence of neurologic complications from femoral-sciatic nerve blocks; 44 of the 45 patients who experienced a complication improved within 4 to 12 weeks. No specific study can be found on the incidence of neurologic complications after ankle block.

For continuous catheter techniques, the incidence of neurologic complications is not well defined, with reported incidence rates for lower extremity blocks ranging from zero for continuous popliteal catheters in Borgeat's study, to 0.4% for continuous femoral nerve blocks in Capdevila's study.

During this period, the patient should be encouraged to report any abnormal sensations and the surgical dressing should be carefully examined to ensure there is no circulatory compromise or nerve compression. In the longer term, the patient should be followed for possible neuroma formation both at the needle insertion and the surgical sites. The natural history of any preexisting neurologic dysfunction should be considered when evaluating any reported complications.

Auroy Y, Narchi P, Messiah A, et al. Serious complications related to regional anesthesia: results of a prospective survey in France. *Anesthesiology* 1997;87:479–486.

Auroy Y, Benhamou D, Bargues L, et al. Major complications of regional anesthesia in France: the SOS regional anesthesia hotline service. *Anesthesiology* 2002;97:1274–1280.

Borgeat A, Blumenthal S, Lambert M, et al. The feasibility and complications of the continuous popliteal nerve block: a 1001-case survey. *Anesth Analg* 2006;103:229–233.

Capdevila X, Pirat P, Bringuier S, et al. Continuous peripheral nerve blocks in hospital wards after orthopedic surgery: a multicenter prospective analysis of the quality of postoperative analgesia and complications in 1,416 patients. *Anesthesiology* 2005;103:1035–1045.

Easley ME. Medicolegal aspects of foot and ankle surgery. *Clin Orthopaed Related Res* 2005;433:77–81.

Fanelli G, Casati A, Garancini P, et al. Nerve stimulator and multiple injection technique for upper and lower limb blockade: failure rate, patient acceptance, and neurologic complications. Study Group on Regional Anesthesia. *Anesth Analg* 1999;88:847–852.

Summary

Although the surgery may be localized to a distal extremity, the anesthetic requirement may be much more extensive. The preoperative evaluation of the patient must be as comprehensive as with any other operations. The anesthetic techniques outlined in the preceding text offers flexibility enough to cover most demands of the surgery, yet ensures the least physiologic disturbance.

CHAPTER 29

Complex Regional Pain Syndromes

SUDHIR A. DIWAN • EDWARD S. RUBIN • VINOD MALHOTRA

A 35-YEAR-OLD MAN

complains of diffuse burning pain in the left arm and hand for the last 6 months. He recalls spraining his left wrist while playing volleyball. His left hand feels colder than the right and his fingertips are blue. He is a recently divorced high-profile executive.

A. Medical Disease and Differential Diagnosis

1. What is the differential diagnosis of pain in this patient?
2. What is complex regional pain syndrome (CRPS)?
3. What are the two types of CRPS?
4. What are the diagnostic criteria for CRPS? What is the incidence of this disease?
5. Define allodynia, hyperalgesia, hyperesthesia, and dysesthesia.
6. What are the associated stages of CRPS?
7. What are the possible etiologies of CRPS?
8. Explain the pathophysiology of the development of CRPS.
9. Define sympathetically maintained pain (SMP) and sympathetically independent pain (SIP).
10. How does CRPS differ from neuralgia?
11. What is central pain? How will you differentiate central pain from CRPS?
12. Is the social history of this patient relevant to the development of chronic pain?

B. Management

1. How will you work up CRPSs type I and II?
2. Describe the sympathetic nerve supply to the arm?
3. Where is the stellate ganglion located?
4. What are the anatomic landmarks used in the stellate ganglion block?
5. What are the clinical signs of stellate ganglion block?
6. What is Horner syndrome?
7. After a stellate ganglion block, this patient reports no significant change in the degree of pain despite Horner syndrome. Is the pain psychogenic in this patient?
8. What types of nerve fibers are interrupted in stellate ganglion block?
9. What is a differential block?

669

10. What are the two major classes of local anesthetics? Describe the major differences in their clinical pharmacology.
11. What factors determine the onset, potency, and duration of a local anesthetic block?
12. How does the addition of epinephrine to commercially available premixed solutions affect the efficacy of local anesthetics?
13. How will you treat this patient?
14. What is the pharmacologic management of CRPS?
15. What is the role of intravenous regional block (Bier method) in diagnosis and treatment of CRPS?
16. What is the role of spinal cord stimulation (SCS) and surgical sympathectomy?

C. Complications

1. What are the complications of stellate ganglion block?
2. What is the systemic toxicity of local anesthetics?
3. How do you treat the systemic toxicity of local anesthetic drugs?

A. Medical Disease and Differential Diagnosis

A.1. What is the differential diagnosis of pain in this patient?

Pain accompanied by burning and temperature change in this patient is most likely due to complex regional pain syndrome (CRPS). The differential diagnosis may also include the following:

1. Peripheral neuropathy
2. Soft tissue injury
3. Vascular insufficiency (Raynaud's disease)
4. Nerve entrapment syndrome (carpal tunnel syndrome)
5. Brachial plexopathy

Over the years, CRPS has been referred to as *reflex sympathetic dystrophy* (RSD), causalgia, sympathetically maintained pain (SMP), and chronic peripheral pain syndrome. The term CRPS was introduced in 1994 by the International Association for the Study of Pain subcommittee on taxonomy. It is subdivided into CRPS type I (formerly described as RSD) and CRPS type II (formerly described as causalgia).

Boas RA. Complex regional pain syndromes: symptoms, signs, and differential diagnosis. In: Janig W, Stanton Hicks M, eds. *Reflex sympathetic dystrophy: a reappraisal. Progress in pain research and management.* Seattle: IASP Press, 1996:79–92.

Merskey H, Bogduk N. *Classification of chronic pain. Task Force on Taxonomy. International Association for the Study of Pain: relatively generalized syndromes*, 2nd ed. Seattle: IASP Press, 1994:39–56.

Stanton-Hicks M, Janis W, Hassenburch S. Reflex sympathetic dystrophy: changing concepts and taxonomy. *Pain* 1995;63:127–133.

A.2. What is complex regional pain syndrome (CRPS)?

CRPS is characterized by pain with sudomotor or vasomotor instability. CRPS is triggered by *noxious stimuli* (type I) or by *nerve injury* (type II). It is not limited to the distribution of a single peripheral nerve and is disproportionate to the inciting event.

Reflex sympathetic dystrophy (RSD), causalgia, algodystrophy, Sudeck's atrophy, and various other conditions are all grouped under CRPS. This diagnosis is better descriptive of the wide range of clinical signs and symptoms and the complexity of the pathophysiology responsible for the clinical picture.

Merskey H, Bogduk N. *Classification of chronic pain. Task Force on Taxonomy. International Association for the Study of Pain: relatively generalized syndromes*, 2nd ed. Seattle: IASP Press, 1994:39–56.

Stanton-Hicks M, Janis W, Hassenburch S. Reflex sympathetic dystrophy: changing concepts and taxonomy. *Pain* 1995;63:127–133.

A.3. What are the two types of complex regional pain syndromes (CRPS)?

CRPS-I is defined as a clinical syndrome triggered by a *noxious stimulus* that is not limited to the distribution of a single peripheral nerve. CRPS-II is defined as a clinical syndrome that is due to a *nerve injury,* and is mostly limited to the distribution of the injured nerve. The diagnostic criteria are the same for CRPS-I and II.

Boas RA. Complex regional pain syndromes: symptoms, signs, and differential diagnosis. *Clin J Pain* 1998;14:48–54.

Janig W, Stanton Hicks M, eds. *Reflex sympathetic dystrophy: a reappraisal. Progress in pain research and management*. Seattle: IASP Press 1996:79–92.

Stanton-Hicks MD, Burton AW, Bruehl SP, et al. An Updated Interdisciplinary clinical pathway for CRPS: report of an expert panel. *Pain Practice* 2000;2(1):1–16.

Veldman PH, Reynen HM, Arntz IE, et al. Signs and symptoms of reflex dystrophy: prospective study of 829 patients. *Lancet* 1993;342:1012–1016.

A.4. What are the diagnostic criteria for complex regional pain syndrome (CRPS)? What is the incidence of this disease?

The diagnosis of CRPS can be made in the following context. A history of trauma to the affected area associated with pain that is disproportionate to the inciting event plus one or more of the following:

- Abnormal function of the sympathetic nervous system
- Swelling
- Movement disorder
- Changes in tissue growth (dystrophy and atrophy)

The main features include pain that is continuous, burning in nature, independent of type and severity of injury, and not limited to a dermatomal distribution. Patients may complain of allodynia, dysesthesia, or hyperalgesia. Movement or stress exacerbates pain. Edema is usually present. Abnormal sudomotor activity, limb discoloration, and local temperature changes are common but inconsistent.

It affects between 200,000 and 1.2 million Americans. This syndrome may follow as many as 5% of all traumatic injuries.

Loeser JD, ed. *Bonica's the management of pain*, 3rd ed. Philadelphia: Lippincott Williams & Wilkins, 2001:388–411.

Merskey H, Bogduk N. *Classification of chronic pain. Task Force on Taxonomy. International Association for the Study of Pain: relatively generalized syndromes*, 2nd ed. Seattle: IASP Press, 1994:39–56.

A.5. Define allodynia, hyperalgesia, hyperesthesia, and dysesthesia.

- *Allodynia.* Pain caused by a stimulus that normally does not provoke pain (i.e., touching with a cotton swab)
- *Hyperalgesia.* An increased response to a stimulus that is normally painful (i.e., increased response to pinprick)
- *Hyperesthesia.* Increased sensitivity to a stimulus either due to a diminished threshold or an increased response to stimuli that are normally recognized. Hyperesthesia includes both allodynia and hyperalgesia
- *Dysesthesia.* An abnormal sensation that is unpleasant to the patient. It may be either spontaneous or evoked (i.e., lumbar radiculopathy)

Loeser JD, ed. *Bonica's the management of pain*, 3rd ed. Philadelphia: Lippincott Williams & Wilkins, 2001:388–411.

A.6. What are the associated stages of complex regional pain syndrome (CRPS)?

Stage I

- Onset of severe pain limited to the site of injury
- Increased sensitivity of skin to touch and light pressure (hyperesthesia)
- Localized swelling
- Muscle cramps
- Stiffness and limited mobility
    At onset, skin is usually warm, red, and dry; then it may change to blue (cyanotic) in appearance and become cold and sweaty.
- Increased sweating (hyperhydrosis)
- In mild cases, this stage lasts a few weeks and then subsides spontaneously or responds rapidly to treatment.

Stage II

- Pain becomes even more severe and more diffuse.
- Swelling tends to spread and it may change from a soft to hard (brawny) type.
- Hair may become coarse then scant, nails may grow faster and become brittle, cracked, and heavily grooved.
- Spotty wasting of bone (osteoporosis) occurs early but may become severe and diffuse.
- Muscle wasting begins.

Stage III

- Marked wasting of tissue (atrophic) eventually becomes irreversible.
- For many patients, the pain becomes intractable and may involve the entire limb.
- A small percentage of patients have developed generalized reflex sympathetic dystrophy (RSD), affecting the entire body.

Loeser JD, ed. *Bonica's the management of pain*, 3rd ed. Philadelphia: Lippincott Williams & Wilkins, 2001:388–411.

A.7. What are the possible etiologies of complex regional pain syndrome (CRPS)?

CRPS may follow relatively minor trauma with or without nerve injury. Causes leading to CRPS include the following:

- Injuries to peripheral tissues (e.g., fractures, dislocations, and postoperative state)
- Inflammatory conditions (e.g., fasciitis, tendonitis, bursitis, and arthritis)
- Immobilization as a result of injury or cast application
- Peripheral nerve injury resulting from direct compression or ischemia (e.g., brachial plexopathy, postherpetic neuralgia, and nerve root injury)
- Central nervous system insults (e.g., head injury, ischemia, and brain tumor)
- Spinal cord lesions
- Idiopathic

Loeser JD, ed. *Bonica's the management of pain*, 3rd ed. Philadelphia: Lippincott Williams & Wilkins, 2001:388–411.

Veldman PH, Reynen HM, Arntz IE, et al. Signs and symptoms of reflex dystrophy: prospective study of 829 patients. *Lancet* 1993;342:1012–1016.

A.8. Explain the pathophysiology of the development of complex regional pain syndrome (CRPS).

Several hypotheses have been postulated but none can explain all the findings and the varying responses to treatment in these patients. These hypotheses include the following:

- Abnormal discharges in sympathetic and nociceptive afferents produced by trauma
- Sensitization of peripheral sensory receptors produced by sympathetic hyperactivity
- Formation of ephapses (artificial synapses) after peripheral nerve injury
- Spontaneous neuronal ectopy at the site of demyelination or axonal injury
- Central reorganization of pain processing

More than one sequence of events likely take place in a patient, giving rise to a mixed clinical picture. Finally, the psychologic component and neuromodulation cannot be discernibly separated.

Campbell JN, Raja SN, Meyer RA, et al. Myelinated afferents signal the hyperalgesia associated with nerve injury. *Pain* 1988;32:89–94.

Payne R. Neuropathic pain syndromes, with special reference to causalgia and reflex sympathetic dystrophy. *Clin J Pain* 1986;2:59–73.

Pleger B. Patterns of cortical reorganization parallel impaired tactile discrimination and pain intensity in complex regional pain syndrome. *Neuroimage* 2006;32:503–510.

Raj PP, ed. *Practical management of pain*, 3rd ed. St. Louis: Mosby, 2000:117–143.

Wall PD, Melzack R, eds. *Textbook of pain*, 5th ed. New York: Churchill Livingstone, 2005: 201–224.

A.9. Define sympathetically maintained pain (SMP) and sympathetically independent pain (SIP).

The pain that is maintained by sympathetic innervation or circulating catecholamines is defined as SMP. It describes a pain mechanism, rather than clinical syndrome. Therefore, by definition, patients with complex regional pain syndrome (CRPS) who report pain relief after a sympathetic block (e.g., stellate ganglion block) have SMP. Conversely, pain conditions that show features of sympathetic overactivity, yet fail to respond to sympathetic blocks, are described as SIP.

Loeser JD ed. *Bonica's the management of pain*, 3rd ed. Philadelphia: Lippincott Williams & Wilkins, 2001:388–411.

Roberts WJ. A hypothesis on the physiologic basis for causalgia and related pains. *Pain* 1986;24:297–311.

A.10. How does complex regional pain syndrome (CRPS) differ from neuralgia?

The chronic pain seen in neuralgia is usually paroxysmal in nature and follows the distribution of nerve. The pain is sharp and shooting without associated vasomotor or sudomotor changes. The chronic pain syndrome of CRPS is a sustained, diffuse, burning pain independent of nerve distribution and is associated with vasomotor and sudomotor changes.

Raj PP, ed. *Practical management of pain*, 3rd ed. St. Louis: Mosby, 2000:117–143.

A.11. What is central pain? How will you differentiate central pain from complex regional pain syndrome (CRPS)?

Central pain is regional pain initiated or caused by a primary lesion or dysfunction in the central nervous system, usually associated with abnormal sensitivity to temperature and to noxious stimulus. Central pain, also referred to as *deafferentation pain*, is a difficult pain syndrome to treat because the pathophysiology is not well understood. Regional pain not relieved by peripheral nerve blocks, either sympathetic or somatic, is more likely to be central pain. Central pain may be associated with various neurologic symptoms and signs such as monoparesis, hemiparesis, or paraparesis.

Abram SE, Haddox JD, eds. *The pain clinic manual*, 2nd ed. Philadelphia: Lippincott Williams & Wilkins, 2000:253–259.

A.12. Is the social history of this patient relevant to the development of chronic pain syndrome?

In patients with complex regional pain syndrome (CRPS), the disproportionate pain and dysfunction, and the absence of clear pathogenesis and pathophysiology have led to examination of potential psychologic etiology. Also noted is the fact that as the CRPS progresses, patients' personality measures such as Minnesota Multiphasic Personality Inventory (MMPI) profiles tend to resemble those of patients experiencing chronic pain and psychologic distress as evidenced by hypochondriasis, depression, and hysteria scales. Certainly, stress has been implicated in increasing sympathetic outflow. The literature suggests that the presence of psychologic disorders, particularly anxiety and depression, may predispose the patient to the development of CRPS.

Bruehl S, Carlson CR. Predisposing psychological factors in the development of reflex sympathetic dystrophy. *Clin J Pain* 1992;8:287–299.

Ciccone DS, Bandilla EB, Wen-hsein W. Psychological dysfunction in patients with reflex sympathetic dystrophy. *Pain* 1997;71:323–333.

B. Management

B.1. How will you work up complex regional pain syndrome (CRPS) type I and II?

CRPS is diagnosed clinically with a detailed history and physical examination. As it is a clinical diagnosis of exclusion, other specific conditions that could account for the degree of pain and dysfunction must be ruled out. Objective signs are variable but almost universally include loss of function of the affected part due to pain. Allodynia and hyperalgesia are extremely common. Change in temperature and sweating may vary depending on the stage of the disease. Several diagnostic studies may aid in the diagnosis of CRPS but are seldom pathognomonic.

Quantitative sweat test may show excessive sweating, and thermography may demonstrate abnormal heat regulation and disparity in temperature between affected and normal regions. Radiologic studies may reveal patchy osteoporosis in early stages. Triple-phase bone scan using technetium Tc 99m may show increased periarticular uptake in the affected extremity. However, negative triple-phase bone scan results do not rule out CRPS. Thermographic, radiologic, or scintigraphic findings can be nonspecific and should be correlated with the clinical findings.

Positive diagnostic sympathetic blocks can confirm the sympathetically mediated component of CRPS.

Betcher AM, Casten DF. Reflex sympathetic dystrophy: criteria for diagnosis and treatment. *Anesthesiology* 1955;6:994–1003.

Merskey H, Bogduk N. *Classification of chronic pain. Task Force on Taxonomy. International Association for the Study of Pain: relatively generalized syndromes*, 2nd ed. Seattle: IASP Press, 1994:39–56.

B.2. Describe the sympathetic nerve supply to the arm?

The preganglionic sympathetic outflow to the upper extremity is derived from T2-9. These fibers synapse with postganglionic neurons in the stellate ganglion. Therefore, a stellate ganglion block interrupts sympathetic outflow to the upper extremity.

Raj PP, ed. *Practical management of pain*, 3rd ed. St. Louis: Mosby, 2000:117–143.

B.3. Where is the stellate ganglion located?

The stellate ganglion is formed by the fusion of the inferior cervical and the first thoracic ganglia. It usually measures 2.5 by 1.5 by 0.5 cm and lies between the base of the transverse process of the seventh cervical vertebra and the neck of the first rib. It is situated behind the carotid sheath, ventral to the longus colli muscle, behind the vertebral artery, and lateral to the body of the vertebra. The vertebral, subclavian, inferior thyroid, and the first intercostals arteries are in close proximity to the ganglion and so is the recurrent laryngeal nerve. The left pleura is 1 to 2 cm below it, whereas the right pleura is in closer proximity.

Miller RD, ed. *Miller's anesthesia*, 6th ed. New York: Churchill Livingstone, 2005:1709.

Raj PP, ed. *Practical management of pain*, 3rd ed. St. Louis: Mosby, 2000:117–143.

B.4. What are the anatomic landmarks used in the stellate ganglion block?

The landmarks used in the stellate ganglion block are the jugular notch of the sternum, the sternocleidomastoid muscle, the cricoid cartilage, and Chassaignac tubercle. In a supine patient with neck extended, a mark placed approximately 3.5 cm from the midline along the jugular notch and the same distance above the clavicle should overlie the transverse process of the seventh vertebra and the medial border of the sternocleidomastoid muscle. This marking is further confirmed by palpating the cricoid cartilage, which lies at the level of the sixth cervical vertebra, and the anterior tubercle on the vertebral transverse process, which is the most prominent tubercle in the neck (Chassaignac tubercle).

Miller RD, ed. *Miller's anesthesia*, 6th ed. New York: Churchill Livingstone, 2005:1709.

Raj PP, ed. *Practical management of pain*, 3rd ed. St. Louis: Mosby, 2000:117–143.

B.5. What are the clinical signs of stellate ganglion block?

A stellate ganglion block results in the following ipsilateral signs:

- *Eye:* ptosis, narrowing of the palpebral fissure, miosis, enophthalmos, conjunctival injection, and lacrimation
- *Face and neck:* anhidrosis, elevated local temperature, and nasal stuffiness
- *Arm:* increased temperature and plethysmographic evidence of improved cutaneous blood flow

Miller RD, ed. *Miller's anesthesia*, 6th ed. New York: Churchill Livingstone, 2005:1709.

Raj PP, ed. *Practical management of pain*, 3rd ed. St. Louis: Mosby, 2000:117–143.

B.6. What is Horner syndrome?

Horner syndrome is a clinical entity characterized by ptosis, miosis, anhidrosis, and enopthalmos, usually seen with a disease process involving the cervical sympathetics and being the classic signs of a stellate ganglion block.

Miller RD, ed. *Miller's anesthesia*, 6th ed. New York: Churchill Livingstone, 2005:2362.

Raj PP, ed. *Practical management of pain*, 3rd ed. St. Louis: Mosby, 2000:117–143.

B.7. After a stellate ganglion block, this patient reports no significant change in the degree of pain despite Horner syndrome. Is the pain psychogenic in this patient?

Not necessarily. Horner syndrome indicates only the interruption of sympathetic supply to the head and neck. Unless it is accompanied by objective changes in the arm, it does not indicate sympathetic nerve block of the upper extremity. Further, sympathetically maintained pain (SMP) will respond to sympathectomy, whereas sympathetically independent pain (SIP) will not.

Raj PP, ed. *Practical management of pain*, 3rd ed. St. Louis: Mosby, 2000:117–143.

Wall PD, Melzack R, eds. *Textbook of pain*, 5th ed. New York: Churchill Livingstone, 2005: 201–224.

B.8. What types of nerve fibers are interrupted in stellate ganglion block?

The stellate ganglion block results in interruption of the preganglionic, thinly myelinated type B fibers, as well as the postganglionic, unmyelinated type C fibers.

Casale R, Glynn CJ, Buonocoe M. Autonomic variations after stellate ganglion block: are they evidence of an autonomic afference? *Funct Neurol* 1990;5:245–246.

B.9. What is a differential block?

The variable effects of local anesthetics on fibers performing different functions are termed *differential block*. The diagnostic distinction can be made by selectively blocking the function of these nerve fibers. The mechanism that results in differential block is best explained by the fiber size and myelination because these factors determine different sensitivities of nerve fibers to local anesthetics. By using different concentrations of local anesthetic, sympathetic, and somatic fibers can be selectively blocked. Differential block may be helpful to differentiate somatic versus sympathetic pain and peripheral versus central pain.

Cousins MJ, Bridenbaugh PO, eds. Neural blockade. *Clinical anesthesia and management of pain*, 3rd ed. Philadelphia: Lippincott Williams & Wilkins, 1998:837–877.

B.10. What are the two major classes of local anesthetics? Describe the major differences in their clinical pharmacology.

The two major classes of clinically employed local anesthetics are esters and amides. The esters are hydrolyzed in the plasma by pseudocholinesterase; the amides are biotransformed in the liver. Although infrequent, local anesthetic toxicity is encountered more commonly in the ester group because of the paraaminobenzoic acid moiety. True allergic reactions to amides are rare and in most instances are caused by preservatives in the solution. Each of the two groups of local anesthetics contains drugs with varying degrees of rate of onset, duration of neural blockade, potency, and toxicity.

Raj PP, ed. *Practical management of pain*, 3rd ed. St. Louis: Mosby, 2000:557–578.

B.11. What factors determine the onset, potency, and duration of a local anesthetic block?

- Onset correlates with pK_a
- Potency correlates with lipid solubility
- Duration correlates with degree of protein binding

The commonly used local anesthetics are weakly basic tertiary amines that are lipid soluble and unstable in water. They are prepared as acidic salts, because the ionized form, which is soluble in water, is stable. Therefore, the aqueous solution contains the ionized (cation) form of the local anesthetic in dissociation equilibrium with the unionized (free base) form depending on the pH of the medium.

$$R \equiv NH^+ \quad \rightleftharpoons \quad R \equiv N + H^+$$
$$\text{Cation} \qquad\qquad \text{Base}$$

When injected into the body, the relative rise in pH will allow the local anesthetic to convert to the uncharged base. The free base, being lipid soluble, will diffuse across the neural membrane and is responsible for neural blockade. With the exception of procaine and chloroprocaine, the commonly employed local anesthetics are highly protein bound, and are therefore longer acting. (Table 29.1)

Table 29.1 **Physiochemical Properties of Commonly Used Local Anesthetics.**

LOCAL ANESTHETIC	pK_a	PROTEIN BINDING (%)
Esters		
Procaine	8.9	5.8
Chloroprocaine	8.7	—
Tetracaine	8.5	75.6
Amides		
Lidocaine	7.9	64.3
Mepivacaine	7.6	77.5
Bupivacaine	8.1	95.6
Etidocaine	7.7	94.0

Cousins MJ, Bridenbaugh PO, eds. Neural blockade. *Clinical anesthesia and management of pain*, 3rd ed. Philadelphia: Lippincott Williams & Wilkins, 1998:56–96.

Raj PP, ed. *Practical management of pain*, 3rd ed. St. Louis: Mosby, 2000:557–578.

B.12. How does the addition of epinephrine to commercially available premixed solutions affect the efficacy of local anesthetics?

The addition of epinephrine to a local anesthetic increases the duration and intensity of a block. However, in commercially available premixed solutions containing epinephrine, antioxidants are added to preserve epinephrine and the result is a lower buffered pH level of the solution. This lowering of the pH level can result in decreased efficacy of the local anesthetic. Best results are achieved by adding the desired concentration of epinephrine to the local anesthetic solution just before injection.

Mooer DC. The pH of local anesthetic solutions: technical communication. *Anesth Analg* 1981;60:833–834.

Raj PP, ed. *Practical management of pain*, 3rd ed. St. Louis: Mosby, 2000:557–578.

B.13. How will you treat this patient?

Early diagnosis and aggressive physical therapy with pharmacologic control of pain form the basis of the treatment of complex regional pain syndrome (CRPS). Physical therapy is widely recommended and accepted as a first line of treatment. The treatment of CRPS will differ depending on whether the pain is sympathetically maintained pain (SMP) or sympathetically independent pain (SIP). A series of sympathetic blocks has been shown effective in treating SMP of CRPS. Multidisciplinary approach including physiotherapy and symptom-specific psychological treatments (e.g., biofeedback and hypnosis) may be beneficial. Many patients have a component of both SMP and SIP, and a combination of sympathectomy and analgesic treatment is recommended. However, no single treatment is consistently successful. Therefore, the treatment plan should be individualized.

Loeser JD, ed. *Bonica's the management of pain*, 3rd ed. Philadelphia: Lippincott Williams & Wilkins, 2001:388–411.

Wall PD, Melzack R, eds. *Textbook of pain*, 5th ed. New York: Churchill Livingstone, 2005: 117–143.

B.14. What is the pharmacologic management of complex regional pain syndrome (CRPS)?

Sympathetically maintained pain (SMP) of CRPS is treated with the drugs that deplete norepinephrine from the sympathetic nerve terminals. Oral sympatholytic agents include phenoxybenzamine, prazosin, and terazosin. Topical clonidine, a selective α_2 agonist, has been successfully used to treat SMP. Tricyclic antidepressants have been effective in approximately half the number of patients and have been recommended as first-line agents. Other drugs that have been successfully used to treat CRPS are anticonvulsants (e.g., gabapentin, pregabalin, carbamazepine, and topiramate), local anesthetics such as lidocaine and mexiletine, calcitonin, corticosteroids, and high-dose opioids. Anecdotal reports suggest that methadone (opioid with anti–*N*-methyl-D-aspartate receptor effect) has been more effective than other opioids. Long-term intrathecal morphine has been reported to produce analgesic effects in CRPS. Nonsteroidal antiinflammatory drugs have also been used successfully.

Abram SE, Haddox JD, eds. *The pain clinic manual*. Philadelphia: Lippincott Williams & Wilkins, 2001:177–184.

Becker WJ, Ablett DP, Harris CJ, et al. Long-term treatment of intractable reflex sympathetic dystrophy with intrathecal morphine. *Can J Neurosci* 1995;22:153–159.

B.15. What is the role of intravenous regional block (Bier method) in diagnosis and treatment of complex regional pain syndrome (CRPS)?

Intravenous regional block (Bier method) with guanethidine, reserpine, bretylium, and phentolamine has been used to achieve temporary sympatholytic effect and relieve sympathetically maintained pain (SMP) of CRPS. Intravenous guanethidine and reserpine have been reported to relieve pain in more than 50% of patients as compared with a control group in one study. However, guanethidine and reserpine are not commercially available in the United States. The combination of bretylium and lidocaine is more effective than lidocaine alone. α-adrenergic blockade with intravenous phentolamine is a sensitive test to identify patients with SMP. Phentolamine has been used as a predictor agent before more invasive sympathetic blocks.

Blanchard J, Ramamurthy S, Walsh N, et al. Intravenous regional sympatholysis: a double blind comparison guanethidine, reserpine and normal saline. *J Pain Symptom Manage* 1990;5:357–361.

Hord AH, Rooks MD, Stephens BO, et al. Intravenous regional bretylium and lidocaine for the treatment of reflex sympathetic dystrophy: a randomized double blind study. *Reg Anesth Pain Med* 1992;74:818–821.

Raja SN, Treede R-D, Davis KD, et al. Systemic alpha-adrenergic blockade with phentolamine: a diagnostic test for sympathetically maintained pain. *Anesthesiology* 1991; 74:691–698.

B.16. What is the role of spinal cord stimulation (SCS) and surgical sympathectomy?

Surgical, chemical, or radiofrequency sympathectomy produces short-term pain relief but long-term results are poor and inconsistent. Delayed failure of sympathectomy may be due to regeneration of ipsilateral nerves or reinnervation from the contralateral sympathetic nerves.

SCS is an effective treatment for the pain of complex regional pain syndrome (CRPS), including recurrent pain after surgical or radiofrequency sympatholysis. Epidural SCS is a simple procedure and carries low morbidity.

Kumar K, Nath RK, Toth C. Spinal cord stimulation is effective in the management of reflex sympathetic dystrophy. *Neurosurgery* 1997;40(3):503–508.

Rocco AG. Radiofrequency lumbar sympatholysis: the evolution of a technique for managing sympathetically maintained pain. *Reg Anesth* 1995;20(1):3–12.

C. Complications

C.1. What are the complications of stellate ganglion block?

Although complications appear infrequently, the more common complications of stellate ganglion block are as follows:

- Intraarterial injection: seizure and hematoma
- Recurrent laryngeal nerve paralysis: hoarseness of voice
- Brachial plexus block: motor weakness
- Accidental epidural or subarachnoid injection
- Esophageal injury
- Pneumothorax: respiratory distress

To avoid complications, aspiration of the needle should be performed before, during, and after administration of local anesthetics to look for (a) air, (b) blood, and (c) cerebrospinal fluid.

Miller RD, ed. *Miller's anesthesia*, 6th ed. New York: Churchill Livingstone, 2005:1710.

Raj PP, ed. *Practical management of pain*, 3rd ed. St. Louis: Mosby, 2000:655–664.

C.2. What is the systemic toxicity of local anesthetics?

The systemic toxic effects of local anesthetics are related to drug levels in blood, and they are manifested mainly in the central nervous system and the cardiovascular system. As a rule, the central nervous system effects precede the cardiovascular toxic manifestations.

Central nervous system effects

Light-headedness, dizziness, tinnitus, visual disturbances, drowsiness, disorientation, slurred speech, muscle twitching, generalized grand mal seizures, and electroencephalographic changes. Blood levels of local anesthetics associated with central nervous system changes in humans are as follows:

- Procaine: 20 μg per mL
- Lidocaine, mepivacaine, and prilocaine: 5 to 10 μg per mL
- Tetracaine, bupivacaine, and etidocaine: 1.5 to 4 μg per mL
- Lowering the Pa_{CO_2} by hyperventilation decreases the convulsive threshold dose of a local anesthetic drug.

Cardiovascular effects (Table 29.2)

Ventricular arrhythmias are reported with intravenous bupivacaine only. Cardiac resuscitation is extremely difficult in patients with bupivacaine-induced cardiac arrhythmias. Ropivacaine

Table 29.2 Cardiovascular Effects of Lidocaine.

BLOOD LEVEL LIDOCAINE (μg/mL)	ELECTROCARDIOGRAPHIC CHANGES	HEMODYNAMIC EFFECTS
<5	—	—
5–10	↑ PR interval ↑ QRS duration Sinus bradycardia	↓ Myocardial contraction ↓ Cardiac output Vasodilatation
>10	↑ PR interval ↑ QRS duration Sinus bradycardia Atrioventricular block Asystole	↓ Myocardial contraction ↓ Cardiac output Circulatory collapse

↑, increase; ↓, decrease.

is less toxic than bupivacaine but more toxic than lidocaine. The mechanism of enhanced cardiotoxicity in pregnant patients is not well understood; nevertheless, 0.75% bupivacaine is no longer recommended in pregnant patients in the United States.

Cousins MJ, Bridenbaugh PO, eds. Neural blockade. *Clinical anesthesia and management of pain*, 3rd ed. Philadelphia: Lippincott Williams & Wilkins, 1998:97–128.

Miller RD, ed. *Anesthesia*, 6th ed. New York: Churchill Livingstone, 2005:573–603.

Raj PP, ed. *Practical management of pain*, 3rd ed. St. Louis: Mosby, 2000:557–578.

C.3. How do you treat the systemic toxicity of local anesthetic drugs?

The principles of treatment include the following:

- Secure and maintain the airway.
- Ensure adequate oxygenation and ventilation.
- Treat hypotension and bradycardia promptly.
- Perform immediate cardiopulmonary resuscitation for profound cardiovascular collapse.
- Perform electrical cardioversion for ventricular tachycardia or fibrillation.

Control seizures with the following:

- Diazepam, 0.1 to 0.2 mg per kg, intravenously
- Thiopental sodium, 1 to 2 mg per kg, intravenously

Cousins MJ, Bridenbaugh PO, eds. Neural blockade. *Clinical anesthesia and management of pain*, 3rd ed. Philadelphia: Lippincott Williams & Wilkins, 1998:97–128.

Miller RD, ed. *Anesthesia*, 6th ed. New York: Churchill Livingstone, 2005:573–603.

Raj PP, ed. *Practical management of pain*, 3rd ed. St. Louis: Mosby, 2000:557–578.

CHAPTER 30

Cancer Pain

SUDHIR A. DIWAN • SHAKIL AHMED

A 44-YEAR-OLD MAN

was referred to the pain clinic for evaluation and management of abdominal pain. He was recently diagnosed with adenocarcinoma of the pancreas with retroperitoneal lymph nodes in the paraaortic region. His pain was localized in the epigastric region and was worse during the night and decreased during the day. He was taking sustained-release morphine sulfate ([MS] Contin), 100 mg orally every 8 hours, and immediate-release MS, 30 mg every 3 hours orally as needed, for breakthrough pain. The patient reported inadequate pain control, nausea, vomiting, and constipation.

A. Medical Disease and Differential Diagnosis

1. What is the definition of pain?
2. How significant is the problem of pain in patients with cancer?
3. What are the components of cancer pain?
4. How does pain contribute to the suffering of patients with cancer?
5. How do psychological factors affect pain in patients with cancer?
6. What are the causes of pain in patients with cancer?
7. How do you classify pain in patients with cancer?
8. What are the characteristics of pancreatic cancer pain?
9. How do you assess pain in patients with cancer?
10. What is the differential diagnosis of abdominal pain?

B. Pharmacologic Treatment of Pain

1. What is the World Health Organization stepladder approach for cancer pain management?
2. Which class of drugs does morphine sulfate (MS) belong to?
3. What is the difference between morphine and synthetic opioids?
4. How does mixed opioid agonist/antagonist differ from opioid agonist?
5. Describe the role of methadone in the management of cancer pain.
6. What are the advantages and disadvantages of methadone?
7. What is the mechanism of action of opioids?
8. What are the side effects of opioid therapy?
9. Define tolerance and physical dependence.
10. How would you treat the side effects of opioid therapy?

11. What is tramadol? Is it an opioid?
12. When would you consider adjuvant analgesics as part of the treatment plan?
13. The patient and his family are worried about addiction. How would you approach this problem?
14. Describe different routes of opioid administration.
15. Describe advantages and complications of patient-controlled analgesia (PCA). What is minimum effective analgesic concentration (MEAC)?
16. What is meperidine? How is it different from other opioids?
17. What is rotation of opioids? When would you consider rotation of opioids?

C. Invasive Therapy

1. Describe the role of peripheral nerve blocks in cancer pain management.
2. Describe the role of a celiac plexus block in cancer pain management.
3. What are the complications of a celiac plexus block?
4. Would you consider neuraxial opioid infusion in this patient? Discuss complications of this procedure.
5. Would you consider neuraxial neurolysis in this patient to manage his pain? Discuss advantages and disadvantages of these blocks.
6. Which neuroablative procedures can be considered in the terminal stage of pancreatic cancer?
7. Describe the role of radiation therapy in cancer pain.

D. Nonpharmacologic Management

1. What are the various nonpharmacologic techniques of cancer pain management?
2. What physical modalities have been successfully tried in cancer pain management?
3. Describe the role of neuromodulation in cancer pain management.
4. What psychological techniques have been promoted for comfort care and pain relief?
5. What are distraction and reframing techniques? What is the role of hypnosis in cancer pain management?

A. Medical Disease and Differential Diagnosis

A.1. What is the definition of pain?

According to the International Association of the Study of Pain, pain is defined as "an unpleasant, sensory and emotional experience associated with actual or potential tissue damage or described in terms of such damage."

Merskey H, Bogduk N, eds. *Classification of chronic pain: descriptions of chronic pain syndromes and definitions of pain terms*, 2nd ed. Seattle: IASP Press, 1994:210.

A.2. How significant is the problem of pain in patients with cancer?

There are 1,382,400 new patients with cancer annually. Cancer causes 560,000 deaths per year, making it the second leading cause of death in the United States. Thirty percent of the patients with cancer have pain at the time of diagnosis, and 65% to 85% of patients with cancer have pain at advanced stages. Thirty-six percent have pain severe enough to impair their ability to function.

Vainio et al. studied 1,840 patients with advanced cancer and found 24% with no pain, 24% with mild pain, 30% with moderate pain, and 21% with severe pain. Daut and Cleeland found pain to be an early symptom of cancer in 48% to 50% of patients with cancer of the breasts, ovary, prostate, colon, and rectum, and in 20% of patients with uterus and cervical cancer.

Bruera E, Kim HN. Cancer pain. *JAMA* 2003;290:2476–2479.

Hewitt DJ. The management of pain in the oncology patient. *Obstet Gynecol Clin North Am* 2001;28:24.

Daut RL, Cleeland CS. The prevalence and severity of pain in cancer. *Cancer* 1982;50:1913.

Vainio A, Auvinen A. Prevalence of symptoms among patients with advanced cancer : an international collaborative study, symptom prevalence group. *J Pain Symptom Manage* 1996;47:5–27.

A.3. What are the components of cancer pain?

The components of cancer pain are (a) sensory, (b) affective, and (c) psychological.
The sensory components could be as follows:

- Nociceptive pain elicited by activation of sensory nerve endings, by mechanical, chemical, radioactive, or thermal energy. Nociceptive pain may be of somatic or visceral origin. Somatic pain may be superficial, well localized, sharp, pricking, burning or deep diffused, dull, and aching. Visceral pain is usually diffused, referred to body surface, and has a sickening quality to it.
- Neuropathic pain is due to pathologic change in the discharge properties of the neurons because of invasion, compression, or damage caused by various cancer treatment modalities.

Loeser JD, ed. *Bonica's management of pain*, 3rd ed. Philadelphia: Lippincott Williams & Wilkins, 2001:623–658.

A.4. How does pain contribute to the suffering of patients with cancer?

Sustained pain on its own can create complex, enduring, unpleasant emotional suffering by its ability to create awareness of the perceived threat to one's life. It causes helplessness in the face of the inevitability of demise as well as exhaustion of hope. Patients with cancer usually identify pain as an indicator of disease progression.

Speigel D, Giese-Davis J. Depression and cancer pain: mechanisms and disease progression. *Biol Psychiatry* 2003;54:269–282.

A.5. How do psychological factors affect pain in patients with cancer?

The ultimate perception of pain depends on the nociceptive stimulus and psychologic fear, anger, anxiety, or depression. Twenty-five percent of patients with cancer meet criteria for major depressive syndromes at some point in their illness, with an overall prevalence of 53% in hospitalized patients with cancer. Psychological factors may significantly exacerbate pain. Symptoms usually include anxiety, restlessness, irritability, sleep disorders, obsessive thinking, slowness in motor responses, and hopelessness.

Speigel D, Giese-Davis J. Depression and cancer pain: mechanisms and disease progression. *Biol Psychiatry* 2003;54:269–282.

A.6. What are the causes of pain in patients with cancer?

Pain in patients with cancer may be due to (a) presence and progression of the tumor itself, for example, bone involvement, viscus obstruction, and nerve compression; (b) indirect effect of the tumor, for example, metabolic imbalance, infection, and venous or lymphatic obstruction; (c) consequence of cancer treatment, such as chemotherapy, radiation therapy, or surgery; or (d) unrelated mechanisms such as migraine and myofascial pain. Grond et al. found in a prospective study of 2,266 patients with cancer that 30% had one pain syndrome, 39% had two pain syndromes, 31% had three pain syndromes, 85% by the cancer itself (bone, 35%; soft tissue, 45%; and visceral, 34%), and 17% by anticancer treatment.

Cherny NI. The management of cancer pain. *CA Cancer J Clin* 2000;50:70–116.

Grond S, Zech D, Diefenbach C, et al. Assessment of cancer pain: a prospective evaluation in 2266 cancer patients referred to a pain service. *Pain* 1996;64:107–114.

A.7. How do you classify pain in patients with cancer?

Pain, in patients with cancer, may be classified on the basis of the following:

- *Chronicity:* acute or chronic
- *Intensity and severity:* visual analog score, numeric pain score, and verbal: mild, moderate, severe, or worst possible pain
- *Pathophysiology and mechanism:* nociceptive or neuropathic, tumor infiltration of nerves, infiltration of soft tissue or hollow organs, serosa, solid organ necrosis, and destruction of bone
- *Individual type and stage of disease:* pancreatic, ovarian, prostatic, breast, or lung
- *Pattern of pain:* incidental pain related to an event or activity; spontaneous pain unrelated to an event or activity and end-of-dose failure
- *Pain syndromes:* tumor invasion of bone, nerves, spinal cord, viscera, blood vessels, postsurgical, and postchemotherapy and postradiation therapy pain.

Caraceni A, Weinstein S. Classification of cancer pain syndromes. *Oncology* 2001;15: 1627–1640.

A.8. What are the characteristics of pancreatic cancer pain?

Pancreatic cancer affects 9 to 10 patients per 100,000 in the Western world, men more than women, and blacks more than whites. Approximately 30% to 60% of patients present with pain, and 80% of the patients with advanced cancer complain of pain. Patients complain of diffuse epigastric pain radiating to the back that is increased on lying down and improved on sitting. Approximately 90% of pancreatic tumors are of the adenocarcinoma type. Cancer in the head of the pancreas usually invades the stomach, duodenum, gallbladder, and peritoneum, whereas tumors in the body spreads to liver, spleen, and lymph nodes and left adrenal gland.

Hawes RH, Xiong Q, Waxman I, et al. A multispecialty approach to the diagnosis and management of pancreatic cancer. *Am J Gastroenterol* 2000;95:17–31.

A.9. How do you assess pain in patients with cancer?

A stepwise approach is required for the assessment of pain. It includes history, physical examination, and data collection ending with clinical diagnosis. It helps the clinician achieve goals of providing pain relief. Assessment involves identifying features of pain, such as location, intensity, quality, timing, exacerbating/relieving factors, response to previous analgesics, and disease-modifying treatments; effects of pain on daily activities and psychological state; associated symptoms; complete physical examination; and laboratory data and imaging.

Loeser JD, ed. *Bonica's management of pain*, 3rd ed. Philadelphia: Lippincott Williams & Wilkins, 2001:650–653.

A.10. What is the differential diagnosis of abdominal pain?

Although abdominal pain could arise from different structures within the peritoneal cavity, the retroperitoneal organs can cause similar pain syndromes. Location and radiation of the pain can give important clues to make the diagnosis. Retroperitoneal structures present with dull or sharp back pain that is increased on lying down and relieved on sitting hunched up. Abdominal tumors are frequently characterized by colicky pain associated with nausea that is worse after eating. Abdominal pain may be referred to distant areas such as shoulder, neck, or back depending on the organ involved. Tumors of the small bowel or large bowel may present with symptoms of obstruction (e.g., abdominal distention, nausea, and bilious vomiting) or hematemesis or melena. Other common causes of abdominal pain include omental metastasis, volvulus of intestine, infectious peritonitis, radiation enteritis, and peritoneal carcinomatosis. Mesenteric ischemia presents with diffuse pain that is increased with meals and weight loss.

Nonmalignant causes of abdominal pain such as appendicitis, cholecystitis, and pancreatitis can occur in patients with cancer coincidentally and may complicate the diagnostic process. Opioid analgesics may not be used in these patients because they may exacerbate symptoms of colicky pain (due to spasm of sphincter of Oddi), nausea, vomiting, paralytic ileus, and constipation.

B. Pharmacologic Treatment of Pain

B.1. What is the World Health Organization stepladder approach for cancer pain management?

The World Health Organization advocated a stepladder approach to manage cancer pain exclusively with oral medications depending on the pain intensity and to some extent the pain mechanism (Fig. 30.1).

Step 1. Manage the pain by nonopioid medications with or without adjuvants.

Step 2. If pain is persisting or increasing, add weak opioids to nonopioid analgesics and adjuvants.

Step 3. Strong opioids are used with nonopioid analgesics and adjuvants until the patient achieves complete analgesia.

At this point, if pain still persists, neurolytic and/or interventional procedures should be employed. Noninvasive routes of drug delivery should be maintained as long as possible, because of their simplicity, convenience, and cost.

Abram SE, Haddox JD, eds. *The pain clinic manual*, 2nd ed. Philadelphia: Lippincott Williams & Wilkins, 2000:293–351.

Max M, ed. *Pain 1999—an update review*. Seattle: IASP Press, 1999:25–35.

B.2. Which class of drugs does morphine sulfate (MS) belong to?

Morphine is classified as a μ-receptor opioid agonist because of its high specificity for activation of μ-receptors. An ideal opioid agonist would have a high specificity for receptors producing

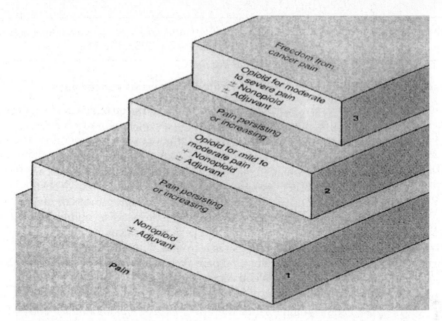

Figure 30.1 World Health Organization–advocated stepladder approach to management of cancer pain.

desirable effects (analgesia and minimal or no specificity for other receptors that cause side effects). Opioids are unique in producing analgesia without loss of consciousness.

Brunton LB, Lazo JS, Parker KL. *Goodman and Gilman's the pharmacological basis of thaerapeutics*, 11th ed. New York: McGraw-Hill, 2006:563–568.

B.3. What is the difference between morphine and synthetic opioids?

Morphine is the principal phenanthrene alkaloid present in opium. It is highly ionized and water-soluble. The most active molecule of morphine is the levorotatory isomer of stereochemical structure. The synthetic opiates contain the phenanthrene nucleus of morphine and are manufactured by synthesis, rather than chemical modification. Clinically, histamine release by morphine differentiates it from the synthetic opioids. This may cause urticaria, allergic reactions, and hemodynamic instability, particularly in volume-depleted patients.

Miller RD, ed. *Anesthesia*, 6th ed. New York: Churchill Livingstone, 2005:401–403.

B.4. How does mixed opioid agonist/antagonist differ from opioid agonist?

The mixed-action opioids bind to μ-receptors, where they are partial agonists or competitive antagonists. Antagonistic properties of these drugs can attenuate the efficacy of subsequently administered opioid agonists and cause withdrawal symptoms in patients already receiving opioid agonists. The advantages of these drugs include low potential for respiratory depression and physical dependence. A dysphoric reaction is very common with mixed-action opioids. Their use is limited because of a ceiling effect whereby progressive escalation in doses does not increase analgesia as with opioid agonists.

Brunton LB, Lazo JS, Parker KL. *Goodman and Gilman's the pharmacological basis of thaerapeutics*, 11th ed. New York: McGraw-Hill, 2006:574–578.

B.5. Describe the role of methadone in the management of cancer pain.

The efficient oral and rectal absorption with prolonged duration of analgesic action of methadone makes it a highly effective and attractive oral drug for cancer pain management.

Methadone is a synthetic opiate drug with a unique agonist/antagonist action. Methadone is a μ-receptor agonist and an *N*-methyl D-aspartate-(NMDA) receptor antagonist. Activation of NMDA receptors is involved in the development of hypersensitivity and central sensitization in neuropathic pain and tolerance to opioids. Because of the antagonistic effect at the NMDA receptor site, methadone is very effective in neuropathic pain secondary to cancer-related pathology and therapeutic interventions. The same antagonistic action of methadone minimizes the development of tolerance to opioids.

Brunton LB, Lazo JS, Parker KL. *Goodman and Gilman's the pharmacological basis of thaerapeutics*, 11th ed. New York: McGraw-Hill, 2006:572–573.

Manfredi PL, Gonzalez GR, Cheville AL, et al. Methadone analgesia in cancer patients on chronic methadone maintenance therapy. *J Pain Symptom Manage* 2001;21:169–174.

B.6. What are the advantages and disadvantages of methadone?

Methadone has several advantages including oral and rectal absorption with bioavailability to 95%, high potency, high lipid solubility, low cost, and no active metabolites. Methadone has a long half-life, and its analgesic effect lasts 6 to 8 hours. However, methadone has been used for a long time for heroin abusers as detoxification and maintenance; it carries a social stigma, which can interfere with adequate pain management. Methadone has an irregular elimination half-life with interindividual variation between 20 and 60 hours. Because of that, the cumulative effect of methadone causes sedation, makes titration difficult, and has led to the concept of individualization of methadone dosing.

Brunton LB, Lazo JS, Parker KL. *Goodman and Gilman's the pharmacological basis of thaerapeutics*, 11th ed. New York: McGraw-Hill, 2006:572–573.

Loeser JD, ed. *Bonica's management of pain*, 3rd ed. Philadelphia: Lippincott Williams & Wilkins, 2001:659–703.

B.7. What is the mechanism of action of opioids?

Opioids act as agonists at stereospecific opioid receptors that are normally activated by endogenous ligands known as *endorphins* in brainstem and spinal cord. Binding of opioid to the receptor inhibits adenylate cyclase activity and causes hyperpolarization of neurons, which results in suppression of spontaneous discharge and evoked potential. Opioids also interfere with transmembrane transport of calcium ion and interfere with the release of neurotransmitters such as acetylcholine, dopamine, norepinephrine, and substance P. Inhibition of acetylcholine release from nerve endings is the basis of analgesic activity of opioids.

Loeser JD, ed. *Bonica's management of pain*. 3rd ed. Philadelphia: Lippincott Williams & Wilkins, 2001:1667–1709.

Miller RD, ed. *Anesthesia*, 6th ed. New York: Churchill Livingstone, 2005:385–397.

B.8. What are the side effects of opioid therapy?

The opioid-related side effects occur because of opioid receptor pharmacodynamics, metabolites, or both. Sedation and respiratory depression are due to μ-receptor activation. Tolerance to these side effects is developed within a very short period of treatment. The dysphoric reaction is due to activation of κ-receptors. Psychotomimetic and depersonalization reactions are due to activation of σ-receptors. Nausea and vomiting are caused by direct stimulation of the chemoreceptor trigger zone. Increased intrabiliary pressure is due to spasm of the sphincter of Oddi. Other side effects commonly observed are constipation, pruritus, and myoclonus. Almost all side effects diminish with time, except constipation and myoclonus. Patients with cancer who develop constipation secondary to opioid therapy are required to be on a regular bowel regimen to avoid subsequent serious consequences. In patients with compromised renal function, metabolites of morphine (M3G, M6G) cause excessive sedation and metabolites of meperidine (normeperidine) lower the seizure threshold.

Miller RD, ed. *Anesthesia*, 6th ed. New York: Churchill Livingstone, 2005:392–400.

Brunton LB, Lazo JS, Parker KL. *Goodman and Gilman's the pharmacological basis of therapeutics*, 11th ed. New York: McGraw-Hill, 2006:547–584.

B.9. Define tolerance and physical dependence.

Tolerance occurs with the development of the need to gradually escalate the dose to achieve the same pain control and it can develop in 2 to 3 weeks. Physical dependence develops after chronic use of opioids, and it is characterized by development of withdrawal syndrome after administration of an opioid antagonist or abrupt discontinuation of the medication. The potential for tolerance is an agonistic effect of opioids.

Streltzer J, Johansen L. Prescription drug dependence and evolving beliefs about chronic pain management. *Am J Psychiatry* 2006;163(4):594–598.

B.10. How would you treat the side effects of opioid therapy?

Oversedation and respiratory depression are treated with a specific μ-receptor antagonist, naloxone, as well as supplemental oxygen. Naloxone, in a 1- to 4-μg per kg intravenous bolus, promptly reverses sedation, respiratory depression, and analgesia. Continuous intravenous infusion at the rate of 2 to 4 μg/kg/hour will reverse only side effects without reversing analgesia. Nausea and vomiting should be managed by antiemetics. Constipation should be treated with a regular bowel regimen of laxatives and stool softener. Peripheral μ-receptor antagonists, for example, alvimopan, which inhibits the μ-receptors in the gut but not in the central nervous system, have been shown in preliminary studies to improve opiate-induced bowel dysfunction without reversing analgesia. Generalized pruritus may respond to one more doses of antihistamine; however, pruritus may not be related to histamine release.

Cherny N, Ripamonti C, Pereira J, et al. Strategies to manage the adverse effects of oral morphine: an evidence based report. *J Clin Oncol* 2001;19:2542–2554.

B.11. What is tramadol? Is it an opioid?

Tramadol (Ultram) is a nonopioid synthetic analgesic with weak μ-receptor agonistic activity and is thought to exert its analgesic effects by inhibition of reuptake of norepinephrine and serotonin. It should be started at 50 to 100 mg every 6 to 8 hours. It may exhibit μ-receptor–related clinical side effects such as respiratory depression and constipation. Prolonged use may lead to physical and psychologic dependence.

Brunton LB, Lazo JS, Parker KL. *Goodman and Gilman's the pharmacological basis of thaerapeutics*, 11th ed. New York: McGraw-Hill, 2006:566–568.

Grond S, Sablotzki A. Clinical pharmacology of tramadol. *Clin Pharmacokinet* 2004; 43:879–923.

B.12. When would you consider adjuvant analgesics as part of the treatment plan?

In cancer pain management, adjuvant drugs are considered to enhance pain relief. The adjuvant analgesics are a heterogeneous group of medications originally developed for purposes other than pain relief. These drugs may become necessary in the multimodal approach to treat pain, the adverse effects of analgesic medications or to treat concomitant psychologic disturbances such as insomnia, anxiety, depression, and psychosis. The most useful adjuvants used clinically to manage cancer pain are as follows:

- Corticosteroids
- Tricyclic antidepressants (e.g., amitriptyline)
- Anticonvulsants (e.g., gabapentin)
- Amphetamines
- NMDA-receptor antagonists (e.g., methadone, ketamine)
- α_2 Agonists (e.g., clonidine)
- antihistamines
- Phenothiazines

Abram SE, Haddox JD, eds. *The pain clinic manual*, 2nd ed. Philadelphia: Lippincott Williams & Wilkins, 2000:293–351.

Loeser JD, ed. *Bonica's management of pain*, 3rd ed. Philadelphia: Lippincott Williams & Wilkins, 2001:659–703.

B.13. The patient and his family are worried about addiction. How would you approach this problem?

Addiction is defined as a persistent pattern of dysfunctional use of opioids that may involve adverse consequences associated with continued use, loss of control over use of opioids, compulsive use of drug, craving for the drug, and a typical drug-seeking behavior. Patients with chronic pain who are using opioids are not at higher risk of addiction than the general population. The goals of treatment including palliation of pain and improvement in the patient's quality of life must be clearly defined and explained to the patient and his relatives. At no time should patients with cancer pain be undertreated because of the fear of addiction. The patient and his family should be educated about the common misconception that addiction is a common outcome of opioid therapy.

Heit HA. Addiction, physical dependence and tolerance: precise definitions to help clinicians evaluate and treat chronic pain patients. *J Pain Palliat Care Pharmacother* 2003;17:15–29.

Table 30.1   Routes of Opioid Administration.

ROUTE OF ADMINISTRATION	AVAILABLE OPIOID PREPARATION
Oral	Morphine
	Hydromorphone (Dilaudid)
	Methadone (Dolophine)
	Oxycodone, hydrocodone
	Codeine, meperidine
	Levorphanol
Rectal	Suppositories containing morphine
	Hydromorphone, oxycodone
Transdermal	Fentanyl patch
Sublingual	Fentanyl, methadone, buprenorphine
Intramuscular/subcutaneous	Morphine, hydromorphone, methadone
	Meperidine, levorphanol
Intravenous	Morphine, meperidine, methadone, fentanyl
	Hydromorphone, oxymorphone
Epidural/intrathecal	Morphine, methadone, hydromorphone
	Fentanyl, meperidine

B.14. Describe different routes of opioid administration.

Oral medications should be used as the first-line approach in most patients with cancer pain who are receiving opioid analgesics. Table 30.1 outlines the routes of opioid administration and available opioid preparations.

The rectal or transdermal route should be chosen before considering invasive therapy for cancer pain. The sublingual route is limited by the inability to deliver large doses.

The intramuscular route is not preferred for long-term administration because it requires repeated painful injections and offers no pharmacodynamic advantages. Intravenous administration provides quick onset and is ideal for painful crises in patients with cancer as patient-controlled analgesia (PCA).

The equianalgesic doses of opioids used orally and parenterally are listed in Table 30.2.

Table 30.2   Opioids Used Orally or Parenterally to Treat Cancer Pain.

DRUG	EQUIANALGESIC DOSE (mg)[a]	
	ORAL	PARENTERAL
Morphine	30	10
Hydromorphone	6	2
Oxycodone	20–30	NA
Methadone	10[b]	10[b]
Levorphanol	2–3[b]	2[b]
Codeine	130[c]	75

NA, not available in the United States.

[a]Suggested doses are guidelines only. Doses are based on chronic opioid use.

[b]Particular care with titration is recommended, as doses may need to be reduced significantly when steady-state levels are reached after 2 to 3 days.

[c]Codeine doses greater than 65 mg may be associated with significant constipation.

Brunton LB, Lazo JS, Parker KL. *Goodman and Gilman's the pharmacological basis of thaerapeutics*, 11th ed. New York: McGraw-Hill, 2006:581–583.

Mercadante S. Expet rev. *Anticancer Ther* 2001;1(3):487–494.

B.15. Describe advantages and complications of patient-controlled analgesia (PAC). What is minimum effective analgesic concentration (MEAC)?

Intravenous PCA is very advantageous for patients with chronic cancer pain because it allows patients to self-administer medication and find their own comfort zone between side effects and pain control within limits set by the physician. The PCA device is a computerized, programmable, lightweight, battery-operated portable pump with the capability of storage and retrieval of data by the microprocessor. The pump is programmed for three modes of drug delivery: (a) continuous per hour rate infusion only, which is preset by the physician and the patient has no control over it; (b) continuous with boluses for breakthrough pain, boluses controlled by the patient; and (c) boluses with lockout time in minutes set by the physician and the patient can control his or her own requirement. If required, the physician or nurse can deliver extra boluses. Intermittent rescue doses for breakthrough pain, along with continuous infusion, decrease the total requirement of opioids. Only rescue-dose delivery mode is safer because patients will not take medication if there is no pain. However, continuous-delivery mode carries risks of oversedation and respiratory depression. The initial cost of the drug-delivery device and training of the health care provider could be expensive. PCA can also be provided by subcutaneous, epidural, or intrathecal route.

MEAC is the minimum effective analgesic concentration of the opioid, which is the lower level of the therapeutic window (Fig. 30.2). The upper level of the therapeutic window represents the serum concentration at which adverse side effects will occur. Neither age, sex, body weight, nor rate of drug elimination appeared to be related to the therapeutic concentration.

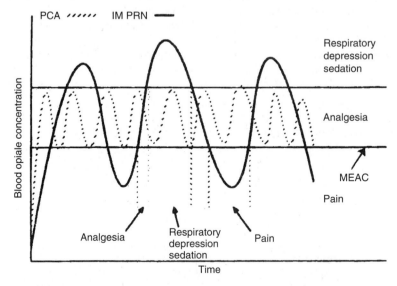

Figure 30.2 The MEAC is the minimum effective analgesic concentration of the opioid, which is the lower level of the therapeutic window. PCA, patient-controlled analgesia; MEAC, minimum effective analgesic concentration. (From Ashburn M, Smith K. The management of postoperative pain. *Surg Rounds* 1991;14:129–134, with permission.)

Loeser JD, ed. *Bonica's management of pain*, 3rd ed. Philadelphia: Lippincott Williams & Wilkins, 2001:766–779.

B.16. What is meperidine? How is it different from other opioids?

Meperidine is a synthetic opioid that pharmacologically resembles morphine. Meperidine is not an ideal drug for chronic pain because of its short duration of action and its high potential for abuse. The byproduct normeperidine is exclusively excreted through the kidney with an elimination half-life of 36 to 40 hours. In patients with compromised renal function, byproduct accumulation has been associated with central nervous system toxicity, including myoclonus, tremulousness, hallucinations, and seizures. Meperidine possesses anticholinergic activity similar to atropine, causing mydriasis, orthostatic hypotension, and tachycardia. Compared with other opioids, meperidine very rarely causes pruritus when given neuraxially. It is extremely effective in the treatment of postoperative shivering. Meperidine also demonstrates local anesthetic actions. It is contraindicated in patients who are receiving monoamine oxidase inhibitors because of the risk of a potentially fatal syndrome characterized by hyperthermia, rigidity, and seizures.

Brunton LB, Lazo JS, Parker KL. *Goodman and Gilman's the pharmacological basis of thaerapeutics*, 11th ed. New York: McGraw-Hill, 2006:568–571.

B.17. What is rotation of opioids? When would you consider rotation of opioids?

The sequential trial of changing one opioid to another when either treatment-limiting toxicity or poor responsiveness develops has become known as *opioid rotation*. The variable response from opioid to opioid in an individual has led to this approach; changing to an alternative opioid may yield a far better balance between side effects and analgesia.

For those patients in whom pain control is inadequate and who have intolerable side effects, different strategies are implemented to improve analgesia. Opioid rotation is a simple strategy that almost all physicians can implement. Depending on equianalgesic potency ratio guidelines, switch is made to other opioids such as methadone or transdermal fentanyl patch. This should be done under close supervision and preferably in an inpatient environment.

Loeser JD, ed. *Bonica's management of pain*, 3rd ed. Philadelphia: Lippincott Williams & Wilkins, 2001:766–779.

C. Invasive Therapy

C.1. Describe the role of peripheral nerve blocks in cancer pain management.

The following nerve blocks can be considered depending on the location and distribution of the thoracic or abdominal pain and the involvement of viscera:

- Intercostal nerve blocks
- Interpleural blockade
- Splanchnic nerve blocks
- Celiac plexus block
- Hypogastric plexus block
- Thoracic and lumbar paravertebral somatic nerve blocks

- Rectus abdominis block
- Iliac crest block
- Ilioinguinal and iliohypogastric nerve block
- Cave of Retzius (space between urinary bladder and symphysis pubis) block

Various combinations of peripheral nerve blocks can be performed to aid in the global comfort of the patient by providing better pain control and reducing the total dose of medications and thereby the side effects. The most useful blocks for the upper abdomen and thorax are intercostal nerve blocks and celiac plexus blocks. The splanchnic nerve block and superior hypogastric blocks are the other two that can be considered depending on the location and involvement of the viscera. Thoracic and lumbar paravertebral blocks are performed to obtain spinal nerve segmental analgesia. The intercostal and thoracic paravertebral nerve blocks carry the risk of pneumothorax due to proximity of the pleura and lung. The peripheral nerve blocks are performed at anatomic sites away from the central neuraxis. More distal blocks have greater chances of incomplete blocks due to spatial distribution, overlap of nerves, and difficulty in blocking multiple branches of arborizing nerve.

DeLeon-Casasola OA. Cancer pain. In: *Pharmacological, interventional and palliative care approaches*. Philadelphia: WB Saunders, 2006:531–533.

Waldman SD, ed. *Interventional pain management*, 2nd ed. Philadelphia: WB Saunders, 2001:541–553.

C.2. Describe the role of celiac plexus block in cancer pain management.

Diagnostic celiac plexus block with a local anesthetic is performed to precisely differentiate sympathetically maintained pain and localize retroperitoneal or upper abdominal pain. A positive result of the diagnostic block is an indication for more definitive neurolysis in chronic cancer and nonmalignant pain. Success rates of celiac plexus neurolysis are lower in patients suffering from chronic nonmalignant abdominal pain than in those suffering from abdominal pain of neoplastic origin. Neurolysis of celiac plexus with alcohol or phenol is performed under fluoroscopic guidance or computed tomography–guided technique and strict sterile condition by using a single-needle periaortic technique, single-needle transaortic technique, single-needle anterior technique or endoscopic ultrasonography (EUS)-guided technique. Individual skills of the treating physician, available facilities, the patient's general condition, and extent of the spread of tumor should be considered in determining the type of technique to use.

Many pain physicians for celiac plexus neurolysis commonly use 40 to 50 mL of 50% to 70% alcohol or 6% to 10% phenol. Smaller volumes are recommended for absolute alcohol and higher concentration of phenol. Neurolysis with phenol is less painful because of its local anesthetic action, whereas alcohol neurolysis is very painful and should be blocked with pretreatment with local anesthetics.

DeLeon-Casasola OA, Cancer pain. In: *Pharmacological, interventional and palliative care approaches* Philadelphia: WB Saunders, 2006:401–416.

Waldman SD, ed. *Interventional pain management*, 2nd ed. Philadelphia: WB Saunders, 2001.

C.3. What are the complications of celiac plexus block?

Serious complications should rarely occur in the hands of a skilled clinician. Hypotension and increased gastrointestinal motility are the most common complications of this block. Neurologic complications include subarachnoid or epidural injection and lumbar nerve root injury, causing long-lasting paresthesia. A potentially severe complication can occur as a result of accidental injection into the nutrient artery of the spinal cord (artery of Adamkiewicz), causing paraplegia. Injury to the kidney may cause temporary hematuria that may not need any treatment. Other complications have been reported due to proximity of other vital structures include pneumothorax, chylothorax, intradisc injection, retroperitoneal hematoma, and failure to ejaculate.

Loeser JD, ed. *Bonica's management of pain*, 3rd ed. Philadelphia: Lippincott Williams & Wilkins, 2001:766–779.

C.4. Would you consider neuraxial opioid infusion in this patient? Discuss complications of this procedure.

In properly selected patients, epidural, intrathecal (subarachnoid), or intraventricular infusions of opioids have the advantage of producing profound analgesia without motor, sensory, or autonomic blockade. These routes are considered to deliver preservative-free medications when pain is not well controlled by noninvasive (oral, subcutaneous, or intravenous) routes and escalation of doses is limited by intolerable side effects. The potency ratio of oral to epidural morphine is 1:30, and that from oral to intrathecal morphine is 1:300. The decrease in the size of dose from oral to intrathecal greatly reduces the side effects and improves pain control and quality of life. The PCA technique can also be employed for epidural routes. Programmable intrathecal pumps can deliver medications at the prescribed dose. Fixed or flexible doses of morphine can deliver through the intrathecal pumps. The recently approved patient-controlled device allows patient-activated doses through the intrathecal pump (Personal Therapy Manager [PTM], Medtronic Neurological, Minneapolis). Morphine is the most commonly used drug. Other opiates, local anesthetics, ziconitide, α agonists etc; can be used as recommended by the polyanalgesic consensus panel.

These routes require a skilled experienced clinician, meticulous technique, and family and facility support in which close monitoring and follow-ups can be done. These procedures are reversible but involve expenses for specialized care and operating room costs. Intraspinal opioids may produce the same side effects of nausea, mental clouding, and sedation as in oral and parenteral dosing. Infection (e.g., meningitis and epidural abscess) and hematoma are potentially devastating complications that can cause permanent neurologic deficit if not dealt with in a timely basis. Pruritus and urinary retention are more common than with oral or parenteral administration.

DeLeon-Casasola OA, Cancer pain. In: *Pharmacological, interventional and palliative care approaches* Philadelphia: WB Saunders, 2006:417–429.

Hassenbusch SJ, Portenoy RK, Cousins M, et al. *Polyanalgesic Consensus Conference 2003: an Update on the Management of Pain By Intraspinal Drug Delivery Report of an Expert Panel*, 2003.

C.5. Would you consider neuraxial neurolysis in this patient to manage his pain? Discuss advantages and disadvantages of these blocks.

Owing to physical separation of motor and sensory nerve roots in the spinal canal and intrathecal space, chemical neurolytic procedures allow sensory blockade without loss of motor functions. Inadequate pain control with intolerable side effects makes this patient an ideal candidate for neuraxial neurolysis; however, complications of the procedure should be weighed against benefits. Epidural or intrathecal (subarachnoid) neurolytic blocks are considered for severe intractable pain from advanced cancer as an adjuvant to relieve pain and suffering and improve quality of life. These blocks are primarily effective in relieving pain of somatic origin and less effective for visceral and neuropathic pain.

In selected patients in whom pain relief is not achieved by less-invasive measures, these blocks can provide rapid analgesia and allow dosage (and side effects) reduction of systemic drugs. However, risks of postural hypotension, bowel and bladder incontinence, and motor and sensory deficit in the lower extremities cannot be overemphasized. These blocks are irreversible and require a skilled clinician to perform the procedure.

DeLeon-Casasola OA, Cancer pain. In: *Pharmacological, interventional and palliative care approaches* Philadelphia: WB Saunders, 2006:501–507.

C.6. Which neuroablative procedures can be considered in the terminal stage of pancreatic cancer?

On the basis of the location and type of pain (somatic, visceral, deafferentation), the general condition of the patient, the stage of tumor and metastasis, the life expectancy, and the expertise available, the following neurosurgical procedures could be considered:

- Peripheral neurectomy
- Dorsal rhizotomy
- Anterolateral cordotomy (spinal tractotomy)
- Commissural myelotomy
- Hypophysectomy

Loeser JD, ed. *Bonica's management of pain*, 3rd ed. Philadelphia: Lippincott Williams & Wilkins, 2001:766–779.

C.7. Describe the role of radiation therapy in cancer pain.

Radiation therapy can relieve pain from metastasis and symptoms from local extension of the disease. Radiation therapy is palliative and complementary to analgesic drug therapies to enhance the effectiveness of pain control. Along with therapeutic effectiveness of radiation treatment, the absence of complete specificity for disease may exacerbate or even cause new pain. The radiation dosage should be administered in the fewest fractions possible to promote pain control during and after treatment.

McQuay HJ, Collins SL, Carroll D, et al. Radiotherapy for the palliation of painful bone metastases. *Cochrane Database Syst Rev* 2000.

Raj PP, ed. *Practical management of pain*, 3rd ed. St. Louis: Mosby, 2000:824–837.

D. Nonpharmacologic Management

D.1. What are the various nonpharmacologic techniques of cancer pain management?

Eisenberg et al. demonstrated that cancer and other chronic pain syndromes such as acquired immune deficiency syndrome and arthritis may get benefit from alternative modalities. The common therapies offered are as follows:

- Physical therapy and physical modalities
- Relaxation and massage
- Chiropractic manipulation

- Spiritual healing
- Biofeedback and hypnosis
- Magnetic and low-power laser therapy
- Transcutaneous electrical nerve stimulation
- Homeopathy
- Acupuncture
- Prayer

Bradley LA, McKendree-Smith NL, Cianfrini LR. Cognitive-behavioral therapy interventions for pain associated with chronic illness: evidence for their effectiveness. *Semin Pain Med* 2003;1:44–54.

Eisenberg DM, Kessler RC, Foster C et al. Unconventional medicine in the United States. *N Engl J Med* 1993;328:246–252.

Raj PP, ed. *Practical management of pain*, 3rd ed. St. Louis: Mosby, 2000:807–814.

D.2. What physical modalities have been successfully tried in cancer pain management?

Physical modalities may help decrease stiffness, increase blood flow to the part, help relax the patient, and reduce the dose of analgesics. They include cutaneous stimulation, superficial heat and cold therapy, massage, vibration, and pressure. Cold therapy (cryotherapy) causes vasoconstriction, reduces inflammation, and decreases muscle spasm. Superficial application of heat (thermotherapy) acts through conduction or convection to increase blood flow to the skin and superficial organs. Heat also decreases joint stiffness and increases muscle flexibility. Physical therapy and exercise help to strengthen weak muscles, mobilize stiff joints, and restore coordination. Exercise may reduce pain by 25%. Weight-bearing exercises are avoided if an impending fracture is suspected.

Santiago-Palma J, Payne R. Palliative care and rehabilitation. *Cancer* 1999;92:1049–1052.

Raj PP, ed. *Practical management of pain*, 3rd ed. St. Louis: Mosby, 2000:807–814.

D.3. Describe the role of neuromodulation in cancer pain management.

Neuromodulation techniques such as spinal cord stimulation and deep brain stimulation have not been popular in cancer pain management. Neuromodulation techniques have variable outcome results with success rates between 18% and 80% depending on the study cited. Much of the literature is about chronic nonmalignant pain syndromes. The consensus among most pain physicians is that neuropathic pain syndromes are more effectively treated as spinal cord syndromes than as nociceptive pain syndromes. Therefore, spinal cord stimulation and deep brain stimulation should offer relief of neuropathic pain syndromes in patients with cancer.

Transcutaneous electrical nerve stimulation and acupuncture are believed to activate endogenous pain-relieving pathways. Low-voltage stimulation to large myelinated peripheral nerves through cutaneous electrodes may significantly reduce pain.

Acupuncture is a neuromodulatory technique that treats pain with insertion of needles in skin and underlying muscles. On the basis of various Chinese scientific principles, acupuncture is becoming very popular in Western medical systems. Many intrinsic factors contribute to the success of acupuncture, and in selected patients, it does control pain.

Nguyen JP, Lefaucher JP, Le Guerinel C, et al. Motor cortex stimulation in the treatment of central and neuropathic pain. *Arch Med Res* 2000;31:263–265.

Oakley J, Prager J. Spinal cord stimulation: mechanism of action. *Spine* 2002;27:2574–2583.

D.4. What psychologic techniques have been promoted for comfort care and pain relief?

Psychologic interventions are an important part of a multimodal approach to pain management in patients with cancer. It helps patients gain a sense of control over pain. Cognitive and behavioral techniques are designed to influence the interpretation of events and bodily sensations. Cognitive techniques help patients think differently about their pain and its management. Behavioral techniques help patients develop skills to cope with pain and help modify their reactions to pain. Patients who undergo psychotherapy report less pain. Relaxation therapy is a well-established modality in managing cancer pain. Several variations of relaxation strategies and techniques have been widely practiced in patients suffering from advanced cancer and have proved effective. Relaxation strategies such as deep breathing, muscle relaxation, and imagery are recommended for the promotion of comfort and relief of pain in hospitalized patients.

Relaxation and imagery are used to achieve a state of mental and physical relaxation, thereby relieving anxiety and muscle tension.

National Institutes of Health. *NIH consensus conference state of the science conference statement on symptom management in cancer: pain, depression and fatigue.* Bethesda: National Institute of Health, 2002.

D.5. What are distraction and reframing techniques? What is the role of hypnosis in cancer pain management?

Distraction and reframing techniques encourage focused attention on stimuli other than pain. This involves singing, talking, praying, and watching television. Reframing helps monitor and evaluate negative thoughts and images while encouraging positive thoughts and behavior.

Hypnosis by a skilled person decreases pain and anxiety in patients who have difficulty managing their pain. It also increases coping skills. This technique allows heightened awareness and focused concentration to manipulate perception of pain and has been effective in the management of cancer-related pain syndromes.

Devine EC. Meta-analysis of the effect of psychoeducational interventions on pain in adults with cancer. *Oncol Nurs Forum* 2003;30:75–89.

Raj PP, ed. *Practical management of pain*, 3rd ed. St. Louis: Mosby, 2000:807–814.

CHAPTER 31

Low Back Pain and Sciatica

David Y. Wang • Jeffrey Y. F. Ngeow

THE PATIENT IS A 57-YEAR-OLD FORMER FACTORY WORKER

who was injured on the job 8 years ago. He experienced severe low back and right leg pain after lifting a heavy piece of equipment and after workup was found to have a herniated L3-4 intervertebral disc with compression of the right L4 nerve root. He underwent a laminectomy and decompression; however, he has continued to complain of back pain.

A. Medical Disease and Differential Diagnosis

1. How great an issue is low back pain in the general population?
2. What are the incidence and prevalence of low back pain?
3. What is the societal cost of low back pain?
4. What are the risk factors for low back pain?
5. What are the potential sources of pain in the spine?
6. What is the anatomy of the intervertebral discs? What is the mechanism of pain from herniated discs?
7. What is that anatomy of the spinal facets? How do the facet joints cause pain?
8. What are the important points of the history and physical examination?
9. Which are the appropriate diagnostic studies for low back pain?
10. What is the differential diagnosis of low back pain?
11. What are the causes of multiple spine surgeries and persistent back pain?

B. Management of Low Back Pain and Sciatica

1. What are the noninterventional treatments available?
2. What are the traditional interventional treatments available and how should they be used?
3. What are some of the recent advances in minimally invasive interventions?
4. When should surgery be considered?
5. What new surgical options are now available for treatment of disc disease?

A. Medical Disease and Differential Diagnosis

A.1. How great an issue is low back pain in the general population?

Disorders of the lumbosacral spine cause pain, disability, suffering, public health, and socioeconomic issues with far greater impact than disorders of any other part of the body.

Most adults will experience several episodes of low back pain during their lifetime. It is estimated that 80% of workers will lose work time due to this particular complaint. On the basis of primary diagnosis only, a National Ambulatory Medical Care Survey (NAMCS) in 1989 to 1990 ranked low back pain as the fifth most frequent reason for adults to visit an office-based medical practice. In surveys employing a wider definition of low back pain, it was found to be the second most frequent symptom prompting physician office visits in the United States.

Fields HL, ed. Core curriculum for professional education. In: *Task force on professional education. Pain*, 2nd ed. Seattle: IASP Press, 1995:75–77.

Fordyce WE, ed. Back pain in the workplace. In: *Task force on pain in the workplace. Management of disability in nonspecific condition*. Seattle: IASP Press, 1995:5–9.

Hart LG, Deyo RA, Cherkin DC. Physician office visits for low back pain. Frequency, clinical evaluation, and treatment patterns from a U.S. national survey. *Spine* 1995;20: 11–19.

Manchikanti L. Epidemiology of low back pain. *Pain Phys* 2000;3:167–192.

A.2. What are the incidence and prevalence of low back pain?

Low back pain usually begins in early life, with the highest frequency of symptoms occurring between ages 35 and 55. Sixty percent to 80% of all adults in industrialized societies are affected at some point in their lives. Work absence and symptom duration increase with aging. An acute episode of low back pain usually resolves within 6 weeks. Up to 50% of all adults report having an episode of low back pain during a given year, and approximately 15% of these patients complain of frequent low back pain or pain lasting longer than 2 weeks during a given year. More persistent pain lasting beyond 3 to 6 months occurred in only 5% to 10% of patients with back pain. The United States Agency for Health Care Policy and Research (AHCPR) reported that 90% of patients with acute low back pain recover their usual activity tolerance within 4 weeks of injury. The remaining 10% of patients who do not recover with time and/or routine therapy go on to develop chronic symptoms and secondary problems. In a cross-sectional study among the Russian workforce published in 1995, Toroptsova et al. reported that the lifetime prevalence of low back complaints was 48.2%; the 1-year prevalence was 31.5% and the point prevalence was 11.5%. Using data from the NHANES II (National Health and Nutrition Examinations Survey II) survey, Deyo et al. reported that 1.6% of adults reported symptoms of both back pain and sciatica (lasting for at least 2 weeks). Only 2.1% of respondents had ever been told they had a "ruptured disc" in the low back. In other clinical studies, it was estimated that as few as 1% to 30% of low back pain can be attributed to nerve root compression.

Deyo RA, Tsui-Wu YJ. Descriptive epidemiology of low back pain and its related medical care in the United States. *Spine* 1987;12:264–268.

Fordyce WE, ed. Back pain in the workplace. In: *Task force on pain in the workplace management of disability in nonspecific condition*. Seattle: IASP Press, 1995: 43–56.

Loney PL, Stratford PW. The prevalence of low back pain in adults. A methodological review of the literature. *Phys Ther* 1999;79:384–396.

Manchikanti L. Epidemiology of low back pain. *Pain Phys* 2000;3:167–192.

Toroptsova NV, Benevolenskaya LI, Karyakin AN, et al. "Cross-Sectional" study of low back pain among workers at an industrial enterprise in Russia. *Spine* 1995;20(3): 328–332.

A.3. What is the societal cost of low back pain?

The cost to society of low back pain is enormous. Robertson et al. indicate that the prevalence of back symptoms and objective impairment to function have been unchanged over the last several decades. It appears, however, that the societal perception of disability has changed dramatically over the same time period. This has resulted in an increased rate and cost of disability and an overutilization of medical care, including surgical treatments. In 1992, the estimates of costs, morbidity and mortality of occupational injury or illness in the United States were $171 billion counting direct costs of $65 billion and indirect costs of $106 billion. Injuries accounted for $145 billion spent and illness $26 billion. It is estimated that 75% or more of these costs can be attributed to the 5% of people who become disabled temporarily or permanently from back pain. Occupational low back pain accounts for at least 33% of all health care and indemnity costs under workers' compensation. These numbers have been confirmed by recent research supported by the National Institute of Arthritis and Musculoskeletal and Skin Disease (NIAMS).

Katz JN. Lumbar disc disorders and low-back pain: socioeconomic factors and consequences. *J Bone Joint Surg* 2006;88(Suppl A):21–24.

Leigh JP, Markowitz SB, Fahs M, et al. Occupational injury and illness in the United States. Estimates of costs, morbidity, and mortality. *Arch Int Med* 1997;157:1557–1568.

Robertson JT. The rape of the spine. *Surg Neurol* 1993;39:5–12.

Volinn E, Turczyn K, Loeser. Theories of back pain and health care utilization. *Neurosurg Clin North Am* 1991;2:739–748.

Williams DA, Feuerstein M, Durbin D, et al. Health care and indemnity costs across the natural history of disability in occupational low back pain. *Spine* 1998;23:2329–2336.

A.4. What are the risk factors for low back pain?

Traditional beliefs suggested that heavy physical jobs required high energy demand and significant stress/strain on the spine, whereas light jobs required low energy demand. Many low-energy jobs, however, are static in nature, which is an inherent risk factor for low back pain. Low back pain, degenerative disc disease and disc herniation are associated with the following:

- Repetitive heavy lifting
- Static work posture (sitting or standing)
- Frequent twisting and bending
- Vibration (operation of motor vehicle or industrial device)
- The common vibration of construction vehicles and industrial devices ranges in frequency from 3.5 to 8.9 Hz.
- Low-frequency vibration, especially around 5 Hz, in conjunction with a prolonged seated position is associated with spine problems.
- The potential for damage to the disc through mechanical resonance is analogous to the high notes of an operatic soprano shattering wine glasses.
- Fatigue of the abdominal and paraspinal muscles has been demonstrated when subjected to 30 minutes of vibration. In the absence of this support, the spine is further susceptible to injury.
- A meta-analysis of 17 studies revealed that whole-body vibration is associated with an increased risk of low back pain, sciatica, and lumbar intervertebral disc disorders.
- Cigarette smoking
- Smoking is linked to low back pain, sciatica, and lumbar disc herniation.
- In an animal model, cigarette smoking significantly affects the vasculature outside the intervertebral disc, where the most pronounced effect is the reduction of solute-exchange capacity, cellular uptake, and metabolism within the disc.

- Cross-country skiing. In a study of skiing and spinal trauma, the diagonal body position required for cross-country skiing was the most common back pain–inducing stance, whereas no skier experienced back pain when only downhill skiing.

The "oxidative stress hypothesis of aging" theory proposed that enhancement of oxygen consumption due to increased physical activity may accelerate degeneration of the disc. On the other hand, strenuous exercises may contribute a positive nutritional effect by facilitating the transport of small solutes into and out of the disc. Generally, it is believed that persons who are physically fit or who maintain a balanced exercise program appear to have a lower risk of chronic low back pain and a more rapid recovery after an episode of acute back pain.

Biering-Sqrensen F, Thosen C. Medical social and occupational history as risk indicators for low-back trouble in a general population. *Spine* 1986;11:720–725.

Bovenzi M, Hulshof CT. An updated review of epidemiologic studies on the relationship between exposure to whole-body vibration and low back pain (1986–1997). *Int Arch Occup Environ Health* 1999;72:351–365.

Frymoyer JW, Pope MH, Clements JH, et al. Risk factors in low back pain. *J Bone Joint Surg* 1983;65-A:213–218.

Frymoyer JW, Pope MH, Kristiansen T. Skiing and spinal trauma. *Clin Sports Med* 1982; 1:309–318.

Holm A, Nachemson A. Nutrition of the intervertebral disc. Acute effects of cigarette smoking. An experimental animal study. *Ups J Med Sci* 1988;93:91–99.

Jerkins RR, Goldfarb A. Introduction. Oxidant stress, aging, and exercise. *Med Sci Sports Exerc* 1993;25:210–212.

Porter RW. Does hard work prevent disc protrusion? *Clin Biomech* 1987;2:196–198.

Sohal RS, Allen RG. Oxidative stress as a causal factor in differentiation and aging: a unifying hypothesis. *Exp Gerontol* 1990;25:499–522.

Wilder DG, Woodworth BB, Frymoyer JW, et al. Vibration and the human spine. *Spine* 1982; 7:243–254.

A.5. What are the potential sources of pain in the spine?

In order to more easily identify the various sources of pain, the spine may be divided into three compartments: anterior, middle, and posterior.

The anterior compartment consists of the vertebral body and intervertebral disc. The anterior unit is bound together by cephalocaudal ligaments: anterior longitudinal ligament (ALL) and posterior longitudinal ligament (PLL). The ALL is anatomically much broader and stronger than the PLL. The PLL is intact throughout the length of the vertebral column until it reaches the lumbar vertebrae. From L1, it becomes progressively narrower until at L5-S1 it is only one half of its original width. This anatomic feature contributes to an inherent structural weakness in the lumbar spine. Hence the lower lumbar spine is the region subjected to the greatest static stress and most spinal movement resulting in the greatest kinetic strain.

The middle (neuraxial) compartment contains all the structures within the bony and ligamentous boundaries of the spinal canal. This includes the PLL, epidural space, meninges, spinal cord, dorsal and ventral nerve roots, root sleeves, dorsal root ganglia, and ligamentum flavum.

The posterior compartment contains the facet joints, laminae, vertebral arches, and structures posterior to the plane of the transverse processes and innervated by the dorsal rami of the spinal nerves. The ligaments are extremely important in stabilizing the vertebral column. The ligamentum flavum (yellow ligament), which connects the laminae of adjacent vertebrae, is the thickest and strongest ligament in the lumbar region. It can contribute to spinal stenosis by folding inward during upright posture, extension of the back, as well as through hypertrophy.

The sinovertebral nerve originates lateral to the neural foramina and enters the spinal canal anterior to the dorsal root ganglion. It is a branch of the somatic ventral nerve root and the sympathetic grey ramus communicans. This specific nerve, also known as the *nerve of Luschka*, innervates the outer annulus of the disc, PLL, epidural membranes and dura at the segmental level of origin and adjacent levels. It is important to note that central low back pain, with or without referred pain to the buttocks, may derive from irritation of the outer part of the annulus fibrosis or the PLL.

In summary, the potential sources of low back and radicular pain include the bony structure of vertebrae, muscles attached to the spine and hips, fasciae, ligaments, discs, facet joints, meninges, vessels, nerve roots, dorsal root ganglia, and nerves in the surrounding areas.

The natural wear and tear on the discs and facet joints results in microtrauma and degeneration. This can induce the release of neurohumoral mediators such as phospholipase A_2, serotonin, H^+, substance P, prostaglandin E_2, and so on, to produce inflammation of the nerve roots or meninges, and sensitize local nociceptors. Furthermore, it has been theorized that material from the nucleus pulposus, sheltered from the immune system by the presence of the annulus fibrosis, might act as a foreign protein and trigger an autoimmune reaction. The recent demonstration of an activated immunocompetent cellular response at the epidural interface of the herniation of the nucleus pulposus (HNP) supports the concept of the immunogenic capacity of the nucleus pulposus. Tissue injury or inflammation can cause a barrage of nociceptive input into the spinal cord. This may lead to a phenomenon called *central sensitization* or *wind-up* of neurons in the dorsal horn of the spinal cord. The release of excitatory amino acids and neuropeptides in the dorsal horn is thought to be the mechanism underlying the phenomenon of central sensitization. At the cellular level, there is an increase in spontaneous discharge and an expansion of neural receptive fields of wide-dynamic-range (WDR) neurons located in Rexed lamina V of the spinal cord. Clinically, this is characterized by sensation of pain when exposed to nonnoxious stimuli (allodynia), significantly increased response to painful input (hyperalgesia), and increased response to repetitive stimulation (hyperpathia).

Bogduk N. The innervation of the lumbar spine. *Spine* 1983;8:286–293.

Bogduk N. *Clinical anatomy of the lumbar spine and sacrum*, 3rd ed. New York: Churchill Livingstone, 1997:43–53.

Cavanaugh JM. Neural mechanisms of lumbar pain. *Spine* 1995;20:1804–1809.

Howe JF, Loeser JD, Calvin WH. Mechanosensitivity of dorsal root ganglia and chronically injured axons: a physiological basis for the radicular pain of nerve root compression. *Pain* 1977;3:25–41.

Jessell TM. Neurotransmitters and CNS disease: pain. *Lancet* 1982;2:1084–1088.

Kang JD, George HI, McIntyre L, et al. Herniated lumbar intervertebral discs spontaneously produce matrix metalloproteinases, nitric oxide, interleukin-6, and prostaglandin E_2. *Spine* 1996;21:271–277.

Manchikanti L. Transforaminal lumbar epidural steroid injection. *Pain Phys* 2000;3:374–398.

Olmarker K, Rydevik B. Pathophysiology of sciatica. *Orthop Clin North Am* 1991;22:223–233.

Olmarker K, Rydevik B, Nordborg C. Autologous nucleus pulposus induces neurophysiologic and histologic changes in porcine cauda equina nerve roots. *Spine* 1993;18:1425–1432.

Saal JS. The role of inflammation in lumbar pain. *Spine* 1995;20:1821–1827.

Williams GW. Low back pain: cost-effective diagnosis and treatment. *Contemp Int Med* 1995;7:27–42.

A.6. What is the anatomy of the intervertebral disc? What is the mechanism of pain from herniated discs?

The intervertebral disc is a ring-like structure composed of a centrally located well-hydrated pliable proteoglycan matrix, the nucleus pulposus, which comprises two thirds of the surface area of the disc. Surrounding the nucleus is a fibrocartilaginous ring composed predominantly of type I collagen, the annulus fibrosus, which makes up the remaining one third of the surface area of the disc. The annulus fibrosus is stronger anteriorly but often defective posteriorly. As a self-contained fluid system, the disc absorbs shock, permits transient compression, and allows movement. It provides a cushion between the vertebral bodies and allow for greater flexibility.

As the disc ages, the number of viable cells in the nucleus pulposus decreases, and the proportion of cells that exhibit necrosis changes from 2% in infancy to 50% in young adults and 80% in the elderly. The water content in the young disc is 80% to 90% in the nucleus pulposus. With aging, the discs tend to dehydrate, losing up to 70% of their water content. As the nucleus pulposus further dehydrates, it becomes more fibrous and less compliant. A disc will usually herniate under strain and pressure. When overstressed, it will protrude along in the path of least resistance, usually posterolaterally. This can cause direct mechanical pressure on the nerve roots resulting in radiculopathy.

In the healthy back, only the outer third of the annulus fibrosus is innervated. In the degenerative or disrupted disc, small unmyelinated nerve fibers grow into the inner third of the annulus fibrosus and even into the nucleus pulposus. Internal disc disruption (IDD) is a condition characterized by a degenerated nucleus pulposus with radial fissures extending into the peripheral annulus fibrosus. Upon rupture of the disc, the release of irritative material near the meninges can induce radiculitis and symptoms of radiculopathy without actual herniated disc material compressing the nerve roots. Under such circumstances, significant disc herniation might not be visualized on magnetic resonance imaging (MRI) or computed tomography (CT) scan. In brief, the proposed mechanisms of radiculopathy include (a) direct pressure on nerve fibers due to compression injury, (b) indirect impact through impairment of microcirculation, chemical irritation and inflammation, immune reaction, edema formation secondary to permeability changes of the intraneural capillaries, and impairment of the nutritional transport to the nerve root.

Compression of the nerve roots is dependent upon the effective space available within the neural foramina, the osseous structures surrounding the neural foramina, and the tethering effects of the intraspinal and extraspinal ligaments. Posterolateral disc herniations can impinge upon the lumbar dorsal root, which then initiates electrical discharges for as long as 25 minutes after the mechanical stimulus has been removed. Radiculopathy can be produced by either biochemical or mechanic stimulation of a swollen, stretched or compressed nerve root. Approximately 3% to 12% of all lumbar disc herniations occur laterally and extend into or beyond the foraminal zone; in this setting, the patients will complain of sudden and severe radicular pain, often with dysesthesia. On the other hand, discogenic pain due to a central disc bulge/herniation stimulates several lumbar tissues such as the outer layer of the annulus fibrosus or posterior longitudinal ligament (PLL). Clinically this is manifested as central low back pain without any radicular symptoms.

Bernick S, Walker JM, Paule WJ. Age changes to the annulus fibrosus in human intervertebral discs. *Spine* 1991;5:520–524.

Bogduk N. *Clinical anatomy of the lumbar spine and sacrum*, 3rd ed. New York: Churchill Livingstone, 1997:171–174.

Buckwalter JA. Aging and degeneration of the human intervertebral disc. *Spine* 1995; 20:1307–1314.

Epstein JA, Epstein BS, Rosenthal AD, et al. Sciatica caused by nerve root entrapment in the lateral recess: the superior facet syndrome. *J Neurosurg* 1972;36:584–589.

Freemont AJ, Peacock TE, Goupille P, et al. Nerve ingrowth into diseased intervertebral disc in chronic back pain. *Lancet* 1997;350:178–181.

Gower WE, Pedrini V. Age-related variations in protein-polysaccharides from human nucleus pulposus, annulus fibrosus and costal cartilage. *J Bone Joint Surg* 1969;51A: 1154–1162.

Kang JD, Geogescu HI, McIntyre-Larkin L, et al. Herniated cervical intervetebral discs spontaneously produce matrix metalloproteinases, nitric oxide, interleukin-6, and prostaglandin E_2. *Spine* 1995;20:2373–2378.

Kuslich SD, Ulstrom CL, Michael CJ. The tissue of origin of low back pain and sciatica. *Orthop Clin North Am* 1991;22:181–187.

Naylor A, Horton WG. The hydrophilic properties of the nucleus pulposus of the intervertebral disc. *Rheumatism* 1955;11:32–35.

Roffe PG. Innervation of the annulus fibrosus and posterior longitudinal ligament. *Arch Neurol Psychiatry* 1940;44:100.

Takebayashi T, Cavanaugh JM, Ozaktay C, et al. Effect of nucleus pulposus on the neural activity of dorsal root ganglion. *Spine* 2001;26:940–945.

Weiner BK, Fraser R. Foraminal injection for lateral lumbar disc herniation. *J Bone Joint Surg* 1997;79-B:804–807.

A.7. What is that anatomy of the spinal facets? How do the facet joints cause pain?

The facet or zygapophysial joints consist of two arthrodial joints superiorly and inferiorly, each lined with synovium, lubricated by synovial fluid, contained within a joint capsule. These synovial joints enhance spinal stability and flexibility. In the upper part of the lumbar spine (L1 3), the facet planes lie in a generally vertical sagittal plane and permit flexion and extension but prevent lateral flexion or bending in the lordotic curve. The lumbosacral facet joints at the level of L5-S1 depart the farthest from the sagittal plane allowing some rotation of the lower part of the lumbar spine. With slight forward flexion, the facets of the other lumbar vertebrae separate and permit a modest degree of lateral movement and rotation. Facet loading, if of a repetitive nature, may play a role in the degeneration of the facet joint. After repeated wear and tear, these joints are susceptible to osteoarthritis and associated synovial cyst formation. Hypertrophic facet joints or cysts can encroach on the spinal canal or the intervertebral foramina and contribute to the development of central spinal or foraminal stenosis.

Hsu KY, Zucherman JF, Shea WJ, et al. Lumbar intraspinal synovial and ganglion cyst (facet cyst), ten-year experience in evaluation and treatment. *Spine* 1995;20: 80–89.

Kuslich SD, Ulstrom CL, Michael CJ. The tissue of origin of low back pain and sciatica. *Orthop Clin North Am* 1991;22:181–187.

Mooney V, Robertson J. The facet syndrome. *Clin Orthop* 1976;115:149–156.

Schwartzer A, Wang S, Bogduk N, et al. Prevalence and clinical features of lumbar zygapophyseal join pain: a study in an Australian population with chronic low back pain. *Ann Rheum Dis* 1995;54:100–106.

Taylor JR, Twomey LT. Age changes in lumbar zygapophyseal joints, observation on structure and function. *Spine* 1986;11:739–745.

A.8. What are the important points of the history and physical examination?

A problem-focused history should include onset, location, intensity (e.g., pain scale 0–10), characteristics (achy, spasmodic, stabbing, burning, shooting, etc.), duration plus aggravating and alleviating factors. The essential step in the initial evaluation is to differentiate patients with serious underlying pathology from those with mild problems.

When the disc is involved, pain increases with activities that increase intradiscal pressure, such as bending, lifting, twisting, and stooping. Patients with a disc problem will usually experience an exacerbation of their symptoms with spinal flexion. By contrast, in the setting of spinal stenosis, standing or walking exacerbates back and leg pain whereas forward flexion may alleviate these symptoms. In moderate to severe spinal stenosis, extension of the spine may cause radicular pain.

Patients with compression fractures typically present with severe back pain relieved by rest, often intense with minimal lateral rotation or with flexion. X-ray is the test of choice to evaluate this problem. On rare occasion, bone scan is required to rule out very small fracture. Back pain in a patient with a history of malignancy should prompt studies to exclude metastatic disease.

A history of bladder, bowel, or sexual dysfunction may indicate compression of the cauda equina or conus medullaris. Unlike sciatica, often with its unilateral nerve root involvement, patients with cauda equina syndrome usually have bilateral involvement. Although motor function may be normal and pain uncommon in those with conus lesions, patients often demonstrate abnormalities of sensation in a saddle distribution, feeling touch or dysesthesiae but neither pain nor temperature. Causes of these symptoms may be a fracture of L1 or L2, tumor, large central disc herniations, or intramedullary cysts affecting the conus. These disorders are considered surgical emergencies and require aggressive evaluation and prompt surgical consultation.

The physical examination should include Lasègue's maneuver (the straight leg raising test), Gower's maneuver (dorsiflexion of the ankle with elevation of the leg), and the crossover test. These clinical tests are considered positive when sciatica is reproduced with elevation of the leg between 30 and 60 degrees. If testing the uninvolved leg produces contralateral symptoms, disc disease should be considered. A positive crossover sign occurs when straight leg raising of the patient's contralateral leg elicits pain on the affected side. It is usually a strong indication of nerve root irritation or compression. Extension of the knee while in a seated position, also known as *distracted straight leg raise*, can test sciatic nerve tension too. The patient with significant nerve root irritation tends to complain of increased pain or lean backward to reduce tension on the nerve. The differential diagnosis of spinal shock, upper motor neuron lesions, and lower neuron lesions is shown in Table 31.1. The nerve root signs are shown in Table 31.2.

Hoppenfeld S. *Orthopaedic neurology: a diagnostic guide to neurologic levels*. Philadelphia: Lippincott-Raven, 1997:93–101.

Simmon SM. Physical examination of the patient in pain. In: Raj PR, ed. *Practical management of pain*, 3rd ed. St. Louis: Mosby, 2000:339–359.

Smith SA, Massie JB, Chesnut R, et al. Straight leg raising. Anatomical effects on the spinal nerve root without and with fusion. *Spine* 1993;18:992–999.

Rowlingson JC. Low back pain and pain of the lower extremity. In: Raj PR, ed. *Practical management of pain*, 2nd ed. St. Louis: Mosby, 1992:296–311.

Table 31.1 Differentiating Spinal Shock, Upper Motor Neuron Lesions, and Lower Motor Neuron Lesions.

DISEASE STATE	DEEP TENDON REFLEX	PATHOLOGICAL REFLEX/PLANTAR RESPONSE	SUPERFICIAL REFLEX (NORMAL)
Spinal shock	Absent	Absent	Absent
Upper motor neuron disease	Increased; rarely may be decreased in the acute setting	Positive/extensor	Decreased or absent
Lower motor neuron disease	Decreased	Negative/flexor	Present

A.9. Which are the appropriate diagnostic studies for low back pain?

In the absence of signs of serious medical disease there is no need for any special studies, because 90% of patients will recover spontaneously within 4 weeks of the onset of pain. Waiting 4 weeks before considering special tests allows these patients to recover spontaneously and avoid unneeded procedures. When pain persists beyond 4 to 6 weeks, plain x-rays of the spine should be considered. Pertinent findings include the height of the intervertebral spaces, the vertebral bodies and bony changes in the endplates. With oblique views, the facet joint space and spondylolysis can also be evaluated. The lateral view can help estimate the severity of spondylolisthesis. A computed tomography (CT) scan can show a herniated disc or fragment in the spinal canal. It can help to identify early epidural hematoma. With contrast, it can help further differentiate tumors, abscesses, and granuloma in central nervous system (CNS). The magnetic resonance imaging (MRI) provides excellent anatomic definition of the disc and its hydration status; it can also show the anatomy of the surrounding soft tissues. An MRI with intravenous gadolinium is the best choice for distinguishing between a recurrent disc herniation and postoperative scar tissue. It is particularly useful in spinal imaging and when distinguishing intrinsic from extramedullary or epidural spinal cord lesions. When MRI is contraindicated, a myelogram may reveal a filling defect at the level of posterior bulging discs. The myelogram in conjunction with a CT scan adds to the imaging of transverse sections of the spinal cord and subarachnoid space. A bone scan is helpful in the diagnosis of bone or bony fractures that may not be visible by x-ray or CT scan.

Electromyelography (EMG) and nerve conduction velocity (NCV) are electrodiagnostic tests that help differentiate diseases of the neuromuscular junction from primary myopathy or

Table 31.2 Nerve Root Signs.

ROOT LEVEL	REFLEX DECREASE	SENSORY DEFECT	MOTOR WEAKNESS
L4	Knee jerk	Anterior thigh, knee, and shin	"Single squat and rise test"; quadriceps (mostly L4)
L5	No easily elicited reflex	Lateral leg and middle dorsal foot	"Heel walk test"; Dorsiflexion of foot and toes (L5 and some L4); especially big toe, extensor hallucis longus (EHL)
S1	Ankle jerk	Posterior calf and sole	"Toe walk test"; gastrocnemius/soleus; "toe flexors"

secondary to denervation. EMG should not be performed earlier than 4 weeks from the onset of symptoms, as results may not be accurate early in the disease process. Somatosensory evoked potentials (SSEPs) are also used to help isolate the level of radiculopathy.

Discography/discogram/discomanometry (discometry) is a specialized diagnostic test specifically indicated to help diagnose discogenic pain. The presence of pain fibers in the outer third of the annulus fibrosus may explain back pain in some individuals with an annulus fracture or internal disc disruption (IDD). The test involves an intradiscal puncture and instillation of contrast into the disc nucleus. It provides direct confirmation of nuclear morphology and integrity of the vertebral endplate and annulus.

Jensen MC, Brant-Zawadzki MN, Obuchowski N, et al. Magnetic resonance imaging of the lumbar spine in people without back pain. *N Engl J Med* 1994;331:69–73.

Mekhail NA, Moufawad S. Discography and discogenic pain. *Tech Regional Anesth Pain Manage* 2000;4:126–131.

Weinstein J, Claverie W, Gibson S. The pain of discography. *Spine* 1988;13:1344–1348.

A.10. What is the differential diagnosis of low back pain?

There are numerous diagnostic labels which all carry the name of low back pain, for example, lumbosacral sprain, lumbar discogenic syndrome, mechanical and chemical consequences of disc herniation, spondylosis, spondylolisthesis, osteoarthritis/facet joint syndrome, myofascial pain syndrome, spinal stenosis, foraminal stenosis, segmental scoliosis, unstable low back, discitis, and failed back surgery syndrome (FBSS). The presence of postural back pain frequently results from reflex muscle spasm secondary to local irritation of structures in the back. When muscle spasm occurs, the normal anatomy may be disturbed and undue force applied to surrounding tissues and structures. A careful history, physical examination, and the appropriate diagnostic studies will help elucidate the "pain generator."

Basmajian JV. Acute back pain and spasm, a controlled multicenter trial of combined analgesic and antispasm agents. *Spine* 1989;14:438–439.

Schwazer AC, Aprill CN, Bogduk N. The sacroiliac joint in chronic low back pain. *Spine* 1995;20:31–37.

Travell JG, Simons DG. *Myofascial pain and dysfunction. The trigger point manual.* Vol.1. Baltimore: Williams & Wilkins, 1983:541–551.

A.11. What are the causes of multiple spine surgeries and persistent back pain?

Persistent back or leg pain after one or several spinal surgeries is called *failed back surgery syndrome (FBSS)* or *postlaminectomy syndrome*. Usually, the cause is a combination of both nociceptive and neuropathic pain. Over time, a strong psychological component can develop with progressive disability as treatments fail. Approximately 37,500 patients are diagnosed with this syndrome annually in the United States.

When pain persists or recurs in a patient with a history of spinal surgery, after recurrent disc herniation and bony stenosis have been ruled out, the most common neuroradiologic finding is usually that of epidural fibrosis and scarring. Patients in this condition often report constant dull, aching, diffuse low back pain with intermittent sharp and intense pain. They also report pain or abnormal sensations with neuropathic characteristics such as burning, shooting, throbbing, stabbing, or pulling. The exact source of these complaints is unclear although scar tissue or arachnoiditis is frequently implicated. When reoperation is performed for the purpose of neurolysis only, a transient improvement of sciatica may be seen, but it usually recurs within the first postoperative year. Success rates for reoperating on FBSS patients have been highly variable, ranging from 25% to 80%. The FBSS patients are perhaps the most challenging of all. They deserve a comprehensive multidisciplinary evaluation including orthopedic and neurosurgical consultations. Further surgical intervention should be avoided in the absence of a neurologic or neurosurgical emergency.

Annertz M, Jonsson B, Sromqvist B, et al. No relationship between epidural fibrosis and sciatica in the lumbar postdiscectomy syndrome. A study with contrast-enhanced magnetic resonance imaging in symptomatic and asymptomatic patients. *Spine* 1995;20: 449–453.

Kim SS, Michelsen CB. Revision surgery for failed back surgery syndrome. *Spine* 1992; 17:957–960.

Richardson J. Editorial: realizing vision. *Br J Anesth* 1999;83:369–371.

Weber H. Lumbar disc herniation: a controlled, prospective study with ten years of observation. *Spine* 1983;8:131–140.

B. Management of Low Back Pain and Sciatica

B.1.   What are the noninterventional treatments available?

The cornerstone of treatment for low back pain and mild sciatica caused by a herniated lumbar disc is conservative care, which includes bed rest, medications, and physical therapy. Patients whose symptoms fail to respond to conservative care may require more invasive treatment.

There is both clinical and epidemiologic evidence that the longer the back pain and work loss persist, the less likely there will be improvement of the pain. The chance for return to work is even lower. Improved early management and greater access to primary care services should greatly reduce the number of patients with simple backache who require referral to hospitals. Over the last decades, there has been a paradigm shift in the treatment of low back pain away from focusing care exclusively on the pain in favor of helping patients improve their activity tolerance and function. An early return to activity seems to be associated with a better outcome than does prolonged bed rest (>4 days).

Treatment varies depending on the cause of pain. In December 1994, the Agency for Health Care Policy and Research (AHCPR) announced the following guidelines for the care of acute low back problems.

- A brief period of rest
- Over-the-counter pain relievers
- Trunk-strengthening exercises
- A single spinal manipulation

Activities and postures that increase stress on the back also tend to aggravate back symptoms. Patients limited by back symptoms can minimize the stress of lifting by keeping any lifted object close to the body at the level of the navel. Activities such as twisting, bending, and reaching while lifting, also increase stress on the back. Prolonged sitting may aggravate back symptoms in discogenic pain patients due to progressive increasing pressure at specific points in the abnormal disc.

In order to avoid becoming debilitated, an incremental, gradually increasing regimen of aerobic exercise (up to 20 to 30 minutes daily) can usually be started within the first 2 weeks of symptom onset. Such activities have been found to stress the back no more than sitting for an equal time period on the side of the bed. The combination of aerobics for general fitness with some specific training to improve the strength and endurance of the back muscles is recommended.

The role of medications in the treatment of low back pain and facet arthropathy is to control pain, facilitate rehabilitation, restore normal sleep patterns and improve mood and/or motivation. Nonsteroidal antiinflammatory drugs (NSAIDs) are an essential part of the treatment of patients with inflammatory back pain, such as that associated with spondylitis. Other medications, which have been shown to be useful, include tricyclic antidepressants and anticonvulsants. Muscle relaxants are often used to decrease muscle spasm and to assist in promoting rest for patients with severe pain. These are usually indicated for short-term treatment and acute relief. Short-term therapy with opioid analgesics may be needed to promote rest as well as maintain activity in the acute phase of low back pain. Long-term use of opioids and muscle relaxants is generally discouraged, but may be required for carefully selected patients.

When recovery does not occur within 6 weeks and no additional pathology is detected, physical therapy is indicated. Patients should be encouraged to increase activity. Body weight optimization and a program that teaches good posture and body mechanics are also important. Neuromuscular reconditioning must be included to ensure a function-specific, task-oriented program. Essential and most importantly, the program must be geared to enhance functional recovery in the affected patient. The exercise training is designed as a step-by-step program to improve patients' function and optimal neutral spine posture. These programs include stabilization training to attain adequate dynamic control of lumbar spine forces and to eliminate repetitive injury. Soft tissue flexibility, joint mobility, abdominal muscle strengthening, and aerobic exercise are also important factors.

Spinal manipulation is controversial and is not recommended in patients with radiculopathy pain, nor is it wise in those for whom a diagnosis has not been established. For appropriately selected patients, if manipulation has not resulted in symptomatic and functional improvement after 4 weeks, it should be stopped and the patient reevaluated.

Cherkin DC, Deyo RA, Battie M, et al. A comparison of physical therapy, chiropractic manipulation, and provision of an educational booklet for the treatment of patients with low back pain. *N Engl J Med* 1998;339:1021–1029.

Deyo RA, Diehl AK, Rosenthal M. How many days of bed rest for acute low back pain? *N Engl J Med* 1986;315:1064–1070.

Faas A, Chavannes AW, van Eijk JTM, et al. A randomized, placebo-controlled trial of exercise therapy in patients with acute low back pain. *Spine* 1993;18:1388–1395.

Malmivaara A, Hakkinen U, Aro T, et al. The treatment of acute low back pain-bed rest, exercise, or ordinary activity? *N Engl J Med* 1996;332:351–355.

Williams GW. Low back pain: cost-effective diagnosis and treatment. *Contemp Int Med* 1995;7:27–42.

B.2. What are the traditional interventional treatments available and how should they be used?

Common traditional interventional treatment includes the following:

- Trigger point injection
- Traditional epidural steroid injection (interlaminar approach)
- Transforaminal epidural steroid injection (transforaminal approach)
- Facet joint intraarticular block or medial branch block

Interventional techniques such as trigger point injections and local infiltration are used to provide pain relief of short duration, so that other activities and physical therapy which might otherwise be severely limited by pain, may be pursued.

Corticosteroids play an important role against inflammation and reduction of edema. Steroids injected into the epidural space have been used for treating low back pain and radiculopathy. Despite widespread use, the results of epidural steroid injection are still in question because the studies evaluating the response to this therapy have been small, poorly controlled and lacking good long-term follow-up. Published studies of the effectiveness of epidural steroid injections have varied from 18% to 90%. The addition of hyaluronidase into the epidural injectate is thought to improve the spread of local anesthetic and steroid through tissue planes. Hyaluronidase acts by cleaving hyaluronic acid, which is found within connective tissue, skin, aorta, vitreous humor of the eye, joint cartilage, and the nucleus pulposus of the disc. Epidural steroid injections can be performed through the interlaminar route, the caudal canal or the intervertebral foramina. The spread of solution in both caudal and interlaminar injection is less controllable due to inconsistent lateral flow into the ventral compartment. This renders the medication less effective as it is diverted away from the vertical compartment depending upon the tightness of the lateral recess and the size of the dural sac. In normal volunteers, the transforaminal method showed good ventral flow, whereas the interlaminar approach showed predominantly dorsal flow, which was far away from the usual site of inflammation.

Patients who suffer from lumbar facet arthropathy may have symptoms including band-like low back pain associated hip, groin, or thigh pain. Pain rarely radiates below the knee. Blockade of the medial branch of the dorsal ramus of the spinal nerve or intraarticular injections of the lumbar facets are effective in short-term alleviation of this type of pain.

Abram SE. Factors that influence the decision to treat pain of spinal origin with epidural steroid injection. *Reg Anesth Pain Med* 2001;26:2–4.

Benzon HT, Molloy RE. Outcomes, efficacy, and complication from management of low back pain. In: Raj PR, ed. *Practical management of pain*. 3rd ed. St. Louis: Mosby, 2000:891–903.

Carette S, Leclaire R, Marcoux S, et al. Epidural corticosteroid injections for sciatica due to herniated nucleus pulposus. *N Engl J Med* 1997;326:1634–1640.

Fanciullo GJ, Hanscom MS, Seville J, et al. An observation study of the frequency and pattern of use of epidural steroid injection in 25,479 patients with spinal and radicular pain. *Reg Anesth Pain Med* 2001;26:5–11.

Farmer JC, Wisneski RJ. Cervical spine nerve root compression. An analysis of neuroforaminal pressures with varying head and arm positions. *Spine* 1994;19:1850–1855.

Manchikanti L. Transforaminal lumbar epidural steroid injection. *Pain Phys* 2000;3:374–398.

Manchikanti L, Singh V, Bakhit C, et al. Interventional techniques in the management of chronic pain: part 1.0. *Pain Phys* 2000;3:7–42.

Manchikanti L, Pampati V, Baktit CE, et al. Effectiveness of lumbar facet joint nerve blocks in chronic low back pain: a randomized clinical trial. *Pain Phys* 2001;4:101–117.

Manchikanti L, Singh V, Kloth D, et al. Interventional techniques in the management of chronic pain: part 2.0. *Pain Phys* 2001;4:24–96.

Nash TP. Facet joints: intra-articular steroid or nerve blocks? *Pain Clin* 1990;3:77–82.

Olmarker K, Brisby H, Yabuki S, et al. The effects of normal, frozen, and hyaluronidase-digested nucleus pulposus on nerve root structure and function. *Spine* 1997;22:471–476.

Olmaker K, Byrod G, Cornefjord M. Effects of methylprednisolone on nucleus pulposus-induced nerve root injury. *Spine* 19994;19:1803–1808.

Rowlingson J. Epidural steroid in treating failed back surgery syndrome. *Anesth Analg* 1999;88:240–242.

Watson D. Hyaluronidase. *Br J Anaesth* 1993;71:422–425.

B.3. What are some of the recent advances in minimally invasive interventions?

There are several recent interventional techniques for the management of low back pain and sciatica that can be applied to appropriately selected patients. These include the following:

- Epidural neuroplasty or epidural adhesiolysis
- Epiduroscopy (spinal canal endoscopy)
- Percutaneous radiofrequency denervation of medial branches for facet joint pain
- Chemonucleolysis
- Automated percutaneous discectomy (APD) or percutaneous automated discectomy (PAD) or percutaneous automated nucleotomy (PAN)
- Percutaneous laser disc decompression (PLDD)
- Intradiscal electrothermal therapy (IDET)
- Percutaneous disc decompression using nucleoplasty
- Percutaneous lumbar discectomy using Dekompressor probe
- Spinal cord stimulation (SCS)
- Intrathecal drug delivery
- Percutaneous vertebroplasty (PV) and percutaneous kyphoplasty (PK)

Epidural neuroplasty or epidural adhesiolysis with hypertonic saline and hyaluronidase is used to lyse epidural adhesions. This technique involves placing a rigid catheter into the epidural space for applying local anesthetic, steroid, hypertonic saline (10%), and hyaluronidase over several days along with manipulation of the catheter to physically break the adhesions.

Epiduroscopy (or spinal canal endoscopy) directly visualizes the epidural space using a combination of both a fiberoptic light source and a flexible fiberoptic catheter. Adhesions are then physically lysed with the catheter; thereafter, better delivery of medications to the target area can be achieved.

Percutaneous radiofrequency denervation of the medial branches of the dorsal (or posterior) rami of segmental spinal nerves offers prolonged pain relief by applying heat to denature the nerves that innervate the painful facet joints. The success rate has been reported variably in the range of 17% to 90% for management of lumbar facet joint pain of a few weeks' to several months' duration. With this technique, the pain may return in several weeks to months after the axons regenerate; repeating the procedure is then indicated.

Chemonucleolysis, first performed by Lyman Smith in 1963, involves the application of chymopapain, a proteolytic enzyme to dissolve the nucleus pulposus. It has an average success rate of 76% to 80%. Unfortunately, chymopapain is indiscriminate in the protein that it will digest, and it may cause neural damage if it comes into contact with neural elements. For example, there is a risk of chymopapain leaking through the adhesions between the disc and the dura mater into the subarachnoid space. The complications include anaphylactic reaction (0.3% allergic reaction), subarachnoid hemorrhage, infection, and transverse myelitis with associated paraplegia.

Percutaneous manual nucleotomy was first presented by Hijikata in 1975. The idea of a percutaneous approach was proposed as a method of preventing the perineural and epidural scar formation by avoidance of entry into the spinal canal. Thereafter, APD or PAD or PAN was designed as a procedure using "nucleotome" (reciprocating suction-cutting probe) for intradiscal pressure decompression by Onik in 1985. The cannula requires a sizable annular incision to reach the nucleus. Its success rate is approximately 70% to 80%.

PLDD is a technique, introduced by Ascher and Choy in 1987, using Nd:YAG laser to "vaporize" a small portion of the nucleus pulposus in an attempt to decompress the involved disc. It has been demonstrated that the inner pressure of the nucleus pulposus drops significantly after the disc ablation. Its success rate is approximately 78%. After 4 to 6 months from this treatment, it was demonstrated that one third of repeat magnetic resonance imaging (MRI) scans showed modest to moderate decrease of disc herniation. There is concern, however, that the potentially hazardous to bone and nerve tissue due to significant rise in temperature, thermal energy transfer and extent of tissue heated.

IDET or annuloplasty, first reported by Saal and Saal in 2000, has been shown to be effective in managing discogenic pain. It is a minimally invasive procedure in which a catheter is inserted into the nucleus pulposus through which an electrode is passed so that a controlled level of heat at a temperature of 90°C (194°F) can be applied to a broad section of the affected disc inner wall. This thermal therapy is postulated to alleviate discogenic pain by shrinking collagen at a target temperature of 65°C (149°F) to 75°C (167°F). Another proposed mechanism is denervation of exposed nociceptor endings in the outer disc annulus starting at 45°C (113°F).

Percutaneous disc decompression using nucleoplasty is a recently developed procedure, first applied in 2000, for disc decompression, for those patients whose symptoms are attributed to radiographically contained discs. By combining tissue removal with thermal treatment, disc decompression can be achieved. It applies a focused "coblation" technique, ablating while advancing deeper into disc versus coagulating (by using bipolar radiofrequency) while withdrawing inside disc, to reach the level of 40°C (104°F) to 70°C (158°F). At this temperature, molecular dissociation is achieved and thought to minimize the potential for surrounding tissue damage.

Percutaneous disc decompression using 17-gauge Dekompressor probe is also a recently developed procedure for disc decompression, for those patients whose symptoms are attributed to radiographically contained discs. By just tissue removal, disc decompression may be achieved It provides objective evidence that disc was removed, the cellular character of that material, and provides a qualitative and quantitative measure.

SCS is a technique where electrodes are passed into the posterior epidural space. Electrical stimulation of the spinal cord has been shown to be effective in the management of certain neuropathic pain syndromes and postlaminectomy syndromes. The exact mechanism by which pain relief is achieved remains controversial.

Intrathecal drug delivery directly (IDET) into the cerebrospinal fluid through an implanted catheter and pump can be used to treat intractable pain from a variety of causes, both nociceptive and neuropathic. A variety of medications and combinations thereof can be used depending upon the type and location of symptoms. Among the experts this is known as *intrathecal polyanalgesia*. This modality is indicated when increasing doses of opioid are required to achieve pain relief but at the expense of disabling side effects. The dose is effectively reduced to approximately 1/300, for example, when converting an oral dose of morphine to its equipotent equivalent delivered intrathecally.

PV and PK are both advanced techniques used in the treatment of painful compression fracture. In the United States, compression fractures occur in approximately 700,000 patients per year, and 80% of these fractures occur in women. The conventional management includes bed rest, analgesics, and bracing. PV was a technique developed in 1984 for the treatment of painful vertebral hemangiomas. It has since become popular for the treatment of osteoporotic vertebral body compression fracture. It involves the application of liquid cement (polymethylmethacrylate), tobramycin, and barium powder (as nonionic contrast) through a special metal needle under fluoroscopy. The cement provides vertebral solidification and buttresses the compressed bone within the vertebral body. The procedure usually takes 45 to 60 minutes and the patient may be discharged several hours later. There are some risks involved with this procedure, such as leakage of cement into surrounding areas (disc, spinal cord, and nerve roots), infection, bleeding, worsened pain, embolism, and paralysis. Overall, more than 80% of treated patients had moderate to marked pain relief.

PK is a recently developed technique similar to PV, which involves the application of an additional inflatable balloon inside the collapsed vertebral body. Thereby, the compressed fracture is expanded, the lost height of the vertebral body is restored, and an inner space/cavity is created for the cement. This procedure was approved by the "U.S. Food and Drug Administration" in 1998. A significant reconstitution of the curvature of the spine can be seen following kyphoplasty. According to Lieberman, in 70% of the collapsed vertebral bodies, the kyphoplasty restored 47% of the lost height. This newer technique offers the additional advantage of realigning the spinal column and restoring height to the fractured vertebrae.

The above two procedures are associated with pain relief in 67% to 100% of cases. Most patients experience significant pain relief within the first 1 to 2 days. There is also a report of 95% improvement in pain and significant improvement in function following treatment by either of the two techniques.

Anderson SR, Racz GB, Heavner J. Evolution of epidural lysis of adhesions. *Pain Phys* 2000;3:262–270.

Brown MD. Update on chemonucleolysis. *Spine* 1996;21:62S–68S.

Choy DS, Ascher PW, Saddekni S, et al. Percutaneous laser disc decompression: a new therapeutic modality. *Spine* 1992;17:949–966.

Dreyfuss P, Halbrook B, Pauza K, et al. Efficacy and validity of radiofrequency neurotomy for chronic lumbar zygapophysial joint pain. *Spine* 2000;25:1270–1277.

Garfin SR, Yuan HA, Reiley MA. New technologies: kyphoplasty and vertebroplasty for the treatment of painful osteoporotic compression fractures. *Spine* 2001;26:1511–1515.

Hayashi K, Thabit G, Bogdanske JJ, et al. The effect of nonablative laser energy on the ultrastructure of joint capsular collagen. *Arthroscopy* 1996;12:474–481.

Heavner JE, Racz GB, Raj P. Percutaneous epidural neuroplasty: prospective evaluation of 0.9% NaCl versus 10% NaCl with or without hyaluronidase. *Reg Anesth Pain Med* 1999;24:202–207.

Lieberman JH, Dudeney S, Reinhardt MK, et al. Initial outcome and efficacy of "kyphoplasty" in the treatment of painful osteoporotic vertebral compression fractures. *Spine* 2001;26:1631–1638.

Lord SM, Barnsley L, Wallis BJ. Percutaneous radio-frequency neurotomy for chronic cervical zygapophyseal-joint pain. *N Engl J Med* 1996;335:721–726.

Onik G, Maroon J, Helms C, et al. Automated percutaneous discectomy: initial patient experience. *Radiology* 1987;162:129–132.

Onik G, Nooney V, Maroon JC, et al. Automated percutaneous discectomy: a prospective multi-institutional study. *Neurosurgery* 1990;26:228–233.

Peh WC, Gilula LA, Peck DD. Percutaneous vertebroplasty for severe osteoporotic vertebral body compression fractures. *Radiology* 2002;223:121–126.

Racz GB, Heavner JE, Raj P. Epidural neuroplasty. *Semin Anesth* 1997;16:302–312.

Saal JA, Saal JS. Nonoperative treatment of herniated lumbar intervertebral disc with radiculopathy, an outcome study. *Spine* 1989;14:431–437.

Saal JS, Saal JA. Management of chronic discogenic low back pain with a thermal intradiscal catheter. *Spine* 2000;25:382–388.

Saberski LR. A retrospective analysis of spinal canal endoscopy and laminectomy outcome data. *Pain Phys* 2000;3:193–196.

Sharps LS, Issac Z. Percutaneous disc decompression using nucleoplasty. *Pain Phys* 2002; 5:121–126.

Singh V. Intradiscal electrothermal therapy: a preliminary report. *Pain Phys* 2000;3:367–373.

Van Kleef M, Barendse GAM, Kessels A, et al. Randomized trial of radiofrequency lumbar facet denervation for chronic low back pain. *Spine* 1999;24:1937–1942.

Watts NB, Harris ST, Genant HK. Treatment of painful osteoporotic vertebral fractures with percutaneous vertebroplasty or kyphoplasty. *Osteoporos Int* 2001;12:429–437.

B.4. When should surgery be considered?

There are several surgeries indicate for low back pain and sciatica. These include laminectomy, macro- or microdiscectomy, foraminotomy, intervertebral body insertion, and spinal fusion.

According to Weber's study, the long-term results appear to be no different in the surgery versus nonsurgery group in the case of low back pain. If the following situations occur, however, surgery should be considered:

- Failure to respond to conservative management for at least 3 months
- A profound or progressing neurologic defect such as a complete foot drop
- Recurring episodes of intractable sciatica involving the same segment—mainly to avoid the cumulative disability of repeated events.

Muscle weakness is a dubious indication for surgery if the paresis is of unknown duration. If the pressure on the nerve root can be relieved immediately after the appearance of the paresis, surgery has been regarded as the therapy of choice. Unfortunately, most patients are unaware of the subtle loss of motor function. The greatest concern and complaints are largely centered around pain, paresthesiae, and immobility.

Within the first 3 months of acute low back symptoms, surgery is considered only when serious spinal pathology or nerve root dysfunction, obviously due to a herniated lumbar disc, is detected. Nerve root decompression can be considered for a patient if all of the following criteria exist:

- Sciatica is both severe and disabling.
- Symptoms of sciatica persist without improvement for longer than 4 weeks or with extreme progression.
- There is strong physiologic evidence of dysfunction of a specific nerve root with intervertebral disc herniation confirmed ipsilaterally at the corresponding level by imaging.

Patients with acute low back pain alone, without findings of serious conditions or significant nerve root compression, rarely benefit from a surgical consultation. With or without surgery, more than 80% of patients with obvious surgical indications eventually recover.

Benzon HT, Molloy RE. Outcomes, efficacy, and complication from management of low back pain. In: Raj PR, ed. *Practical management of pain*, 3rd ed. St. Louis: Mosby, 2000:891–903.

Kim SS, Michelsen CB. Revision surgery for failed back surgery syndrome. *Spine* 1992; 17:957–960.

McCulloch JA. Focus issue on lumbar disc herniation: macro- and microdiscectomy. *Spine* 1996;21:45S–56S.

Weber H. Lumbar disc herniation: a controlled, prospective study with ten years of observation. *Spine* 1983;8:131–140.

Zdeblick TA. A prospective, randomized study of lumbar fusion. *Spine* 1993;18:983–991.

B.5. What new surgical options are now available for treatment of disc disease?

- Artificial disc replacement (ADR)
- Interspinous process decompression system (X STOP)

In the mid-1980s, Drs. Schellnack and Buttner, two German orthopedic surgeons, developed a metal and plastic prosthesis, which has been in clinical use for more than 17 years. The prosthesis is known as the *SB CHARITÉ*. The prosthesis design is currently in its third generation. There are other prosthetic discs available including Prodisc, Maverick and FlexiCore and Kineflex. In October 2004, the CHARITÉ artificial disc became the first to be approved for disc replacement in the United States. It is composed of two metallic endplates and a polyethylene core that moves between them (Figs. 31.1–31.4). Traditional spinal fusion does change the mechanics of the segment that is fused. Adjacent segment degeneration can develop at approximately 3% per year (or 16.5% at 5 years, 36.1% at 10 years). One major theoretic advantage of ADR over spine fusion is that it results in no change in the biomechanics of the lower spine, thereby allowing the spine to maintain its normal range of motion and reducing or eliminating the risk of degeneration in the adjacent segments of the spine. The indications for ADR are similar to that for an anterior lumbar interbody fusion (ALIF) using interbody cages. The contraindications for ADR include infection, spinal stenosis, spondylolisthesis (or other types of instability in the spine, such as fracture or tumor), scoliosis, facet joint osteoarthritis, significant radiculopathy, osteoporosis and pregnancy. Artificial discs are not perfect. The potential disadvantage of ADR is a limited durability. Because disc injury is a common cause of back pain in younger adults, an artificial disc in such patients needs to last for decades. The demands on that disc will be very great and it may not outlast the lifetime of the patient, who may need revision surgery later. Revision ADR can be very dangerous because of scar tissue from the original surgery in nearby vascular structures. In addition, there is a 1% to 3% of complication of retrograde ejaculation in the male.

The interspinous process decompression system (X STOP) is a titanium metal implant made to fit between the lumbar spinous processes of the vertebrae (Figs. 31.5 and31.6). It is designed to relieve narrowing of the spinal canal and neural foramen during extension and thereby reducing the symptoms of neurogenic intermittent claudication (NIC). The indications include spinal stenosis and degenerative lumbar spondylolisthesis.

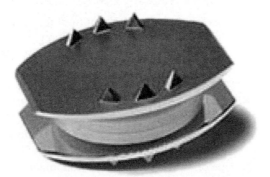

Figure 31.1 Charité disc.

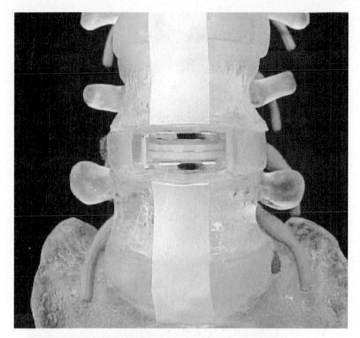

Figure 31.2 Charité disc.

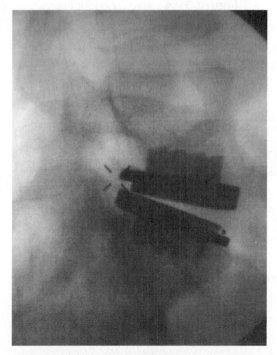

Figure 31.3 L5-S1 artificial disc replacement (ADR), lateral fluoroscopic view.

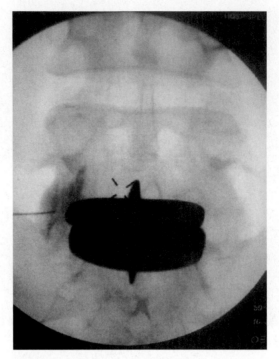

Figure 31.4 Anteroposterior fluoroscopic view of artificial disc replacement (ADR).

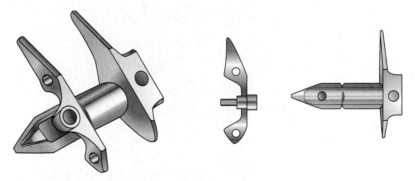

Figure 31.5 Interspinous process decompression system (X STOP).

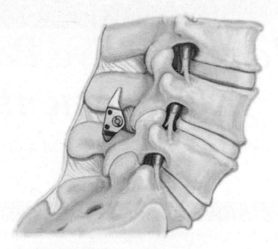

Figure 31.6 Interspinous process decompression system (X STOP).

Anderson PA, Tribus CB, Kitchel SH. Treatment of neurogenic claudication by interspinous decompression: application of the X STOP device in patients with lumbar degenerative spondylolisthesis. *J Neurosurg Spine* 2006;4(6):463–471.

Blumenthal SL, McAfee PC, Guyer RD et al. *A prospective, randomized investigational device exemptions study of lumbar total disc replacement with the Charité™ artificial disc versus lumbar fusion: part I: evaluation of clinical outcomes.*

Geisler FH, Blumenthal SL, Guyer RD, et al. Neurological complications of lumbar artificial disc replacement and comparison of clinical results with those related to lumbar arthrodesis in the literature: results of a multicenter, prospective, randomized investigational device exemption study of Charité™ intervertebral disc. *J Neurosurg Spine* 2004;1(2):143–154.

Ghiselli G, Wang JC, Bhatai NN, et al. Adjacent segment degeneration in the lumbar spine. *J Bone Joint Surg* 2004;86-A7:1497–1503.

Kulkarni V, Rajshekhar V, Raghuram L. Accelerated spondylotic changes adjacent to the fused segment following central cervical corpectomy: magnetic resonance imaging study evidence. *J Neurosurg* 2004;100:2–6.

Van Ooij A, Oner FC, Verbout AJ. Complications of artificial disc replacement: a report of 27 patients with the SB Charite disc. *J Spinal Disord Tech* 2003;16(4):369–383.

Zucherman JF, Hsu KY, Hartjen CA, et al. A multicenter, prospective, randomized trial evaluating the X STOP interspinous process decompression system for the treatment of neurogenic intermittent claudication: two-year follow-up results. *Spine* 2005; 1530(12):1351–1358.

CHAPTER 32

Perioperative Pain Management

Narinder Rawal • Vinod Malhotra

A 60-YEAR-OLD-MAN

with a smoking history of a packet of cigarettes a day for approximately 40 years and chronic obstructive pulmonary disease (COPD) is scheduled for thoracotomy for removal of carcinoma in his right middle lobe.

A. Perioperative Pain Management for Thoracotomy

1. What would be your advice to the patient about the planned thoracotomy and postoperative pain relief?
2. How will you decide about the choice of anesthetic technique?
3. What is chronic postthoracotomy pain syndrome (PTPS)? Does video-assisted thoracic surgery (VATS) reduce the risk of chronic pain after thoracotomy?
4. What would be your perioperative analgesic strategy?
5. Does the choice of analgesic technique influence postoperative outcome?
6. Does it matter if the tip of epidural catheter is at the thoracic or lumbar level?
7. Does the choice of drugs influence the efficacy or safety of thoracic epidural analgesia (TEA)?
8. What are the usual doses and concentrations of the anesthetic combinations commonly employed in epidural analgesia?
9. If accidental dural puncture occurs during placement of the epidural needle, what steps should be taken?
10. What are the alternatives to TEA?
11. What is the usual clinical regimen for intravenous patient-controlled analgesia (IV-PCA) and is special patient monitoring required during its use?
12. What are the side effects and complications of epidural technique?
13. What recommendations for placement and removal of the epidural catheter will you make if this patient is on antiplatelet or anticoagulant therapy or thromboprophylaxis is planned?

> ### A 70-YEAR-OLD WOMAN
>
> with breast cancer and metastasis is being treated for the last 6 months with transdermal fentanyl (Duragesic patch) for her cancer pain. She is currently on a 100-μg per hour patch every 72 hours. She is now scheduled for surgery for hip fracture after a fall. The patient was very dissatisfied with postoperative pain management after her breast surgery 3 months earlier.

B. Chronic Opioid Therapy and Perioperative Pain Management

1. How does chronic opioid therapy influence postoperative pain management?
2. What are the causes for increased postoperative pain and opioid consumption in patients chronically using opioids?
3. What are the main differences between a chronic opioid-consuming patient and a patient who abuses or is addicted to opioids?
4. What issues need to be considered in the opioid-tolerant patient who is scheduled for surgery?
5. What would be your strategy regarding preoperative information and choice of anesthesia technique?
6. What are the choices for perioperative pain management in opioid-tolerant patients?
7. What issues need to be considered before discharging an opioid-tolerant patient?

> ### A 38-YEAR-OLD ASA II PATIENT
>
> scheduled for ambulatory laparoscopic cholecystectomy demands to see the anesthesiologist preoperatively to discuss her postoperative analgesia strategy. She experienced severe pain at home for several days after a previous ambulatory gynaecologic laparoscopic procedure

C. Perioperative Pain Management for Ambulatory Surgery

1. What would be your preoperative considerations and patient advice?
2. What are the consequences of inadequate pain management after ambulatory surgery?
3. What is the role of premedication or preoperative analgesic?
4. Does the choice of anesthetic technique influence postoperative pain?
5. Are nonsteroidal antiinflammatory drugs (NSAIDs) effective? If so, does the choice of drug matter?
6. There are three types of pain after laparoscopic cholecystectomy—incisional, subphrenic, and shoulder pain. What is the role of surgical technique in influencing postoperative pain?
7. What would be your strategy for pain control after discharge home?

> ### MANY PATIENTS
>
> experience moderate to severe pain after surgery, as shown in several surveys including a recent one from the United States. What can we do to address this longstanding problem?

D. The Role of Acute Pain Service

1. What is the extent of the problem and which patients are at greater risk of undertreatment?

2. What are the consequences of inadequate postoperative pain relief?

3. What is the role of Acute Pain Services (APSs) in improving postoperative pain management?

4. Does an APS improve postoperative outcome?

A. Perioperative Pain Management for Thoracotomy

A.1. What would be your advice to the patient about the planned thoracotomy and postoperative pain relief?

It is essential that patients undergoing thoracotomy be informed about what to expect after surgery, as an understanding of the procedure as well as realistic expectations of pain and rehabilitation can promote recovery and return to normal activity. Patients undergoing thoracotomy may suffer from severe acute postoperative pain if analgesia is not managed appropriately. Pulmonary function is impaired as a result of thoracic surgery, and may be worsened by the effects of pain. Therefore during the early postoperative period, pain control and maintenance of pulmonary function are the major goals. For preoperative improvement of pulmonary function, patients should be given intermittent physiotherapy of the lung and general physical exercises, and be advised to stop smoking.

Educational resources, such as www.youranaesthetic.info and www.asahq.org/patientEducation.htm can inform patients about their forthcoming anesthetic procedure and provide specific advice about the different anesthetic and pain relief techniques for surgery.

Early postoperative pain may be intense, and can delay rehabilitation and mobilization unless appropriately treated. Different techniques may be used to manage different levels of pain immediately following surgery, within the first postoperative day and thereafter. Pain management often involves a step-down approach from regional anesthesia or systemic opioids to oral medication. The following issues need to be addressed:

- Information must be given on the hospital policy for pain assessment, for example, the use of visual analog scores.
- Patients require a realistic expectation of the intensity and duration of postoperative pain.
- Pain management techniques that require patient involvement (intravenous patient-controlled analgesia, patient-controlled epidural analgesia) need to be properly demonstrated.

Information resources such as postoperative pain guidelines may be useful:
www.oqp.med.va.gov/cpg/cpg.htm (Rosenquist 2003) and *http://www.nhmrc.gov.au/publications/files/cp104.pdf* (Australian and New Zealand College of Anaesthetists and Faculty of Pain Medicine).

www.postoppain.org (PROSPECT—procedure-specific evidence-based and recommendations for thoracotomy by an international panel of anesthesiologists and surgeons).

A.2. How will you decide about the choice of anesthetic technique?

The decision about which anesthetic technique to use for an individual patient is based on a review of their overall medical condition and any medication that they are taking. General, epidural, and spinal anesthesia, and combinations of these, have separate risks and benefits, which vary according to the patient's comorbidity and medications. Other factors such as surgical and anesthetic experience and practice, local ward or institutional protocols for postoperative pain relief and patient mobilization will also influence the choice of anesthetic technique. Intraoperative use may be desirable as an adjunct to general anesthesia, to ensure epidural catheter function and to facilitate a comfortable transition to the immediate postoperative period.

The use of intra- and postoperative thoracic epidural technique has become a widely used technique for management of pain associated with thoracic and major abdominal surgery. Many experimental and clinical studies have shown that thoracic epidural anesthesia may have effects far beyond pain relief. Transient thoracic sympathectomy by thoracic epidural analgesia (TEA) is believed to offer protective cardiac, pulmonary, and gastrointestinal effects in addition to positive immunologic and coagulation effects. A common anesthetic technique is a combination of preoperative thoracic epidural and general anesthesia. Administration of local anesthetic into the epidural catheter results in several postoperative benefits such as reduced risk of pulmonary complications, improved bowel recovery, and a significant reduction in the incidence of myocardial infarction.

Ballantyne JC, Carr DB, DeFerranti S, et al. The comparative effects of postoperative analgesia therapies on pulmonary outcome: cumulative meta-analyses of randomized, controlled trials. *Anesth Analg* 1998;86(3):598–612.

Beattie WS, Badner NH, Choi P. Epidural analgesia reduces postoperative myocardial infarction: a meta-analysis. *Anesth Analg* 2001;93(4):853–858.

Jørgensen H, Wetterslev J, Møiniche S, et al. Epidural local anaesthetics versus opioid-based analgesic regimens for postoperative gastrointestinal paralysis, PONV and pain after abdominal surgery 2001. *Cochrane Database Syst Rev* 1, art no CD001893.D01:10.1002/14651858.CD001893.

A.3. What is chronic postthoracotomy pain syndrome (PTPS)? Does video-assisted thoracic surgery (VATS) reduce the risk of chronic pain after thoracotomy?

Chronic PTPS is defined as pain that recurs or persists along a thoracotomy scar at least 2 months after surgery and is not related to the recurrence of a tumor or an infection. PTPS is generally neuropathic in nature and varies in severity, with a reported incidence of 44% to 80%. Several studies suggest that poor perioperative pain management may contribute to chronic PTPS and that aggressive management of early postoperative pain with epidural analgesia may reduce its incidence.

Although used with increasing frequency, thoracoscopic approaches have not had the favorable impact on pain that many had anticipated. Surprisingly, VATS is associated with a prevalence of chronic pain comparable to that of open procedures, with rates of pain ranging from 22% to 63% which is probably due to intercostal nerve and muscle damage from trocar insertion.

Lung volumes after thoracic surgery may be reduced by up to 50% and aggressive analgesic therapy leads to improvements in pulmonary function not observed with standard therapy.

Bertrand PC, Regnard JF, Spaggiari L, et al. Immediate and long-term results after surgical treatment of primary spontaneous pneumothorax by VATS. *Ann Thorac Surg* 1996;61:1641–1645.

Gottchalk A, Cohen SP, Yang S, et al. Preventing and treating pain after thoracic surgery. *Anesthesiology* 2006;104:594–600.

International Association for the Study of Pain, Subcommittee of Taxonomy. Classification of chronic pain. *Pain* 1986;24(Suppl 3):S138–S139.

Katz J, Jackson M, Kavanagh BP, et al. Acute pain after thoracic surgery predicts long-term post-thoracotomy pain. *Clin J Pain* 1996;12(1):50–55.

Landreneau RJ, Mack MJ, Hazelrigg SR, et al. Prevalence of chronic pain after pulmonary resection by thoracotomy or video-assisted thoracic surgery. *J Thorac Cardiovasc Surg* 1994;107:1079–1085.

Ng JM, Hartigan PM. Pain management strategies for patients undergoing extrapleural pneumoectomy. *Thorac Surg Clin* 2004;14:585–592.

Perttunen K, Tasmuth K, Kalso E. Chronic pain after thoracic surgery: a follow-up study. *Acta Anaesthesiol Scand* 1999;43(5):563–567.

Senturk M, Ozcan PE, Talu GK, et al. The effects of three different analgesia techniques on long-term postthoracotomy pain. *Anesth Analg* 2002;94(1):11–15.

Tiippana E, Nilsson E, Kalso E. Post-thoracotomy pain after thoracic epidural analgesia: a prospective follow-up study. *Acta Anaesthesiol Scand* 2003;47(4):433–438.

A.4. What would be your perioperative analgesic strategy?

A multimodal approach would be preferable; this takes into account the multiple pathways by which nociceptive input is conveyed to the central nervous system, the number of pharmacologically distinct mechanisms of modulating this input, the need for effective analgesia throughout the perioperative period and after discharge, and the importance of minimizing side effects, particularly respiratory depression.

Thoracic epidural analgesia (TEA) is the mainstay of recommended therapy, with alternative interventions for situations where TEA is not suitable. When epidural catheters fail intraoperatively, intercostal nerve blocks (ICNBs) or paravertabral blocks may supplant epidural analgesia or serve as a bridge to the immediate postoperative period when an epidural catheter can be safely replaced. The analgesic plan should consider the entire perioperative period.

Intravenous nonsteroidal antiinflammatory drugs (NSAIDs) are useful for treating shoulder pain refractory to epidural analgesia and, given their effectiveness as analgesic adjuncts, patients using patient-controlled epidural analgesia should receive oral or IV NSAIDs. Although the limited effect on platelets of drugs that specifically inhibit cyclooxygenase 2 (COX-2) may be important, the potential of these drugs in the setting of thoracic surgery awaits resolution of their cardiovascular safety. Regular administration of paracetamol (acetaminophen) may also be useful for treating shoulder pain and can be used in addition to NSAIDs. For analgesic continuity when making the transition to oral opioid analgesics, the first oral dose should be administered at the time patient-controlled epidural analgesia is discontinued.

www.postoppain.org (PROSPECT—procedure specific evidence-based and recommendations for thoracotomy by an international panel of anesthesiologists and surgeons).

A.5. Does the choice of analgesic technique influence postoperative outcome?

Recent large meta-analyses strongly suggest that epidural analgesia is associated with lower rates of perioperative pulmonary and cardiac complications. Compared with systemic opioids, epidural opioids decreased the incidence of postoperative atelectasis; epidural local anesthetics increased PaO_2 and decreased the incidence of pulmonary infections and pulmonary complications overall. Effective pain control with epidural technique leads to improved pulmonary function, more effective coughing, earlier mobilization, and improved cooperation with respiratory physiotherapy.

Postoperative myocardial infarction rates are reduced when thoracic epidural analgesia (TEA) is incorporated into the anesthesia and extended at least 24 hours into the postoperative period. Supraventricular tachyarrhythmias, which are the most common form of cardiac morbidity after pulmonary resection and occur in up to 25% of cases, are reduced by TEA, even when compared with alternative analgesic regimens that confer equivalent pain control. The cardioprotective mechanism of TEA is believed to relate to its sympatholytic effects.

A meta-analysis found that epidural analgesia provided superior postoperative analgesia compared with intravenous patient-controlled analgesia (IV-PCA).

Wu CL, Cohen SR, Richman JM, et al. Efficacy of postoperative patient-controlled and continuous infusion epidural analgesia versus intravenous patient-controlled analgesia with opioids: a meta-analysis. *Anesthesiology* 2005;103(5):1079–1088; quiz 1109–1110.

A.6. Does it matter if the tip of epidural catheter is at the thoracic or lumbar level?

Thoracic epidural analgesia (TEA) is currently the standard for analgesia for thoracic surgery and, in the absence of contraindications, all patients undergoing major open thoracic surgical procedures should have a thoracic epidural catheter placed preoperatively. The tip of the catheter should reside at the dermatome along which the incision will be made.

Thoracic (versus lumbar) placement of the epidural catheter is dose saving, with possibly fewer consequent side effects at equianalgesia and superior postoperative recovery. Thoracic placement also reduced motor block of the lower extremities, which may delay postoperative ambulation. Even lumbar placement can be efficacious, particularly when used with hydrophilic opioids such as morphine.

Grant GJ, Zakowski M, Ramanthan S, et al. Thoracic versus lumbar administration of epidural morphine for postoperative analgesia after thoracotomy. *Reg Anesth* 1993;18:351–355.

Sandler AN, Stringer D, Panos L, et al. A randomized, double-blind comparison of lumbar epidural and intravenous fentanyl infusions for postthoracotomy pain relief: Analgesic, pharmacokinetic, and respiratory effects. *Anesthesiology* 1992;77:626–634.

A.7. Does the choice of drugs influence the efficacy or safety of thoracic epidural analgesia (TEA)?

Effective postoperative pain control may be achieved by delivering an opioid, local anesthetic, or a combination of both into the thoracic epidural space. Combinations are the standard, because the synergy between opioids and local anesthetic agents enable an appropriate balance in the mixture to minimize blockade of motor function of the thorax and dynamic consequences of sympatholysis. Common components include the opioids morphine, fentanyl, and sufentanil and local anesthetic agents such as bupivacaine, levobupivacaine, and ropivacaine. Systemic absorption effects (e.g., sedation) tend to be more common with the lipophilic opioids, such as fentanyl, whereas hydrophilic opioids, such as morphine, produce a wider dermatomal band of analgesia and are associated with more minor side effects, such as nausea, and vomiting. Of the three local anesthetic agents, bupivacaine possesses the least favorable cardiac safety profile, whereas ropivacaine has differential sensory and motor blocking effects. When used in dilute concentrations in combination with opioids, it seems unlikely that any advantage of one agent over the other will be apparent.

Ng JM, Hartingan PM. Pain management strategies for patients undergoing extrapleural pneumonectomy. *Thorac Surg Clin* 2004;14:585–592.

Rawal N. Intraspinal opioids. In: Rowbotham DJ, Macintyre PE, eds. *Acute pain*. Arnold, 2003:241–266.

A.8. What are the usual doses and concentrations of the anesthetic combinations commonly employed in epidural analgesia?

Before the initiation of patient-controlled epidural analgesia, a test dose of 3 mL of 1.5% lidocaine with epinephrine 1:200,000 is usually employed to rule out intrathecal or intravascular placement of catheter.

Commonly employed combinations of epidural drugs vary from institution to institution. However, in the interest of patient safety, compliance, auditing, and quality assurance, standardization within the institution is recommended.

For example, at our institution the following drugs and drug combinations are used at an infusion rate of 4 mL per hour with each demand bolus of 3 mL as needed.

- Bupivacaine 0.0625% with fentanyl 5 μg per mL with a lockout period of 10 minutes between boluses.
- Fentanyl 10 μg per mL with a lockout period of 10 minutes.
- Bupivacaine 0.0625% with dilaudid 100 μg per mL with a lockout period of 20 minutes.
- Morphine sulphate 100 μg per mL with a lockout period of 30 minutes.

(See sample order form [Fig.32.1].)

A.9. If accidental dural puncture occurs during placement of the epidural needle, what steps should be taken?

If accidental dural puncture occurs during placement of epidural needle, the general practice is to remove the needle and place the epidural catheter at adjacent intervertebral spaces. The likelihood of intrathecal spread should be carefully assessed with the test dose. Epidural infusion may be started at the usual rate. Frequent monitoring for sensory and sympathetic block should continue in a controlled setting until the efficacy and safety of the epidural analgesia is established. The patient should be informed of the dural puncture and the potential for postdural puncture headache.

A.10. What are the alternatives to thoracic epidural analgesia (TEA)?

There are times when for technical, medical, or other reasons thoracic epidural catheter placement is unsuccessful, undesirable, or not possible. Alternatives to mid-TEA include lower thoracic and lumbar epidural catheter placement, intercostal nerve blocks (ICNBs), paravertebral blocks, intrapleural catheters, local anesthetic infiltration, and systemic analgesia with one or more agents.

Even lumbar placement can be efficacious, particularly when used with hydrophilic opioids such as morphine. ICNBs can be performed percutaneously or under direct vision, using single injections or placement of an intercostal catheter. However, unpredictable spread of local anesthetic and rapid local anesthetic absorption make it less effective than epidural analgesia. Furthermore, indwelling intercostal catheters do not adequately control pain after posterolateral thoracotomy because posterior primary rami and sympathetic fibers are not blocked. Percutaneous positioning and securing of intercostal catheters may be technically problematic.

Paravertebral block results in ipsilateral somatic and sympathetic nerve blockade in multiple contiguous thoracic dermatomes above and below the site injection. Paravertebral analgesia has been found to produce good pain relief and preservation of pulmonary function after thoracotomy and is the only serious contender to challenge epidural analgesia. Because the concomitant sympathetic blockade is unilateral, the incidence of adverse effects, such as hypotension and urinary retention, is lower. Paravertebral blocks can be performed as single injections or through a paravertebral catheter. Paravertebral catheters can be placed percutaneously or intraoperatively

NewYork-Presbyterian
The University Hospital of Columbia and Cornell

45171

EPIDURAL ANALGESIA ORDER SHEET
PAIN MANAGEMENT

IF NO PLATE, PRINT NAME, SEX AND MEDICAL RECORD NO.

DATE: / / TIME: am/pm	ORDER POSTED	CHECKED BY RN
1) Analgesia by epidural infusion (using the PCA infuser).		
2) The patient **MUST NOT** receive any supplemental narcotics, sedatives and/or antiemetics while receiving Epidural Analgesic unless orders are written by the Pain Management Service.		
3) Narcotic (Specify drug, # of mgs, volume, and diluent and concentration):		
4) Initial Bolus given by Pain Service M.D. (Dose given _____)ml		

5) Initial Machine Settings: **Epidural Mode** (circle one) Continuous / Bolus / Both Program in ml.
   a) **Program in ml.**
   b) Bolus/Demand Dose _____ ml per attempt.
   c) Bolus/Demand Lockout _____ minutes.
   d) Continuous Rate _____ ml per hour.
   e) Limit _____ ml per four hours.		

6) If pain is not controlled at the above settings (pain ≥ 6), the nurse may administer a PRN rescue / loading dose_____ml every 10 minutes until the patient is comfortable.
 The maximum rescue / loading dose is_____ml Increase pump settings to:
   a) Bolus/Demand Dose _____ ml per attempt.
   b) Bolus/Demand Lockout _____ minutes.
   c) Continuous Rate _____ ml per hour.
   d) Limit _____ ml per four hours.		

7) A) For oversedation (sedation scal ≥ 4/R4) and respiratory rates 10–14 minute, notify Acute Pain Service, and decrease pump settings to:
   a) Bolus/Demand Dose _____ ml per attempt.
   b) Bolus/Demand Lockout _____ minutes
   c) Continuous Rate _____ ml per hour.
   d) Limit _____ ml per four hours
 B) For respiratory rate less than 10/minute, stop infusion and call the Acute Pain Servive (X-66700, beeper 16664),
 C) For respiratory rate less than 8/minute, obtain naoxone (0.4 mg/ml and administer 0.1 mg (0.25 ml) IV bolus q2 minutes until respiratry rate is 8/minute or greater, stop Infusion, and notify Pain mangement Service (X-66700, beeper 16664).		

8) Upon initiation and after every loading dose, obtain BP, pulse, respiratory rate, sedation scale and sensory motor function q30 min × 2 hours then q1 h × 2 then q4 hours. Pain analog q4 hours, Temp q12 hours).		
9) If no maintenance IV solution is ordered, IV to med lock.		
10) For Nausea (Specify drug and dosing):		
11) For Sleep (Specify drug and dosing):		
12) Activity level per surgical/medical orders.		
13) For questions or problems, call the Pain Management Service at X-62960 or page: X-66700, beeper 16664.		
14) Please call Unit Coordinator when the pump is discontinued.		

M.D Signature   Print Name   Code   Beeper Number

50306 (6/01)

Figure 32.1 Epidural analgesia order sheet.

under direct vision and are more suitable than epidural catheters when coagulopathy is of concern. In some studies, paravertebral blocks have been shown to be as effective as TEA with respect to pain control and preservation of pulmonary function after thoracotomy.

A preoperative single bolus of spinal morphine as part of multianalgesic regimen may be preferable to intravenous patient-controlled analgesia (IV-PCA) when epidural or paravertebral techniques are not possible.

Although systemic opioids have been well documented to reduce postthoracotomy pain, their adverse effects on the respiratory system after general anesthesia, even using patient-controlled delivery systems, and their inability to provide optimal dynamic pain relief favor regional anesthetic techniques in postthoracotomy patients. Compared with systemic opioids, meta-analyses demonstrate a tendency toward reduced pulmonary complications with epidural opioids or local anesthetic agents.

Systemic analgesics are the main alternative to more invasive techniques, can be adjuncts to these techniques, and become the mainstay of analgesic therapy, when invasive approaches are discontinued.

Cohen E, Neustein SM. Intrathecal morphine during thoracotomy, part I: effect on intraoperative enfluence requirements. *J Cardiothorac Vasc Anesth* 1993;7(2):1546.

Debreceni G, Molnar Z, Szelig L, et al. Continuous epidural or intercostal analgesia following thoracotomy: a prospective randomized double-blind clinical trial. *Acta Anaesthesiol Scand* 2003;47:1091–1095.

Etches RC. Respiratory depression associated with patient-controlled analgesia: a review of eight cases. *Can J Anaesth* 1994;41(2):125–132.

Liu N, Kuhlman G, Dalibon N, et al. A randomized, double-blinded comparison of intrathecal morphine, sufentanil and their combination versus IV morphine patient-controlled analgesia for thoracotomy pain. *Anesth Analg* 2001;92(1):31–36.

Neustein SM, Cohen E. Intrathecal morphine during thoracotomy, part II: effect on postoperative meperidine requirements and pulmonary function tests. *J Cardiothorac Vasc Anesth* 1993;7(2):1579.

Perttunen K, Nilsson E, Heinonen J, et al. Extra-dural, paravertebral and intercostal nerve blocks for post-thoracotomy pain. *Br J Anaesth* 1995;75:541–547.

A.11. What is the usual clinical regimen for intravenous patient-controlled analgesia (IV-PCA) and is special patient monitoring required during its use?

Clinical regimens for IV-PCA vary among institutions but the two most commonly used opioids are morphine and dilaudid. Continuous delivery of the drug is commonly avoided to decrease the likelihood of respiratory depression. Boluses of morphine sulphate 2 mg or dilaudid 0.2 mg are given per demand with a lockout period of 10 minutes. Incremental boluses may be given by the nurse if pain is not controlled. The dose may be decreased or the opioid discontinued if respiratory depression occurs. Close monitoring and rescue strategies must be in place to ensure patient safety. (See Sample Order Form [Fig. 32.2].)

A recent workshop of the Anesthesia Patient Safety Foundation (APSF) looked at the issue of dangers of postoperative opioids. The workshop was held in October 2006 and focused on the issue of improved detection of postoperative opioid-induced respiratory depression. The premise of the workshop was that "the available evidence suggests that there is a significant and underappreciated risk of serious injury from PCA and neuraxial opioids in the postoperative period." The incidence of respiratory depression is 0.1% to 1.0% and increases to 3.2% in those older than 80 years. Patients with obstructive sleep apnea and the elderly are at a higher risk

⌐ NewYork-Presbyterian
⌐ The University Hospital of Columbia and Cornell

45171

PATIENT CONTROLLED ANALGESIA (PCA) ADULT ORDER SHEET

	ORDERED POSTED	CHECKED BY RN
DATE: / / TIME: am/pm		
1) Analgesia by Patient Controlled Analgesia (PCA).		
2) The patient **MUST NOT** receive any supplemental narcotics, sedatives and/or antiemetics while receiving PCA unless approved the Pain Management Service or House Officer		
3) Narcotics (Specify drug, # of mgs, volume, and diluent)		
4) Initial Loading: Dose_____mg every 5 minutes until the patient is comfortable. Maximum total load_____mg.		
5) Initial Machine Settings: **PCA Mode** (circle one) Continous / PCA / Both a) **Program in mg.** b) Continous Rate_____mg per hour. c) PCA Dose_____mg per demand. d) PCA Lockout_____minutes. e) Limit_____mg per four hours.		
6) If pain is not controlled at the above settings (pain ≥ 6), the nurse may administer a PRN recue / loading dose_____every 5 minutes until the patient is comfortable. The maximum rescue / loading dose is_____mg. Increase pump settings to: a) PCA Dose_____mg per demand. b) Continous Rate_____mg per hour. c) PCA Lockout_____minutes. d) Limit_____mg per four hours.		
7) For over sedation (sedation > 4/R4) and respiratory rate < 14, decrease pump settings to: a) PCA Dose_____mg per demand. b) Continous Rate_____mg per hour. c) PCA Lockout_____minutes. d) Limit_____mg per four hours. For respiratory rate of 10 or lower, stop the pump and call the Pain Management Service (X66700, beeper 16664) or House Officer.		
8) Upon initiation, and after every loading dose given, obtain respiratory rate, heart rate and blood pressure. Repeat qh X 2, q4h X 3, and then heart rate and blood pressure per unit routine or as otherwise ordered. Monitor repiratory rate, pain analog and sedation scale q4h.		
9) Note: For patients who receive intrathecal/Epidural Morphine intraoperatively and have PCA initiated within 12 hours, monitor blood pressure, pulse, respiratory rate, pain analog/sedation q30minutes X 2h, qh X2 and then q4 hours X3, Then, BP per unit routine, Monitor respiratory rate, pain analog/sedation of 4hr.		
10) If no maintenance IV is odered, infuse D5 1/2NS at 40 ml/h via PCA Extension Set.		
11) For Nausea (Specify drug and dosing):		
12) For Sleep (Specify drug and dosing):		
13) For questions or problems, call the Pain Management Service at X62960 or page X66700, beeper 16664		
14) Please call the Unit Coordinator when the pump is discontinued.		
15)		

M.D. Signature   Print Name   Code   Beeper Number

50305 (6/01)

Figure 32.2 Patient-controlled analgesia (PCA) adult order sheet.

of opioid-induced respiratory depression but there is still a low and unpredictable incidence of life-threatening respiratory depression in young, healthy patients. The workshop highlighted the argument that in the United States the Joint Commission's emphasis on pain as the "fifth vital sign" has had the unintended consequence of creating an expectation among patients that they will have no pain after surgery. As a result, more patients may be receiving excessive amounts of analgesics. The current monitoring technologies are unreliable in that they often give both false-positive and false-negative alarms. The APSF does not accept the status quo and advocates the routine use of continuous respiratory monitoring in at-risk patients receiving PCA or neuraxial opioids.

The workshop also argued that the use of supplemental oxygen may mask cases of serious cases of hypoventilation and that a fall in oximetry is a late sign of respiratory depression. The pulse oximeter is an effective method of detecting hypoventilation when the patient is breathing room air. The workshop recommendations were that there should be zero tolerance of postoperative respiratory depression; continuous monitoring of oxygenation and ventilation could prevent a significant number of case of patient harm; any monitoring system should be centrally linked so that a competent health care professional can be summoned in a timely manner; programs should be instituted to educate providers and patients about the risks of opioid-associated life-threatening respiratory depression; governmental agencies and nongovernmental entities should provide increased support for scientific research in this area; treatment of postoperative, opioid-induced depression is important, but prevention may be a more effective strategy. The full text of the article can be found in the winter 2006 to 2007 Journal of the APSF newsletter at www.Apsf.org.

Weinger MB. Dangers of post operative opioids. APSF workshop and white paper address prevention of postoperative respiratory complications. *APSF Newsl Winter* 2006–2007;21(4):61–67.

A.12. What are the side effects and complications of epidural technique?

Depending on the extent of blockade thoracic epidural analgesia (TEA) interferes with sympathetic outflow and produces hypotension through cardiodepressant action and a reduction in systemic vascular resistance. The use of dilute local anesthetic solutions had led to clinically insignificant motor blockade. Opioid-related side effects include sedation, nausea and vomiting, pruritus, delayed gastrointestinal motility, urinary retention, and respiratory depression. The incidence of delayed respiratory depression after administration of epidural opioids is very low, and epidural opioid analgesia can be used safely on hospital wards. All patients who receive epidural analgesia should have standard orders for the treatment of breakthrough pain and side effects.

The overall catheter-related complication rate is low and includes such complications as dural puncture, unsuccessful catheter placement, paresthesia, and neurologic injury. Paraplegia associated with epidural analgesia may result from epidural hematoma, or less commonly epidural abscess.

The potentially catastrophic complications of epidural or intraspinal hematoma are best prevented by realization that motor blockade should not occur with dilute local anesthetic solutions, and postoperative motor weakness should trigger immediate imaging evaluation (magnetic resonance imaging [MRI]) and neurosurgical consultation. Clearly, concerns about coagulopathy can limit epidural catheter placement.

Rawal N. Intraspinal opioids. In: Rowbotham DJ, Macintyre PE, eds. *Acute pain*. Arnold, 2003:241–266.

A.13. What recommendations for placement and removal of epidural catheter will you make if this patient is on antiplatelet or anticoagulant therapy or thromboprophylaxis is planned?

On the basis of current literature and second consensus statement for regional anesthesia in the anticoagulated patient developed by the American Society of Regional Anesthesia (ASRA), the following guidelines may be helpful.

Prophylactic unfractionated heparin

In the setting of twice-daily subcutaneous prophylaxis, there is no contraindication to the use of neuraxial techniques. The clinician should keep in mind, however, that subcutaneous heparin reaches peak effect 1 to 2 hours after administration.

Recommendations

- Subcutaneous heparin should be administered *after* block placement. The current agreement with the surgical services is to wait for 30 minutes after epidural catheter placement to administer heparin.
- In a small subset of patients (2% to 4%), subcutaneous heparin dosing may exert a therapeutic effect. If the patient has been receiving subcutaneous heparin in the hospital, we recommend checking the partial thromboplastin time (PTT) before neuraxial block.
- Because heparin-induced thrombocytopenia may occur during heparin administration, patients receiving heparin for more than 4 days should have a platelet count check before neuraxial block placement and catheter removal.
- An epidural catheter may be removed 4 or more hours after the last heparin dose.
- Inpatients may already be receiving prophylactic heparin on the floor. The clinician should take this into account when considering neuraxial blockade. It may be prudent to hold the dose before block placement.

Therapeutic intravenous unfractionated heparin

Neuraxial techniques combined with intraoperative anticoagulation (excluding the full anticoagulation of cardiac surgery) are acceptable with certain precautions as described in the subsequent text.

Recommendations

- Risk/benefit determinations are needed, especially in patients receiving anticoagulant medications such as antiplatelet agents, Coumadin, and low molecular weight heparin (LMWH). These medications may increase the risk of bleeding complications.
- Heparin administration should be delayed for 1 hour after block placement.
- Epidural catheters may be removed 2 to 4 or more hours after the last heparin dose and the laboratory coagulation values have been reevaluated.
- Bloody or difficult block placement may increase the risk of epidural hematoma formation in the setting of intraoperative anticoagulation.

Preoperative low molecular weight heparin

The clinician needs to take into account any other antiplatelet or oral anticoagulant medications in combination with low molecular weight heparin (LMWH). This combination increases the risk of spinal and epidural hematoma formation in the setting of neuraxial blockade.

- *Prophylactic LMWH.* An example of a prophylactic dose is enoxaparin 40 mg qd or 30 mg q12 hours. Block placement should occur no sooner than 12 hours after the last dose of LMWH.

- *Treatment Dose LMWH.* An example of a treatment dose is enoxaparin 1.5 mg per kg qd or 1 mg per kg q12 hours. Block placement should occur no sooner than 24 hours after the last dose of LMWH.

Postoperative low molecular weight heparin

- *Prophylactic LMWH, twice-daily dosing.* This dosing regimen may be associated with an increased risk of hematoma. The first dose of LMWH should be administered no sooner than 24 hours postoperatively. Epidural catheters should not be maintained in this situation, and should be removed at least 2 hours before the first LMWH dose.
- *Prophylactic LMWH, single-daily dosing.* Epidural catheters may be maintained in this situation, but only after a thorough risk/benefit analysis. The first dose of LMWH should be given 6 to 8 hours postoperatively. The second dose should be given no sooner than 24 hours after the first dose. The epidural catheter should be removed 12 hours after the last dose of LMWH, and the subsequent dose should be given no sooner than 2 hours after catheter removal.
- *Treatment dose LMWH.* Epidural catheters should not be maintained in this situation. The first dose of LMWH should be given 24 hours after catheter removal.

Oral anticoagulants

- *Aspirin.* There is no contraindication to neuraxial anesthesia in patients taking aspirin alone (81 mg or 325 mg).
- *Nonsteroidal antiinflammatory drugs (NSAIDs).* There is no contraindication to neuraxial anesthesia in patients taking NSAIDs alone.
- *Preoperative Coumadin*
  a. Coumadin should be stopped 4 to 5 days before a neuraxial block.
  b. The prothrombin time/international normalized ratio (PT/INR) should be measured before the block.
  c. An epidural may be placed if the INR is less than or equal to 1.2.
  d. A spinal may be placed if the INR is less than or equal to 1.3
  e. For patients receiving an initial preoperative coumadin dose, the PT/INR should be checked before neuraxial block if the first dose was given more than 24 hours earlier, or a second dose has been given.
- Postoperative Coumadin
  a. Epidural catheters may be maintained in patients on Coumadin for up to 36 hours after the first postoperative dose. The PT/INR should be monitored daily and assessed before catheter removal.
  b. Epidural catheters can be removed if the INR is less than 1.5.
  c. If the INR is greater than 1.5, fresh frozen plasma (FFP) administration followed by a repeat coagulation profile should be considered before epidural catheter removal.
- Preoperative clopidogrel (Plavix) and ticlopidine (Ticlid)
  a. Plavix must be held for a minimum of 7 days before neuraxial block placement.
  b. If Plavix is combined with other antiplatelet agents such as aspirin or NSAIDs, these medications should be held a minimum of 10 days before neuraxial block placement.
  c. Ticlid must be held for a minimum of 14 days before neuraxial block placement.

Dehring DJ, Arens JF. Pulmonary thromboembolism: disease recognition and patient management. *Anesthesiology* 1990;73:146–164.

Horlocker TT, Wedel DJ, Benzon H, et al. Regional anesthesia in the anticoagulated patient: defining the risks. Second consensus conference on neuraxial anesthesia and anticoagulation. April 25–28, 2002, www.asra.com. *Reg Anesth Pain Med* 2004; 29(2 Suppl 1):1–11.

Liu SS, Mulroy MF. Neuraxial anesthesia and analgesia in the presence of standard heparin. *Reg Anesth Pain Med* 1998;23(6 Suppl 2):157–163.

B. Chronic Opioid Therapy and Perioperative Pain Management

B.1. How does chronic opioid therapy influence postoperative pain management?

In recent years, a greater emphasis has been placed on pain as an important health problem. Consequently opioids now play a greater role in the treatment of chronic pain of various causes. This has resulted in a rapid increase in the annual sales of opioid analgesics. For example, between 1999 and 2003, the annual sales of outpatient opioid analgesics in the United States increased by approximately 130%, more than doubling the sales recorded in the previous decade. Because more patients are treated chronically with opioids, every anesthesiologist is likely to be confronted with acute pain management issues in these patients. Chronic opioid-consuming patients can experience significant postoperative pain given that health care professionals are not accustomed to their markedly increased opioid requirements.

Patients on long-term opioid therapy are more likely to require surgery and higher doses of opioids postoperatively. Although the prevalence of chronically opioid-consuming patients who present for surgery is not known, the growing use of opioids is likely to increase the number of such patients. High levels of postoperative pain have been associated with an increased risk of chronic pain as a consequence of surgery. Therefore, the aggressive treatment of postoperative pain may be important in patients with chronic pain because they may represent a population that is particularly vulnerable to complications or are at risk for chronic postsurgical pain.

Although available data are limited, the management of postoperative pain seems to be more difficult in chronically opioid-consuming patients even when they consume only a modest daily opioid dose. Tolerance to any one opioid preparation results in clinically measurable insensitivity to most others.

Carroll IA, Angst MS, Clark JD. Management of perioperative pain in patients chronically consuming opioids. *Reg Anesth Pain Med* 2004;29:576–591.

Mehta V, Langford RM. Acute pain management for opioid dependent patients. *Anaesthesia* 2006;61:269–276.

Mitra S, Sinatra RS. Perioperative management of acute pain in the opioid-dependent patient. *Anesthesiology* 2004;101:212–227.

Rapp SE, Ready LB, Nessly ML. Acute pain management in patients with prior opioid consumption: a case controlled retrospective review. *Pain* 1995;61:195–201.

Swenson JD, Davis JJ, Johnson KB. Postoperative care of the chronic opioid-consuming patient. *Anesthesiol Clin North America* 2005;23:37–48.

B.2. What are the causes for increased postoperative pain and opioid consumption in patients chronically using opioids?

Chronic exposure to opioids may result in a need to increase the dose over time to maintain the desired analgesic effect. The need for escalating the dose is often attributed to the development of tolerance. However, dose escalation can be the result of other factors, such as the progression of the underlying disease that causes the chronic pain.

More recent evidence points to an opioid-induced hyperalgesia (OIH) as an alternative neuropharmacologic phenomenon to explain the need to escalate the opioid dose over time. Paradoxically, administration of opioids may induce an increased sensitivity to pain (hyperalgesia). Further complicating matters, the phenomena of tolerance and hyperalgesia can coexist.

Clinical surveys of long-term opioid use in patients with both cancer and nonmalignancy-associated pain have not shown escalating drug dosage to be inevitable; however, some degree of dose increase over time is often observed.

Carroll IA, Angst MS, Clark JD. Management of perioperative pain in patients chronically consuming opioids. *Reg Anesth Pain Med* 2004;29:576–591.

Mitra S, Sinatra RS. Perioperative management of acute pain in the opioid-dependent patient. *Anesthesiology* 2004;101:212–227.

B.3. What are the main differences between a chronic opioid-consuming patient and a patient who abuses or is addicted to opioids?

Patients undergoing surgery may not admit that they are actively abusing pain medications; difficulties in achieving adequate postoperative pain control may provide a hint to such abuse.

Many of the issues with respect to chronically opioid-consuming patients also apply to patients who abuse or are addicted to opioids. However, several important differences exist. First, the daily dose of opioid consumed by opioid-abusing patients before surgery is typically larger. Second, opioid-abusing or opioid-addicted patients often suffer from coexisting psychiatric diseases. For example, heroin addicts have an elevated prevalence of depression, anxiety, psychosis, and personality disorders. Depression and anxiety are independent predictors of severe pain after surgery and may complicate the management of postoperative pain. Third, the attitude of health care providers toward the use of opioids for controlling pain may be influenced by the abuse history, which makes these patients particularly vulnerable to inadequate postoperative pain control.

De Moja CA. Longitudinal survey of anxiety and depression in drug users and addicts. *Psychol Rep* 1992;70(3 pt 1):738.

Von Limbeek J, Wouters L, Kaplan CD, et al. Prevalence of psychopathology in drug-addicted Dutch. *J Subst Abuse Treat* 1992;9:43–52.

B.4. What issues need to be considered in the opioid-tolerant patient who is scheduled for surgery?

Tolerance develops at different rates to desired (analgesia) and undesired effects (sedation, nausea, euphoria, constipation). Long-term use of opioids results in tolerance to some opioid effects such as analgesia, nausea, sedation, and respiratory depression but not to miosis or constipation (4). Cross-tolerance with other opioids also occurs. Opioid-tolerant patients may require about three times more opioid than their opioid-naive counterparts. Opioid-tolerant patients report higher pain scores at rest and on movement and also remained longer under the care of Acute Pain Services (APSs) than other patients. The incidence of opioid-induced nausea and vomiting may be lower in opioid-tolerant patients.

Jage J, Bey T. Postoperative analgesia in patients with substance use disorders: part I. *Acute Pain* 2000; 3:141–156.

de Leon-Casasola OA, Myers DP, Donaparthi S, et al. A comparison of postoperative epidural analgesia between patients with chronic cancer taking high doses of oral opioids versus opioid-naïve patients. *Anesth Analg* 1993;76:302–307.

Rapp SE, Ready BL, Nessly ML. Acute pain management in paients with prior opioid consumption: a case-controlled retrospective review. *Pain* 1995;61:195–201.

B.5. What would be your strategy regarding preoperative information and choice of anesthesia technique?

Acute pain management in opioid-dependent patients is a complex issue. There has been a tendency to use opioids sparingly, resulting in both poor pain management and withdrawal phenomena. Patients may react with a degree of suspicion, mistrust, or even hostility.

They need to be reassured that their drug history and dependence will not be an obstacle to the relief of pain. During assessment, care should be exercised to maintain privacy and confidentiality.

Despite the increasing prevalence of opioid dependency, there are few controlled studies available to guide the anesthesiologist in optimizing anesthetic and analgesic care. Because the minimum daily opioid dose that significantly increases postoperative opioid requirements and pain is not known, all patients should be informed about the potential for severe pain and increased opioid requirements during the postoperative period. Patients should be informed about alternative analgesic techniques that complement opioids.

The selection of anesthesia technique has to be done on an individual basis because there are no data available favoring general, regional, or combined anesthesia for this specific patient population. Although there is no evidence indicating superiority of regional anesthesia for chronic pain patients, individual consideration may favor regional anesthesia.

Expert opinion suggests that opioid-tolerant patients should be offered regional anesthesia or analgesia, particularly for procedures performed on the extremities. Advantages of a regional anesthetic and analgesic approach include reduction in opioid requirements and improvement in distal perfusion as a result of sympathetic blockade.

Iocolano CF. Perioperative pain management in the chemically dependent patient. *J Perianesth Nurs* 2000;15:329–347.

Kopf A, Banzhaf A, Stein C. Perioperative management of the chronic pain patient. *Best Pract Res Clin Anaesthesiol* 2005;19:59–76.

B.6. What are the choices for perioperative pain management in opioid-tolerant patients?

Management of these patients should focus on three main goals: (a) prevention of withdrawal, (b) effective analgesia, and (c) symptomatic treatment of psychological affective disorders such as anxiety. Preexisting opioid medication has to be continued throughout the perioperative period to avoid withdrawal. This applies for general anesthesia as well as regional anesthesia. During surgery, the required opioid dose consists of the daily opioid dose taken before surgery and the opioid dose necessary for the surgical intervention. The use of a continuous infusion of opioid may be the best way to provide a steady serum concentration if the oral route is unavailable perioperatively.

Catching up on the opioid dose in the postoperative period can be difficult because of inevitable delays in obtaining and administering opioids at the bedside, the high levels of pain that patients may experience, and a possible reluctance of recovery room staff to administer a sufficiently large opioid dose. Requirements for individual patients are difficult to predict; however, patients who use even modest opioid doses (<50 mg/day oral morphine equivalent) before surgery may often require their baseline opioid dose plus two or more times the amount of opioids typically used for adequate pain control in opioid-naive patients.

Regional anesthesia techniques have many benefits and may be particularly useful in chronically opioid-consuming patients because they provide excellent analgesia to patients prone to severe postoperative pain experiences, and avoid certain difficulties due to the reduced effectiveness of opioids.

However, opioid-dependent patients need their daily systemic opioid dose to prevent withdrawal. Opioid requirements by the epidural route and by the intravenous route for alleviating breakthrough pain are higher in chronically opioid-consuming patients than in opioid-naive patients. Also, the use of potent lipophilic opioids seems superior to the use of hydrophilic compounds such as morphine.

Nevertheless, chronically opioid-consuming patients treated with regional techniques for postoperative pain control should also have access to systemic opioids by the intravenous or oral route for preventing opioid withdrawal. Intravenous patient-controlled analgesia (IV-PCA) is a useful modality for pain relief in opioid-tolerant patients, provided that pain intensity and opioid consumption are monitored and background requirements are provided if the patient cannot take their usual opioid; larger bolus doses will often be needed. Opioid rotation (i.e., using an opioid that is different from their preadmission opioid) may be of use.

Withdrawal from opioids should be prevented by maintenance of normal preadmission opioid regimens where possible, or appropriate substitutions with another opioid or the same opioid through another route. It may be of benefit to check preadmission opioid doses with the patient's doctor or pharmacist; the use of unauthorized additional opioids (licit or illicit) or of lower doses than prescribed, may affect both pain relief and the risk of adverse effects.

Neuraxial opioids have been used effectively in opioid-tolerant patients, although higher doses may be required and may not result in an increase in adverse effects. Effective analgesia using intrathecal or epidural opioids will not necessarily prevent symptoms of opioid withdrawal.

Ketamine may reduce opioid requirements in opioid-tolerant patients. Although multimodal analgesic regimens (e.g., non-steroidal antiinflammatory drugs [NSAIDs], paracetamol, ketamine, and regional analgesia) will be of benefit, opioid-tolerant patients are at risk of opioid withdrawal if a purely nonopioid analgesic regimen or tramadol is used. For this reason, opioid antagonists (naloxone, naltrexone) or mixed agonist-antagonists (e.g., buprenorphine, pentazocine) should also be avoided as their use precipitates acute withdrawal reactions.

Australian and New Zealand College of Anaesthetists and Faculty of Pain Medicine. *Acute pain management: scientific evidence, Chapter 10 (The opioid tolerant patient).* Australian and New Zealand College of Anaesthetists and Faculty of Pain Medicine, 2005.

de Leon-Casasola OA, Lema MJ. Epidural bupivacaine/sufentanil therapy for postoperative pain control in patients tolerant to opioid and unresponsive to epidural bupivacaine/ morphine. *Anesthesiology* 1993;80:302–307.

Macintyre PE, Ready LB. *Acute pain management: a practical guide,* 2nd ed. London: WB Saunders, 2001.

B.7. What issues need to be considered before discharging an opioid-tolerant patient?

Discharge planning must take into account the potential for prescribed opioids to be abused or misused. Appropriate use of nonopioid analgesic where possible, communication with the primary physician and patient education and support must all be considered.

Chronically opioid-consuming patients typically require significantly higher postoperative opioid doses for adequate pain control than they received before surgery for their chronic pain symptoms. Attempting to discharge chronically opioid-consuming patients on the same opioid regimen they adhered to before surgery often results in inadequate pain control. Whatever the final oral dose the chronically opioid-consuming patients are stabilized on at discharge, a slow tapering from this dose toward the preoperative opioid dose over 2 to 4 weeks is often a reasonable goal. In the case under consideration, the transdermal fentanyl patch should be left in place to provide the preexisting opioid requirement and additional short-acting analgesics should be prescribed for postoperative pain.

The anesthesiologist plays a key role in maintaining baseline opioid requirements, administering supplemental intraoperative and postoperative opioids, and providing nonopioid analgesics and neural blockade. Delivering a patient who has severe pain to the postanesthesia care unit (PACU) is unacceptable practice and often results in an extremely difficult and time-consuming management issue. Awareness and administration of appropriate doses of analgesics as well as continuous clinical monitoring remain the keys to successful perioperative pain management in this special group of patients.

C. Perioperative Pain Management for Ambulatory Surgery

C.1. What would be your preoperative considerations and advice to the patient?

Adequate postoperative pain management is often the limiting factor when determining whether a patient can have surgery performed as an ambulatory surgical procedure. Ensuring that the patient has appropriate expectations of the outcome of laparoscopic cholecystectomy is critical for a successful conclusion to the procedure, especially with regard to postoperative pain. Unrealistic expectations for no pain at all can be met with anger, disappointment, and the fear and anxiety that something has gone wrong. Failure to meet unrealistic expectations can even lead to litigation.

Planning for postoperative pain management should begin in the preoperative period. Patient education regarding the degree of pain that she might expect, the pain assessment tools, and the modalities of pain treatment that might be utilized should reduce the patient's anxiety and the fear of unrelieved pain. Reduced patient anxiety reduces the incidence of postoperative pain. In addition, patients have to be made aware of the importance of communicating their analgesic needs. They may benefit from an explanation of how much and what type of pain can be expected following their procedure. Patients should receive instruction on the importance of coughing, deep breathing, ambulation, and postoperative rehabilitation. Patient information on acute postoperative pain management is available from public sources.

Details of the complications of laparoscopic cholecystectomy given to patients vary between countries and cultures. The most relevant for postoperative pain is to mention the risk of conversion to open laparotomy in a small percentage of cases, which will be associated with a significantly larger wound, more pain and longer period of hospitalization. An expectation of the degree of pain that might be experienced—generally mild or moderate in the case of laparoscopic cholecystectomy (although even with laparoscopic cholecystectomy this can be severe and it can sometimes last for several days).

Patients need to be informed that there may be three types of pain: (a) incisional, (b) visceral, and (c) shoulder pain. It is also necessary to have a separate discussion of the discomfort, rather than significant pain that might be felt in the region of the shoulders, and reassurance that this is related to the laparoscopy and not their heart or chest are necessary. The patient should be informed that there is a relatively high risk of postoperative nausea and vomiting after laparoscopic cholecystectomy (~30% to 50%) and what will be done to prevent and treat it (a history of previous postoperative nausea and vomiting should alert the anesthesiologist to administer 1 to 2 antiemetics before extubation).

Predischarge patient information should also include the following: (a) that patients will receive analgesic and antiemetic medication (or prescription or both) for management of pain and postoperative nausea and vomiting at home, (b) that the hospital (surgeon or nurse) will make a (3- to -5-minute follow-up call) and, (c) that they will get contact telephone numbers in case there are problems or questions.

American Academy of Family Physicians. *Pain control after surgery: pain medicines*. Available at: http://www.familydocotr.org/handsouts/259.html. Accessibility verified June 24, 2002.

Crews JS. Multimodal pain management strategies for office-based and ambulatory procedures. *JAMA* 2002;288:629–632.

Joshi GP, White PF. Postoperative pain management: day surgery. In: David J Rowbotham and Pamela McIntyre, eds. *Clinical pain management—acute pain*. Arnold, 2003:329–340.

Laparoscopic cholecystectomy. www.postoppain.org. Accessed March 2007.

Payne FB, Ghia JN, Wilkes NC. The relationship of preoperative and intraoperative factors on the incidence of pain following ambulatory surgery. *Ambul Surg* 1996;3:127–130.

Rawal N. Analgesia for day-case surgery. *Br J Anaesth* 2001;87:73–87.

C.2. What are the consequences of inadequate pain management after ambulatory surgery?

In the ambulatory setting, the type of surgery is a significant predictor of severity of postoperative pain. Recent clinical studies indicate that postoperative pain is not always effectively treated. Rawal et al. reported that 30% to 35% of patients undergoing ambulatory surgery experienced moderate to severe pain at home.

Uncontrolled pain may be associated with an increased incidence of postoperative nausea, agitation, prolonged postanesthesia care unit (PACU) stay, delayed discharge from an ambulatory facility, and unanticipated hospital admission. Inadequate postoperative pain control was also the most frequent reason for patients to contact their family practitioner after discharge from the hospital. Importantly, the presence of postoperative symptoms including pain contributes to patient dissatisfaction with their surgical experience (see Table 32.1).

Anderson R, Krohg K. Pain as a major cause of postoperative nausea. *Can Anaesth Soc J* 1976;23:366–369.

Chung F, Ritchie E, Su J. Postoperative pain in ambulatory surgery. *Anesth Analg* 1997; 85:808–816.

Rawal N, Hylander J, Nydahl PA, et al. Survey of postoperative analgesia following ambulatory surgery. *Acta Anaesthesiol Scand* 1997;41:1017–1022.

Tong D, Chung F, Wong D. Predictive factors in global and anesthesia satisfaction in ambulatory surgical patients. *Anesthesiology* 1997;87:856–864.

Table 32.1 Consequences of Inadequate Pain Management After Ambulatory Surgery.

Increased postanesthesia care unit stay
Increased phase II unit stay
Delayed discharge at home
Unanticipated hospital admission
Increased contact with family practitioner
Delayed return to daily living function
Decreased patient satisfaction

C.3. What is the role of premedication or preoperative analgesic?

Preoperative administration of opioid or nonopioid analgesics reduces analgesic requirements and pain scores in the immediate postoperative period. However, opioid premedication is controversial in the ambulatory setting because it may increase the incidence of opioid-related side effects and even delay recovery. Premedication with oral nonsteroidal antiinflammatory drug (NSAIDs) given 60 to 90 minutes before surgery can reduce the degree of postoperative pain, analgesic requirements, and discharge times.

Preemptive analgesia refers to the concept that an analgesic medication or intervention administered before surgical tissue injury may produce a greater effect than the same medication or intervention administered following surgical tissue injury. This preemptive analgesic effect has been demonstrated for several different medications in animal models, but collecting definitive clinical data in postoperative patients has been more challenging.

Preoperative administration of opioid or nonopioid analgesics reduces analgesic requirements and pain scores in the immediate postoperative period. However, opioid premedication is controversial in the ambulatory setting because it may increase the incidence of opioid-related side effects and even delay recovery. Premedication with oral NSAIDs given 60 to 90 minutes before surgery can reduce the degree of postoperative pain, analgesic requirements, and discharge times.

Analgesic medication should be instituted in time to secure sufficient analgesia when the patient is waking following the procedure.

For laparoscopic cholecystectomy there is no strong evidence that preincisional timing of analgesic administration (preemptive analgesia) decreases the intensity or duration of postoperative pain, when compared with postoperative administration.

A systematic review (Moiniche 2002) confirms that there is no overall clinical benefit of preoperative analgesia on postoperative pain in a large number of studies that examined a variety of analgesic techniques in different surgical procedures.

Cholecystectomy. www.postoppain.org. Accessed March 2007.

Joshi GP, White PF. Postoperative pain management: day surgery. In: David J Rowbotham and Pamela McIntyre, eds. *Clinical pain management—acute pain*. Arnold, 2003:329–340.

Katz J. Pre-emptive analgesia: evidence, current status and future directions. *Eur J Anaesthesiol Suppl* 1995;10:8–13.

Møiniche S, Kehlet H, Dahl JB. A qualitative and quantitative systematic review of preemptive analgsia for postoperative pain relief: the role of timing of analgesia. *Anesthesiology* 2002;96:725–741.

Woolf CJ, Chong MS. Preemptive analgesia—treating postoperative pain by preventing the establishment of central sensitization. *Anesth Analg* 1993;77:362–379.

C.4. Does the choice of anesthetic technique influence postoperative pain?

The choice of the anesthetic technique has been shown to have a significant influence on postoperative analgesia in patients undergoing ambulatory surgery. Regional anesthesia techniques offer a number of advantages in outpatient surgery, including prolonged postoperative analgesia.

Opioids still remain the primary drugs used to provide intraoperative analgesia. As a result of the faster recovery from ultrashort-acting opioids such as remifentanil, it is necessary to administer longer-acting opioid or nonopioid analgesics to achieve adequate postoperative pain control. However, the role of opioids in ambulatory surgery remains controversial. The use of opioids may be associated with a dose-dependent increase in adverse effects, including nausea, vomiting, sedation, bladder dysfunction, and respiratory depression, all of which may contribute to a delayed recovery.

Only one study has examined the effect of anesthetic regime on postoperative pain management in patients with laparoscopic cholecystectomy. This study examined combined epidural and general anesthesia (CEGA) versus total intravenous anesthesia (TIVA) it showed a benefit for reducing postoperative pain scores for CEGA versus TIVA. However, epidural technique is not recommended for routine anesthetic management in patients undergoing laparoscopic cholecystectomy as the risks outweigh the benefits. Nevertheless, in certain high-risk pulmonary patients, CEGA can be justified.

TIVA offers an alternative to inhalational anesthesia, and although rapid recovery from anesthesia and reduction in nausea and vomiting are recognized benefits, the analgesic components of TIVA have a very short duration and do not contribute to improved postoperative analgesia.

There is specific evidence in the literature to support the use of incisional local anesthetic infiltration is recommended at end of surgery; combined incisional/intraperitoneal local anesthetics are also recommended.

Infiltration of the surgical wound with local anesthetic can provide excellent analgesia that outlasts the duration of action of the local anesthetics. Installation or aerosol application of local anesthetics in the surgical wound has also been found to provide long-lasting analgesia.

Another simple and effective method of reducing the intensity of postlaparoscopic pain is intraperitoneal instillation of local anesthetic drugs. Recent studies have reported significant pain relief after laparoscopic cholecystectomy when 15 to 20 mL of 0.5% bupivacaine was administered into the hepatodiaphragmatic space, near and above the hepatoduodenal ligament and above the gallbladder or gallbladder bed.

Albrecht S, Schuttler J, Yarmush J. Postoperative pain management after intraoperative remifentanil. *Anesth Analg* 1999;89:S40–S45.

Alexander JI. Pain after laparoscopy. *Br J Anaesth* 1997;78:369–378.

Alexander DJ, Ngoi SS, Lee L, et al. Randomized trial of periportal peritoneal bupivacaine for pain relief after laparoscopic cholecystectomy. *Br J Surg* 1996;83:1223–1225.

Dahl JB, Moiniche S, Kehlet H. Wound infiltration with local anesthetics for postoperative pain relief. *Acta Anaesthesiol Scand* 1994;38:7–14.

Gupta A, Thörn SE, Axelsson K, et al. Postoperative pain relief using intermittent injections of 0.5% ropivacaine via an intra-abdominal catheter following laparoscopic cholecystectomy. *Anesth Analg* 2002;95:450–456.

Kehlet H, Gray AW, Bonnet F, et al. A procedure-specific systematic review and consensus recommendations for postoperative analgesia following laparoscopic cholecystectomy. *Surg Endosc* 2005;19:1396–1415.

Luchetti M, Palomba R, Sica G, et al. Effectiveness and safety of combined epidural and general anesthesia for laparoscopic cholecystectom. *Reg Anesth* 1996;21(5):465–469.

Mraovic B, Jurisic T, Kogler-Majeric V, et al. Intra-peritoneal bupivacaine for analgesia after laparoscopic cholecystectomy. *Acta Anaesthesiol Scand* 1997;41:193–196.

Pasqualucci A, de Angelis V, Contardo R, et al. Pre-emptive analgesia: intraperitoneal local anesthetic in laparoscopic cholecystectomy. A randomized, double-blind, placebo-controlled study. *Anesthesiology* 1996;85:11–20.

Sinclair R, Cassuto J, Hogstrom S, et al. Topical anesthesia with lidocaine aerosol in the control of postoperative pain. *Anesthesiology* 1988;68:895–901.

C.5. Are nonsteroidal antiinflammatory drugs (NSAIDs) effective? If so, does the choice of drug matter?

The opioid-sparing effects of NSAIDs lower the risk of postoperative nausea and vomiting, thereby improving patient comfort and allowing for an earlier discharge.

The introduction of a parenteral preparation of NSAID and the widespread acceptance of the concept of multimodal ("balanced") analgesia has increased the popularity of NSAIDs in the management of perioperative pain. NSAIDs available for intravenous use include ketorolac, diclofenac, indomethacin, ketoprofen, tenoxicam, lornoxicam, and parecoxib.

However, NSAIDs have weaker analgesic properties than opioids or local anesthetics and also exhibit a "ceiling effect" with respect to their maximum analgesic effect. Despite their limitations, NSAIDs may decrease the risk of breakthrough pain because of their more prolonged duration of action and are valuable adjuvants when used in combination with opioids and local anesthetics.

There is no documented evidence of superiority of any particular NSAID for perioperative use. Therefore, the choice of NSAID would depend upon the route of administration, the duration of the analgesia, propensity for side effects, and the cost.

The oral availability of most NSAIDs is high, whereas that after rectal administration is low; therefore NSAIDs should be preferably administered orally if patients can swallow. Overall, NSAIDs appear to be safe and well tolerated in patients undergoing ambulatory surgery.

Cyclooxygenase (COX) 2 inhibitors have been demonstrated in multiple clinical trials to produce analgesic efficacy equal to that of the traditional nonselective NSAIDs without the COX-1 mediated adverse effects of inhibition of platelet aggregation or gastroduodenal ulceration, although there is some controversy about the latter. COX-2 inhibitors used over a short period of time for postoperative analgesia have not been demonstrated to cause any major adverse events in healthy patients.

Gupta A. Analgesic techniques for day cases. In: Paola Lemos and Beverly Phillips, eds. *Day surgery-development and practice*. International Association for Ambulatory Surgery (IAAS), 2006:209–227.

Joshi GP, White PF. Postoperative pain management: day surgery. In: David J Rowbotham and Pamela McIntyre, eds. *Clinical pain management—acute pain*. Arnold, 2003:329–340.

Kehlet H, Gray AW, Bonnet F, et al. A procedure-specific systematic review and consensus recommendations for postoperative analgesia following laparoscopic cholecystectomy. *Surg Endosc* 2005;19:1396–1415.

Kehlet H, Mather LE. The value of non-steroidal antiinflammatory drugs in postoperative pain. *Drugs* 1992;44:1–63.

Tong D, Chung F. Postoperative pain control in ambulatory surgery. *Surg Clin North Am* 1999;79:401–430.

Tramer MR, Williams JE, Carroll D, et al. Comparing analgesic efficacy of non-steroidal anti-inflammatory drugs given by different routes in acute and chronic pain: a quantitative systematic review. *Acta Anaesthesiol Scand* 1998;42:71–79.

C.6. There are three types of pain after laparoscopic cholecystectomy: incisional, subphrenic and shoulder pain. What is the role of surgical technique in influencing postoperative pain?

The pain after laparoscopic procedures is primarily visceral in origin. Factors responsible for this pain may be related to surgical incisions, carbon dioxide insufflation, and the intraabdominal pressures maintained during the laparoscopic procedure. Higher insufflation pressures should be avoided, as they can significantly increase the severity of postoperative pain. Subphrenic and shoulder pain after laparoscopic procedures appears to arise from diaphragmatic and phrenic nerve irritation due to insufflated carbon dioxide. This pain tends to be aggravated by ambulation and may persist for several days after surgery. Residual insufflating gas can also increase the intensity of postlaparoscopic pain. Therefore, the abdomen should be actively deflated at the end of the laparoscopic procedure.

Recommendations based on literature review (*www.postoppain.org*) of laparoscopic cholecystectomy specific evidence are as follows:

- Low pressure CO_2 pneumoperitoneum was superior to conventional CO_2 pneumoperitoneum in three out of three controlled studies.
- No evidence to recommend warmed CO_2 pneumoperitoneal for reducing postoperative pain.
- Peritoneal lavage after CO_2 pneumoperitoneum is recommended to reduce postoperative pain.
- Helium pneumoperitoneum has no advantage versus CO_2 pneumoperitoneum.

Alexander JI. Pain after laparoscopy. *Br J Anaesth* 1997;79:369–378.

Cholecystectomy. www.postoppain.org. Accessed March 2007.

C.7. What would be your strategy for pain control after discharge home?

After discharge, oral paracetamol (acetaminophen), nonsteroidal antiinflammatory drug (NSAIDs), or opioids, either alone or in combination, are frequently used to provide postoperative pain relief.

Given that acetaminophen has a similar efficacy and a better side-effect profile than NSAIDs, it should be considered as an alternative to NSAIDs. Recently, coadministration of acetaminophen and NSAIDs has been advocated.

Codeine and its derivatives are the most commonly used oral opioid analgesics after ambulatory surgery. Oxycodone and hydrocodone are orally active derivatives of codeine with higher analgesic potency. Controlled-release preparations of oxycodone have longer duration of action and fewer side effects than the older formulations and have been shown to be highly effective postoperatively. However, there has been some recent concern over the misuse of time-release oxycodone in the Oxycontin formulation. This tablet is a nondigestible matrix that is then filled with large amounts of oxycodone and slowly time released by diffusion out the matrix. If the matrix is crushed and ingested, the entire drug contained in the preparation is immediately released, providing the user with a euphoric state. This preparation has also been the cause of a number of deaths due to accidental overdose. Providers should exercise caution when prescribing this medication because of its high potential for abuse. The administration of oral medications is usually not appropriate immediately postoperatively in patients who have received general anesthesia—this is because general anesthesia often results in impaired consciousness and postoperative nausea and vomiting, which can lead to aspiration.

Joshi GP, White PF. Postoperative pain management: day surgery. In: David J Rowbotham and Pamela McIntyre, eds. *Clinical pain management—acute pain*. Arnold, 2003:329–340.

Rawal N. Analgesia for day-case surgery. *Br J Anaesth* 2001;87:73–87.

Sunshine A, Olson NZ, Rivera J, et al. Analgesic efficacy of controlled-releae oxycodone in postoperative pain. *J Clin Pharmacol* 1996;36:595–603.

Cholecystectomy. www.postoppain.org.

D. The Role of Acute Pain Service

D.1. What is the extent of the problem and which patients are at greater risk of undertreatment?

Pain relief after surgery continues to be a major medical challenge. Despite a significant improvement over the last decade in our understanding of acute (and chronic) pain mechanism and the establishment of Acute Pain Services (APSs), recently updated studies continue to report that postoperative pain management is not satisfactory. In addition, publications of guidelines for acute pain management, the introduction of "pain as the fifth vital sign", and the incorporation of the standards advocated by the Joint Commission for Accreditation of Health Care Organization (JCAHO) have apparently not been effective and have not translated into improved postoperative analgesia.

More than 30% patients have moderate to severe pain in these studies (in some surveys these numbers are considerably higher). Certain patient subpopulations are at greater risk of undertreatment, these include infants and children, the elderly, ethnic minorities, and patients with psychiatric illness or those unable to communicate.

ANZCA (Australian and New Zealand College of Anaesthetists). *Acute pain management: scientific evidence*. Available at: www.anzca.edu/au/publications/acutepain.htm, accessed 24 July, 2005.

Apfelbaum JL, Chen C, Shilpa S, et al. Postoperative pain experience: results from a national survey suggest postoperative pain continues to be undermanaged. *Anesth Analg* 2003;97:534–540.

Ashburn MA, Caplan A, Carr DB, et al. Practice guidelines for acute pain management in the perioperative setting. *Anesthesiology* 2004;100:1573–1581.

Dolin SJ, Cashman JN, Bland JM. Effectiveness of acute postoperative pain management: evidence from published data. *Br J Anaesth* 2002;89:409–423.

International Association for the Study of Pain (IASP). *Core curriculum third revision*. IASP Press, www.iasp-pain.org. 2005.

Rawal N. Acute pain services revisited—good from far, far from good? *Reg Anesth Pain Med* 2002;27:117–121.

Werner MU, Søholm L, Rotbøll-Nielsen P, et al. Does an acute pain service improve postoperative outcome? *Anesth Analg* 2002;95:1361–1372.

D.2. What are the consequences of inadequate postoperative pain relief?

Evidence suggests that inadequate relief of postoperative pain may result in harmful physiologic and psychological consequences that lead to significant morbidity, which may delay recovery and the return to daily living. In addition, the presence of postoperative symptoms, including pain, significantly contributes to patients' dissatisfaction with their anesthesia and surgical experience. The autonomic overactivity results in an increased heart rate, peripheral vascular resistance, increased blood pressure, and myocardial contractility, all of which culminate in increased myocardial oxygen consumption from increased cardiac work. Postoperative pain has been found to be an important cause for long-lasting postoperative temper tantrums and untoward behavioral changes in children.

Recently, persistent pain after surgery, also referred to as *chronic postsurgical pain syndrome*, has been recognized as a major factor in delaying recovery and return to normal daily living.

Long-lasting pain has been reported after several surgical procedures including thoracotomy, mastectomy, hernia repair, and limb amputation. Predisposing risk factors include the severity of pre- and postoperative pain, intraoperative nerve injury and psychological vulnerability. Specific early analgesic interventions may reduce the incidence.

Ballantyne JC, Carr DB, de Ferranti S, et al. The comparative effects of postoperative analgesic therapies on pulmonary outcome: cumulative meta-analyses of randomized, controlled trials. *Anesth Analg* 1998;86:598–612.

Joshi GP, Ogunnaike BO. Consequences of inadequate postoperative pain relief and chronic persistent postoperative pain. *Anesthesiol Clin North America* 2005;23:21–36.

Kotiniemi LH, Ryhanen PT, Moilanen IK. Behavioral changes in children following day-case surgery: a 4-week follow-up of 551 children. *Anaesthesia* 1997;52:970–976.

Liu SS, Block BM, Wu CL. Effects of perioperative central neuraxial analgesia on outcome after coronary artery bypass surgery: a meta-analysis. *Anesthesiology* 2004;101:153–161.

Liu SS, Carpenter RL, Mackey DC, et al. Effects of perioperative analgesic technique on rate of recovery after colon surgery. *Anesthesiology* 1995;83:757–765.

Macrae WA. Chronic pain after surgery. *Br J Anaesth* 2001;87:88–98.

Wu CL, Naqibuddin M, Rowlingson AJ, et al. The effect of pain on health-related quality of life in the immediate postoperative period. *Anesth Analg* 2003;97:1078–1085.

D.3. What is the role of Acute Pain Services (APSs) in improving postoperative pain management?

It is generally accepted that the solution to the problem of inadequate pain relief lies not so much in the development of new analgesic drugs or technologies but in the development of an appropriate organization to utilize existing expertise.

More effective acute pain management will result from education and organizational structure for the delivery of pain relief rather than the analgesic techniques themselves. Even simple methods of pain relief can be more effective if proper attention is given to education, analgesic drug orders, documentation, monitoring of patients and the provision of appropriate policies, protocols, and guidelines. In some institutions, APSs assume responsibility for managing more advanced methods of pain relief such as patient-controlled analgesia (PCA) and epidural analgesia.

It is generally accepted that an organized APS that supervises the quality of pain management within an institution and documents institutional performance, ensures the quality of this organization and if shortfalls arise the APS recognizes them and prevents their recurrence.

Agency for Health Care Policy and Research. *Acute pain management: operative and medical procedures and trauma*. Rockville: US Department of Health and Human Services, Publication # 92-0032. AHCPR Publications, 1992.

American Society of Anesthesiologists. Practice guidelines for acute pain management in the perioperative setting: an updated report by American Society of Anesthesiologists, Task Force on Acute Pain Management. *Anesthesiology* 2004;100:1573–1581.

Joint Commission on Accreditation of Healthcare Organizations. *1992 Hospital accreditation standards*. Oakbrook Terrace: JCAHO, 2001.

Rawal N. Acute pain services revisited—good from far, far from good? (Editorial). *Reg Anesth Pain Med* 2002;27:117–121.

Rawal N. Organization, function, and implementation of Acute pain service. *Anesthesiol Clin North America* 2005;23:211–225.

Royal College of Surgeons and College of Anaesthetists Working Party on Pain after Surgery. *Pain after surgery*. London: Royal College of Surgeons, 1990.

Werner MU, Søholm L, Rotbøll-Nielsen P, et al. Does an acute pain service improve postoperative outcome? *Anesth Analg* 2002;95:1361–1372.

D.4. Does an Acute Pain Service (APS) improve postoperative outcome?

It is believed that the introduction of an APS has led to an increase in the appropriate use of specialized analgesic techniques, such as intravenous patient-controlled analgesia (IV-PCA) opioid and epidural and perineural analgesia. The implementation of these techniques is an advance in improving analgesia and patient well-being and in reducing postoperative morbidity. In addition, an APS may reduce "analgesic gaps" that can occur during the transition from IV-PCA or epidural analgesia to oral analgesic therapy. Although evaluating the safety of analgesic techniques is an important objective of an APS, its role in preventing and reducing adverse events has not been well established.

In a recent literature review, Werner et al. evaluated the effects of an APS on postoperative outcome in 44 audits and 4 clinical trials, which included 84,097 postoperative patients. The authors found that the implementation of an APS was associated with a significant decrease in pain intensity. In addition, the introduction of an APS might have been associated with less postoperative nausea and vomiting and urinary retention. However, the authors could not draw clear conclusions about the side effects of analgesic modalities, patient satisfaction, or postoperative morbidity because of a large variability in the studies regarding an APS function and the services provided.

Rawal N. Organization, function, and implementation of Acute pain service. *Anestehsiol Clin North Am* 2005;23:211–225.

Werner MU, Søholm L, Rotbøll-Nielsen P, et al. Does an acute pain service improve postoperative outcome? *Anesth Analg* 2002;95:1361–1372.

CHAPTER 33

Acupuncture

YUAN-CHI LIN

A 66-YEAR-OLD WOMAN

was scheduled for arthroscopic surgery of her right knee. She experienced severe postoperative nausea and vomiting in the postanesthesia care unit. Despite the use of conventional therapies, her nausea and vomiting persisted. Her past medical history was significant for mastectomy due to breast cancer, headache, chronic neck pain, osteoarthritis in her knees, peptic ulcer disease, and allergy to Novocain. What role can acupuncture therapy play in her care?

A. Acupuncture as a Complementary Medical Therapy
  1. What is acupuncture?
  2. How is acupuncture practiced?
  3. What are the mechanisms of acupuncture analgesia?
  4. What were the conclusions of the National Institute of Health Consensus Conference about acupuncture?

B. Acupuncture for the Treatment of Chronic Conditions
  1. Can acupuncture be used for the treatment of postoperative nausea and vomiting?
  2. Can acupuncture be used for the treatment of chemotherapy-induced nausea and vomiting?
  3. How effective is acupuncture for the management of chronic headache?
  4. Can acupuncture be used for the treatment of chronic neck pain?
  5. Can acupuncture be used for the treatment of osteoarthritis?
  6. What role can acupuncture play in the care of patients with cancer?

C. Complications
  1. What are the complications of acupuncture treatment?

A. Acupuncture as a Complementary Medical Therapy

A.1. What is acupuncture?

The word acupuncture is derived from the Latin words *acus*, "needle," and *punctura*, "a pricking." The original Chinese term for acupuncture is *Jin Jiao* which describes the practice of "acupuncture and moxibustion." Moxibustion, which is the burning of moxa (*artemisia vulgaris*) over the acupuncture points, can also be used for the treatment of various illnesses.

Acupuncture is one of the treatment modalities of comprehensive Traditional Chinese Medicine. The history of Traditional Chinese Medicine can be traced back 3,000 years. The "Yellow

Emperor's Classic of Internal Medicine" from the 4th century BC described the practice of puncturing the body for pain relief. Traditional Chinese medicine is a system of thoughts and practices that are based on the investigations of nature, causes, and effects. It takes the principles of realism and ethics, and employs them for the prevention and healing of illnesses.

The theory of "yin and yang" underlies the theoretical framework of acupuncture. Yin and yang are two opposite dynamics cannot exist in isolation. Rather, they are in a constant state of dynamic balance. If yin and yang are not balanced, illnesses occur in the body.

The human body is controlled by a vital force called "Qi." "Qi" circulates throughout the body and defends the body parts. There are 365 identified acupuncture points in the body that fall along 12 principal and eight extrameridian systems. "Qi" was postulated to flow through these meridians in the body.

A.2. How is acupuncture being practiced?

Acupuncture utilizes a technique of inserting very fine needles into strategic points in the body called *acupuncture points*. Acupuncture needles vary from $1/2$ to 5 in. in length and from 36 to 42 gauge. There is a wide variety of needles currently available. In *"Huang Di Nei Jing"* (*"The Yellow Emperor's Internal Classic"*), Lingf Shu described nine shapes of acupuncture needles. Sterile disposable stainless steel acupuncture needles are the current standard for acupuncture treatment.

The acupuncture needle is inserted through the epidermis. Following placement of the needle, stimulation of the acupuncture point may be achieved manually or by the use of low voltage electrodes introduced to the needle in a method called *electroacupuncture*.

Each acupuncture point has a prescribed depth of insertion. Manual techniques may involve the lifting and thrusting of the needle and/or twisting and twirling. "De-Qi" is a typical sensation that is associated with proper acupuncture needle position. Patients describe the sensation as a feeling of soreness, numbness, warmth, heaviness, or pressure around the area where the needle is inserted. The "De-Qi" sensation is mediated through nonmyelinated C fibers. Many practitioners consider this sensation to be crucial in achieving the effects of acupuncture. Electroacupuncture achieves a similar effect through the use of high or low frequency electricity. There is very little pain associated with the introduction of acupuncture, as most acupuncturists are quite skilled in the painless insertion of needles. For various conditions, multiple acupuncture treatment sessions over an extended period of time may be required to achieve its greatest effectiveness.

Auricular, hand, or scalp acupuncture can be utilized as microsystems of acupuncture. For example, for the auricular acupuncture, the upper region of the external ear is used to alleviate conditions in the leg and feet. The middle region of the external ear represents chest and back pain. The lower regions are utilized to relieve headache and neurologic conditions. Auricular acupuncture can also be utilized for preoperative anxiety control.

Chernyak GV, Sessler DI. Perioperative acupuncture and related techniques. *Anesthesiology* 2005;102(5):1031–1049; quiz 1077–1038.

Vincent CA, Richardson PH, Black JJ, et al. The significance of needle placement site in acupuncture. *J Psychosom Res* 1989;33(4):489–496.

A.3. What are the mechanisms of acupuncture analgesia?

Acupuncture inhibits the transmission of pain according to the gate-control theory. It may act by stimulating sensory A-β fibers, thereby directly inhibiting the spinal transmission of pain by a smaller A-δ and C fibers.

Acupuncture stimulates the production of endogenous opioid peptides, such as the endorphins, enkephalins, and stimulation of the endogenous descending inhibitory pathways. In human

studies, analysis of cerebrospinal fluid (CSF) showed elevated levels of serotonin, endorphins, and enkephalins following acupuncture treatments. Acupuncture analgesia is mainly achieved by the activation of the endogenous antinociceptive system to modulate pain transmission and pain response. Low frequency (2 Hz) and high frequency (100 Hz) electrical acupuncture selectively induces the release of enkephalins and dynorphins in both experimental animals and humans. Acupuncture analgesia may be reversed by naloxone.

Functional magnetic resonance (fMRI) has been utilized to investigate the effect of acupuncture in normal volunteers. Acupuncture needle manipulation on the LI 4 (Hegu) point modulates the activity of the limbic system and subcortical structure revealed in fMRI. There is individual variation of the cortical activation patterns elicited by electrical acupuncture stimulation. Real acupuncture elicited significantly higher activation than sham acupuncture over the hypothalamus and primary somatosensory-motor cortex and deactivation over the rostral segment of anterior cingulated cortex.

Abraham MK, Menon SS, Bindumole PS. Thoracoscopic repair of eventration of diaphragm. *Indian Pediatr* 2003;40(11):1088–1089.

He L. Involvement of endogenous opioid peptides in acupuncture analgesia. *Pain* 1987;31:99–121.

Hui K, Liu J, Makris N, et al. Acupuncture modulates the limbic system and subcortical gray structures of the human brain: evidence from fMRI studies in normal subjects. *Hum Brain Mapp* 2000;9:13–25.

Lewith G, Kenyon JN. Physiological and psychological explanations for the mechanism of acupuncture as a treatment for chronic pain. *Soc Sci Med* 1984;19(12):1367–1378.

Mayer D, Price D, Raffii A. Antagonism of acupuncture analgesia in man by the narcotic antagonist naloxone. *Brain Res* 1977;121:368–372.

Sjolund B, Terenius L, Eriksson M. Increased cerebrospinal fluid levels of endorphins after electro-acupuncture. *Acta Physiol Scand* 1977;100:382–384.

Ulett G, Han S, Han J. Electroacupuncture: mechanisms and clinical application. *Biol Psychiatry* 1998;44:129–138

Wu M, Sheen J, Chuang K, et al. Neuronal specificity of acupuncture response: a fMRI study with electroacupuncture. *Neuroimage* 2002;16:1028–1037.

A.4. What were the conclusions of the National Institute of Health Consensus Conference about acupuncture?

A National Institute of Health Consensus Conference concluded that acupuncture is an effective therapeutic intervention that is widely practiced in the United States. Promising results have emerged, for example, showing clear evidence that supports the efficacy of acupuncture in adult postoperative and chemotherapy-related nausea and vomiting, and in postoperative dental pain. There are other conditions, such as addiction, stroke rehabilitation, headache, menstrual cramps, tennis elbow, fibromyalgia, myofascial pain, osteoarthritis, low back pain, carpal tunnel syndrome, and asthma, in which acupuncture may also be useful as an adjunct treatment, as an acceptable alternative, or when included in a comprehensive management program. Further research is expected to uncover additional areas in which acupuncture interventions will be useful.

NIH Consensus conference: Acupuncture. *JAMA* 1988;280:1518–1524.

B. Acupuncture for the Treatment of Chronic Conditions

B.1. Can acupuncture be used for the treatment of postoperative nausea and vomiting?

Postoperative nausea and vomiting are frequent occurrences following surgery, and are best avoided whenever possible. Acupuncture is a commonly used therapy for the treatment of these symptoms. Stimulation of the acupuncture PC-6 (*Nei Guan acupuncture point; Chinese means Gate of the Internal Organ*) points by acupuncture needles, electrical apparatus, pressure, or magnets is utilized to achieve nausea and vomiting relief. The pc-6 acupuncture point is located 2 in. above the transverse crease of the wrist, between the tendons of the long palmar muscle and the radial flexor muscle.

Studies support the use of acupuncture for the treatment of postoperative nausea and vomiting. A systemic review was conducted of 33 randomized controlled trials of acupuncture and acupressure. The results were positive in 27 of these trials. A randomized controlled trial of pediatric patients undergoing tonsillectomy utilizing electroacupuncture in the conscious patients showed significant reduction in the occurrence of nausea compared with those in the sham and control groups. The efficacy of acupuncture for postoperative nausea and vomiting prevention is similar to commonly used pharmacotherapies. A double-blind, randomized, placebo-controlled study revealed that hand acupressure is an effective method for reducing postoperative vomiting in children after strabismus repair.

PC-6 acupressure is a noninvasive method that may have a place as prophylactic antiemetic therapy during gynecologic surgery. Alkaissi et al. did a prospective randomized controlled trial of acupressure in the prevention of postoperative nausea and vomiting for women undergoing general anesthesia for elective gynecologic surgery, with positive results.

Alkaissi A, Evertsson K, Johnsson VA, et al. P6 acupressure may relieve nausea and vomiting after gynecological surgery: an effectiveness study in 410 women. *Can J Anaesth* 2002;49(10):1034–1039.

Chu YC, Lin SM, Hsieh YC, et al. Effect of BL-10 (tianzhu), BL-11 (dazhu) and GB-34 (yanglinquan) acuplaster for prevention of vomiting after strabismus surgery in children. *Acta Anaesthesiol Sin* 1998;36(1):11–16.

Macario A, Weinger M, Carney S, et al. Which clinical anesthesia outcomes are important to avoid? The perspective of patients. *Anesth Analg* 1999;89(3):652–658.

Rusy LM, Hoffman GM, Weisman SJ. Electroacupuncture prophylaxis of postoperative nausea and vomiting following pediatric tonsillectomy with or without adenoidectomy. *Anesthesiology* 2002;96(2):300–305.

Schlager A, Boehler M, Puhringer F. Korean hand acupressure reduces postoperative vomiting in children after strabismus surgery. *Br J Anaesth* 2000;85(2):267–270.

Vickers A. Can acupuncture have specific effects on health? A systematic review of acupuncture antiemetic trials. *J R Soc Med* 1996;89:303–311.

B.2. Can acupuncture be used for the treatment of chemotherapy-induced nausea and vomiting?

Acupressure at the PC-6 acupuncture point has been shown to have a protective effect on people experiencing chemotherapy-induced nausea. A review of 11 randomized controlled trials studying the effectiveness of acupuncture point stimulation on chemotherapy-induced nausea and vomiting revealed that electroacupuncture reduced chemotherapy-induced acute vomiting.

Ezzo JM, Richardson MA, Vickers A, et al. Acupuncture-point stimulation for chemotherapy-induced nausea or vomiting. *Cochrane Database Syst Rev* 2006;(2):CD002285.

B.3. How effective is acupuncture for the management of chronic headache?

Acupuncture therapy for migraine headaches has been reported to be effective in several adult studies. In a randomized controlled trial of 168 women with migraine, acupuncture was proved to be an adequate migraine prophylaxis. Relative to flunarizine, acupuncture treatment exhibited greater efficiency in the first months of therapy and better patient tolerance. A systemic review of 22 trials, including a total of 1,042 patients, suggests that acupuncture has a role in the treatment of recurrent headaches. As added benefit, in a randomized controlled trial of 401 patients with chronic migraine headache, it was also shown that, through 12 months of follow up, acupuncture is relatively cost-effective. Compared with the patients in the control groups, patients receiving acupuncture used 15% less medication, made 25% fewer visits to general practitioners, and took 15% fewer sick days from work.

Allais G, De Lorenzo C, Quirico P, et al. Acupuncture in the prophylactic treatment of migraine without aura: a comparison with flunarizine. *Headache* 2002;42(9):855–861.

Dowson D, Lewith GT, Machin D. The effects of acupuncture versus placebo in the treatment of headache. *Pain* 1985;21(1):35–42.

Loh L, Nathan PW, Schott GD, et al. Acupuncture versus medical treatment for migraine and muscle tension headaches. *J Neurol Neurosurg Psychiatry* 1984;47(4):333–337.

Melchart D, Linde K, Fischer P, et al. Acupuncture for recurrent headaches: a systematic review of randomized controlled trials. *Cephalalgia* 1999;19(9):779–786.

Vickers AJ, Rees RW, Zollman CE, et al. Acupuncture for chronic headache in primary care: large, pragmatic, randomised trial. *Br Med J* 2004;328(7442):744.

B.4. Can acupuncture be used for the treatment of chronic neck pain?

In a randomized controlled trial of 177 patients with chronic neck pain, the effectiveness of acupuncture, massage, and "sham" laser acupuncture were compared. A study followed 14,161 patients with chronic neck pain for a period of more than 6 months. The patients in the acupuncture group received up to 15 acupuncture sessions over 3 months. The reported neck pain levels and disability scores of the members of the acupuncture group were improved over those of the control group. Treatment success was followed and maintained for 6 months.

Irnich D, Behrens N, Molzen H, et al. Randomised trial of acupuncture compared with conventional massage and "sham" laser acupuncture for treatment of chronic neck pain. *Br Med J* 2001;322(7302):1574–1577.

Witt CM, Jena S, Brinkhaus B, et al. Acupuncture for patients with chronic neck pain. *Pain* 2006;125:98–106.

B.5. Can acupuncture be used for the treatment of osteoarthritis?

There is evidence of the efficacy of acupuncture for reducing the pain and dysfunction of osteoarthritis. In a study of 300 patients with chronic osteoarthritis of the knee, participants were randomly assigned to acupuncture, minimal acupuncture, or wait list control group. After

8 weeks of treatment, pain and joint function were improved more with acupuncture than with minimal or no acupuncture.

In another randomized controlled trial of 570 patients with osteoarthritis of the knee, the acupuncture group received 23 true acupuncture sessions over 26 weeks. Acupuncture was shown to provide improvement in function and pain relief as an adjunctive therapy for osteoarthritis of the knee when compared with credible sham acupuncture and education control groups.

In a trial of thirty patients with symptomatic osteoarthritis of the knee, participants were randomized into one of three treatment groups. One group of patients had acupuncture alone, another group of patients had acupuncture, but continued on their symptomatic medication, and the third group of patients used their symptomatic medication for the first 5 weeks and then had a course of acupuncture added. The patients receiving acupuncture were treated twice weekly over 5 weeks. The results of this study concluded that manual and electroacupuncture causes a significant improvement in the symptoms of osteoarthritis of the knee, either alone or as an adjunct therapy, and with no loss of benefit after 1 month.

Berman BM, Lao L, Langenberg P, et al. Effectiveness of acupuncture as adjunctive therapy in osteoarthritis of the knee: a randomized, controlled trial. *Ann Intern Med* 2004;141(12):901–910.

Tukmachi E, Jubb R, Dempsey E, et al. The effect of acupuncture on the symptoms of knee osteoarthritis–an open randomised controlled study. *Acupunct Med* 2004;22(1): 14–22.

Witt C, Brinkhaus B, Jena S, et al. Acupuncture in patients with osteoarthritis of the knee: a randomised trial. *Lancet* 2005;366(9480):136–143.

B.6. What role can acupuncture play in the care of patients with cancer?

A report of a randomized controlled trial of 90 patients with cancer pain revealed clear benefit from auricular acupuncture for cancer patients experiencing pain, despite stable analgesic treatment. It is reasonable to use acupuncture for the management of chronic cancer-related pain management. It is also reasonable to use acupuncture in conjunction with standard antiemetics to control chemotherapy-related nausea and vomiting.

Alimi D, Rubino C, Pichard-Leandri E, et al. Analgesic effect of auricular acupuncture for cancer pain: a randomized, blinded, controlled trial. *J Clin Oncol* 2003;21(22): 4120–4126.

Ezzo JM, Richardson MA, Vickers A, et al. Acupuncture-point stimulation for chemotherapy-induced nausea or vomiting. *Cochrane Database Syst Rev* 2006;(2): CD002285.

C. Complications

C.1. What are the complications of acupuncture treatment?

Acupuncture is safe. Occasionally, although rarely, a patient may have some bruising at an acupuncture site, which is quickly resolved. The principal risk is infection from the use of improperly sterilized needles. This can be avoided by using disposable sterile acupuncture needles and through the practice of proper insertion of the needles. There have also been extremely rare reports of pneumothorax caused by improperly inserted acupuncture needles.

A study of the adverse effects of 32,000 acupuncture consultations in the United Kingdom revealed that the most common adverse events were bleeding, needling pain and aggravation of symptoms. None of these events were serious. Similarly, a review of nine surveys showed that the most common adverse events were needle pain, tiredness, and bleeding. Feelings of faintness and syncope were uncommon. Feelings of relaxation were reported by as many as 86% of patients. The report of pneumothorax were extremely rare, occurring only twice in nearly a quarter of a million treatments.

A study was conducted involving a prospective postal audit of treatments performed by 1,848 professional acupuncturists in the United Kingdom over a 4-week period. They reported 43 minor adverse events, a rate of 1.3 per 1,000 treatments. The events report included severe nausea and fainting, prolonged aggravation of the symptoms, and pain and bruising. The overall frequency of acupuncture-related adverse events is extremely low, and prospective studies have indicated that even minor adverse events are uncommon. Acupuncture is considered to be a very safe intervention when applied appropriately and adverse effects of acupuncture are extremely rare.

Ernst E, White A. Prospective studies of the safety of acupuncture: a systemic review. *Am J Med* 2001;110:481–485.

MacPherson H, Thomas K, Walters S, et al. The York acupuncture safety study: prospective survey of 34 000 treatments by traditional acupuncturists. *Br Med J* 2001; 323(7311):486–487.

Von Riedenauer WB, Baker MK, Brewer RJ, Video-assisted thoracoscopic removal of migratory acupuncture needle causing pneumothorax. *Chest* 2007;131:899–901.

SECTION VI

The Endocrine System

CHAPTER 34

Thyrotoxicosis

Dana L. Gurvitch

A 48-YEAR-OLD MAN

presented with diffuse neck swelling. History of present illness was significant for dyspnea, dysphagia, weight loss, paroxysmal palpitations, and heat intolerance. His blood pressure was 160/100 mm Hg and his heart rate was 120 beats per minute; his hematocrit level was 29%.

A. Medical Disease and Differential Diagnosis
1. What diagnosis is compatible with these symptoms?
2. Describe the synthesis, release, and peripheral conversion of triiodothyronine (T_4) and thyroxine (T_3).
3. What is the role of the hypothalamic–pituitary axis in thyroid function?
4. Describe the effects of thyroid hormone.
5. What are the causes of hyperthyroidism?
6. What are the clinical signs and symptoms of thyrotoxicosis?
7. How would you distinguish thyroid storm from thyrotoxicosis?
8. What can precipitate thyroid storm?
9. Discuss innervation of the larynx.

B. Preoperative Evaluation and Preparation
1. Are there anatomic problems associated with an enlarged thyroid gland?
2. Describe the signs and symptoms of superior vena cava syndrome.
3. How would you assess the possibility of airway obstruction?
4. Discuss the laboratory assessment of thyroid function.
5. Describe medical strategies for achieving an euthyroid state.
6. What are the benefits of adrenergic blockade?

7. When is the hyperthyroid patient ready for elective surgery?

8. How would you premedicate this patient?

9. How would you prepare the thyrotoxic patient for emergent surgery?

C. Intraoperative Management

1. How would you monitor this patient?

2. How would you induce anesthesia?

3. Is endotracheal intubation necessary for this operation? Discuss the type and length of tube you would use.

4. How would you maintain anesthesia?

5. Intraoperatively the patient became hyperthermic and tachycardic. Discuss the differential diagnosis of malignant hyperthermia and thyroid storm. How would you intervene?

6. How would you extubate this patient?

D. Postoperative Management

1. The patient became stridulous and dyspneic in the recovery room. What was your differential diagnosis and intervention strategy?

2. When does thyroid storm most often present?

A. Medical Disease and Differential Diagnosis

A.1. What diagnosis is compatible with these symptoms?

These signs and symptoms are classic for hyperthyroidism. Differential diagnosis includes other hypermetabolic states such as pheochromocytoma, carcinoid, carcinoma, chronic infection, anxiety states, lethal catatonia, exertional heat stroke, strychnine poisoning, and certain drugs such as inhalation anesthetics, sympathomimetic agents, serotonin antagonists, antipsychotic agents, and compounds exhibiting anticholinergic properties.

Braunwald E, Fauci AS, Hauser S, et al. eds. *Harrison's principles of internal medicine*, 16th ed. New York: McGraw-Hill, 2005:2069–2074.

Hadad E, Wehbroum AA, Ben-Abraham R. Drug induced hyperthermia and muscle rigidity: a practical approach. *Eur J Emerg Med* 2003;10:149–154.

Rakel RE, ed. *Saunders manual of medical practice.* Philadelphia: WB Saunders, 2000: 638–641.

A.2. Describe the synthesis, release, and peripheral conversion of triiodothyronine (T_3) and thyroxine (T_4).

The synthesis of thyroid hormone is dependent on iodine. Sufficient amounts of iodine must come from dietary intake or from the deiodination of preexisting thyroid hormone. Iodine is actively transported into thyroid cells and concentrated in the form of iodide. Organification occurs as iodine binds to tyrosine residues of thyroglobulin, the receptor protein for iodine. Coupling of iodinated tyrosine residues results in the formation of T_4 and T_3. Once cleaved from thyroglobulin as regulated by thyroid-stimulating hormone, thyroid hormone is released into the circulation. Ninety percent of the hormone secreted from the thyroid gland is T_4, whereas only 10% is T_3, the biologically active form with a much shorter half-life. However, in the peripheral tissues, most of the T_4 is converted to T_3. T_4 can also be converted to reverse T_3, an inactive metabolite. In the circulation, most of the T_4 and T_3 binds to plasma proteins; mainly thyronine binding globulin. A small amount binds to albumin and prealbumin and less than 1% is unbound in the plasma.

Braunwald E, Fauci AS, Hauser S, et al. eds. *Harrison's principles of internal medicine*, 16th ed. New York: McGraw-Hill, 2005:2105–2106.

Goldman D. Surgery in patients with endocrine dysfunction. *Med Clin North Am* 1987;71:502–504.

Guyton A, Hall J. *Textbook of medical physiology*, 11th ed. Philadelphia: WB Saunders, 2006:934–935.

Mitchell J. Thyroid disease in the emergency department. *Emerg Med Clin North Am* 1989;7:885–888.

Reid JR, Wheeler SF. Hyperthyroidism: diagnosis and treatment. *Am Fam Physician* 2005;72(4):635–636.

A.3. What is the role of the hypothalamic–pituitary axis in thyroid function?

The hypothalamus secretes thyroid-releasing hormone, which in turn stimulates the synthesis and release of thyroid-stimulating hormone (TSH) by the anterior pituitary gland. TSH stimulates the synthesis and secretion of thyroid hormones by the thyroid gland. Within pituitary cells, T_4 is converted to T_3. The intracellular level of T_3 within pituitary cells regulates the pituitary release of TSH. Low levels of T_3 stimulate the release of TSH, whereas increased levels of thyroid hormone decrease TSH secretion.

Braunwald E, Fauci AS, Hauser SL, et al. eds. *Harrison's principles of internal medicine*, 16th ed. New York: McGraw-Hill, 2005:2060–2061.

Guyton A, Hall J. *Textbook of medical physiology*, 11th ed. Philadelphia: WB Saunders, 2006:734.

A.4. Describe the effects of thyroid hormone.

Thyroid hormone has effects at the cellular, organ, and systemic levels.

Cellular effects

- Thyroid hormone regulates the nuclear transcription of messenger ribonucleic acid (mRNA) in all cells. T_3 binds to a deoxyribonucleic acid (DNA) domain named the "thyroid response element." Once bound, T_3 initiates the transcription of an array of biochemical enzymes that regulate tissue metabolism. T_3 is also postulated to bind to mitochondrial T_3-binding proteins with resultant transcription and synthesis of cytochromes. The basal metabolic rate can increase as much as 60% to 100% when large quantities of thyroid hormones are secreted. One ubiquitous enzyme that is transcribed in response to thyroid hormone stimulation is Na, K-ATPase.
- In addition to its role in enzyme transcription, thyroid hormone regulates cellular energy use. It stimulates cellular glucose use by increasing glucose absorption from the gastrointestinal tract, glycogenolysis, gluconeogenesis, insulin secretion, and cellular uptake of glucose. Thyroid hormone increases free fatty acid availability by increasing lipid mobilization from adipocytes. Conversely, thyroid hormone decreases plasma levels of cholesterol, phospholipids, and triglycerides by increasing the rate of cholesterol secretion into the bile.

Organ effects

- Thyroid hormone is believed to have a direct effect on the heart by increasing heart rate and contractility with resultant increases in cardiac output.
- Thyroid hormone increases oxygen consumption and carbon dioxide production with a compensatory increase in respiratory rate and tidal volume.

- Thyroid hormone increases bone formation and catabolism with resultant changes in parathyroid hormone levels.

Systemic effects

- Increased cellular metabolism and production of metabolic end products result in vasodilation and enhanced tissue blood flow.

Braunwald E, Fauci AS, Hauser S, et al. eds. *Harrison's principles of internal medicine*, 16th ed. New York: McGraw-Hill, 2005:2105–2106.

Guyton A, Hall J. *Textbook of medical physiology*, 11th ed. Philadelphia: WB Saunders, 2006:858–860.

Mitchell J. Thyroid disease in the emergency department. *Emerg Med Clin North Am* 1989;7:885–888.

Smallridge R. Metabolic and anatomic thyroid emergencies. *Crit Care Med* 1992;20:276–291.

Tietgens S, Leinung M. Thyroid storm. *Med Clin North Am* 1995;79:169–178.

A.5. What are the causes of hyperthyroidism?

Graves disease accounts for 90% of all cases of hyperthyroidism. The next most common cause is thyroiditis. Less commonly, toxic multinodular goiter, toxic solitary nodule, and excessive exogenous iodide consumption, and side effects of certain medications can cause hyperthyroidism. Trophoblastic tumors (e.g., hydatidiform mole and choriocarcinoma) are infrequent causes of hyperthyroidism.

Surreptitious overdosing (factitious thyrotoxicosis) is occasionally seen.

Kaplan MM, Meier DA, Dworkin HJ. Treatment of hyperthyroidism with radioactive iodine. *Endocrinol Metab Clin North Am* 1998;27(1):205–214.

Reid JR, Wheeler SF. Hyperthyroidism: diagnosis and treatment. *Am Fam Physician* 2005;72(4):623–630.

de los Santos E, Mazzaferri E. Thyrotoxicosis results and risks of current therapy. *Postgrad Med* 1990;87:277–294.

Smallridge R. Metabolic and anatomic thyroid emergencies. *Crit Care Med* 1992;20:276–291.

A.6. What are the clinical signs and symptoms of thyrotoxicosis?

The clinical presentation depends on the severity of thyrotoxicosis, the duration of the disease, patient susceptibility to excess thyroid hormone, and the patients' age. Nonspecific constitutive signs such as sweating, heat intolerance, weakness, and restlessness are common clinical signs and symptoms of thyrotoxicosis. Weight loss occurs despite a normal or increased appetite resulting from the increased metabolic rate. Fine tremor is a frequent finding as is lid retraction, causing a staring appearance, as a result of sympathetic overactivity.

Cardiovascular involvement is a prominent feature of thyrotoxicosis with resulting increased cardiovascular morbidity and mortality, primarily due to heart failure and thromboembolism. Alterations include tachyarrhythmias, increased stroke volume, increased cardiac output, increased oxygen consumption, and decreased systemic and pulmonary vascular resistance. In addition, patients demonstrate increased myocardial contractility, automaticity, and excitability. Pulse pressure can be widened with an increase in systolic blood pressure. In patients with coronary atherosclerosis, angina may be precipitated or worsened. Young adults usually tolerate hyperthyroidism without cardiovascular decompensation. However, high-output congestive heart failure can occur in older patients and those with a previously damaged heart. Thyrotoxic patients may present with sinus tachycardia, atrial fibrillation, complete heart block, or ventricular dysrhythmias.

Hypercarbia and increased oxygen consumption resulting from the hypermetabolic state result in a compensatory increased minute ventilation with tachypnea and elevated tidal volumes. Vital capacity often decreases because of weak muscles and decreased compliance, whereas diffusing capacity remains normal. Exercise results in increased ventilation and increased oxygen uptake.

Neurologic manifestations include anxiety, agitation, tremors, insomnia, muscle weakness, and changes in cognition such as confusion and delirium. This can progress in severe cases to stupor, obtundation, and coma. Other manifestations include myopathies, periodic paralysis, seizures, chorea, and a fine resting tremor. On electroencephalogram, these patients may show an increase in fast-wave activity.

Thyrotoxicosis shortens gastrointestinal tract transit time and a secretory diarrhea may develop. Weight loss caused by increased caloric requirements is often observed. Acid secretion occasionally decreases (parietal cell antibodies in 30%), thereby potentially affecting drug absorption.

Hematologic derangements include anemia, neutropenia, and thrombocytopenia. Red blood cell mass increases because of the increased oxygen requirement.

Regarding renal involvement, tubular reabsorption and secretion are increased, leading to eventual decreased potassium excretion and increased sodium excretion.

Braunwald E, Fauci AS, Hauser SL, et al. eds. *Harrison's principles of internal medicine*, 16th ed. New York: McGraw-Hill, 2005:2105–2106.

Felig P, Frohman LA. The thyroid: physiology, thyrotoxicosis, hypothyroidism and the painful thyroid. In: *Endocrinology and metabolism*, 4th ed. New York: McGraw-Hill, 2001.

Jameson JL, Weetman AP. Disorders of the thyroid gland. In: Kasper DL, ed. *Harrison's principles of internal medicine*, 16th ed. Chapter 320, New York: McGraw-Hill, 2005.

Pronovost P, Parris K. Perioperative management of thyroid disease. *Postgrad Med* 1995;98:83–96.

Ruffi M, Cattaneo F, Tupol EJ. Thyrotoxicosis and the cardiovascular system: subtle but serious effects. *Cleve Clin J Med* 2003;70(1):57–63. Jan

Stoelting RK, Miller RD. *Anesthesia and co-existing disease*, 4th ed. New York: Churchill Livingstone, 2002:412–416.

A.7. How would you distinguish thyroid storm from thyrotoxicosis?

Thyrotoxicosis refers to all disorders of increased thyroid hormone concentrations. The clinical spectrum ranges from asymptomatic biochemical abnormalities to life-threatening crises with multisystem dysfunction and a high mortality rate. Thyroid storm exists when a patient's metabolic, thermoregulatory, and cardiovascular compensatory mechanisms fail. The clinical picture is characterized by four main features: fever, tachycardia or supraventricular arrhythmias, central nervous system symptoms, and gastrointestinal symptoms. Early recognition and aggressive treatment are fundamental in limiting morbidity and mortality. No laboratory test differentiates between thyroid storm and thyrotoxicosis. Thyroid function tests should be given. However, once thyroid storm is suspected, treatment should be immediately instituted and not delayed for test results. Goals include: reduction of circulating thyroid hormone levels; inhibition of the peripheral effects of circulating thyroid hormones; supportive care, and treatment of the underlying precipitating event.

Migneco A, Ojetti V, Testa A, et al. Management of thyrotoxic crisis. *Eur Rev Med Pharmacol Sci* 2005;9(1):69–74.

Smallridge R. Metabolic and anatomic thyroid emergencies. *Crit Care Med* 1992;20:276–291.

A.8. What can precipitate thyroid storm?

Thyroid storm has an abrupt onset and can be precipitated by conditions that cause a rapid rise in thyroid hormone levels such as thyroid surgery, withdrawal of antithyroid drug therapy, radioiodine therapy, iodinated contrast dyes, and vigorous thyroid manipulation. Nonthyroid illnesses such as nonthyroid surgery, infection, cerebral vascular accident, congestive heart failure, bowel infarction, pulmonary embolism, pregnancy, parturition, diabetic ketoacidosis, trauma, or administration of iodine containing materials (amiodarone) can also precipitate thyroid storm. It is the acute change of thyroid hormone levels, rather than the absolute levels, which precipitates thyroid storm.

Burch H, Wartofsky L. Life threatening thyrotoxicosis. *Endocrinol Metab Clin North Am* 1993;22:263–274.

Migneco A, Ojetti V, Testa A, et al. Management of thyrotoxic crisis. *Eur Rev Med Pharmacol Sci* 2005;9(1):69–74.

Nicoloff J. Thyroid storm and myxedema coma. *Med Clin North Am* 1985;69:1005–1012.

Stoelting RK, Miller RD. *Anesthesia and co-existing disease*, 4th ed. New York: Churchill Livingstone, 2002:412–416.

A.9. Discuss innervation of the larynx.

Innervation of the larynx is from two branches of the vagus nerve: the superior laryngeal and the recurrent laryngeal nerve. The superior laryngeal nerve divides just superficial to the thyrohyoid membrane into the internal laryngeal nerve (sensory and autonomic) and external laryngeal nerve (motor). The internal laryngeal nerve pierces the thyrohyoid membrane and supplies sensory fibers to the larynx superior to the vocal cords. The external laryngeal nerve remains superficial to the thyrohyoid membrane to supply the cricothyroid muscle and a portion of the transverse arytenoid muscle. The recurrent laryngeal nerve supplies motor innervation to all of the remaining intrinsic muscles of the larynx and sensory innervation to the larynx inferior to the vocal cords.

The cricothyroid muscle is the only tensor muscle of the larynx. Bilateral recurrent laryngeal nerve injury will result in motor paralysis of all the intrinsic muscles of the larynx except the cricothyroid muscle and part of the transverse arytenoid muscle. Respiratory obstruction occurs as the vocal cords become approximated at midline. However, the cords are flaccid, not tense. The cricothyroid muscle requires resistance from the other intrinsic muscles to tense the cords. Unilateral recurrent laryngeal nerve injury results in one midline flaccid cord with the other cord being normal. Hoarseness and risk of aspiration are more problematic than respiratory obstruction.

Barash P, Cullen B, Stoelting R, eds. *Clinical anesthesia*, 5th ed. Philadelphia: Lippincott Williams & Wilkins, 2006.

Grenvik A, Ayres S, Shoemaker W, et al. eds. *Textbook of critical care*, 5th ed. Philadelphia: WB Saunders, 2005.

Moore KL, Dalley AF. *Clinically oriented anatomy*, 5th ed. Baltimore: Lippincott Williams & Wilkins, 2006:1083–1087.

B. Preoperative Evaluation and Preparation

B.1. Are there anatomic problems associated with an enlarged thyroid gland?

The thyroid gland incompletely encircles the trachea and esophagus. Glandular enlargement can cause tracheoesophageal compression with symptoms such as dyspnea and dysphagia. The anatomic location of the thyroid, suprasternal versus substernal, has important implications. Airway involvement can include deviation, compression, or luminal narrowing. With muscle relaxation, an enlarged substernal thyroid can cause unanticipated tracheal compression after the administration of agents that result in loss of respiratory muscle tone. Tracheal invasion or intratracheal hemorrhage can occur with thyroid carcinomas.

The anatomic position of the superior vena cava in the thorax makes it vulnerable to compression by mediastinal masses.

Acute respiratory insufficiency secondary to bilateral vocal cord paralysis from recurrent laryngeal nerve compression has been reported in patients with intrathoracic goiter.

Braunwald E, Fauci AS, Hauser S, et al. eds. *Harrison's principles of internal medicine*, 16th ed. New York: McGraw-Hill, 2005:2120.

Peters K, Nance P, Wingard D. Malignant hyperthyroidism or malignant hyperthermia. *Anesth Analg* 1981;60:613–615.

Smallridge R. Metabolic and anatomic thyroid emergencies. *Crit Care Med* 1992;20:276–291.

Steenerson R, Barton R. Mediastinal goiter and superior vena cava syndrome. *Laryngoscope* 1978;88:1688–1690.

B.2. Describe the signs and symptoms of superior vena cava syndrome.

Superior vena cava syndrome is an insidious gradual compression/obstruction of the superior vena cava. The low-flow, low-pressure, thin-walled superior vena cava is susceptible to compression from expanding mediastinal masses. The low intravascular pressure also allows for the possibility of thrombus formation, such as catheter induced thrombus. The obstruction of venous drainage from the upper thorax results in interstitial edema and retrograde collateral flow and produces face, neck, and upper extremity edema, dilation of collateral veins of the upper thorax and neck, and symptoms of headache and vertigo. Because of the predominance of right-sided thyromegaly, compression of the right innominate vein is more common. As the superior vena cava becomes obstructed, collaterals such as the azygous, internal mammary, vertebral, and lateral thoracic venous plexuses form. Venography is the "gold standard" for anatomic delineation.

Ulreich S, Lowman R, Stern H. Intrathoracic goiter: a cause of the superior vena cava syndrome. *Clin Radiol* 1977;28:663–665.

Walton A. Superior vena cava syndrome: an education sheet for patients. *Clin J Oncol Nurs* 2005;9(4):479–480.

B.3. How would you assess the possibility of airway obstruction?

Chest radiograph and computed tomography scanning of the neck are helpful in evaluating tracheal position and airway obstruction.

Pulmonary function testing is a noninvasive method used to evaluate patients with airway obstruction. Flow–volume loop analysis determines the extent and location of airway obstruction. Flow–volume loops are generated by inhaling to total lung capacity, exhaling to residual volume,

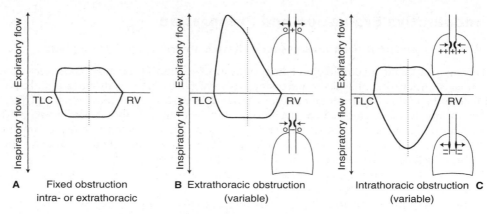

Figure 34.1 Flow–volume curves in fixed and variable obstruction. **A:** Fixed obstruction, intrathoracic or extrathoracic. **B:** Extrathoracic obstruction (variable). **C:** Intrathoracic obstruction (variable). RV, residual volume; TLC, total lung capacity. (From Benumof J. *Anesthesia for thoracic surgery,* 2nd ed. Philadelphia: WB Saunders, 1995:536, with permission.)

and then inhaling back to total lung capacity. Differing patterns in flow–volume loops can distinguish intrathoracic versus extrathoracic airway obstructions (Fig. 34.1).

Fixed lesions of the upper airway, which include tracheal tumors, subglottic stenosis, and goiters, will produce plateaus in both the inspiratory and expiratory cycle of the flow–volume loop (Fig. 34.1A).

Variable extrathoracic lesions are most often caused by vocal cord paralysis, vocal cord neoplasms, and neoplasms in the neck. The inspiratory limb of the flow–volume loop plateaus. During inhalation, the generation of negative intrathoracic pressure pulls the extrathoracic airway closed. During exhalation, airflow maintains the patency of the airway (Fig. 34.1B).

Variable intrathoracic lesions, which include endobronchial tumors, tracheal tumors, and tracheomalacia, produce plateau of the expiratory cycle only. Inhalation is unimpaired because negative intrathoracic pressure will stent the airway. During exhalation, positive intrathoracic pressure narrows the airway and results in plateau of the expiratory limb of the flow–volume loop (Fig. 34.1C). These patients will have preserved forced vital capacity but marked reductions of forced expiratory volume in 1 second.

Benumof J. *Anesthesia for thoracic surgery*, 2nd ed. Philadelphia: WB Saunders, 1995:536.

Lunn W, Sheller J. Flow volume loops in the evaluation of upper airway obstruction. *Otolaryngol Clin North Am* 1995;28:721–729.

B.4. Discuss the laboratory assessment of thyroid function.

Thyroid function tests are divided into three categories:

- Direct tests of thyroid function
- Tests related to concentration and binding of thyroid hormones
- Tests of homeostatic control of thyroid function

Direct tests of thyroid function involve administration of radioactive iodine and measurement of its uptake by the thyroid. Radioactive iodine uptake is measured 24 hours after administration of the isotope. Uptake will vary inversely with the plasma iodide concentration and vary directly with thyroid function.

Table 34.1 Serum Thyroid Hormone Tests in Health and Disease.

	TOTAL T₄	T₃	FREE T₄ INDEX	FREE T₄	T₃	REVERSE T₃	TSH
Euthyroid	N	N	N	N	N	N	N
Hyperthyroid	↑	↑	↑	↑	↑	↑	↓
Hypothyroid	↓	↓	↓	↓	N, ↓	↓	↑
TBG excess	↑	↓	N	N	↑	↑	N
TBG deficiency	↓	↑	N	N, ↓	↓	↓	N
Nonthyroidal illness	N, ↓	↑	N, ↓	↑, N, ↓	↓	↑	N, ↓
FDH	↑	N	↑	N	N	N	N

T_4, thyroxine; T_3, triiodothyronine; TSH, thyroid-stimulating hormone; ↑, increased; ↓, decreased; N, normal; TBG, thyroxine-binding globulin; FDH, familial dysalbuminemic hyperthyroxinemia.
From Smallridge RC. Metabolic and anatomic thyroid emergencies: a review. *Crit Care Med* 1992;20:276, with permission.

Tests related to hormone concentration and binding in serum include measurements of T_4 and T_3. Radioimmunoassays of both free and total T_3 and T_4 are available. Although some centers measure the percent of T_4 or T_3 that is dialyzable or free, most use an *in vitro* uptake test. Serum is enriched with labeled T_4 or labeled T_3 and is then incubated with a resin that binds free hormone. Labeled T_3 will bind to unoccupied hormone-binding sites. If these sites are already occupied by endogenous thyroid hormone, such as during hyperthyroidism, labeled T_3 will be picked up by the resin. T_3 uptake will also be elevated when thyroid-binding sites are decreased, as in low-protein states such as malnutrition, nephrotic syndrome, and liver cirrhosis. T_3 uptake is low during hypothyroidism or when thyroid-binding globulin sites are increased, such as during pregnancy, with use of oral contraceptives, and in infectious hepatitis.

Though nonspecific, serum creatinine phosphokinase, lactate dehydrogenase, and aspartate aminotransferase levels are slightly depressed in hyperthyroidism.

Tests of homeostatic control include measurement of serum TSH and thyrotropin-releasing hormone stimulating test. TSH levels will vary inversely with thyroid hormone levels. The thyrotropin-releasing hormone stimulation test assesses the hypothalamic–pituitary–thyroid axis.

Serum thyroid hormone tests in health and disease are listed in Table 34.1.

Braunwald E, Fauci AS, Hauser S, et al. eds. *Harrison's principles of internal medicine*, 16th ed. New York: McGraw-Hill, 2005:2108.

de los Santos E, Mazzaferri E. Thyrotoxicosis results and risks of current therapy. *Postgrad Med* 1990;87:277–294.

Smallridge RC. Metabolic and anatomic thyroid emergencies: a review. *Crit Care Med* 1992;20:276.

Surks M, Chopra I, Mariash C, et al. American Thyroid Association guidelines for use of laboratory tests in thyroid disorders. *JAMA* 1990;263:1529–1532.

B.5. Describe medical strategies for achieving an euthyroid state.

Medical strategy is directed at blocking the production of thyroid hormone, the release of thyroid hormone, and the adrenergic effects of excessive hormonal levels.

Initial therapy is directed at blocking thyroid hormone synthesis using antithyroid drugs such as methimazole and propylthiouracil. These drugs are iodinated within the thyroid gland, therefore diverting iodine away from new thyroid hormone synthesis. They do not block the release of thyroid hormone and are not effective until thyroid hormone stores are depleted. Propylthiouracil also inhibits peripheral conversion of T_4 to T_3. In addition to blocking thyroid hormone biosynthesis, these drugs lower concentrations of thyroid-stimulating hormone receptor antibodies and increase activity of suppressor T cells, suggesting they have an immunosuppressive effect. Side effects of antithyroid medications include fever, urticaria, arthralgias, arthritis, leukopenia, agranulocytosis, and rarely toxic hepatitis. Glucocorticoids inhibit peripheral conversion of T_4 to T_3, and they have an additive effect when given with propylthiouracil.

After initiation of antithyroid drug therapy, iodides, such as potassium iodide, are useful to inhibit thyroid hormone synthesis and to block the conversion of T_4 to T_3, thereby lowering thyroid hormone levels in the blood. Onset of action occurs within 24 hours. Iodine can also be given for 8 to 10 days preoperatively to decrease the vascularity of the thyroid gland. Iodine therapy requires 2 weeks for maximal effect. A euthyroid state should be achieved with antithyroid drugs before initiating iodine therapy, otherwise the exogenous iodine can be used as substrate for the synthesis of new thyroid hormone. Exogenous iodine administration destroys functioning thyroid cells and blocks the binding of intrinsic iodine. This Wolff–Chaikoff effect lasts only a few days. Thereafter, formation of thyroid hormone resumes despite the continued high intake of iodine. Iodides are mainly useful for thyroid crisis and for emergency surgery in hyperthyroid patients. Iodine is contraindicated, in children, pregnancy, and women who are breast-feeding; pregnancy is reportedly safe 4 months or more after treatment.

β-Antagonists are useful to block the peripheral adrenergic manifestations of hyperthyroidism. Patients become clinically euthyroid; however, without additional intervention, they will remain chemically hyperthyroid. Propranolol is the most commonly used β-adrenergic antagonist because it additionally inhibits peripheral conversion of T_4 to T_3. In thyrotoxic patients, larger doses of β-antagonists may be required because of the accelerated metabolism. Central-acting adrenergic antagonists such as reserpine or guanethidine can be used in patients who cannot take β-blockers as can calcium channel blockade with diltiazem. Finally, cholestyramine or colestipol will bind T_4 in the gut during enterohepatic circulation and may help to bring down the T_4 level more quickly.

Braunwald E, Fauci AS, Hauser S, et al. eds. *Harrison's principles of internal medicine*, 16th ed. New York: McGraw-Hill, 2005:2115–2117.

Falk S. The management of hyperthyroidism. *Otolaryngol Clin North Am* 1990;23:361–362.

Greenspan FS, Gardner DG. *Endocrine emergencies. Basic and clinical endocrinology*, 7th ed. Chapter 24. McGraw-Hill, 2004.

Kaplan MM, Meier DA, Dworkin HJ. Treatment of hyperthyroidism with radioactive iodine. *Endocrinol Metab Clin North Am* 1998;27(1):205–214.

de los Santos E, Mazzaferri E. Thyrotoxicosis results and risks of current therapy. *Postgrad Med* 1990;87:277–294.

Smallridge R. Metabolic and anatomic thyroid emergencies. *Crit Care Med* 1992;20:276–291.

Stoelting RK, Miller RD. *Anesthesia and co-existing disease*, 4th ed. New York: Churchill Livingstone, 2002:412–416.

B.6. What are the benefits of adrenergic blockade?

Catecholamines contribute to the symptoms of thyrotoxicosis. Pharmacologic agents that deplete stores or block the action of catecholamines will decrease heart rate, cardiac output, and cardiac irritability. Drugs used in the treatment of thyrotoxic symptoms include β-antagonists, combined α–β-antagonists, and central-acting agents such as reserpine and guanethidine. Side effects associated with use of these drugs include hypotension, sedation, depression, myocardial depression, bronchospasm, and diarrhea.

Ingbar S. Management of emergencies, thyrotoxic storm. *N Engl J Med* 1966;274:1252–1254.

Stoelting RK, Miller RD. *Anesthesia and co-existing disease*, 4th ed. New York: Churchill Livingstone, 2002:412–416.

B.7. When is the hyperthyroid patient ready for elective surgery?

Emphasis should be placed on relief of symptoms. The patient should demonstrate a return of normal heart rate, pulse pressure, and sinus rhythm, as well as a resolution of recent-onset cardiac murmurs. Tremors, anxiety, palpitations, dyspnea, and heat intolerance should be relieved.

B.8. How would you premedicate this patient?

The goal of premedication of the thyrotoxic patient is to relieve anxiety and prevent the activation of the sympathetic nervous system. Benzodiazepines such as oral diazepam (5 to 10 mg) or central adrenergic blockers such as clonidine (3 to 5 μg/kg orally) are appropriate. Antimuscarinics such as atropine and scopolamine are not recommended, because they cause tachycardia and interfere with normal heat regulation.

Smallridge R. Metabolic and anatomic thyroid emergencies. *Crit Care Med* 1992;20:276–291.

Stoelting RK, Miller RD. *Anesthesia and coexisting disease*, 4th ed. New York: Churchill Livingstone, 2002:412–416.

B.9. How would you prepare the thyrotoxic patient for emergent surgery?

When surgery is emergent, measures should be taken to prevent thyroid storm. Reduction of the hyperadrenergic state, along with decreased conversion of T_4 to T_3, can be attempted with propranolol. Esmolol, as an alternative, may offer some advantages because of its β_1 specificity and short half-life. However, esmolol has not been shown to decrease peripheral conversion. Antithyroid drugs should be given to prevent further thyroid hormone synthesis. Either propylthiouracil, 200 to 400 mg orally every 6 hours, or methimazole, 20 to 40 mg orally every 6 hours, should be administered as soon as possible. Methimazole in an aqueous solution, but not propylthiouracil, can be administered rectally. Propylthiouracil and glucocorticoids can also block peripheral conversion of T_4 to T_3, and together, they have an additive effect. Intravenous dexamethasone (2 mg every 6 hours) or hydrocortisone (40 mg every 6 hours) can be administered. Saturated solution of potassium iodide (five drops orally every 6 hours) or Lugol solution (30 drops orally every 6 to 8 hours) can be given to acutely inhibit release of T_4 and T_3. Parasympatholytics such as atropine and pancuronium should be avoided, because unopposed sympathetic activity may result.

Therapy should also be directed at correcting systemic decompensation. Fluids and electrolytes must be replaced. Invasive monitoring may be needed to guide the administration of inotropes and vasopressors when hypotension is unresponsive to fluids.

Fink NP, Abraham E, Vincent JL, et al. *Textbook of critical care*, 5th ed. Philadelphia: WB Saunders, 2005:1510–1511.

Gavin L. Thyroid crises. *Med Clin North Am* 1991;75:179–190.

Grenvik A, Ayres S, Shoemaker W, et al. eds. *Textbook of critical care*, 4th ed. Philadelphia: WB Saunders, 2000:790–793.

Pronovost P, Parris K. Perioperative management of thyroid disease. *Postgrad Med* 1995;98:83–96.

Stoelting RK, Miller RD. *Anesthesia and co-existing disease*, 4th ed. New York: Churchill Livingstone, 2002:412–416.

Tietgens S, Leinung M. Thyroid storm. *Med Clin North Am* 1995;79:169–178.

C. Intraoperative Management

C.1. How would you monitor this patient?

Once blood pressure, end-tidal carbon dioxide, pulse oximetry, electrocardiogram, and core temperature monitors are in place, the thyrotoxic patient is monitored to manage any cardiac decompensation and to recognize increased thyroid and adrenergic activity. If the patient presents to the operating room in thyroid storm, large-bore peripheral intravenous lines and an arterial line should be placed. If the patient is currently in or has a history of congestive heart failure, myocardial ischemia, renal failure, or hypotension, placement of a central venous or a pulmonary artery catheter is warranted. Invasive monitors should be placed before skin incision is made. Once surgery has begun, access for placement of monitors will be difficult.

C.2. How would you induce anesthesia?

Induction and intubation can proceed with standard techniques if airway obstruction is not suspected. Patients with orthopnea, dyspnea, stridor, wheezing, or hoarseness require further preoperative evaluation. Preoperative studies, as described in section B.3, need to be reviewed. At a minimum, the chest x-ray film must be evaluated by the anesthesiologist. Airway obstruction necessitates awake fiberoptic intubation or spontaneous inhalational induction. Inhalational induction using halothane or sevoflurane will maintain spontaneous respiration and airway patency. Isoflurane and desflurane may be too irritating to the airway for inhalational induction. Intubation should be attempted only after a deep plane of anesthesia is achieved. Patients with severe obstruction may require awake intubation, which will require anesthetizing the glossopharyngeal, superior laryngeal, and recurrent laryngeal nerves. Judicious use of small amounts of amnestic or anxiolytic agents may be necessary to prevent the precipitation of thyroid storm.

A rigid bronchoscope should be available in the event of airway collapse. Emergency tracheotomies are difficult to perform because of anatomic distortion and an increase in tissue vascularity. Small reinforced endotracheal tubes should be available.

C.3. Is endotracheal intubation necessary for this operation? Discuss the type and length of tube you would use.

Endotracheal intubation is necessary for thyroid surgery. If tracheal obstruction is suspected, a reinforced anode endotracheal tube should be used to prevent airway collapse. The length of the tube should be sufficient to extend beyond the thyroid gland.

C.4. How would you maintain anesthesia?

Maintenance of anesthesia should avoid sympathetic nervous system activation. Muscle relaxants are not necessary. Narcotics such as fentanyl or morphine should be given only in small amounts to ensure an alert patient who can maintain the airway after extubation. Treatment of hypotension with sympathomimetic drugs must take into account possible exaggerated responses. Because of the high level of circulating endogenous catecholamines, direct sympathomimetics (such as epinephrine or norepinephrine), or α-agonists (such as phenylephrine) are more appropriate than indirect sympathomimetics (such as ephedrine or metaraminol).

C.5. Intraoperatively, the patient became hyperthermic and tachycardic. Discuss the differential diagnosis of malignant hyperthermia and thyroid storm. How would you intervene?

Differential diagnosis includes hyperthyroid storm, malignant hyperthermia, pheochromocytoma, and carcinoid crisis. Many of the clinical manifestations of malignant hyperthermia and thyroid storm are compensatory mechanisms for hyperthermia. However, malignant hyperthermia will result in metabolic acidosis, profound hypercarbia, and muscle rigidity, which are not present during thyroid storm. Hyperthyroidism decreases the level of creatinine phosphokinase to about half the normal level, whereas creatinine phosphokinase levels are increased during malignant hyperthermia. Both disorders progress rapidly and intervention is urgent.

Once thyroid storm is suspected, treatment must start immediately. Goals of intervention include the following:

- *Diagnosis and treatment of inciting event.* Without treatment of the underlying cause, therapy will be less effective.
- *Supportive measures.* Replace fluids, glucose, and electrolytes. Reduce temperature with acetaminophen, cold lavage of body cavities, cooling blankets, ice packs, and reduction of ambient temperature. Aspirin should not be used as an antipyretic. It displaces thyroid hormones from binding proteins, thereby raising free hormone levels. Inotropes, diuretics, and supplemental oxygen may be needed for acute congestive heart failure.
- *Reduce secretion and production of thyroid hormones.* Antithyroid drugs prevent iodide binding in the thyroid within the hour. One hour after the administration of methimazole or propylthiouracil, iodide can be started.
- *Block the metabolic effects of thyroid hormones.* Metabolic manifestations can be treated with β-adrenergic blockers such as propranolol or catecholamine-depleting agents such as reserpine or guanethidine.

Peters K, Nance P, Wingard D. Malignant hyperthyroidism or malignant hyperthermia. *Anesth Analg* 1981;60:613–615.

Stoelting RK, Miller RD. *Anesthesia and co-existing disease,* 4th ed. New York: Churchill Livingstone, 2002:412–416.

C.6. How would you extubate this patient?

If tracheomalacia is suspected, direct visualization of airway patency is suggested. The fiberoptic bronchoscope can be used to assess for airway collapse and vocal cord movement as the endotracheal tube and bronchoscope together are slowly pulled back. If tracheal collapse is noted, the endotracheal tube and bronchoscope should be immediately readvanced. Vocal cord assessment must be done. If any question exists of the patient's ability to protect his airway, leave the endotracheal tube in place. A tracheostomy set, endotracheal tubes, and laryngoscope should be readily available at bedside.

D. Postoperative Management

D.1. The patient became stridulous and dyspneic in the recovery room. What was your differential diagnosis and strategy of intervention?

Causes of respiratory failure include hemorrhage, respiratory obstruction, recurrent laryngeal nerve palsies, tracheomalacia, pneumothorax, and hypocalcemia.

Signs of airway obstruction require emergent evaluation. Hematomas can cause compressive airway obstruction and restrict venous and lymphatic drainage of tracheal mucosa. Hematoma evacuation requires opening and drainage of incision sites. However, tracheal obstruction from mucosal edema may still persist. Patients should be intubated early before airway edema from compromised lymphatic and venous return occurs. Initially, patients should be seated upright at 45 degrees to facilitate venous drainage. Steroids and racemic epinephrine through nebulization should be used to decrease laryngeal edema. If dyspnea worsens, the patient should be intubated.

Injury to bilateral recurrent laryngeal nerves results in respiratory obstruction. Patients demonstrate paramedian position of both of the true vocal cords. These patients require emergent airway intervention including intubation or tracheotomy. Patients with unilateral recurrent laryngeal nerve paralysis present with hoarseness and minimal signs of airway obstruction.

If dissection is carried down to the mediastinum, pneumothorax must be ruled out as a cause of postoperative respiratory deterioration.

Hypocalcemia secondary to inadvertent excision of parathyroid tissue manifests within the first 3 days postoperatively. Acute airway obstruction in the immediate postoperative period is uncommon. The patient will complain of circumoral numbness and tingling of the hands and feet. If calcium is not supplemented, the patient can develop stridor and airway obstruction secondary to muscle weakness. Severe hypocalcemia can also be associated with seizures and tetany.

Netterville J, Aly A, Ossoff R. Evaluation and treatment of complications of thyroid and parathyroid surgery. *Otolaryngol Clin North Am* 1990;23:529–550.

Stoelting RK, Miller RD. *Anesthesia and co-existing disease*, 4th ed. New York: Churchill Livingstone, 2002:412–416.

D.2. When does thyroid storm most often present?

Thyroid storm most often occurs 6 to 18 hours postoperatively, rather than intraoperatively. Treatment with the same regimen as outlined for emergency surgery is indicated (see section B.9). Supportive measures with fluids, oxygen, and a cooling blanket are important. Aspirin should not be used as an antipyretic, because it displaces thyroid hormones from binding proteins and thereby raises free hormone levels.

Stoelting RK, Miller RD. *Anesthesia and co-existing disease*, 4th ed. New York: Churchill Livingstone, 2002:412–416.

CHAPTER 35

Pheochromocytomas

GREGORY E. KERR • MANUEL L. FONTES

THE PATIENT IS A 49-YEAR-OLD WOMAN

with a history of recurrent headaches, diaphoresis, and severe hypertension. During a physical examination, she was found to have an exceptionally high blood pressure (BP) of 220/140 mm Hg with a heart rate (HR) of 108 beats per minute. The patient denied any other medical problems except occasional anxiety. Further studies were obtained to evaluate the etiology of her high BP and headaches.

A. Medical Disease and Differential Diagnosis

1. What are some common problems that should be included in a differential diagnosis for hypertension?
2. What is a pheochromocytoma?
3. Trace the embryology of the adrenal gland and describe its normal anatomy.
4. What substances do the adrenal medulla excrete?
5. What are the mechanisms of action of epinephrine and norepinephrine?
6. What is the pathway for synthesis and breakdown of catecholamines?
7. What does the adrenal cortex secrete?
8. What are the metabolic actions of the glucocorticoids and the mineralocorticoids?
9. What are some clinical features associated with a pheochromocytoma?
10. In whom do we find pheochromocytoma?
11. What is the incidence of pheochromocytoma?
12. What is a reasonable diagnostic pathway in evaluating a patient with a pheochromocytoma?

B. Preoperative Evaluation and Preparation

1. How can you diagnose and localize the tumor preoperatively?
2. How do you pharmacologically prepare the patient with a pheochromocytoma for surgery?
3. What other aspects of preoperative management are important?

C. Intraoperative Management

1. What drugs should be avoided during the operation?
2. How would you monitor this patient?
3. Describe acceptable options for administering anesthesia to this patient.
4. What are some methods of controlling the effects of catecholamine stimulation during surgery?

767

5. What are some management issues after the tissue is removed?
6. If a pheochromocytoma is found complicating pregnancy, does magnesium sulfate (MnSo₄) have a role in managing the hypertension?
7. What are some of the issues one must be aware of with a laparoscopic adrenalectomy?

D. Postoperative Management

1. What is the significance of postoperative hypotension? How is it treated?
2. What other problems can arise in the postoperative period?

A. Medical Disease and Differential Diagnosis

A.1. What are some common problems that should be included in a differential diagnosis for hypertension?

There are many reasons why blood pressure (BP) would become elevated during surgery. The following is a partial list of reasons:

- *Essential hypertension.* Unknown etiology
- *Primary renal disease.* Nephritis, renal artery stenosis, and renal infarction
- *Endocrine.* Adrenocortical hyperfunction, thyroid disease, pheochromocytoma, and acromegaly
- *Hemodynamic alterations.* Decreased peripheral vascular resistance and increased intravascular volume
- *Sympathetic stimulation.* Light anesthesia, hypoxia, and hypercarbia
- *Neurogenic.* Seizure activity, elevated intracranial pressure, and denervation of the carotid sinus
- *Miscellaneous.* Malignant hyperthermia, neuroleptic malignant syndrome, carcinoid syndrome, and toxemia of pregnancy

---

Hickler R, Vandam LD. Hypertension. *Anesthesiology* 1970;33:219.

Kasper DL, Braunwald E, Fauci AS, et al. eds. *Harrison's principles of internal medicine*, 16th ed. New York: McGraw-Hill, 2005:1463.

A.2. What is a pheochromocytoma?

Pheochromocytomas are catecholamine-secreting tumors of chromaffin tissue. They are usually located in the adrenal medullae or sympathetic paraganglia, but may be found anywhere chromaffin tissue exists. These locations extend from the base of the skull to the anus. Although most pheochromocytomas are found in the medulla portion of the adrenal gland, 10% of these tumors are located elsewhere.

Pheochromocytomas are entities that only account for 0.1% of all cases of hypertension. They occur in only 0.005% to 0.1% of people. When unsuspected or improperly managed during surgery, the physiologic effects of the released catecholamines can be profound.

The word pheochromocytoma is derived from the Greek words for dusky, *phaios*, and color, *chroma*. In 1912, Pick noted that these tumors stained a deep rust color when treated with chromium salts.

Artusio J. Anesthesiology for pheochromocytoma. In: Malhotra V, ed. *Anesthesia for renal and genito-urologic surgery*, 1st ed. New York: McGraw-Hill, 1996:80.

Hull CJ. Pheochromocytoma. *Br J Anaesth* 1986;58:1453–1468.

Manger WM. An overview of pheochromocytoma: history, current concepts, vagaries, and diagnostic challenges. *Ann N Y Acad Sci* 2006;1073:1–20.

Pullerits J, Ein S, Balfe JW. Anesthesia for pheochromocytoma. *Can J Anaesth* 1988;35(5): 526–534.

Townsend CM, ed. *Sabiston textbook of surgery*, 17th ed. Philadelphia: WB Saunders, 2004: 1052–1057.

A.3. Trace the embryology of the adrenal gland and describe its normal anatomy.

The adrenal cortex and medulla have separate embryologic origins. The medullary portion is derived from the chromaffin ectodermal cells of the neural crest. These cells are split off very early from the sympathetic ganglion cells and migrate further ventrally, so as to lie ventrolateral to the aorta, where they form the paraganglia. Several such nodules near the cranial end of the gonads combine into a larger mass of cells lying between the dorsal aorta and the dorsomedial border of the mesonephros. Here they come into approximation with a group of mesodermal cells destined to become the adrenal cortex. These latter cells are derived principally from a narrow strip of coelomic mesothelium lying between the dorsal mesentery and the genital ridge. These cells, arising in numerous places in the suprarenal ridge, lose their connection with the mesothelium and form a complete layer of mesoderm around the ectodermal cells derived from the sympathetic ganglia. The chromaffin cells become enclosed within the cortex to form the medulla. The organs of Zuckerkandl are paraganglia around the aorta at the level of the kidney anterior to the inferior aorta. Accessory areas for the occurrence of pheochromocytoma are in the mediastinum, in the bladder, occasionally in the neck, in the sacrococcygeal region, or in the anal or vaginal areas.

Schwartz SI, Shires GT, Daly JM, et al. eds. *Principles of surgery*, 7th ed. New York: McGraw-Hill, 1998:1561.

Townsend CM, ed. *Sabiston textbook of surgery*, 17th ed. Philadelphia: WB Saunders, 2004:1052–1057.

A.4. What substances do the adrenal medulla excrete?

The adrenal medulla primarily secretes three substances, all of which are catecholamines. The catecholamines are epinephrine, norepinephrine, and dopamine. These three compounds are found in the chromaffin cells of the sympathetic nervous system, which includes the adrenal medulla, aberrant tissue along the sympathetic chain, and paraganglia. Both norepinephrine and dopamine are found at the endings of the postganglionic fibers of the sympathetic nervous system and in the central nervous system (CNS).

Brunicardi FC, Andersen DK, Billiar TR, et al. eds. *Schwartz's principles of surgery*, 8th ed. New York: McGraw-Hill, 2005:140–1462.

Townsend CM, ed. *Sabiston textbook of surgery*, 17th ed. Philadelphia: WB Saunders, 2004; 1052–1057.

A.5. What are the mechanisms of action of epinephrine and norepinephrine?

These catecholamines exert their effects by acting on β-adrenergic and α-adrenergic receptors. It is believed that the results of β-receptor stimulation are largely mediated by the stimulation of adenylate (adenylyl) cyclase, which results in the production and activation of cyclic

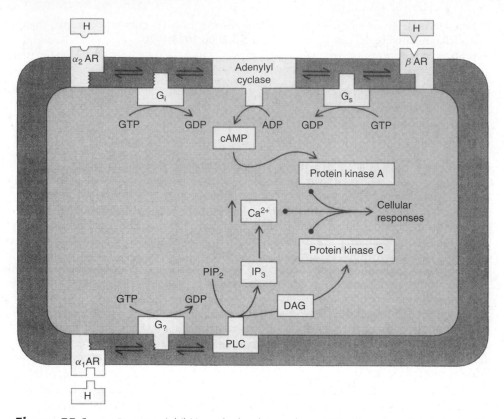

Figure 35.1 α_2 Receptor inhibition of adenylate cyclase. ADP, adenosine diphosphate; AR, adrenergic receptor; cAMP, cyclic adenosine monophosphate; Ca^{2+}, calcium; DAG, diacylglycerol; G_i, regulatory protein that, along with GTP, inhibits adenylate cyclase; G_s, regulatory protein that interacts with liganded β-adrenergic receptor to stimulate adenylate cyclase; GDP, guanosine diphosphate; GTP, guanosine triphosphate; H, neurotransmitter or hormone; IP_3, inositol triphosphate; PIP_2, phosphatidyl inositol biphosphate. (Reprinted with permission from Goodman AG, Rall TW, Nies AS, et al. eds. *The pharmacologic basis of therapeutics*, 8th ed. New York: MacMillan, 1993:109.)

adenosine monophosphate (cAMP). The stimulation of cAMP eventually leads to an increased inward calcium (Ca^{2+}) flux, thereby increasing cytoplasmic Ca^{2+} concentrations. The increased availability of Ca^{2+} ultimately results in enhanced actin and myosin interactions. The stimulation of α_1 receptors creates an increased inward flux of Ca^{2+} and also affects the formation of inositol triphosphate. The stimulation of α_2 receptors inhibits the action of adenylate cyclase (Fig. 35.1).

The pharmacologic response is dependent on the location of the receptors throughout the body. The distribution and density of the receptors will determine the predominant response to each catecholamine.

Hardman JG, Limbird LE, eds. *Goodman and Gillman's the pharmacologic basis of therapeutics*, 11th ed. New York: MacMillan, 2006:237–242.

Stoelting RK, ed. *Pharmacology and physiology in anesthetic practice*, 4th ed. Philadelphia: Lippincott Williams & Wilkins, 2005.

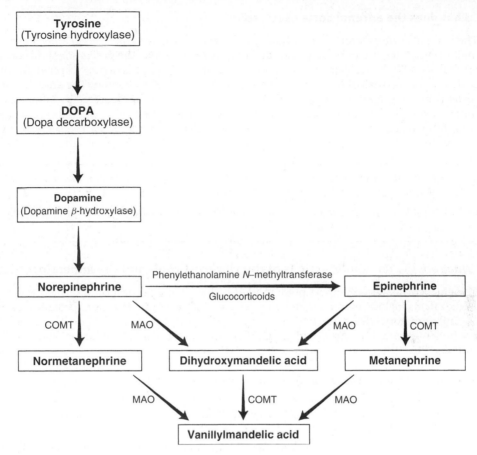

Figure 35.2 Synthesis and metabolism of endogenous catecholamine. COMT, catechol-*O*-methyltransferase; MAO, monoamine oxidase. (Reprinted with permission from Pullerits J, Ein S, Balfe JW. Anesthesia for phaeochromocytoma. *Can J Anesth* 1988;35(5): 526–534.)

A.6. What is the pathway for synthesis and breakdown of catecholamines?

The synthesis of endogenous catecholamines begins with the active transport of the amino acid tyrosine from the circulation into postganglionic sympathetic nerve endings. The hydroxylation of tyrosine is generally regarded as the rate-limiting step of the pathway (Fig. 35.2). Any drug containing the 3,4-dihydroxybenzene (catecholamine) structure is rapidly inactivated by catechol-*O*-methyltransferase (COMT) or monoamine oxidase (MAO). The most important aspect of the termination of the biologic activity of these catecholamines is reuptake into the nerve endings.

Oeltmann T, Carson R, Shannon JR, et al. Assessment of O-methylated catecholamine levels in plasma and urine for diagnosis of autonomic disorders. *Autonom Neurosci Basic Clin* 2004;116(1–2):1–10.

Schulz C, Eisenhofer G, Lehnert H. Principles of catecholamine biosynthesis, metabolism and release. *Front Horm Res* 2004;31:1–25.

A.7. What does the adrenal cortex secrete?

The adrenal cortex secretes more than 30 different corticosteroids. These can be divided into two major classes, the mineralocorticoids and the glucocorticoids. The precursor of all corticosteroids is cholesterol. Aldosterone is the most important mineralocorticoid secreted by the adrenal cortex, whereas cortisol is the most important glucocorticoid secreted. The adrenal cortex is also responsible for secreting sex steroids. Each of these substances is secreted by different zones—the mineralocorticoids are secreted by the zona glomerulosa, the glucocorticoids are secreted by the zona fasciculata, and the sex steroids (the androgens and estrogens) are secreted by the zona reticularis.

Hardman JG, Limbird LE, eds. *Goodman and Gillman's the pharmacologic basis of therapeutics*, 11th ed. New York: MacMillan, 2000; 1587,1593–1610.

Stoelting RK, ed. *Pharmacology and physiology in anesthetic practice*, 4th ed. Philadelphia: Lippincott Williams & Wilkins, 2005.

A.8. What are the metabolic actions of the glucocorticoids and the mineralocorticoids?

The glucocorticoids have their predominant mechanism of action on intermediary metabolism. These effects include increased gluconeogenesis, fatty acid mobilization, protein catabolism, and antiinflammatory effects. Cortisol may improve cardiac function by improving responsiveness of β-adrenergic receptors. Approximately 95% of the glucocorticoid activity is from the secretion of cortisol. The mineralocorticoids have their predominant action on the body minerals, sodium, and potassium. By conserving sodium ions they sustain extracellular fluid volume. They also help maintain normal potassium plasma concentrations.

Barnes PJ. Molecular mechanisms and cellular effects of glucocorticosteroids. *Immunol Allergy Clin North Am* 2005;25(3):451–468.

Czock D, Keller F, Rasche FM, et al. Pharmacokinetics and pharmacodynamics of systemically administered glucocorticoids. *Clin Pharmacokinet* 2005;44(1):61–98.

Hardman JG, Limbird LE, eds. *Goodman and Gillman's the pharmacologic basis of therapeutics*, 11th ed. New York: MacMillan, 2006:1593–1596.

A.9. What are some clinical features associated with a pheochromocytoma?

The classic triad is severe headache, diaphoresis, and palpitations. One or more of the following often signal the presence of a pheochromocytoma: sudden severe headaches, perspiration, weight loss, paroxysmal hypertension, pallor, palpitations, diabetes-like syndrome with elevated fasting blood sugar, nausea, vomiting, fever, encephalopathy, anxiety, myocardial infarction, stroke, or acute renal failure. Although hypertension can be paroxysmal, 65% of adults demonstrate sustained hypertension. The aforementioned symptoms are usually paroxysmal in nature. These "attacks" may last from a few moments to hours.

A pressor response to particular drugs suggests the presence of this tumor. These drugs include histamine, glucagon, droperidol, tyramine, metoclopramide, cytotoxic drugs, saralasin, tricyclic antidepressant, and phenothiazines.

Artusio J. Anesthesiology for pheochromocytoma. In: Malhotra V, ed. *Anesthesia for renal and genito-urologic surgery*, 1st ed. New York: McGraw-Hill, 1996:80.

Table 35.1   Multiple Endocrine Adenomatosis.

Type IIa (Sipple's syndrome)	Parathyroid adenoma/hyperplasia Medullary carcinoma of thyroid Pheochromocytoma
Type IIb	Medullary carcinoma of the thyroid Mucosal adenomas Marfanoid appearance Pheochromocytoma
von Hippel-Landau syndrome	Haemangioblastoma of the retina, cerebellum, or other parts of the CNS, pheochromocytoma
Neurofibroma	Neurofibromas, café'-au- lait spots, axillary or inguinal freckling, optic nerve glioma

Manger WM. An overview of pheochromocytoma: history, current concepts, vagaries, and diagnostic challenges. *Ann N Y Acad Sci* 2006;1073:1–20.

Townsend CM, ed. *Sabiston textbook of surgery*, 17th ed. Philadelphia: WB Saunders, 2004:1052–1057.

A.10. In whom do we find it?

Pheochromocytomas occur in both sexes with peak incidence in the third to fifth decades of life. Approximately 5% of cases of pheochromocytomas are inherited as an autosomal dominant trait either alone or as part of the neoplastic syndrome, multiple endocrine adenomatosis (MEA) (Table 35.1).

Artusio JF Jr. Anesthesia for Pheochromocytoma. In: Malhotra V, ed. *Anesthesia for renal and genito-urologic surgery* New York: McGraw-Hill, 1996:80.

Nguyen-Martin M, Hammer G. *Hospital physician*. February, 2006:17–24.

Pullcrits J, Ein S, Balfe JW. Anesthesia for pheochromocytoma. *Can J Anaesth* 1988;35(5): 526–534.

Widimsky J Jr. Recent advances in the diagnosis and treatment of pheochromocytoma. *Kidney Blood Press Res* 2006;29(5):321–326.

Young WF Jr. Clinical practice. The incidentally discovered adrenal mass. *N Engl J Med* 2007;356(6):601–610.

A.11. What is the incidence of pheochromocytoma?

It is estimated that one to eight cases of pheochromocytoma occur per million persons annually. It seems that the incidence increases with advancing age. It also appears that there is a genetic predisposition with 10% to 20% of diagnosed patients with the disease having had a family history.

Manger WM. An overview of pheochromocytoma: history, current concepts, vagaries, and diagnostic challenges. *Ann N Y Acad Sci* 2006;1073:1–20.

Nguyen-Martin M, Hammer G. *Hospital physician*. February, 2006:17–24.

B. Preoperative Evaluation and Preparation

B.1. How can you diagnose and localize the tumor preoperatively?

The laboratory tests for pheochromocytoma are shown in Table 35.2. The biochemical diagnosis is based on the fact that pheochromocytomas release an excessive amount of catecholamines and metabolites. Urinary specimens that can be measured include urinary norepinephrine, epinephrine, dopamine, total metanephrines and vanillylmandelic acid (VMA) which are collected during a 24-hour period. The total metanephrines have given the highest true-positive results, approximately 98% to 99%.

In theory, the hydroxy-methoxy-mandelic acid (often misnamed VMA) level should be the most reliable laboratory test because it is the final common product of both catecholamine metabolic pathways. In practice, however, the intermediate metanephrines have proved to be better discriminators of pheochromocytomas. VMA is often used as an initial "case-finding" test because it has "acceptable" specificity and sensitivity and is relatively inexpensive.

Historically, 24-hour urine tests were generally considered superior to plasma tests in the diagnosis of pheochromocytomas because the tumor secretes catecholamines only intermittently and the catecholamines have a short half-life. These combined factors could result in relatively normal plasma catecholamine levels in the presence of an active tumor. Some authors have demonstrated that plasma-free metanephrines constitute the best test for excluding or confirming the presence of pheochromocytomas and should be the test of first choice for diagnosis of the tumor. Chromaginin A, a monomeric acidic protein found in the adrenal medulla, is secreted along with the catecholamines. It has been reported to have a sensitivity of 83% and a specificity of 96%. Measuring its plasma level may be useful along with the plasma levels of the catecholamines in making a diagnosis. High-pressure liquid chromatographic and radioenzyme methods for measuring levels in the plasma have also been known to improve diagnostic accuracy.

The clonidine-suppression test (which is still occasionally used) may be helpful in distinguishing the patient with a pheochromocytoma whose hypersecretion of norepinephrine does not respond to the drug from the patient without the tumor whose high basal plasma concentration is decreased to normal by the drug.

Computed tomography (CT) with or without iodine 131 (^{131}I) labeled metaiobenzyl-guanadine (MIGB) is extremely accurate in diagnosing and localizing the tumor. Use of arteriography, once popular, should be performed cautiously because dye can stimulate catecholamine release. CT scanning and magnetic resonance imaging (MRI) scanning are excellent imaging techniques that visualize normal adrenal glands when the diagnosis is equivocal. CT scanning has a sensitivity of 98%, whereas MRI is greater than 99%. For extraadrenal locations and in pregnant patients, MRI scanning may be a more desirable choice. MIBG has also been useful in localizing extraadrenal tumors as well as recurrent pheochromocytomas. MIBG has a specificity of greater than 95%, but a sensitivity of only 77%.

Artusio JF Jr. Anesthesiology for pheochromocytoma. In: Malhotra V, ed. *Anesthesia for renal and genito-urologic surgery*. New York: McGraw-Hill, 1996:84.

Brunicardi FC, Andersen DK, Billiar TR, et al. eds. *Schwartz's principles of surgery*, 8th ed. New York: McGraw-Hill, 2005:140–1462.

Hull CJ. Phaeochromocytoma. *Br J Anaesth* 1986;58:1453–1468.

Lenders J, Pacak K, Walther MM, et al. Biochemical diagnosis of pheochromocytomas. *JAMA* 2002;287(11):1427–1434.

Nguyen-Martin M, Hammer G. *Hospital physician*, February, 2006:17–24.

Widimsky J Jr. Recent advances in the diagnosis and treatment of pheochromocytoma. *Kidney Blood Press Res* 2006;29(5):321–326.

Witteles BA, Kaplan EL, Roizen MF. Sensitivity of diagnosis and localization tests for pheochromocytoma in clinical practice. *Arch Intern Med* 2000;160:2521–2524.

B.2.   How do you pharmacologically prepare the patient with a pheochromocytoma for surgery?

The major goal is to partially block the responses to catecholamines and to avoid the pressor effects of the catecholamines. Although surgery remains the only definitive therapy, the above goals must be obtained as soon as the diagnosis is made by using pharmacologic methods.

Administration of α-adrenergic blockers has been the cornerstone of management. The most commonly used agents have been phenoxybenzamine (POB) (Dibenzyline 10 to 20 mg, three to four times per day orally), prazosin (2 to 5 mg two times per day orally) and phentolamine as a constant infusion. Phenoxybenzamine has been most widely used because of its relatively long duration of action and ease of administration. It irreversibly alkylates α_1-adrenergic receptors on vascular smooth muscle, thereby making them nonfunctional. It may cause postural hypotension and reflex tachycardia. These may be avoided with the careful administration of fluid volume as well as β-blockers. Be sure not to start β-blockade until the α-blockers have been started, otherwise congestive heart failure may be precipitated. Many feel that β-blockers should only be used when tachycardia or arrhythmias exist.

Prazosin has been used but does not seem to adequately prevent perioperative hypertensive episodes. Prazosin as well as magnesium sulfate ($MnSo_4$), β-blockers, angiotensin-converting enzyme (ACE) inhibitors and calcium channel blockers have been used in combination with POB to attain hemodynamic stability.

α-Methyl-paratyrosine inhibits tyrosine hydroxylase. It may be given orally, gradually increasing the dose from 0.5 g per day to 4 g per day. This may decrease the catecholamine

Table 35.2   Laboratory Tests for Pheochromocytoma.

DIAGNOSTIC TEST	NORMAL VALUES	PHEOCHROMOCYTOMA
Blood		
Plasma catecholamines	<1,000 pg/mL	>2,000 pg/mL
Urine (24-hr collection)		
Catecholamines	<125 μg	>1,200 μg
Norepinephrine	<100 μg	Increased
Epinephrine	<1 μg	Increased
Metanephrines	<1.6 mg	>2.5 mg
Vanillylmandelic acid	<8 mg	>10 mg
Confirmation if test results are equivocal		
Clonidine suppression of norepinephrine secretion	Suppressed in essential hypertensive patients	Not suppressed
Localization of tumor		
Magnetic resonance imaging		
Computed tomography		
Scintigraphy with metaiodobenzyl guanidine (MIBG)		
Selective adrenal venous catheterization and sampling		

From Artusio J. Anesthesiology for pheochromocytoma. In: Malhotra V, ed. *Anesthesia for renal and genito-urologic surgery.* New York: McGraw-Hill, 1996:84, with permission.

synthesis by 40% to 80%. It is very effective, but may cause diarrhea, sedative fatigue, anxiety, or agitated depression or tumors.

A study from the Cleveland Clinics suggests that preoperative use of α-blocking agents may not necessarily decrease the incidence of intraoperative hypertension or tachycardia. In fact, patients who did not receive preoperative POB had a few advantages. Eighty percent of these patients did not require vasopressors in the postanesthesia care unit (PACU), although the rest did so for a very short period of time. Similarly, 79% of patients received no vasodilators in the PACU. There was no difference in intensive care unit (ICU) length of stay between those patients who received preoperative POB/prazosin versus those who did not.

It is possible that advances in anesthetic and monitoring techniques as well as the availability of fast-acting drugs capable of correcting sudden changes in hemodynamics has eliminated the need to use preoperative POB or prazosin in the preoperative period for those patients who are about to undergo surgery for a pheochromocytoma resection.

Artusio JF Jr. Anesthesiology for pheochromocytoma. In: Malhotra V, ed. *Anesthesia for renal and genito-urologic surgery*. New York: McGraw-Hill, 1996:80.

Boutros AR, Bravo EL, Zanettin G, et al. Perioperative management of 63 patients with pheochromocytoma. *Cleve Clin J Med* 1990;57(7):613–617.

Connery LE, Coursin DB. Assessment and therapy of selected endocrine disorders. *Anesthesiol Clin North America* 2004;22(1):93–123.

Prys-Roberts C, Farndon JR. Efficacy and safety of doxazosin for perioperative management of patients with pheochromocytoma. *World J Surg* 2002;26(8):1037–1042.

B.3. What other aspects of preoperative management are important?

The circulating blood volume is decreased in many patients with pheochromocytomas. Therefore, many clinicians support the idea of administering volume (frequently blood) before surgery while patients receive α-blockade. One must be very careful with patients who have decreased myocardial function to avoid congestive heart failure. Many other clinicians feel volume loading is not necessary. They feel that if the patient has been on α-blockers for 2 weeks or more, then the volume has been restored.

Sedation for the preoperative period is considered by many clinicians to be important before surgery. Sedation may obviate the need to use high doses of antihypertensive agents before surgery.

Artusio JF Jr. Anesthesiology for pheochromocytoma. In: Malhotra V, ed. *Anesthesia for renal and genito-urologic surgery*. New York: McGraw-Hill, 1996:80.

Connery LE, Coursin DB. Assessment and therapy of selected endocrine disorders. *Anesthesiol Clin North America* 2004;22(1):93–123.

Prys-Roberts C, Farndon JR. Efficacy and safety of doxazosin for perioperative management of patients with pheochromocytoma. *World J Surg* 2002;26(8):1037–1042.

C. Intraoperative Management

C.1. What drugs should be avoided during the operation?

As there are many agents to choose from, but many whose use is controversial, the controversial agents should be avoided (Table 35.3). This appears to be secondary to the inhibition of

Table 35.3 Suggested Drugs to Avoid in Patients with Pheochromocytoma.

Droperidol
Morphine
Atracurium
Pancuronium
Ketamine
Ephedrine
Halothane
Cocaine
Metoclopramide
curare

catecholamine reuptake. Atropine exacerbates the chronic effects of epinephrine by vagal inhibition. All drugs that release histamine (i.e., morphine, curare, atracurium) might be avoided because histamine has been known to provoke pheochromocytomas. Agents that cause an indirect increase in catecholamine levels (i.e., pancuronium, ketamine, ephedrine) should be avoided. It should be noted that morphine, curare, atracurium, and pancuronium have all been used with clinical reports documenting their safe use.

Artusio JF Jr. Anesthesiology for pheochromocytoma. In: Malhotra V, ed. *Anesthesia for renal and genito-urologic surgery*. New York: McGraw-Hill, 1996:84.

Connery LE, Coursin DB. Assessment and therapy of selected endocrine disorders. *Anesthesiol Clin North America* 2004;22(1):93–123.

Kinney MA, Narr BJ, Warner MA. Perioperative management of pheochromocytoma. *J Cardiothorac Vasc Anesth* 2002;16(3):359–369.

Myklejord DJ. Undiagnosed pheochromocytoma: the anesthesiologist nightmare. *Clin Med Res* 2004;2(1):59–62.

C.2. How would you monitor this patient?

Monitoring in these patients should include an electrocardiogram (ECG) with a V_5 lead, core temperature, pulse oximetry, intraarterial blood pressure (BP) monitoring along with central venous pressure monitoring and a urinary catheter. For patients with known or suspected myocardial dysfunction, a pulmonary artery catheter should be considered. One may also want to consider noninvasive techniques for assessing cardiac function.

Kinney MA, Narr BJ, Warner MA. Perioperative management of pheochromocytoma. *J Cardiothorac Vasc Anesth* 2002;16(3):359–369.

C.3. Describe acceptable options for administering anesthesia to this patient.

Either general anesthesia, regional anesthesia, or a combination of the two are considered acceptable. For all techniques, it is important to avoid wide swings in blood pressure (BP).

For general anesthesia, induction with thiopental has been most commonly used, but induction with propofol has recently been reported to be a safe technique. One can lessen the response to intubation by administering 1.5 μg per kg lidocaine intravenously 2 minutes before laryngoscopy. Other measures to attenuate hemodynamic responses to intubation are described in Chapter 12,

Table 35.4   Drugs to Manage High Blood Pressure.

DRUG	ROUTE	DOSE
Diltiazem	IV	Load with 5- to 10-mg boluses and infuse at 0.25–0.5 μ/kg/min
Esmolol	IV	5- to 10-mg boluses or infusion
Hydralazine	IV	5- to 10-mg boluses every 30 min
Labetalol	IV	10-mg boluses to total 150 mg
Magnesium sulfate	IV	2-g boluses; be cautious in patients with renal failure and neuromuscular blockade
Nitroprusside	IV	Infuse initially with 0.5–1.5 μg/kg/min to maximum of 8 μg/kg/min over 1–3 hr
Nicardipine	IV	Infuse initially at 5 mg/hr; may alter rate by 2.5 mg/hr every 15 min; to maximum of 15 mg/hr
Phentolamine	IV	1–5 mg every 5 min or infuse initially with 1 mg/min
Propanolol	IV	1-mg boluses to total 10 mg

sections C.5. and C.6. General anesthesia has been maintained with most of the inhalation agents, but most commonly with isoflurane. Clinicians also seem o to like the concomitant use of narcotics with the inhalation agent. Some authors advocate the avoidance of halothane because of its ability to increase the incidence of arrhythmias. Recently, the safety of desflurane was demonstrated. It was effective at controlling hypertensive surges in well-prepared patients, although it is known to cause sympathetic stimulation.

Kinney MA, Narr BJ, Warner MA. Perioperative management of pheochromocytoma. *J Cardiothorac Vasc Anesth* 2002;16(3):359–369.

Whalley DG, Berrigan MJ. Anesthesia for radical prostatectomy, cystectomy, nephrectomy, pheochromocytoma, and laparoscopic procedures. *Anesthesiol Clin North America* 2000;18(4):899–917.

C.4. What are some methods of controlling the effects of catecholamine stimulation during surgery?

Drugs used to control intraoperative hypertension are listed in Table 35.4.

Phentolamine, a short acting α-blocking agent, can be given as a continuous infusion to control blood pressure (BP). Phentolamine along with isoflurane may maintain an appropriate BP. Sodium nitroprusside (solution 0.01%) has become the most commonly used agent for control of high BP during pheochromocytoma surgery. Many clinicians are becoming more comfortable with nicardipine as a way to control elevated BP.

Magnesium sulfate ($MgSO_4$) is another agent that is commonly used as an adjunct vasodilator. β-blockers are helpful during the preoperative period to control BP as well as heart rate (HR) and possible arrhythmias. Lidocaine should also be considered for the control of arrhythmias.

Diamond JA. Pheochromocytoma in a symptomatic patient with severe hypertension upon anesthesia induction. *Am J Hypertens* 2001;14(7 Pt 1):729–730.

Kinney MA, Narr BJ, Warner MA. Perioperative management of pheochromocytoma. *J Cardiothorac Vasc Anesth* 2002;16(3):359–369.

Minami T, Adachi T, Fukuda K. An effective use of magnesium sulfate for intraoperative management of laparoscopic adrenalectomy for pheochromocytoma in a pediatric patient. *Anesth Analg* 2002;95(5):1243–1244.

Poopalalingam R, Chin EY. Rapid preparation of a patient with pheochromocytoma with labetolol and magnesium sulfate. *Can J Anaesth* 2001;48(9):876–880.

C.5. What are some management issues after the tissue is removed?

It is important to be aware of the fact that blood pressure (BP) may fall very quickly after the blood supply of the tumor is interrupted. BP may be maintained by administering norepinephrine as well as by administering fluids. Blood should be administered if the blood loss is substantial.

Kinney MA, Narr BJ, Warner MA. Perioperative management of pheochromocytoma. *J Cardiothorac Vasc Anesth* 2002;16(3):359–369.

Pullerits J, Ein S, Balfe JW. Anesthesia for phaeochromocytoma. *Can J Anaesth* 1988;35(5): 526–534.

C.6. If a pheochromocytoma is found complicating pregnancy, does magnesium sulfate (MgSO₄) have a role in managing the hypertension?

Reports indicate that $MgSO_4$ can be used in conjunction with several potent inhalation anesthetics to control blood pressure (BP). Hypomagnesemia may be present in the pregnant patient and should be corrected preoperatively. Where an adequate level of magnesium can be achieved, its use may be ideal as an adjunct to anesthetic management because it has been shown that the use of magnesium to control BP is not deleterious to the fetus.

Bullough A, Karadia S, Watters M. Phaeochromocytoma: an unusual cause of hypertension in pregnancy. *Anaesthesia* 2001;56(1):43–46.

Grodski S, Jung C, Kertes P, et al. Phaeochromocytoma in pregnancy. *Int Med J* 2006;36(9): 604–606.

James MF, Cronje L. Pheochromocytoma crisis: the use of magnesium sulfate. *Anesth Analg* 2004;99(3):680–686.

Widimsky J Jr. Recent advances in the diagnosis and treatment of pheochromocytoma. *Kidney Blood Press Res* 2006;29(5):321–326.

C.7. What are some of the issues you must be aware of with a laparoscopic adrenalectomy?

Owing to the relatively recent advancement of imaging techniques, such as computed tomography (CT), ^{131}I metaiodo-benzylguanidine (MIBG) scintigraphy, magnetic resonance imaging (MRI), and positron emission tomography, localization of the tumor has become fairly accurate. These techniques allow for the selective surgical approach seen in laparoscopic surgery. Therefore, it is important to understand the issues associated with this form of adrenalectomy.

Creation of the pneumoperitoneum and, not surprisingly, manipulation of the tumor has been associated with an elevation in catecholamine and vasopressin levels in patients undergoing laparoscopic adrenalectomies. With this elevation in the catecholamine levels, there is an associated increase in cardiac output and blood pressure (BP). Insufflation of CO_2 into the peritoneum causes hypercarbia which can in turn increase sympathetic tone. Studies show that intraoperative hemodynamic values during laparoscopic surgery are in fact comparable to those of traditional surgery. But the decreased postoperative pain and the quicker postoperative recovery in patients who have undergone laparoscopic surgery make it an attractive alternative.

Gumbs AA, Gagner M. Laparoscopic adrenalectomy. *Best Pract Res Clin Endocrinol Metab* 2006;20(3):483–499.

Joris JL, Hamoir EE, Hartstein GM, et al. Hemodynamic changes and catecholamine release during laparoscopic adrenalectomy for pheochromocytoma. *Anesth Analg* 1999; 88:16–21.

Lombardi CP, Raffaelli M, De Crea C, et al. Role of laparoscopy in the management of adrenal malignancies. *J Surg Oncol* 2006;94(2):128–131.

Sprung J, O'Hara JF Jr, Gill IS, et al. Anesthetic aspects of laparoscopic and open adrenalectomy for pheochromocytoma. *Urology* 2000;55 (3):339–343.

Wilhelm SM, Prinz RA, Barbu AM, et al. Analysis of large versus small pheochromocytomas: operative approaches and patient outcomes. *Surgery* 2006;140(4):553–559.

D. Postoperative Management

D.1. What is the significance of postoperative hypotension? How is it treated?

Postoperative hypotension is often seen after the excision of the tumor. This may be due to hypovolemia and/or persistent fatigue of the vasoconstrictor mechanism. Once the excess catecholamines are diminished after the removal of the tumor, the response by the vascular bed to maintain pressure may be sluggish. Hypotension is rarely seen in patients who have been adequately volume-expanded and α-blocked preoperatively. If it does occur, it should be treated with volume administration and, if needed, norepinephrine. Be cognizant of the fact that persistent hypotension may be secondary to bleeding.

Artusio JF Jr. Anesthesiology for pheochromocytoma. In: Malhotra V, ed. *Anesthesia for renal and genito-urologic surgery*. New York: McGraw-Hill, 1996:84.

Malhotra SK, Ramprabu K, Dutta A, et al. An unusual cause of respiratory distress and hypotension following removal of a pheochromocytoma. *Can J Anaesth* 2002;49(10): 1099–1100.

Tan SG, Koay CK, Chan ST. The use of vasopressin to treat catecholamine-resistant hypotension after phaeochromocytoma removal. *Anaesth Intensive Care* 2002;30(4): 477–480.

D.2. What other problems can arise in the postoperative period?

For the first 48 hours after surgery, these patients may be very somnolent. This is possibly due to the sudden removal of activating catecholamines. Frequently, this results in decreased narcotic requirements.

Be aware that these patients are also prone to significant hypoglycemia, which alone can make a patient somnolent. In more severe cases, hypoglycemia may cause loss of consciousness and respiratory arrest. The hypoglycemia results from the fact that the suppression of β-cell function disappears after removal of the tumor. Hence the plasma insulin level rises. Neoglycogenesis and glycogenolysis, which had sustained the high blood sugar, are no longer present. Therefore, one should consider switching to a glucose-containing intravenous fluid after removal of the tumor and monitor the glucose levels very closely for at least 24 hours in the postoperative period.

Persistent hypertension after removal of a pheochromocytoma occasionally signifies that a residual pheochromocytoma tumor is present. Be aware that plasma catecholamine levels may not decrease to normal levels for many days after removal of the tumor.

Davies MJ, McGlade DP, Banting SW. A comparison of open and laparoscopic approaches to adrenalectomy in patients with phaeochromocytoma. *Anaesth Intensive Care* 2004;32(2):224–229.

Wilhelm SM, Prinz RA, Barbu AM, et al. Analysis of large versus small pheochromocytomas: operative approaches and patient outcomes. *Surgery* 2006;140(4):553–559; discussion 559–560

CHAPTER 36

Diabetes Mellitus

Klaus Kjaer • Vinod Malhotra

A 45-YEAR-OLD WOMAN

has a known history of diabetes for 30 years. Her diabetes is normally controlled with a combination regimen of neutral protamine hagedorn (NPH) and regular insulin: NPH 32 units and regular 16 units before breakfast, and NPH 12 units and regular 12 units before dinner. She is scheduled for emergency surgery for ovarian abscess. Her blood glucose level is 350 mg per dL.

A. Medical Disease and Differential Diagnosis

1. What is the prevalence of diabetes mellitus (DM) in the general population?
2. What are the factors in the etiology of the disease?
3. How do you classify DM?
4. What are the complications of DM?
5. How would you treat the different forms of this illness?
6. How do you adequately monitor control of the disease?
7. What are some of the factors that alter insulin requirements?
8. What are the principles of management of diabetic ketoacidosis?
9. What is nonketotic hyperosmolar coma?

B. Preoperative Evaluation and Preparation

1. How would you evaluate this patient preoperatively?
2. How would stiff joint syndrome affect her airway management?
3. What are the signs and implications of autonomic neuropathy in the diabetic patient?
4. How would you prepare this patient for anesthesia and surgery?
5. For elective surgery, how do you manage the insulin and glucose requirements on the day of surgery?
6. How would you premedicate this patient? Why?

C. Intraoperative Management

1. What is the effect of anesthesia and surgery on insulin and glucose metabolism?
2. What anesthetic techniques would you employ?
3. How would you monitor this patient?
4. How would you treat hyperglycemia intraoperatively?
5. How would you recognize and treat hypoglycemic shock intraoperatively?

D. Postoperative Management

1. How would you control diabetes in this patient postoperatively?

2. What are the common postoperative complications you expect in a diabetic patient?
3. Does diabetes increase perioperative risk? Is it necessary to achieve tight perioperative control of blood glucose?

A. Medical Disease and Differential Diagnosis

A.1. What is the prevalence of diabetes mellitus (DM) in the general population?

The estimated prevalence of DM in the United States varies depending on the criteria used to define the disease (Table 36.1). The fasting plasma glucose level is the most reliable and convenient test. Routine screening with the oral glucose tolerance test is not recommended. As of 2005, it was estimated that 20.8 million people in the United States met the diagnostic criteria for DM, representing approximately 7% of the population. The prevalence of impaired glucose tolerance is significantly higher. In 2005, 1.5 million new cases of DM were diagnosed in people aged 20 years or older.

More than 90% of diabetic patients in the United States have type 2 DM. Most of these patients tend to be elderly and overweight. The prevalence of type 2 DM is rising, most likely due to increased obesity and decreased activity levels in the general population. Other risk factors include family history, minority ethnicity, and low socioeconomic status. In addition, 3% to 5% of pregnant women develop gestational diabetes.

American Diabetes Association. *Diabetes 4-1-1: facts, figures, and statistics at a glance.* American Diabetes Association, 2005.

Kasper D, Braunwald E, Fauci A, et al. eds. *Harrison's principles of internal medicine,* 16th ed. New York: McGraw-Hill, 2005:2152–2180.

A.2. What are the factors in the etiology of the disease?

The pathogenesis of DM appears to involve the combination of genetic susceptibility and an environmental trigger. The process is almost certainly autoimmune. Viral infection is a suggested etiology, but noninfectious causes are possible. Although the role of genetic factors in the development of the disorder is undisputed, the exact mode of inheritance remains controversial. Studies on monozygotic twins show a concordance rate for type 1 DM of 30% to 70%, indicating that factors other than genetics are involved in the development of the disease. Meanwhile, 80% of type 1 DM occurs in children with no family history of diabetes. In view of such diverse findings, it is reasonable to assume a polygenic transmission modified by environmental factors. Factors that underline the significance of immune factors in the pathogenesis of the disease include histopathologic studies, elevated human leukocyte antigen (HLA) titers, the presence of insulin antibodies, and the association of type 1 DM with certain well-known autoimmune diseases such as thyroiditis and myasthenia gravis. At least 17 different genetic loci confer susceptibility to type 1 DM, including HLA-DR3 and HLA-DR4, located on the short arm of chromosome 6.

Table 36.1 Diagnostic Criteria for Diabetes Mellitus by American Diabetes Association.

1. Symptoms of diabetes plus random plasma glucose level >200 mg/dL
2. Fasting plasma glucose level >126 mg/dL
3. Two-hour plasma glucose level >200 mg/dL during oral glucose tolerance test

Although major genes that predispose to type 2 DM have not yet been identified, the concordance rate in twins is between 70% and 90%, suggesting a strong genetic component.

Virus β-cell interactions have been postulated in the pathogenesis of type 1 DM, with supportive evidence of antiviral antibody titers implicating several common viruses such as Coxsackie and rubella. A typical scenario for onset of type 1 DM, then, might be a genetically susceptible individual with an exposure to a virus that causes inflammation of the pancreatic islet cells and lymphocytic infiltration. This in turn triggers the autoimmune response, resulting in the destruction of β cells. Type 2 DM results from a combination of insulin resistance, β-cell failure, and excessive hepatic glucose production.

Ahmed Z, Lockhart CH, Weiner M, et al. Advances in diabetic management: implications for anesthesia. *Anesth Analg* 2005;100(3):666–669.

Kasper D, Braunwald E, Fauci A, et al. eds. *Harrison's principles of internal medicine*, 16th ed. New York: McGraw-Hill, 2005:2152–2180.

Miller RD, ed. *Miller's anesthesia*, 6th ed. Philadelphia: Churchill Livingstone, 2005:1776–1781.

A.3. How do you classify diabetes mellitus (DM)?

The current classification of DM is based on the pathogenesis of the disease, rather than age at onset or type of therapy. Type 1 DM results from pancreatic β-cell failure and ensuing insulin deficiency. Onset is typically before age 30 but can occur at any time, and insulin is required for control of glucose. Type 1 DM is believed to be caused by an autoimmune mechanism. Type 2 DM is a milder form of the disease, affects all ages, and results from a combination of insulin deficiency, insulin resistance, and increased glucose production. Most patients with type 2 DM are managed with diet, exercise, and oral hypoglycemic agents. A significant number eventually require insulin for adequate glucose control as the disease progresses, but type 2 diabetic patients are not at risk of diabetic ketoacidosis if they do not receive insulin. Obesity and older age are the main risk factors for type 2 DM. Two other types of diabetes are gestational diabetes, which sometimes may require insulin, and secondary diabetes, which can occur as a result of various endocrine disorders or drugs such as steroids.

Kasper D, Braunwald E, Fauci A, et al. eds. *Harrison's principles of internal medicine*, 16th ed. New York: McGraw-Hill, 2005:2152–2180.

Miller RD, ed. *Miller's anesthesia*, 6th ed. Philadelphia: Churchill Livingstone, 2005:1019–1027.

A.4. What are the complications of diabetes mellitus (DM)?

The long-term complications of DM are the result of end-organ pathology due to chronic hyperglycemia. Diabetic nephropathy is the leading cause of end-stage renal disease (ESRD) in the United States, accounting for 44% of new cases in 2002. Strict blood pressure control, especially with angiotensin-converting enzyme (ACE) inhibitors, may slow the decline in renal function once diabetic nephropathy is diagnosed. Cardiovascular changes include coronary artery disease, hypertension, cardiac autonomic neuropathy, and microangiopathic cardiomyopathy. Myocardial infarction is the most common cause of death in the elderly diabetic patient. The American Heart Association recently designated DM as a major risk factor for cardiovascular disease, along with smoking, hypertension, and hyperlipidemia. Coronary artery disease occurs in 3% of diabetic patients aged 18 to 44 , 14.3% of patients aged 45 to 64 , and 20% of patients older than 65 years. It affects women as often as men and is more often fatal in women due to atypical presentation. Stroke occurs in 2% of diabetic patients aged 18 to 44 , 8.4% of patients aged 45 to 64 , and 12.7% of patients older than 65 years. Lower extremity pulse deficits are present in more than 10% of diabetic patients, nephropathy in more than 40%, and distal polyneuropathy in more than 50%. Stiff joint syndrome can occur as a result of glycation of collagen tissues. In gestational diabetes, additional risks include late intrauterine demise, traumatic birth injury, cephalopelvic disproportion, neonatal hypoglycemia, neonatal respiratory distress syndrome, and postpartum maternal hypoglycemia.

In the case of a type 1 diabetic patient such as this one, the common life-threatening complications are mainly caused by poor control and include hypoglycemia, hyperglycemia, diabetic ketoacidosis, and nonketotic hyperosmolar coma. The mortality rate for type 1 diabetic patients is five times greater than that for the general population. For patients with type 2 DM, mortality is twice that for the general population. Tight control of blood glucose levels reduces the risk of chronic complications from diabetes.

American Diabetes Association. *Diabetes 4-1-1: facts, figures, and statistics at a glance*. American Diabetes Association, 2005.

Datta S, ed. *Anesthetic and obstetric management of high-risk pregnancy*, 3rd ed. New York: Springer-Verlag New York, 2004:157–158.

Kasper D, Braunwald E, Fauci A, et al. eds. *Harrison's principles of internal medicine*, 16th ed. New York: McGraw-Hill, 2005:2152–2180.

A.5. How would you treat the different forms of this illness?

The type 1 diabetic patient, who has the severe form of the disease, is dependent on insulin both for control of glucose and for prevention of diabetic ketoacidosis. Several preparations of insulin have become available over the last few years, many produced by recombinant DNA technology. The onset and duration of action of these agents in diabetic patients by subcutaneous injection are shown in Table 36.2. In healthy persons, the onset of regular insulin is within 15 minutes when given intravenously as compared to 30 minutes when given subcutaneously. Maximal action of regular insulin occurs at 2 hours when given intravenously, and duration is 6 to 8 hours.

Treatment for patients with type 2 DM centers around weight loss and diet control. Patients whose diabetes is not well controlled on this regimen require drug therapy. There are four broad categories of glucose-lowering agents: (a) insulin secretagogues, such as the sulfonylureas, which stimulate insulin secretion by interacting with the adenosine triphosphate (ATP)-sensitive

---

Table 36.2   Onset and Duration of Action of Subcutaneous Insulin Types.

TYPE	ONSET	PEAK ACTIVITY	DURATION
Rapid acting (Lispro/Aspart)	15–30 min	30–90 min	3–4 hr
Short acting (regular insulin)	30–60 min	2–4 hr	6–10 hr
Intermediate acting (NPH Lente)	1–4 hr	4–12 hr	12–24 hr
Long acting			
Ultralente	1–2 hr	8–20 hr	24–30 hr
Glargine	1 hr	3–20 hr	24 hr

NPH, neutral protamine hagedorn.
(Ahmed Z, Lockhart CH, Weiner M, et al. Advances in diabetic management: implications for anesthesia. *Anesth Analg* 2005;100(3):666–669.)

Table 36.3 Onset and Duration of Action of Oral Hypoglycemic Agents.

DRUG CLASS	DRUG NAME	ONSET	DURATION
First-generation sulfonylureas	Tolbutamide	1 hr	12 hr
	Acetohexamide	3 hr	24 hr
	Tolazamide	4 hr	16 hr
	Chlorpropamide	2 hr	24 hr
Second-generation sulfonylureas	Glyburide	30 min	24 hr
	Glipizide IR	30 min	24 hr
	Glipizide ER	2–4 hr	24 hr
	Glimepiride	2–3 hr	24 hr
Biguanides	Metformin	1–3 hr	17 hr
α-Glucosidase inhibitor	Acarbose	2 hr	4 hr
	Miglitol	2–3 hr	NA
Thiazolidinediones	Pioglitazone	2 hr	NA

IR, immediate release; ER, extended release; NA, not available.
(From Angelini G, Ketzler JT, Coursin DB. Perioperative care of the diabetic patient. *ASA Refresher Courses Anesthesiol* 2001;29:1–10, with permission.)

potassium channel on the β cell; (b) biguanides, such as metformin, which reduce hepatic glucose production and improve peripheral glucose utilization; (c) α-glucosidase inhibitors, such as miglitol, which reduce postprandial hyperglycemia by delaying glucose absorption; and (d) thiazolidinediones, such as pioglitazone, which reduce insulin resistance by binding to receptors in the nucleus of adipocytes.

Oral glucose-lowering agents by themselves may not lower blood glucose levels to the normal range, and therefore, many type 2 diabetic patients require exogenous insulin therapy. Alternatively, oral hypoglycemics from different classes may be used to increase the success rate of noninsulin drug therapy. Metformin has been used successfully with newer sulfonylureas such as glyburide. However, metformin should not be used in the setting of renal failure, as it may cause lactic acidosis. The newer sulfonylureas have a long duration of action and are rarely associated with hypoglycemia; however, when hypoglycemia occurs, it can be severe and prolonged. The onset and duration of action of oral glucose-lowering agents are shown in Table 36.3. The risks of intense medical regimens to keep blood sugar levels in the normal range always must be weighed against the risk of hypoglycemia, which can be fatal.

Other therapies currently under investigation include the following:

- New and more potent insulin secretagogues
- Inhaled insulin
- Aminoguanidine to prevent excessive glycation of tissues
- Pancreatic transplant
- Islet cell transplant

Ahmed Z, Lockhart CH, Weiner M, et al. Advances in diabetic management: implications for anesthesia. *Anesth Analg* 2005;100(3):666–669.

Angelini G, Ketzler JT, Coursin DB. Perioperative care of the diabetic patient. *ASA refresher courses in anesthesiology.* Park Ridge: American Society of Anesthesiologists, 2001: 1–10.

Kasper D, Braunwald E, Fauci A, et al. eds. *Harrison's principles of internal medicine,* 16th ed. New York: McGraw-Hill, 2005:2152–2180.

Vreven R, De Kock M. Metformin lactic acidosis and anaesthesia: myth or reality? *Acta Anaesthesiol Belg* 2005;56(3):297–302.

A.6. How do you adequately monitor control of the disease?

Patients with mild diabetes and those with well-controlled diabetes are usually self-monitored by a daily urine test for reducing sugars and ketones. In acute management of hyperglycemia, or in situations in which the insulin requirement is altered (as in the aforementioned patient secondary to infection), the best control is achieved with regular insulin and frequent monitoring of blood glucose levels, because the changes in urinary sugar levels appear after a lag period. Present technology allows for nearly painless collection of blood samples and quick electronic measurement of the glucose level at the bedside.

Increasing evidence indicates that most of the end-organ complications of diabetes are the result of chronic hyperglycemia. Therefore, maintaining as close to a euglycemic state as possible is the goal. Most patients who follow their blood glucose level can do so at home using readily available kits. Endocrinologists frequently measure glycated hemoglobin, hemoglobin A_{1C} (Hb A_{1C}), to monitor long-term control. Hb A_{1C} (normal value, 6%) is increased in patients with poorly controlled diabetes, because its synthesis depends on glycation (formerly referred to as *nonenzymatic glycosylation*). Hb A_{1C} reflects plasma glucose control over the preceding 6 weeks and can reach values of up to 20%.

Ahmed Z, Lockhart CH, Weiner M, et al. Advances in diabetic management: implications for anesthesia. *Anesth Analg* 2005;100(3):666–669.

Angelini G, Ketzler JT, Coursin DB. Perioperative care of the diabetic patient. *ASA refresher courses in anesthesiology*. Park Ridge: American Society of Anesthesiologist, 2001:1–10.

Kasper D, Braunwald E, Fauci A, et al. eds. *Harrison's principles of internal medicine*, 16th ed. New York: McGraw-Hill, 2005:2152–2180.

A.7. What are some of the factors that alter insulin requirement?

Factors commonly known to increase the insulin requirement include a high-carbohydrate diet, infection, sepsis, stress, and certain frequently employed drugs, namely, corticosteroids, thyroid preparations, oral contraceptives, and thiazide diuretics. Exercise and alcohol commonly result in decreased requirements. Certain drugs such as Coumadin may also result in decreased requirements by interfering with the metabolism of oral glucose-lowering agents.

Kasper D, Braunwald E, Fauci A, et al. eds. *Harrison's principles of internal medicine*, 16th ed. New York: McGraw-Hill, 2005:2152–2180.

A.8. What are the principles of management of diabetic ketoacidosis?

Diabetic ketoacidosis is an acute medical emergency characterized by an absolute or relative deficiency of insulin, resulting in an accumulation of ketone acids in the blood. The main disturbances are hyperglycemia, glucosuria, intracellular dehydration, acidosis, and electrolyte imbalance. Conventionally, severe ketoacidosis implies levels of ketone acids in the blood of generally more than 7 mmol per L, a decrease in serum bicarbonate to less than 10 mEq per L, or a decrease in pH level to less than 7.25. The initial physical examination should be supported with urinalysis, venous blood analysis for glucose, electrolytes and determination of anion gap, serum ketone estimation, urea nitrogen level, and complete blood cell count. Reagent strips may be used to electronically determine the blood glucose and ketones quickly so therapy can be initiated. An arterial blood gas sample should be analyzed to determine acid–base imbalance. The mainstay of treatment includes fluids, insulin, bicarbonate, and potassium.

- *Fluids:* Most patients are dehydrated and the loss of water exceeds that of salt. Therefore, a hypotonic saline solution (0.45% sodium chloride) is considered optimal. Five percent dextrose should be instituted once the serum glucose level falls to less than 300 mg per dL to prevent hypoglycemia secondary to insulin therapy. A central venous pressure measurement and urine output are good guidelines for fluid therapy.
- *Insulin:* All patients in ketoacidosis are in immediate need of insulin. Therefore, a rapid-onset short-acting insulin should be employed to attain better control. Insulin, 10 to 20 units, is given intravenously initially, and an infusion of insulin at a rate of 1 to 2 units per hour is started depending on blood glucose levels. Initial bolus dose may be repeated depending on the severity of ketoacidosis and hyperglycemia, as well as the glucose-lowering response to the initial dose. Blood glucose level should be reduced at a rate of no more than 50 mg/dL/hour, as a faster reduction rate can lead to cerebral edema.
- *Bicarbonate:* Sodium bicarbonate should be used to correct severe metabolic acidosis (with a pH level of <7.20) as guided by determinations of arterial blood pH level, Pco_2, and bicarbonate. Overcorrection should be avoided.
- *Potassium:* After acidosis, osmotic diuresis, and vomiting, body potassium stores are depleted by 5 to 10 mEq per kg of body weight. Serum potassium level, although initially normal, usually decreases as a result of hemodilution, and because the correction of hyperglycemia and acidosis results in movement of potassium from extracellular space to intracellular space. Therefore, potassium should be added to the intravenous infusion 3 to 4 hours after initiating the therapy, provided the renal function is adequate. Frequent laboratory data and clinical findings should dictate the dose and frequency regimen of the treatment. Supportive therapy for associated problems should continue, and overcorrection should be avoided.

Angelini G, Ketzler JT, Coursin DB. Perioperative care of the diabetic patient. *ASA refresher courses in anesthesiology*. Park Ridge: American Society of Anesthesiologists, 2001: 1–10.

Kasper D, Braunwald E, Fauci A, et al. eds. *Harrison's principles of internal medicine*, 16th ed. New York: McGraw-Hill, 2005:2152–2180.

Kitabchi AE. Low dose insulin therapy in diabetic ketoacidosis: fact or fiction? *Diabetes Metab Rev* 1989;5:337–363.

A.9. What is nonketotic hyperosmolar coma?

Nonketotic hyperosmolar coma is a syndrome of profound dehydration usually seen in patients with type 2 DM when they are unable to drink enough to keep up with urinary fluid losses secondary to glycosuria. No ketoacidosis is present. Patients present with extreme hyperglycemia, hyperosmolality, volume depletion, and mental status changes. Plasma glucose level is generally approximately 1,000 mg per dL, approximately twice the value seen in diabetic ketoacidosis. The mortality rate is greater than 50%. The most important aspect of treatment is rapid administration of large amounts of intravenous fluid, but as with diabetic ketoacidosis, insulin, dextrose, and potassium are necessary as well.

Kasper D, Braunwald E, Fauci A, et al. eds. *Harrison's principles of internal medicine*, 16th ed. New York: McGraw-Hill, 2005:2152–2180.

B. Preoperative Evaluation and Preparation

B.1. How would you evaluate this patient preoperatively?

A complete preoperative evaluation includes a history and physical examination supported by the following laboratory data:

- Electrocardiogram
- Urinalysis for detecting sugar and ketones
- Venous blood estimation of complete blood cell count, serum electrolytes, urea nitrogen, sugar, and ketones (serum osmolality if available)
- Arterial blood gas analysis to determine acid–base status

Of great pertinence is the history of the last intake of meal and the last dose of insulin. Nausea and vomiting in this patient will affect her state of hydration, acid–base status, and electrolyte balance significantly. As diabetic nephropathy progresses, protein appears in the urine before the creatinine level rises. The patient should be questioned and examined for stiff joint syndrome. The prayer sign, a classic feature of stiff joint syndrome, is demonstrated when a patient is unable to approximate their fingers and palms while pressing their hands together.

Alberti KGMM. Diabetes and surgery. *Anesthesiology* 1991;74:209–211.

Angelini G, Ketzler JT, Coursin DB. Perioperative care of the diabetic patient. *ASA refresher courses in anesthesiology*. Park Ridge: American Society of Anesthesiologist, 2001: 1–10.

Hirsh IB, McGill JB, Cryer PE, et al. Perioperative management of surgical patients with diabetes mellitus. *Anesthesiology* 1991;74:346–359.

B.2. How would stiff joint syndrome affect her airway management?

Stiff joint syndrome has been reported as frequently as approximately one of four adolescent diabetic patients. In addition to stiff joints, typical manifestations include short stature and tight waxy skin. These changes are due to the glycation of collagen tissues, the same process that results in an increase in Hb A_{1C}, frequently used to monitor the adequacy of control of diabetes. If this involves the temporomandibular joint, atlantooccipital joint, or cervical spine, the resultant limitation of head and neck mobility may make endotracheal intubation difficult.

Angelini G, Ketzler JT, Coursin DB. Perioperative care of the diabetic patient. *ASA refresher courses in anesthesiology*. Park Ridge: American Society of Anesthesiologist, 2001:1–10.

Salzarulo HH, Taylor LA. Diabetic "stiff joint syndrome" as a cause of difficult endotracheal intubation. *Anesthesiology* 1986;64:366–368.

B.3. What are the signs and implications of autonomic neuropathy in the diabetic patient?

Autonomic neuropathy occurs in approximately 1 of every 10 diabetic patients. In the older population, especially those with coexisting hypertension, the incidence increases fourfold to fivefold. Signs of autonomic neuropathy include lack of sweating, early satiety, orthostatic hypotension, gastric reflux, and lack of change in pulse rate with deep inspiration. Impotence and urinary symptoms of dysautonomic bladder may be evident.

The implication of autonomic neuropathy is increased morbidity and mortality. Orthostatic hypotension in the perioperative period is common and may be severe immediately postoperatively.

Myocardial ischemia is often painless with risks of cardiorespiratory arrest. Gastroparesis predisposes these patients to nausea, vomiting, regurgitation, and aspiration.

Angelini G, Ketzler JT, Coursin DB. Perioperative care of the diabetic patient. *ASA refresher courses in anesthesiology*. Park Ridge: American Society of Anesthesiologist, 2001: 1–10.

Charleson MC, Mackenzie CR, Gold JP. Preoperative autonomic function abnormalities in patients with diabetes mellitus and patients with hypertension. *J Am Coll Surg* 1994;179:1–10.

B.4. How would you prepare this patient for anesthesia and surgery?

The preoperative evaluation will determine the preparation of this patient, the principles of which are as follows:

Hydration

- Poor oral intake secondary to malaise and abdominal pain, concomitant vomiting (if present), and osmotic diuresis resulting from glucosuria will make dehydration quite likely in this patient. Any dehydration that is present, therefore, should be rapidly corrected. Normal or half-normal saline is a preferred intravenous solution because the blood glucose level is already elevated in this instance.

Insulin

- Infection and stress are known to increase insulin requirements, which explains hyperglycemia in this patient. Insulin can be given to this patient either in small doses (5–10 units intravenously) every hour or as a continuous infusion at 1 to 2 units per hour using a pump. Hourly blood and urine glucose and acetone measurements should be used to adequately monitor this therapy. Acid–base and electrolyte correction should be carried out as dictated by blood test results.

Antibiotics

- Antibiotics should be instituted once appropriate culture samples are obtained.

Angelini G, Ketzler JT, Coursin DB. Perioperative care of the diabetic patient. *ASA refresher courses in anesthesiology*. Park Ridge: American Society of Anesthesiologist, 2001:1–10.

Hirsh IB, McGill JB, Cryer PE, et al. Perioperative management of surgical patients with diabetes mellitus. *Anesthesiology* 1991;74:346–359.

B.5. For elective surgery, how do you manage the insulin and glucose requirements on the day of surgery?

A large number of protocols exist for managing insulin and glucose requirements in the diabetic patient taking insulin. For the type 2 diabetic patient not taking insulin, the morning dose of oral glucose-lowering agent is omitted, and for most surgical procedures, glucose-containing intravenous solutions can be avoided. Metformin should be continued 24 hours before surgery. Lactated RINGER's solution may predispose to hyperglycemia, as lactate is converted to glucose. On the basis of blood sugar determinations, regular insulin can be used to treat hyperglycemia. For extensive procedures and when the patient is not expected to resume oral intake for a few days, glucose should be given in the intravenous solution as a substrate for the increased metabolic demand, thereby providing a protein-sparing effect. Parenteral regular insulin is best suited to control hyperglycemia in that situation. For the diabetic patient taking insulin, the problem is more acute and none of the commonly followed protocols offers a complete solution (Table 36.4).

Frequent blood sugar determination is the key to tailoring insulin therapy for patients taking insulin. It is recommended that blood glucose be measured the morning of surgery. For cases scheduled for surgery later in the day, it can be repeated before anesthesia. The blood sugar should be less than 250 mg per dL before the start of surgery. In pediatric patients, rapid-acting insulin may be given using a correction factor based on the "rule of 1500": Divide 1,500 by the patient's total daily dose of insulin; this is the amount, in mg per dL, by which 1 unit of insulin is expected to lower the blood glucose. The goal should be to bring the blood glucose down to 150. (e.g., in someone taking 50 units of insulin daily, 1 unit of insulin is expected to reduce the blood glucose by 1,500/50 = 30 mg/dL.)

For procedures greater than 2 hours in duration, patients on insulin may benefit from simultaneous infusion of dextrose and insulin. In pediatric patients, a solution of 10% dextrose and 0.5 normal saline at the appropriate maintenance rate (4 mL/kg/hr for the first 10 kg, 2 mL/kg/hr for the next 11–20 kg, and 1 mL/kg/hr >20 kg) is appropriate. The accompanying insulin rate should be 1 unit per 5 g dextrose in children 12 years or older, and 1 unit per 3 g dextrose in children older than 12 years. In adults, dextrose can be given as an infusion providing 5 to 10 g per hour, and insulin started at 1 unit per hour. Intraoperatively, blood sugar should be measured every 1 to 2 hours, or more frequently if necessary.

Hirsh IB, McGill JB, Cryer PE, et al. Perioperative management of surgical patients with diabetes mellitus. *Anesthesiology* 1991;74:346–359.

Rhodes ET, Ferrari LR, Wolfsdorf JI. Perioperative management of pediatric surgical patients with diabetes mellitus. *Anesth Analg* 2005;101(4):986–999.

Stoelting RK, Dierdorf SF. *Anesthesia and co-existing disease*, 4th ed. Philadelphia: Churchill Livingstone, 2002:395–411.

D.6. How would you premedicate this patient? Why?

We would premedicate these patients with 10 mg of metoclopramide given orally approximately 1 hour before surgery. Metoclopramide has been shown to be very effective in improving gastric emptying in the diabetic patient with gastroparesis. This should decrease the likelihood of regurgitation, aspiration, nausea, and vomiting.

Angelini G, Ketzler JT, Coursin DB. Perioperative care of the diabetic patient. *ASA refresher courses in anesthesiology*. Park Ridge: American Society of Anesthesiologist, 2001:1–10.

C. Intraoperative Management

C.1. What is the effect of anesthesia and surgery on insulin and glucose metabolism?

Both sevoflurane and isoflurane impair glucose tolerance to the same degree, independent of surgical stimulation. No studies have examined the effects of nitrous oxide on glucose tolerance.

Surgery results in a stress response, accompanied by a catabolic state. The extent of this metabolic response is related to the severity of the operation and other concomitant factors, such as sepsis in this patient and shock, if present. The well-recognized hormonal changes include increased catecholamines, adrenocorticotropic hormone, and cortisol secretions, as well as plasma cyclic adenosine monophosphate and glucagon levels. As a result, blood glucose levels

Table 36.4   Perioperative Insulin Therapy Protocols in the Diabetic Patient.

PROTOCOL	LIMITATIONS	COMMENTS
No insulin or glucose on the day of surgery	Not suitable for insulin-dependent diabetic patients	Acceptable for noninsulin-dependent diabetic patients and minor surgical procedures
	Patient's stores of glucose are used to meet increased metabolic demands	Frequent blood sugar monitoring and insulin therapy, as necessary, are recommended
	Unacceptable in severe diabetic patients for even a short period	
	Patients taking long-acting oral hypoglycemics predisposed to hypoglycemia	
Partial-dose NPH insulin on morning of surgery, 5% dextrose solution IV 125 mL/hr	Insulin requirements vary in perioperative period	Has been shown to have the lowest therapeutic ratio in a controlled study
	Onset and peak effect may not correlate with glucose administration or start of surgery	Frequent blood glucose monitoring recommended
	Predisposes to hypoglycemia, especially in afternoon	
Constant IV infusion of insulin using special pumps, D_5 W given	Insulin requirements vary greatly intraoperatively	Frequent blood glucose monitoring recommended
	Insulin is adsorbed to bottles, IV tubing	
	Predisposes to hypoglycemia	
	Setting up pump or drips is a tedious process	
IV bolus injection of regular insulin	Difficult to control preoperatively on patient floors	Frequent blood glucose monitoring recommended
	Best suited for intraoperative and immediate postoperative period	Results in comparable blood glucose control when compared with constant IV infusion of insulin
Subcutaneous regular insulin based on sliding scale	Perioperative changes in regional blood flow resulting from heating, cooling, anesthesia, intrinsic or extrinsic catecholamines, vasoconstriction caused by pain, hypovolemia, anxiety, and shivering, result in unpredictable absorption of subcutaneous insulin	Frequent blood sugar monitoring and appropriate IV insulin therapy
Continuation of patient's insulin infusion pump	Insulin requirements vary greatly intraoperatively	Frequent blood glucose monitoring recommended

NPH, neutral protamine hagedorn.

are known to increase during surgery, whereas plasma insulin levels remain constant. There is also a phase of relative insulin resistance after surgery. All these changes increase insulin requirements acutely in the diabetic patient.

Insulin treatment started before surgery, along with a glucose infusion to maintain normoglycemia, results in lowering of cortisol levels immediately after surgery. Epidural block also reduces the release of stress hormones.

Breaking the preoperative fasted state shortly before surgery with liquid oral carbohydrates has been shown to reduce postoperative insulin resistance. The benefits of such intake should be weighed against the increased risk of aspiration.

Angelini G, Ketzler JT, Coursin DB. Perioperative care of the diabetic patient. *ASA refresher courses in anesthesiology*. Park Ridge: American Society of Anesthesiologist, 2001:1–10.

Ljungqvist O, Nygren J, Soop M, et al. Metabolic perioperative management: novel concepts. *Curr Opin Crit Care* 2005;11(4):295–299.

Tanaka T, Nabatame H, Tanifuji Y. Insulin secretion and glucose utilization are impaired under general anesthesia with sevoflurane as well as isoflurane in a concentration-independent manner. *J Anesth* 2005;19(4):277–281.

C.2. What anesthetic techniques would you employ?

A general anesthetic with intubation of the trachea will be a satisfactory choice for airway protection. After adequate preoxygenation, a rapid-sequence induction/intubation with cricoid pressure should be employed to prevent aspiration for emergency surgery in the diabetic patient. There is no significant difference among the commonly employed general anesthetics regarding their effect on diabetic control. Close monitoring will be necessary to provide cardiovascular stability and adequate control of diabetes.

Angelini G, Ketzler JT, Coursin DB. Perioperative care of the diabetic patient. *ASA refresher courses in anesthesiology*. Park Ridge: American Society of Anesthesiologist, 2001:1–10.

Hirsh IB, McGill JB, Cryer PE, et al. Perioperative management of surgical patients with diabetes mellitus. *Anesthesiology* 1991;74:346–359.

C.3. How would you monitor this patient?

In addition to continuous monitoring of pulse oximeter, electrocardiogram, blood pressure, capnogram, and temperature, frequent determinations of both blood and urine glucose should be made. The blood glucose level can be estimated easily in the operating room with the use of standard bedside electronic equipment, or the iSTAT, which will then dictate further insulin therapy.

Angelini G, Ketzler JT, Coursin DB. Perioperative care of the diabetic patient. *ASA refresher courses in anesthesiology*. Park Ridge: American Society of Anesthesiologist, 2001:1–10.

Hirsh IB, McGill JB, Cryer PE, et al. Perioperative management of surgical patients with diabetes mellitus. *Anesthesiology* 1991;74:346–359.

C.4. How would you treat hyperglycemia intraoperatively?

Intraoperative hyperglycemia (blood glucose level >250 mg/dL) should be treated with intravenous regular insulin. Small doses (up to 10 units) of insulin may be used reliably and effectively as single intravenous injections. In adults, a useful rule of thumb is that each unit of regular insulin lowers the blood sugar level by approximately 30 mg per dL. Blood sugars monitored every 1 to 2 hours further dictate the continuation of therapy. Although the half-life of intravenous insulin is short, hypoglycemia as late as 3 hours after an injection has been observed.

Another way to control hyperglycemia intraoperatively is to use a continuous infusion of insulin, starting at 1 unit per hour; if preoperatively, the patient requires 20 units or less of NPH insulin daily. In this patient, a starting rate of 2 units per hour, further dictated by frequent blood and urine glucose estimations, will be a reasonable regimen. The use of an infusion pump with a plastic syringe affords a 90% recovery of insulin due to limited adsorption. The keystone to intraoperative diabetes management is the measurement of blood glucose concentration.

Angelini G, Ketzler JT, Coursin DB. Perioperative care of the diabetic patient. *ASA refresher courses in anesthesiology*. Park Ridge: American Society of Anesthesiologist, 2001:1–10.

Hirsh IB, McGill JB, Cryer PE, et al. Perioperative management of surgical patients with diabetes mellitus. *Anesthesiology* 1991;74:346–359.

C.5. How would you recognize and treat hypoglycemic shock intraoperatively?

It is virtually impossible to differentiate hypoglycemic shock from other forms of shock intraoperatively unless supported by low blood glucose concentrations measured concomitantly. Treatment lies in administration of glucose, which may be given as a bolus of 50% glucose, followed by a 10% dextrose-insulin infusion. Blood sugar level increases approximately 30 mg per dL for each 7.5-g bolus of dextrose in a 70-kg adult.

Angelini G, Ketzler JT, Coursin DB. Perioperative care of the diabetic patient. *ASA refresher courses in anesthesiology*. Park Ridge: American Society of Anesthesiologist, 2001:1–10.

D. Postoperative Management

D.1. How would you control diabetes in this patient postoperatively?

Infusion of 10% dextrose-insulin-potassium, as determined by blood glucose and potassium every 4 to 6 hours, should be continued. Alternatively, NPH insulin may be replaced by regular insulin in divided doses. An additional 20% of insulin may be required because infection is present. As the patient totally resumes her controlled diet, the original preoperative regimen should be restored.

Hirsh IB, McGill JB, Cryer PE, et al. Perioperative management of surgical patients with diabetes mellitus. *Anesthesiology* 1991;74:346–359.

D.2. What are the common postoperative complications you expect in a diabetic patient?

In addition to the usual complications, the common problems in a diabetic patient include poor diabetes control and infection. Hyperglycemia is associated with delayed wound healing, decreased leukocyte function, and greater likelihood of brain damage in the setting of cardiorespiratory arrest. A higher incidence of cardiovascular and renal problems, in combination with autonomic neuropathy, can also result in postural hypotension and urinary retention. Overall morbidity and mortality are increased.

Angelini G, Ketzler JT, Coursin DB. Perioperative care of the diabetic patient. *ASA refresher courses in anesthesiology*. Park Ridge: American Society of Anesthesiologist, 2001:1–10.

Hirsh IB, McGill JB, Cryer PE, et al. Perioperative management of surgical patients with diabetes mellitus. *Anesthesiology* 1991;74:346–359.

D.3. Does diabetes increase perioperative risk? Is it necessary to achieve tight perioperative control of blood glucose?

Diabetes itself may not be as important to perioperative outcome as its end-organ effects. Diabetic and nondiabetic patients who are matched for type of surgery, age, sex, weight, and complicating diagnoses have similar complication rates. As noted previously, however, diabetic patients have complicating diagnoses much more frequently than nondiabetic patients, particularly obesity (see Chapter 62). Therefore, the average diabetic patient presents a higher perioperative risk than the average nondiabetic patient. Sepsis and complications of atherosclerosis are the leading causes of death in these patients. Other changes, such as nephropathy and autonomic neuropathy (e.g., urinary retention, gastroparesis, and painless myocardial ischemia), contribute to increased morbidity. Episodes of hyperglycemia, hypoglycemia, and diabetic ketoacidosis, conditions not generally encountered in the healthy population, carry a higher than normal risk of perioperative morbidity.

Glycemic control, particularly in the diabetic patient taking insulin, is a critical factor in the perioperative outcome. Although controversy has existed in the past about how tightly blood sugar levels should be controlled chronically in diabetic patients, the preponderance of recent data suggests that the long-term benefits of such tight control include delayed onset and limitation of complications of diabetes. It is also known that hyperglycemia may worsen neurologic outcome after intraoperative cerebral ischemia. Studies also suggest that hyperglycemia with a blood glucose level of more than 250 mg per dL inhibits polymorphonuclear cell activity. Increased incidence of infection, decreased wound healing, and a higher incidence of end-organ damage should prompt us to achieve tight perioperative control of blood sugar in diabetic patients. In this population, patients with poor intraoperative glycemic control (four consecutive blood glucose measurements >200 mg/dL despite insulin therapy) during cardiac surgery have been shown to have higher rate of cardiovascular, respiratory, infectious, renal, and neurologic complications following surgery.

Clark CM, Lee DA. Jr Prevention and treatment of the complications of diabetes mellitus. *N Engl J Med* 1995;332:1210–1217.

The Diabetic Control and Complications Trial Research Group. The effect of intensive treatment of diabetes on the development and progression of long term complications for insulin dependent diabetes mellitus. *N Engl J Med* 1993;329:977–987.

Ljungqvist O, Nygren J, Soop M, et al. Metabolic perioperative management: novel concepts. *Curr Opin Crit Care* 2005;11(4):295–299.

Miller RD, ed. *Anesthesia*, 6th ed. Philadelphia: Churchill Livingstone, 2005:1019–1027, 1776–1781.

Ouattara A, Lecomte P, Le Manach Y, et al. Poor intraoperative blood glucose control is associated with a worsened hospital outcome after cardiac surgery in diabetic patients. *Anesthesiology* 2005;103(4):687–694.

The Genitourinary System

CHAPTER 37

Transurethral Resection of the Prostate

FUN-SUN F. YAO • VINOD MALHOTRA • VIJAYENDRA SUDHEENDRA

A 79-YEAR-OLD MAN

with benign prostatic hypertrophy was scheduled for transurethral resection of the prostate (TURP). Past medical history included myocardial infarction (MI) complicated by congestive heart failure (CHF) 7 months earlier. The patient had been taking diuretics, β-blockers, and calcium channel blocker.

A. Medical Disease and Differential Diagnosis

1. Are there differences in morbidity and mortality rates between transurethral resection of the prostate (TURP) and suprapubic or retropubic prostatectomy?
2. What chronic medical conditions are common in patients who have undergone TURP?
3. Does a history of prior myocardial infarction (MI) increase the patient's risk of perioperative reinfarction?
4. In patients with a history of recent MI, would you recommend that the surgery be postponed for a certain period? If so, why?

B. Preoperative Evaluation and Preparation

1. How would you evaluate the patient's cardiac condition? What laboratory tests would you like to have done? Would you recommend that the patient undergo coronary angiography before surgery?

2. Are patients with a Q-wave infarction at greater risk of reinfarction than those with a non–Q-wave infarction?

3. Would you discontinue any antihypertensives or any medications for angina?

C. Intraoperative Management

1. What monitors would you use for this patient?

2. What anesthetic technique is preferable for patients undergoing TURP and why?

3. Is regional anesthesia associated with a lower incidence of perioperative mortality than general anesthesia?

4. What intravenous fluid would you use during TURP?

5. After administration of midazolam, 2 mg intravenously, a patient scheduled for TURP received spinal anesthesia with bupivacaine, 10 mg. The level of anesthesia was T-10. Approximately 40 minutes after the surgery had started, the patient became restless, the blood pressure started to rise, and the heart rate decreased. Two more milligrams of midazolam was given. Shortly thereafter, the patient became cyanotic and obtunded, blood pressure fell precipitously, and pupils became dilated and unresponsive to light. What is the differential diagnosis of this set of clinical signs during TURP?

6. What are the important characteristics of irrigation solutions used during TURP?

7. Why is plain distilled water rarely used for irrigation during TURP? What types of irrigation solutions are available?

8. What is the effect of continuous bladder irrigation during TURP on body temperature?

9. What are the definition and signs and symptoms of the TURP syndrome?

10. How does the patient absorb irrigation solution during TURP? How much irrigation solution is typically absorbed?

11. How can one estimate the volume of irrigation solution absorbed during TURP?

12. What is the relation between the duration of surgery and the incidence of TURP syndrome?

13. What factors increase the incidence of TURP syndrome?

14. What is the effect of excessive absorption of irrigation solution during TURP on cardiopulmonary, renal, and central nervous system (CNS) functions?

15. What is the cause of CNS dysfunction in patients who have undergone TURP?

16. What is the physiologic role of sodium ions in the body? What is the effect of excessive absorption of irrigation solution on serum sodium level?

17. What is the relation between serum sodium level and the incidence of neurologic symptoms in patients who have undergone TURP?

18. What is the effect of acute hyponatremia on the cardiovascular system?

19. What prophylactic measures may reduce the incidence of TURP syndrome?

20. What therapeutic measures are recommended for patients with TURP syndrome?

21. Is saline administration always necessary to correct hyponatremia? What are the risks of rapid correction of hyponatremia?

22. What are the toxic effects of glycine? Is there an antidote to glycine toxicity? What are the metabolic byproducts of glycine?

23. What are the symptoms and clinical course of TURP-induced hyperammonemia?

24. Why do some patients who have undergone TURP develop hyperammonemia and others do not? Is there a preventive treatment against hyperammonemia in these patients?

25. What are the clinical characteristics, causes, and prognosis of TURP-related blindness?

26. What gynecologic procedure has been associated with a syndrome similar to TURP syndrome?

27. What are the causes of excessive bleeding during TURP?

28. What triggers disseminated intravascular coagulopathy in patients undergoing TURP? How would you treat it?

29. What are the causes, signs, and treatment of bladder perforation during TURP?

30. What are the causes, symptoms, and preventive measures of bladder explosion during TURP?

31. What are the causes of hypotension during TURP?

D. Postoperative Management

1. What is the source of postoperative bacteremia in patients who have undergone TURP? What factors increase the incidence of bacteremia?

2. What are the signs of post-TURP septicemia? What preventive measures are recommended?

3. What bacteria-related cause may possibly lead to sudden postoperative shock in patients who have undergone TURP?

4. Is postoperative hypothermia a risk factor for myocardial ischemia?

5. How would you make a diagnosis of perioperative MI?

E. Laser Prostatectomy

1. What is laser prostatectomy? What are its advantages?

A. Medical Disease and Differential Diagnosis

A.1. Are there differences in morbidity and mortality rates between transurethral resection of the prostate (TURP) and suprapubic or retropubic prostatectomy?

TURP is considered by many to be a simpler and safer procedure than "open" prostatectomy. However, despite many improvements in anesthesia and surgery, 7% of patients who have undergone TURP sustain major complications and approximately 1% die perioperatively. No differences are seen in mortality rates between patients who have undergone TURP and those who have undergone retropubic or suprapubic prostatectomy.

Fox M, Hammonds JC, Copland RF. Prostatectomy in patients of 70 and over. *Eur Urol* 1981;7:27–30.

Malhotra V. Transurethral resection of prostate. *Anesthesiol Clin North America* 2000;18: 883–897.

Melchior J, Valk WL, Foret JD, et al. Transurethral prostatectomy: computerized analysis of 2,223 consecutive cases. *J Urol* 1974;112:634–642.

Nanninga JB, O'Coner VJ. Jr Suprapubic prostatectomy: a review, 1966–1970. *J Urol* 1972; 108:453–454.

A.2. What chronic medical conditions are common in patients who have undergone transurethral resection of the prostate (TURP)?

Patients who have undergone TURP are often elderly and suffer from cardiac, pulmonary, vascular, and endocrinologic disorders. The incidence of cardiac disease is 67%; cardiovascular disease, 50%; abnormal electrocardiogram (ECG), 77%; chronic obstructive pulmonary disease,

29%; and diabetes mellitus, 8%. Occasionally, these patients are dehydrated and depleted of essential electrolytes because of long-term diuretic therapy and restricted fluid intake.

Fox M, Hammonds JC, Copland RF. Prostatectomy in patients of 70 and over. *Eur Urol* 1981;7:27–30.

Gravenstein D. Transurethral resection of the prostate (TURP) syndrome: a review of the pathophysiology and management. *Anesth Analg* 1997;84:438–446.

Malhotra V. Transurethral resection of prostate. *Anesthesiol Clin North America* 2000;18: 883–897.

A.3. Does a history of prior myocardial infarction (MI) increase the patient's risk of perioperative reinfarction?

Yes, a history of prior MI is an intermediate predictor of preoperative cardiac morbidity.(See sections A.1 and A.7 in Chapter 15)

A.4. In patients with a history of recent myocardial infarction (MI), would you recommend that the surgery be postponed for a certain period? If so, why?

The American Heart Association/American College of Cardiology Task Force on Perioperative Evaluation of the Cardiac Patient Undergoing Noncardiac Surgery has advocated an MI of less than 6 weeks as the group at highest risk, whereas after that period, risk stratification is based on the presentation of disease (i.e., those with active ischemia being at highest risk). Multiple studies have demonstrated an increased incidence of reinfarction if the MI was within 6 months of surgery. With improvements in perioperative care, this difference has decreased.

Eagle KA, Berger PB, Calkins H, et al. American Heart Association. ACC/AHA guideline update for perioperative cardiovascular evaluation for noncardiac surgery-executive summary. A report of the American College of Cardiology/American Heart Association Task Force on Practice Guidelines (Committee to Update the 1996 Guidelines on Perioperative Cardiovascular Evaluation for Noncardiac Surgery). *J Am Coll Cardiol* 2002;39:542–543.

B. Preoperative Evaluation and Preparation

B.1. How would you evaluate the patient's cardiac condition? What laboratory tests would you like to have done? Would you recommend the patient to undergo coronary angiography before surgery?

In addition to the routine history and physical examination of all organ systems, special attention should be paid to circulatory functions. Minimally, routine electrocardiogram (ECG) and chest radiograph should be obtained to evaluate the presence of myocardial ischemia and/or infarction, as well as congestive heart failure (CHF). Functional capacity of the patient is best evaluated by initial history. If the patient presents with signs and symptoms of CHF, further cardiac testing should be considered.

American Heart Association Task Force on Practice Guidelines. ACC/AHA guideline updates for perioperative cardiovascular evaluation for noncardiac surgery—executive summary. A report of the American College of Cardiology/American Heart Association Task Force on Practice Guidelines. *Anesth Analg* 2002;94:1052–1064.

B.2. Are patients with a Q-wave infarction at greater risk of reinfarction than those with a non–Q-wave infarction?

Recent studies suggest that patients who survive a non–Q-wave infarction are at greater risk of reinfarction than those who survive a Q-wave infarction. (See section B.4 in Chapter 15.)

B.3. Would you discontinue any antihypertensives or any medications for angina?

All antihypertensive and antianginal drugs, especially β-blockers, should be continued until the time of surgery to prevent rebound hypertension and tachycardia that may result from sudden withdrawal of these drugs.

American Heart Association Task Force on Practice Guidelines. ACC/AHA guideline updates for perioperative cardiovascular evaluation for noncardiac surgery–executive summary. A report of the American College of Cardiology/American Heart Association Task Force on Practice Guidelines. *Anesth Analg* 2002;94:1052–1064.

Fleisher LA, Beckman JA, Brown KA, et al. ACC/AHA 2006 guideline update on perioperative cardiovascular evaluation for noncardiac surgery: focused update on perioperative beta-blocker therapy—A report of ACC/AHA task force on practice guidelines. *Anesth Analg* 2007;104:15–26.

C. Intraoperative Management

C.1. What monitors would you use for this patient?

The following monitors would be used for this patient.

- Electrocardiogram (ECG)—simultaneous leads V_5 and II, multiple-lead ST-segment analysis if available
- Blood pressure—noninvasive automatic
- Pulmonary artery catheter if there is evidence of left ventricular dysfunction or pulmonary hypertension
- Central venous pressure line—if the patient has good left ventricular function
- Temperature
- End-tidal CO_2 analyzer—if general anesthesia is administered
- Pulse oximeter for arterial oxygenation

C.2. What anesthetic technique is preferable for patients undergoing transurethral resection of the prostate (TURP) and why?

Regional anesthesia is the anesthetic technique of choice for patients undergoing TURP because of the following reasons:

- It allows monitoring of the patient's mentation and thereby early detection of signs of TURP syndrome.
- It promotes vasodilation and peripheral pooling of blood and thereby reduces the severity of circulatory overloading.

- It reduces blood loss by reducing the blood pressure during surgery.
- It provides postoperative analgesia and thereby reduces the incidence of postoperative hypertension and tachycardia, which often accompanies recovery from general anesthesia.

Barash PG, Cullen BF, Stoelting RK, eds. *Clinical anesthesia*, 5th ed. Philadelphia: Lippincott Williams & Wilkins, 2006:1026–1029.

Madsen RE, Madsen PO. Influence of anesthesia on blood loss in transurethral prostatectomy. *Anesth Analg* 1967;46:330–332.

Malhotra V. *Anesthesia for renal and genituourologic surgery*. New York: McGraw-Hill, 1996: 265–275.

Malhotra V. Transurethral resection of prostate. *Anesthesiol Clin North America* 2000; 18:883–897.

Miller RD, ed. *Miller's anesthesia* 6th ed. Philadelphia: Churchill Livingstone 2005: 2175–2207.

C.3. Is regional anesthesia associated with a lower incidence of perioperative mortality than general anesthesia?

Although spinal anesthesia offers certain distinct advantages over general anesthesia for transurethral resection of the prostate (TURP) surgery, mortality, and many markers of patient outcome have been similar for both groups. The 30-day mortality rate associated with TURP is reported to be between 0.2% and 0.8%. Mortality rates are reported to be similar in patients receiving regional anesthesia or general anesthesia. Increased morbidity was found in patients with resections exceeding 90 minutes, gland size greater than 45 g, acute urinary retention, and age older than 80 years. The incidence of postoperative complications, namely, myocardial infarction (MI), pulmonary embolism, cerebrovascular accidents, transient ischemia attacks, renal failure, hepatic insufficiency, and the need for prolonged ventilation, is similar when comparing patients receiving regional anesthesia with those receiving general anesthesia.

Barash PG, Cullen BF, Stoelting RK, eds. *Clinical anesthesia*, 5th ed. Philadelphia: Lippincott Williams & Wilkins, 2006:1026–1029.

Malhotra V. Transurethral resection of prostate. *Anesthesiol Clin North America* 2000;18: 883–897.

Miller RD. *Miller's anesthesia*, 6th ed. Philadelphia: Churchill Livingstone, 2005:2175–2207.

C.4. What intravenous fluid would you use during transurethral resection of the prostate (TURP)?

Because dilutional hyponatremia commonly occurs in patients undergoing TURP, the intravenous fluid of choice perioperatively is normal saline which contains sodium, 154 mEq per L. It is important, however, to remember that circulatory overloading from absorbed irrigant is common in patients who have undergone TURP; therefore, the amount of intravenous fluid administered during surgery should be carefully monitored.

Barash PG, Cullen BF, Stoelting RK, eds. *Clinical anesthesia*, 5th ed. Philadelphia: Lippincott Williams & Wilkins, 2006:1026–1029.

C.5. After administration of midazolam, 2 mg intravenously, a patient scheduled for transurethral resection of the prostate (TURP) received spinal anesthesia with bupivacaine, 10 mg. The level of anesthesia was T-10. Approximately 40 minutes after the surgery had started, the patient became restless, blood pressure started to rise, and the heart rate decreased. Two more milligrams of midazolam was given. Shortly thereafter, the patient became cyanotic and obtunded, blood pressure fell precipitously, and pupils became dilated and unresponsive to light. What is the differential diagnosis of this set of clinical signs during TURP?

Restlessness and incoherence during TURP are particularly ominous signs of TURP syndrome. These are often caused by subtle pulmonary edema, hypoxemia, and cerebral edema. These signs must not be misinterpreted as signs of inadequate anesthesia. The administration of sedatives or general anesthesia in the presence of TURP syndrome is often fraught with severe complications and even death.

Aasheim GM. Hyponatremia during transurethral surgery. *Can Anaesth Soc J* 1973;20: 274–280.

Gravenstein D. Transurethral resection of the prostate (TURP) syndrome: a review of the pathophysiology and management. *Anesth Analg* 1997;84:438–446.

C.6. What are the important characteristics of irrigation solutions used during transurethral resection of the prostate (TURP)?

TURP irrigation solutions are either isotonic or nearly isotonic, electrically inert, nontoxic, and transparent. Hypotonic solutions are avoided because they can cause hemolysis. Electrolyte-containing solutions are also avoided because they can conduct electrical current from the resectoscope to the surrounding tissues and cause burns. Because significant absorption of irrigation solution occurs during TURP, only solutions with nontoxic solutes are used. Also, the solution must be transparent to allow the surgeon to visualize the surgical site.

Barash PG, Cullen BF, Stoelting RK, eds. *Clinical anesthesia*, 4th ed. Philadelphia: Lippincott Williams & Wilkins, 2006:1026–1029.

Gravenstein D. Transurethral resection of the prostate (TURP) syndrome: a review of the pathophysiology and management. *Anesth Analg* 1997;84:438–446.

Madsen PO, Madsen RE. Clinical and experimental evaluation of different irrigating fluids for transurethral surgery. *Invest Urol* 1965;3:122–129.

Malhotra V. Transurethral resection of prostate. *Anesthesiol Clin North America* 2000;18: 883–897.

C.7. Why is plain distilled water rarely used for irrigation during transurethral resection of the prostate (TURP)? What types of irrigation solutions are available?

Distilled water is totally transparent and electrically inert and in the past was regularly used for irrigation during TURP. However, because it is extremely hypotonic, when absorbed by the patient, it may cause hemolysis, shock, and renal failure.

Over the years, a number of isotonic and nearly isotonic irrigation solutions have been introduced and they almost totally replaced plain distilled water. The more commonly used solution currently is glycine (1.2% and 1.5%). Mannitol (3%), glucose (2.5% to 4%), Cytal (a mixture of sorbitol 2.7% and mannitol 0.54%), and urea (1%) solutions are also occasionally used. To maintain their transparency, these solutions are purposely prepared moderately hypotonic.

Barash PG, Cullen BF, Stoelting RK, eds. *Clinical anesthesia*, 5th ed. Philadelphia: Lippincott Williams & Wilkins, 2006:1026–1029.

Gravenstein D. Transurethral resection of the prostate (TURP) syndrome: a review of the pathophysiology and management. *Anesth Analg* 1997;84:438–446.

Madsen PO, Madsen RE. Clinical and experimental evaluation of different irrigating fluids for transurethral surgery. *Invest Urol* 1965;3:122–129.

Malhotra V. Transurethral resection of prostate. *Anesthesiol Clin North America* 2000;18:883–897.

Miller RD. *Miller's anesthesia*, 6th ed. Philadelphia: Churchill Livingstone, 2005:2175–2207.

C.8. What is the effect of continuous bladder irrigation during transurethral resection of the prostate (TURP) on body temperature?

Several liters of irrigation solution pass through the bladder during TURP, which can reduce body temperature at the rate of 1°C per hour (Fig. 37.1). Approximately half the number of patients undergoing TURP become hypothermic and shiver at the conclusion of surgery.

Allen TD. Body temperature changes during prostatic resection as related to the temperature of the irrigating solution. *J Urol* 1973;110:433–435.

Barash PG, Cullen BF, Stoelting RK, eds. *Clinical anesthesia*, 5th ed. Philadelphia: Lippincott Williams & Wilkins, 2006:1026–1029.

Malhotra V. Transurethral resection of prostate. *Anesthesiol Clin North America* 2000;18:883–897.

Miller RD. *Miller's anesthesia*, 6th ed. Philadelphia: Churchill Livingstone, 2005:2175–2207.

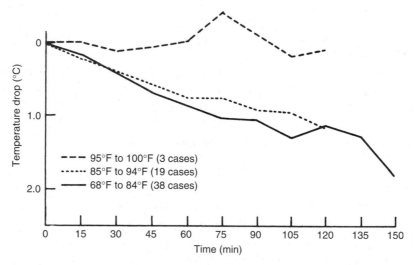

Figure 37.1 The decrease in body temperature during transurethral resection of the prostate (TURP) is related to the temperature of the irrigating solution and to the duration of surgery. (From Allen TD. Body temperature changes during prostatic resection as related to the temperature of the irrigating solution. *J Urol* 1973;110:433–435, with permission.)

C.9. **What are the definition and signs and symptoms of the transurethral resection of the prostate (TURP) syndrome?**

Rapid absorption of a large-volume irrigation solution during TURP can lead to TURP syndrome. The TURP syndrome is characterized by intravascular volume shifts and plasma-solute (osmolarity) effects. The signs and symptoms of the TURP syndrome are as follows:

Cardiopulmonary
  Hypertension
  Bradycardia
  Dysrhythmia
  Respiratory distress
  Cyanosis
  Hypotension
  Shock
  Death
Hematologic and renal
  Hyperglycinemia
  Hyperammonemia
  Hyponatremia
  Hypoosmolality
  Hemolysis/anemia
  Acute renal failure
  Death
Central nervous system (CNS)
  Nausea/vomiting
  Confusion/restlessness
  Blindness
  Twitches/seizures
  Lethargy/paralysis
  Dilated/nonreactive pupils
  Coma
  Death

The TURP syndrome can occur as early as a few minutes after surgery has started and as late as several hours after surgery. The patient begins to complain of dizziness, headaches, nausea, tightness in the chest and throat, and shortness of breath. He then becomes restless, confused, and starts to retch. Some patients complain of abdominal pain. The blood pressure rises (both systolic and diastolic), and the heart rate decreases (Fig. 37.2). If not treated promptly, the patient becomes cyanotic and hypotensive and ultimately sustains cardiac arrest.

Occasionally, the TURP syndrome starts with neurologic signs. The patient first becomes lethargic and then unconscious and the pupils dilate and react sluggishly to light. This can be followed by short episodes of tonic-clonic seizures and then coma that lasts from a few minutes to many hours.

If the patient is under general anesthesia, the presenting signs of the TURP syndrome are typically a rise and then a fall in blood pressure, respiratory arrest, and severe refractory bradycardia. The electrocardiogram (ECG) may show nodal rhythm, ST-segment changes, U waves, and widening of the QRS complex. Recovery from general anesthesia is usually delayed.

Barash PG, Cullen BF, Stoelting RK, eds. *Clinical anesthesia*, 5th ed. Philadelphia: Lippincott Williams & Wilkins, 2006:1026–1029.

Gravenstein D. Transurethral resection of the prostate (TURP) syndrome: a review of the pathophysiology and management. *Anesth Analg* 1997;84:438–446.

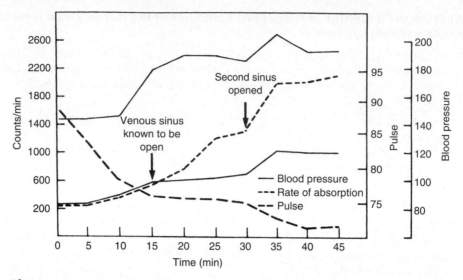

Figure 37.2 The blood pressure, heart rate, and absorption rate of radioactively tagged irrigation solution during transurethral resection of the prostate. (From Taylor RO, Maxson ES, Carter FH, et al. Volumetric gravimetric and radioisotopic determination of fluid transference in transurethral prostatectomy. *J Urol* 1958;79:490–499, with permission.)

Henderson DJ, Middleton RG. Coma from hyponatremia following transurethral resection of prostate. *Urology* 1980;15:267–271.

Hurlbert BJ, Wingard DW. Water intoxication after 15 minutes of transurethral resection of the prostate. *Anesthesiology* 1979;50:355–356.

Malhotra V. Transurethral resection of prostate. *Anesthesiol Clin North America* 2000;18: 883–897.

Miller RD. *Miller's anesthesia*, 6th ed. Philadelphia: Churchill Livingstone, 2005:2175–2207.

Roesch RP, Stoelting RK, Lingeman JE, et al. Ammonia toxicity resulting from glycine absorption during a transurethral resection of the prostate. *Anesthesiology* 1983;58: 577–579.

Still AJ, Modell JA. Acute water intoxication during transurethral resection of the prostate using glycine solution for irrigation. *Anesthesiology* 1973;38:98–99.

C.10. How does the patient absorb irrigation solution during transurethral resection of the prostate (TURP)? How much irrigation solution is typically absorbed?

The irrigation solution enters the bloodstream directly through open prostatic venous sinuses and accumulates in the periprostatic and retroperitoneal spaces. The latter occurs primarily when the prostatic capsule is violated during surgery.

Reports in the literature suggest that as many as 8 L of irrigation solution can be absorbed by the patient during TURP. The average rate of absorption is 20 mL per minute and may reach 200 mL per minute; the average weight gain by the end of surgery is 2 kg (Fig. 37.3).

Barash PG, Cullen BF, Stoelting RK, eds. *Clinical anesthesia*, 5th ed. Philadelphia: Lippincott Williams & Wilkins, 2006:1026–1029.

Masloff JI, Milam JH, Bunts RC. Fluid and electrolyte changes associated with transurethral prostatic resection. *South Med J* 1966;59:1203–1208.

Oester A, Madsen PO. Determination of absorption of irrigating fluid during transurethral resection of the prostate by means of radioisotope. *J Urol* 1969;102:714–719.

C.11. How can one estimate the volume of irrigation solution absorbed during transurethral resection of the prostate (TURP)?

A practical method to estimate the absorbed volume of irrigation solution during TURP is based on the following equation:

$$\text{Volume absorbed} = \frac{\text{preoperative [Na}^+]}{\text{postoperative [Na}^+]} \times \text{extracellular fluid} - \text{extracellular fluid}$$

To use this equation, serum sodium level ([Na$^+$]) is determined at the beginning of surgery and again at the time of estimation of the volume absorbed. The extracellular fluid (ECF) volume is assumed to be 20% to 30% of body weight. For example, if the patient's preoperative body weight is 60 kg and the ECF is assumed to constitute 20% of the patient's body weight, then a decrease in serum sodium level from 140 to 100 mEq per L would suggest an absorption of 4.8 L:

$$140/100 \times \text{ECF} - \text{ECF} = 1.4\ \text{ECF} - \text{ECF} = 0.4\ \text{ECF} = 0.4 \times 60 \times 20\% = 4.8\text{L}$$

Henderson DJ, Middleton RG. Coma from hyponatremia following transurethral resection of prostate. *Urology* 1980;15:267–271.

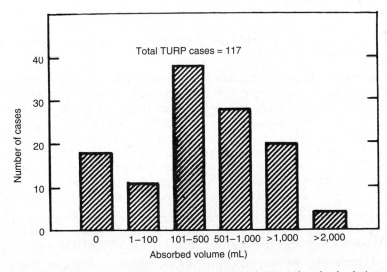

Figure 37.3 The volume of irrigation solution absorbed during transurethral resection of the prostate. (From Madsen PO, Madsen RE. Clinical and experimental evaluation of different irrigating fluids for transurethral surgery. *Invest Urol* 1965;3:122–129, with permission.)

C.12. What is the relation between the duration of surgery and the incidence of the transurethral resection of the prostate (TURP) syndrome?

Many believe that the duration of surgery is the most important determinant of incidence of TURP syndrome. However, several studies in the literature report severe TURP syndrome occurring as early as 15 to 20 minutes after surgery has started. In general, poor correlation is seen between the duration of surgery and the amount of irrigation solution absorbed. In one large series, morbidity and mortality of patients undergoing TURP did not correlate with length of surgery, except when surgery lasted more than 150 minutes. Similarly, the incidence and severity of hyponatremia did not correlate with the duration of surgery.

Aasheim GM. Hyponatremia during transurethral surgery. *Can Anaesth Soc J* 1973;20: 274–280.

Barash PG, Cullen BF, Stoelting RK, eds. *Clinical anesthesia*, 5th ed. Philadelphia: Lippincott Williams & Wilkins, 2006:1026–1029.

Desmond J. Serum osmolality and plasma electrolytes in patients who develop dilutional hyponatremia during transurethral resection. *Can J Surg* 1970;13:116–121.

Hurlbert BJ, Wingard DW. Water intoxication after 15 minutes of transurethral resection of the prostate. *Anesthesiology* 1979;50:355–356.

Malhotra V. Transurethral resection of prostate. *Anesthesiol Clin North America* 2000;18: 883–897.

Melchior J, Valk WL, Foret JD, et al. Transurethral prostatectomy: computerized analysis of 2,223 consecutive cases. *J Urol* 1974;112:634–642.

Miller RD. *Miller's anesthesia*, 6th ed. Philadelphia: Churchill Livingstone, 2005:2175–2207.

Oester A, Madsen PO. Determination of absorption of irrigating fluid during transurethral resection of the prostate by means of radioisotope. *J Urol* 1969;102:714–719.

Osborn DE, Rao PN, Green MJ, et al. Fluid absorption during transurethral resection. *Br Med J* 1980;281:1549–1550.

C.13. What factors increase the incidence of the transurethral resection of the prostate (TURP) syndrome?

TURP syndrome is more likely to occur if the prostatic gland is particularly large, the prostatic capsule is violated during surgery, or the hydrostatic pressure of the irrigation solution is excessively high. Large prostatic glands have rich venous networks that promote intravascular absorption of irrigation solution. The violation of the prostatic capsule during surgery promotes entry of irrigation solution into the periprostatic and retroperitoneal spaces. The hydrostatic pressure of the irrigation solution is an important determinant of the solution absorption rate of the patient. This pressure depends primarily on the height of the irrigation solution pole. When the height of the pole exceeds 60 cm, the absorption of irrigation solution is greatly enhanced. Also, an excessively distended bladder during surgery facilitates absorption.

Gravenstein D. Transurethral resection of the prostate (TURP) syndrome: a review of the pathophysiology and management. *Anesth Analg* 1997;84:438–446.

Hulten J, Bengtsson M, Engberg A, et al. The pressure in the prostatic fossa and fluid absorption. *Scand J Urol Nephrol* 1984;82(Suppl):33–43.

Logie JRC, Keenan RA, Whiting PH, et al. Fluid absorption during transurethral prostatectomy. *J Urol* 1980;52:526–528.

Madsen PO, Naber KG. The importance of the pressure in the prostatic fossa and absorption of irrigation fluid during transurethral resection of prostate. *J Urol* 1973;109:446–452.

Malhotra V. Transurethral resection of prostate. *Anesthesiol Clin North America* 2000;18: 883–897.

Miller RD. *Miller's anesthesia*, 6th ed. Philadelphia: Churchill Livingstone, 2005:2175–2207.

C.14. What is the effect of excessive absorption of irrigation solution during transurethral resection of the prostate (TURP) on cardiopulmonary, renal, and central nervous system (CNS) functions?

Excessive absorption of irrigation solution during TURP causes hypervolemia and hypertension and may provoke angina and pulmonary edema (Fig. 37.4). It may also have an adverse effect on renal function. An inverse relation has been observed between the amount of irrigation solution absorbed during surgery and postoperative urinary output.

Some patients with TURP syndrome exhibit neurologic signs resulting from water intoxication. They assume a decerebrate posture, exhibit clonus and positive Babinski's reflex, and eventually convulse and lapse into coma. Examination of the eyes reveals papilledema and dilated and

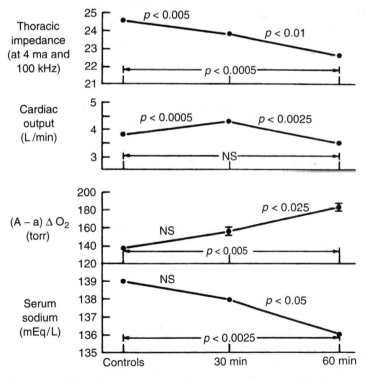

Figure 37.4 Mean changes in thoracic impedance, cardiac output, alveolar–arterial oxygen tension difference, and serum sodium level during transurethral resection of the prostate. NS, nonsignificant. (From Casthely P, Ramanathan S, Chalon J, et al. Decrease in electric impedance during transurethral resection of the prostate: an index of early water intoxication. *J Urol* 1981;125:347–349, with permission.)

sluggishly reacting pupils. The electroencephalogram (EEG) shows low-voltage bilaterally. The patients remain in coma from a few hours to several days.

Barash PG, Cullen BF, Stoelting RK, eds. *Clinical anesthesia*, 5th ed. Philadelphia: Lippincott Williams & Wilkins, 2006:1026–1029.

Casthely P, Ramanathan S, Chalon J, et al. Decrease in electric impedance during transurethral resection of the prostate: an index of early water intoxication. *J Urol* 1981;125:347–349.

Charlton AJ. Cardiac arrest during transurethral prostatectomy after absorption of 1.5% glycine. A case report and review of the literature. *Anaesthesia* 1980;35:804–806.

Desmond J. Serum osmolality and plasma electrolytes in patients who develop dilutional hyponatremia during transurethral resection. *Can J Surg* 1970;13:116–121.

Gravenstein D. Transurethral resection of the prostate (TURP) syndrome: a review of the pathophysiology and management. *Anesth Analg* 1997;84:438–446.

Hahn R, Berlin T, Lewenhaupt A. Rapid massive irrigating fluid absorption during transurethral resection of the prostate. *Acta Chir Scand* 1986;530(Suppl):63–65.

Henderson DJ, Middleton RG. Coma from hyponatremia following transurethral resection of prostate. *Urology* 1980;15:267–271.

Malhotra V. Transurethral resection of prostate. *Anesthesiol Clin North America* 2000;18:883–897.

Miller RD. *Miller's anesthesia*, 6th ed. Philadelphia: Churchill Livingstone, 2005:2175–2207.

C.15. What is the cause of central nervous system (CNS) dysfunction in patients who have undergone transurethral resection of the prostate (TURP)?

The crucial physiologic derangement of CNS function is not hyponatremia *per se*, but acute hypoosmolality. This is predictable because the blood–brain barrier is essentially impermeable to sodium but freely permeable to water. Cerebral edema caused by acute hypoosmolality can increase intracranial pressure, which results in bradycardia and hypertension by the Cushing reflex. Furthermore, cerebral edema is not caused by decreased serum colloid oncotic pressure, but by decreased osmolality. Apparently, the hypervolemia and hyponatremia that often accompany TURP promote cerebral edema and this in turn raises intracranial pressure and provokes neurologic symptoms. The rise in intracranial pressure is directly related to the gain in body weight during TURP.

Barash PG, Cullen BF, Stoelting RK, eds. *Clinical anesthesia*, 5th ed. Philadelphia: Lippincott Williams & Wilkins, 2006:1026–1029.

Gravenstein D. Transurethral resection of the prostate (TURP) syndrome: a review of the pathophysiology and management. *Anesth Analg* 1997;84:438–446.

Malhotra V. Transurethral resection of prostate. *Anesthesiol Clin North America* 2000;18:883–897.

C.16. What is the physiologic role of sodium ions in the body? What is the effect of excessive absorption of irrigation solution on serum sodium level?

Sodium is a ubiquitous electrolyte that is essential for proper function of excitatory cells, particularly those of the heart and brain. Extreme reduction in serum sodium level alters brain function, as well as cardiac and renal function.

During transurethral resection of the prostate (TURP), serum sodium level typically falls 3 to 10 mEq per L. However, the correlation between the severity of the hyponatremia and the amount of irrigation solution absorbed during surgery is inconsistent. Apparently, the fall in serum sodium level depends primarily on the rate at which the irrigation solution is absorbed rather than the total amount absorbed.

Barash PG, Cullen BF, Stoelting RK, eds. *Clinical anesthesia*, 5th ed. Philadelphia: Lippincott Williams & Wilkins, 2006:1026–1029.

Desmond J. Serum osmolality and plasma electrolytes in patients who develop dilutional hyponatremia during transurethral resection. *Can J Surg* 1970;13:116–121.

Hahn RG. Relations between irrigation absorption rate and hyponatraemia during transurethral resection of the prostate. *Acta Anaesthesiol Scand* 1988;32:53–60.

Malhotra V. Transurethral resection of prostate. *Anesthesiol Clin North America* 2000;18: 883–897.

Rhymer JC, Bell TJ, Perry KC, et al. Hyponatremia following transurethral resection of the prostate. *Br J Urol* 1985;57:450–452.

C.17. What is the relation between serum sodium level and the incidence of neurologic symptoms in patients who have undergone transurethral resection of the prostate (TURP)?

Acute severe hyponatremia is often associated with abnormal neurologic symptoms, and it can lead to irreversible brain damage. The neurologic signs may be accompanied by electroencephalogram (EEG) abnormalities such as loss of α-wave activity and irregular discharge of high-amplitude slow-wave activity. However, the correlation between the severity of the hyponatremia and the incidence of neurologic symptoms is inconsistent because hyponatremia may not be the sole or even the primary cause of the neurologic manifestations of TURP syndrome. The crucial derangement of central nervous system (CNS) function is not hyponatremia *per se*, but acute hypoosmolarity. In some cases, moderate hyponatremia is associated with severe neurologic symptoms; in others, severe hyponatremia causes no symptoms at all. Apparently, the determining factor is the rate at which the serum sodium level falls rather than the total fall. The faster the fall in serum sodium level the greater the incidence of neurologic symptoms. A slow fall in serum sodium level apparently allows the CNS to adapt to the hyponatremia.

Barash PG, Cullen BF, Stoelting RK, eds. *Clinical anesthesia*, 5th ed. Philadelphia: Lippincott Williams & Wilkins, 2006:1026–1029.

Gravenstein D. Transurethral resection of the prostate (TURP) syndrome: a review of the pathophysiology and management. *Anesth Analg* 1997;84:438–446.

Henderson DJ, Middleton RG. Coma from hyponatremia following transurethral resection of prostate. *Urology* 1980;15:267–271.

Malhotra V. Transurethral resection of prostate. *Anesthesiol Clin North America* 2000;18: 883–897.

C.18. What is the effect of acute hyponatremia on the cardiovascular system?

When serum sodium level falls to less than 120 mEq per L, signs of cardiovascular depression can occur. A decrease to less than 115 mEq per L causes bradycardia, widening of the QRS complex, ST-segment elevation, ventricular ectopic beats, and T-wave inversion. Patients with a serum sodium level of less than 110 mEq per L can develop respiratory and cardiac arrest.

Barash PG, Cullen BF, Stoelting RK, eds. *Clinical anesthesia*, 5th ed. Philadelphia: Lippincott Williams & Wilkins, 2006:1026–1029.

Logie JRC, Keenan RA, Whiting PH, et al. Fluid absorption during transurethral prostatectomy. *J Urol* 1980;52:526–528.

Malhotra V. Transurethral resection of prostate. *Anesthesiol Clin North America* 2000;18: 883–897.

Mebust WK, Brady TW, Valk WL. Observations on cardiac output, blood volume, central venous pressure, fluid and electrolyte changes in patients undergoing transurethral prostatectomy. *J Urol* 1970;103:632–636.

Osborn DE, Rao PN, Green MJ, et al. Fluid absorption during transurethral resection. *Br Med J* 1980;281:1549–1550.

Stoelting RK, Dierdorf SF. *Anesthesia and co-existing disease*, 4th ed. New York: Churchill Livingstone, 2002:367–371.

Surawicz B. Relationship between electrocardiogram and electrolytes. *Am Heart J* 1967; 73:814–834.

C.19. What prophylactic measures may reduce the incidence of transurethral resection of the prostate (TURP) syndrome?

The incidence of TURP syndrome depends primarily on the surgeon's technical skills. However, if the patient is properly prepared before surgery and closely monitored during surgery, the incidence and severity of the syndrome can be reduced.

Fluid and electrolyte imbalance should be corrected preoperatively and special attention paid to the serum sodium level during surgery. Patients with preoperative CHF should be treated vigorously with diuretics and fluid restriction. A conservative surgical approach should be considered in critically ill patients. A simple canalization or balloon dilation of the urethra or a staged TURP is less likely to provoke TURP syndrome.

The most important preventive measure during surgery is preservation of the prostatic capsule. Another preventive measure is limiting the hydrostatic pressure of the irrigation solution to 60 cm H_2O. This can be accomplished by limiting the height of the irrigation pole to 60 cm. Also, the bladder should not be allowed to overdistend and the duration of surgery should be restricted.

If a sudden significant decrease in serum sodium level occurs, the surgeon should be informed and therapeutic measures immediately instituted. If the sodium blood level decreases to less than 120 mEq per L, surgery should be terminated as soon as possible.

Intravenous fluids should be cautiously administered during TURP. A microdrip is recommended particularly in patients with cardiac or renal disease. If regional anesthesia causes hypotension, a small dose of a vasoconstrictor is recommended to raise the blood pressure, rather than rapid infusion of intravenous fluids.

Gale DW, Notley RG. TURP without TURP syndrome. *Br J Urol* 1985;57:708–710.

Gravenstein D. Transurethral resection of the prostate (TURP) syndrome: a review of the pathophysiology and management. *Anesth Analg* 1997;84:438–446.

Malhotra V. *Anesthesia for renal and genituourologic surgery*. New York: McGraw-Hill, 1996: 93–109.

Watkins-Pitchford JM, Payne SR, Rennie CD, et al. Hyponatremia during transurethral resection. Its practical prevention. *Br J Urol* 1984;56:676–678.

C.20. What therapeutic measures are recommended for patients with transurethral resection of the prostate (TURP) syndrome?

When symptoms of TURP syndrome appear, the following therapeutic measures are recommended:

- Terminate surgery as soon as possible.
- Administer furosemide, 20 mg intravenously.
- Administer oxygen by nasal cannula or face mask.
- If the patient develops pulmonary edema, consider tracheal intubation and positive pressure ventilation with oxygen.
- Draw a sample of arterial blood for blood gas and serum sodium analysis.
- If the serum sodium level is abnormally low and clinical signs of hyponatremia are seen, intravenous administration of hypertonic saline (3% to 5%) may be recommended. The hypertonic solution should be given at a rate no faster than 100 mL per hour. In most cases, no more than 300 mL of saline is needed to correct the hyponatremia.
- If the patient develops seizures, a short-acting anticonvulsant agent such as diazepam, 5 to 20 mg, or midazolam, 2 to 10 mg, can be administered intravenously. If this does not stop the seizures, a barbiturate or phenytoin can be added. As a last resort, a muscle relaxant may also be used.
- If pulmonary edema or hypotension develops, invasive hemodynamic monitoring is recommended. This will serve as a guide for pharmacologic support and fluid administration.
- If significant blood loss is suspected, the administration of packed red blood cells should be considered. In general, intravenous fluids should be administered cautiously because of the propensity of these patients to develop pulmonary edema.

Barash PG, Cullen BF, Stoelting RK, eds. *Clinical anesthesia*, 5th ed. Philadelphia: Lippincott Williams & Wilkins, 2006:1026–1029.

Malhotra V. Transurethral resection of prostate. *Anesthesiol Clin North America* 2000;18: 883–897.

Miller RD. *Miller's anesthesia*, 6th ed. Philadelphia: Churchill Livingstone, 2005:2175–2207.

C.21. Is saline administration always necessary to correct hyponatremia? What are the risks of rapid correction of hyponatremia?

The administration of hypertonic saline to correct hyponatremia is not always necessary and can sometimes be detrimental. Unless the patient develops clinical signs of hyponatremia, saline administration is not recommended. Spontaneous or induced diuresis usually corrects the hyponatremia within a few hours.

Patients who have undergone transurethral resection of the prostate (TURP) often sustain circulatory overloading during surgery, so saline administration in these patients can provoke pulmonary edema. In addition, rapid administration of hypertonic saline has been associated with central pontine myelinolysis (osmotic demyelination syndrome)—a poorly understood and fatal neurologic complication.

To reduce the hazards of saline administration, serum osmolarity should be monitored and corrected aggressively only until symptoms substantially resolve; then hyponatremia should be corrected at a rate no faster than 1.5 mEq/L/hour.

Day JO. Acute water intoxication complicating transurethral resection of the prostate. *J Med Assoc Ga* 1983;72:845–846.

Gravenstein D. Transurethral resection of prostate (TURP) syndrome: a review of pathophysiology and management. *Anesth Analg* 1997;84:438–446.

Rothenberg DM, Berns AS, Ivankovich AD. Isotonic hyponatremia following transurethral prostate resection. *J Clin Anesth* 1990;2:48–53.

Sterns RH, Riggs JE, Schochet SS Jr. Osmotic demyelinization syndrome following correction of hyponatremia. *N Engl J Med* 1986;314:1535–1542.

C.22. What are the toxic effects of glycine? Is there an antidote to glycine toxicity? What are the metabolic byproducts of glycine?

Glycine is an inhibitory neurotransmitter similar to γ-aminobutyric acid in the spinal cord and brain. When absorbed by the patient in large amounts, glycine has direct toxic effects on the heart and retina. In patients who have undergone transurethral resection of the prostate (TURP), glycine absorption has been shown to cause an average decrease of 17.5% in cardiac output. In animal studies, the administration of the amino acid arginine reversed the myocardial depressing effect of glycine. Neither the mechanism by which glycine depresses cardiac function nor the one by which arginine protects the heart is known.

Hyperglycinemia may cause transient visual disturbance (blindness) during TURP. However, glycine toxicity in patients who have undergone TURP is uncommon, probably because most of the absorbed glycine is retained in the periprostatic and retroperitoneal spaces, where access to the circulation is limited.

The most common metabolites of glycine are ammonia and glyoxylic and oxalic acids (Fig. 37.5). In some patients, excessive absorption of glycine during TURP leads to hyperammonemia. Hyperoxaluria could compromise renal function in patients with coexisting renal disease, as is often present in elderly patients undergoing TURP.

Glycine may cause encephalopathy and seizures through its ability to potentiate the effects of *N*-methyl D-aspartate (NMDA), an excitatory neurotransmitter. Magnesium exerts a negative control on the NMDA receptor, and hypomagnesemia caused by dilution may increase the

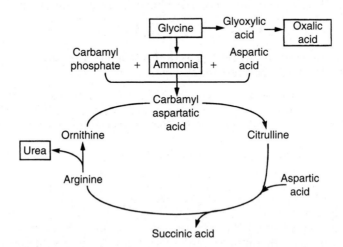

Figure 37.5 Metabolic pathways of glycine. (From McGilvery RW, Goldstein GW. *Biochemistry: a functional approach,* 3rd ed. Philadelphia: WB Saunders, 1983:584, with permission.)

susceptibility to seizures. For this reason, a trial of magnesium therapy may be indicated in patients who develop seizures during TURP.

Barash PG, Cullen BF, Stoelting RK, eds. *Clinical anesthesia,* 5th ed. Philadelphia: Lippincott Williams & Wilkins, 2006:1026–1029.

Gravenstein D. Transurethral resection of the prostate (TURP) syndrome: a review of the pathophysiology and management. *Anesth Analg* 1997;84:438–446.

Handler P, Kamin H, Harris JS. The metabolism of parenterally administered amino acid, I: glycine. *J Biol Chem* 1949;179:283–301.

Malhotra V. Transurethral resection of prostate. *Anesthesiol Clin North America* 2000;18: 883–897.

McGilvery RW, Goldstein GW. *Biochemistry: a functional approach,* 3rd ed. Philadelphia: WB Saunders, 1983:584.

Miller RD. *Miller's anesthesia*, 6th ed. Philadelphia: Churchill, Livingstone, 2005:2175–2207.

Ovassapian A, Joshi CW, Brumer EA. Visual disturbances: an unusual symptom of transurethral prostatic resection reaction. *Anesthesiology* 1982;57:332–334.

Wang JM, Wong KC, Creel DJ, et al. Effects of glycine on hemodynamic responses and visual evoked potentials in the dog. *Anesth Analg* 1985;64:1071–1077.

C.23. What are the symptoms and clinical course of transurethral resection of the prostate (TURP)-induced hyperammonemia?

The signs and symptoms of hyperammonemia usually appear within 1 hour of surgery. Typically, the patient becomes nauseated, vomits, and then becomes comatose. Blood ammonia level rises to more than 500 mmol per L. The patient remains comatose for 10 to 12 hours and eventually awakens when ammonia blood level decreases to less than 150 mmol per L. The hyperammonemia tends to linger postoperatively, probably because glycine absorption from the periprostatic space continues after surgery.

Malhotra V. Transurethral resection of prostate. *Anesthesiol Clin North America* 2000;18: 883–897.

Oester A, Madsen PO. Determination of absorption of irrigating fluid during transurethral resection of the prostate by means of radioisotope. *J Urol* 1969;102:714–719.

C.24. Why do some patients who have undergone transurethral resection of the prostate (TURP) develop hyperammonemia and others do not? Is there a preventive treatment against hyperammonemia in these patients?

Because ammonia is metabolized primarily in the liver, it has been speculated that hyperammonemia after TURP is a result of liver dysfunction. However, no liver dysfunction has been found in these patients. Further, there is no evidence that patients with a known liver dysfunction are susceptible to hyperammonemia after TURP.

A more plausible explanation for the hyperammonemia is arginine deficiency. Normally, the ornithine cycle in the liver converts ammonia to urea (Fig. 37.5). Arginine is an important intermediate product of this cycle. Apparently, patients who have undergone TURP while having arginine deficiency cannot detoxify the excess ammonia produced from glycine metabolism and therefore develop hyperammonemia. The time necessary to deplete the endogenous arginine stores may be as brief as 12 hours, which approximates the preoperative fasting time.

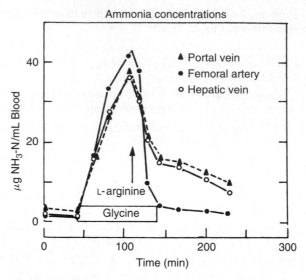

Figure 37.6 Ammonia blood levels during glycine administration in dogs before and after arginine supplementation. (From Nathans D, Fahey JL, Ship AG. Sites of origin and removal of blood ammonia formed during glycine infusion: effect of l-arginine. *J Lab Clin Med* 1958;51:124–133, with permission.)

Several studies support this hypothesis. In dogs, the administration of arginine concurrently with glycine reduced the secretion of ammonia by the liver (Fig. 37.6). In humans, prophylactic administration of arginine or ornithine prevents hyperammonemia that otherwise follows rapid intravenous administration of glycine. Routine administration of arginine in patients undergoing TURP, however, is not recommended because they rarely develop hyperammonemia.

Fahey JL. Toxicity and blood ammonia rise resulting from intravenous amino acid administration in man: the protective effect of l-arginine. *J Clin Invest* 1957;36:1647–1655.

Fahey JL, Perry RS, McCoy PF. Blood ammonia elevation and toxicity from intravenous L-amino acid administration to dogs: the protection role of L-arginine. *Am J Physiol* 1958;192:311–317.

Gravenstein D. Transurethral resection of the prostate (TURP) syndrome: a review of the pathophysiology and management. *Anesth Analg* 1997;84: 438–446.

Nathans D, Fahey JL, Ship AG. Sites of origin and removal of blood ammonia formed during glycine infusion: effect of L-arginine. *J Lab Clin Med* 1958;51:124–133.

Roesch RP, Stoelting RK, Lingeman JE, et al. Ammonia toxicity resulting from glycine absorption during a transurethral resection of the prostate. *Anesthesiology* 1983;58: 577–579.

Ryder KW, Olson JF, Khanoski RJ, et al. Hyperammonemia after transurethral resection of the prostate: a report of 2 cases. *J Urol* 1984;132:995–997.

C.25. What are the clinical characteristics, causes, and prognosis of transurethral resection of the prostate (TURP)-related blindness?

Transient blindness is one of the more alarming complications of TURP. The patient complains of blurred vision and of seeing halos around objects. This can occur either during surgery or later in the recovery room. Although it is sometimes accompanied by other TURP-related complications, the blindness usually occurs as an isolated symptom. Examination of the eyes reveals dilated and unresponsive pupils. Postoperatively, TURP-related blindness gradually resolves and the eyesight returns to normal within 8 to 48 hours of surgery.

The cause of TURP-related blindness is not clear. The intraocular pressure and optic discs remain normal. In the past, edema of the cerebral optical cortex was suspected; however, the clinical signs of TURP-related blindness are consistent with retinal rather than cortical dysfunction. Unlike cortical blindness, TURP-related blindness allows perception of light and the blink reflex is preserved. TURP-related blindness is most likely caused by a toxic effect of glycine on the retina. This theory is supported by the fact that glycine is a known inhibitory neurotransmitter. In animals, glycine has been shown to inhibit neuronal visual pathways. Also, the severity of TURP-related blindness is directly related to glycine blood level. Postoperatively, the vision gradually improves as the glycine blood level declines.

Appelt GL, Benson GS, Corrier JN Jr. Transient blindness: unusual initial symptom of transurethral prostatic resection reaction. *Urology* 1979;13:402–404.

Defalque RJ, Miller DW. Visual disturbances during transurethral resection of the prostate. *Can Anaesth Soc J* 1975;22:620–621.

Gravenstein D. Transurethral resection of the prostate (TURP) syndrome: a review of the pathophysiology and management. *Anesth Analg* 1997;84:438–446.

Kaiser R, Adragna MG, Weis FR Jr, et al. Transient blindness following transurethral resection of the prostate in an achondroplastic dwarf. *J Urol* 1985;133:685.

Korol S, Leunberger PM, Englert U, et al. *In vivo* effects of glycine on retinal ultrastructure and averaged electroretinogram. *Brain Res* 1975;97:235–251.

Malhotra V. Transurethral resection of prostate. *Anesthesiol Clin North America* 2000;18:883–897.

Ovassapian A, Joshi CW, Brumer EA. Visual disturbances: an unusual symptom of transurethral prostatic resection reaction. *Anesthesiology* 1982;57:332–334.

Wang JM, Wong KC, Creel DJ, et al. Effects of glycine on hemodynamic responses and visual evoked potentials in the dog. *Anesth Analg* 1985;64:1071–1077.

C.26. What gynecologic procedure has been associated with a syndrome similar to transurethral resection of the prostate (TURP) syndrome?

Hysteroscopy has been associated with symptoms not unlike those of TURP syndrome. The procedure involves visualization of the interior lining of the uterus for diagnostic purposes and on occasion for transcervical resection of the endometrium or submucous myomectomy. The latter often requires electrical cauterization. As with TURP, hysteroscopy requires irrigation with nonionic isotonic solutions. Commonly used solutions contain either glucose or glycine. Side effects such as hyponatremia, hyperglycemia, circulatory overloading, and coagulopathy have been reported.

Carson SA, Hubert GD, Schriock ED, et al. Hyperglycemia and hyponatremia during operative hysteroscopy with 5% dextrose in water distention. *Fertil Steril* 1989;51:341–343.

Goldenberg M, Zolti M, Seidman DS, et al. Transient blood oxygen desaturation, hypercapnia, and coagulopathy after operative hysteroscopy with glycine used as the distending medium. *Am J Obstet Gynecol* 1994;170:25–29.

C.27. What are the causes of excessive bleeding during transurethral resection of the prostate (TURP)?

Patients undergoing TURP commonly bleed perioperatively. One possible cause is dilutional thrombocytopenia resulting from excessive absorption of irrigation solution. Another possible cause is local release fibrinolytic agents (plasminogen and urokinase) from the mucosa of the lower urinary tract. During and immediately after TURP, these agents cause local fibrinolysis and promote bleeding from the raw surfaces of the prostatic gland. The existence of a local fibrinolytic mechanism is supported by the observation that prophylactic administration of ϵ-aminocaproic acid (an antifibrinolytic agent) reduces bleeding from the prostatic bed.

Systemic coagulopathy can also occur during TURP. Contrary to common misconception, the coagulopathy is due to disseminated intravascular coagulation (DIC), rather than primary fibrinolysis. Characteristically, the platelet count and fibrinogen blood level are abnormally low. At autopsy, multiple microthrombi are observed in various parts of the body. The high level of fibrin-degradation products found in the blood of these patients is caused by secondary fibrinolysis, which commonly accompanies DIC.

Barash PG, Cullen BF, Stoelting RK, eds. *Clinical anesthesia*, 5th ed. Philadelphia: Lippincott Williams & Wilkins, 2006:1026–1029.

Ladehoff AA, Rasmussen J. Fibrinolysis and thromboplastic activities in relation to hemorrhage in transvesical prostatectomy. *Scand J Clin Lab Invest* 1961;13:231–244.

Ljungner H, Bergquist D, Isacson S. Plasminogen activator activity in patients undergoing transvesical and transurethral prostatectomy. *Eur Urol* 1983;9:24–27.

Malhotra V. Transurethral resection of prostate. *Anesthesiol Clin North America* 2000;18: 883–897.

Miller RD. *Miller's anesthesia*, 6th ed. Philadelphia: Churchill Livingstone, 2005:2175–2207.

Smith RB, Riach P, Kaufman JJ. Epsilon aminocaproic acid and the control of post-prostatectomy bleeding: a prospective double blind study. *J Urol* 1984;131:1093–1095.

C.28. What triggers disseminated intravascular coagulopathy in patients undergoing transurethral resection of the prostate (TURP)? How would you treat it?

Apparently disseminated intravascular coagulation (DIC) is triggered during TURP by prostatic particles rich in thromboplastin that enter the bloodstream during surgery. The recommended treatment for DIC is replacement of blood loss and administration of platelets, cryoprecipitates, and fresh frozen plasma. Heparin administration is controversial.

Friedman NJ, Hoag MS, Robinson AJ, et al. Hemorrhagic syndrome following transurethral prostatic resection for benign adenoma. *Arch Intern Med* 1969;124:341–349.

Ladehoff AA, Rasmussen J. Fibrinolysis and thromboplastic activities in relation to hemorrhage in transvesical prostatectomy. *Scand J Clin Lab Invest* 1961;13:231–244.

Malhotra V, ed. *Anesthesia for renal and genito-urologic surgery*. New York: McGraw-Hill, 1996:108.

Malhotra V. Transurethral resection of prostate. *Anesthesiol Clin North America* 2000;18: 883–897.

C.29. What are the causes, signs, and treatment of bladder perforation during transurethral resection of the prostate (TURP)?

The incidence of bladder perforation during TURP is approximately 1%. The causes are trauma by surgical instrumentation, overdistention of the bladder, and rarely explosion of traces of hydrogen gas inside the bladder.

An early sign of bladder perforation is a sudden decrease in return of irrigation solution from the bladder. This sign often goes unnoticed until a significant amount of irrigation solution accumulates in the abdomen and causes abdominal distress. Other clinical signs are hypotension, followed by hypertension and nausea. Reflex-type movements of the limbs have been observed under both general and regional anesthesia. When the perforation is intraperitoneal, the symptoms develop faster; they include severe shoulder pain caused by diaphragmatic irritation.

Diagnosis of bladder perforation is confirmed using cystourethrography. Treatment is immediate suprapubic cystotomy.

Barash PG, Cullen BF, Stoelting RK, eds. *Clinical anesthesia*, 5th ed. Philadelphia: Lippincott Williams & Wilkins, 2006:1026–1029.

Hansen RI, Iverson P. Bladder explosion during uninterrupted transurethral resection of the prostate: a case report and experimental model. *Scand J Urol Nephrol* 1979;13:211–212.

Malhotra V. Transurethral resection of prostate. *Anesthesiol Clin North America* 2000;18: 883–897.

C.30. What are the causes, symptoms, and preventive measures of bladder explosion during transurethral resection of the prostate (TURP)?

A rare but extremely dangerous complication of TURP is gas explosion inside the bladder during surgery. Various explosive gases, particularly hydrogen, are generated by the cauterization of prostatic or bladder tissue during TURP. The explosion is triggered by the hot metal loop of the resectoscope. After a loud thump, the patient complains of sudden abdominal pain. This is accompanied by an abrupt decline in the return of irrigation solution. Usually, the concentration of oxygen in the bladder is too low to support combustion or explosion. However, if air is allowed to enter the irrigation system during surgery, the oxygen concentration in the bladder will rise and this in turn may support an explosion.

Strict precautions should be taken to prevent entry of air into the bladder during TURP. If air is observed in the bladder at the beginning of surgery, it must be evacuated before cauterization starts. The bladder should be emptied often to avoid accumulation of explosive gases during surgery.

Hansen RI, Iverson P. Bladder explosion during uninterrupted transurethral resection of the prostate: a case report and experimental model. *Scand J Urol Nephrol* 1979;13:211–212.

C.31. What are the causes of hypotension during transurethral resection of the prostate (TURP)?

The more common causes of hypotension during TURP are circulatory overloading with CHF, myocardial infarction (MI) or myocardial ischemia, severe anemia resulting from blood loss, and severe hyponatremia and water intoxication.

D. Postoperative Management

D.1. What is the source of postoperative bacteremia in patients who have undergone transurethral resection of the prostate (TURP)? What factors increase the incidence of bacteremia?

The prostatic gland often harbors large amounts of various bacteria. TURP facilitates the entry of these bacteria into the bloodstream, leading to postoperative bacteremia. Also, a preoperative indwelling catheter promotes bacterial growth in the urethra. Approximately 30% of patients undergoing TURP have infected urine preoperatively, and half of them sustain bacteremia postoperatively.

Surgical disruption of the prostatic venous sinuses and excessive hydrostatic pressure of the irrigation solution facilitate the entry of bacteria into the bloodstream.

Barash PG, Cullen BF, Stoelting RK, eds. *Clinical anesthesia*, 5th ed. Philadelphia: Lippincott Williams & Wilkins, 2006:1026–1029.

Kidd EE, Kennedy B. Bacteremia, septicemia, and intravascular haemolysis during transurethral resection of the prostate gland. *Br J Urol* 1965;37:551–559.

Malhotra V. Transurethral resection of prostate. *Anesthesiol Clin North America* 2000;18: 883–897.

Murphy DM, Stassen L, Carr ME, et al. Bacteremia during prostatectomy and other transurethral operations: influence of timing of antibiotic administration. *J Clin Pathol* 1984;37:673–676.

D.2. What are the signs of post–transurethral resection of the prostate (TURP) septicemia? What preventive measures are recommended?

The signs of septicemia usually appear postoperatively in the postanesthesia care unit. They include fever, chills, low blood pressure, and tachycardia.

Antibiotics administered prophylactically before TURP do not sterilize the urine because they do not easily penetrate the prostatic gland. Nevertheless, the preoperative administration of antibiotics is recommended to render the bloodstream hostile to bacteria. The prophylactic administration of antibiotics in patients undergoing TURP is particularly important because of the grave prognosis of septicemia in these patients.

If sepsis is suspected postoperatively in a patient who has undergone TURP, broad-spectrum antibiotics should be immediately started without waiting for blood culture results.

Barash PG, Cullen BF, Stoelting RK, eds. *Clinical anesthesia*, 5th ed. Philadelphia: Lippincott Williams & Wilkins, 2006:1026–1029.

Malhotra V. Transurethral resection of prostate. *Anesthesiol Clin North America* 2000;18: 883–897.

Robinson MRG, Cross RJ, Shetty MB, et al. Bacteremia and bacteriogenic shock in district hospital urological practice. *Br J Urol* 1980;52:10–14.

D.3. What bacteria-related cause may possibly lead to sudden postoperative shock in patients who have undergone transurethral resection of the prostate (TURP)?

On occasion, patients who have undergone TURP develop a short episode of hypotension, severe chills, and fever postoperatively. These symptoms last only a few hours, and then the patient recovers uneventfully. The cause of these symptoms is not clear; however, absorption of bacterial endotoxins has been suspected. Experimentally, the administration of bacterial endotoxins in humans provoked symptoms similar to those described.

Bennett IL. Pathogenesis of fever. *Bull N Y Acad Med* 1961;37:440–447.

Malhotra V. Transurethral resection of prostate. *Anesthesiol Clin North America* 2000;18: 883–897.

D.4. Is postoperative hypothermia a risk factor for myocardial ischemia?

Yes. Unintentional hypothermia is associated with a significantly higher incidence of postoperative myocardial ischemia. Therefore, it is important to maintain normothermia during the perioperative period. (See section D.4 in Chapter 15.)

D.5. How would you make a diagnosis of perioperative myocardial infarction (MI)?

An intraoperative MI can be totally silent, or it may be called to the attention of the anesthesiologist by a sudden decrease in blood pressure. The sudden decrease in blood pressure may be accompanied by tachycardia, which is indistinguishable from the hypovolemic hypotension resulting from acute blood loss.

   The electrocardiogram (ECG) is a good monitor of the adequacy of the coronary circulation. Only the appearance of Q waves more than 0.03 seconds in width is diagnostic of definite MI. However, the Q waves usually appear postoperatively instead of intraoperatively. Postoperative measurements of the myocardial isoenzymes of creatine phosphokinase may confirm the diagnosis. (See section D.5 in Chapter 15.)

E. Laser Prostatectomy

E.1. What is laser prostatectomy? What are its advantages?

Laser prostatectomy has found renewed interest among urologists and is being conducted in several centers. On the basis of initial experience, it promises to replace conventional transurethral resection of the prostate (TURP) in the very near future. The neodymium: yttrium-aluminum-garnet (Nd-YAG) laser, holmium laser, and potassium-titanyl-phosphate (KTP) laser are commonly used. These lasers produce varying degrees of coagulation and vaporization of prostate tissue. The main advantages over conventional TURP include minimal blood loss (as little as 50 to 70 mL) and minimal fluid absorption, which should nearly eliminate these two major complications of TURP; however, other potential complications are introduced, including coagulation through the prostatic fossa and sloughing of prostatic debris in the postoperative period, with subsequent urinary obstruction and urinary retention. Protective eyewear should be used, as well as a means to evacuate the smoke plume. In critically ill patients, caudal anesthesia has been successfully used for laser prostatectomy because the use of continuous irrigation combined with minimal bleeding obviates the need for copious irrigation and minimizes bladder distention.

Shingleton WB, Farabaugh P, May W. Three-year follow-up of laser prostatectomy versus transurethral resection of the prostate in men with benign prostatic hyperplasia. *Urology* 2002;60:305–308.

Tan AH, Gilling PJ. Holmium laser prostatectomy: current techniques. *Urology* 2002;60: 152–156.

CHAPTER 38

Kidney Transplant

PANCHALI DHAR • FUN-SUN F. YAO

A 40-YEAR-OLD MAN

with a 10-year history of type 1 diabetes mellitus and hypertension is scheduled to have a living donor renal transplant. He has been on hemodialysis for 5 years.

A. Medical Diseases and Differential Diagnosis

1. What are the common causes of end-stage renal disease (ESRD)?
2. What are the common clinical manifestations of ESRD?
3. What hematologic issues are important in patients with ESRD?
4. How does chronic anemia affect blood oxygen-carrying capacity?
5. Do patients with ESRD and anemia need to be transfused at any point?
6. What solute and water disturbances may exist in a patient with ESRD?
7. How can hyponatremia be evaluated and treated?
8. How can hypernatremia be evaluated and treated?
9. What are the etiologies, clinical signs, and management of hyperkalemia?
10. What other electrolyte imbalances occur in patients with impaired renal function? Specifically magnesium, phosphate, and calcium.
11. When would you correct the metabolic acidosis? What are the dangers of overzealous correction?
12. Are patients with ESRD at increased risk of cardiovascular disease?
13. What categories of immunosuppressant agents are used in patients who undergo transplantation?
14. How are immunosuppressive agents in a transplant recipient managed?
15. Who are expanded criteria kidney donors?
16. What are the contraindications to receiving a kidney transplant?
17. How are donors and recipients matched for transplant?
18. What new surgical techniques are available for donor nephrectomy?
19. How are donor kidneys preserved before transplant?
20. Describe the operative procedure of kidney transplantation.

B. Preoperative Evaluation and Preparation

1. What preoperative workup would you order for a kidney recipient?
2. What medications might the patient have been receiving before kidney transplant? What medications are administered in the preoperative period?
3. What are the normal values for blood urea nitrogen (BUN) and serum creatinine concentration? How is glomerular filtration rate (GFR) measured? Is there a risk of renal impairment in living donors?

C. Intraoperative Management

1. What type of anesthetic techniques can be used for renal transplant?
2. Is central venous monitoring required for the procedure?
3. Is an arterial line required for the transplant procedure?
4. Is a pulmonary artery catheter required for the transplant procedure?
5. How would you conduct the anesthesia induction?
6. Is succinylcholine contraindicated in renal failure patients?
7. How are the nondepolarizing muscle relaxants affected by renal failure?
8. What unusual situations can prolong neuromuscular (NM) blockade?
9. How would you maintain anesthesia during the case? What anesthetic agents would you use?
10. What are the effects of inhalation anesthetics on renal blood flow (RBF), glomerular filtration, and urine output?
11. What are the nephrotoxic effects of inhalation anesthetics? What are the nephrotoxic metabolites of inhalation anesthetics?
12. How does renal failure affect the pharmacology of opiods?
13. Discuss the intraoperative fluid management during a renal transplant.
14. What severe reactions can occur with the administration of polyclonal and monoclonal antibodies intraoperatively?
15. Describe the differential diagnosis of oliguria.
16. How does renal failure affect the dosing of neuromuscular reversal agents?

D. Postoperative Management

1. What are some side effects of immunosuppressive agents anesthesiologists should be aware of?
2. How is the diagnosis of acute transplant rejection made?

A. Medical Disease and Differential Diagnosis

A.1. What are the common causes of end-stage renal disease (ESRD)?

The common causes of ESRD are diabetes mellitus (40%), hypertension (27%), chronic glomerulonephritis (13%), cystic kidney disease (3.5%), interstitial nephritis (4%), and other diseases (12%) such as obstructive uropathy, lupus nephritis and human immunodeficiency virus (HIV). Despite the diversity of causes, the pathophysiology and clinical manifestations of progressive kidney disease are quite similar across the spectrum. The 5-year survival after kidney transplantation is approximately 70% compared with the 5-year survival of 30% for patients receiving dialysis. The key to long-term graft survival is early transplantation. Less time on dialysis is enhanced through living donor transplant.

Kasper DL, Braunwald E, Fauci AS, et al. *Harrison's principles of internal medicine*, 16th ed. New York: McGraw-Hill, 2005:1654.

A.2. What are the common clinical manifestations of end-stage renal disease (ESRD)?

The common problems related to ESRD are the following:

- *Electrolytes.* Volume expansion, hyponatremia, hyperkalemia, metabolic acidosis, hyperurecemia, hyperphosphatemia, hypocalcemia

- *Cardiovascular.* Accelerated atherosclerosis, systemic hypertension, left ventricular hypertrophy (LVH), congestive heart failure, pulmonary edema, cardiomyopathy, pericarditis, hyperdynamic circulation
- *Hematologic.* Anemia, B- and T-cell dysfunction, qualitative platelet dysfunction, bleeding diathesis
- *Musculoskeletal.* Muscle weakness
- *Neurologic.* Encephalopathy, loss of memory, seizures, peripheral neuropathy, myoclonus, asterixis
- *Gastrointestinal.* Gastroparesis, uremic gastroenteritis, nausea, vomiting, peptic ulcer disease, gastrointestinal bleeding, pancreatitis
- *Endocrine.* Vitamin D deficiency, secondary hyperparathyroidism, carbohydrate intolerance, hypertriglyceridemia

Kasper DL, Braunwald E, Fauci AS, et al. *Harrison's principles of internal medicine*, 16th ed. New York: McGraw-Hill, 2005:1654.

Obrador GT, Pereira BJG. Systemic complications of chronic kidney disease: pinpointing clinical manifestations and best management. *Postgrad Med* 2002;111(2):115–123.

A.3. What hematologic issues are important in patients with end-stage renal disease (ESRD)?

Anemia is often a consequence of progressive renal insufficiency. The anemia is due to several factors including chronic blood loss, hemolysis, marrow suppression by uremic factors, and reduced renal production of erythropoietin. The decreased production of erythropoietin is the result of a reduction in functioning renal mass. This manifests as a normochromic normocytic anemia. These patients may have hemoglobin levels of 5 to 7 g per dL corresponding to a hematocrit of 15% to 25%.

Untreated anemia can lead to physiologic abnormalities such as decreased tissue oxygen delivery and utilization, increased cardiac output, cardiac enlargement, ventricular hypertrophy, angina, congestive heart failure, decreased cognition and mental acuity, and impaired host defenses against infection. Additional factors which contribute to anemia are iron and folate deficiency, aluminum toxicity, hemolysis, bone marrow fibrosis due to hyperparathyroidism, chronic infection, and hemoglobinopathies. Patients can also be treated with darbopoetin-α, which is an analog of recombinant human erythropoietin but has greater biologic activity and a prolonged half-life.

Chronic renal disease (CRD) also leads to abnormalities with hemostasis and coagulation. This is primarily associated with prolonged bleeding time, decreased activity of platelet factor III, abnormal platelet aggregation and adhesion, and impaired prothrombin consumption. Patients with CRD also have a greater susceptibility to thromboembolic complications, especially if the underlying disease has a nephritic manifestation. In light of these hemostasis problems, the anesthesiologists must weigh the risk versus benefit of epidural placement in a patient with uremia.

Patients with a nephrotic syndrome may have thromboembolic complications because of urinary loss of antithrombin, altered levels and/or activity of protein C and S, hyperfibrinogenemia, impaired fibrinolysis, and increased platelet aggregability.

Kasper DL, Braunwald E, Fauci AS, et al. *Harrison's principles of internal medicine*, 16th ed. New York: McGraw-Hill, 2005:1658,1685.

A.4. How does chronic anemia affect blood oxygen-carrying capacity?

A normochromic normocytic anemia of chronic disease is usually present with renal failure. The red blood cells compensate for the lower oxygen-carrying capacity with higher levels of 2, 3 diphospoglycerate (2,3 DPG). The increased DPG and the presence of metabolic acidosis shifts the oxygen dissociation curve to the right. A right-shifted curve indicates a decreased affinity of hemoglobin for oxygen. An increased cardiac output and a hyperdynamic circulation help increase oxygen delivery to peripheral tissues. Therefore, patients can adapt to a low hematocrit of 15% to 25%. Currently, recombinant erythropoietin and darbopoietin help maintain a higher hematocrit. The National Kidney Foundation-Kidney Disease Outcomes Quality Initiative (NKF-K/DOQI) recommends a hemoglobin level of 11 to 12 g per dL for patients with end-stage renal disease (ESRD) receiving hemodialysis. This has decreased the requirement for transfusion.

Collins AJ, Brenner RM, Ofman JJ. Epoetin alpha use in patients with ESRD: an analysis of recent US prescribing patterns and hemoglobin outcomes *Am J Kidney Dis* 2005;46(3): 481–488.

A.5. Do patients with end-stage renal disease (ESRD) and anemia need to be transfused at any point?

Blood transfusions should be avoided if possible. Routine transfusion of patients with ESRD results in sensitization to human leukocyte antigens (HLA) antigens in the population. This may decrease the success of the graft. The frequency of transfusion has decreased with recombinant erythropoietin/darbopoietin therapy. The goal of erythropoietin therapy is to maintain the hematocrit between 36% and 40%. There is no clinical data supporting preoperative transfusion to improve outcome. Occasionally during surgery blood transfusion may be required for hypotension or hematocrit level less than 15%. It is best to use packed, washed red blood cells (leukocyte-poor) that are irradiated and cytomegalovirus (CMV) negative. This will help decrease leukocyte antigen exposure that can induce the development of alloantibodies predisposing to rejection of the implanted kidney.

Stoelting RK, Dierdorf SF. *Anesthesia and co-existing disease*, 4th ed. Philadelphia: Churchill Livingstone, 2002:347–348.

A.6. What solute and water disturbances may exist in a patient with end-stage renal disease (ESRD)?

Volume overload is a common concern in patients with ESRD. The extracellular fluid (ECF) compartment is 20% of the body weight and is subdivided by intravascular fluid (IVF = 4%) and interstitial fluid (ISF = 16%). The intracellular fluid (ICF) compartment is 40% of the body weight. The normal osmolality of the ECF and ICF compartments is 290 ± 10 mOsm per kg H_2O energy (adenosine triphosphate [ATP]) is used to pump potassium into the cell and sodium out of the cell.

The accumulation of nonsodium solutes in the ECF or ICF contributes to the osmolality of that compartment. For example, high glucose and/or urea concentration have the following effect:

$$P_{osm} = 2 \times [Na] + \frac{BUN \ (mg/dL)}{2.8} + \frac{Glucose \ (mg/dL)}{18}$$

(The constants 2.8 and 18 convert the blood urea nitrogen [BUN] and glucose from mg/L to mmol/L.)

Glucose is mainly restricted to the ECF. The increase in ECF osmolality shifts water from the ICF to the ECF. This dilutes the ECF while increasing the ICF solute concentration and osmolality. The water shift continues until the ECF and ICF osmolality are equal. Each 100 mg per dL increase in glucose will reduce the serum Na concentration by 1.4 mEq per L. The opposite effect occurs when hyperglycemia is corrected shifting water from the ECF to ICF. Urea does not contribute to water shift across cell membranes because it is not confined to either compartment.

In patients with ESRD the total body contents of Na and H_2O may be increased. This can be due to glomerular disease promoting Na retention, or excessive ingestion of Na leading to ECF expansion. The ECF expansion contributes to hypertension. A patient not on dialysis may be treated with loop diuretics and salt restriction.

The renal mechanisms for conserving Na and H_2O could also be impaired in ESRD. Coupled with additional fluid loss (vomiting, fever), patients are likely to become volume depleted. The usual indices of prerenal azotemia (high urine osmolality, low urine Na, low FeNa) are not applicable because the kidneys cannot conserve Na or H_20. These patients have to be hydrated carefully with normal saline.

Gennari FJ. Serum osmolality. Uses and limitations. *N Engl J Med* 1984;310:102–105.

Kasper DL, Braunwald E, Fauci AS, et al. *Harrison's principles of internal medicine*, 16th ed. New York: McGraw-Hill, 2005:252,1655.

Lin M, Lui SJ, Lim IT. Disorders of water imbalance. *Emerg Med Clin North Am* 2005;23: 749–770.

A.7. How can hyponatremia be evaluated and treated?

Hyponatremia can be categorized as hyperosmolar, isoosmolar or hypoosmolar.

Hyperosmolar hyponatremia can be caused by hyperglycemia. Water moves from the intracellular fluid (ICF) into the extracellular fluid (ECF) diluting sodium concentration. Quantitatively, the measured sodium concentration decreases 1.4 mEq per L for every 100 mg per dL rise in serum glucose.

Isoosmolar hyponatremia can be caused when massive volumes of sodium free irrigant (glycine) are systemically absorbed or high levels of lipids (hypertriglyceridemia) decreases the total sodium content per unit volume of serum.

Hypoosmolar hyponatremia is categorized on the basis of intravascular volume. It indicates an excess of total body water relative to total body solute. The low ECF osmolality means that ICF osmolality is also reduced. Table 38.1 helps in evaluation of hypoosmolar hyponatremia.

In hypovolemic hyponatremia, normal saline administration increases the delivery of sodium and fluid to the distal tubules and also inhibits antidiuretic hormone (ADH) release. This produces

Table 38.1 Three Types of Hypoosmolar Hyponatremia.

HYPONATREMIA	HYPOVOLEMIC	EUVOLEMIC	HYPERVOLEMIC
Clinical etiology	GI fluid losses, third spacing, burns	SIADH, hypothyroidism, cortisol deficiency	Congestive heart failure, cirrhosis, renal failure
Urinary sodium	<10 mEq/L	>10 mEq/L	<10 mEq/L
Urine osmolality	High	High	High
BUN	Elevated	Decreased	Elevated

GI, gastrointestinal; SIADH, syndrome of inappropriate antidiuretic hormone; BUN, blood urea nitrogen.

a water diuresis that corrects the hyponatremia. Euvolemic hyponatremia can be corrected with water restriction. Hypervolemic hyponatremia has low effective arterial blood volume. Salt intake must be reduced and loop diuretics promote naturiesis and reduce the maximal renal concentrating ability.

Acute symptomatic hyponatremia may be associated with nausea, vomiting, irritability, mental confusion, seizures, coma, and death. Neurologic symptoms occur primarily if Na concentration falls below 120 mEq per L or decreases rapidly. In severe conditions, hypertonic saline (3% = 517 mEq/L) may be used to increase serum sodium. Rapid correction of chronic hyponatremia can result in osmotic demyelination syndrome. This occurs when water moves too rapidly out of brain cells as hypertonic solution is administered. The rate of sodium correction should be 1.5 to 2 mEq/L/hour for severe symptoms and less than 0.5 mEq/L/hour for mild symptoms. Loop diuretic use can increase free water excretion and prevent ECF volume overload. The total increase in serum sodium should not exceed 10 to 12 mEq per L in 24 hours. The total body sodium deficit is calculated with the following equation:

$$\text{Sodium deficit (mEq)} = 0.6^* \times \text{weight (kg)} \times (\text{desired Na} - \text{actual Na})$$

*0.5 may be used for women.

Adrogue HJ. Hyponatremia. *N Engl J Med* 2000;342:1581–1589.

Lin M, Lui SJ, Lim IT. Disorders of water imbalance. *Emerg Med Clin North Am* 2005;23: 749–770.

A.8. How can hypernatremia be evaluated and treated?

Plasma sodium greater than 145 mEq per L defines hypernatremia. Hypernatremia may occur from either water deficit or sodium gain.

Water loss may due to diarrhea, nasogastric suctioning, vomiting, third spacing, fever, burns, and mechanical ventilation. Reduced water intake due to impaired thirst or access to water may contribute. Clinical symptoms of hypernatremia due to water deficit include flat neck veins, orthostatic hypotension, tachycardia, poor skin turgor, dry mucous membranes, lethargy, weakness, irritability, seizures, coma, or death. The symptoms reflect the severity and rapidity of the development of hypernatremia. Therapy requires hypotonic fluid and correction of the underlying disorder. The water deficit can be calculated as follows:

$$\text{Water deficit (liter)} = 0.6^* \times \text{weight (kg)} \times [(\text{Na}/140) - 1]$$

* 0.5 may be used for women

The sodium concentration should be lowered 0.5 to 1 mEq/L/hour with a maximum decrease of 10 mEq/L/24 hours. Hypernatremia may occasionally result from administration of $NaHCO_3$ during cardiopulmonary resuscitation, or hypertonic dialysis solutions. In such cases the patient is volume expanded. Clinical symptoms may include pulmonary edema or congestive heart failure. Treatment involves diuretics and free water replacement. For patients with severe renal failure, naturesis is achieved by dialysis.

Adrogue HJ, Madias NE. Hypernatremia *N Engl J Med* 2000;342:1493–1499.

Lin M, Lui SJ, Lim IT. Disorders of water imbalance. *Emerg Med Clin North Am* 2005;23: 749–770.

Table 38.2 Drug Treatment for Hyperkalemia.

DRUG	DOSE
Calcium chloride	5 mL of 10% solution IV over 2 min (monitor for bradycardia)
Calcium gluconate	10 mL of 10% solution IV over 2 min (monitor for bradycardia)
Insulin	5–10 units regular insulin with 1–2 amps D50W IV bolus
Sodium bicarbonate	1 mEq/kg slow IV push or continuous drip; not to exceed 50–100 mEq
β agonists (albuterol)	2.5 mg mixed with 3 mL isotonic saline through nebulizer q 20 min as tolerated
Diuretic (furosemide)	20–40 mg IV push
Magnesium	1–2 gm IV over 30–60 sec; repeat q 5–15 min as required or 3–10 mg/min IV infusion

A.9. What are the etiologies, clinical signs, and management of hyperkalemia?

Potassium is the principal cation of the intracellular fluid (ICF), where its concentration is 150 mEq per L. The concentration of K+ in the extracellular fluid (ECF) and plasma is lower, between 3.5 and 5.0 mEq per L. Adults ingest approximately 50 to 100 mEq of potassium daily and excrete an equal quantity in the urine. Chronic hyperkalemia is usually caused by impaired renal potassium excretion. In patients with end-stage renal disease (ESRD) or transplant recipients, hyperkalemia can be exacerbated by excessive dietary intake, hemolysis, hemorrhage, massive blood transfusion, metabolic acidosis, β-adrenergic blockade, angiotensin-converting enzyme inhibitors, angiotensin receptor blockers, insulin deficiency/resistance, hyperosmolality, hyperglycemia, rhabdomyolysis, succinylcholine, digoxin overdose, potassium sparing diuretics, and cyclosporine.

Metabolic acidosis is associated with an efflux of potassium from the ICF to ECF. It is common in ESRD as these patients have a reduced ability to produce ammonia. Hyperkalemia further depresses urinary ammonium excretion. As a general rule, for every 0.1 unit change in blood pH the potassium level increases approximately 0.6 mEq per L. Treatment of hyperkalemia improves the acidosis as well.

Severe hyperkalemia increases cardiac and skeletal muscle excitability. The earliest changes begin with levels above 6.5 mEq per L. The electrocardiogram (ECG) shows peaked T waves, flattened P waves, lengthened PR interval, disappearance of P waves, and a widened QRS complex that can progress to a "sine wave", ventricular asystole or ventricular fibrillation. The correlation between serum potassium and ECG changes is not definite because there may be few ECG abnormalities in the presence of severe hyperkalemia. Muscle weakness can cause respiratory failure. Membrane excitability is in fact more dependent on the rate of increase in potassium than on potassium concentration per se.

Treatment involves (a) antagonizing the cardiac toxic effects and stabilizing the cardiac membrane with intravenous calcium salts; magnesium can be given for acute suppression of torsade de pointes and (b) shifting the ECF potassium into cells by administering glucose, insulin, β-adrenergic agonists (albuterol), and sodium bicarbonate (Table 38.2). Of note, calcium can potentiate digitalis toxicity. In such circumstances, the calcium gluconate should be added to 100 mL of D5W and infused over 20 to 30 minutes. The anesthesiologist may also institute hyperventilation in mechanically ventilated patients. Loop diuretics can increase potassium elimination (nonanuric). Hemodialysis or peritoneal dialysis is the definitive treatment for patients with chronic renal failure.

Esposito C, Bellotti N, Fasoli G, et al. Hyperkalemia induced ECG abnormalities in patients with reduced renal function. *Clin Nephrol* 2004;62:465–468.

Kasper DL, Braunwald E, Fauci AS, et al. *Harrison's principles of internal medicine*, 16th ed. New York: McGraw-Hill, 2005:1656.

Schaefer TJ, Wolford RW. Disorders of potassium. *Emerg Med Clin North Am* 2005;23: 723–747.

A.10. What other electrolyte imbalances occur in patients with impaired renal function? Specifically magnesium, phosphate and calcium.

Chronic renal insufficiency and end-stage renal disease (ESRD) are associated with impaired excretion and balance of electrolytes.

Hypermagnesemia can accompany chronic renal failure, especially when the glomerular filtration rate (GFR) decreases to less than 10 mL per minute. High blood magnesium levels cause dose-dependent neuromuscular (NM) toxicity. Symptoms include diminished deep tendon reflexes, flaccid paralysis which may progress to respiratory failure. An increased sensitivity to depolarizing and nondepolarizing NM agents is noted. Bradycardia, hypotension, and heart block are due to the calcium channel blocking effects of magnesium. The acute toxicity can be antagonized by intravenous infusion of calcium. Hemodialysis or peritoneal dialysis can normalize blood magnesium levels.

Phosphate retention occurs when GFR begins to decline. Retained phosphate promotes secondary hyperparathyroidism by lowering ionized plasma calcium levels, decreasing renal formation of calcitriol (1,25 dihydroxyvitamin D), and stimulating parathyroid hormone gene expression.

Ionized and protein-bound calcium levels are lower in uremic patients. This is the result of hyperphosphatemia, and reduced gastrointestinal absorption secondary to the decreased production of vitamin D.

Goodman WG. Calcium and phosphorus metabolism in patients who have chronic kidney disease. *Med Clin North Am* 2005;89:631–647.

Kasper DL, Braunwald E, Fauci AS, et al. *Harrison's principles of internal medicine*, 16th ed. New York: McGraw-Hill, 2005:1657.

A.11. When would you correct the metabolic acidosis? What are the dangers of overzealous correction?

A mild to moderate acidosis is commonly noted when the glomerular filtration rate (GFR) decreases to less than 20% to 25% of normal. The decreased renal mass results in decreased NH_4^+ production and excretion of proton load. The plasma bicarbonate concentration ranges between 12 and 22 mEq per L, and blood pH remains greater than 7.20. This does not routinely require correction. It may gradually evolve into a high anion gap acidosis when the GFR is below 20 mL per minute. Some patients with end-stage renal disease (ESRD) maintain close to normal acid–base parameters even when renal function is severely compromised. However, when exposed to an increased dietary acid load these patients may have decreased ability to increase bicarbonate generation. Chronic acidosis promotes muscle wasting, reduces albumin synthesis, impairs bone formation, and decreases insulin sensitivity. There are no guidelines requiring the correction of acidosis to normal pH. Each case should be treated on an individual basis. The recommendations in regard to the amount of bicarbonate to be administered to the patient with acidosis is based on the space of distribution of bicarbonate, which in metabolic acidosis is 70% of lean body weight, and the maximum desired level of plasma bicarbonate, which is 24 mEq per L. The bicarbonate required can be calculated as follows:

$$HCO_3^- \text{ replacement} = 0.7 \times \text{ weight in kg} \times (24 - \text{serum } HCO_3^-)$$

Only half of the calculated bicarbonate is given because doses exceeding 1 mEq/kg/minute may lead to alkaline overshoot. Serial blood gases should be followed to monitor the response to treatment. Overzealous use of sodium bicarbonate may cause volume overload, promote metastatic calcification by decreasing the solubility of calcium phosphate, and decrease ionized calcium. For each 0.1 increase in pH, oxygen availability may decrease by 10% because of the shift of the oxygen-hemoglobin dissociation curve to the left. Severe symptomatic acidosis (pH <7.20) that is resistant to bicarbonate administration requires dialysis.

Kasper DL, Braunwald E, Fauci AS, et al. *Harrison's principles of internal medicine*, 16th ed. New York: McGraw-Hill, 2005:267,1656.

Kraut JA, Kurtz I. Metabolic acidosis of CKD: diagnosis, clinical characteristics, and treatment. *Am J Kidney Dis* 2005;45(6):978–993.

A.12. Are patients with end-stage renal disease (ESRD) at increased risk of cardiovascular disease?

Cardiac disease accounts for almost 50% of deaths among patients with ESRD. The process of cardiovascular damage starts in the early stages of renal disease. Ischemic heart disease, dilated cardiomyopathy, congestive heart failure, left ventricular hypertrophy (LVH), and pulmonary hypertension occur in dialysis patients.

Accelerated arteriosclerosis is promoted by diabetes and dyslipidemias. In one study coronary angiography was performed on 30 new ESRD patients with no known cardiac history. It was noted that 16 of 30 patients (53.3%) had significant coronary artery stenotic lesions. Among diabetic patients, 10 of 12 patients (83.3%) had significant stenosis.

Hypertension almost invariably develops in patients with chronic renal disease (CRD), and is usually due to volume overload. High levels of renin-angiotensin secondary to relative intravascular volume depletion contribute to hypertension. Administration of erythropoietin may raise blood pressure and increase the requirement for antihypertensive drugs in patients with ESRD. Aggressive management of blood pressure and controlling modifiable cardiovascular risk factors can slow the progression of kidney disease. The goal is to achieve a blood pressure of less than 130/85 mm Hg. A blood pressure target of less than 125/75 mm Hg is recommended for patients with proteinuric renal disease (urinary protein ≥1 g/24 hour).

Uremic cardiomyopathy results from volume and pressure overload. The expansion of the extracellular volume, high blood flow through arteriovenous (AV) fistulas, and anemia leads to volume overload. Arterial hypertension causes pressure overload. Eccentric hypertrophy is a response to volume overload, and the concentric changes are a response to pressure overload.

Anemia is strongly linked to cardiac morbidity. The risk of LVH increases with decreasing hemoglobin concentration. An increase in cardiac output is the natural response to chronic anemia. Treatment of anemia with erythropoietin (Epo) therapy improves cardiac oxygen supply, reduces cardiac output, increases peripheral vascular resistance, and ameliorates LVH.

The pulmonary vasculature is also affected by chronic renal failure. A unique *"low pressure" pulmonary edema* can result from increased permeability of alveolar capillary membranes. Pulmonary congestion and edema may occur in the absence of volume overload and is associated with normal or mildly elevated intracardiac and pulmonary wedge pressures. The chest radiograph is characterized by a "butterfly wing" pattern. This entity responds promptly to dialysis. There is a 40% incidence of unexplained *pulmonary hypertension* in patients receiving long-term hemodialysis through an AV fistula that does not occur in those receiving peritoneal dialysis. The pulmonary pressures decrease to normal after renal transplant.

Pericarditis was once a common finding but is seen much less often now because dialysis is usually started before it appears. Uremic pericardial fluid is hemorrhagic. Classic signs and symptoms include pericardial pain with respiratory accentuation, a multicomponent friction rub, PR interval depression, and diffuse ST-segment elevation. It may progress to cardiac tamponade. Treatment of this condition includes invasive dialysis and the use of nonsteroidal antiinflammatory drugs.

Exercise tolerance testing is recommended in patients with diabetes and patients older than 50. Many dialysis patients are unable to exercise adequately. Noninvasive testing such as dipyridamole thallium/sestamibi (DTS) or dobutamine stress echocardiography (DSE) can be done but the results should be interpreted based on the patient's clinical status. One study evaluated 126 renal transplant candidates, performing coronary angiography as well as both key noninvasive tests. The primary finding was that DTS has a sensitivity and specificity of only 58% and 67% respectively, and DSE had a sensitivity of 44% and specificity of 87%. The number of false-negative tests is high because these patients have a high pretest probability of disease. Coronary angiography is the best method for determining cardiac risk in patients with ESRD who are 50 years or older or have a high number of coronary risk factors. If definitive treatment of coronary obstruction is required, coronary artery bypass surgery is preferred because restenosis rates of up to 70% to 80% have been reported following coronary angioplasty.

DeLima JJ, Sabbaga E, Vieira ML, et al. Coronary angiography is the best predictor of events in renal transplant candidates compared to noninvasive testing. *Hypertension* 2003;42:263–268.

Eckardt K. Cardiovascular consequences of renal anemia and erythropoietin therapy. *Nephrol Dial Transplant* 1999;14(5):1317–1323.

Lemmens HJM. Kidney transplantation: recent developments and recommendations for anesthetic management. *Anesthesiol Clin North America* 2004;22:651–662.

Obrador GT, Pereira BJG. Systemic complications of chronic kidney disease: pinpointing clinical manifestations and best management. *Postgrad Med* 2002;111(2):115–123.

Ohtake T, Kobayashi S, Moriya H, et al. High prevalence of occult coronary artery stenosis in patients with chronic kidney disease at the initiation of renal replacement therapy: an angiographic examination. *J Am Soc Nephrol* 2005;16:1141–1148.

Vanholder R, Massy Z, Argiles A, et al. Chronic kidney disease as cause of cardiovascular morbidity and mortality. *Nephrol Dial Transplant* 2005;20:1048–1056.

Yigla M, Nakhoul F, Sabag A, et al. Pulmonary hypertension in patients with end stage renal disease. *Chest* 2003;123(5):1577–1582.

A.13. What categories of immunosuppressant agents are used in transplant patients?

The following drugs are used for immunosuppression:

- Steroids
- Calcineurin inhibitors (CNI)
  Cyclosporin (Sandimmune, Neoral)
  Tacrolimus (Prograf)
- Target of Rapamycin (TOR) inhibitors
  Sirolimus (Rapamune)
  Everolimus
- Polyclonal antibodies
  Antilymphocyte globulin (Atgam, Thymoglobulin)
- Monoclonal antibodies
  Interleukin 2 (IL-2) receptor blockers (CD25)
  Daclizumab (Zenapax)

Basiliximab (Simulect)
OKT3 (anti-CD3, monomurab)
- Purine synthesis inhibitors
  Azathioprine (Imuran)
  Mycophenolate mofentil (MMF, CellCept)

Halloran PF. Immunosupressive drugs for kidney transplantation. *N Engl J Med* 2004; 351(26):2715–2729.

Wong W, Venetz JP, Rubin NT, et al. 2005 Immunosuppressive strategies in kidney transplantation: which role for calcineurin inhibitors? *Transplantation* 2005;80:289–296.

A.14. How are immunosuppressive agents in a transplant recipient managed?

To decrease the incidence of graft rejection, several regimens of immunosuppressive agents have been devised. Centers throughout the world may use different combinations of these drugs, but the basic idea behind their use remains the same. The use of immunosuppression for kidney transplant is divided into three periods.

The first period is induction therapy. Induction therapy involves administration of medications that provide marked immune suppression before and during the first week of posttransplantation. Induction agents include thymoglobulin, OKT3, daclizumab, or basiliximab.

The second period is the maintenance period. Maintenance therapy involves administration of agents continuously for 3 to 6 months to prevent acute rejection. These medications are also given to induce tolerance. Tolerance means unresponsiveness by the recipient to the kidney graft in the absence of maintenance immunosuppression. Tolerance can decrease the use of long-term medications, reduce adverse effects, and improve the quality of life.

The third period beyond 6 months is when long-term immunosuppression is established. The regimen will be maintained for the rest of the life of the transplant recipient.

Halloran PF. Immunosuppressive drugs for kidney transplantation. *N Engl J Med* 2004; 351(26):2715–2729.

A.15. Who are expanded criteria kidney donors?

There are an increasing number of persons awaiting a kidney transplant. The ideal donor is aged 5 to 49 years, a nonhypertensive whose cause of death was not cerebrovascular accident and whose creatinine was less than or equal to 1.5 mg per dL. The term *expanded criteria donor* (ECD) is one that has been introduced as part of an effort to increase the use of kidneys that might otherwise have been discarded, and to minimize the length of cold ischemia to which they are subjected. ECDs are defined as donors older than 60 or 50 to 59 years with two additional risk factors, including a history of hypertension, death as a result of cardiovascular accident, or serum creatinine greater than or equal to 1.5 mg per dL. ECD kidneys account for approximately 15% of deceased donor kidneys, but have at least a 70% increased risk of failure within 2 years when compared with standard criteria kidneys. The long-term survival of single or dual kidney grafts from donors older than 60 is excellent, provided that the grafts are evaluated histologically before implantation. ECD kidneys are offered only to patients willing to accept them. Oftentimes this decision must be made within 2 hours. This has increased the number of transplants anesthesiologists encounter.

Danovitch GM. *Handbook of kidney transplantation*, 4th ed. Philadelphia: Lippincott Williams & Wilkins, 2005:70,159.

Remuzzi G, et al. Long term outcome of renal transplantation from older donors. *N Engl J Med* 2006;354(4):343–352.

A.16. What are the contraindications to receiving a kidney transplant?

The major contraindications to a kidney transplant are as follows:

Absolute contraindications:

- Recent or metastatic malignancy
- Untreated current infection
- Severe irreversible extrarenal disease
- Recalcitrant treatment nonadherence
- Psychiatric illness impairing consent and adherence
- Current recreational drug abuse
- Limited, irreversible rehabilitative potential
- Active infection: Note that some centers now include recipients with hepatitis and even human immunodeficiency virus (HIV) infection under strict protocols to determine whether the risks and benefits favor transplantation over dialysis. Patients who have serologic evidence of hepatitis C or B, but without evidence of active hepatic inflammation or cirrhosis, are acceptable transplant candidates.

Relative contraindications

- Presence of vesical or urethral abnormalities
- Aortoiliac occlusive disease
- Morbid obesity
- Smoking

Brunicardi FC, Andersen DK, Billiar TR, et al. *Schwartz's principles of surgery*, 8th ed. New York: McGraw-Hill, 2005:306.

Danovitch GM. *Handbook of kidney transplantation*, 4th ed. Philadelphia: Lippincott Williams & Wilkins, 2005:158.

Kasper DL, Braunwald E, Fauci AS, et al. *Harrison's principles of internal medicine*, 16th ed. New York: McGraw-Hill, 2005:1668–1673.

A.17. How are donors and recipients matched for transplant?

The three sources of donor kidneys are living related donor, living unrelated donor, and deceased donor.

- *ABO blood group.* The blood group antigen compatible means the recipient and donor have no mismatched ABO antigens. For example, a person with blood type A may donate to a person with blood type A or AB. Identical means the recipient and donor have the exact same ABO phenotype. The cadaver kidney should be ABO identical to the recipient. An A donor should be placed in an A type recipient. A live donor kidney may be either ABO identical or compatible. For example, a donor kidney of either A, B, or O type can be placed in an AB recipient. It is possible to place an ABO-incompatible organ in a recipient using protocol such as plasmapheresis and immunoabsorption to overcome rejection. The Rh system is not expressed on graft tissue.
- *Tissue typing.* The human major histocompatibility complex is a cluster of genes on chromosome 6 that encoded human leukocyte antigens (HLA). Before any transplant, specific

HLA antigens are identified in all donors and recipients. Individuals are typed by DNA-based methods. Outcome is best with a perfect HLA matched donor and recipient. Graft survival is similar with a partial HLA-matched or -mismatched kidney. Of course, the kidney with the least number of mismatches is preferred. Again because of improvement in immunosuppression protocols, recipients can receive an organ from a donor with a less than perfect match.

- *Cross-matching.* A cross-match test determines if the recipient has serum antibodies directed against donor HLA lymphocyte antigens. These may arise as a result of exposure through pregnancies or blood transfusions in the past. A positive cross-match is a relative contraindication to transplant, as it will cause rejection of the graft. Currently, there are methods to reduce HLA allosensitization using intravenous immunoglobulin and plasmapheresis.

Danovitch GM. *Handbook of kidney transplantation*, 4th ed. Philadelphia: Lippincott Williams & Wilkins, 2005:43–71.

Kaihara S, Okamoto M, Akioka S, et al. Improved graft survival in ABO-incompatible living donor kidney transplantation. *Transplant Proc* 2005;37:1804–1085.

A.18. What new surgical techniques are available for donor nephrectomy?

The number of living donors has exceeded the number of cadaver donors partly as a consequence of widespread availability of laparoscopic living donor nephrectomy. The minimally invasive approach allows a significant reduction in postoperative pain, decreased length of hospital stay, shorter recovery time, and enhanced cosmesis.

Recently robotic hand assisted donor nephrectomy has increased in popularity. The robotics system provides considerable potential benefits to minimally invasive surgery when compared with standard laparoscopic approaches. In particular, the system restores the three-dimensional vision lost in the laparoscopic approach and enhances the ability of the surgeon to perform complex tasks in a laparoscopic environment.

Horgan S, Benedetti E, Moser F. Robotically assisted donor nephrectomy for kidney transplant. *Am J Surg* 2004;188:45S–51S.

A.19. How are donor kidneys preserved before transplant?

Deceased donor kidneys are preserved using hypothermia and pharmacologic inhibition to slow down metabolic processes. A temperature decrease from $37°C$ ($98.6°F$) to $4°C$ ($39.2°F$) slows metabolism approximately 12-fold. Cold storage solutions are agents that do not readily permeate the cell membrane and have an electrolyte composition similar to the intracellular environment (low sodium, high potassium), thereby preventing loss of cellular potassium. Cold ischemic times should be kept below 36 to 40 hours after which delayed graft function significantly increases. The retrieved kidney is flushed with cold storage solution and packed in a sterile container with ice. The kidney is transported in a machine that pumps preservation solution through the organ until the moment of graft placement.

Kidneys from living donors may be flushed with preservation solution or iced Ringer's lactate solution containing heparin and mannitol. The ischemic time during implantation is usually 20 to 30 minutes because the transplant operation takes place immediately. Some practices place the living donor kidney in a pulsatile preservation machine that maintains organ viability for longer periods of time.

Brunicardi FC, Andersen DK, Billiar TR, et al. *Schwartz's principles of surgery*, 8th ed. New York: McGraw-Hill, 2005:305.

Salahudeen AK, Haider N, May W. Cold ischemia and the reduced long-term survival of cadaveric renal allografts. *Kidney Int* 2004;65(2):713–718.

A.20. Describe the operative procedure of kidney transplantation.

Before the induction of anesthesia, a large bore peripheral intravenous line (18 gauge or 16 gauge) is required. Following induction of anesthesia, a triple-lumen central line may be placed either in the internal jugular or subclavian route. A Foley catheter is placed in the bladder and the bladder is irrigated with an antibiotic solution. Fluids are infused liberally through the central line and intravenous line.

The transplanted kidney is placed in a heterotopic position. Retroperitoneal placement is preferred, to allow easy access for percutaneous renal biopsy. The standard location is either the right or left iliac fossa. The right kidney is usually placed in the left groin and *vice versa*. The internal or external renal artery can be used as an inflow vessel to the donor kidney renal artery. The donor renal vein is anastomosed to the external iliac vein. In the event that the patient weighs less than 20 kg, the kidney is placed intraabdominally posterior to the right colon. The aorta and vena cava may be the major vessels employed for revascularization. Urinary continuity is restored by attaching the ureter in well-described techniques that prevent reflux during voiding. In deceased donor kidney transplant, before the release of the arterial clamp and following completion of the anastomosis, an intraarterial injection of verapamil or papaverine may be given by direct push into the renal artery to prevent arterial vasospasm. In addition, furosemide (200 mg) is frequently given immediately after revascularization.

In dual kidney transplantation, two kidneys from a donor are placed into one recipient. Such kidneys have usually been refused for single kidney transplantation. Dual kidney transplant is done at the extremes of donor age. It is a reflection of donor shortage and reluctance to discard potentially functional organs. For donors younger than 2 years of age, both kidneys are transplanted *en bloc* with the donor aorta and vena cava. The creatinine clearance should be less than 70 mL per minute in a donor 60 years of age or older. A dual kidney transplant procedure is of longer duration, involves more third spacing, greater volume requirements and blood loss.

Brunicardi FC, Andersen DK, Billiar TR, et al. *Schwartz's principles of surgery*, 8th ed. New York: McGraw-Hill, 2005:307.

Danovitch GM. *Handbook of kidney transplantation*, 4th ed. Philadelphia: Lippincott Williams & Wilkins, 2005:199–201.

The New York Hospital- Cornell Medical Center Kidney Transplantation Protocol 2005, New York, NY

B. Preoperative Evaluation and Preparation

B.1. What preoperative workup would you order for a kidney recipient?

The transplant recipient should have routine systemic tests such as electrocardiogram (ECG), chest radiograph, blood counts, platelet count, electrolytes, serum glucose, blood urea nitrogen (BUN), creatinine concentration, prothrombin time, partial thromboplastin time, liver function enzymes (aspartine transaminase, alanine transaminase), bilirubin, and albumin. Dialysis, if indicated, is done within 24 hours of the operation. It is best to avoid overzealous ultrafiltration, as expanded filling pressures are desired. A urinalysis and urine culture should be performed on all urinating patients.

Dialysis-related problems such as dialysis dementia, disequilibrium syndrome after dialysis (cerebral edema), hypovolemia (hypotension after anesthetic induction following recent dialysis), peritonitis (peritoneal dialysis), systemic anticoagulation (after dialysis) should be evaluated. It is important to know the time of the last dialysis. The dialysis records should be reviewed for pre- and postdialysis weight. The loss of more than 2 kg during dialysis suggests intravascular volume depletion, which may result in severe hypotension during or after anesthetic induction.

Sprung J, Kapural L, Bourke DL, et al. Anesthesia for kidney transplant. *Anesthesiol Clin North America* 2000;18 (4):919–951.

B.2. What medications might the patient been receiving before transplant? What medications are administered in the preoperative period?

Patients awaiting transplant often have comorbidities such as hypertension and diabetes. The variety of medications used to treat these conditions may include β-adrenergic blockers, angiotensin-converting enzyme inhibitors, angiotensin receptor blockers, oral hypoglycemic agents or insulin. The antihypertensive drugs should be continued until the time of surgery. NPH insulin subcutaneous at half the total morning dose is given the morning of transplant. Oral hypoglycemic agents should be held on the morning of surgery. A sliding scale insulin regimen may be used intraoperatively if high blood glucose levels are measured. Antibiotic prophylaxis for infectious complications includes a first-generation cephalosporin (cefazolin 1 gm 30 minutes before surgery) or if penicillin allergic, vancomycin (1 gm intravenous [IV]).

Induction of immunosuppression is started before entering the operating room. At the New York Presbyterian Hospital, a steroid-sparing regimen is usually followed. Before entering the operating room, patients are given methylprednisone (SoluMedrol 500 mg), and mycophenolate mofentil (CellCept 500 to 1000 mg). Diphenhydramine and acetaminophen are given as prophylaxis before thymoglobulin infusion. In the operating room, the rabbit antithymocyte globulin is run peripherally at 1.5 mg per kg over 12 hours, maximum dose is 150 mg (1.5 mg/kg/day for 5 days total). The peripheral administration of thymoglobulin may decrease the incidence of allergic reaction. Under specific circumstances, basiliximab (Simulect) is substituted for thymoglobulin. This is practiced if the patient has a history of reaction to thymoglobulin or is a perfect match to the donor kidney. No prophylactic premedication is required with basiliximab. Patients receive only five doses of methylprednisolone; steroids are then discontinued. In the steroid protocol, patients are continued on prednisone.

Anxiolytics should be titrated carefully as these patients may have increased sensitivity to premedication drugs. For example, diazepam is highly bound to albumin, but with decreased albumin levels the effect of the drug is increased. Midazolam is water soluble, less affected by albumin levels, and useful before induction.

The New York Hospital-Cornell Medical Center Kidney Transplantation Protocol 2005, New York.

B.3. What are the normal values for blood urea nitrogen (BUN) and serum creatinine concentration? How is glomerular filtration rate (GFR) measured? Is there a risk of renal impairment in living donors?

Normal values for BUN range from 8 to 20 mg per dL and creatinine levels range from 0.5 to 1.2 mg per dL. Creatinine is produced by hepatic conversion of skeletal muscle creatine. The plasma concentration of creatinine remains stable with age. Creatinine is freely filtered and not reabsorbed, and is minimally secreted by the kidneys. Creatinine clearance is used to estimate the GFR—the standard by which kidney function is assessed. The creatinine clearance test compares the level of creatinine in urine with the creatinine level in the blood. Ideally the test is based on measurements of a 24-hour urine sample and a blood sample drawn at the end of the 24-hour period. Clearance is often measured as milliliters per minute (mL/min). The following formula provides an estimate of creatinine clearance. This formula is applicable only if the serum creatinine is stable.

$$\text{Creatinine clearance (mL/min)} = \frac{140 - age \times \text{weight(kg)}}{\text{Plasma Cr (mg/dL)} \times 72}$$

This value should be multiplied by 0.85 for women, because a lower fraction of the body weight is composed of muscle. Kidney donors experience a 25% increase in serum creatinine level. This level should return near baseline by 3 months after the operation. There may be an increased risk for hypertension, mild proteinuria, and some increased risk for developing renal insufficiency beginning approximately 20 to 25 years after surgery.

Davis CL. Evaluation of the living donor kidney: current perspectives. *Am J Kidney Dis* 2004; 43(3):508–530.

Kalble T, Lucan M, Nicita G, et al. European association of urology guidelines on renal transplantation. *Eur Urol* 2005;47:156–166.

C. Intraoperative Management

C.1. What type of anesthetic techniques can be used for renal transplant?

General anesthesia is the preferred technique for renal transplantation. The use of epidural or combined spinal-epidural anesthesia is controversial. If the decision is made to use regional anesthesia, there are certain factors the anesthesiologist should consider.

It is important to note that uremic bleeding tendency combined with the effects of residual heparin given during dialysis increase the risk of hemorrhage into the epidural space. Underlying hepatic disease can also alter platelet function and decrease coagulation factor levels. Studies have not demonstrated higher plasma concentrations of local anesthetic due to hyperdynamic circulation or acid–base changes in renal patients.

The duration of surgery is the major determinant of anesthetic technique. Epidural anesthesia has been used successfully in renal transplant surgery. Studies have shown no overall difference in mortality or major morbidity between patients randomly assigned to general anesthesia or to combined spinal-epidural anesthesia for renal transplantation. The advantages of the combined technique are rapid onset and good muscle relaxation from the subarachnoid block, with the ability to supplement analgesia through the epidural catheter during and after the surgery. With longer operative times, general anesthesia is preferred.

Brunicardi FC, Andersen DK, Billiar TR, et al. *Schwartz's principles of surgery*, 8th ed. New York: McGraw-Hill, 2005:307.

Hadimioglu N, Ertug Z, Bigat M, et al. A randomized study comparing combined spinal or general anesthesia for renal transplant surgery. *Transplant Proc* 2005;37:2020–2022.

C.2. Is central venous monitoring required for the procedure?

Adequate hydration is an important part of the anesthetic management in renal transplant. Measuring the central venous pressure (CVP) is not an absolute requirement. The CVP or pulmonary artery pressure (only in patients with left ventricular dysfunction) can be used to guide fluid therapy. Adequate hemodialysis should be performed within 48 hours of surgery. These postdialysis patients have intravascular volume depletion. To decrease the incidence of postoperative acute tubular necrosis (ATN), a liberal hydration policy is employed intraoperatively. The systolic blood pressure is maintained between 130 and 160 mm Hg, and the CVP is maintained between 12 and 14 mm Hg. Maintaining adequate CVP is especially important in pediatric recipients because reperfusion of an adult size kidney graft may divert a significant amount of their own blood volume.

In a randomized prospective study where patients were divided into groups with (n = 31) or without (n = 30) central venous monitoring, the onset of graft function within the first 3 postoperative days was significantly more frequent in the group with CVP monitoring than in the group without (62% versus 30%) despite absence of difference in the measurable warm and cold ischemic periods. Administering mannitol and furosemide is helpful in maximizing reperfusion to the kidney graft. Mannitol and furosemide have never been shown to improve organ recovery or decrease reperfusion injury. Furosemide maintains a nonoliguric state to ease postoperative care.

CVP may decline 1 to 2 hours after revascularization despite aggressive fluid management in the operating room. The decline in CVP is similar in recipients of both cadaveric and living related donor kidneys. It may decline 25% to 50% below the CVP measured in the operating room at reperfusion of the transplanted kidney. The reason for the decline is not clear but may be multifactorial such as redistribution of fluids, changes in vascular permeability, or increased nitric oxide levels. This is why postoperative hydration is an essential factor in maintaining renal function. Increased hydration likely works by atrial distension and the subsequent release of atrial natriuretic peptide, and increased renal perfusion. The patient should receive an equal amount of fluid replacing the urine output.

Ferris RL, Kittur DS, Wilasrusmee C, et al. Early hemodynamic changes after renal transplantation: determinants of low central venous pressure in the recipients and correlation with acute renal dysfunction. *Med Sci Monit* 2003;9(2):CR61–CR66.

Thomsen HS, Lokkegaard H, Munke O. Influence of normal central venous pressure on set of function in renal allografts. *Scand J Urol Nephrol* 1987;21(2):143–145.

C.3. Is an arterial line required for the transplant procedure?

An arterial line is not absolutely required for the transplant procedure, but many transplant surgeons now require placement. It should be placed if a patient has an advanced comorbid condition(s) that requires close monitoring of blood pressure or acid–base status. Occasionally placement of an intraarterial line is difficult as many recipients have poor arterial access secondary to diabetes, peripheral vascular disease, arteriovenous (AV) fistulas and shunts. Major swings in blood pressure may occur, with hypotension (49.6%) being more likely than hypertension (26.8%). Administration of induction drugs and maintenance agents should be titrated carefully. The main utility of instantaneous blood pressure reading is toward the end of the procedure. Hypotension may occur after unclamping of the iliac vessels and/or from partial systemic absorption of the vasodialator (verapamil or papaverine) injected by the surgeon into the graft vessels. Hypotension must be avoided during this period as it can lead to delayed graft function and/or renal vein thrombosis.

Miller RD. *Miller's anesthesia*, 6th ed. Philadelphia, Churhill Livingstone, 2005:2240–2241.

C.4. Is a pulmonary artery catheter required for the transplant procedure?

A pulmonary artery catheter is not routinely placed for kidney transplantation. Patients with severe comorbid conditions, such as symptomatic coronery artery disease (CAD), left ventricular dysfunction, congestive heart failure, valvular heart disease, or severe chronic obstructive pulmonary disease can be monitored precisely with a pulmonary artery catheter. A transesophageal echocardiography can help determine if hypotension is caused by hypovolemia or myocardial dysfunction.

Miller RD. *Miller's anesthesia* 6th ed. Philadelphia, Churchill Livingstone, 2005:2240–2241.

C.5. How would you conduct the anesthesia induction?

The circumstances for renal transplant can vary between a scheduled or emergent procedure. Living donor transplants are scheduled surgical cases. Patients receiving cadaver kidneys may learn of the surgical procedure under short notice.

Standard anesthesia monitors are required before induction. The central venous line and/or arterial line are usually placed after induction.

The induction of general anesthesia and intubation of the trachea can be safely accomplished with several of the commonly used drugs. The induction drugs should be given slowly to minimize the chance of drug-induced hypotension. Regardless of blood volume status, these patients often respond to induction of anesthesia as if they were hypovolemic. The sympathetic nervous system response may be attenuated by antihypertensive therapy or diabetic autonomic neuropathy. A blunted sympathetic response impairs compensatory peripheral vasoconstriction. In addition, the central nervous system (CNS) may exhibit an increased sensitivity to the induction drugs. Low serum protein and albumin levels can increase the level of unbound drug crossing the blood–brain barrier into CNS receptors. Uremia can also disrupt the blood–brain barrier. The dose of induction agent may need to be adjusted based on volume status, acidic pH and comorbidities. Propofol, thiopental, or etomidate can be used in routine circumstances. A reduced induction dose of propofol or thiopental may be considered because lower plasma protein levels and postdialysis hypovolemia can exaggerate their cardiodepressant effects. Some studies have noted higher propofol dose requirements in patients with end-stage renal disease (ESRD) compared to normal patients. Renal failure patients required a higher dose of propofol to reach the clinical end point of hypnosis and bispectral index (BIS) of 50. The hyperdynamic circulation from uremia and higher plasma volume from anemia can counteract the effect of low serum albumin explaining the higher dose requirement. Ketamine pharmacokinetics is not significantly changed by renal disease, but its hypertensive effects make it undesirable in patients with underlying hypertension. Etomidate is well tolerated and preserves hemodynamic stability.

Large fluctuations in blood pressure and heart rate may occur in patients with preexisting hypertension during intubation. Underlying coronary artery disease is a major consideration. Opioids can blunt the response to laryngoscopy. Fentanyl, 5 μg per kg, can be used, but there is a risk of hypotension after induction and lack of stimulation. Remifentanil is also effective for heart rate control. A short acting β-blocker such as esmolol (0.5 to 1.0 mg/kg) can blunt the response to intubation.

A number of neuromuscular (NM) blocking agents can be used to facilitate tracheal intubation. Patients with uremia and diabetes may have gastroparesis. Pretreatment with a clear, nonparticulate antacid such as 30 mL of sodium citrate raises gastric pH. A rapid sequence induction with cricoid pressure using either succinylcholine or rocuronium may be required to prevent reflux and aspiration. Succinylcholine can be used safely as potassium release is not exaggerated in patients with chronic renal failure. If the preoperative potassium is in the high normal range or if there is underlying metabolic acidosis, the additional increase of 0.5 to 1.0 mEq per L should be considered. When choosing a nondepolarizing agent for maintenance it is better to use ones that are independent of renal clearance mechanisms (cisatracurium, atracurium, mivacurium).

Goyal P, Puri GD, Pandey CK, et al. Evaluation of induction doses of propofol: comparison between end stage renal disease and normal renal function patients. *Anaesth Intensive Care* 2002;30:584–587.

Miller RD. *Miller's anesthesia*, 6th ed. Philadelphia: Churchill Livingstone, 2005:2241.

Stoelting RK, Dierdorf SF. *Anesthesia and co-existing disease*, 4th ed. Philadelphia: Churchill Livingstone, 2002:353.

C.6. Is succinylcholine contraindicated in renal failure patients?

Normally succinylcholine causes an increase in serum potassium of 0.5 to 1.0 mEq per L within 3 to 5 minutes of intravenous administration, and lasts less than 10 to 15 minutes. Succinylcholine can be used safely in patients with chronic renal failure if the potassium concentration is less than 5.5 mEq per L and repeated doses are avoided. Potassium flux after administration of succinylcholine in patients with renal failure does not differ from normal patients. Plasma cholinesterase activity has been reported to be below normal in more than 20% of end-stage renal disease (ESRD) patients whether they are receiving any form of dialysis. Values are rarely so low that they cause a prolonged block.

Miller RD. *Miller's anesthesia*, 6th ed. Philadelphia: Churchill Livingstone, 2005:2184–2185, 2241.

Thapa S, Brull SJ. Succinylcholine-induced hyperkalemia in patients with renal failure: an old question revisited. *Anesth Analg* 2000;91(1):237–241.

C.7. How are the nondepolarizing muscle relaxants affected by renal failure?

The prolonged duration of action to nondepolarizing agents is primarily due to slow renal clearance (Table 38.3). Mivacurium metabolism is affected by decreased activity of pseudocholinesterase. Atracurium and cisatracurium mainly undergo Hoffman elimination that is not altered in patients with chronic kidney disease. Renal failure may delay clearance of laudanosine, the principal metabolite of atracurium and cisatracurium. Laudanosine does not have effect at the neuromuscular (NM) junction, but at high plasma levels may act as a central

Table 38.3 Pharmacokinetics of Neuromuscular Blocking Agents in Normal and Anephric Patients.

DRUG	RENAL EXCRETION	NORMAL t1/2	ANEPHRIC t1/2
Pancuronium	85%	132 min	258 min
Rocuronium	10%	42 min	58 min
Vecuronium	40%–50%	54 min	84 min
Atracurium	10%–40%	18 min	24 min
Cisatracurium	16%	34 min	No effect
Mivacurium	<5%	1.8 min	3.6 min
Succinylcholine	<25%	1 min	1 min

nervous system (CNS) stimulant. A long-acting muscle relaxant such as pancuronium is not suitable for use as the kidneys excrete most of the drug and its metabolite. The prolonged effect of a nondepolarizing agent may not be apparent after a single small dose. After a small dose, the termination of action is by redistribution rather than elimination. It is only after a single large dose, repeated dosing, or prolonged infusion that the increased elimination half-life becomes clinically apparent. Maintenance doses for patients with decreased renal function should be smaller and the interval between doses should be increased. Monitoring of NM blockade with a nerve stimulator is recommended.

McLeskey CH. Geriatric anesthesiology 2nd ed. *Relaxants and their reversal agents*. Springer, 2007. In press

Miller RD. *Miller's anesthesia*, 6th ed. Philadelphia: Churchill Livingstone, 2005:2184–2185.

Robertson EN, Driessen JJ, Booij LH. Pharmacokinetics and pharmacodynamics of rocuronium in patients with and without renal failure. *Eur J Anesthesiol* 2005;22(1): 4–10.

C.8. What unusual situations can prolong neuromuscular (NM) blockade?

Drugs

- *Antibiotics*. The amnioglycosides (e.g., gentamycin) and tetracycline decrease the presynaptic release of acetylcholine by blocking the influx of calcium. Antagonism of antibiotic potentiated NM blockade by an anticholinesterase drug or calcium is unpredictable. Penicillins and cephalosporins do not have any NM effects.
- *Local anesthetics*. Small doses of local anesthetics enhance NM blockade, and large doses block NM transmission. Depending on the dose, local anesthetics interfere with the prejunctional release of acetylcholine, stabilize postjunctional membranes, and directly depress skeletal muscle.
- *Cardiac antidysrhythmic drugs*. Lidocaine can augment preexisting NM blockade. Quinidine interferes with the prejuctional release of acetylcholine and potentiates depolarizing and nondepolarizing drugs.
- *Diuretics*. Furosemide, 1 mg per kg, enhances nondepolarizing agents by inhibiting cyclic adenosine monophosphate (cAMP) production, leading to decreased prejunctional release of acetylcholine. Large doses of furosemide can inhibit phosphodiesterase, increasing cAMP levels leading to antagonism of nondepolarizing drugs.
- *Phenytoin*. Treatment with phenytoin causes resistance to nondepolarizing drugs.
- *Lithium*. This drug can enhance the effects of nondepolarizing and depolarizing drugs.
- *Calcium channel blockers*. Verapamil enhances nondepolarizing agents and may produce difficulty with obtaining adequate reversal.

Electrolytes

- *Potassium*. An acute decrease in potassium levels increases the transmembrane potential, causing hyperpolarization of cell membranes. This leads to resistance to depolarizing drugs and increased sensitivity to nondepolarizing drugs. An acute increase in potassium has the opposite effect by lowering the resting transmembrane potential and partial depolarizing the cell membrane. This increases the effect of depolarizing drugs and opposes the action of nondepolarizing drugs.
- *Magnesium*. Hypermagnesemia enhances nondepolarizing agents by decreasing the prejunctional release of acetylcholine and postjunctional sensitivity to acetylcholine. Phase II block may occur more readily when succinylcholine is administered in the presence of elevated plasma concentrations of magnesium

Acid-base imbalance

- Respiratory acidosis enhances d-tubocurarine (d-Tc) - and pancuronim-induced NM blockade and opposes their reversal with neostigmine.
- The effects of metabolic acidosis, respiratory and metabolic alkalosis are inconsistent.

Temperature

- *Hypothermia.* A decrease in temperature reduces hepatic enzyme activity responsible for metabolizing d-Tc and pancuronium, prolonging drug effect. Hypothermia can have a direct mechanical effect on the muscle, slowing contraction and relaxation and thereby enhancing the block.

Stoelting RK, Hillier SC. *Pharmacology and Physiology in Anesthetic Practice.* 4th ed. Philadelphia: Lippincott Williams & Wilkins, 2006:224–227

C.9. How would you maintain anesthesia during the case? What anesthetic agents would you use?

General anesthesia is the preferred technique for kidney transplantation. Volatile agents, opioids, and a muscle relaxant are required to provide optimal operating conditions.

The choice of inhaled anesthetic includes desflurane, isoflurane, and sevoflurane. The metabolism of sevoflurane has been implicated in renal toxicity due to production of fluoride, and compound A. Desflurane and isoflurane do not have any nephrotoxic potential secondary to fluoride accumulation.

Opioids such as fentanyl, sufentanil, alfentanil, and remifentanil can be used during the procedure. Morphine and meperidine have metabolites that depend on renal clearance and can accumulate. A muscle relaxant that is not dependent on renal clearance such as atracurium, cisatracurium, and mivacurium should be used.

Lemmens HJM. Kidney transplantation: recent developments and recommendations for anesthetic management. *Anesthesiol Clin North America* 2004;22:651–662.

Miller RD. *Anesthesia*, 6th ed. Philadelphia: Churchill Livingstone, 2005:2241–2242.

C.10. What are the effects of inhalation anesthetics on renal blood flow (RBF), glomerular filtration, and urine output?

All volatile anesthetics produce a dose-related transient and reversible decrease in RBF, glomerular filtration rate (GFR), urine output, and the urinary excretion of sodium. This is primarily in response to a decline in systemic blood pressure and cardiac output. Reduced RBF, loss of renal autoregulation, and neurohumoral and neuroendocrine factors also contribute. Specific differences among the agents on renal function are to be noted. Halothane does not alter autoregulation of RBF and decreases renal vascular resistance and perfusion pressure proportionally. Isoflurane minimally alters RBF with light levels of anesthesia (1 MAC) and significantly decreases renal vascular resistance. As the depth of anesthesia with isoflurane is increased, RBF decreases because of a greater decrease in perfusion pressure than in vascular resistance.

Miller RD. *Miller's anesthesia* 6th ed. Philadelphia: Churchill Livingstone, 2005:2183.

Stoelting RK, Dierdorf SF. *Anesthesia and co-existing disease*, 4th ed. Philadelphia: Churchill Livingstone, 2002:352.

C.11. What are the nephrotoxic effects of inhalation anesthetics? What are the nephrotoxic metabolites of inhalation anesthetics?

Fluoride-induced nephrotoxicity is a potential hazard following metabolism of volatile anesthetics. It is commonly stated that a serum fluoride concentration of 50 μmol per L is the peak value that is nephrotoxic. However, there is no evidence that this peak value is a valid indicator of renal dysfunction. Sevoflurane and enflurane undergo biodegradation to inorganic fluoride. Although the conventional measurements of renal function (blood urea nitrogen [BUN], creatinine) are not altered, there is evidence of transient impairment of renal concentrating ability and renal tubular injury in patients receiving sevoflurane or enflurane. It has not been confirmed if administration of sevoflurane in patients with preexisting renal disease could further deteriorate renal function. Fluoride levels after isoflurane and halothane increase by 3 to 5 μM per L and 1 to 2 μM per L, respectively. These agents do not pose a risk of nephrotoxicity. Desflurane is resistant to biodegradation because fluorine is the only halogen in the desflurane molecule. Mean inorganic fluoride concentration after 1 MAC hour exposure to desflurane is less than 1 μmol per L. Prolonged exposure to desflurane (7.0 MAC hours) has been associated with normal renal function in patients without renal disease. Neither desflurane nor isoflurane lead to a deterioration of creatinine clearance in patients with preexisting renal impairment.

Sodium or barium hydroxide lime absorbents react with sevoflurane, resulting in a byproduct called *compound A*. The nephrotoxic potential of compound A has been noted in animals and is inconclusive in human studies. The concentrations that occur in humans are far below the nephrotoxic levels in animals. A fresh gas flow of 1 L per minute or higher is recommended to minimize the accumulation of compound A in the breathing circuit. Low flow sevoflurane (1 L/minute) has been used on many occasions with no effect on renal function. Carbon dioxide absorbents that contain calcium hydroxide and calcium chloride do not result in compound A formation when exposed to sevoflurane. The U.S. Food and Drug Administration (FDA) recommends the use of sevoflurane with fresh gas flow rates at least 1 L per minute for exposures up to 1 hour and at least 2 L per minute for exposures greater than 1 hour. However, it is important to note that other countries have not recommended such limitations on the clinical use of sevoflurane and problems have not been noted.

Gentz BA, Malan TP Jr. Renal toxicity of sevoflurane: a storm in a teacup? *Drugs* 2001; 61(15):2155–2162.

Litz RJ, Hubler M, Lorenz W, et al. Renal response to desflurane and isoflurane in patients with renal insufficiency. *Anesthesiology* 2002;97:1133–1136.

Miller RD. *Anesthesia*, 6th ed. Philadelphia: Churchill Livingstone, 2005:2183.

Stoelting RK, Dierdorf SF. *Anesthesia and co-existing disease*, 4th ed. Philadelphia: Churchill Livingstone, 2002:352.

C.12. How does renal failure affect the pharmacology of opioids?

The effect of renal failure on individual opioids varies; one must consider the effect of renal failure on drug metabolites as well as the parent compound.

Morphine is metabolized in the liver to morphine-6-glucuronide (M6G) (10%), morphine-3-glucuronide (M3G) (55%) and normorphine (4%), all of which are excreted by the kidneys, along with approximately 10% of the parent compound, in subjects with normal renal function. M6G has been reported to mediate central nervous system (CNS) and respiratory depression when it accumulates in renal failure. Meperidine is metabolized in the liver to normeperidine, also excreted by the kidneys. Accumulation of this metabolite may lead to excitatory CNS effects such as convulsions. Fentanyl is metabolized by the liver, with only 7% excreted unchanged in the urine. Fentanyl is suitable for use during surgery and is safe in the short term. There are reports of the parent compound accumulating during renal failure, but clinical experience is that there are no adverse effects. However, if being used long term in renal failure patients, the pharmacodynamic effects should be monitored carefully. The clearance and half-life of sufentanil and alfentanil are not significantly different in patients with reduced renal function. Remifentanil is metabolized by blood and tissue esterases. The principal metabolite of remifentanil (GR90291) is eliminated by the kidney. The reduced renal elimination of this metabolite is not of clinical significance because the potency is 1/4,000 of the parent compound. Alfentanil metabolism occurs by inducible cytochrome *c* enzymes in the liver making it suitable for renal failure patients.

Dean M. Opioids in renal failure and dialysis patients. *J Pain Symptom Manage* 2004;28 (5):497–504.

Miller RD. *Anesthesia* 6th ed. Philadelphia: Churchill Livingstone, 2005:2183,2241.

C.13. Discuss the intraoperative fluid management during a renal transplant.

The administration of normal saline and normal saline-based fluids (5% albumin) is the standard of care for fluid management in patients undergoing renal transplant surgery. This practice is primarily based on avoidance of potassium-containing fluids that can contribute to intraoperative hyperkalemia. The typical fluid requirement for a 70-kg adult is approximately 3,000 to–4,000 mL. In addition, 500 mL of 5% albumin is given. The recipient's blood is usually type and screened, but blood loss is minimal so transfusion is unlikely. The anesthesiologist should attempt to maintain a systolic blood pressure range of 130 to 160 mm Hg, central venous pressure (CVP) between 10 to 14 cm H_2O and mean pulmonary artery pressure of 18 to 20 mm Hg.

Hypotension may occur after unclamping the iliac vessels and reperfusion of the graft. It is important to maintain the blood pressure because renal function is critically dependent on adequate perfusion. It is critical that the patient is adequately hydrated throughout surgery in preparation for reperfusion of the graft. Close monitoring of the CVP, and lightening the level of anesthesia during this period can prevent hypotension. Vasopressors with α agonist action should be avoided, as they can comprise blood flow to the transplanted organ. Additional fluid may be required to maintain blood pressure and replace urine output. Furosemide or mannitol can enhance urine output. Loop diuretics block the Na/K channels in the thin ascending loop of Henle. This prevents reabsorption of electrolytes in this part of the nephron. The high osmolar fluid then prevents reabsorption of water in the distal tubule. A large volume of fluid with high electrolyte content is excreted. Mannitol is freely filtered in the glomerulus, but not reabsorbed. It causes osmotic expansion of urine volume.

The estimated blood loss during the case ranges between 200 and 500 mL. In some cases, greater blood loss may require transfusion of packed red cells. Packed red cells should be cytomegalovirus (CMV) negative. At the end, patients undergoing surgery can be given reversal agents and extubated promptly. Patients are then transferred to the postanesthesia care unit (PACU) for continued monitoring of urine output and electrolytes.

The intravenous administration of adequate volumes of fluid is associated with earlier onset of graft function, lower postoperative serum creatinine, higher postoperative creatinine clearance, reduced incidence of delayed graft function, and improved graft survival.

O' Malley CMN, Frument RJ, Bennett EG. Intravenous fluid therapy in renal transplant recipients: results of a US survey. *Transplant Proc* 2002;34:3142–3145.

The New York Hospital-Cornell Medical Center Kidney Transplantation Protocol 2005, New York, NY

C.14. What severe reactions can occur with the administration of polyclonal and monoclonal antibodies intraoperatively?

Thymoglobulin is a product of heterologous sera and has the potential to produce type 1 hypersensitivity such as anaphylaxis. Thymoglobulin is made by immunization of rabbits with human lymphoid tissue. In the case of thymoglobulin, which is available in the United States, thymocytes are used; in the case of anti–T-lymphocyte immunoglobulin (ATG), which is available in Europe, an activated T-cell line is used. The side effects of polyclonal antibodies are related to the fact they are foreign protein. Chills, fever, and arthralgias are common. Objective evidence of an anaphylactic reaction should prompt cessation of ATG administration. The treatment is primarily supportive. This includes continued ventilation with 100% oxygen, support of blood pressure with epinephrine, steroids, and antihistamines. Patients on β-adrenergic blocking agents or angiotensin-converting enzyme inhibitors may not tolerate an anaphylactic event, or respond to its treatment, as well as other patients.

Other adverse reactions possible with polyclonal antibodies include pruritis, rash, nausea, vomiting, diarrhea, back or flank pain, hemolytic anemia, thrombocytopenia, leukopenia, or serum sickness. Phlebitis can occur when administered through a peripheral vein.

The monoclonal antibody, OKT3, may be administered intraoperatively. A rapidly developing noncardiogenic pulmonary edema may occur after the first dose.

The initial side effects of monoclonal antibody (muromonab-CD3, OKT3) are similar to that of antilymphocyte globulin. It includes high fever and hypotension. To prevent this, acetaminophen, an antihistamine, and a steroid usually are administered before injection. Because this agent is also associated with high frequency of pulmonary edema, it should not be given to any patient who has more than 3% body weight gain during the week before therapy.

Millar MM, Grammer LC. Case reports of evaluation and desensitization for anti-thymocyte globulin hypersensitivity. *Ann Allergy Asthma Immunol* 2000;85:311–316.

Min DI, Monaco AP. Complications associated with immunosuppressive therapy and their management. *Pharmacotherapy* 1991;11(5):119S–125S.

C.15. Describe the differential diagnosis of oliguria?

Immediate urine production is seen in over 90% of living donor kidney transplants and between 40% and 70% of cadaveric transplants. In addition to maintaining intraoperative hydration, mannitol, loop diuretics, and occasionally dopamine can all enhance urine production. Oliguria is defined as urine output of less than 0.3 mL/kg/hour. Glomerular filtration is directly dependent on renal perfusion. Renal perfusion is dependent on arterial pressure and renal vascular resistance. Renal vascular resistance is a response to autoregulation and the renin-angiotensin-aldosterone system. Low urine output indicates a dramatic reduction in glomerular filtration rate (GFR) or the presence of mechanical obstruction. Oliguria can be divided into prerenal, renal and postrenal etiologies.

Prerenal oliguria

- *Decreased intravascular volume.* This may be a result of inadequate hydration that can result in systemic hypotension. The autoregulation curves are shifted to the right in patients who have chronic hypertension and renal vascular disease. Therefore a greater arterial pressure may be required to ensure adequate renal perfusion. A fluid challenge can correct the volume depletion. The urine sediment is normal in hypovolemic prerenal failure.

- *Relative decrease in blood volume.* An example is vasodilatation of capacitance vessels from volatile agents. The response to mannitol or furosemide is brisk when blood pressure and hydration are adequate.

Renal oliguria

- *Structural causes.* Impedance to renal blood flow (RBF) can occur from renal artery thromboembolism or renal vein thrombosis. Drugs such as cyclosporine, tacrolimus, and angiotensin-converting enzyme inhibitors cause intrarenal vasoconstriction through the afferent arterioles.
- *Acute tubular necrosis (ATN).* This is the end result of all of the factors listed in the preceding text, but may be due to nephrotoxic agents such as antibiotics or contrast. The urine sediment may contain coarse granular casts and tubular epithelial casts. Red cell casts indicate glomerular disease. Eosinophiluria indicates interstitial nephritis or atheroembolic disease.

Postrenal olguria

- Mechanical obstruction. If urine output declines during surgical wound closure impingement of the graft vessels or ureter may be the reason. The Foley catheter should be irrigated to ensure that clot or tissue is not blocking patency. Intraoperative ultrasound can examine the flow in the arterial and venous anastomosis. No casts or sediment is seen in the urine.

Various indices are used to distinguish between prerenal and renal oliguria. The most useful are the urine osmolality, urine sodium, the fractional excretion of sodium (FeNa*), and urine to serum creatinine ratio. The comparison is noted in the Table 38.4.

Subramanian S, Ziedalski TM. Oliguria, volume overload, Na balance and diuretics. *Crit Care Clin* 2005;21:291–303.

C.16. How does renal failure affect the dosing of neuromuscular (NM) reversal agents?

The dose of neostigmine depends on the intensity of the NM blockade, which is determined by the total amount of muscle relaxant given, the frequency of administration, and the time of last dose. A normal healthy adult patient requires 1.5 to 3.0 mg of neostigmine to antagonize a nondepolarizing block. The maximum dose is up to 5 mg (0.6 to 0.8 mg/kg). Larger doses of neostigmine may enhance NM blockade acting as an agonist. The pharmacokinetics of anticholinesterase drugs in renal failure is similar to that in normal patients. Normally, the continued renal elimination of NM blocking agents prevents the reappearance of residual muscle weakness and offsets waning effects of the anticholinesterase drugs. Renal excretion accounts for approximately 50% of the clearance of neostigmine, and approximately 75% of the elimination of edrophonium and pyridostigmine. Renal failure allows some protection against residual NM blockade because renal elimination half times of anticholinesterase drugs is prolonged. The plasma clearance of anticholinesterase drug is longer than that of nondepolarizing NM blocking drugs.

Table 38.4   The Difference between Prerenal and Renal Oliguria.

INDEX	PRERENAL	RENAL
Urine osmolarity (mOsm/L)	>500	<400
Urine sodium (mEq/L)	<20	>40
Urine/Serum creatinine	>40	<20
BUN/creatinine ratio	>20	<10−15
Fe Na* (%)	<1	>2

*FeNa $= [U_{Na}/S_{Na}]/[U_{Cr}/S_{Cr}]$.

Stoelting R, Dierdorf SF. *Anesthesia and co-existing disease*, 4th ed. New York: Churchill Livingstone, 2002:355.

D. Postoperative Management

D.1. What are some side effects of immunosuppressive agents anesthesiologists should be aware of?

Some of the side effects may be encountered if a posttransplant patient presents for other surgeries, and are pertinent to anesthetic care:

- *Calcineurin inhibitors (cyclosporin, tacrolimus).* Nephrotoxicity, hypertension, hyperchloremic acidosis, hyperkalemia, hypomagnesemia, hypocalcemia, glucose intolerance, coarse tremor, dysesthesia, headache, seizure, prolonged QT interval, hypercoagulability, acute microvascular disease (similar to thrombotic thrombocytopenic purpura)
- *Mycophenolate mofentil.* Nausea, vomiting, cytopenia (leukopenia, anemia, thrombocytopenia), leukocytosis
- *Target of Rapamycin (TOR) inhibitors (sirolimus, everolimus).* Mucocutaneous ulceration, hypokalemia, hypomagnesemia, impaired wound healing, interstitial pneumonia, cytopenia
- *Azathioprine.* Cytopenia, hepatitis

Danovitch GM. *Handbook of kidney transplantation*, 4th ed. Philadelphia: Lippincott Williams & Wilkins, 2005:72–134.

van Hoof JP, Christiaans MHL, van Duijnhoven, EM. Tacrolimus and posttransplant diabetes mellitus in renal transplantation. *Transplantation* 2005;79:1465–1469.

D.2. How is the diagnosis of acute transplant rejection made?

Hyperacute rejection occurs within minutes of a transplanted organ being reperfused. It is due to preformed antibodies in the recipient that are specific to the donor. The antibodies may be directed against donor human leukocyte antigens (HLAs) or they may be antiABO blood group antibodies. It leads to ischemic necrosis of the graft resulting in a swollen and darkened graft. This type of rejection is not reversible.

Accelerated acute rejection occurs within a few days of transplant. It is both a cell- and antibody-mediated injury. The process involves an immunologic memory response when a recipient has been sensitized by previous exposure to antigens present in the donor.

Acute rejection is usually seen within days to a few months of the transplant. The diagnosis is made with a renal biopsy. It is a cell-mediated process involving lymphocytes. In patients with prolonged delayed graft function, surveillance biopsies can detect or exclude acute rejection episodes. The process is associated with systemic symptoms such as fever, chills, malaise, and arthralgias. However, with current immunosuppressive drugs, most acute rejection episodes are generally asymptomatic. Laboratory data note a rapid increase in creatinine of 10% to 25% over baseline with or without a decrease in urine output.

Brunicardi FC, Andersen DK, Billiar TR, et al. *Schwartz's principles of surgery*, 8th ed. New York: McGraw-Hill, 2005:298.

Ponticelli C. Renal transplantation 2004: where do we stand today? *Nephrol Dial Transplant* 2004;19:2937–2947.

CHAPTER 39

Laparoscopic Surgery

Judith Weingram

A 72-YEAR-OLD MAN

with biopsy-proved carcinoma of the prostate had a prostate-specific antigen (PSA) of 22 ng per mL but negative pelvic computed tomography (CT) and bone scans. He weighed 100 kg. Despite hypertension and a 50 pack-year smoking history, he was vigorous and active, and he was anxious to begin definitive treatment. First, he was scheduled for staging by laparoscopic pelvic lymph node dissection.

A. Medical Disease and Differential Diagnosis

1. What is the incidence of carcinoma of the prostate?
2. How is prostate cancer diagnosed?
3. How is prostate cancer treated?
4. Our patient is scheduled for pelvic lymph node dissection. What are the indications for this procedure and by which techniques can it be performed?
5. What other types of cancer can be staged by laparoscopic lymph node dissection?
6. Define laparoscopy.
7. What are the three major forces that uniquely alter the patient's physiology during laparoscopy?
8. What are the advantages and disadvantages of laparoscopy?
9. What are the contraindications to laparoscopic surgery? Is pregnancy a contraindication to laparoscopic surgery?
10. What other specialties commonly perform laparoscopic or minimally invasive surgery?
11. What are the differences in pulmonary function after laparoscopic cholecystectomy compared with open cholecystectomy?
12. Why is carbon dioxide the gas of choice for laparoscopy? What are its disadvantages?
13. How much endogenous CO_2 is produced at basal level and at maximal exercise?
14. How much CO_2 is stored in the body? Where is it stored? Of what significance is this to laparoscopy?
15. Describe the diffusion and solubility properties of CO_2 and their significance in laparoscopy.
16. Is CO_2 soluble in blood? Why?

B. Preoperative Evaluation and Preparation

1. What do you want to know about this patient's history and physical condition that may affect whether or not you clear him for laparoscopic surgery?
2. What factors increase this patient's risk of pulmonary complications?
3. What laboratory tests should be performed preoperatively?

4. What specific information should the patient be given about laparoscopic surgery before obtaining informed consent?

5. What additional procedures should be done before surgery?

6. What three general areas should you be concerned about in your attempt to minimize or prevent complications during laparoscopy?

C. Intraoperative Management

1. What monitors and devices would you apply to the patient? Why?

2. What intravenous (IV) solution and how much fluid volume do you plan to deliver?

3. How would the patient be positioned?

4. What are the respiratory and circulatory effects of the Trendelenburg position?

5. What is the anesthetic technique of choice for laparoscopy? Why?

6. Can a laryngeal mask airway (LMA) be used?

7. What anesthetic agents or adjuvant drugs are recommended for laparoscopy? Are any anesthetic agents contraindicated?

8. Should N_2O be used during laparoscopy? What are the pros and cons? Does N_2O cause bowel distention during laparoscopy? Does N_2O cause nausea and vomiting after laparoscopy?

9. Can laparoscopy be performed under local anesthesia or regional anesthesia?

10. What two techniques are available for initial laparoscopic access to the peritoneal cavity? What anesthetic problems can arise during insufflation?

11. What is the purpose of the heparinized saline irrigation-suction device used by the surgeon and why should you be concerned with it?

12. Under what circumstances should laparoscopy be converted to laparotomy?

13. What is the mechanism of increase in shunting resulting from embolization?

14. What are the arterial to end-tidal CO_2 gradients ($Paco_2$–$PETCO_2$) in the normal awake patient? What is the cause of the gradient? Does the gradient change during laparoscopy? Why?

15. Is an arterial line necessary? Why? Does end-tidal CO_2 tension accurately reflect arterial CO_2 tension? Under what circumstances may the $PETCO_2$ exceed the $Paco_2$? Why?

16. What are the possible causes of hypercarbia?

17. What factors play a role in the unusually rapid and marked elevation of CO_2 that is sometimes seen in laparoscopy?

18. How rapidly does the $Paco_2$ rise in the apneic patient (endogenous CO_2)? How rapidly does the $Paco_2$ rise if 5% CO_2 gas is inhaled (exogenous)? How rapidly can the CO_2 rise during laparoscopy? What factors explain the differences?

19. What are the direct and indirect effects of hypercarbia on the cardiovascular system? How are these effects altered by increased intraabdominal pressure and patient position?

20. What are the direct and indirect effects of hypercarbia on the respiratory system? How does the Trendelenburg position and the increased intraabdominal pressure of pneumoperitoneum alter these effects?

21. What are the direct and indirect effects of hypercarbia on the central nervous system?

22. What are the neuroendocrine changes that occur during laparoscopy?

23. What are the direct and indirect effects of laparoscopy on the renal system?

24. What is the effect of hypercarbia and laparoscopy on the bowel and gastrointestinal system?

25. How would you recognize CO_2 embolism during laparoscopy? How does this differ from air embolism? Why should N_2O be discontinued during suspected embolization? Will N_2O increase the size of the CO_2 emboli?

26. How is gas embolism (CO_2 or air) treated?

27. What are the causes of pneumothorax or pneumomediastinum during laparoscopy? How would you diagnose it? How would you treat it?

28. How would you decide when to extubate?

D. Postoperative Management

1. What are some of the unique complications of laparoscopy?

2. What postoperative orders will you write? When would you remove the Foley catheter and arterial line? Under what circumstances would you order a chest x-ray film?

3. What is the incidence of postoperative nausea and vomiting?

A. Medical Disease and Differential Diagnosis

A.1. What is the incidence of carcinoma of the prostate?

Carcinoma of the prostate is the second most common cause of death from cancer in American men. In 1983, the incidence of carcinoma of the prostate was approximately 75,000 new cases along with 25,000 deaths of old cases. In 2006, the American Cancer Society estimates that the incidence will be 234,460 new cases, along with 27,350 deaths.

This "epidemic" increase in carcinoma of the prostate is believed to result from new methods for early detection rather than from a true rise in incidence of the disease. Undetected microscopic prostate cancer cells are believed to be present in 30% to 40% of men over the age of 50, and in 75% of men over the age of 75, but it is estimated that only approximately 8% of these will become clinically significant. It has been stated that more men die *with* prostate cancer than *from* it. Therefore, it is not yet known whether early detection of subclinical disease, much of which may have remained clinically insignificant, will improve survival.

Carcinoma of the prostate is rare in Asian men, whereas African-American men have about twice the incidence as white American men.

Dugan JA, Bostwick DG, Myers RP, et al. The definition and preoperative prediction of clinically insignificant prostate cancer. *JAMA* 1996;275:288–294.

Potosky AL, Miller BA, Albertsen PC, et al. The role of increasing detection in the rising incidence of prostate cancer. *JAMA* 1995;273:548–552.

Sarma AV, Schottenfeld D. Prostate cancer incidence, mortality, and survival trends in the United States: 1981–2001. *Semin Urol Oncol* 2002;20:3–9.

A.2. How is prostate cancer diagnosed?

The most reliable methods for diagnosis include digital rectal examination plus the serum prostate-specific antigen (PSA) level. Palpation of a tumor or indurated area and finding an elevated PSA should be followed by prostatic needle biopsies, perhaps under transrectal ultrasound (TRUS) guidance.

Gann PH, Hennekens CH, Stampfer MJ. A prospective evaluation of plasma prostate-specific antigen for detection of prostatic cancer. *JAMA* 1995;273:289–294.

Oesterling JE. Prostate-specific antigen: improving its ability to diagnose early prostate cancer [Editorial]. *JAMA* 1992;267:2236–2238.

A.3. How is prostate cancer treated?

Treatment choices vary not just with the stage of the disease but also with the patient's age and life expectancy, associated medical conditions, and lifestyle. In patients with negative lymph nodes, treatment choices include "watchful waiting", brachytherapy (in which radioactive seeds are implanted in the prostate gland), external beam radiation, and surgery. Surgical options include open radical prostatectomy, or laparoscopic radical prostatectomy which can be hand-assisted or robot-assisted.

A patient with positive lymph nodes can choose to be treated with radiation, hormones, chemotherapy, or other nonsurgical options, or even to have no treatment.

Menon N, Shrivastava A, Tewari A. Laparoscopic radical prostatectomy: conventional and robotic. *Urology* 2005;66(5):101–104.

Rozet F, Galiano M, Cathelineau X, et al. Extraperitoneal laparoscopic radical prostatectomy: a prospective evaluation of 600 cases. *J Urol* 2005;174(3):908–911.

A.4. Our patient is scheduled for pelvic lymph node dissection. What are the indications for this procedure and by which techniques can it be performed?

Histologic examination of the pelvic lymph nodes is necessary to accurately stage the tumor and select the appropriate treatment. Our patient is older, has multisystem disease, has a suspiciously high prostate-specific antigen (PSA), and has chosen to be treated nonsurgically.

Pelvic lymph node dissection can be performed by several techniques. Before laparoscopic surgery was introduced, each patient underwent major open abdominal surgery. The laparoscopic approach to the pelvic lymph nodes can be transabdominal (i.e., entering the peritoneum anteriorly, then opening the posterior peritoneum for access), or it can be done directly extraperitoneally. In either case, laparoscopy avoids a large incision, is less painful, has less morbidity and quicker recovery, and offers about the same nodal yield as open surgery. The chief disadvantage of the laparoscopic approach is the longer duration.

Allaf ME, Bhayani SB, Link RE, et al. Laparoscopic retroperitoneal lymph node dissection: duplication of open technique. *Urology* 2005;65(3):575–577.

Jarrard DF, Chodak GW. Prostate cancer staging after radiation utilizing laparoscopic pelvic lymphadenectomy. *Urology* 1995;46:538–541.

Kava BR, Dalbagni G, Conlon KC, et al. Results of laparoscopic pelvic lymphadenectomy in patients at high risk for nodal metastases from prostate cancer. *Ann Surg Oncol* 1998; 5:173–180.

Kozlowski PM, Winfield HN. Laparoscopic lymph node dissection: pelvic and retroperitoneal. *Semin Laparosc Surg* 2000;7:150–159.

Patel R, Stifelman MD. Hand-assisted laparoscopic devices: the second generation. *J Endurol* 2004;18(7):649–653.

Wolf JS. Indications, technique, and results of laparoscopic pelvic lymphadenectomy. *J Endourol* 2001;15:427–435. Discussion 447–448.

A.5. What other types of cancer can be staged by laparoscopic lymph node dissection?

Laparoscopic lymph node dissections have been performed in association with carcinomas of the prostate, bladder, urethra, testis, and penis. In addition, laparoscopic dissections of bilateral aortic and pelvic lymph nodes are used for staging of gynecologic malignancies, especially cervical and ovarian. Diagnostic laparoscopy, in conjunction with computed tomography (CT), has been used to detect and confirm positive lymph nodes and distant metastases in many other surgical specialties, thereby potentially resulting in altered treatment and prognosis.

Albqami N, Janetschek G. Laparoscopic retroperitoneal lymph-node dissection in the management of clinical stage I and II testicular cancer. *J Endourol* 2005;19(6):683–692.

Heath EI, Kaufman HS, Talamini MA, et al. The role of laparoscopy in preoperative staging of esophageal cancer. *Surg Endosc* 2000;14:495–499.

Kohler C, Klemm P, Schau A, et al. Introduction of transperitoneal lymphadenectomy in a gynecological oncology center: analysis of 650 laparoscopic pelvic and/or paraaortic transperitoneal lymphadenectomies. *Gynecol Oncol* 2004;95(1):52–61.

Whalley DG, Berrigan MJ. Anesthesia for radical prostatectomy, cystectomy, nephrectomy, pheochromocytoma, and laparoscopic procedures. *Anesthesiol Clin North America* 2000; 18(4):899–917.

A.6. Define laparoscopy.

Laparoscopy (or peritoneoscopy) is a "minimally invasive" procedure allowing endoscopic access to the peritoneal cavity after insufflation of a gas (CO_2) to create space between the anterior abdominal wall and the viscera. The space is necessary for the safe manipulation of instruments and organs. Laparoscopic surgery can also be extraperitoneal. It can also be gasless with abdominal wall retraction, and, more recently, it may be hand-assisted.

Seifman BD, Wolf JS. Technical advances in laparoscopy: hand assistance, retractors, and the pneumodissector. *J Endourol* 2000;14:921–928.

Weingram J. Laparoscopic and laser surgery. In: Malhotra V, ed. *Anesthesia for renal and genito-urologic surgery*. New York: McGraw-Hill, 1996:151–176.

Wolf JS. Indications, technique, and results of laparoscopic pelvic lymphadenectomy. *J Endourol* 2001;15:427–435.

A.7. What are the three major forces that uniquely alter the patient's physiology during laparoscopy?

- The increase in intraabdominal pressure and volume (pneumoperitoneum).
- Extremes of patient positioning
- Carbon dioxide and hypercarbia

It is vital that the anesthesiologist have a thorough understanding of the physiologic consequences of changes in these three forces. Separately or in combination, they have profound effects on the patient's hemodynamic, respiratory, and metabolic functions. The early gynecologic laparoscopies were usually brief, and they were performed on young healthy women who tolerated these physiologic trespasses with nearly insignificant changes. These same three forces, however, may produce significant physiologic changes in long, complex laparoscopies in older sicker patients unable to compensate.

Henny CP, Hofland J. Laparoscopic surgery: pitfalls due to anesthesia, positioning, and pneumoperitoneum. *Surg Endosc* 2005;19(9):1163–1171.

Hirvonen EA, Poikolainen EO, Paakkonen ME, et al. The adverse hemodynamic effects of anesthesia, head-up tilt, and carbon dioxide pneumoperitoneum during laparoscopic cholecystectomy. *Surg Endosc* 2000;14(3):272–277.

O'Malley C, Cunningham AJ. Physiologic changes during laparoscopy. *Anesthesiol Clin North America* 2001;19(1):1–19.

Ost MC, Tan BJ, Lee BR. Urologic laparoscopy: basic physiologic considerations and immunological consequences. *J Urol* 2005;174(4):1183–1188.

Sosa RE, Weingram J. Physiologic considerations in laparoscopic surgery. *J Endourol* 1992; 6:285–287.

A.8. What are the advantages and disadvantages of laparoscopy?

The advantages include the cosmetic results of small, non–muscle-splitting incisions, decreased blood loss, less postoperative pain and ileus, shorter hospitalization and convalescence, and ultimately lower cost. Postoperative respiratory muscle function returns to normal more quickly than in open surgery, especially in laparoscopic cholecystectomy and other upper abdominal procedures. Wound complications such as infection and dehiscence are less frequent, and host defense mechanisms may be greater in laparoscopic than in open surgery.

The disadvantages include the long learning curve for the surgeon (most complications occur during the first 10 laparoscopies), the narrowed two-dimensional visual field on video, the need for general anesthesia, and the often longer duration. Ideally, surgeons should have more advanced laparoscopic skills, especially in knot tying, suturing, and working two instruments simultaneously. The use of simulators to enhance these skills has been advocated.

Collet D, Vitale GC, Reynolds M, et al. Peritoneal host defenses are less impaired by laparoscopy than by open operation. *Surg Endosc* 1995;9:1059–1064.

Conacher ID, Soomro NA, Rix D. Anaesthesia for laparoscopic urological surgery. *Br J Anaesth* 2004;93(6):859–864.

Rovina N, Bouros D, Tzanakis N, et al. Effects of laparoscopic cholecystectomy on global respiratory muscle strength. *Am J Respir Crit Care Med* 1996;153:458–461.

A.9. What are the contraindications to laparoscopic surgery? Is pregnancy a contraindication to laparoscopic surgery?

Increasing experience with the laparoscopic technique has made most contraindications relative not absolute. However, it is probably best to avoid or to use extreme caution in patients with coagulopathy, diaphragmatic hernia, severe cardiovascular or pulmonary disease (including bullae), increased intracranial pressure or space-occupying masses, impending renal shutdown, a history of extensive surgery or adhesions, sickle cell disease (because sickle crisis may be precipitated by acidosis), peritonitis, a large intraabdominal mass, tumor of the abdominal wall, or hypovolemic shock. Patients with shunts (e.g., ventriculoperitoneal) are at risk for gas emboli, shunt obstruction, and intracranial hypertension, all of which may occur during laparoscopy and may require intracranial pressure monitoring and ventricular drainage if laparoscopic surgery is necessary. In summary, most of the contraindications concern patients who are unable to tolerate extremes of position, pneumoperitoneum and/or hypercarbia.

Although pregnancy has been considered a contraindication to laparoscopic surgery in the past, an increasing number of such procedures are being performed in the parturient. Laparoscopic cholecystectomy is now more frequent than open cholecystectomy in the pregnant patient. The overall objective of laparoscopic as well as open surgery is to preserve fetal and maternal well-being and to prevent premature labor. In addition to the general problems of anesthesia for the parturient, the anesthesiologist must also consider the specific problems that result from the interplay between the anatomic and physiologic changes of pregnancy and the anatomic and physiologic triad of pneumoperitoneum, hypercarbia, and positional changes.

Factors to consider in the management of the pregnant patient include awareness of her increased blood volume, increased cardiac output, decreased systemic vascular resistance (SVR), hypercoagulability, the supine hypotensive syndrome, increased respiratory minute volume, decreased residual volume, decreased functional residual capacity (FRC), increased oxygen consumption, mild hypocapnia, increased risk of aspiration, and decreased anesthetic requirement.

This combination of factors tends to promote hypercarbia and hypoxemia. However, extreme hyperventilation may result in decreased uteroplacental perfusion. Arterial blood gas monitoring has been suggested to detect fetal acidosis because capnography may not reveal a large arterial to end-tidal difference in CO_2. In all cases, preoperative and postoperative fetal and uterine monitoring is essential.

Cunningham AJ, Schlanger M. Intraoperative hypoxemia complicating laparoscopic cholecystectomy in a patient with sickle hemoglobinopathy. *Anesth Analg* 1992;75: 838–843.

Society of Gastrointestinal Endoscopic Surgeons. Guidelines for laparoscopic surgery during pregnancy. Society of Gastrointestinal Endoscopic Surgeons. *Surg Endosc* 1998; 12:189–190.

Lachman E, Schienfeld A, Voss E, et al. Pregnancy and laparoscopic surgery. *J Am Assoc Gynecol Laparosc* 1999;6:347–351.

Ravaoherisoa J, Meyer P, Afriat R, et al. Laparoscopic surgery in a patient with ventriculoperitoneal shunt: monitoring of shunt function with transcranial Doppler. *Br J Anaesth* 2004;92(3):434–437.

Rosen MA. Management of anesthesia for the pregnant surgical patient. *Anesthesiology* 1999;91:1159–1163.

Shankar KB, Mushlin PS. Arterial to end-tidal gradients in pregnant subjects. *Anesthesiology* 1997;87:1596–1598.

Steinbrook RA, Bhavani-Shankar K. Hemodynamics during laparoscopic surgery in pregnancy. *Anesth Analg* 2001;93:1570–1571.

Uzzo RG, Bilsky M, Mininberg DT, et al. Laparoscopic surgery in children with ventriculoperitoneal shunts: effect of pneumoperitoneum on intracranial pressure—preliminary experience. *Urology* 1997;49:753–757.

A.10. What other specialties commonly perform laparoscopic or minimally invasive surgery?

Laparoscopic procedures in urology have become standard, especially for prostatectomy, uncomplicated adrenalectomy and nephrectomy including live donor nephrectomy. Laparoscopic gynecologic surgery includes tubal surgery (sterilization, treatment of ectopic pregnancy, etc.), cystectomies, hysterectomies, various ablations (endometriosis), and so on. Laparoscopy is performed in pregnancy and also in pediatrics. Complications include bladder and ureteral injuries and fistulae, but apparently these are not more prevalent than in standard surgery.

Laparoscopic general surgery includes cholecystectomy, hernia repair, antireflux procedures, splenectomy, appendectomy, bowel surgery including bariatric procedures, and various other upper and lower abdominal procedures.

Thoracoscopic surgery and neurosurgical intracranial surgery using modified laparoscopic instruments, but without the need for gas insufflation, are two of the more recent areas of minimally invasive surgery. Lumbar discectomies and other types of spinal surgery have also been done laparoscopically through an anterior approach. Even autopsies have been attempted laparoscopically. The list continues to grow.

Brown SL, Biehl TR, Rawlins MC, et al. Laparoscopic live donor nephrectomy: a comparison with the conventional open approach. *J Urol* 2001;165:766–769.

Lindgren L, Koivusalo AM, Kellokumpu I. Conventional pneumoperitoneum compared with abdominal wall lift for laparoscopic cholecystectomy. *Br J Anaesth* 1995;75:567–572.

Mage G, Masson FM, Canis M, et al. Laparoscopic hysterectomy. *Curr Opin Obstet Gynecol* 1995;7:283–289.

Pennant JH. Anesthesia for laparoscopy in the pediatric patient. *Anesthesiol Clin North America* 2001;19(1):69–88.

Zelko JR, Misko J, Swanstrom L, et al. Laparoscopic lumbar discectomy. *Am J Surg* 1995; 169:496–498.

A.11. What are the differences in pulmonary function after laparoscopic cholecystectomy compared with open cholecystectomy?

Pulmonary function is substantially impaired after a large upper abdominal incision, as in open cholecystectomy. Marked diaphragmatic dysfunction occurs postoperatively, caused by both reflex diaphragmatic changes and incisional pain. Vital capacity and functional residual capacity (FRC) may be reduced by 20% to 40% of preoperative values, and they may not return to normal until 2 to 3 days after surgery. The mini incision of laparoscopic cholecystectomy results in far less pulmonary and diaphragmatic loss of function, as well as less ileus.

Bablekos GD, Michaelides SA, Roussou T, et al. Changes in breathing control and mechanics after laparoscopic vs open cholecystectomy. *Arch Surg* 2006;141(1):16–22.

Cunningham AJ, Brull SJ. Laparoscopic cholecystectomy: anesthetic implications [Review]. *Anesth Analg* 1993;76:1120–1133.

Gunnarsson L, Lindberg P, Tokics L, et al. Lung function after open versus laparoscopic cholecystectomy. *Acta Anaesthesiol Scand* 1995;39:302–306.

Hong SJ, Cho EJ, Lee JY, et al. The physiologic response to laparoscopic cholecystectomy: CO(2) pneumoperitoneum vs wall lift. *Can J Anaesth* 2003;50(2):200–201.

Koivusalo AM, Lindgren L. Effects of carbon dioxide pneumoperitoneum for laparoscopic cholecystectomy. *Acta Anaesthesiol Scand* 2000;44(7):834–841.

A.12. Why is carbon dioxide the gas of choice for laparoscopy? What are its disadvantages?

Carbon dioxide is the insufflating gas of choice because it is nonflammable, does not support combustion, readily diffuses across membranes, is rapidly removed in the lungs, and is highly soluble because of rapid buffering in blood. The risk of CO_2 embolization is small. As much as 200 mL of CO_2 injected directly into a peripheral vein may not be lethal, whereas only 20 mL of air may prove to be so. In addition, CO_2 levels in blood and expired air can easily be measured, and its elimination can be augmented by increasing ventilation. As long as oxygen requirements are met, a high concentration of blood CO_2 can be tolerated. Also, medical grade CO_2 is readily available and inexpensive.

It is for these reasons that the following gases are unsatisfactory for pneumoperitoneum: nitrous oxide (does not cause pain intraabdominally but does not suppress combustion), oxygen (flammable), helium, air and nitrogen (each has no hemodynamic or acid-base sequelae, but can cause gas emboli), argon (adverse effect on hepatic blood flow, emboli).

It should be emphasized, however, that carbon dioxide plays a duel role in the body, and it is not inert. Under normal circumstances it is a waste product of metabolism. Under the circumstances of laparoscopies, it acts as a drug, often present in quantities far larger than the body is capable of generating from even the most extreme exercise or hypermetabolic state.

The disadvantages mainly stem from the fact that carbon dioxide is not inert, and it has contradictory roles as an endogenous chemical and as an exogenous foreign substance. Changes in its concentration and tensions have enormous biochemical and physiologic consequences. Changes at the local tissue level are often at odds with the overall systemic effect. It causes direct peritoneal irritation and pain during laparoscopy under local anesthesia because it transiently forms carbonic acid when in contact with the moist peritoneum. In addition, CO_2 is not very soluble in the absence of red blood cells, and, therefore, it can remain in gaseous form intraperitoneally after laparoscopy, causing referred shoulder pain. Hypercarbia and respiratory acidosis occur when the buffering capacity of blood is temporarily exceeded. In addition, CO_2 exerts widespread local and (often contradictory) systemic effects that may manifest overall as hypertension, tachycardia, cerebral vasodilation, hypercarbia, and respiratory acidosis.

Menes T, Spivak H. Laparoscopy: searching for the proper insufflation gas. *Surg Endosc* 2000;14(11):1050–1056.

Tsereteli Z, Terry ML, Bowers SP, et al. Prospective randomized clinical trial comparing nitrous oxide and carbon dioxide pneumoperitoneum for laparoscopic surgery. *J Am Coll Surg* 2002;195(2):173–180.

Weingram J. Laparoscopic and laser surgery. In: Malhotra V, ed. *Anesthesia for renal and genito-urologic surgery*. New York: McGraw-Hill, 1996:157.

A.13. How much endogenous CO_2 is produced at basal level and at maximal exercise?

Carbon dioxide and water are the major end products of aerobic metabolism in the mitochondria of the cells. Carbonic acid, the major acid produced in the body, is uniquely volatile, and, therefore, it must be largely eliminated by the lungs. (Other acids are eliminated by the kidney.)

At basal rate, an average adult manufactures approximately 200 mL of CO_2 per minute (while consuming 250 mL of O_2) or 12 L of CO_2 (35 g) per hour. At maximal metabolic rate, it is estimated that the body can produce, transport, and excrete 90 to 100 L/hour, an increase of 800% over basal rate.

Kinney JM. Transport of carbon dioxide in the blood. *Anesthesiology* 1960;21:615–619.

Lumb AB. *Nunn's applied respiratory physiology*, 6th ed. Philadelphia: Butterworth-Heinemann, 2005:148–154.

A.14. How much CO_2 is stored in the body? Where is it stored? Of what significance is this to laparoscopy?

The body contains approximately 120 L of carbon dioxide. (This is approximately 100 times the amount of stored oxygen.) CO_2 in the blood is in equilibrium with CO_2 in different tissues. The rate of uptake and distribution of CO_2 from the blood depends on the perfusion and storage capacity of those different tissues. The well-perfused tissues, including blood, brain, and kidney, come to rapid equilibrium. The medium-perfused compartment consists mainly of resting skeletal muscle. The slowly perfused compartment, mainly fat and bone, has the largest CO_2 storage capacity. In contrast to rapidly changing oxygen levels, CO_2 levels reach equilibrium more slowly.

These storage sites serve to buffer and stabilize blood CO_2 levels because they provide a place for excess CO_2 to "park" until ventilation can catch up and restore equilibrium. The increase in CO_2 storage during laparoscopy is illustrated clinically by the decelerating rate of rise in $PETCO_2$ despite continuing insufflation. Blood or end-tidal CO_2 levels increase rapidly at first, then plateau at between 15 and 35 minutes, despite continuing low flow insufflation. At constant ventilation, CO_2 levels increase, but not as much as if no simultaneous storage processes were occurring. But if ventilation is increased to keep CO_2 constant, then the increase needed is only approximately 40% of the predicted volume of ventilation because of the drain-off of CO_2 into the storage sites.

Farhi LE, Rahn H. Dynamics of changes in carbon dioxide stores. *Anesthesiology* 1960;21: 604–614.

Lumb AB. *Nunn's applied respiratory physiology*, 6th ed. Philadelphia: Butterworth-Heinemann, 2005:158.

Seed RF, Shakespeare TF, Muldoon MJ. Carbon dioxide homeostasis during anaesthesia for laparoscopy. *Anaesthesia* 1970;25:223–231.

A.15. Describe the diffusion and solubility properties of CO_2 and their significance in laparoscopy.

Diffusion describes the process by which gases travel from an area of higher partial pressure to one of lower partial pressure. For a gaseous environment, Graham's law states that the rate of diffusion of a gas is inversely proportional to the square root of its density (i.e., the smaller the molecule the more easily it will diffuse).

When that same gas molecule arrives at an aqueous membrane (e.g., a gas–liquid interface), the solubility of that gas in water now becomes the major factor in determining its diffusing capacity, as shown in Table 39.1. The water solubility of CO_2 is 24 times that of O_2, whereas the diffusion capacity of CO_2 is 20.5 times that of O_2. The capacity of a gas to diffuse across a membrane is directly proportional to its solubility in water and inversely proportional to its molecular weight. However, the actual movement of that gas across the aqueous membrane depends not only on its diffusing capacity but, more importantly, on the pressure gradient across that membrane.

The fate of CO_2 gas insufflated into the peritoneal cavity is the same that would occur in any other closed but distensible cavity. The pressure obtained within the cavity varies directly with the volume of gas insufflated and indirectly with the compliance of the closed cavity.

Table 39.1 Influence of Physical Properties on the Diffusion of Gas through a Gas/Liquid Interface.

GAS	MOLECULAR WEIGHT	DENSITY RELATIVE TO O_2	SOLUBILITY RELATIVE TO O_2	WATER DIFFUSION CAPACITY RELATIVE TO O_2
O_2	32	1.0	1.0	1.0
N_2	28	0.88	0.515	0.55
CO_2	44	1.37	24.0	20.5
N_2O	44	1.37	16.3	14.0
He	4	0.125	0.37	1.05

Therefore, the ability of CO_2 to move from the closed peritoneal cavity to the lungs for excretion is dependent on its intrinsic diffusion and solubility properties, the rate of continuing CO_2 insufflation, the surface area of the cavity, and the partial pressure difference across membranes.

Lumb AB. *Nunn's applied respiratory physiology*, 6th ed. Philadelphia: Butterworth-Heinemann, 2005:148–152.

McHoney M, Corizia L, Eaton S, et al. Carbon dioxide elimination during laparoscopy in children is age dependent. *J Pediatr Surg* 2003;38(1):105–110.

A.16. Is CO₂ soluble in blood? Why?

Carbon dioxide is relatively insoluble in plasma, interstitial fluid, and water. The solubility of CO_2 in water at $37°C$ ($98.6°F$) is 0.03 mmol/L/mm Hg. This must be contrasted to the very high solubility of CO_2 in blood. This extremely important distinction exists because of a zinc-containing enzyme, carbonic anhydrase, that exists only within the erythrocyte and not at all in plasma.

$$H_2O + CO_2 \xrightarrow{\text{carbonic anhydrase}} H_2CO_3 \rightarrow H^+ + HCO_3^-$$

In the equation shown, carbonic anhydrase catalyzes only the left side of the equation i.e., the hydration of CO_2 to H_2CO_3). Once formed, carbonic acid is unstable and quickly dissociates into H^+ and HCO_3^-. It is estimated that without carbonic anhydrase it would take 200 seconds at $38°C$ ($100.4°F$) for the previous reaction to come to 10% equilibrium. Because blood travels through the pulmonary capillaries in less than 1 second, carbonic anhydrase speeds up the reaction by a factor of 7,500 times.

Christian G, Greene NM. Blood carbonic anhydrase activity in anesthetized man. *Anesthesiology* 1962;23:179–186.

Lumb AB. *Nunn's applied respiratory physiology*, 6th ed. Philadelphia: Butterworth-Heinemann, 2005:148–158.

B. Preoperative Evaluation and Preparation

B.1. What do you want to know about this patient's history and physical condition that may affect whether or not you clear him for laparoscopic surgery?

Because of his advanced age it is best to form one's own observations of his mental and physical condition. Is he confused, short of breath, kyphoscoliotic, and so forth? A glimpse at where and how this patient's body weight is distributed means more than just knowing that he weighs 100 kg. Ask about wheezing or any change in exercise tolerance, cough, or recent upper respiratory infection. In 2007, the patient safety goals of the Joint Commission on Accreditation of Hospitals (JCAHO) include the timely administration, redosing and discontinuation of prophylactic antibiotics to reduce surgical site infections. Consult with the surgeon regarding the need for appropriate preoperative antibiotics. If you have any doubts, acquire the history and perform the physical examination yourself, or get consultations.

Efron DT, Bender JS. Laparoscopic surgery in older adults. *J Am Geriatr Soc* 2001;49:658–663.

B.2. What factors increase this patient's risk of pulmonary complications?

- *The laparoscopic procedure itself.* The basic laparoscopic Trendelenburg position and the increased intraperitoneal volumes and pressures in a paralyzed, mechanically ventilated patient cause respiratory dysfunction. Insufflation pressures should not exceed 12 to 15 mm Hg. Lower pressures are especially advantageous in American Society of Anesthesiologists (ASA) class III and IV patients with diminished cardiopulmonary reserve. In addition, an increased CO_2 load might call for respiratory minute volumes that are so large that further cardiopulmonary compromise occurs.
- *Age.* Pulmonary function declines with age, especially in a patient older than age 70.
- *Smoking/chronic obstructive pulmonary disease (COPD).* Smokers have increased tracheobronchial secretions with decreased ciliary transport function. They may already have significant pulmonary dysfunction, which may be manifested by diminished exercise tolerance. The forced vital capacity (FVC) may be diminished in restrictive pulmonary disease, whereas the forced expired volume in 1 second (FEV_1) is likely to be decreased in obstructive pulmonary disease.
- *Obesity.* Obesity compounds the problems of increased intraabdominal pressure in the Trendelenburg position. Excessive weight and pressure on the diaphragm and lung bases can lead to marked ventilation and perfusion abnormalities, difficulty in inserting trocars, upward displacement of the carina (leading to possible endobronchial intubation), barotrauma, and so forth.
- *Overhydration.* Patients often experience oliguria during laparoscopy. This may be interpreted as insufficient hydration, and a relative overtransfusion may ensue. Unless frank pulmonary edema occurs, this cause of mild or moderate respiratory distress in the postanesthesia care unit (PACU) may not be recognized without a chest x-ray film.

Kendell AP, Bhatt S, Oh TE. Pulmonary consequences of carbon dioxide insufflation for laparoscopic cholecystectomies. *Anaesthesia* 1995;50:286–289.

B.3. What laboratory tests should be performed preoperatively?

Basic tests should include complete blood count (CBC), urinalysis, clotting functions, electrocardiogram (ECG), and blood typing and screening. In addition, baseline electrolytes, chemistries, and renal function tests (blood urea nitrogen [BUN], creatinine) should be obtained because of the possibility of oliguria during a long laparoscopy. Baseline pulmonary function tests, arterial blood gas measurement, and oxygen saturation values while breathing room air would be helpful in this patient. Markedly abnormal values might suggest the need for bronchodilators, antibiotics, postural drainage, and delay in surgery until pulmonary function is optimal for this particular patient. Baseline chest films are necessary not only to rule out active disease but also for postoperative comparison of acute changes such as subcutaneous or mediastinal emphysema, pneumothorax, or interstitial or pulmonary edema. The presence of bullae on preoperative chest x-ray films may represent a contraindication to laparoscopic surgery because of the accompanying large tidal volumes and high intrathoracic pressures.

Miller RD, ed. *Anesthesia*, 6th ed. Philadelphia: Churchill Livingstone, 2005:2285–2306.

B.4. What specific information should the patient be given about laparoscopic surgery before obtaining informed consent?

In addition to the usual general complications of the planned surgery and anesthesia, the patient must also be told of the complications unique to laparoscopy, and consent for possible laparotomy must be obtained. Emergency laparotomy may be required in the event of such complications as hemorrhage or organ perforation or because of anatomic or technical reasons. The patient should also be advised of the possibility of postoperative referred shoulder pain.

B.5. What additional procedures should be done before surgery?

Although the surgery is described as minimally invasive, the patient must be ready for maximally invasive surgery if necessary. Therefore, the patient must comply with preoperative orders regarding:

- Diet—it should consist of clear liquids the day before surgery. Nothing orally after midnight.
- A complete bowel preparation is necessary.
- Preoperative antibiotics, as per surgeon.

B.6. What three general areas should you be concerned about in your attempt to minimize or prevent complications during laparoscopy?

- Pneumoperitoneum and problems related to its creation, maintenance, and consequences
- Carbon dioxide, including its chemical and physical properties, and its local and systemic effects
- Position on the operating table, which in this case will be Trendelenburg with alternating side elevations

C. Intraoperative Management

C.1. What monitors and devices would you apply to the patient? Why?

The usual intraoperative monitors including standard 5-lead electrocardiogram (ECG) with ST trending; systemic blood pressure (BP) using automated oscillometry; pulse oximetry; capnography; a nerve stimulator; and indicators of inspired oxygen fraction, minute ventilation, and peak airway pressures are necessary. An esophageal probe may be used for both temperature monitoring (optimal at the distal esophagus) and for breath, heart, and murmur sound monitoring (at heart level). Body temperature should be maintained with a forced warm air heating blanket, warmed intravenous fluids, or other means. Rarely, central venous pressure (CVP), pulmonary artery pressure, pulmonary capillary wedge pressure (PCWP), and cardiac output may be measured in patients with severe cardiac or pulmonary abnormalities. A bispectral index (BIS) monitor may be used. Other possibilities include Doppler, transesophageal echocardiography, and noninvasive assessment of cardiac output by thoracic bioimpedance or thoracic ultrasound. An arterial line is suggested during longer, more complex laparoscopic procedures in sicker (American Society of Anesthesiologists [ASA] class III and IV) patients.

Intermittent sequential compression antiembolic stockings should be applied. Shoulder braces are used for support in the Trendelenburg position. After the patient is asleep, a nasogastric or orogastric tube and a Foley catheter is inserted for decompression of stomach and bladder. Use of an orogastric tube is not optional. In addition to the danger of regurgitation from the increased abdominal pressure, reports have been made of stomach perforation by trocars. The orogastric tube should not be clamped after initial placement, and intermittent suctioning should continue because CO_2 gas continues to diffuse into the stomach and distend it.

In addition to mechanical monitoring, visual and tactile monitoring are necessary during laparoscopy. Skin color, skin turgor, and capillary refill should be monitored periodically, because they can change abruptly. The head, neck, and upper chest may assume a purplish color in the dependent position, especially during hypercarbia. The upper chest wall should be checked periodically for subcutaneous emphysema. The cornea and conjunctiva should be checked periodically for edema, especially in the Trendelenburg position, and also whenever oliguria occurs because the extent of the edema may influence your decision on when to extubate.

It is extremely important to maintain accurate data on the volume of fluids infused, and the patient's hourly or half-hourly urine output, along with observations on its color and concentration. Despite adequate hydration, oliguria frequently occurs during pneumoperitoneum, especially at intraabdominal pressures approaching or exceeding 15 mm Hg. Diuresis usually occurs rapidly on release of intraabdominal pressure.

Jacobs VR, Morrison JE, Mettler L, et al. Measurement of CO2 hypothermia during laparoscopy and pelviscopy: how cold it gets and how to prevent it? *J Am Assoc Gynecol Laparosc* 1999;6:289–295.

Ogunnaike BO, Jones SB, Jones DB, et al. Anesthetic considerations for bariatric surgery. *Anesth Analg* 2002;95(6):1793–1805.

Tournadre JP, Chassard D, Berrada KR, et al. Effect of pneumoperitoneum and Trendelenburg position on lower oesophageal sphincter pressure. *Br J Anaesth* 1996;76: 130–132.

Weingram J. Laparoscopic and laser surgery. In: Malhotra V, ed. *Anesthesia for renal and genito-urologic surgery*. New York: McGraw-Hill, 1996:166–168.

C.2. What intravenous (IV) solution and how much fluid volume do you plan to deliver?

Large-bore intravenous catheters should be placed because of the possibility of major hemorrhage. The amount of IV fluid infused is of vital importance, especially in older adults. Transient oliguria during laparoscopy is common. In our early cases, we increased our infusion rate in response to waning urine output, and we hydrated intraperitoneal laparoscopic cases as if they were open intraperitoneal cases. After several cases of "unexplained" pulmonary edema in the postanesthesia care unit (PACU), we concluded that the oliguria seen in laparoscopy is not related to volume depletion, and we have decreased our fluid replacement to approximately 4 mL/kg/hour of Ringer's lactate solution, depending on the patient's preoperative hemodynamic status and the volume of intraperitoneal irrigation fluid used by the surgeon. In calculating fluid requirements during laparoscopy, it is important to remember that much less "third-spacing" occurs than in open surgery, no fluid loss is caused by evaporation, and the volume of retained intraperitoneal saline (used for irrigation by the surgeon) should be added to the final total volume of infused IV fluids. In addition, the intraabdominal humidification of the insufflated dry CO_2 gas results in only a negligible insensible water loss.

After pneumoperitoneum is ended, diuresis occurs promptly and renal function quickly returns to normal (see section C.23).

Gomez Dammeier BH, Karanik E, et al. Anuria during pneumoperitoneum in infants and children: a prospective study. *J Pediatr Surg* 2005;40(9):1454–1458.

London ET, Ho HS, Neuhaus AM, et al. Effect of intravascular volume expansion on renal function during prolonged CO2 pneumoperitoneum. *Ann Surg* 2000;231:195–201.

Muzii L, Bellati F, Manci N, et al. Ringer's lactate solution remains in the peritoneal cavity after laparoscopy longer than expected. *Fertil Steril* 2005;84(1):148–153.

Olsson J, Svensen CH, Hahn RG. The volume kinetics of acetated Ringer's solution during laparoscopic cholecystectomy. *Anesth Analg* 2004;99(6):1854–1860.

Sjostrand F, Hahn RG. Volume kinetics of glucose 2.5% solution during laparoscopic cholecystectomy. *Br J Anaesth* 2004;92(4):485–492.

Tittel A, Schippers E, Grablowitz V, et al. Intraabdominal humidity and electromyographic activity of the gastrointestinal tract. Laparoscopy versus laparotomy. *Surg Endosc* 1995;9:786–790.

Weingram J, Sosa RE, Stein B. Oliguria during laparoscopic pelvic lymph node dissection. *Anesth Analg* 1996;82:S484.

C.3. How would the patient be positioned?

Our patient will be in the supine Trendelenburg position with both arms tucked in at the sides. The side to be worked on is usually elevated, enabling gravity to assist in separating the organs and allowing blood to pool away from the operative field. Therefore, the patient may be supine, in the Trendelenburg position (with possible lateral rotation) for urology; in dorsolithotomy for gynecology; in the head-up position for upper gastrointestinal and biliary tract surgery; and in the lateral decubitus position for thoracoscopy, nephrectomy, and adrenalectomy.

C.4. What are the respiratory and circulatory effects of the Trendelenburg position?

Respiratory

Vital capacity and functional residual capacity (FRC) are reduced. The abdominal contents restrict movement of the diaphragm, especially in the obese and in older adults. Decreased compliance, increased ventilation-perfusion abnormalities, and cephalad displacement of the mediastinum commonly occur.

Circulatory

In healthy patients, Trendelenburg position results in minimal circulatory changes. Venous return and cardiac output are increased, whereas central venous pressure (CVP), pulmonary capillary wedge pressure (PCWP), systemic vascular resistance (SVR), and heart rate are essentially unchanged. In patients with cardiovascular disease, the Trendelenburg position may result in increased CVP, PCWP, and decreased cardiac output. The increase in venous return and myocardial oxygen demand that occurs in severe cardiovascular disease can precipitate acute heart failure.

Battillo JA, Hendler MA. Effects of positioning during anesthesia. *Int Anesthesiol Clin* 1993;31:67–86.

Freeza EE. The lithotomy versus the supine position for laparoscopic advanced surgeries: a historical review. *J Laparoendosc Adv Surg Tech A* 2005;15(2):140–144.

Maartin JT, Warner MA, eds. *Positioning in anesthesia and surgery*, 3rd ed. Philadelphia: WB Saunders, 1997; 95–123.

C.5. What is the anesthetic technique of choice for laparoscopy? Why?

The technique of choice for laparoscopy is general anesthesia with a cuffed endotracheal tube and controlled positive pressure ventilation, because of the following reasons:

- Duration may be long.
- Patient may be anxious.
- The Trendelenburg position may cause respiratory compromise and dyspnea in the awake or in the spontaneously breathing patient with abdominal contents under pressure. The obese patient may be especially uncomfortable in this position.

- A nasogastric or orogastric tube, difficult to insert in a conscious patient, is necessary to decompress the stomach and minimize the risk of aspiration or perforation by trocars. Carbon dioxide, as with N_2O, diffuses into the stomach.
- However, perhaps the most important reason relates to muscle relaxation. Muscle relaxation and paralysis are necessary because the increase in intraabdominal pressure and splinting of the diaphragm make spontaneous breathing difficult. It provides a quieter surgical field and better surgical exposure. "Bucking" increases negative pressure in the chest, which increases the risk of pneumothorax or gas dissection. Coughing can further increase pressure in the abdomen and cause movement of, and perforation by, intraabdominal instruments. Moreover, muscle relaxation is necessary to control and augment ventilation to compensate for the hypercarbia and respiratory acidosis that results from absorption of CO_2.

Brull SJ. Anesthetic considerations for laparoscopic procedures. *ASA refresher courses in anesthesiology.* Vol. 23. Park Ridge: American Society of Anesthesiologists, 1995:15–28.

Chassard D, Berrada K, Tournadre J-P, et al. The effects of neuromuscular block on peak airway pressure and abdominal elastance during pneumoperitoneum. *Anesth Analg* 1996;82:525–527.

Chui PT, Gin T, Oh TE. Anaesthesia for laparoscopic general surgery. *Anaesth Intensive Care* 1993;21:163–171.

C.6. Can a laryngeal mask airway (LMA) be used?

Although successful use of the LMA has been reported by several British groups for very brief laparoscopic procedures in healthy patients, its use is not recommended. LMA does not protect against aspiration. It also limits the ability to apply positive pressure ventilation, and it interferes with use of an orogastric tube.

Bapat PP, Verghese C. Laryngeal mask airway and the incidence of regurgitation during gynecological laparoscopies. *Anesth Analg* 1997;85:139–143.

Brimacombe J, Keller C, Berry A. Gastric insufflation with the ProSeal laryngeal mask. *Anesth Analg* 2001;92(6):1614–1615.

C.7. What anesthetic agents or adjuvant drugs are recommended for laparoscopy? Are any anesthetic agents contraindicated?

Almost any combination that provides amnesia, analgesia, and paralysis is suitable. Because closure of a laparoscopic procedure may be abrupt, because patients may be discharged soon after surgery, and because a large painful (stimulating) incision is absent, the most common combination probably includes an inhalation agent, a medium-duration narcotic, and an intermediate-acting muscle relaxant.

Use of an antiemetic is recommended to counteract the nausea resulting from peritoneal stimulation and bowel distention (secondary to diffusion of CO_2 into the bowel). Droperidol had been used effectively because it potentiated sedation, was long acting, could be given early in the procedure, and as an α-blocker helped counteract the hypertensive effects of systemic CO_2. Newer antiemetics include such $5-HT_3$ receptor antagonists as ondansetron and dolasetron. These may be combined with dexamethasone.

Propofol also has an HT_3 antiemetic effect. However, a propofol-based maintenance anesthetic, when combined with neuromuscular block, may not adequately prevent patient awareness. A bispectral index monitor (BIS) may be helpful in that situation.

A vagolytic drug should be at hand because acute stretching of the peritoneum may cause reflex bradycardia. This is more likely to occur in young women than in older adults.

Halothane is the only anesthetic that should probably be avoided because it can cause arrhythmias in the presence of hypercarbia. Hypnotics and sedatives should be used cautiously in older adults because their duration is often prolonged.

Seed RF, Shakespeare TF, Muldoon MJ. Carbon dioxide homeostasis during anaesthesia for laparoscopy. *Anaesthesia* 1970;25:223–231.

Scuderi PE, D'Angelo R, Harris L, et al. Small-dose propofol by continuous infusion does not prevent postoperative vomiting in females undergoing outpatient laparoscopy. *Anesth Analg* 1997;84:71–75.

C.8. Should N_2O be used during laparoscopy? What are the pros and cons? Does N_2O cause bowel distention during laparoscopy? Does N_2O cause nausea and vomiting after laparoscopy?

The use of N_2O has been considered controversial. The controversies surrounding laparoscopic use of N_2O center on the causes of bowel distention during surgery and nausea and vomiting postoperatively.

In examining the issue of bowel distention with N_2O, note the following. The diffusion capacity of N_2O is approximately 15 times that of O_2 and 30 times that of nitrogen. Therefore, in a closed space that contains air, N_2O enters faster than N_2 can leave, thereby increasing the size of the closed space. It has been calculated that the volume of an enclosed air pocket can be doubled by inhalation of 50% N_2O and quadrupled by inhalation of 75% N_2O after several hours.

However, during laparoscopy, we are concerned about CO_2 pockets not air pockets. N_2O, which has a diffusion capacity almost as great as CO_2, will diffuse from the bloodstream into the intraperitoneal pocket of 100% CO_2 at a rate determined by its solubility in water, its diffusing capacity through an aqueous membrane, and its pressure gradients, as discussed in section A.15. Similarly, CO_2 will leave the peritoneal cavity according to its pressure gradients and solubility and diffusion characteristics. Eventually, the amount of N_2O found in the peritoneal cavity can be significant, and theoretically it can form an ignition hazard. (However, Hunter states that it is necessary for methane or hydrogen to occupy at least 5.5% of the gas volume for nitrous oxide to support combustion, a condition that does not naturally occur.)

In the situation of an air pocket in the bowel, it is well known that N_2O will diffuse in according to its gradients, thereby enlarging the pocket. However, few realize that even in the absence of N_2O, CO_2 will also diffuse into this pocket and expand it in a manner that is clinically indistinguishable from N_2O.

N_2O is often blamed for a distended bowel during laparoscopy, not realizing that CO_2 is equally capable of diffusing into and distending the bowel. In a double-blinded study of bowel distention in patients undergoing laparoscopic cholecystectomy with either isoflurane 70% N_2O-O_2 or isoflurane-air-O_2, the surgeon was able to identify the use of N_2O correctly only 44% of the time. In addition, postoperative nausea and vomiting was independent of the use of N_2O, because the incidence was similar in both groups. Another study found no difference in the incidence of postoperative nausea and vomiting between groups receiving propofol-air-O_2 or propofol-N_2O-O_2 in gynecologic laparoscopy. In fact, the propofol-N_2O-O_2 group had the advantages of significantly more rapid emergence, use of 30% less propofol, additional analgesia, and less risk of awareness.

Because of these issues, it is recommended that nitrous oxide, if used, be limited to not more than 50% of the inspired mixture during laparoscopy.

Arellano RJ, Pole ML, Rafuse SE, et al. Omission of nitrous oxide from a propofol-based anesthetic does not affect the recovery of women undergoing outpatient gynecological surgery. *Anesthesiology* 2000;93(2):332–339.

Diemunsch PA, Torp KD, Van Dorsselaer T, et al. Nitrous oxide fraction in the carbon dioxide pneumoperitoneum during laparoscopy under general inhaled anesthesia in pigs. *Anesth Analg* 2000;90:951–953.

Diemunsch PA, Van Dorsselaer T, Torp KD, et al. Calibrated pneumoperitoneal venting to prevent N2O accumulation in the CO2 pneumoperitoneum during laparoscopy with inhaled anesthesia: an experimental studying pigs. *Anesth Analg* 2002;94:1014–1018.

Eger EI II, Saidman LJ. Hazards of nitrous oxide anesthesia in bowel obstruction and pneumothorax. *Anesthesiology* 1965;26:61–66.

Hunter JG, Staheli J, Oddsdottir M, et al. Nitrous oxide pneumoperitoneum revisited. Is there a risk of combustion?. *Surg Endosc* 1995;9:501–504.

Neuman GG, Sidebotham G, Negoianu E, et al. Laparoscopic explosion hazards with N_2O. *Anesthesiology* 1993;78:875–879.

Sukhani R, Lurie J, Jabamoni R. Propofol for ambulatory gynecologic laparoscopy: does omission of nitrous oxide alter postoperative emetic sequelae and recovery?. *Anesth Analg* 1994;78:831–835.

Taylor E, Feinstein R, White PF, et al. Anesthesia for laparoscopic cholecystectomy. Is nitrous oxide contraindicated? *Anesthesiology* 1992;76:541–543.

C.9. Can laparoscopy be performed under local anesthesia or regional anesthesia?

Yes. However, under local anesthesia, CO_2 causes pain intraperitoneally which is also referred to the shoulder. It is for this reason that N_2O, which is nonirritating to the peritoneum, has been used as the insufflating gas for brief diagnostic laparoscopy under local anesthesia without cautery. However, rapid peritoneal distention causes nausea, which may be worsened without a nasogastric tube. Because of patient discomfort, the surgeon may obtain suboptimal visualization of the surgical field. Also the possibility, although remote, of having to open the abdomen speaks against local anesthesia.

Regional anesthesia can be used for laparoscopy. However, it too has serious drawbacks. It requires a high level of sensory block, possibly causing dyspnea in the Trendelenburg position. A nasogastric tube may not be tolerated. Hyperventilation in response to hypercarbia may cause too much movement in the surgical field, and spontaneous ventilation may be inadequate to compensate for hypercarbia in the Trendelenburg position. Because the systemic response to hypercarbia is mediated primarily through sympathetic stimulation, the sympathetic denervation resulting from high regional anesthesia will result in hypotension and decreased cardiac output rather than the hypertension and increased cardiac output usually seen with general anesthesia.

Use of IV analgesics or propofol may result in respiratory depression or obstruction, especially in Trendelenburg position. Hypoxia in the presence of hypercarbia may have serious consequences.

Collins LM, Vaghadia H. Regional anesthesia for laparoscopy. *Anesthesiol Clin North America* 2001;19(1):43–55.

Fishburne JI. Anesthesia for laparoscopy: considerations, complications and techniques. *J Reprod Med* 1978;21:37–40.

Vaghadia H, Solylo MA, Henderson CL, et al. Selective spinal anesthesia for outpatient laparoscopy. II: epinephrine and spinal cord function. *Can J Anaesth* 2001;48:261–266.

C.10. What two techniques are available for initial laparoscopic access to the peritoneal cavity? What anesthetic problems can arise during insufflation?

Pneumoperitoneum can be achieved by a "blind" or closed technique of percutaneous insertion of the 2-mm diameter hollow Veress needle, which, after verification of correct positioning, is connected to the CO_2 insufflator. (After Veress needle insertion, the first trocar is also inserted blindly.)

Alternatively, if previous surgery or adhesions are to be avoided, an "open" approach is taken. A mini incision is created, and the blunt-tipped Hasson cannula is inserted without prior pneumoperitoneum. The laparoscope is then inserted through the trocar to verify the intraabdominal position before insufflation begins.

During insufflation, abdominal distention should be evenly distributed in all four quadrants. Respiratory variations of intraperitoneal pressure should be visible, and peak inspiratory pressures will gradually increase as the abdomen distends. It is at this time that the anesthesiologist should be alert to the possibility of vagally mediated reflexes. Bronchospasm, bradycardia, and even sinus arrest have been reported, especially in young women. Visceral and vascular perforations are also well-reported complications, especially with the blind technique. Cardiovascular collapse and gas emboli have been reported when CO_2 has been inadvertently insufflated directly into a blood vessel.

Merlin TL, Hiller JE, Maddern GJ, et al. Systematic review of the safety and effectiveness of methods used to establish pneumoperitoneum in laparoscopic surgery. *Br J Surg* 2003;90(6):688–679.

Mori T, Bhoyrul S, Way LW, eds. *Fundamentals of laparoscopic surgery.* New York: Churchill Livingstone, 1995:79–154.

Schwartz ML, Drew RL, Andersen JN. Induction of pneumoperitoneum in morbidly obese patients. *Obes Surg* 2003;13(4):601–604.

Teoh B, Sen R, Abbott J. An evaluation of four tests used to ascertain Veress needle placement at closed laparoscopy. *J Minim InvasiveGynecol* 2005;12(2):153–158.

Vilos GA, Vilos AG. Safe laparoscopic entry guided by Veress needle CO2 insufflation pressure. *J Am Assoc Gynecol Laparosc* 2003;10(3):415–420.

C.11. What is the purpose of the heparinized saline irrigation-suction device used by the surgeon and why should you be concerned with it?

The heparinized saline solution (2,000 to 5,000 U/L delivered by a bag pressurized to 300 mm Hg) is used by the surgeons to retard clot formation in the abdomen, to remove blood from the field, and to remove smoke from electrocautery. It takes the place of lap pads and sponges in open surgery. If the tip of the suction device is not kept under the fluid level, CO_2 gas will be aspirated and exposure of the field will be lost.

Its further significance to the anesthesiologist is twofold. First, the difference between the volume of saline missing from the irrigation bag and the volume in the suction collection bottle must be considered as part of the patient's fluid intake. Second, the temperature of the saline solution intraperitoneally can alter the patient's body temperature.

Moore SS, Green CR, Wang FL, et al. The role of irrigation in the development of hypothermia during laparoscopic surgery. *Am J Obstet Gynecol* 1997;176:598–602.

C.12. Under what circumstances should laparoscopy be converted to laparotomy?

Laparotomy should be performed immediately in cases of bleeding or major organ damage. Other circumstances include persistent problems with inadequate exposure, procedure beyond the surgeon's capability, procedure taking too long, inability to create or maintain pneumoperitoneum, patient deterioration, equipment failure, and discovery of other unsuspected disease.

Tabboush ZS. When hypotension during laparoscopic cholecystectomy indicates termination of the laparoscopy [Letter]. *Anesth Analg* 1994;79:195–196.

C.13. What is the mechanism of increase in shunting resulting from embolization?

Emboli in the pulmonary capillaries cause an increase in pulmonary vascular resistance (PVR) (vasoconstriction), which leads to increased pulmonary artery, right ventricle, and right atrium pressures and opening of pulmonary precapillary arteriovenous anastomoses, resulting in shunt and hypoxemia.

Lumb AB. *Nunn's applied respiratory physiology*, 6th ed. Philadelphia: Butterworth-Heinemann, 2005:116.

C.14. What are the arterial to end-tidal CO_2 gradients ($PaCO_2 - PETCO_2$) in the normal awake patient? What is the cause of the gradient? Does the gradient change during laparoscopy? Why?

In the awake person at rest, the normal arterial to end-tidal PCO_2 difference is small, perhaps ranging from 2 to 6 mm Hg. The gradient and its variations are measures of the alveolar dead space. The gradient is the sum of the difference between the arterial and alveolar CO_2 plus the difference between the alveolar and end-tidal CO_2. It is commonly increased in emphysema. The difference is increased when underperfused alveoli are ventilated, as often occurs during hyperventilation in laparoscopy.

The total physiologic dead space consists of the anatomic dead space (passageways that do not participate in gas exchange, approximately 150 mL) and the alveolar dead space (i.e., underperfused alveoli). The alveolar dead space gas is expired at the same time as the alveolar ideal gas from well-perfused alveoli in equilibrium with pulmonary capillary blood. The dilution of the ideal alveolar gas by the alveolar dead space gas is represented by the end-tidal CO_2.

Some of the factors resulting in a relative increase in ventilation-to-perfusion ratio include mechanical ventilation, hyperventilation, rapid or shallow ventilation, and Trendelenburg or lateral decubitus position.

Some of the factors resulting in a relative decrease in perfusion-to-ventilation ratio include hypotension, decreased cardiac output anesthesia and myocardial depression, pulmonary emboli, high positive airway pressure, and ablation of the hypoxic pulmonary vasoconstriction reflex.

Christensen MA, Bloom J, Sutton KR. Comparing arterial and end-tidal carbon dioxide values in hyperventilated neurosurgical patients. *Am J Crit Care* 1995;4:116–121.

Lumb AB. *Nunn's applied respiratory physiology*, 6th ed. Philadelphia: Butterworth-Heinemann, 2005:157–158, 318–319.

C.15. Is an arterial line necessary? Why? Does end-tidal CO_2 tension accurately reflect arterial CO_2 tension? Under what circumstances may the $PETCO_2$ exceed the $PaCO_2$? Why?

An arterial line is recommended whenever the laparoscopic procedure is unusually complex or long or when the patient has significant cardiopulmonary disease. In such cases, ventilation-perfusion abnormalities, intraoperative hypoxemia, marked hypercarbia, or high airway pressures may be expected. During these situations, and possibly in all laparoscopies, an unsteady state exists with respect to CO_2, and the assumption that $PETCO_2$ may accurately reflect a predictable relationship to $PaCO_2$ is not valid.

End-tidal CO_2 tension can either estimate $PaCO_2$; or, more often, it may underestimate $PaCO_2$; or, less often, it may even exceed $PaCO_2$. Furthermore, the values for these two measurements do not always change proportionally, nor do they always change in the same direction. The relationship between $PETCO_2$ and $PaCO_2$ varies during the course of the procedure. At the beginning of insufflation, $PETCO_2$ can be used as a rough estimate of $PaCO_2$. However, when redistribution of the excess CO_2 from the well-perfused tissues to the less well-perfused tissues begins, $PETCO_2$ begins to underestimate the $PaCO_2$. Characteristically, the arterial to end-tidal CO_2 difference progressively increases as hyperventilation (and dead space) increases.

Especially during strenuous exercise when metabolic CO_2 production is increased and during laparoscopy when excess exogenous CO_2 must be excreted, the $PETCO_2$ may be found to exceed the $PaCO_2$. This condition has also been reported in a hyperventilating patient at cesarean section. This occurs because the $PaCO_2$ fluctuates during each deep breath and may not represent the highest value at that instant, whereas the $PETCO_2$ shows the maximal value (i.e., because of tidal ventilation and pulsatile blood flow in exercise, $PETCO_2$ may exceed mean alveolar and arterial CO_2).

Bhavani-Shankar K, Steinbrook RA, Brooks DC, et al. Arterial to end-tidal carbon dioxide difference during laparoscopic surgery in pregnancy. *Anesthesiology* 2000;93(2): 370–373.

Gravenstein JS, ed. *Gas monitoring and pulse oximetry.* Boston: Butterworth-Heinemann, 1990:106–116.

Jones NL, Robertson DG, Kane JW. Difference between end-tidal and arterial PCO_2 in exercise. *J Appl Physiol* 1979;47:954–960.

Lee T-S. End-tidal partial pressure of carbon dioxide does not accurately reflect $PaCO_2$ in rabbits treated with acetazolamide during anaesthesia. *Br J Anaesth* 1994;73:225–226.

Lumb AB. *Nunn's applied respiratory physiology*, 6th ed. Philadelphia: Butterworth-Heinemann, 2005:157–158, 318–319.

Scheid P, Meyer M, Piper J. Arterial-expired PCO_2 differences in the dog during acute hypercapnia. *J Appl Physiol* 1979;47:1074–1078.

Shankar KB, Moseley H, Kumar Y, et al. Arterial to end-tidal carbon dioxide tension difference during caesarean section anaesthesia. *Anaesthesia* 1986;41:698–702.

Wulkan ML, Vasudevan SA. Is end-tidal CO_2 an accurate measure of arterial CO_2 during laparoscopic procedures in children and neonates with cyanotic congenital heart disease?. *J Pediatr Surg* 2001;36(8):1234–1236.

C.16. What are the possible causes of hypercarbia?

- Hypoventilation.
- CO_2 in the inspired gas—rebreathing endogenous CO_2 will increase $Paco_2$ by 3 to 6 mm Hg per minute.
- Increased CO_2 supply or production—occurring in the hypermetabolic states of malignant hyperpyrexia, fever, and hyperthyroidism; laparoscopy; or following administration of bicarbonate or lactate (1 ampule of 50 mEq of bicarbonate liberates more than 1 L of CO_2).
- Increased dead space (rare) as in pulmonary embolism, ventilation of a lung cyst, or in advanced chronic obstructive pulmonary disease (COPD).

Lumb AB. *Nunn's applied respiratory physiology*, 6th ed. Philadelphia: Butterworth-Heinemann, 2005:140, 328.

Wolf JS Jr, Clayman RV, Monk TG, et al. Carbon dioxide absorption during laparoscopic pelvic operation. *J Am Coll Surg* 1995;180:555–560.

C.17. What factors play a role in the unusually rapid and marked elevation of CO_2 that is sometimes seen in laparoscopy?

- Patients with significant cardiopulmonary disease
- Intraabdominal pressure greater than 15 mm Hg
- Presence of subcutaneous emphysema
- Retroperitoneal rather than intraperitoneal approach
- Long duration of laparoscopy

Bozkurt P, Kaya G, Yeker Y, et al. Arterial carbon dioxide markedly increases during diagnostic laparoscopy in portal hypertensive children. *Anesth Analg* 2002;95(5):1236–1240.

Liem KS, Kallewaard JW, deSmet AM, et al. Does hypercarbia develop faster during laparoscopic herniorrhaphy than during laparoscopic cholecystectomy? Assessment with continuous blood gas monitoring. *Anesth Analg* 1995;81:1243–1249.

C.18. How rapidly does the $Paco_2$ rise in the apneic patient (endogenous CO_2)? How rapidly does the $Paco_2$ rise if 5% CO_2 gas is inhaled (exogenous)? How rapidly can the CO_2 rise during laparoscopy? What factors explain the differences?

In the apneic patient, $Paco_2$ rises at the rate of 3 to 6 mm Hg per minute. Rebreathing, or inhalation of 5% CO_2 in oxygen, causes a much more rapid rise in $Paco_2$, up to 8 to 10 mm Hg per minute. The difference in rate of rise between endogenous and exogenous CO_2 is explained by the presence of large body stores of CO_2. Approximately 120 L of CO_2 exist in the body (100 times the amount for CO_2) distributed among well-perfused tissue (e.g., blood, brain), moderately perfused tissue (e.g., muscle), and poorly perfused tissue (e.g., fat, bone). These storage places adjust slowly to acute CO_2 changes. In the steady state, the amount of CO_2 produced metabolically in the body is equal to the amount expired through the lungs, and there is no change in the body stores of CO_2. During laparoscopy an unsteady state exists, with the rate of rise of Pco_2 being greatest during the first 20 to 30 minutes. After that time, new equilibrium levels are reached between the different compartments, and the Pco_2 rate of rise is slower.

Frumin et al. studied the hypercarbic state during their classic study of apneic oxygenation. In paralyzed apneic intubated denitrogenated patients receiving only thiopental for amnesia, Frumin et al. demonstrated at least a 3-mm Hg average rise in $Paco_2$ per minute and an ultimate

Pa_{CO_2} as high as 250 mm Hg (pH 6.72) with 98% to 100% CO_2 saturation after 53 minutes of apnea. They also found that the hypercarbia was accompanied by hypertension (mean arterial pressure rise of 26%, followed by fall of 14% on return of respirations and normocarbia). Other features accompanying apneic hypercarbic hypertension included normal sinus rhythm with an essentially unchanged rate, rising arterial epinephrine and norepinephrine concentrations, and rising arterial potassium levels (which rose still further after ventilation and normocarbia resumed) with unchanged sodium levels.

Frumin J, Epstein RM, Cohen G. Apneic oxygenation in man. *Anesthesiology* 1959;20: 789–798.

Lumb AB. *Nunn's applied respiratory physiology*, 6th ed. Philadelphia: Butterworth-Heinemann, 2005:160, 318–319.

C.19. What are the direct and indirect effects of hypercarbia on the cardiovascular system? How are these effects altered by increased intraabdominal pressure and patient position?

The effects of hypercarbia on the circulatory system are complex and often contradictory. At the cellular level, hypercarbia is a direct depressor of myocardial contractility and rate of contraction, and it is also a direct stimulant of myocardial irritability and arrhythmicity. These effects may be enhanced by the reduced pH caused by hypercarbia.

The direct effect of hypercarbia on isolated or denervated blood vessels is a diminished responsiveness to catecholamines and vasodilation especially on the venous side, leading to peripheral pooling, decreased venous return, and decreased cardiac output. The exception to the dilatory effect of hypercarbia and acidosis on blood vessels exists in the pulmonary vessels, which undergo vasoconstriction. It appears, however, that the effects on the pulmonary vessels are actually due to acidosis rather than hypercarbia because if the pH is kept constant while the P_{CO_2} rises, then pulmonary vascular resistance (PVR) does not change.

In the patient, however, the direct or local effects of CO_2 can be overshadowed by a variety of systemic effects. Simultaneous with these local or direct effects, hypercarbia causes profound systemic changes secondary to stimulation of the central nervous system and sympathoadrenal system. The net effect usually includes an increase in cardiac output, heart rate, force of myocardial contraction, blood pressure (BP), central venous pressure (CVP), vasoconstriction in the pulmonary (capacitance) vessels, and decreased peripheral resistance. The rise in cardiac output of up to 50% exceeds the rise in BP, because of the drop in peripheral resistance and increase in blood flow primarily in the cerebral and coronary circulations. This net stimulatory effect accompanies the elevation of P_{CO_2} up to approximately 90 mm Hg. Above this level, further increases in CO_2 cause a marked drop in response.

In a normal anesthetized human breathing 7% to 15% inspired CO_2, these stimulatory changes were shown to correspond primarily to rising plasma concentrations of epinephrine and norepinephrine. When the sympathoadrenal response was prevented by subarachnoid block, ganglioplegics, or α-adrenergic blockers, the cardiovascular response to inhaled CO_2 was hypotension and decreased cardiac output. The stimulatory response is also diminished by general anesthesia.

Hypercarbia can cause arrhythmias during epinephrine infiltrations or in the presence of halothane but not other anesthetics. Other than in these two circumstances, hypercarbia is not arrhythmogenic unless hypoxia is also present.

The full range of possible effects of hypercarbia on the cardiovascular system are subject to many influences. Healthy (American Society of Anesthesiologists [ASA] class I) patients are less likely than ASA class III patients to undergo extreme changes. Similarly, a brief surgical duration, head-up positioning, low intraabdominal pressures, and intraperitoneal (rather than extraperitoneal) surgery can limit the range of physiologic and metabolic responses to near-normal.

In the patient with marginal cardiovascular function, however, peritoneal insufflation can result in significant increase in cardiac workload. In this situation, transesophageal echocardiography may provide a useful noninvasive method of estimation of left ventricular function.

Arrhythmias such as bradycardia, nodal rhythm, or even asystole can follow rapid peritoneal distention and vagal stimulation. In general, BP, pulse, cardiac output, and CVP will increase up to an intraabdominal pressure of 15 mm Hg. At insufflation pressures of 20 to 30 mm Hg, a decrease in BP, cardiac output, and CVP will occur because of pressure on the inferior vena cava and decreased venous return. Pneumoperitoneum may also induce changes in the cardiac electrical axis which may affect interpretation of the ECG seen on the monitor during the operation.

Gannedahl P, Odeberg S, Brodin LA, et al. Effects of posture and pneumoperitoneum during anaesthesia on the indices of left ventricular filling. *Acta Anaesthesiol Scand* 1996;40:160–166.

Hirvonen EA, Nuutinen LS, Kauko M. Hemodynamic changes due to Trendelenburg positioning and pneumoperitoneum during laparoscopic hysterectomy. *Acta Anaesthesiol Scand* 1995;39:949–955.

Hofer CK, Zalunardo MP, Klaghofer R, et al. Changes in intrathoracic blood volume associated with pneumoperitoneum and positioning. *Acta Anaesthesiol Scand* 2002;46:303–308.

Irwin MG, Ng JK. Transesophageal acoustic quantification for evaluation of cardiac function during laparoscopic surgery. *Anaesthesia* 2001;56:623–629.

Joshi GP, Hein HA, Mascarenhas WL, et al. Continuous transesophageal echo-Doppler assessment of hemodynamic function during laparoscopic cholecystectomy. *J Clin Anesth* 2005;17(2):117–121.

Lumb AB. *Nunn's applied respiratory physiology*, 6th ed. Philadelphia: Butterworth-Heinemann, 2005:330–331.

Rist M, Hemmerling TM, Rauh R, et al. Influence of pneumoperitoneum and patient positioning on preload and splanchnic blood volume in laparoscopic surgery of the lower abdomen. *J Clin Anesth* 2001;13:244–249.

Suzuki M, Koda S, Nakamura Y, et al. The relationship between cardiac output measured by the thermodilution method and that measured by the carbon dioxide rebreathing technique during laparoscopic surgery. *Anesth Analg* 2005;100:1381–1383.

C.20. What are the direct and indirect effects of hypercarbia on the respiratory system? How does the Trendelenburg position and the increased intraabdominal pressure of pneumoperitoneum alter these effects?

Hypercarbia and acidosis stimulate the respiratory center both directly and indirectly through chemoreceptors, hormones, and autonomic nerves. In the conscious patient breathing oxygen, the maximal stimulating effect occurs at 100 to 150 mm Hg, producing minute volumes of up to 75 L. Above these levels, CO_2 becomes a respiratory depressant. Current anesthetics blunt the stimulatory respiratory response to CO_2. (Diethyl ether, however, the only volatile anesthetic known to stimulate respiration, is reported to have caused a patient to continue to breathe spontaneously at an inadvertent PCO_2 of 234 mm Hg.)

In the awake patient, each mm Hg increase in $PaCO_2$ increases ventilation by 2 to 3 L per minute (if PaO_2 is constant). This response is diminished by anesthesia. Hypercarbia also produces bronchodilatation; acidosis, rather than hypercarbia *per se*, causes pulmonary vascular constriction.

General anesthesia with intubation and mechanical ventilation results in a decrease in functional residual capacity (FRC), which is caused by loss of muscle tone, diaphragmatic displacement, and loss of thoracic volume. Lung compliance drops, airway pressures increase, and $\dot{V}/\dot{Q}$ abnormalities occur. However, most patients have no difficulty tolerating these changes. These changes are exaggerated in the Trendelenburg position, especially in older adults, the obese, and those with preexisting cardiopulmonary disease. Intrathoracic, peak inspiratory, and plateau pressures increase and then increase even further when pneumoperitoneum creates an increase in pressure and volume. Endobronchial intubation can occur as a result of cephalad movement of the carina, and it should be ruled out if hypoxemia occurs.

Andersson LE, Baath M, Thorne A, et al. Effect of carbon dioxide pneumoperitoneum on development of atelectasis during anesthesia, examined by spiral computed tomography. *Anesthesiology* 2005;102(2):293–299.

Kendall AP, Bhatt S, Oh TE. Pulmonary consequences of carbon dioxide insufflation for laparoscopic cholecystectomies. *Anaesthesia* 1995;50:286–289.

Lobato EB, Paige GB, Brown MM, et al. Pneumoperitoneum as a risk factor for endobronchial intubation during laparoscopic gynecologic surgery. *Anesth Analg* 1998;86: 301–303.

Lumb AB. *Nunn's applied respiratory physiology*, 6th ed. Philadelphia: Butterworth-Heinemann, 2005:330.

Meininger D, Byhahn C, Mierdl S, et al. Positive end-expiratory pressure improves arterial oxygenation during prolonged pneumoperitoneum. *Acta Anesthesiol Scand* 2005;49(6):778–783.

Obeid F, Saba A, Fath J, et al. Increases in intra-abdominal pressure affect pulmonary compliance. *Arch Surg* 1995;130:544–547.

Rauh R, Hemmerling TM, Rist M, et al. Influence of pneumoperitoneum and patient positioning on respiratory system compliance. *J Clin Anesth* 2001;13:361–365.

Sprung J, Whalley DG, Falcone T, et al. The effects of tidal volume and respiratory rate on oxygenation and respiratory mechanics during laparoscopy in morbidly obese patients. *Anesth Analg* 2003;97:268–274.

Whalen FX, Gajic O, Thompson GB, et al. The effects of the alveolar recruitment maneuver and positive end-expiratory pressure on arterial oxygenation during laparoscopic bariatric surgery. *Anesth Analg* 2006;102:298–305.

C.21. What are the direct and indirect effects of hypercarbia on the central nervous system?

The brain is particularly sensitive to changes in P_{CO_2}. Slight elevations of CO_2 cause direct cortical depression and increase the threshold for seizures. Higher levels of CO_2 (25% to 30%) stimulate subcortical hypothalamic centers, resulting in increased cortical excitability and seizures. This hyperexcitability level is enhanced by adrenal cortical and medullary hormones released secondary to hypercarbia-induced stimulation of the hypothalamus. Further elevations of CO_2 cause an anesthetic-like state of cortical and subcortical depression.

Carbon dioxide was first used as an anesthetic by Hickman in 1824 and reintroduced by Leake and Waters in 1928. CO_2 caused an N_2O-like narcosis at approximately 90 to 120 mm Hg. However, hypercarbia also causes increased excitability of neurons so that seizures occurred shortly afterward. In dogs, however, general anesthesia is achieved at the higher level of P_{CO_2}, approximately 245 mm Hg, probably by intracellular derangements caused by low pH.

Carbon dioxide, not H^+, crosses the blood—brain barrier and the brain cell membrane and affects the cell metabolism. Therefore, a change in P_{CO_2} also causes a rapid change in cerebrospinal fluid (CSF) pH. CO_2 is the most important factor in regulating cerebral blood flow (CBF). The relation between CBF and P_{CO_2} is essentially linear from 20 to 100 mm Hg, with maximal vasodilatation at approximately 120 mm Hg. Normal CBF is approximately 20% of cardiac output, or 50 mL/100 g/minute. For each 1 mm Hg increase in P_{CO_2} between 25 and 100 mm Hg, CBF increases by 2% to 4%. Hypercarbia decreases cerebral vascular resistance, causing CBF to increase.

Hypercarbia causes an increase in intracranial pressure, probably secondary to vasodilatation. When the patient is placed in the Trendelenburg position, venous congestion of the head and neck occurs. Additional increases in intraabdominal and intrathoracic pressures contribute to further increases in intracranial and CSF pressures.

Therefore, an acute rise in intraabdominal pressure (pneumoperitoneum) causes an immediate rise in intracranial pressure. This occurs through intermediary steps that include compression of the inferior vena cava (resulting in decreased drainage in the lumbar plexus), increased continuous venous pressure (CVP), increased mean arterial pressure, increased intrathoracic pressure, increased venous stasis and increased pressure in the sagittal sinus, and decreased resorption of CSF. Hypercarbia contributes to the increased intracranial pressure, but hyperventilation will not decrease the elevated intracranial pressure until the elevated intraabdominal pressure is released.

Halverson A, Buchanan R, Jacobs L, et al. Evaluation of mechanism of increased intracranial pressure with insufflation. *Surg Endosc* 1998;12:266–269.

Irgau I, Koyfman Y, Tikellis JI. Elective intraoperative intracranial pressure monitoring during laparoscopic cholecystectomy. *Arch Surg* 1995;130:1011–1013.

Kirkinen P, Hirvonen E, Kauko M, et al. Intracranial blood flow during laparoscopic hysterectomy. *Acta Obstet Gynecol Scand* 1995;74:71–74.

Lumb AB. *Nunn's applied respiratory physiology*, 6th ed. Philadelphia: Butterworth Heinemann, 2005:328–330.

Moncure M, Salem R, Moncure K, et al. Central nervous system metabolic and physiologic effects of laparoscopy. *Am Surg* 1999;65:168–172.

Rosenthal RJ, Friedman RL, Chidambaram A, et al. Effects of hyperventilation and hypoventilation on Pa_{CO_2} and intracranial pressure during acute elevations of intraabdominal pressures with CO_2 pneumoperitoneum: large animal observations. *J Am Coll Surg* 1998;187:32–38.

Huettemann E, Terborg C, Sakka SG, et al. Preserved CO2 reactivity and increase in middle cerebral arterial blood flow velocity during laparoscopic surgery in children. *Anesth Analg* 2002;94:255–258.

C.22. What are the neuroendocrine changes that occur during laparoscopy?

Excessive intraabdominal pressure and hypercarbia may activate the sympathoadrenal axis, resulting in increased plasma levels of epinephrine and norepinephrine. Renin, cortisol, aldosterone, antidiuretic hormone (ADH), and atrial natriuretic peptide levels are also increased. In awake patients in the Trendelenburg position, increased secretion of atrial natriuretic peptide occurs, probably in response to increased venous return and atrial stretch. During pneumoperitoneum, however, secretion of atrial natriuretic factor diminishes, suggesting interference with venous return.

Hirvonen EA, Nuutinen LS, Vuolteenaho O. Hormonal responses and cardiac filling pressures in head-up or head-down position and pneumoperitoneum in patients undergoing operative laparoscopy. *Br J Anaesth* 197;78:128–133.

Mann C, Boccara G, Pouzeratte Y, et al. The relationship among carbon dioxide pneumoperitoneum, vasopressin release, and hemodynamic changes. *Anesth Analg* 1999;89: 278–283.

Mikami O, Fujise K, Matsumoto S, et al. High intra-abdominal pressure increases plasma catecholamine concentrations during pneumoperitoneum for laparoscopic procedures. *Arch Surg* 1998;133:39–43.

O'Leary E, Hubbard K, Tormey W, et al. Laparoscopic cholecystectomy: haemodynamic and neuroendocrine responses after pneumoperitoneum and changes in position. *Br J Anaesth* 1996;76:640–644.

Sood J, Jayaraman L, Kumra VP, et al. Laparoscopic approach to pheochromocytoma: is a lower intraabdominal pressure helpful? *Anesth Analg* 2006;102:637–641.

C.23. What are the direct and indirect effects of laparoscopy on the renal system?

Oliguria has been frequently observed during laparoscopy despite adequate hydration. Although prerenal causes such as hypovolemia, positive pressure ventilation, and positive end-expiratory pressure (PEEP) contribute to oliguria, it is believed that neurohumoral changes (e.g., antidiuretic hormone [ADH] secretion) secondary to hypercarbia and increased intraabdominal pressure secondary to insufflation may be responsible. Sympathetic stimulation causes a release of catecholamines, resulting in decreased renal cortical blood flow with shunting of blood to the adrenal medulla, constriction of glomerular afferent arterioles, and decreased glomerular filtration rate. It has recently been shown that when intraperitoneal insufflation reaches a pressure of 15 mm Hg, renal cortical blood flow decreases approximately 60%, and a reversible 50% drop in urine volume occurs. In contrast, no decrease in urine output occurred when the abdominal wall was lifted with a force of 15 mm Hg during "gasless laparoscopy." It has also been shown that pneumoretroperitoneum, which causes a more gradual increase in intraabdominal pressure, also caused a more gradual decrease in renal perfusion. Finally, it has been shown that unilateral retroperitoneal insufflation causes decreased renal cortical perfusion of only the ipsilateral kidney if the intraabdominal pressure is not elevated.

Ben-David B, Croituru M, Gaitini L. Acute renal failure following laparoscopic cholecystectomy: a case report. *J Clin Anesth* 1999;11:486–489.

Chiu AW, Chang LS, Birkett DH. The impact of pneumoperitoneum, pneumoretroperitoneum, and gasless laparoscopy on the systemic and renal hemodynamics. *J Am Coll Surg* 1995;181:397–406.

Hazebroek EJ, deVosNederveen CR, Cappel R, et al. Antidiuretic hormone release during laparoscopic donor nephrectomy. *Arch Surg* 2002;137:600–605.

Hunter JG. Laparoscopic pneumoperitoneum: the abdominal compartment syndrome revisited [Editorial]. *J Am Coll Surg* 1995;181:469–470.

Lumb AB. *Nunn's applied respiratory physiology*, 6th ed. Philadelphia: Butterworth-Heinemann, 2005:331.

Nguyen NT, Perez RV, Fleming N, et al. Effect of prolonged pneumoperitoneum on intraoperative urine output during laparoscopic gastric bypass. *J Am Coll Surg* 2002;195: 476–483.

Nishio S, Takeda H, Yokoyama M. Changes in urinary output during laparoscopic adrenalectomy. *BJU Int* 1999;83:944–947.

C.24. What is the effect of hypercarbia and laparoscopy on the bowel and gastrointestinal system?

Although CO_2 directly causes vasodilatation of the splanchnic capillary beds, the increased intraabdominal pressure of laparoscopy decreases perfusion, increases systemic vascular resistance, impairs gastric submucosal perfusion and metabolism, and may cause bowel hypoxia at high pressures. On release of intraabdominal pressure, residual CO_2 again causes vascular dilation, allowing additional CO_2 to enter the blood stream. Myoelectric activity and recovery from ileus is faster after laparoscopic than after open surgery. The combined effect of the increase in abdominal pressure, stretching of the peritoneum by insufflation, and diffusion of CO_2 into bowel is probably responsible for any postoperative nausea.

Bohm B, Milsom JW, Fazio VW. Postoperative intestinal motility following conventional and laparoscopic intestinal surgery. *Arch Surg* 1995;130:415–419.

Eleftheriadis E, Kotzampassi K, Papanotas K, et al. Gut ischemia, oxidative stress, and bacterial translocation in elevated abdominal pressure in rats. *World J Surg* 1996; 20:11–16.

Koivusalo AM, Kellokumpu I, Ristkari S, et al. Splanchnic and renal deterioration during and after laparoscopic cholecystectomy: a comparison of the carbon dioxide pneumoperitoneum and the abdominal wall lift method. *Anesth Analg* 1997;85:886–891.

Meierhenrich R, Gauss A, Vandenesch P, et al. The effects of intraabdominally insufflated carbon dioxide on hepatic blood flow during laparoscopic surgery assessed by transesophageal echocardiography. *Anesth Analg* 2005;100:340–347.

Schwarte LA, Scheeren TW, Lorenz C, et al. Moderate increase in intraabdominal pressure attenuates gastric mucosal oxygen saturation in patients undergoing laparoscopy. *Anesthesiology* 2004;100:1081–1087.

Takagi S. Hepatic and portal vein blood flow during carbon dioxide pneumoperitoneum for laparoscopic hepatectomy. *Surg Endosc* 1998;12:427–431.

C.25. How would you recognize CO_2 embolism during laparoscopy? How does this differ from air embolism? Why should N_2O be discontinued during suspected embolization? Will N_2O increase the size of CO_2 emboli?

Gas embolism can occur whenever the internal pressure of an open vessel is less than the external pressure. Gas embolism may cause increased ventilatory dead space, increased pulmonary vascular resistance (PVR), increased pulmonary artery pressure, and decreased cardiac output. Early signs include a rapid drop in end-tidal CO_2 and PaO_2 and increased $PaCO_2$. During laparoscopy, insufflation of a large amount of CO_2 directly into a blood vessel can occur initially after blind Veress needle insertion, especially at high pressures. This should be suspected if the abdominal cavity does not distend equally in all four quadrants despite insufflation of several liters of CO_2. Hypotension, hypoxia, cyanosis, or cardiac arrest can occur. If the gas volume is large enough, a "mill-wheel" murmur may be heard through a precordial or esophageal stethoscope. If ventilation is kept constant, a sudden decrease in end-tidal CO_2 may be noted. The most sensitive means to detect gas emboli are the precordial and transesophageal Doppler and transesophageal echocardiography. Aspiration of foamy blood from a central venous catheter is diagnostic.

Table 39.2   Differences Between Air and Carbon Dioxide Emboli.

EMBOLISM	AIR	CO$_2$
Composition	79% N$_2$, 21% O$_2$	100% CO$_2$
Position	Sitting upright	Any
Origin	Vein open to air	No contact with air
Pressure source	Hydrostatic	Insufflator
Solubility	Negligible	Large
Effect of N$_2$O	Enlarged	Not enlarged

Carbon dioxide embolism, however, must be distinguished from air embolism, a far more ominous event, as shown in Table 39.2. Carbon dioxide, being extremely soluble in the presence of red blood cells, is much less life threatening than an identically sized intravascular bolus of air. It has been reported that the lethal volume of intravascular CO$_2$ gas in cats is 30 times greater than the lethal volume of intravascular air.

Air emboli are likely to be entrained in open veins above the level of the heart, a condition that can exist during head and neck or neurosurgery. Other gases that are present, nitrous oxide, for example, will diffuse into that air space according to their diffusion capacities and pressure gradients. Therefore, nitrous oxide will diffuse in, oxygen will be consumed and/or diffuse out, and the size or pressure of the bubble will increase. It is estimated that inhalation of 50% N$_2$O will double the size of an air (i.e., nitrogen) bubble in 10 minutes, whereas inhalation of 75% N$_2$O will quadruple its size. A gas bubble composed of 100% CO$_2$, however, will not enlarge in a patient inhaling 50% or even 75% N$_2$O because more CO$_2$ will move out or be absorbed or buffered (also more quickly) than N$_2$O will move in. This is not to deny that CO$_2$ gas has caused fatal embolisms or that N$_2$O should be discontinued if embolism is suspected. A recent study using transesophageal echocardiography in 16 patients undergoing laparoscopic cholecystectomy reported gas embolism in 11 of the 16 patients (5 during peritoneal insufflation and 6 during gallbladder dissection), but all were subclinical with no signs of cardiorespiratory instability. In addition, conditions for creating CO$_2$ embolism differ from conditions for air embolism. Other than direct insufflation of CO$_2$ into a vein, as during Veress needle insufflation, the capillaries and veins within the abdomen are collapsed by the positive pressure within the abdomen.

Derouin M, Couture P, Boudreault D, et al. Detection of gas embolism by transesophageal echocardiography during laparoscopic cholecystectomy. *Anesth Analg* 1996;82:119–124.

Ishiyama T, Hanagata K, Kashimoto S, et al. Pulmonary carbon dioxide embolism during laparoscopic cholecystectomy. *Can J Anaesth* 2001;48:319–320.

Kunkler A, King H. Comparison of air, oxygen, and carbon dioxide embolization. *Ann Surg* 1959;449:95–99.

Junghans T, Bohm B, Meyer E. Influence of nitrous oxide anesthesia on venous gas embolism with carbon dioxide and helium during pneumoperitoneum. *Surg Endosc* 2000;14:1167–1170.

C.26. How is gas embolism (CO$_2$ or air) treated?

- Nitrous oxide should be discontinued, and the F$_{IO_2}$ should be increased to 1.0.
- Identify and occlude the air entrainment site. Insufflation (in the case of CO$_2$) should be halted, and the pneumoperitoneum should be released immediately.

- An increase in the rate and volume of controlled ventilation with positive end-expiratory pressure (PEEP) has been suggested as a method of minimizing air entrainment. However, this may decrease the cardiac output and excessively increase the airway pressure and pulmonary vascular resistance (PVR) (and can lead to paradoxical air embolization).
- If possible, the patient should be placed in steep left lateral decubitus Trendelenburg position to prevent obstruction of the pulmonary outflow tract and right ventricular failure.
- A central venous pressure (CVP) catheter is useful for diagnosis and for therapeutic aspiration of air. Radial artery cannulation is useful to track improvement or deterioration.
- Therapy is essentially supportive and may include fluids, vasopressors, and Swan-Ganz catheterization. A large bolus of gas may form a gas lock in the right atrium, decreasing the CO. Smaller bubbles can lodge in the lungs, causing pulmonary hypertension, right ventricular failure, and pulmonary edema. Venous gas emboli may also enter the arterial circulation through an atrial septal defect or open foramen ovale, a condition that may exist in 20% of patients.

Beck DH, McQuillan PJ. Fatal carbon dioxide embolism and severe haemorrhage during laparoscopic salpingectomy. *Br J Anaesth* 1994;72:243–245.

Gravenstein N, ed. *Manual of complications during anesthesia.* Philadelphia: JB Lippincott, 1991:332–345.

C.27. What are the causes of pneumothorax or pneumomediastinum during laparoscopy? How would you diagnose it? How would you treat it?

Pneumothorax can result from migration of the laparoscopic gas under pressure or from direct pulmonary barotrauma.

During laparoscopy, CO_2 under pressure can pass from the abdominal cavity into the pleural and pericardial spaces through anatomic or congenital paths (e.g., the hiatus around the esophagus) or through acquired defects in the diaphragm. (Embryologically, before formation of the diaphragm, the peritoneal and pleural cavities derived from one sac.) CO_2 gas insufflated retroperitoneally gains rapid direct access to a vast space, and may result in widespread subcutaneous emphysema.

Pneumothorax can be diagnosed by a sudden decrease in pulmonary compliance, an increase in airway pressure, an increase in $PetCO_2$ and $PaCO_2$, an unchanged or decreased PaO_2, an unchanged or decreased blood pressure (BP), abnormal motion of the involved side hemidiaphragm, and absence of breath sounds without wheezing on the affected side. The shape of the capnogram is usually unchanged. Fiberoptic bronchoscopy will rule out endobronchial intubation, and intraoperative chest fluoroscopy or x-ray film will confirm the diagnosis.

Pneumothorax caused by laparoscopic gas is easily treated or it can resolve spontaneously. One study reports an incidence of pneumothorax in 7 of 46 patients undergoing laparoscopic fundoplication for repair of hiatus hernia. In these cases, intraoperative treatment consisted of positive end-expiratory pressure (PEEP) and increased minute ventilation to reinflate the lung and increased pressure to decrease the gradient from abdomen to pleural cavity and possibly to seal the tear.

Alternatively, pneumothorax may be undetected until the patient wakes up and exhibits respiratory distress and restlessness, which can be misinterpreted as pain or inadequate reversal of the muscle relaxant. Treatment consists of 100% oxygen by mask. CO_2 will quickly diffuse out, as can be easily seen by serial blood gases and x-ray films, and invasive treatment is unnecessary.

Because of the increased volumes and pressures in the lung during laparoscopy, pneumothorax can also result from barotrauma. This cause of pneumothorax is far more serious and may require tube thoracostomy. Attempts at hyperventilating to decrease the $PetCO_2$ can result in overdistention and rupture of alveoli, with subsequent dissection of the anesthetic gases into the perivascular sheaths, mediastinum, pleura, and fascial planes of the head and neck. Large tidal volumes and rapid ventilator rates can be especially dangerous in patients with COPD or bullae because insufficient emptying time may increase air trapping.

Bartelmaos T, Blanc R, DeClaviere G, et al. Delayed pneumomediastinum and pneumothorax complicating laparoscopic extraperitoneal inguinal hernia repair. *J Clin Anesth* 2005;17:209–212.

Batra MS, Driscoll JJ, Coburn WA, et al. Evanescent nitrous oxide pneumothorax after laparoscopy. *Anesth Analg* 1983;62:1121–1123.

Joris JL, Chiche J-D, Lamy ML. Pneumothorax during laparoscopic fundoplication: diagnosis and treatment with positive end-expiratory pressure. *Anesth Analg* 1995; 81:993–1000.

Streich B, Decailliot F, Perney C, et al. Increased carbon dioxide absorption during retroperitoneal laparoscopy. *Br J Anaesth* 2003;91:793–796.

C.28. How would you decide when to extubate?

In addition to the usual criteria for extubation, prolonged laparoscopy in the Trendelenburg position requires other considerations.

Delay extubation if the patient has edema, venous congestion, and duskiness of the head and neck. Sometimes the tongue becomes edematous. If unsure, check the eyes for conjunctival and lid edema, and keep the patient in head-up position until the conjunctivae no longer seem raised or watery.

Causes of edema include dependent stasis from the Trendelenburg position, resistance from elevated abdominal and thoracic pressures, and temporary fluid overload from oliguria or anuria. In some cases it is best to leave the patient intubated until diuresis has begun, especially because postanesthesia care unit (PACU) pulmonary edema is not rare.

D. Postoperative Management

D.1. What are some of the unique complications of laparoscopy?

Injuries from instruments

Improper placement of Veress needle or trocars can cause abdominal wall bleeding, blood vessel or visceral puncture, subcutaneous emphysema, peritonitis, wound infections, hernia at the trocar site, and hemorrhage. Thermal injuries may occur from cautery or laser use. Staples and clips can cause nerve entrapment.

Complications of pneumoperitoneum

Increased intraabdominal pressure can result in bowel ischemia, omental or bowel herniation, gastric regurgitation, excessive compression of vena cava, decreased venous return, venous stasis in legs, hypotension, increased intrathoracic pressure, mediastinal and subcutaneous emphysema, pneumothorax, barotrauma, CO_2 gas embolism, atelectasis, nausea and vomiting, bradyarrhythmias from vagal stimulation of trocar insertion and peritoneal distention, dysfunction of ventriculoperitoneal shunts, and shoulder pain from retained CO_2.

Systemic effects of CO_2 absorption

Among the systemic effects of CO_2 absorptions are hypercarbia, acidosis, increased sympathoad-renal stimulation, hypertension, tachycardia, increased intracranial pressure, embolization, and sickle cell crisis. Arrhythmias can occur from hypercarbia, hypoxia, and catecholamines and in combination with halothane.

Trendelenburg position

Venous congestion of head and neck, increased venous pressure, increased intracranial pressure, retinal hemorrhage, retinal detachment, increased intraocular pressure and glaucoma attack, endobronchial intubation and hypoxemia, ventilation-perfusion mismatch and hypoxia, neuropathy, corneal and conjunctival edema, edema of airway including larynx, airway obstruction and closure, brachial plexus injury from shoulder braces, femoral nerve and peroneal neuropathies, and an assortment of respiratory complications have been reported with use of the Trendelenburg position.

Late complications

Among the late complications are bowel obstruction from injury, cautery burn, intestine or omentum herniation through the trocar site, adhesions, deep vein thrombosis, and nerve injury resulting from improper padding. Fever may indicate infection from bowel necrosis. Cutaneous metastasis can occur at the port site.

Bangma CH, Kirkels WJ, Chadha S, et al. Cutaneous metastasis following laparoscopic pelvic lymphadenopathy for prostatic carcinoma. *J Urol* 1995;153:1635–1636.

Bolder PM, Norton ML. Retinal hemorrhage following anesthesia. *Anesthesiology* 1984; 61:595–597.

Childers JM, Caplinger P. Spontaneous pneumothorax during operative laparoscopy secondary to congenital diaphragmatic defects. A case report. *J Reprod Med* 1995; 40:151–153.

Fahlenkamp D, Rassweiler J, Fornara P, et al. Complications of laparoscopic procedures in urology: experience with 2,407 procedures at 4 German centers. *J Urol* 1999; 162:765–771.

Fuller J, Ashar BS, Carey-Corrado J. Trocar-associated injuries and fatalities: an analysis of 1399 reports to the FDA. *J Minim Invasive Gynecol* 2005;12:302–307.

Joshi GP. Complications of laparoscopy. *Anesthesiol Clin North America* 2001;19:89–105.

Miele VJ, Bendok B, Bloomfield SM. Ventriculoperitoneal shunt dysfunction in adults secondary to conditions causing a transient increase in intraabdominal pressure: report of three cases. *Neurosurgery* 2004;55:434.

Nishikawa K, Nagashima C, Shimodate Y, et al. Migration of the endotracheal tube during laparoscopy-assisted abdominal surgery in young and elderly patients. *Can J Anaesth* 2004;51:1053–1054.

Santana A, Crausman RS, Dubin HG. Late onset of subcutaneous emphysema and hypercarbia following laparoscopic cholecystectomy. *Chest* 1999;115:1468–1471.

D.2. What postoperative orders will you write? When would you remove the Foley catheter and arterial line? Under what circumstances would you order a chest x-ray film?

Immediate chest x-ray film is ordered if respiratory distress, subcutaneous emphysema, and actual or suspected pneumothorax occurred; the case was prolonged and retroperitoneal; the patient was oliguric despite adequate hydration; intraabdominal pressure was greater than 15 mm Hg; or the patient has a history of cardiac or pulmonary disease.

Do not remove the arterial line until the patient is stable and blood gas values are normal. Check urine volumes. Expect an immediate diuresis. Do not remove the Foley catheter until the patient is stable, with fluid intake and volume output stable. Order IV fluids. Check voiding after the catheter is removed. Appropriate medications for nausea and pain control must be written. For ambulatory patients, an adult escort must be available to take them home.

Pavlin DJ, Chen C, Penaloza DA, et al. Pain as a factor complicating recovery and discharge after ambulatory surgery. *Anesth Analg* 2002;95:627–634.

D.3. What is the incidence of postoperative nausea and vomiting?

The incidence of nausea and vomiting after laparoscopy has been reported to be as high as 42%. It is the most important factor in causing an overnight admission after ambulatory surgery. IV antiemetics such as ondansetron, often with dexamethasone may be given, preferably during surgery. The cause of nausea and vomiting is believed to be rapid peritoneal distention. Neurogenic pathways are activated by traction reflexes and by splanchnic pressure and manipulation.

Green G, Jonsson L. Nausea: the most important factor determining length of stay after ambulatory anaesthesia. A comparative study of isoflurane and/or propofol techniques. *Acta Anaesthesiol Scand* 1993;37:742–746.

Sukhani R, Lurie J, Jabamoni R. Propofol for ambulatory gynecologic laparoscopy: does omission of nitrous oxide alter postoperative emetic sequelae and recovery?. *Anesth Analg* 1994;78:831–835.

Wilson EB, Bass CS, Abrameit W, et al. Metoclopramide versus ondansetron in prophylaxis of nausea and vomiting for laparoscopic cholecystectomy. *Am J Surg* 2001;181:138–141.

SECTION VIII

The Reproductive System

CHAPTER 40

Peripartum Hemorrhage

Klaus Kjaer • Eric Cappiello

A 40-YEAR-OLD WOMAN

gravida 5 para 4, presents to your hospital with painless vaginal bleeding at 38 weeks' gestation. She had one episode of painless vaginal bleeding at 28 weeks' gestation which resolved spontaneously. She has a past surgical history of three cesarean sections. Her obstetrician wants to take her back for a cesarean section now for continued vaginal bleeding. Her vital signs are as follows: blood pressure 90/36 mm Hg, heart rate 112 beats per minute, respiratory rate 22 per minute, and SpO$_2$ 97% on room air. Her hematocrit is 25%.

A. Medical Disease and Differential Diagnosis

1. What are the leading causes of maternal mortality?
2. Discuss anesthesia-related maternal mortality.
3. You saw this patient at 28 weeks' gestation. What is the differential diagnosis for antepartum hemorrhage?
4. How would you diagnose placenta previa in this patient?
5. What are the different types of placenta previa and describe the management of these patients?
6. Who is at a greater risk for placenta previa and what are the associated conditions with placenta previa?
7. What is a double setup and what anesthetic would you use for this patient?
8. How is placental abruption diagnosed?

881

9. What are the risk factors for the development of a placental abruption?
10. What complications are associated with placental abruption?
11. Who is at risk for uterine rupture and how is uterine rupture diagnosed?
12. What is the treatment for uterine rupture?
13. What is vasa previa, how is it diagnosed, and what is the management?
14. What are the different types of placenta accreta?
15. How is placenta accreta diagnosed?

B. Preoperative Evaluation and Preparation

1. Of what significance to the anesthesiologist are the changes in maternal respiratory function at term?
2. What are the maternal cardiovascular changes of pregnancy?
3. What laboratory data do you need before taking this patient to the operating room (OR)?
4. What is the supine hypotensive syndrome?
5. What is the relative anemia of pregnancy?
6. Would you transfuse this patient preoperatively?
7. What invasive monitors should be used during management of severe hemorrhage?
8. What are the maternal gastrointestinal changes of pregnancy?
9. What anatomic changes of pregnancy may contribute to a difficult airway?
10. What preoperative medications would you administer to this patient?
11. Would evaluation of fetal maturity be indicated in this patient?

C. Intraoperative Management

1. What is the anesthetic management for placenta accreta?
2. After delivery of the fetus and placenta you notice generalized oozing from the surgical site. What is disseminated intravascular coagulation (DIC)?
3. You suspect DIC in this patient. Discuss the use of additional blood products in patients who develop DIC.
4. After how many units of packed red blood cells (PRBCs) should you give fresh frozen plasma (FFP) and platelets?
5. What is the role of emergency release blood and how does this change your future management?
6. What is the role of activated factor VII in obstetric patients?
7. You are called to see a 27-year-old woman who just delivered and is continuing to hemorrhage. What is the definition and differential diagnosis of postpartum hemorrhage?
8. What are the anesthetic considerations of postpartum hemorrhage?
9. What laboratory tests should be ordered during the resuscitation of this patient?
10. What are the treatment options for uterine atony?
11. The patient is hemorrhaging after removal of her placenta using excessive traction. How is uterine inversion treated?
12. Discuss retained placenta and treatment options.
13. Define amniotic fluid embolism and discuss treatment.
14. What is the role of cell savage in obstetric patients?
15. How do you treat the Jehovah's Witness with postpartum hemorrhage or a known placenta accreta?

16. What is the role for uterine artery balloon placement and uterine artery embolization?

D. Postoperative Management

1. When do you remove an epidural in patients who have just been treated for DIC?

2. You have successfully treated the patient with DIC and her laboratory values have returned to normal. Her central venous pressure (CVP) is normal and urine output is normal. The patient is still hypotensive despite her intravascular volume replacement. What is your concern in this case?

A. Medical Disease and Differential Diagnosis

A.1. What are the leading causes of maternal mortality?

Maternal mortality is defined as the number of deaths per 100,000 maternity cases. Maternal mortality has decreased significantly over the last 100 years. In 1900 there were approximately 850 deaths per 100,000 live births. Pregnancy-related mortality surveillance in the United States was observed for the period of 1991 to 1999. The overall mortality ratio was 11.8 deaths per 100,000 live births over this period. The leading causes of maternal mortality were embolism (19.6%), hemorrhage (17.2%), and pregnancy-induced hypertension (15.7%). Maternal age was also associated with an increased mortality risks. The risk ratio for patients aged 35 to 39 was found to be 2.5 and the risk ratio for patients older than 40 was found to be 5.3.

In the United Kingdom, the maternal mortality decreased from 70 per 100,000 in 1952 to 1954 to 11 per 100,000 in 1994 to 1996. The leading direct causes of maternal morbidity in the United Kingdom were thrombosis, hypertension, early pregnancy loss, hemorrhage, amniotic fluid embolism, and genital tract sepsis. Fifty percent of the hemorrhage-related deaths were due to placental abruption and placenta previa, with the remaining 50% linked to postpartum hemorrhage.

Chang J, Elam-Evans L.D., Berg C.J., et al. Pregnancy-related mortality surveillance–United States, 1991–1999. *Morb Mortal Wkly Rep* 2003;52:(SS02):1–8.

de Swiet M. Maternal mortality: confidential enquiries into maternal deaths in the United Kingdom. *Am J Obstet Gynecol* 2000;182(4):760–766.

A.2. Discuss anesthesia-related maternal mortality.

Anesthesia-related maternal mortality has decreased from 4.3 per million live births during 1979 to 1981 to 1.7 per million live births during 1988 to 1990. Most deaths occurred during general anesthesia for cesarean sections, with 73% arising from airway problems (aspiration, induction, or intubation problems; inadequate ventilation; or respiratory failure). Since 1984, use of regional anesthesia has been correlated with a decrease in the number of maternal deaths, whereas general anesthesia–related maternal deaths have remained unchanged during the 1979 to 1990 period.

Hawkins JL, Koonin LM, Plamer SK, et al. Anesthesia-related deaths during obstetric delivery in the United States, 1979–1990. *Anesthesiology* 1997;86:277–284.

Ross Brian K. ASA closed claims in obstetrics: lessons learned. *Anesthesiol Clin North America* 2003;21:183–197.

de Swiet M. Maternal mortality: confidential enquiries into maternal deaths in the United Kingdom. *Am J Obstet Gynecol* 2000;182(4):760–766.

A.3. You saw this patient at 28 weeks' gestation. What is the differential diagnosis for antepartum hemorrhage?

Antepartum hemorrhage is vaginal bleeding after 24 weeks' gestation and before the onset of labor. Approximately 3% to 4% of all pregnancies are affected by antepartum hemorrhage.

The most common causes of antepartum hemorrhage are placenta previa and placental abruption. Placenta previa is the abnormal implantation of the placenta in front of the fetal presenting part. Placental abruption is separation of the placenta from the deciduas basalis before delivery of the fetus.

Patients who have had previous uterine surgery have a higher risk for a placenta previa. There is a strong association between a previous uterine scar and the development of placenta previa. In a study performed by Clark et al. 97,799 patients were retrospectively reviewed and 292 (0.3%) patients were found to have a placenta previa. The risk for previa was found to be 0.26% with an unscarred uterus. The association of placenta previa and previous cesarean sections appears to be linear with a frequency of 10% with four or more previous cesarean sections.

Other less common causes of antepartum bleeding include uterine rupture, vasa previa, and local genital tract lesions. There are also a number of patients who have no identifiable cause for antepartum hemorrhage.

Bender S. Placenta previa and previous lower segment cesarean section. *Surg Gynecol Obstet* 1954;98:625.

Clark SL, Koonings PP, Phelan JP. Placenta previa/accreta and prior cesarean section. *Obstet Gynecol* 1985;66(1):89–92.

Norwitz ER, Lee-Parritz A. Obstetric complications. In: Lobo RA, ed. *Obstetrics and gynecology*, Castile Connolly Graduate Medical Publishing, 2003:22–23.

A.4. How would you diagnose placenta previa in this patient?

Patients who present with placenta previa usually have painless bleeding in either the second or third trimester. Placenta previa occurs in up to 1% of all full term pregnancies. The first event of bleeding typically occurs preterm, is not associated with increased uterine activity, and generally resolves spontaneously. If placenta previa is suspected, then a vaginal examination is avoided due to the risk of massive hemorrhage. Ultrasonography is most frequently used to diagnose placenta previa. Not only can it help to localize the placenta but it also can be used to rule out a placental abruption which may also be present. Magnetic resonance imaging (MRI) may also be used to help with the diagnosis of placenta previa, but it is not the first modality chosen due to cost and availability.

Mayer DC, Spielman FJ, Bell EA. Antepartum and postpartum hemorrhage. In: Chestnut DH, ed. *Obstetric anesthesia: principles and practice*, 3rd ed. Mosby, 2004:662.

Sarna MC, Hess P, Takoudes TC, et al. Postpartum hemorrhage. In: Datta S, ed. *Anesthetic and obstetric management of high-risk pregnancy*, 3rd ed. New York: Springer, 2004: 111–132.

Stoelting RK, Dierdorf SF. *Anesthesia and co-existing disease*, 4th ed. Churchill Livingstone, 2002:676–677.

Wali A, Suresh MS, Gregg AR. Antepartum hemorrhage. In: Datta S, ed. *Anesthetic and obstetric management of high-risk pregnancy*, 3rd ed. New York: Springer, 2004:87–110.

A.5. What are the different types of placenta previa and describe the management of these patients?

Placenta previa is classified on the basis of placental relation to the cervix. Placenta previa can be complete, partial, or marginal. A complete placenta previa covers the internal cervical os, a partial previa partially covers the internal cervical os, and a marginal previa lies close to but does not cover the cervical os.

Obstetric management is dependent on maternal and fetal well-being. If the mother and fetus are stable and the bleeding is minimal, conservative management is typically recommended. The mother is placed on bed rest and the bleeding is monitored. Serial hematocrits are followed until the bleeding has stabilized. The fetus is monitored to ensure well-being.

If the bleeding continues or there is instability of the mother or fetus, then delivery may be expedited by cesarean section due to the location of the placenta.

The patient should have adequate IV access due to the risk of continued bleeding. Laboratory results should be obtained which include a complete blood count (CBC), coagulation profile, and a type and crossmatch. If there are no coagulation problems then a regional technique could be performed.

There is a known association between placenta previa and placenta accreta. General anesthesia should be considered if there is a suspected placenta accreta.

Mayer DC, Spielman FJ, Bell EA. Antepartum and postpartum hemorrhage. In: Chestnut DH, ed. *Obstetric anesthesia: principles and practice*, 3rd ed. Mosby, 2004:662.

Norwitz ER, Lee-Parritz A. Obstetric complications. In: Lobo RA, ed. *Obstetrics and gynecology*. Castile Connolly Graduate Medical Publishing, 2003:22–23.

A.6. Who is at a greater risk for placenta previa and what are the associated conditions with placenta previa?

The risk for developing placenta previa increases with multiparity, advanced maternal age, prior placenta previa, and prior cesarean sections.

There is a strong association between prior uterine surgery, placenta previa, and the development of placenta accreta. If the patient has placenta previa and an unscarred uterus there is a 5% risk of placenta accreta. If a patient has a placenta previa and one previous cesarean section there is a 24% risk of placenta accreta. The risk of placenta accreta goes up to 67% if the patient has a placenta previa and has had four or more cesarean sections.

Clark SL, Koonings PP, Phelan JP. Placenta previa/accreta and prior cesarean section. *Obstet Gynecol* 1985;66(1):89–92.

Wali A, Suresh MS, Gregg AR. Antepartum hemorrhage. In: Datta S,ed. *Anesthetic and obstetric management of high-risk pregnancy*, 3rd ed. Springer, New York, 2004:94–98.

A.7. What is a double setup and what anesthetic would you use for this patient?

If there is a suspected placenta previa, then a vaginal examination is usually avoided due to the possibility of massive hemorrhage. Most cases can be diagnosed by ultrasonography or magnetic resonance imaging (MRI) and therefore a double setup will be utilized less frequently. If a vaginal examination needs to be performed a double setup will be carried out in the operating room (OR). The entire obstetric team needs to be present (anesthesiologist, obstetrician, pediatrician, nurse, and surgical technician). The patient should have two large-bore intravenous lines, standard monitoring, and blood available in the OR. The patient is positioned and the abdomen is prepped and draped for a cesarean section. The obstetrician then executes a careful vaginal examination and if either bleeding worsens or it is determined that there is a complete previa with a mature fetus then a cesarean section is performed.

For a patient who has massive hemorrhage, a general anesthetic will often be the anesthetic of choice. A general anesthetic may also be preferred if a placenta accreta is suspected. If the situation is less emergent and the patient is hemodynamically stable then a regional anesthetic may be preferred by some anesthesiologists.

Mayer DC, Spielman FJ, Bell EA. Antepartum and postpartum hemorrhage. In: Chestnut DH, ed. *Obstetric anesthesia: principles and practice*, 3rd ed. Mosby, 2004:662.

A.8. How is placental abruption diagnosed?

Placental abruption usually presents with painful vaginal bleeding. It is typically associated with uterine tenderness and increased uterine activity. The amount of bleeding is not always easy to quantify. Much of the bleeding can be confined behind the placenta, making an estimate of blood loss difficult. Placental abruption can be diagnosed with ultrasonography or magnetic resonance imaging (MRI).

Mayer DC, Spielman FJ, Bell EA. Antepartum and postpartum hemorrhage. In: Chestnut DH, ed. *Obstetric anesthesia: principles and practice*, 3rd ed. Mosby, 2004:662.

Wali A, Suresh MS, Gregg AR. Antepartum hemorrhage. In: Datta S, ed. *Anesthetic and obstetric management of high-risk pregnancy*, 3rd ed. New York: Springer, 2004:89–94.

A.9. What are the risk factors for the development of a placental abruption?

Approximately 33% of third trimester bleeding is caused by placental abruption. The incidence of placental abruption is increased with high parity and uterine anomalies.

There are several risk factors associated with placental abruption. Any pregnant patient who has experienced trauma should be ruled out for placental abruption. The risk of placental abruption is increased with exposure to cocaine, methadone, and tobacco. Patients with hypertension and superimposed preeclampsia, severe preeclamptics, and patients with a fibroid uterus are also at an increased risk of developing a placental abruption.

Stoelting RK, Dierdorf SF. *Anesthesia and co-existing disease*, 4th ed. Churchill Livingstone, 2002:662.

Wali A, Suresh MS, Gregg AR. Antepartum hemorrhage. In: Datta S, ed. *Anesthetic and obstetric management of high-risk pregnancy*, 3rd ed. New York: Springer, 2004:89–94.

A.10. What complications are associated with placental abruption?

Severe abruption can be associated with anemia, varying degrees of coagulopathy including disseminated intravascular coagulopathy, acute renal failure, postpartum hemorrhage, uterine atony, and Sheehan's syndrome. Placental abruption can lead to either fetal distress or fetal demise.

Wali A, Suresh MS, Gregg AR. Antepartum hemorrhage. In: Datta S, ed. *Anesthetic and obstetric management of high-risk pregnancy*, 3rd ed. New York: Springer, 2004:89–94.

A.11. Who is at risk for uterine rupture and how is uterine rupture diagnosed?

Uterine rupture is a rare occurrence with an incidence of 1 in 15,000 patients who have an unscarred uterus. However, the risk for uterine rupture or dehiscence is increased in patients with a previous uterine scar. Similarly, in patients attempting vaginal birth after cesarean section (VBAC), use of prostaglandins have been shown to increase the relative risk of uterine rupture by a factor of 15. Additional risk factors associated with uterine rupture include uterine trauma, a tumultuous labor, midforceps delivery, breech version and extraction, inappropriate uterotonic use, uterine anomalies, placenta percreta, tumors, fetal macrosomia, and fetal malposition. The most consistent sign of uterine rupture is fetal distress. Other signs that may be present include hypotension, vaginal bleeding, abdominal pain, change in the uterine contour, changes in the uterine contraction pattern, and cessation of labor. True diagnosis is made either during manual inspection of the uterus or during a laparotomy.

ACOG. *Practice Bulletin Clinical Management Guidelines for Obstetrician-Gynecologists*. July 2004; 54.

Mayer DC, Spielman FJ, Bell EA. Antepartum and postpartum hemorrhage. In: Chestnut DH, ed. *Obstetric anesthesia: principles and practice*, 3rd ed. Mosby, 2004:667–668.

Plauche WC. Surgical problems involving the pregnant uterus. Uterine inversion, uterine rupture, and leiomyomas. *Surgical obstetrics*. Philadelphia: WB Saunders, 1989:224.

Stoelting RK, Dierdorf SF. *Anesthesia and co-existing disease*, 4th ed. Churchill Livingstone, 2002:678.

Wali A, Suresh MS, Gregg AR. Antepartum hemorrhage. In: Datta S, ed. *Anesthetic and obstetric management of high-risk pregnancy*, 3rd ed. New York: Springer, 2004:104–105.

A.12. What is the treatment for uterine rupture?

If the rupture occurs antepartum, then an emergent laparotomy is performed with delivery of the fetus and concurrent stabilization of the mother. After delivery of the fetus the uterus can either be repaired, the uterine arteries can be ligated, or a hysterectomy can be performed depending on the size of the rupture and the patient's condition. A rupture that occurs in an unscarred uterus is usually associated with a greater amount of blood loss and requires more intense management. A general anesthetic will usually be performed due to the rapid decompensation of the patient and anticipated massive hemorrhage that will occur. A regional technique can be utilized if the patient's condition is stable and if the uterine rupture is suspected in a previous low-transverse uterine scar, where the risk of massive hemorrhage is decreased. Swift treatment needs to be performed to decrease maternal and fetal mortality. Invasive monitoring such as an arterial line, a central venous pressure (CVP) line, and a Foley catheter should be utilized to help guide the patient's resuscitation. Laboratory data including hematocrit, coagulation profile, and electrolytes should be sent to further guide the management of the patient.

Hepner DL, Gutsche BB. Obstetric hemorrhage. *Curr Rev Clin Anesth* 1998;18(22):213–224.

Mayer DC, Spielman FJ, Bell EA. Antepartum and postpartum hemorrhage. In: Chestnut DH, ed. *Obstetric anesthesia: principles and practice*, 3rd ed. Mosby, 2004:667–668.

Stoelting RK, Dierdorf SF. *Anesthesia and co-existing disease*, 4th ed. Churchill Livingstone, 2002:678.

Wali A, Suresh MS, Gregg AR. Antepartum hemorrhage. In: Datta S, ed. *Anesthetic and obstetric management of high-risk pregnancy*, 3rd ed. New York: Springer, 2004:104–105.

A.13. What is vasa previa, how is it diagnosed, and what is the management?

Vasa previa develops when the intramembranous fetal vessels overlie the cervical os in front of the fetal presenting part. The patient usually presents with painless vaginal bleeding and decreased fetal movement. Fetal mortality is high because the bleeding is from a fetal source and can lead to fetal hemorrhage. The incidence of vasa previa was found to be 1.6 per 10,000 pregnancies in a study that looked at 93,874 patients.

Diagnosis is made by either palpation or ultrasonography. Color Doppler ultrasonography can be used to help with the diagnosis. If blood is present then it can be tested by either a Wright's stain or an Apt test. A Wright's stain is conducted to look for fetal nucleated red blood cells (RBCs). An Apt test is performed by adding an alkaline solution to the blood. Adult RBCs will rupture in this environment and turn the solution brown as opposed to fetal RBCs, which will remain bright red.

If a vasa previa is suspected then the patient should have an emergent cesarean section. Owing to the small blood volume of the fetus delay in delivery could lead to fetal demise. Because the bleeding is primarily from a fetal source the mother is usually hemodynamically stable. A regional or a general anesthetic could be selected and should be based on maternal factors in addition to the need for a rapid surgical anesthetic.

Lee W, Lee VL, Kirk JS, et al. Vasa previa: prenatal diagnosis, natural evolution, and clinical outcome. *Obstet Gynecol* 2000;95(4):572–576.

Mayer DC, Spielman FJ, Bell EA. Antepartum and postpartum hemorrhage. In: Chestnut DH, ed. *Obstetric anesthesia: principles and practice*, 3rd ed. Mosby, 2004:662.

Norwitz ER, Lee-Parritz A. Obstetric complications. In: Lobo RA, ed. *Obstetrics and gynecology*. Castile Connolly Graduate Medical Publishing, 2003:22–23.

Wali A, Suresh MS, Gregg AR. Antepartum hemorrhage. In: Datta S, ed. *Anesthetic and obstetric management of high-risk pregnancy*, 3rd ed. New York: Springer, 2004:97–98, 100–101.

A.14. What are the different types of placenta accreta?

Placenta accreta is identified on the basis of invasion of the myometrium. If the placenta is affixed to the myometrium but does not invade the uterine muscle then this is placenta accreta vera. Placenta increta grows into the myometrium. Placenta percreta grows through the uterine muscle and invades the uterine serosa with possible invasion of other pelvic structures including bowel or bladder.

Mayer DC, Spielman FJ, Bell EA. Antepartum and postpartum hemorrhage. In: Chestnut DH, ed. *Obstetric anesthesia: principles and practice*, 3rd ed. Mosby, 2004:673–674.

A.15. How is placenta accreta diagnosed?

The frequency of placenta accreta is between 1 in 1,667 and 1 in 70,000. Antepartum diagnosis of placenta accreta would be preferred so that management could be appropriately planned. Unfortunately this is often not the case and diagnosis of placenta accreta is made postpartum when separation of the placenta does not occur, hematuria develops, uterine inversion occurs, or massive hemorrhage follows placental removal. Patients with a prior uterine scar who present with previa should be suspected as possibly having placenta accreta. Patients at a high risk could have gray-scale ultrasonography, color Doppler ultrasonography, or MRI to help identify placenta accreta. The diagnosis can be confirmed during laparotomy.

Mayer DC, Spielman FJ, Bell EA. Antepartum and postpartum hemorrhage. In: Chestnut DH, ed. *Obstetric anesthesia: principles and practice*, 3rd ed. Mosby, 2004:673–674.

Wali A, Suresh MS, Gregg AR. Antepartum Hemorrhage. In: Datta S, ed. *Anesthetic and obstetric management of high-risk pregnancy*, 3rd ed. New York: Springer, 2004:102–104.

B. Preoperative Evaluation and Preparation

B.1. Of what significance to the anesthesiologist are the changes in maternal respiratory function at term?

A number of maternal respiratory changes are seen at term:

- Capillary engorgement of the mucosa is found throughout the respiratory tract, causing swelling of the vocal cords and oral pharynx, larynx, and trachea.
- Increased minute ventilation (45%), tidal volume (45%), respiratory rate (no change), and oxygen consumption (30% to 40%)
- Arterial $Paco_2$ decrease (to 30 mm Hg)
- Arterial pH increase (to 7.44)
- Functional residual capacity (FRC) decrease (20%)

Following rapid sequence induction, the combination of decreased FRC and increased oxygen consumption makes the onset of hypoxemia very rapid. Administering 100% oxygen for 3 to 5 minutes while taking normal tidal breaths, or for four vital capacity breaths, leads to effective nitrogen washout of FRC, such that maximal maternal oxygen reserves are attained before induction and more time can be spent securing the airway before attempting intubation.

The reduced FRC increases the rapidity of changes in the depth of anesthesia while employing an inhaled anesthetic technique. In addition, the minimum alveolar concentration (MAC) of inhaled anesthetic agents has been found to be decreased in pregnancy.

Benumof JL. Preoxygenation: best method for both efficacy and efficiency. *Anesthesiology* 1999;91(3):603–605.

Chestnut DH, ed. *Obstetric anesthesia, principles and practice*, 3rd ed. Philadelphia: Mosby, 2004:16–17.

B.2. What are the maternal cardiovascular changes of pregnancy?

Cardiovascular changes of pregnancy at term include the following:

- Intravascular fluid volume increases 45%.
- Plasma volume increases 55%.
- Red blood cell (RBC) volume increases 30%.
- Cardiac output increases 50%.
- Stroke volume increases 25%.
- Heart rate increases 25%.
- Systolic blood pressure is minimally affected by pregnancy.
- Diastolic blood pressure decreases up to 20% by midpregnancy, but returns to its prepregnant level at term.
- Systemic vascular resistance decreases 20%.
- CVP remains unchanged.

During labor, cardiac output rises 10% during the early first stage, 25% during the late first stage, and 40% during the second stage. Each uterine contraction increases cardiac output an additional 15% to 25%. The greatest increase in cardiac output occurs immediately after delivery, when the cardiac output is 80% higher than prelabor values.

In addition, the following coagulation factors are increased at term: factors I, VII, VIII, IX, X, and XII. Plasminogen is also increased. Factors II and V are unchanged, and factors XI and XIII are decreased. Overall, the result is a decrease in both the prothrombin time (PT) and partial thromboplastin time (PTT) of 20%. The platelet count is typically unchanged at term, but may fall to below 100×10^9 per L in close to 1% of patients. In most women, pregnancy is associated with a hypercoagulable state.

Burrows RF, Kelton JG. Thrombocytopenia at delivery: a prospective survey of 6715 deliveries. *Am J Obstet Gynecol* 1990;162(3):731–734.

Chestnut DH, ed. *Obstetric anesthesia, principles and practice*, 3rd ed. Philadelphia: Mosby, 2004:18–23.

B.3. **What laboratory data do you need before taking this patient to the operating room (OR)?**

At a minimum, this patient needs to have a type and cross, for anticipated transfusion of blood products, as well as a complete blood count (CBC) with platelets, performed immediately. A prothrombin time (PT) and partial thromboplastin time (PTT) should also be performed. The platelet count may fall during significant hemorrhage, and the PT/PTT may rise. If this is happening, the patient may not be a good candidate for regional anesthesia due to an increased risk of epidural hematoma.

Regional anesthesia may in many cases be safer than general anesthesia even at platelet counts below 100×10^3 per μL. In such patients, and in patients on anticoagulation medication such as low molecular weight heparin (LMWH), the risk of epidural hematoma associated with regional anesthesia is difficult to assess. The bleeding time is no longer considered relevant in assessing the risk of clinical bleeding. Thromboelastography (TEG) is a simple test that provides information about the interaction between clotting factors and platelets, clot strength, and clot stability in a short time. It has been used in pregnant women with thrombocytopenia or on LMWH to determine adequacy of hemostasis before regional anesthesia. However, further studies are required to determine the ability of TEG to predict risk of epidural hematoma.

In the setting of LMWH, the anti-Xa level is not predictive of the risk of bleeding after regional anesthesia. The American Society of Regional Anesthesia and Pain Medicine (ASRA) Consensus Conference concluded that in patients receiving preoperative LMWH for thromboprophylaxis, needle placement should occur at least 10 to 12 hours after the last dose. In patients receiving higher doses of LMWH, needle placement should not occur until at least 24 hours after the last dose.

Chestnut DH, ed. *Obstetric anesthesia, principles and practice*, 3rd ed. Philadelphia: Mosby, 2004:770–777.

Datta S, ed. *Anesthetic and obstetric management of high-risk pregnancy*, 3rd ed. New York: Springer-Verlag, 2004:157–158.

Horlocker TT, Wedel DJ, Benzon H, et al. Regional anesthesia in the anticoagulated patient: defining the risks (the second ASRA Consensus Conference on Neuraxial Anesthesia and Anticoagulation). *Reg Anesth Pain Med* 2003;28(3):172–197.

Klein SM, Slaughter TF, Vail PT, et al. Thromboelastography as a perioperative measure of anticoagulation resulting from low molecular weight heparin: a comparison with anti-Xa concentrations. *Anesth Analg* 2000;91(5):1091–1095.

B.4. What is the supine hypotensive syndrome?

Supine hypotensive syndrome, or aortocaval compression, may be caused by compression of the abdominal aorta and inferior vena cava in the supine position. Compression of the inferior vena cava occurs as early as 13 to 16 weeks' gestation. At term, 40% of women experience a fall in femoral artery pressure, consistent with compression of the aorta. Symptoms typically include weakness, lightheadedness, nausea, dizziness, and syncope. However, the syndrome may occur without maternal symptoms. For this reason, all patients at term should be positioned with left uterine displacement.

Aortocaval compression leads to a decrease in uteroplacental perfusion by three mechanisms. First, it decreases maternal venous return, with a concomitant drop in maternal arterial blood pressure. Second, direct compression of the internal iliac arteries may drop uterine artery pressure even further. Third, obstruction of uterine venous drainage causes a decrease in uterine perfusion pressure.

Chestnut DH, ed. *Obstetric anesthesia, principles and practice*, 3rd ed. Philadelphia: Mosby, 2004:19–20, 422–424.

Datta S, ed. *Anesthetic and obstetric management of high-risk pregnancy*, 3rd ed. New York: Springer-Verlag, 2004:157–158.

B.5. What is the relative anemia of pregnancy?

With pregnancy, blood volume increases by 45% during the first half of pregnancy. But although plasma volume increases approximately 55%, red blood cell (RBC) volume increases by only approximately 30%. This disproportionate increase in plasma volume leads to hemodilution, and may be an essential adaptive mechanism for maintaining the patency of the uteroplacental vascular bed.

By midgestation, hematocrit has typically fallen approximately 15% below prepregnant levels, to approximately 34%. As RBC mass continues to build in late gestation, this relative anemia tends to become slightly less severe, rising to approximately 35.5% by term.

Chestnut DH, ed. *Obstetric anesthesia, principles and practice*, 3rd ed. Philadelphia: Mosby, 2004:21.

B.6. Would you transfuse this patient preoperatively?

During rapid bleeding, the hematocrit may not accurately reflect the amount of blood loss due to lack of equilibration with other fluid compartments. Tachycardia is often the earliest indicator of hypovolemia, but in the typical parturient it may not be apparent until blood loss is in excess of 2 L. The ideal blood product should be type-specific, crossmatched whole blood; however, during massive blood loss, there may not be sufficient time to allow for typing and crossmatching. In this setting, O Rh-negative blood may be administered.

If the patient is bleeding profusely and is hemodynamically unstable, attempts to fully correct blood loss before surgery begins may not be feasible. Frequently, blood loss will tend to outpace blood replacement until surgical control of bleeding is established. If normovolemia cannot

Table 40.1   The Physical Findings in Relation to Percentage of Blood Loss.

BLOOD LOSS (%)	PHYSICAL FINDINGS
<15–20	None
20–25	Tachycardia (>100 beats/min)
	Mild hypotension
	Peripheral vasoconstriction
25–35	Tachycardia (100–120 beats/min)
	Hypotension (systolic blood pressure 80–100 mm Hg)
	Restlessness
	Oliguria
>35	Tachycardia (>120 beats/min)
	Hypotension (systolic blood pressure <60 mm Hg)
	Altered consciousness
	Anuria

be established before surgery, general anesthesia will typically be the technique of choice. The physical findings in relation to percentage of blood loss are listed in Table 40.1.

Chestnut DH, ed. *Obstetric anesthesia, principles and practice*, 3rd ed. Philadelphia: Mosby, 2004:662–665.

Naef RW, Washburne JF, Martin RW. Hemorrhage associated with cesarean delivery: when is transfusion needed. *J Perinatol* 1995;15:32–35.

B.7.   What invasive monitors should be used during management of severe hemorrhage?

A Foley catheter should be placed to assess adequacy of urine output. Urine output below 0.5 mL/kg/hour, despite adequate volume replacement, merits placing a central venous line. A radial arterial line permits rapid detection of sudden drops in systemic blood pressure. It also simplifies the process of obtaining serial blood samples for following the hematocrit, platelet count, prothrombin time (PT), partial thromboplastin time (PTT), fibrinogen, and acid–base status, all of which can fluctuate unpredictably during volume resuscitation.

Datta S, ed. *Anesthetic and obstetric management of high-risk pregnancy*, 3rd ed. New York: Springer-Verlag, 2004:157–158.

B.8.   What are the maternal gastrointestinal changes of pregnancy?

Gastrointestinal changes during pregnancy make parturients vulnerable to aspiration of gastric contents. Gastric emptying of liquid and solid materials is not altered at any time during pregnancy. However, due to upward displacement of the stomach by the gravid uterus, lower esophageal sphincter tone is decreased. As a result, the incidence of heartburn increases dramatically during pregnancy, from 22% in the first trimester to 72% in the third trimester. Recent work suggests that gastric acid secretion is not increased in pregnancy.

In nonlaboring women, it is primarily the decrease of lower esophageal pressure, combined with an unpredictable need for cesarean delivery without preoperative fasting, that leads to an increased risk of aspiration. During labor, gastric emptying is slowed and mean gastric volume is increased. This further increases the risk of aspiration in the event of unplanned cesarean delivery.

Chestnut DH, ed. *Obstetric anesthesia, principles and practice*, 3rd ed. Philadelphia: Mosby, 2004:23–24.

Chiloiro M, Darconza G, Piccioli E, et al. Gastric emptying and orocecal transit time in pregnancy. *J Gastroenterol* 2001;36(8):538–543.

B.9. What anatomic changes of pregnancy may contribute to a difficult airway?

Failed intubation is approximately 10 times more likely to occur during induction of general anesthesia in pregnant patients than in general surgical patients. When pulmonary aspiration of gastric contents occurs, it is usually in the setting of failed intubation. Anatomic changes of pregnancy, which contribute to failed intubation, include edema of the tongue and larynx, and capillary engorgement causing friability and bleeding of the airway mucosa. Epistaxis is more likely to occur, and nasal intubation is relatively contraindicated. In addition, mammary hyperplasia and the resultant shortening of the distance from the chest to the chin can make insertion of a laryngoscope difficult. Proper attention to head and neck positioning during induction can make laryngoscope insertion easier.

Careful assessment of the airway in all obstetric patients is essential. Most cases of failed intubation occur during emergency cesarean deliveries, at off-peak hours, and with less experienced anesthesia personnel.

Barnardo PD, Jenkins JG. Failed tracheal intubation in obstetrics: a 6-year review in a UK region. *Anaesthesia* 2000;55:685–694.

Chestnut DH, ed. *Obstetric anesthesia, principles and practice*, 3rd ed. Philadelphia: Mosby, 2004:21.

B.10. What preoperative medications would you administer to this patient?

Patients at increased risk for aspiration should receive a nonparticulate oral antacid such as sodium citrate in the 30 minutes before induction of general anesthesia. Intravenous metoclopramide may also be given preoperatively, as it raises lower esophageal sphincter tone and accelerates gastric emptying. Premedication with sedatives or opioids are relatively contraindicated immediately before delivery because of their depressant effects on the neonate.

Chestnut DH, ed. *Obstetric anesthesia, principles and practice*, 3rd ed. Philadelphia: Mosby, 2004:424–440.

B.11. Would evaluation of fetal maturity be indicated in this patient?

In a patient with placenta previa who is bleeding profusely, fetal maturity does not impact the decision to proceed with immediate cesarean delivery. Patients with a small, self-limited episode of bleeding and a premature fetus can be treated conservatively with bed rest and corticosteroids to accelerate fetal lung maturity. Once the patient is closer to term, cesarean delivery is performed. With the use of antenatal corticosteroids and exogenous surfactant to prevent respiratory distress syndrome, neonatal survival is now greater than 80% after 26 weeks' gestation and approximates 100% after 32 weeks' gestation.

Chestnut DH, ed. *Obstetric anesthesia, principles and practice*, 3rd ed. Philadelphia: Mosby, 2004:605–606.

C. Intraoperative Management

C.1. What is the anesthetic management for placenta accreta?

Postpartum hemorrhage can occur with placenta accreta due to inadequate constriction of the spiral arteries at the implantation site. Removal of the placenta can worsen bleeding due to the exposure of large sinuses in the myometrium. If placenta accreta is suspected or known before delivery then discussions should occur with the team that is managing the patient and fetus. Decisions may center around placement of preoperative internal iliac arterial balloons. The balloons could be inflated after delivery of the fetus, which will decrease blood flow to the uterus and provide time for appropriate management of the placenta accreta. The most common cause of obstetric hysterectomy is placenta accreta. Owing to the possibility of massive hemorrhage adequate intravenous access is required, which should include two large-bore intravenous lines. Arterial access is also helpful due to the possibility of acute hemodynamic compromise. Central monitoring can be a useful guide during the resuscitation. Baseline laboratory values allow you to follow the changes that will occur during the resuscitation and should include a hematocrit as well as the starting coagulation status. The patient is typed and crossmatched for four units of packed red blood cells (PRBCs) and the case does not start until blood is available in the operating suite. Epidurals could be placed in patients with a known or suspected placenta accreta who are going to have balloon placements. Often the blood loss can be controlled with the use of the internal iliac balloons, and depending on the stability of the patient, the epidural could be used during the case. If blood control is not adequate or stability of the patient is not maintained a conversion to a general anesthetic may be necessary. Such concern should be discussed with the patient and obstetric team before surgery. On the other hand, if the patient has a suspected percreta, and general anesthetic is usually choice for the operative hysterectomy. Likewise, if the patient presents emergently with severe postoperative hemorrhage a general anesthetic is preferred.

Alamia V, Meyer BA. Controversies in labor management. *Obstet Gynecol Clin North America* 1999;26(2):385–398.

Mayer DC, Spielman FJ, Bell EA. Antepartum and postpartum hemorrhage. In: Chestnut DH, ed. *Obstetric anesthesia: principles and practice*, 3rd ed. Mosby, 2004:662.

Sarna MC, Hess P, Takoudes TC, et al. Postpartum hemorrhage. In: Datta S, ed. *Anesthetic and obstetric management of high-risk pregnancy*, 3rd ed. New York: Springer, 2004: 112–120, 123–125.

C.2. After delivery of the fetus and placenta you notice generalized oozing from the surgical site. What is disseminated intravascular coagulation (DIC)?

DIC occurs when consumption of the coagulation factors, platelets, and fibrinogen occurs with deposition of thrombi in the microcirculation. The thrombi can diminish the blood flow to organs, which may ultimately lead to multisystem organ failure. At the same time, fibrinolysis occurs with the formation of fibrin split products. Owing to the inappropriate consumption of the factors and platelets bleeding can be difficult to control. Coagulation can be impaired to the level of spontaneous bleeding from any disturbed area including the uterus and intravenous sites. Often DIC occurs in the setting of postpartum hemorrhage, which worsens an already tenuous situation. DIC can develop rapidly in the peripartum period. DIC is seen in up to 10% of placental abruptions and it occurs more frequently when there is fetal demise. Patients who also have developed pregnancy-induced hypertension or amniotic fluid embolism are at risk for developing DIC. DIC is also seen in patients with sepsis, severe trauma, solid tumors, and hematologic cancers. Laboratory data can help to guide management and should include prothrombin time/partial thromboplastin time/international normalized ratio (PT/PTT/INR), platelets, fibrin degradation products, and fibrinogen. Differentiation between DIC and dilutional coagulopathy can sometimes be done by observing the fibrinogen levels. Treatment should center on taking care of the underlying disorder and supporting the patient. Low doses of unfractionated heparin at a rate of 300 to 500 units per hour may be helpful in treating DIC. Antifibrinolytic drugs are not recommended for patients in DIC due to the fact that the patients already have inadequate fibrinolysis.

American Society of Anesthesiologists Committee on Transfusion Medicine. *Questions and answers about transfusion practices*. 3rd ed. American Society of Anesthesiologists Committee on Transfusion Medicine, 1998.

Mayer DC, Spielman FJ, Bell EA. Antepartum and postpartum hemorrhage. In: Chestnut DH, ed. *Obstetric anesthesia: principles and practice*, 3rd ed. Mosby, 2004:678–679.

Stoelting RK, Dierdorf SF. *Anesthesia and co-existing disease*, 4th ed. Churchill Livingstone, 2002:496–497.

Wali A, Suresh MS, Gregg AR. Antepartum hemorrhage. In: Datta S, ed. *Anesthetic and obstetric management of high-risk pregnancy*, 3rd ed. New York: Springer, 2004:93–95.

C.3. You suspect disseminated intravascular coagulation (DIC) in this patient. Discuss the use of additional blood products in patients who develop DIC.

The airway should be secured if the patient is not already intubated. During the course of the resuscitation third spacing will occur and airway edema will worsen. Respiratory compromise may develop due to pulmonary edema. Replacement of the factors and platelets needs to be done in order to correct the DIC. Crystalloid and/or colloid should be given to treat the hypotension and hypovolemia until the blood products are available. Owing to ongoing blood loss packed red blood cells (PRBCs) should be given based on the amount of blood loss observed and the hematocrit levels. Fresh frozen plasma (FFP) should be given based on clinical bleeding and prothrombin time/partial thromboplastin time (PT/PTT) levels. FFP should be given when PT/PTT levels are 1.5 times normal or when factor V or VIII levels are low. Platelets should be given as needed secondary to the consumption that occurs in DIC and should be infused based on clinical bleeding and platelet levels. Platelets should be replaced if platelet levels are under 50×10^3 per μL or platelet levels are between 50 and 100×10^3 per μL and clinical bleeding is continuing. Cryoprecipitate, which contains higher levels of fibrinogen, should also be given due to the consumption of fibrinogen. It is important to anticipate the needs of the patient. Blood products should be ordered early, especially FFP and cryoprecipitate which need to thaw.

American Society of Anesthesiologists Committee on Transfusion Medicine. *Questions and Answers About Transfusion Practices*. 3rd ed. American Society of Anesthesiologists Committee on Transfusion Medicine, 1998.

Mayer DC, Spielman FJ, Bell EA. Antepartum and postpartum hemorrhage. In: Chestnut DH, ed. *Obstetric anesthesia: principles and practice*, 3rd ed. Mosby, 2004:678–679.

Stoelting RK, Dierdorf SF. *Anesthesia and co-existing disease*, 4th ed. Churchill Livingstone, 2002:496–497.

Wali A, Suresh MS, Gregg AR. Antepartum hemorrhage. In: Datta S, ed. *Anesthetic and obstetric management of high-risk pregnancy*, 3rd ed. New York: Springer, 2004:93–95.

C.4. After how many units of packed red blood cells (PRBCs) should you give fresh frozen plasma (FFP) and platelets?

The administration of blood products should not be formulaic. Blood products should be given based on the clinical situation and laboratory values. Coagulation factors have to fall below

20% of normal before clinical bleeding is experienced. The likelihood of this occurring increases when more than one blood volume is transfused. If the prothrombin time (PT) and partial thromboplastin time (PTT) are greater then 1.5 times normal than factors may need to be replaced using FFP. Platelets should be replaced if they are less than 50×10^9 per L with microvascular bleeding or under 100×10^9 per L with continued bleeding.

American Society of Anesthesiologists Committee on Transfusion Medicine. *Questions and answers about transfusion practices*, 3rd ed. American Society of Anesthesiologists Committee on Transfusion Medicine, 1998.

C.5. What is the role of emergency release blood and how does this change your future management?

Obstetric patients can deteriorate rapidly in postpartum hemorrhage situations or at times when disseminated intravascular coagulation (DIC) develops. Patients are supported with crystalloid and colloid solutions until blood is typed and crossmatched. Emergency release of O Rh-negative red blood cells (RBCs) should be performed when there is significant hemodynamic deterioration that potentially poses risks to the patient. This is a relatively safe practice due to the low incidence of antibodies in patients that have either been transfused (1%) or not (0.1%). There is some confusion as to when it is safe to switch back to the patient's native blood type. The American Society of Anesthesiologists (ASA) states that after patients have received two units of group O Rh-negative whole blood, which contains antibodies to type A and type B blood, one should not switch back to the patient's specific blood type. Further testing by the blood bank should be performed before switching back to the patients native blood type or one should continue with group O blood. Additive solution RBCs (packed red blood cells [PRBCs]), on the other hand, have very little plasma in each unit and therefore a minimal amount of antibodies. Patients who have received additive solution RBCs can therefore receive many more units without concern for antibody reactions. Individual centers have different approaches as to the maximum number of uncrossmatched units that can be given before switching back to the patient's specific cell type. Most centers do recommend switching to the patient's native blood type as soon as possible in order to conserve the emergency supply of group O Rh-negative RBCs. Recommendations should be received from your local blood bank representative.

American Society of Anesthesiologists Committee on Transfusion Medicine. *Questions and answers about transfusion practices*, 3rd ed. American Society of Anesthesiologists Committee on Transfusion Medicine, 1998.

C.6. What is the role of activated factor VII in obstetric patients?

Recombinant factor VII (rFVIIa) has been used to facilitate control of bleeding in patients with hemophilia, other coagulopathies, and trauma. There are several case reports of rFVIIa being used in obstetric cases after massive hemorrhage with symptoms suggesting disseminated intravascular coagulation (DIC). rFVIIa binds onto tissue factor at the sites of exposed vascular injury. The complex that forms initiates coagulation and allows a fibrin clot to develop. The rFVIIa may be used in situations where bleeding continues even after replacement therapy. Ninety to 100 μg per kg is the dose that has been used with success.

Segal S, Shemesh IY, Blumenthal R, et al Treatment of obstetric hemorrhage with recombinant activated factor VII. *Arch Gynecol Obstet* 2003;268:266–267.

C.7. **You are called to see a 27-year-old woman who just delivered and is continuing to hemorrhage. What is the definition and differential diagnosis of postpartum hemorrhage?**

Postpartum hemorrhage can develop in as many as 5% to 10% of deliveries. It has been classically defined as greater than 500 mL of blood loss in the first 24 hours postdelivery. It is accepted that accurate measurement of blood loss is difficult and may be misleading. The American College of Obstetrics and Gynecology has defined postpartum hemorrhage as greater than a 10% decrease in the hematocrit level or the need for a blood transfusion in the postpartum period. Patients with unexplained hypotension, tachycardia, or low urine output should be suspected as having a postpartum hemorrhage and resuscitation should commence.

The most common cause of postpartum hemorrhage is uterine atony, which accounts for up to 80% of the cases. Other uterine causes include retained products of conception, placental accreta, uterine inversion, and uterine rupture. Nonuterine causes include genital tract lesions, genital tract hematomas, intraabdominal lacerations, pelvic lacerations, and coagulopathies.

Mayer DC, Spielman FJ, Bell EA. Antepartum and postpartum hemorrhage. In: Chestnut DH, ed. *Obstetric anesthesia: principles and practice*, 3rd ed. Mosby, 2004:668–671.

Sarna MC, Hess P, Takoudes TC, et al. Postpartum hemorrhage. In: Datta S, ed. *Anesthetic and obstetric management of high-risk pregnancy*, 3rd ed. New York: Springer, 2004: 112–114.

C.8. **What are the anesthetic considerations of postpartum hemorrhage?**

Specific anesthetic considerations will vary depending on the source of the postpartum hemorrhage. A team approach should be instituted with early recognition and treatment. In the report out of Great Britain titled "Why Mothers Die," poor communication between specialties was believed to have mostly contributed to maternal death. In addition, there were several cases related to hemorrhage in which delays in obtaining blood from the blood bank and therefore a delay in treatment could be partially responsible for an increase in maternal mortality. If postpartum hemorrhage is occurring, then the patient should be moved to either an intensive care unit (ICU) or operating room (OR) setting. This will allow the anesthesiologist to appropriately monitor the patient, have the resources to place additional lines, and be able to provide a general anesthetic in a safe environment. The obstetric team will also have the resources to manage the postpartum hemorrhage.

The patient should have large-bore intravenous access. An arterial line should be placed to allow continuous hemodynamic monitoring and a central access should be considered to facilitate the resuscitation. Fluid warmers should be used when large amounts of fluids or blood products are anticipated. Hypothermia can also be avoided by maintaining an appropriate room temperature and utilizing a warming blanket. If there is ongoing blood loss crystalloids or colloids should be used to replace blood loss until blood becomes available. It is important that blood and blood products be ordered early and direct discussions should be had with the blood bank concerning the urgency of the situation. If massive hemorrhage continues or the patient is unable to protect her airway, she should have a general anesthetic.

Massive transfusion is the replacement of greater than one blood volume within several hours. In the setting of massive transfusion, the patient should be left intubated and transferred to the ICU for continued monitoring once the postoperative hemorrhage is treated and the patient is stabilized.

Lewis G, Drife J. *Why mother die 1997–1999–The fifth report of the confidential enquires into maternal deaths in the United Kingdom*. London: RCOG Press, 2001:134–150.

Sarna MC, Hess P, Takoudes TC, et al. Postpartum hemorrhage. In: Datta S, ed. *Anesthetic and obstetric management of high-risk pregnancy*, 3rd ed. New York: Springer, 2004: 123–126.

C.9. What laboratory tests should be ordered during the resuscitation of this patient?

Baseline labs should be sent as soon as possible and should include a hematocrit level, platelet count, coagulation status (partial thromboplastin time [PTT], prothrombin time [PT], international normalized ratio [INR], and fibrinogen levels), and an arterial blood gas. During resuscitation, the above labs should be sent periodically to help guide treatment including blood component therapy. If massive transfusion has occurred, then electrolytes will also need to be followed, including a potassium and calcium level. Patients can develop hyperkalemia due to the elevated potassium levels in transfused blood and are also at risk of hyperkalemia due to the cellular shifts caused by acidosis. Patients can develop hypocalcemia from citrate toxicity. Citrate is the anticoagulant found in transfused blood. Arterial blood gases should also be frequently monitored to evaluate the acidosis that may have developed due to poor tissue perfusion. Depending on the shelf-life of the stored blood (>14 days), preexisting acidosis can be exacerbated by multiple transfusions of "old" blood.

American Society of Anesthesiologists Committee on Transfusion Medicine. *Questions and answers about transfusion practices*, 3rd ed. American Society of Anesthesiologists Committee on Transfusion Medicine, 1998.

C.10. What are the treatment options for uterine atony?

Initially, physical compression of the uterus by bimanual compression or uterine massage should be initiated for atony. During this time, oxytocin is started as an intravenous infusion. Synthetic oxytocin (Pitocin, Syntocinon) is the drug of choice that is given once the fetus is born and the placenta is delivered. The uterus increases the number of oxytocin receptors throughout pregnancy, peaking at near term. Oxytocin differs from antidiuretic hormone (ADH) by only two amino acids and is produced in the posterior pituitary. It may exhibit a small antidiuretic effect but clinically this does not seem to be concerning unless very large doses are given. In this situation, systemic and/or pulmonary hypertension, and water intoxication can occur. If a bolus of oxytocin is given, then hypotension can follow and should be treated with appropriate vasopressors (ephedrine or phenylephrine). The hypotension is caused by a decrease in peripheral vascular resistance. Patients may also exhibit tachycardia and arrhythmias. Once the oxytocin binds onto the receptors, the frequency and duration of the uterine contractions increase. The contractions are most likely mediated through an increase in intracellular calcium levels.

Ergot alkaloids (ergonovine and methylergonovine) can be used to treat uterine atony. The agent is usually given intramuscularly and has an effect in 2 to 5 minutes. The ergot alkaloids produce tetanic contractions of the uterus, which is probably mediated through α-adrenergic receptors. The agents have many potential side effects. Hypertension can be prominent due to vasoconstriction such that these agents should be avoided in chronic hypertensive patients or in patients with pregnancy-induced hypertension. The ergot alkaloids may have other cardiovascular affects including coronary artery spasm leading to myocardial infarction, arrhythmias, or cerebrovascular accidents. Pulmonary complications have been reported with the ergot alkaloids including pulmonary artery vasoconstriction and pulmonary hypertension. The ergot alkaloids are also associated with side effects such as headache, dizziness, and nausea and vomiting.

Prostaglandins increase through labor reaching a peak level after the placenta is delivered. The prostaglandins cause the intracellular levels of calcium to increase, leading to an increase in myosin light-chain kinase activity and then uterine contraction. Side effects with the prostaglandins include nausea and vomiting, fever, and diarrhea. 15-Methyl prostaglandin F2-α (carboprost, Hemabate) can be given either intramuscularly or intramyometrially. The prostaglandins should be avoided in patients with reactive airway disease due to the bronchospasm that can develop. Prostaglandin E_1 (Misoprostol) can be given rectally to help when uterine atony is persistent. A review of randomized controlled trials comparing misoprostol (PO/rectal) verses injectable (IV/IM) uterotonics (oxytocin/ergotamine/combination) found that misoprostol was less effective than injectable uterotonics.

Mayer DC, Spielman FJ, Bell EA. Antepartum and postpartum hemorrhage. In: Chestnut DH, ed. *Obstetric anesthesia: principles and practice*, 3rd ed. Elsevier Mosby, 2004:670–671.

Sarna MC, Hess P, Takoudes TC, et al. Postpartum hemorrhage. In: Datta S, ed. *Anesthetic and obstetric management of high-risk pregnancy*, 3rd ed. New York: Springer, 2004: 114–116.

Villar J, Gulmezoglu AM, Hofmeyr GJ, et al. Systemic review of randomized controlled trials of misoprostol to prevent postpartum hemorrhage. *Am Coll Obstet Gynecol* 2002;100(6):1301–1312.

C.11. The patient is hemorrhaging after removal of her placenta using excessive traction. How is uterine inversion treated?

Uterine inversion is a complication that is associated with postpartum hemorrhage. The incidence of uterine inversion is between 1 in 2,000 to 1 in 10,000 pregnancies. The risk factors include uterine atony, uterine anomalies, inappropriate fundal pressure, and umbilical cord traction. Diagnosis is made when the patient develops acute hemorrhage and pain. Uterine inversion is confirmed by loss of fundal height and a mass in the vagina. Frequently, the uterus can be replaced with manual pressure before the cervical ring contracts down.

Occasionally relaxation of the cervix and uterus will need to be performed in order to replace the uterus. Agents such as nitroglycerin or terbutaline can be used to provide the appropriate relaxation. Nitroglycerin in 50 μg boluses up to 200 μg may be helpful in this situation. The patient's vital signs should be monitored during administration of these agents due to the hypotension and tachycardia that can develop in an already compromised patient.

Pain relief should also be offered either in the form of regional anesthesia or intravenous analgesia. If the uterus remains inverted, then a general anesthetic may provide the relaxation needed to reposition the uterus. Once the uterus is repositioned and the placenta is removed, uterotonics will be given in order to stop the hemorrhage and keep the uterus in position. Prostaglandins and oxytocin in addition to bimanual compression of the uterus should be used to help the uterus contract. Patients who are undergoing a general anesthetic should have the halogenated agent turned down at this point to allow the uterus to become firm. The patient can be placed on 70% nitrous oxide while maintaining a low level of halogenated agent and resuscitation should be continued. The addition of an amnestic such as midazolam can be given to prevent awareness. Occasionally, the inversion will need to be corrected surgically by performing a hysterectomy in cases of protracted hemorrhage.

Mayer DC, Spielman FJ, Bell EA. Antepartum and postpartum hemorrhage. In: Chestnut DH, ed. *Obstetric anesthesia: principles and practice*, 3rd ed. Mosby, 2004:674–675.

Sarna MC, Hess P, Takoudes TC, et al. Postpartum hemorrhage. In: Datta S, ed. *Anesthetic and obstetric management of high-risk pregnancy*, 3rd ed. New York: Springer, 2004: 123–124.

C.12. Discuss retained placenta and treatment options.

Retained placenta occurs when there is abnormal separation of the placenta from the uterus. If there is partial separation of the placenta, the uterine arterioles may become exposed and hemorrhage may ensue. Manual extraction may need to be performed in order to properly remove the placenta. If the patient already has an epidural in place, she may require a bolus of local anesthetic for pain relief during the extraction. If no epidural is in place and the patient is stable, a spinal could be performed. Another option is to provide intravenous analgesia with midazolam (1 to 2 mg), ketamine (10 mg bolus up to 0.5 mg/kg), or fentanyl (50 to 100 μg). The patient's vital signs should be monitored throughout the removal of the placenta. The patient should also be given a nonparticulate antacid before any analgesic. If the uterus has started to contract and the placenta is unable to be removed, uterine relaxation needs to be performed. The uterus can be relaxed with the use of intravenous nitroglycerin in 50 μg increments. Another option is to perform a general anesthetic and use a high dose of volatile anesthetic.

Mayer DC, Spielman FJ, Bell EA. Antepartum and postpartum hemorrhage. In: Chestnut DH, ed. *Obstetric anesthesia: principles and practice*, 3rd ed. Mosby, 2004:672–673.

Sarna MC, Hess P, Takoudes TC, et al. Postpartum hemorrhage. In: Datta S, ed. *Anesthetic and obstetric management of high-risk pregnancy*, 3rd ed. New York: Springer, 2004: 121–122.

C.13. Define amniotic fluid embolism and discuss treatment.

Amniotic fluid embolism can occur when there is direct communication between the amniotic fluid and the maternal circulation. This most likely occurs in multiparous patients who are experiencing a complicated labor. The communication can occur at the level of the endocervical vessels, at the level of the placenta, or at a uterine trauma site. The patients may experience sudden onset of hypotension, dyspnea, hypoxemia, cyanosis, loss of consciousness, and possible seizures. The symptoms are due in part to mechanical blockage of the pulmonary vasculature and then subsequent pulmonary vasoconstriction, which may be mediated through the release of substances such as prostaglandins, histamine, serotonin, or leukotrienes. The patients may develop acute cor pulmonale and right heart failure. More than 80% of these patients experience cardiopulmonary arrest. The patients are at a high risk for developing disseminated intravascular coagulation (DIC). The patients need to have their airway secured and their ventilation supported. Application of positive end-expiratory pressure may help to oxygenate the patients. An arterial line should be placed to monitor hemodynamics. Central monitoring may help to evaluate fluid requirements. The blood pressure should be supported with vasopressors and DIC should be treated as discussed previously. The mortality of patients who develop an amniotic fluid embolism is higher than 80%. Amniotic fluid embolism is often a diagnosis of exclusion. Diagnosis is usually based on clinical signs and symptoms. Blood aspirated from pulmonary artery catheters would often show squamous cells, fat, and mucin.

Stoelting RK, Dierdorf SF. *Anesthesia and co-existing disease*, 4th ed. Churchill Livingstone, 2002:678–680.

C.14. What is the role of cell salvage in obstetric patients?

The safety of cell salvage used during cesarean section has been questioned due to the theoretic risk of developing an amniotic fluid embolism. The fear is that amniotic fluid components will be administered to the patient and cause an amniotic fluid embolism. Cell salvage could be very helpful in some obstetric situations such as postpartum hemorrhage or in Jehovah's Witnesses. Cell saver may decrease the risk of blood born infections associated with transfusion of banked red blood cells (RBCs) and may also decrease the risk of alloimmunization. The risks of transfusion reactions and transfusion-related acute lung injury would also be reduced if autologous blood was used instead of banked blood. Unfortunately the pathophysiology of amniotic fluid embolism has been unidentified and therefore knowing what to remove from salvaged blood is also unknown. Also, the incidence of amniotic fluid embolism is between 1 in 8,000 to 1 in 80,000 cases. Although several studies have not shown an increased risk of amniotic fluid embolism during cell salvage, most are statistically underpowered assess such risk. In one historic cohort study by Rebarber et al., 139 patients were identified who had autologous blood collection and autotransfusion during cesarean section. They found no increased risk of complications in the patients who received cell salvaged blood transfusions during cesarean sections. Several studies have looked at the processing of blood collected during cesarean sections. One of the concerns is the reinfusion of particulate decontaminants that may be involved in the development of amniotic fluid embolism. Waters et al. showed that by washing the blood and then filtering it using a leukocyte reduction filter, contaminants are reduced to a level comparable to maternal venous blood. Also, it has been shown that debris may be decreased by using a separate suction for aspiration of amniotic fluid.

Camann W. Cell salvage during cesarean delivery: is it safe and valuable? Maybe, maybe not!. *Int J Obstet Anesth* 1999;8:75–76.

Catling SJ, Williams S, Fielding AM. Cell salvage in obstetrics: an evaluation of the ability of cell salvage combined with leukocyte depletion filtration to remove amniotic fluid from operative blood loss at caesarean section. *Int J Obstet Anesth* 1999;8:79–81.

Rainaldi MP, Tazzari PL, Scagliarini G, et al. Blood salvage during Caesarean section. *Br J Anaesth* 1998;80:195–198.

Waters JH, Biscotti C, Potter PS. Amniotic fluid removal during cell salvage in the Cesarean section patient. *Anesthesiology* 2000;92:1531–1536.

C.15. How do you treat the Jehovah's Witness with postpartum hemorrhage or a known placenta accreta?

In a study done by Singla et al., Jehovah's Witnesses were shown to be at a 44-fold increased risk for maternal death secondary to hemorrhage. Jehovah's Witnesses have religious beliefs that restrict them from receiving blood transfusions. The beliefs are based on several passages from the Bible as follows: "Everything that lives and moves will be food for you .... But you must not eat meat that has its lifeblood still in it" (Genesis 9:3-6) and "If anyone ... partakes of any blood, I will set My face against the person who partakes of the blood" (Leviticus 17:10, 11). Jehovah's Witnesses avoid the transfusion of whole blood, packed red blood cells (PRBCs), plasma, and platelet administration based on these passages. Their religious interpretation does not "absolutely prohibit" albumin, immune globulins, and hemophiliac preparations. The Jehovah's Witness website states that each Witness needs to decide individually if they can accept these products. They believe that blood that has left the body should be disposed of and therefore will not allow autologous transfusions. If the blood is kept in line, then most Jehovah's Witnesses will agree to this type of treatment, which may include cardiopulmonary bypass, dialysis, intraoperative salvage (where the circulation is uninterrupted), and possibly normovolemic hemodilution. Jehovah's Witnesses will allow certain medical treatments that may help to prevent blood transfusion. The Jehovah's Witness website (www.watchtower.org) discusses the acceptable use of hypotensive anesthesia, erythropoietin, dextran, and hetastarch. The anesthesiologist needs to have a discussion with the patient concerning their individual beliefs and their treatment options. Appropriate consents will also need to be discussed and signed before anesthetic intervention.

Singla AK, Lapinski RH, Berkowitz RL, Are women who are Jehovah's witnesses at risk of maternal death? *Am J Obstet Gynecol* 2001;185(4):893–895.

C.16. What is the role for uterine artery balloon placement and uterine artery embolization?

Uterine artery balloon placement and uterine artery embolization have both been used in the peripartum setting due to either anticipated or ongoing obstetric hemorrhage. Owing to the improved imaging modalities and known associations with abnormal placentation, prophylactic internal iliac artery occlusion balloon catheters or embolization catheters can be placed preoperatively. The balloon catheters may help reduce the bleeding associated with abnormal placentation or uterine anomalies (e.g., arteriovenous malformation, atony). Abnormal placentation is often associated with collateral circulation and balloon dilation may not completely stop bleeding. It has been suggested that the use of balloon dilation may reduce the overall blood loss in these cases and may provide a more stable surgical situation. Although balloon placement with or without embolization may help to control bleeding, a hysterectomy may still have to be performed for definitive control of blood loss. Prophylactic catheterization may allow the patient to avoid a general anesthetic and all the complications associated with general anesthesia. It must be understood that conversion to a general anesthetic may need to be performed during the case, if continuing resuscitation is needed and airway control is required.

In an emergent situation, arterial embolization may help control hemorrhage. Some patients may experience complications due to emergent embolization including thrombosis of the left popliteal artery, vaginal necrosis, and paresthesia of the right leg.

Fuller AJ, Carvalho B, Brummel C. Epidural anesthesia for elective Cesarean delivery with intraoperative arterial occlusion balloon catheter placement. *Anesth Analg* 2006;102: 585–587.

Ojala K, Perala J, Kariniemi J, et al. Arterial embolization and prophylactic catheterization for the treatment for severe obstetric hemorrhage. *Acta Obstet Gynecol Scand* 2005; 84:1075–1080.

Uterine Artery Embolization. ACOG committee opinion number 293. American college of obstetricians and gynecologists. *Obstet Gynecol* 2004;103:403–404.

D. Postoperative Management

D.1. When do you remove an epidural in patients who have just been treated for disseminated intravascular coagulation (DIC)?

Sprung et al. made recommendations about the removal of epidural catheters after DIC. First, they recommended frequent evaluation of the neurologic status and treatment of the coagulopathy. Removal of the catheter should occur if there is no indication of intraspinal bleeding due to the risk of catheter migration into a vessel. They also state that the catheter should be left in place if bleeding is occurring around the catheter insertion site with the possibility of epidural or subarachnoid bleeding due to a tamponade effect that may be caused by the catheter. Also, any neurologic deficits should be immediately evaluated for the possibility of surgical decompression.

Often, it is difficult to evaluate the patient's neurologic status due to postoperative intubation and sedation. The catheter should be left in place until neurologic assessment can be established. The coagulation status of the patient will also guide the removal of the catheter. Remember that an epidural hematoma can develop at the time of insertion as well as during removal of the catheter; therefore, coagulation needs to be optimized before removal.

ASRA consensus conference Second Consensus Conference on Neuraxial Anesthesia and Anticoagulation, April 25–28, 2002.

Sprung J, Cheng EY, Patel S. When to remove an epidural catheter in a parturient with disseminated intravascular coagulation? *Reg Anesth* 1992;17(6):351–354.

Vandermeulen EP, Van Aken H, Vermylen J. Anticoagulants and spinal-epidural anesthesia. *Anesth Analg* 1994;79:1165–1177.

D.2.   **You have successfully treated the patient with disseminated intravascular coagulation (DIC) and her laboratory values have returned to normal. Her central venous pressure (CVP) is within normal limits and urine output is appropriate. The patient is still hypotensive despite her intravascular volume replacement and support with vasopressors. What is your concern in this case?**

The patient has just been resuscitated due to massive hemorrhage. She may have developed Sheehan's syndrome, which is pituitary infarction. The infarction is usually associated with hypotension or hemorrhage. The conditions that are linked with Sheehan's syndrome consist of hypotension that is unrelieved by fluid resuscitation or vasopressors. Patients may also present with failure to lactate, fatigue, or cold intolerance. Patients with any of the above conditions and a history of hemorrhage or hypotension in the peripartum period should be suspected of having Sheehan's syndrome.

Roizen RF, Fleisher LA. Anesthetic implications of concurrent diseases. In: Miller RH, ed. *Miller's anesthesia*, 6th ed. Churchill Livingstone, 2005:1052.

CHAPTER 41

Hypertensive Disorders of Pregnancy

SHARON ABRAMOVITZ • BARBARA LEIGHTON

A 39-YEAR-OLD FEMALE

gravida 1 para 0000 at 29 weeks' gestation was admitted to the hospital because of an elevated blood pressure (182/111 mm Hg), headache, and proteinuria (6 g over a 24-hour period).

A. Medical Disease and Differential Diagnosis

1. What is the classification of hypertension disorders in pregnancy as defined by the American College of Obstetricians and Gynecologists?
2. What is preeclampsia?
3. What is severe preeclampsia?
4. What is eclampsia?
5. What are the risk factors for developing preeclampsia?
6. What is the mortality associated with preeclampsia?
7. Discuss the pathogenesis of preeclampsia.
8. Discuss the pathologic alterations of preeclampsia.
9. Which component of blood pressure best predicts the occurrence of preeclampsia?
10. What is the significance of increased pulse wave velocity during pregnancy? How does this relate to birthweight?
11. What are some of the complications associated with preeclampsia?

B. Preoperative Evaluation and Preparation

1. What initial laboratory studies are recommended for patients with preeclampsia?
2. What are the important routine monitors for patients with preeclampsia? When is a central venous pressure monitor indicated?
3. What conditions mandate immediate delivery, regardless of the gestational age?
4. Discuss the obstetric management of preeclampsia.
5. In the United States, what drug therapy is the treatment of choice for seizure prophylaxis?
6. Discuss the treatment of magnesium sulfate toxicity.
7. Discuss the mechanism of action of magnesium sulfate.
8. What are the fetal effects of magnesium sulfate therapy?
9. Discuss the treatment of eclampsia.

C. Intraoperative Management

1. What is your choice of analgesia/anesthesia for patients with preeclampsia?
2. What is the advantage of prehydration?
3. How should patients be hydrated before epidural analgesia/anesthesia for labor and delivery?
4. Discuss bleeding time and platelet count evaluation during preoperative assessment of a patient with preeclampsia requesting epidural analgesia/anesthesia for labor and delivery.
5. What level of analgesia/anesthesia is required for labor and delivery?
6. Discuss the commonly used local anesthetics for labor analgesia.
7. Is the addition of epinephrine to local anesthetics advisable in preeclamptic patients?
8. What is the treatment for the abnormal fetal heart rate pattern seen with maternal hypotension after epidural analgesia/anesthesia is instituted?
9. What would you do after an accidental spinal tap? How do you treat postdural puncture headache?
10. How would you manage total spinal anesthesia?
11. Should ergonovine be given to preeclamptic patients?
12. When and how would you give spinal anesthesia?
13. Discuss a general anesthesia technique for the patient with preeclampsia presenting for cesarean delivery.
14. What agents can be used to prevent hypertension during the induction of general anesthesia for cesarean delivery?
15. What is HELLP syndrome?

D. Postoperative Management

1. Discuss the postpartum management of preeclamptic patients.

A. Medical Disease and Differential Diagnosis

A.1. What is the classification of hypertension disorders in pregnancy as defined by the American College of Obstetricians and Gynecologists?

Hypertensive disorders of pregnancy are classified as follows:
Gestational hypertension
Preeclampsia
- Mild
- Severe

HELLP (hemolysis, elevated liver enzymes, low platelets) syndrome
Chronic hypertension preceding pregnancy
Chronic hypertension with superimposed preeclampsia

American College of Obstetricians and Gynecologists. *Hypertension in pregnancy, ACOG practice bulletin*, No. 33. Washington, DC: American College of Obstetricians and Gynecologists, January 2002.

A.2. What is preeclampsia?

Preeclampsia is a multiorgan disease characterized by the development of hypertension with proteinuria after the 20th week of gestation. It is a disorder of unknown etiology affecting approximately 8% of all pregnancies, with most cases occurring in the first pregnancy. Hypertension is defined as a sustained systolic blood pressure of at least 140 mm Hg or a diastolic blood pressure of at least 90 mm Hg. Proteinuria is defined as 300 mg or more of protein in a 24-hour urine collection. Edema may manifest as a recent, rapid weight gain.

American College of Obstetricians and Gynecologists. *Hypertension in pregnancy, ACOG practice bulletin*, No. 33.Washington, DC: American College of Obstetricians and Gynecologists, January 2002.

Cunningham FG, MacDonald PC, Grant NF, et al. eds. *Williams obstetrics*, 20th ed. Stamford: Appleton & Lange, 1997:693–744.

Sibai BM, Gordon T, Thom E, et al. Risk factors for preeclampsia in healthy nulliparous women: a prospective multicenter study. *Am J Obstet Gynecol* 1995;172:642–648.

A.3. What is severe preeclampsia?

Severe preeclampsia includes at least one of the following features:

- Blood pressure: systolic BP 160 mm Hg or higher or diastolic BP 110 mm Hg or higher on two occasions at least 6 hours apart; diagnosis not delayed if the diastolic blood pressure exceeds 110 mm Hg
- Proteinuria: 5 g of protein or more in a 24-hour urine specimen (or 3+ to 4+ on semiquantitative urinalysis)
- Oliguria: urine output less than 500 mL in 24 hours
- Cerebral or visual disturbances: headache, blurred vision, or altered consciousness
- Pulmonary edema or cyanosis
- Epigastric or right upper quadrant pain, which may be caused by stretching of Glisson's capsule by hepatic edema
- Hepatic rupture: rare complication
- Impaired liver function
- Thrombocytopenia: resulting from platelet adhesion to exposed collagen at sites of endothelial damage
- HELLP syndrome: hemolysis, elevated liver enzymes, low platelets
- Evidence of fetal compromise (e.g., intrauterine growth retardation, oligohydramnios) or placental abruption

Chestnut DH, ed. *Obstetric anesthesia: principles and practice*, 3rd ed. Philadelphia: Mosby, 2004:794–835.

Stoelting RK, Dierdorf SF. *Anesthesia and co-existing disease*, 4th ed. New York: Churchill Livingstone, 2002:658.

A.4. What is eclampsia?

Eclampsia is defined as convulsions and/or coma not caused by coincidental neurologic disease (e.g., epilepsy), which occurs during pregnancy or the puerperium in a woman whose condition also meets the criteria for preeclampsia.

Broughton-Pipkin F. The hypertensive disorders of pregnancy. *Br Med J* 1995;311:609–613.

Chestnut DH, ed. *Obstetric anesthesia: principles and practice*, 3rd ed. Philadelphia: Mosby, 2004:794–835.

Stoelting RK, Dierdorf SF. *Anesthesia and co-existing disease*, 4th ed. New York: Churchill Livingstone, 2002:658.

A.5. What are the risk factors for developing preeclampsia?

The risk factors for developing preeclampsia are as follows:

Hypertensive disease

- Previous preeclampsia
- Systolic hypertension during early pregnancy
- History of chronic hypertension
- Family history of hypertension during pregnancy
- Increase in pulse pressure during the first trimester

Coexisting vascular and endothelial disease

- Chronic renal disease
- Lupus erythematosus
- Protein S deficiency
- Activated protein C resistance
- Circulating anticardiolipin antibodies

Obstetric factors

- African-American race
- Angiotensinogen gene *T*235
- Nulliparity
- Age older than 40 years
- History of smoking
- Obesity
- Increased trophoblastic mass (e.g., multiple gestation, molar pregnancy)
- Large for gestational age fetus
- Diabetes
- Erythroblastosis fetalis
- Polyhydramnios, particularly in young primigravidas

Boxer LM, Malinow AM. Preeclampsia and eclampsia. *Curr Opin Anesth* 1997;10:188–198.

Chestnut DH, ed. *Obstetric anesthesia: principles and practice*, 3rd ed. Philadelphia: Mosby, 2004:794–835.

A.6. What is the mortality associated with preeclampsia?

Hypertensive disorders of pregnancy account for 15% to 19% of maternal deaths in the United States and the United Kingdom.

American College of Obstetricians and Gynecologists. *Hypertension in pregnancy, ACOG Practice Bulletin*, No. 33. Washington, DC: American College of Obstetricians and Gynecologists, January 2002.

Berg CJ, Atrash HK, Koonin LM, et al. Pregnancy-related mortality in the United States, 1987–1990. *Obstet Gynecol* 1996;88:161–167.

Hibbard BM, Anderson MM, O'Driffe JO, et al. *Report on confidential enquiries into maternal deaths in the United Kingdom, 1991–1993*. London: HMSO, 1996:1–31.

A.7. Discuss the pathogenesis of preeclampsia.

Preeclampsia is most likely a disease of heterogeneous causes of both maternal and placental origin.

Immunologic factors

Immunologic disorders may arise from an abnormal maternal–fetal antigen–antibody response or from the contents of seminal fluids; spermatozoa may cause antibody formation or prostaglandins may initiate uterine vasoconstriction. The fetus acquires 50% of its genes from the father, which represents in part a paternal allograft that interacts with maternal tissue as fetal trophoblast migrates into the maternal decidua after implantation. Migration normally occurs in two phases. Trophoblasts displace the muscular structure of the maternal spiral arteries before 20 weeks of gestation, causing their adrenergic denervation and converting them from high-resistance to low-resistance vessels. At the same time, biochemical adaptations occur in the maternal vasculature, with an increased dominance of endothelium-dependent vasodilators, prostacyclin (prostaglandin I [PGI]), and nitric oxide (NO). In preeclampsia, the second wave of trophoblastic migration fails. This failure can result in a high-resistance, low-flow uteroplacental circulation and consequent placental ischemia and hypoxia. These changes may represent an aberrant immunologic mechanism.

Genetic factors

A familial tendency toward preeclampsia exists in some populations, and it may result from a recessive genetic inheritance.

Endothelial factors

Vascular endothelial damage or dysfunction is the common pathologic feature of preeclampsia and occurs in the placental decidual vessels and renal microvasculature. Endothelial cell dysfunction in response to unknown factors may cause a hormonal imbalance in women with preeclampsia (Fig. 41.1).

The metabolic end products of normal vascular endothelium include PGI_2 and endothelium-derived relaxing factor (EDRF), which is either NO or a related nitrosyl substance. Both PGI_2 and EDRF are potent vasodilators. In patients with preeclampsia, the failure of trophoblast to invade the uteroplacental vascular bed may encourage an increased production of free radicals and lipid peroxides by the decidual lymphoid tissue. As a result, an imbalance occurs between the production of the vasoconstrictor thromboxane A_2 (TXA_2), which is derived from platelets, and the production of endothelium-derived PGI_2. This imbalance results in a reduced perfusion of the intervillous space. Some investigators have concluded that hypoxia-induced impairment of NO production by the syncytiotrophoblast results in uteroplacental insufficiency and production of a toxin responsible for the clinical manifestations of preeclampsia.

It has been shown that production of endothelin 1(ET-1), which is the most potent endogenous vasoconstrictor and produced mainly by vascular smooth muscle cells as well as by the vascular endothelium, is markedly increased in preeclampsia and correlates inversely with NO production. Therefore, the imbalance between NO and ET-1 may play a significant role in the pathophysiology of preeclampsia,

Fetoplacental blood vessels, namely, the human placental chorionic plate arteries, constrict in response to ET-1. Moreover, there is now some evidence that amniotic concentrations of ET-1 is elevated in pregnancies associated with preeclampsia. Margarit et al. found a statistically significant increase in ET-1 concentration in the aminionic fluid of women at 17 weeks' gestation who developed preeclampsia as compared to those who did not develop preeclampsia. By the second trimester, higher levels of ET-1 have also been shown in the amniotic fluid of women with preterm premature rupture of the membranes.

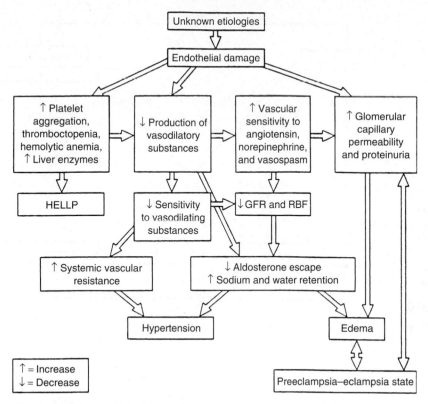

Figure 41.1 Endothelial cell dysfunction in response to unknown factors may cause a hormonal imbalance in women with pregnancy-induced hypertension. GFR, glomerular filtration rate; HELLP, hemolysis, elevated liver enzymes, low platelets; RBF, renal blood flow (From Chestnut DH, ed. *Obstetric anesthesia: principles and practice,* 3rd ed. Philadelphia: Mosby, 2004:798, with permission.)

Platelet factors

In mild preeclampsia, serotonin (5-HT) released from aggregating platelets interacts with endothelial 5-HT_1 receptors, resulting in the release of prostacyclin and NO (EDRF). The released prostacyclin induces angiotensin II release, improving uteroplacental perfusion. In early-onset severe preeclampsia, damaged uteroplacental vessels cannot respond to 5-HT_1 effects. Instead, serotonin interacts with 5-HT_2 receptors on vascular smooth muscle cells, inducing vasoconstriction. Platelet-derived serotonin also activates 5-HT_2 platelet receptors, establishing a positive feedback loop and intensifying platelet aggregation. The loss of 5-HT_1 receptors prevents stimulation of angiotensin II release (Fig. 41.2).

Calcium

In normal pregnancy, the intracellular free calcium concentration increases slowly, but this increase is significantly greater in the third trimester in women with preeclampsia. The increase in cytoplasmic calcium levels is enhanced by angiotensin II, and the enhancement is greater in women with preeclampsia compared with normotensive women. This response to angiotensin II occurs long before signs of preeclampsia become evident and is a sensitive indicator of its subsequent development.

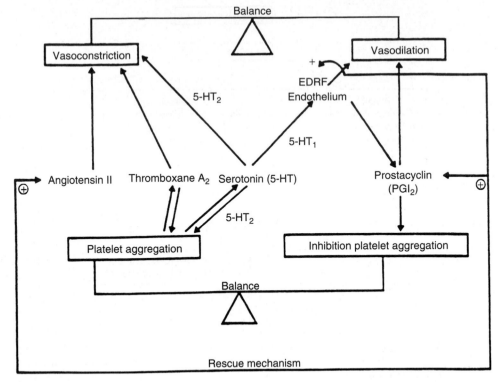

Figure 41.2 The loss of 5-HT$_1$ receptors prevents stimulation of angiotensin II release. EDRF, endothelium-derived relaxing factor. (From Chestnut DH, ed. *Obstetric anesthesia: principles and practice,* 3rd ed. Philadelphia: Mosby, 2004:797, with permission.)

Coagulation factors

Platelet activation in preeclampsia is surface mediated. Women with preeclampsia have an increased tendency toward thromboembolism, which may result in part from an alteration in the plasma ratio between von Willebrand factor and factor VIII coagulant activity.

Fatty acid metabolism

Altered handling of fatty acids by the liver is a key factor in the pathogenesis of preeclampsia. Both increased hepatic uptake of free fatty acids and hypertriglyceridemia are seen more frequently in women who develop preeclampsia.

Markers of angiogenesis

Preeclamptic patients have elevated plasma levels of endoglin and soluble FLT-1, the receptor for vascular endothelial growth factor (VEGF), throughout gestation. Recent research suggests that these molecules are not just disease markers but are involved in the pathogenesis of preeclampsia.

Baksu B, Davas I, Baksu A, et al. Plasma nitric oxide, endothelin -1 and urinary nitric oxide and cyclic guanosine monophosphate levels in hypertensive pregnant women. *Int J Gynaecol Obstet* 2005;90(2):112–117.

Broughton-Pipkin F, Rubin PC. Preeclampsia: the "disease of theories." *Br Med Bull* 1994;50:381–396.

Chestnut DH, ed. *Obstetric anesthesia: principles and practice*, 3rd ed. Philadelphia: Mosby, 2004:794–835.

DeJong CL, Dekker GA, Sibai BM. The renin-angiotensin-aldosterone system in preeclampsia: a review. *Clin Perinatol* 1991;18:683–711.

Dekker GA, Sibai BM. Etiology and pathogenesis of preeclampsia: current concepts. *Am J Obstet Gynecol* 1998;179:1359–1375.

Lindoff C, Ingemarsson I, Martinsson G, et al. Preeclampsia is associated with a reduced response to activated protein C. *Am J Obstet Gynecol* 1997;176:457–460.

Margarit L, Griffiths A, Tsapanos V, et al. Second trimester amniotic fluid endothelin concentration. A possible predictor for pre-eclampsia. *J Obstet Gynaecol* 2005;25(1): 18–20.

Venkatesha S, Toporsian M, Lam C, et al. Soluble endoglin contributes to the pathogenesis of preeclampsia. *Nat Med* 2006;12:642–649.

Zeeman GG, Dekker GA. Pathogenesis of preeclampsia: a hypothesis. *Clin Obstet Gynecol* 1992;35:317–337.

Zuspan FP. New concepts in the understanding of hypertensive diseases during pregnancy: an overview. *Clin Perinatol* 1991;18:653–659.

A.8. Discuss the pathologic alterations of preeclampsia.

Cardiovascular changes

- *Blood pressure.* Increase in blood pressure results from an increase in peripheral vascular resistance secondary to a state of sympathetic overactivity. Alternatively, systolic blood pressure increases as a result of increased cardiac output (increased plasma volume—typical of pregnancy) and a noncompliant aorta. In such case, the systemic vascular resistance(SVR), which is predominantly determined by the smaller arterioles, is not increased but due to aortic stiffness, the ejected stroke volume causes the systolic component to rise significantly.
- *Blood volume.* Reduction in blood volume causes a greater degree of hemoconcentration.

Hemodynamic changes

- Three hemodynamic subsets exist:
- *Hyperdynamic* with increased cardiac output, normal, or slightly increased SVR, and normal or slightly decreased blood volume and filling pressures
- *High SVR* with normal cardiac output and lower filling pressures
- *Markedly increased SVR* with decreased blood volume and depressed left ventricular function
- Poor correlation between central venous pressure (CVP) and pulmonary artery (PA) occlusion pressure
- Decreased colloid oncotic pressure (COP) in pregnancy with further reduction in preeclampsia. The low COP, coupled with increased vascular permeability and the loss of intravascular fluid and protein into interstitial tissues, increases the risk of pulmonary edema.

Hematologic changes

- Hypercoagulable state (Table 41.1)
- Platelet activation: Thrombocytopenia occurs in 15% to 30% of women with preeclampsia or eclampsia. Preeclampsia may be associated with a significant defect in *both* platelet function and platelet number. Thrombocytopenia without other coagulation abnormalities but with

---

Table 41.1   Changes that Imply Hypercoagulation in Preeclampsia.

↑ Common pathway activity
↓ Fibrinogen
↑ Fibrin-degradation products
D-Dimer positive
↑ Fibrinopeptide A
↑ Factor VIII antigen; factor VIII activity
↓ Antithrombin-III
↑ Antithrombin-III/antithrombin complex
↓ Platelets
↑ β-Thromboglobulin
↑ Platelet aggregability
↓ Sensitivity to prostacyclin

Source: From Chestnut DH. *Obstetric anesthesia: principles and practice,* 3rd ed. Philadelphia: Mosby, 2004:803, with permission.

evidence of hemolysis and increased liver enzymes characterizes HELLP (hemolysis, elevated liver enzymes, low platelets) syndrome.

Renal changes

- Glomerular enlargement results in ischemia, leading to decreased glomerular filtration rate (GFR).
- Proteinuria occurs as a result of an increased permeability to most large molecular weight proteins.
- Urate clearance decreases and serum uric acid concentrations increase. Hyperuricemia may provide an early indication of preeclampsia.
- Oliguria parallels the severity of preeclampsia.

Endocrine changes

In women with preeclampsia, a breakdown of the normal balance between vasodilators (PGI_2, nitric oxide [NO]) and vasoconstrictors (angiotensin II, thromboxane A_2 [TXA_2], serotonin, endothelin) occurs. There is also a decrease in plasma renin concentration and a suppression of the renin–angiotensin–aldosterone system.

Respiratory changes

- Pharyngeal and laryngeal edema may make airway management difficult, necessitating the use of smaller endotracheal tubes.
- Pulmonary edema occurs in 3% of cases, with some cases occurring postpartum.

Hepatic changes

- Serum transaminase levels frequently increase in patients with mild preeclampsia.
- Epigastric or subcostal pain is an ominous symptom that is typically caused by distension of the liver capsule by edema or subcapsular or parenchymal bleeding. Hepatic swelling produces epigastric pain.
- Liver rupture is associated with a more than 80% mortality.

Neurologic changes

- The classic manifestations of preeclampsia include severe headache, visual disturbances, central nervous system (CNS) hyperexcitability, and hyperreflexia.

- The occurrence of seizures indicates eclampsia until proved otherwise. Etiologies of seizures include hypertonic encephalopathy, vasospasm, microinfarctions and punctate hemorrhages, thrombosis, and cerebral edema.
- Postpartum eclampsia may occur up to 10 days after delivery.

Uteroplacental perfusion

- Uteroplacental perfusion is decreased in preeclampsia with the potential for intrauterine growth retardation.

Benigni A, Orisio S, Gaspari F, et al. Evidence against a pathogenic role for endothelin in preeclampsia. *Br J Obstet Gynaecol* 1992;99:798–802.

Chestnut DH, ed. *Obstetric anesthesia: principles and practice*, 3rd ed. Philadelphia: Mosby, 2004:794–835.

DeJong CL, Dekker GA, Sibai BM. The renin–angiotensin–aldosterone system in preeclampsia: a review. *Clin Perinatol* 1991;18:683–711.

Inayatulla A, Chemtob S, Nuwayhid B, et al. Responses of placental arteries from normotensive and preeclamptic women to endogenous vasoactive agents. *Am J Obstet Gynecol* 1993;168:869–874.

Perry KG, Martin JN. Abnormal hemostasis and coagulopathy in preeclampsia and eclampsia. *Clin Obstet Gynecol* 1992;35:338–350.

Seligman SP, Buyon JP, Clancy RM, et al. The role of nitric oxide in the pathogenesis of preeclampsia. *Am J Obstet Gynecol* 1994;171:944–948.

A.9. Which component of blood pressure best predicts the occurrence of preeclampsia?

Pregnancy induces several cardiovascular responses and adaptation that include increase in vascular and extravascular volume, higher cardiac output, and marked reduction in peripheral resistance that effectively causes a relatively lower blood pressure by the second trimester of pregnancy. Multiple attempts have been made to correlate first and second trimester systolic, diastolic and mean arterial pressures (MAP) with development of preeclampsia. Unfortunately, there is significant variability in the aforementioned components of blood pressure throughout pregnancy complicated further by factors such as ethnicity, age, nulliparous versus multiparous state, and gestational differences at the time of measurements. In addition, the anxiety component of office visit (white-coat effect) frequently contributes to variability in measures of blood pressure, limiting their predicatibility of preeclampsia. Ravi et al., reported that although systolic, diastolic, and MAP were elevated in women who developed hypertensive disorder of pregnancy as compared to normotensive women, these parameters did not correlate with ensuing preeclampsia. Conversely, elevations in pulse pressure at 7 to 15 weeks of gestation, was a significant predictor of preeclampsia but not of gestational hypertension. In fact, for every 1 mm Hg increase in pulse pressure, the associated risk of preeclampsia increased by 6%.

A.10. What is the significance of increased pulse wave velocity (PWV) during pregnancy? How does this relate to birthweight?

Similar to increase in pulse pressure, PWV can be a marker of arterial stiffness. In normal pregnancy, arterial stiffness decreases during the first trimester and remains low until the end of pregnancy due to either reduced smooth muscle tone or vessel wall remodeling. However, there is a wide range in arterial stiffness even in normal pregnancy, suggesting varying degree of cardiovascular adaptation. Maladaptation may lead to retardation in fetal growth as measured by

birthweight and by postnatal catch-up growth. Elvan-Taspinar et al., found a significant relation between PWV during the last trimester of pregnancy and fetal birhtweight and postnatal catch-up growth independent of mean arterial pressures (MAP). For example, an increase in PWV of 1 m per second was associated with a decrease in birthweight by 17.6%. Similarly, a strong link was found between pulse pressure and birthweight, with an incrcase of 10 mm Hg in pulse pressure being associated with an 11.8% decrease in weight. Both PWV and pulse pressure appear to offer superior circulatory as well as prognostic information relating fetal and neonatal outcome.

Elvan-Taspinar A, Franx A, Bots ML, et al. Arterial stiffness and fetal growth in normotensive pregnancy. *Am J Hematol* 2005;18:337–341.

Lurbe E, Torro I, Alvarez V, et al. The impact of birth weight on pulse pressure during adolescence. *Blood press monit* 2004;9:187–192.

Spasojevic M, Smith S, Morris J, et al. Peripheral arterial pulse wave analysis in women with preeclampsia and gestational hypertension. *Int J Gynaecol Obstet* 2005;112:1475–1478.

A.11. What are some of the complications associated with preeclampsia?

Maternal complications include disseminated intravascular coagulation, congestive heart failure with pulmonary edema, placental abruption, postpartum hemorrhage, acute renal failure, rupture of the liver, cerebrovascular accident, and septic shock. The leading cause of maternal death is intracranial hemorrhage.

Fetal complications includc prematurily with respiratory distress, intrauterine growth retardation, oligohydramnios, intracranial hemorrhage, small for gestational age, and aspiration of meconium. The leading cause of intrauterine morbidity and mortality is uteroplacental insufficiency caused by placental infarcts, followed by placental abruption, and chorioamnionitis.

Datta S, ed. *Anesthetic and obstetric management of high-risk pregnancy*, 3rd ed. New York: Springer, 2004:270–281.

B. Preoperative Evaluation and Preparation

B.1. What initial laboratory studies are recommended for patients with preeclampsia?

- Complete blood cell count
- Platelet count and aggregation when available
- Coagulation assay including activated partial thromboplastin time, prothrombin time, fibrinogen, D-dimer
- Serum electrolytes
- Blood urea nitrogen, creatinine, and uric acid concentration
- Liver function tests
- Urinalysis, microscopy, 24-hour specimen for protein and creatinine clearance
- Type and screen (cross-match if antibodies present)

Chestnut DH, ed. *Obstetric anesthesia: principles and practice*, 3rd ed. Philadelphia: Mosby, 2004:794–835.

Stoelting RK, Dierdorf SF. *Anesthesia and co-existing disease*, 4th ed. New York: Churchill Livingstone, 2002:658–643.

B.2. What are the important routine monitors for patients with preeclampsia? When is a central venous pressure (CVP) monitor indicated?

Important routine monitors are as follows:

- Noninvasive blood pressure
- Maternal respiratory function assessment with oxygen saturation
- Hourly deep tendon reflexes
- Muscle strength
- Serial magnesium sulfate levels
- Foley catheter for assessing urine output
- Uterine contraction monitor
- Continuous fetal heart rate monitoring
- Consider invasive blood pressure monitoring with an arterial line when severe refractory hypertension is present, when rapid acting vasodilators, such as sodium nitroprusside (SNP) or nicardipine, are used, or when noninvasive blood pressure measurement proves difficult (e.g., obesity).
- A CVP monitor or a pulmonary artery (PA) catheter may be indicated for the following conditions:
  Persistent oliguria
  Difficulty in fluid management therapy in antepartum and/or postpartum period
  Presence of pulmonary edema

A survey on the use of invasive hemodynamic monitoring among anesthesiologists who care for patients with preeclampsia indicate that central monitoring is used in 7.5% of patients. When invasive hemodynamic monitoring is used, 56% of anesthesiologists use an arterial line, 26% use an arterial line and central monitoring and 20% use central monitoring only. Also, 92% of respondents use a CVP monitor whereas only 8% use a PA catheter. The etiology of pulmonary edema, however, may be due to an increase in capillary permeability as well as from diastolic dysfunction, complicating assessment of cardiac function and volume status. Only in severe forms of preeclampsia is left ventricular systolic function markedly reduced. Further, there may be technical difficulties with placing the PA catheter that are both patient related (awake, anxious, short neck with poorly visible landmarks, coagulopathy) and physician related (inexperience with central venous catheterization), which may alter the balance between benefit and risk of invasive monitoring. Whenever possible, a bedside transthoracic echocardiogram may be obtained; however, there may be limited windows for imaging due to the gravid uterus—causing distension of the abdomen.

Birnbach DJ, Gatt SP, Datta S, eds. *Textbook of obstetric anesthesia*, 1st ed. New York: Churchill Livingstone, 2000:546.

Ross VH, Moore CH, Fragneto RY, et al. Invasive hemodynamic monitoring in the management of PIH: a survey of practicing anesthesiologists. *Anesthesiology* 2000;92: A89.

B.3. What conditions mandate immediate delivery, regardless of the gestational age?

- Severe hypertension that persists after 24 to 48 hours
- Progressive thrombocytopenia
- Liver dysfunction
- Progressive renal dysfunction (including severe oliguria)
- Premonitory signs of eclampsia
- Evidence of fetal jeopardy
- Persistent headache or other neurologic sequelae of preeclampsia

Datta S, ed. *Anesthetic and obstetric management of high-risk pregnancy*, 3rd ed. New York: Springer, 2004:407–408.

B.4. Discuss the obstetric management of preeclampsia.

The goal of therapy is to stabilize the mother and to safely deliver the fetus and placenta.

- Improve intravascular volume.
- Administer seizure prophylaxis with magnesium sulfate.
- Administer antihypertensives for blood pressure control.

Labetalol is a commonly used antihypertensive agent that decreases maternal systemic vascular resistance (SVR) without increasing maternal heart rate or decreasing cardiac index, uterine blood flow, or fetal heart rate when it is given in a total dose of less than 1 mg per kg. When given in an initial intravenous bolus dose of 10 to 20 mg, it has a faster onset of action than hydralazine and, if necessary, the dose may be doubled every 10 minutes. It is useful in the management of refractory hypertension. If a second agent must be administered (e.g., hydralazine, sodium nitroprusside [SNP] or nicardipine), labetalol helps to prevent reflex tachycardia. It is important to note that the mechanism of hypertension is mediated greatly by circulating catecholamines, making labetalol a preferred antihypertensive agent that will antagonize the vasoconstrictive effects of norepinephrine, in particular. Other agents may reduce the blood pressure as reflected by a peripheral blood pressure monitor; however, unopposed vasoconstriction at the central and at the microcirculatory levels may cause end organ injury.

Hydralazine is another antihypertensive agent that can be used because of its direct vasodilating effect. The full extent of its effect is evident in 20 minutes; therefore, if sufficient time is not allowed between injections, severe hypotension will be seen. It is used in 5- to 10-mg increments intravenously every 20 to 30 minutes until the diastolic blood pressure is decreased, with a cumulative dose of 20 mg. Hydralazine directly decreases peripheral vascular resistance. Reflex sympathetic activity can result in tachycardia and increased stroke volume and cardiac output. Tachycardia can be treated with labetalol, 10 to 20 mg intravenously. The patient may complain of headache and flushing of the face during therapy.

Nitroglycerin (NTG) causes vascular smooth muscle relaxation by means of its intracellular degradation to NO. The primary effect of NTG is venodilation, but it is less effective in prehydrated patients. NTG readily crosses the placenta. The drug is most useful for short-term treatment (e.g., to control the pressor response to tracheal intubation). Small doses, 50 to 100 μg, may be given intravenously, or NTG may be given sublingually in a 400-μg metered spray.

SNP relaxes the arterial vessels, thereby reducing afterload. However, SNP also reduces venous return. The drug is most useful for short-term treatment, similar to NTG. Cyanide toxicity is proposed to be more likely with prolonged infusion rates that exceed 4 μg/kg/minute over several hours to days; however, Naulty et al. demonstrated that intravenous infusion of nitroprusside solution in pregnant ewes, maintained at a rate sufficient to decrease mean maternal arterial pressure by 20% for 1 hour, resulted in equilibration of maternal and fetal levels of nitroprusside at the 20-minute sample. Five of the eight animals exhibited tachyphylaxis to nitroprusside, and their fetuses died *in utero* with lethal levels of cyanide. No significant changes were observed in uterine blood flow. There have been attempts to counteract the cyanide toxicity of nitroprusside by coadministration of sodium thiosulfate. Curry et al. administered sodium thiosulfate and nitroprusside to pregnant ewes and only nitroprusside to a control group. Although control ewes and fetuses suffered progressive increases in red cell cyanide concentrations into the toxic range, experimental ewes and fetuses never developed toxic red cell cyanide levels. These results suggest that coadministration of sodium thiosulfate with SNP to pregnant women at doses currently in use for nonpregnant patients will prevent fetal, as well as maternal, cyanide toxicity. Unfortunately, it is not known whether these findings are transferable to humans, raising major concern over ongoing clinical use of nitroprusside in obstetrics when safer drugs such as nicardipine and labetalol are available.

Nifedipine is a calcium entry blocker that affects predominantly arterial and arteriolar smooth muscle. Common maternal side effects include facial flushing, headache, and tachycardia. Nifedipine rapidly lowers blood pressure after oral or sublingual administration. After an initial dose of 10 mg sublingually, it may be repeated in 30 minutes and subsequently given in a maintenance dose of 10 to 20 mg every 3 to 6 hours. Caution must be exercised in the patient receiving both magnesium sulfate and calcium entry blockers because of the risk of myocardial depression and resultant pulmonary edema.

Chestnut DH, ed. *Obstetric anesthesia: principles and practice*, 3rd ed. Philadelphia: Mosby, 2004:794–835.

Curry SC, Carlton MW, Raschke RA. Prevention of fetal and maternal cyanide toxicity from nitroprusside with coinfusion of sodium thiosulfate in gravid ewes. *Anesth Analg* 1997;84(5):1121–1126.

Lopez-Jaramillo P, Narvaez M, Calle A, et al. Cyclic guanosine 3′5′ monophosphate concentrations in preeclampsia: effects of hydralazine. *Br J Obstet Gynaecol* 1996;103: 33–38.

Naulty J, Cefalo RC, Lewis PE. Fetal toxicity of nitroprusside in the pregnant ewe. *Am J Obstet Gynecol* 1981;139(6):708–711.

B.5. In the United States, what drug therapy is the treatment of choice for seizure prophylaxis?

Magnesium sulfate is the initial therapy for seizure prophylaxis. The Eclampsia Trial Collaborative Group compared magnesium sulfate, phenytoin, and diazepam administration for the prevention of recurrent seizures in women with preeclampsia. They found that magnesium sulfate was more effective in preventing recurring seizures than either phenytoin or diazepam.

An initial bolus of 4 to 6 g of magnesium sulfate is administered over 20 minutes and followed with an intravenous infusion of 1 to 2 g per hour. Urine output, respiratory rate, and patellar reflexes are monitored during magnesium therapy. The serum magnesium sulfate concentration should be measured at least 4 hours after initiation of therapy. The therapeutic range for serum magnesium sulfate concentrations is between 4 and 6 mEq per L. Loss of deep tendon reflexes occurs at 10 mEq per L with evidence of prolonged P-Q intervals and widening QRS complexes. Respiratory arrest occurs at 15 mEq per L, and asystole occurs at 20 mEq per L.

Eclampsia Trial Collaborative Group. Which anticonvulsant for women with eclampsia? Evidence from the collaborative eclampsia trial. *Lancet* 1995;345:1455–1463.

B.6. Discuss the treatment of magnesium sulfate toxicity.

Magnesium sulfate is excreted by the kidneys. Therefore, urine output must be followed closely and serial serum concentrations of magnesium sulfate must be checked, especially in women with renal dysfunction. If magnesium sulfate toxicity is suspected, the magnesium sulfate infusion should be immediately discontinued. Intravenous calcium gluconate, 1 g, or calcium chloride, 300 mg, should be administered if needed to antagonize the effects of magnesium sulfate. If respiratory distress occurs, the patient may require endotracheal intubation and mechanical ventilation.

Chestnut DH, ed. *Obstetric anesthesia: principles and practice*, 3rd ed. New York: Churchill Livingstone, 2004:808–809.

B.7. Discuss the mechanism of action of magnesium sulfate.

Magnesium has the following effects:

- It is a central nervous system (CNS) depressant and anticonvulsant.
- It inhibits the release of acetylcholine at the neuromuscular junction, decreases the sensitivity of the motor endplate to acetylcholine, and decreases muscle membrane excitability, thereby potentiating the effects of nondepolarizing and depolarizing muscle relaxants.
- It decreases uterine hyperactivity by its mild relaxant effect on vascular and uterine smooth muscle; it may improve uterine blood flow.
- It is a mild vasodilator in vascular beds (including small-diameter cerebral vessels) by a direct or indirect (calcium-competing) effect; and it has a mild antihypertensive effect.

Chestnut DH, ed. *Obstetric anesthesia: principles and practice*, 3rd ed. Philadelphia: Mosby, 2004:808–809.

B.8. What are the fetal effects of magnesium sulfate therapy?

Magnesium sulfate crosses the placenta. There can be evidence of decreased beat-to-beat variability in the fetal heart rate. Neonatal depression (e.g., respiratory depression and hyporeflexia) can also occur.

Chestnut DH, ed. *Obstetric anesthesia: principles and practice*, 3rd ed. Philadelphia: Mosby, 2004:808–809.

B.9. Discuss the treatment of eclampsia.

- Stop the convulsions (thiopental, 50 to 100 mg intravenously).
- Establish an airway.
- Turn patient to the left side; apply jaw thrust.
- Attempt bag and mask ventilation.
- Insert oropharyngeal airway if necessary.
- Maintain ventilation and oxygenation.
- Continue bag and mask ventilation.
- Apply pulse oximeter and monitor.
- Maintain circulation.
- Secure intravenous access.
- Check blood pressure at frequent intervals.
- Monitor electrocardiographic (ECG) recordings.
- Administer magnesium sulfate.
- Treat hypertension.
- Deliver the baby expeditiously.

Chestnut DH, ed. *Obstetric anesthesia: principles and practice*, 3rd ed. Philadelphia: Mosby, 2004:808–809.

C. Intraoperative Management

C.1. What is your choice of analgesia/anesthesia for patients with preeclampsia?

Most anesthesiologists and obstetricians consider epidural analgesia the preferred form of pain relief for labor and delivery in preeclamptic women. Epidural analgesia provides the following advantages:

- Epidural analgesia provides pain relief that is superior to all other analgesic methods.
- Epidural analgesia attenuates the exaggerated hypertensive response to pain of preeclamptic women.
- Epidural analgesia reduces circulating levels of catecholamines and stress-related hormones, which facilitates blood pressure control.
- Epidural analgesia may improve intervillous blood flow in preeclamptic women.
- Epidural analgesia results in stable cardiac output.
- Preeclamptic women are at increased risk of cesarean delivery compared with normal parturients, and early administration of epidural analgesia for labor facilitates the subsequent administration of epidural anesthesia for emergent cesarean delivery.

Benedetto C, Zonca M, Marozio L, et al. Blood pressure patterns in normal pregnancy and in pregnancy-induced hypertension, preeclampsia, and chronic hypertension. *Obstet Gynecol* 1996;88:503–510.

Cunningham FG, Lindheimer MD. Hypertension in pregnancy. *N Engl J Med* 1992;326: 927–932.

C.2. What is the advantage of prehydration?

Prehydration helps compensate for reductions in preload and afterload during the administration of epidural analgesia/anesthesia. Two studies have investigated the effects of intravenous volume loading with crystalloid on atrial natruretic peptide (ANP) secretion in preeclamptic women. ANP is a vasodilator secreted from the cardiac atria in response to an acute volume load, and this response is more pronounced in preeclamptic women. ANP has properties that counteract vasospasm and improve renal elimination of excess extracellular fluid. These studies support the use of volume expansion before administration of regional anesthesia in preeclamptic women.

Chestnut DH, ed. *Obstetric anesthesia: principles and practice*, 3rd ed. Philadelphia: Mosby, 2004:814.

C.3. How should patients be hydrated before epidural analgesia/anesthesia for labor and delivery?

Most preeclamptic patients may receive prehydration with crystalloid in a 10 mL per kg bolus. Attention must be given to evidence of recent excessive weight gain or a fluid balance chart suggesting overhydration. Also, one must monitor for the development of pulmonary edema. Additional crystalloid (e.g., 250 to 500 mL) can be infused if hypotension ensues during epidural analgesia/anesthesia.

Datta S, ed. *Anesthetic and obstetric management of high-risk pregnancy*, 3rd ed. New York: Springer, 2004:285–286.

C.4. Discuss bleeding time and platelet count evaluation during preoperative assessment of a patient with preeclampsia requesting epidural analgesia/anesthesia for labor and delivery.

The bleeding time does not specifically measure platelet function, and it can be abnormal in a number of coagulation disorders, such as factor deficiencies. No evidence suggests that the skin bleeding time predicts the potential for bleeding from a traumatized epidural vein in a woman with severe preeclampsia. Therefore, the bleeding time should not be used to measure platelet function. A specific platelet count that predicts the risk of complications from regional anesthesia has not been determined. The *trend* in platelet count is important to note, as preeclampsia is a dynamic disorder, and a rapid decrease in platelet count in a short interval may warrant concern.

Many anesthesiologists will place an epidural anesthetic at a platelet count of 80,000 per μL and some at lower platelet counts. The patient must be individualized and a thorough bleeding history, along with the trend in platelet count, should be considered.

Beilin Y, Zahn J, Comerford M. Safe epidural analgesia in thirty parturients with platelet counts between 69,000 and 98,000 mm(-3). *Anesth Analg* 1997;85:385–388.

Chestnut DH, ed. *Obstetric anesthesia: principles and practice*, 3rd ed. Philadelphia: Mosby, 2004:814–815.

C.5. What level of analgesia/anesthesia is required for labor and delivery?

First stage of labor: T10-L1
Second stage of labor: S2-4

Chestnut DH, ed. *Obstetric anesthesia: principles and practice*, 3rd ed. Philadelphia: Mosby, 2004:288–292.

C.6. Discuss the commonly used local anesthetics for labor analgesia.

Bupivacaine, ropivacaine, and levobupivacaine (amide local anesthetics) are commonly used because they provide potent analgesia. They provide analgesia with less motor block than an equipotent concentration of lidocaine. Moreover, dilute solutions cause less hypotension than more concentrated solutions.

Bupivacaine is four times more potent than lidocaine. It is 90% to 95% bound to maternal plasma protein. It is known to be more cardiotoxic than lidocaine. The mechanism relates to its action on cardiac sodium channels. Bupivacaine and lidocaine both block sodium channels to the nerves and to the heart. They are similar because they both cause a rapid block of cardiac sodium channels on depolarization. They differ in their recovery from block. The lidocaine block is complete within less than 1 second, whereas bupivacaine takes five times longer. Bupivacaine is a "fast-in, slow-out" agent. Its main advantage is that it has a longer duration and a weak motor block when given in analgesic concentrations.

Ropivacaine is a homolog of mepivacaine and bupivacaine, but it is formulated as a single levorotatory isomer rather than as a racemic mixture. It appears to be less cardiotoxic than bupivacaine.

Levobupivacaine is also a single levorotatory isomer formulation of a local anesthetic. Levobupivacaine appears to be less cardiotoxic than bupivacaine.

2-Chloroprocaine is an ester type of local anesthetic. It is hydrolyzed by plasma cholinesterase, and it has a rapid metabolism, allowing for a very quick onset of action.

Chestnut DH, ed. *Obstetric anesthesia: principles and practice*, 3rd ed. Philadelphia: Mosby, 2004:192–193.

Mazoit JX, Boico O, Samii K. Myocardial uptake of bupivacaine, II: pharmacokinetics and pharmacodynamics of bupivacaine enantiomers in the isolated perfused rabbit heart. *Anesth Analg* 1993;77:477–482.

Valenzuela C, Snyders DJ, Bennett PB, et al. Stereoselective block of cardiac sodium channels by bupivacaine in guinea pig ventricular myocytes. *Circulation* 1995;92:3014–3024.

C.7. Is the addition of epinephrine to local anesthetics advisable in preeclamptic patients?

Clinical evidence supports the safety of epidural administration of an epinephrine-containing local anesthetic in preeclamptic women. However, care must be taken when using epinephrine-containing local anesthetic solutions in severe preeclamptic women as inadvertent intravascular injection may result in acute severe hypertension.

Chestnut DH, ed. *Obstetric anesthesia: principles and practice*, 3rd ed. Philadelphia: Mosby, 2004:819.

Dror A, Abboud TK, Moore J, et al. Maternal hemodynamic responses to epinephrine-containing local anesthetics in mild preeclampsia. *Reg Anesth* 1988;13:107–111.

Heller PJ, Goodman C. Use of local anesthetics with epinephrine for epidural anesthesia in preeclampsia. *Anesthesiology* 1986;65:224–226.

C.8. What is the treatment for the abnormal fetal heart rate pattern seen with maternal hypotension after epidural analgesia/anesthesia is instituted?

- Administration of oxygen with face mask
- Left uterine displacement
- Increased hydration
- Elevation of lower extremities to facilitate venous return
- Administration of small increments of ephedrine, 2.5 to 5 mg or phenylephrine, 50 to 100 μg intravenously, if the blood pressure falls more than 20% of baseline.

Chestnut DH, ed. *Obstetric anesthesia: principles and practice*, 3rd ed. Philadelphia: Mosby, 2004:337.

Vercateren M. Obstetric spinal analgesia and anesthesia. *Curr Opin Anesthesiol* 2003;16:503–507.

C.9. What would you do after an accidental spinal tap? How do you treat postdural puncture headache?

Accidental spinal tap can be treated in one of two ways. First, the epidural needle may be repositioned in another interspace. Local anesthetic must be administered slowly because now there is a direct communication with the intrathecal space through the dural hole, and thereby, a more profound analgesic/anesthetic block may appear. The incidence of a postdural puncture headache after an accidental wet tap with an epidural needle is more than 50%. After delivery of the fetus, the catheter should be removed. Intravenous and oral caffeinated beverages should be encouraged. An abdominal binder may be used. Intravenous caffeine and oral analgesics may be used as well. If symptoms worsen (e.g., tinnitus, blurry vision, neck pain, and difficulty sitting or standing), one should consider an epidural blood patch. Immediate relief occurs in 95% of patients on first attempt and 99% of patients on second attempt. Transient side effects include backache and neck pain. Second, an epidural catheter (20 gauge) can be inserted intrathecally for use as a continuous spinal catheter. After delivery, one can remove the catheter and follow the guidelines as listed earlier, or one can consider maintaining the intrathecal catheter in place for 24 hours to allow for an inflammatory reaction to develop around the intrathecal catheter. This inflammatory reaction may decrease the leakage of cerebrospinal fluid and thereby the incidence of postdural puncture headache.

Birnbach DJ, Gatt S, Datta S, eds. *Textbook of obstetric anesthesia*, 1st ed. New York: Churchill Livingstone, 2000:498–500.

C.10. How would you manage total spinal anesthesia?

- High spinal anesthesia may occur several minutes after an epidural injection of local anesthetic. It is vitally important to communicate with the patient. Agitation, dyspnea, and difficulty speaking may herald the onset of total spinal anesthesia.
- Avoid aortocaval compression.
- Administer 100% oxygen to the mother.
- Provide positive pressure ventilation, preferably through an endotracheal tube.
- Monitor maternal blood pressure, electrocardiographic (ECG) recordings, and fetal heart rate.
- Support maternal circulation with intravenous fluids and ephedrine as needed. Do not hesitate to give epinephrine if needed.

Chestnut DH, ed. *Obstetric anesthesia: principles and practice*, 3rd ed. Philadelphia: Mosby, 2004:339–340.

C.11. Should ergonovine be given to preeclamptic patients?

Preeclampsia is a relative contraindication to the use of ergot alkaloids because of the risk of inducing a hypertension crisis. In preeclamptic patients, uterine atony unresponsive to oxytocin may be treated with 15-methylprostaglandin $F_{2\alpha}$.

Secher NJ, Arnsbro P, Wallin L. Haemodynamic effects of oxytocin and methyl ergometrine on the systemic and pulmonary circulations of pregnant anaesthetized women. *Acta Obstet Gynecol Scand* 1978;57:97–103.

C.12. When and how would you give spinal anesthesia?

Spinal anesthesia may be used for cesarean delivery, even in a patient with severe preeclampsia. Hyperbaric bupivacaine 0.75% in a dose of 11.25 mg to 12 mg with or without fentanyl, 15 to 20 μg, or morphine, 100 to 200 μg, may be given.

Advantages of spinal anesthesia in severe preeclampsia include:

- Avoidance of general anesthesia and risks of difficulty with an edematous airway
- Elimination of risk of severe hypertensive response to laryngoscopy and endotracheal intubation
- More reliable anesthesia than with an epidural anesthetic technique
- Smaller needle size than an epidural and therefore possibly less risk of trauma to epidural veins

A recent study noted that the risk of hypotension was almost six times less in severely preeclamptic women than in healthy pregnant women receiving spinal anesthesia for elective cesarean section.

Chestnut DH, ed. *Obstetric anesthesia: principles and practice,* 2nd ed. Philadelphia: Mosby, 2004:820–824.

Stoelting RK, Dierdorf SF. *Anesthesia and co-existing disease*, 4th ed. New York: Churchill Livingstone, 2002:663–664.

C.13. Discuss a general anesthesia technique for the patient with preeclampsia presenting for cesarean delivery.

- Aspiration prophylaxis. Acceptable methods include 30 mL of an oral nonparticulate antacid, and/or an H_2-blocker intravenously and possibly metoclopramide, 10 mg intravenously.
- Preoxygenation and denitrogenation with 100% oxygen through face mask
- Induction of anesthesia with cricoid pressure and sodium pentothal, 4 to 6 mg per kg
- Succinylcholine, 1.5 mg per kg, for effective intubation conditions
- Use a smaller endotracheal tube (6.0 or 6.5 mm internal diameter) because of airway edema.
- May consider use of nondepolarizing muscle relaxants for maintenance of neuromuscular block once the patient has demonstrated recovery from succinylcholine. Magnesium sulfate potentiates the effects of both depolarizing and nondepolarizing muscle relaxants.
- Use two thirds of the minimum alveolar concentration of inhalation agent of the nonpregnant adult to ensure an adequate depth of anesthesia.
- Continue magnesium sulfate administration during intraoperative and postoperative periods
- Consider arterial line placement before induction in patients with severe preeclampsia for continuous blood pressure measurement. The transient but severe hypertension that accompanies tracheal intubation in preeclamptic women can significantly increase maternal intracranial pressure (ICP), with the attendant risks of cerebrovascular accident.
- Antihypertensive drugs can be given as required.

Chestnut DH, ed. *Obstetric anesthesia: principles and practice,* 3rd ed. Philadelphia: Mosby, 2004:824–825.

C.14. What agents can you use to prevent hypertension during induction of general anesthesia for cesarean delivery?

Before induction, labetalol, 5-mg increments, nitroglycerin (NTG), 50-μg increments, or sodium nitroprusside (SNP), 50-μg increments, can be used to attenuate the pressor response to laryngoscopy and intubation. SNP should be used only in conjunction with an arterial line.

Chestnut DH, ed. *Obstetric anesthesia: principles and practice,* 3rd ed. Philadelphia: Mosby, 2004:824–825.

C.15. What is HELLP syndrome?

HELLP syndrome is a severe form of preeclampsia characterized by hemolysis (*H*), elevated liver enzymes *(EL)*, and low platelets *(LP)*. It can occur antepartum or postpartum. Delivery represents the only definitive treatment of HELLP syndrome. HELLP syndrome is associated with maternal and neonatal morbidity and mortality. Hemolysis is defined by an abnormal peripheral blood smear and an increased bilirubin level (1.2 mg/dL or greater). Elevated liver enzymes are defined as an increased serum glutamic-oxaloacetic transaminase (aspartate aminotransferase) of at least 70 U per L and a lactate dehydrogenase level of more than 600 U per L. A low platelet count is defined as a count of less than 100,000 per mm³. Patients with HELLP syndrome have a high incidence of serious maternal complications including disseminated intravascular coagulation, placental abruption, need for blood transfusion, pleural effusion, acute renal failure, and wound infection.

Audibert F, Friedman SA, Frangieh AY, et al. Clinical utility of strict diagnostic criteria for the HELLP (hemolysis, elevated liver enzymes, and low platelets) syndrome. *Am J Obstet Gynecol* 1996;175:460–464.

Chestnut DH, ed. *Obstetric anesthesia: principles and practice,* 3rd ed. New York: Churchill Livingstone, 2004:812–813.

Sibai BM. The HELLP syndrome (hemolysis, elevated liver enzymes, and low platelets): much ado about nothing. *Am J Obstet Gynecol* 1990;162:311–316.

Stoelting RK, Dierdorf SF. *Anesthesia and co-existing disease,* 4th ed. New York: Churchill Livingstone, 2002:658–659.

D. Postoperative Management

D.1. Discuss the postpartum management of preeclamptic patients?

- Provide adequate analgesia.
- Maintain strict intake/output for at least 24 hours postpartum or until diuresis develops.
- Continue magnesium sulfate for at least 24 hours postpartum or until evidence of diuresis.
- Maintain hemodynamic control with antihypertensives if necessary.

Chestnut DH, ed. *Obstetric anesthesia: principles and practice,* 3rd ed. Philadelphia: Mosby, 2004:825.

CHAPTER 42

Transverse Lie, Fetal Distress, and Mitral Stenosis

Jill Fong

A 20-YEAR-OLD UNREGISTERED PRIMIGRAVIDA

at 38 weeks of gestation presented to the labor room contracting with transverse fetal lie. The patient had a history of rheumatic fever. On physical examination, she had a diastolic murmur and an opening snap. She reported that now she gets short of breath when climbing two flights of stairs. She was attached to an external fetal heart rate (FHR) monitor and tocodynamometer; severe variable decelerations without any beat-to-beat variability were noted. Simultaneously, the patient was found to have a prolapsed umbilical cord with meconium-stained amniotic fluid. She was rushed to the operating room for an emergency cesarean section. Her blood pressure was 100/60 mm Hg; regular pulse, 100 beats per minute; respiratory rate, 18 breaths per minute.

A. Medical Disease and Differential Diagnosis

1. How are fetal lie, presentation, and position defined and determined?
2. What is the approximate frequency of the various lies and presentations at or near term?
3. What is the proposed etiology of transverse lie?
4. What are the problems associated with transverse lie?
5. What is the usual obstetric management for patients with transverse lie?
6. What are the different types of breech presentation, and what is their incidence?
7. What is the cause of breech presentation?
8. What are the problems associated with breech presentation?
9. What is the incidence of heart disease in pregnancy?
10. What are maternal and fetal mortality rates with maternal cardiac disease?
11. What is the functional classification of heart disease by the New York Heart Association (NYHA)?
12. What are the cardiovascular changes of pregnancy?
13. What changes may normally occur in heart sounds during pregnancy?
14. What are the normal electrocardiographic and echocardiographic changes seen during pregnancy?

15. What causes rheumatic heart disease?
16. What are the physiologic consequences of mitral stenosis?
17. What are the ausculatory findings associated with mitral stenosis?
18. What may be seen on the electrocardiogram in patients with mitral stenosis?
19. What are the echocardiographic findings associated with mitral stenosis?
20. What is the effect of the physiologic changes of pregnancy on patients with mitral stenosis?
21. If mitral stenosis is first recognized during pregnancy and symptoms develop, how would you treat the patient?
22. What are the determinants of fetal oxygenation?
23. What are the determinants of uterine blood flow?

B. Preoperative Evaluation and Preparation

1. How is fetal well-being assessed during labor?
2. How are fetal heart rate (FHR) and maternal contractions monitored?
3. What is the normal FHR with beat-to-beat variability?
4. What are transient or periodic decelerations?
5. How accurate is FHR monitoring in predicting fetal well-being?
6. In the fetus with a nonreassuring FHR pattern, what other modalities can be used to assess whether hypoxia has led to acidosis? What are the normal values of fetal blood gases?
7. Can fetal scalp capillary blood pH sampling give false signals?
8. What are the causes of acute fetal distress?
9. What is the significance of meconium-stained amniotic fluid?
10. What is meconium aspiration syndrome?
11. What are the usual noninvasive tests used to evaluate the pregnant cardiac patient?
12. What preoperative medications would you give this patient?

C. Intraoperative Management

1. What monitors would you use in the New York Heart Association (NYHA) Class II patient during her cesarean section?
2. When would you use invasive monitoring in a pregnant patient with cardiac disease?
3. What are the hemodynamic goals of intraoperative management of the pregnant patient with mitral stenosis?
4. What anesthetic technique would you use for emergency cesarean section?
5. What technique could you use for general anesthesia in this patient?
6. If you had unexpectedly been unable to intubate this patient, how would you have managed the airway?
7. Would this patient benefit from the use of β-blockade?
8. What is the effect of the inhalation agents on uterine contractility?
9. What is the Apgar scoring system?
10. What is the significance of Apgar scores?
11. At birth, what should be done to minimize the infant's risk of meconium aspiration syndrome?
12. The Apgar score of the newborn was 3 at 1 minute. How would you treat the newborn?

D. Postoperative Management

1. Immediately after the baby was delivered, the patient's oxygen saturation decreased. What is the differential diagnosis?

A. Medical Disease and Differential Diagnosis

A.1. How are fetal lie, presentation, and position defined and determined?

- Fetal lie is the relation of the long axis of the fetus to the long axis of the mother. Longitudinal, transverse, and oblique lies exist. Longitudinal lies are either cephalic or pelvic (breech), depending on which fetal structure enters the maternal pelvis. Oblique lie results when the long axis of the fetus is at an acute angle to that of the mother. It is usually only transitory and converts to a transverse or longitudinal lie when labor begins.
- Presentation describes the part of the fetus that is lowermost in the pelvis: cephalic, breech, or shoulder. Cephalic presentations are further subdivided into vertex, brow, and face presentations.
- Position of the presenting part is described as a relationship between a certain pole of the presenting part and the surrounding pelvis.
- Fetal lie, presentation, and position can often be determined by manual pelvic and abdominal examination. Ultrasonography is also useful, particularly when palpation is inconclusive, as can occur with multiple gestations, placenta previa, and hydramnios.

Cunningham FG, Leveno KJ, Bloom SL, et al. eds. *Williams Obstetrics*, 22nd ed. New York: McGraw-Hill, 2005:410–411.

A.2. What is the approximate frequency of the various lies and presentations at or near term?

Cephalic presentation, 97%; breech presentation, 3% to 5%; transverse lie, 0.3%; and face presentation, 0.5%.

Cunningham FG, Leveno KJ, Bloom SL, et al. eds. *Williams Obstetrics*, 22nd ed. New York: McGraw-Hill, 2005:410.

A.3. What is the proposed etiology of transverse lie?

The exact etiology of transverse lie is unknown, but certain factors are associated with this lie, including abdominal wall relaxation from high parity with a pendulous maternal abdomen, prematurity, placenta previa, uterine anomalies, excessive amniotic fluid, pelvic contraction. Prematurity is often a factor with this abnormal lie, reported in approximately 2% of pregnancies at 32 weeks. The persistence of transverse lie beyond 37 weeks requires an assessment and management plan because the incidence of fetal and maternal morbidity is increased.

Cunningham FG, Leveno KJ, Bloom SL, et al. eds. *Williams Obstetrics*, 22nd ed. New York: McGraw-Hill, 2005:510.

Gabbe SG, Niebyl JR, Simpson JL, eds. *Obstetrics–normal and problem pregnancies*, 4th ed. New York: Churchill Livingstone, 2002:473–475.

Gemer O, Segal S. Incidence and contribution of predisposing factors to transverse lie presentation. *Int J Gynaecol Obstet* 1994;44:219.

A.4. What are the problems associated with transverse lie?

There is an increased incidence of prolapsed umbilical cord with ensuing fetal distress. Therefore, the mother's membranes are not ruptured while in the transverse lie.

Savage EW. Prolapse of the umbilical cord. *Obstet Gynecol* 1970;35:502.

A.5. What is the usual obstetric management for patients with transverse lie?

An external cephalic version can be attempted to convert the lie to longitudinal with a vertex presentation before labor ensues. External cephalic version is often used in patients with fetuses in a transverse lie or breech presentation. The reported success rate varies from 50% to 75% with a similar percentage remaining in the vertex presentation during labor. Ylikorkula and Hartikainen-Sorri found that before 34 weeks' gestation many breech infants will spontaneously convert to cephalic, and few will do so after that time. Successful version is more common in parous than nulliparous women and more successful between 37 and 39 weeks than after 40 weeks. Tocolysis has been shown to be variably effective in improving version success rates. Epidural anesthesia during version has been shown by Schorr et al. and Mancuso et al. to improve the success rate of external cephalic version. If the version is successful, labor and vaginal delivery may proceed. If, however, the version of a fetus in the transverse lie is unsuccessful, a cesarean section is done.

Cunningham FG, Leveno KJ, Bloom SL, et al. eds. *Williams Obstetrics*, 22nd ed. New York: McGraw-Hill, 2005:510.

Gabbe SG, Niebyl JR, Simpson JL, eds. *Obstetrics–normal and problem pregnancies*, 4th ed. New York: Churchill Livingstone, 2002:491–493.

Mancuso KM, Yancey MK, Murphy JA, et al. Epidural anesthesia for cephalic version: a randomized trial. *Obstet Gynecol* 2000;95(5):648.

Phelan JP. The role of external version in the intrapartum management of the transverse lie presentation. *Am J Obstet Gynecol* 1985;151:297.

Schorr SJ, Speights SE, Rose EL, et al. A randomized trial of epidural anesthesia to improve external cephalic version success. *Am J Obstet Gynecol* 1997;177:1133.

Skupski DW, Harrison-Restelli C, Dupont RB. External cephalic version: an approach with few complications. *Gynecol Obstet Invest* 2003;56(2):83.

Ylikorkula O, Hartikainen-Sorri A. Value of external version in fetal malpresentation in combination with use of ulrtrasound. *Acta Obstet Gynecol Scand* 1977;56:63.

A.6. What are the different types of breech presentation, and what is their incidence?

- *Frank breech:* Both fetal lower extremities are flexed at the hips and extended at the knees. The incidence is approximately 60% of breech presentations.
- *Complete breech:* The knees are flexed, as are the hips. The incidence is approximately 10%.
- *Incomplete or footling breech:* One or both hips are extended and a foot or knee hangs below the breech. The incidence is approximately 30%.

Gabbe SG, Niebyl JR, Simpson JL, eds. *Obstetrics–normal and problem pregnancies*, 4th ed. New York: Churchill Livingstone, 2002:482.

A.7. What is the cause of breech presentation?

The etiology of breech is unknown, but certain factors are associated with this presentation including prematurity, hydramnios, uterine relaxation associated with high parity, multiple fetuses, oligohydramnios, hydrocephaly, anencephaly, previous breech delivery, uterine anomalies, pelvic tumors, and cornual–fundal placenta implantation.

Cunningham FG, Leveno KJ, Bloom SL, et al. eds. *Williams Obstetrics*, 22nd ed. New York: McGraw-Hill, 2005:566.

A.8. What are the problems associated with breech presentation?

There is an increased incidence of prolapsed cord, perinatal morbidity and mortality resulting from difficult delivery, low birth weight and/or growth restriction from preterm delivery, fetal anomalies, placenta previa, and uterine anomalies.

Cunningham FG, Leveno KJ, Bloom SL, et al. eds. *Williams Obstetrics*, 22nd ed. New York: McGraw-Hill, 2005:566.

A.9. What is the incidence of heart disease in pregnancy?

The incidence varies from 0.4% to 4.1%. Congenital heart disease, not rheumatic heart disease, is now the major cause of heart disease in pregnancy in the developed world.

Burrow GN, Duffy TP, eds. *Medical complications during pregnancy*, 5th ed. Philadelphia: WB Saunders, 1999:111.

Chestnut DH, ed. *Obstetric anesthesia: principles and practice*, 3rd ed. 2004:707.

Hibbard LT. Maternal mortality due to cardiac disease. *Clin Obstet Gynecol* 1975;18: 27–36.

Hughes SC, Levinson G, Rosen MA, eds. *Shnider and Levinson's anesthesia for obstetrics*, 4th ed. Philadelphia: Lippincott Williams & Wilkins, 2002:456.

A.10. What are maternal and fetal mortality rates with maternal cardiac disease?

Both maternal and fetal mortality rates are increased in patients with cardiac disease. Maternal outcome seems to correlate well with the New York Heart Association (NYHA) functional classifications. Class I or II patients have less than 1% maternal mortality rate whereas class III and IV patients have between 5% and 15% mortality rate. Fetal mortality also correlates with the mother's functional class. Class III and IV patients have a perinatal loss rate of 20% to 30%. Fetal mortality generally exceeds that of the mother.

Exceptions to this functional classification correlation exist and include patients with pulmonary hypertension, significant left ventricular dysfunction and severe Marfan's syndrome. Patients with these lesions have a high mortality rate regardless of functional class.

Chestnut DH, ed. *Obstetric anesthesia: principles and practice*, 3rd ed. Philadelphia: Mosby, 2004:707.

Hughes SC, Levinson G, Rosen MA, eds. *Shnider and Levinson's Anesthesia for Obstetrics*, 4th ed. Philadelphia: Lippincott Williams & Wilkins, 2002:455.

A.11. What is the functional classification of heart disease by the New York Heart Association (NYHA)?

The NYHA classification of a complete diagnosis of cardiovascular disease is not widely used now. The grading of dyspnea and/or fatigue resulting from heart failure is, however, often still classified using the old functional NYHA classification.

- *Class I:* no limitation of physical activity
- *Class II:* slight limitation of physical activity; symptoms with ordinary activity
- *Class III:* marked limitation of physical activity; symptoms with less than ordinary activity
- *Class IV:* unable to carry on any physical activity without discomfort; symptoms may be present at rest

On the basis of an analysis of 562 pregnant patients with heart disease, Siu et al. expanded on the NYHA classification and developed a system for predicting complications during pregnancy. Their predictors of cardiac complications included the following:

1. Prior heart failure, arrhythmia, transient ischemic attack, or stroke.
2. A baseline NYHA III classification or more or cyanosis.
3. A left-sided heart obstruction defined as a mitral valve area less than 2 cm^2, aortic valve area less than 1.5 cm^2, or an echocardiographically demonstrated peak left ventricular outflow tract gradient more than 30 mm Hg.
4. A less than 40% ejection fraction

With one of these factors, the risk of sustained arrhythmia, pulmonary edema, stroke, or cardiac death was increased and even more so if two or more factors exist.

Cunningham FG, Leveno KJ, Bloom SL, et al. eds. *Williams Obstetrics*, 22nd ed. New York: McGraw-Hill, 2005:1019.

Siu SC, Sermer M, Colman JM, et al Prospective multicenter study of pregnancy outcomes in women with heart disease. *Circulation* 2001;104:515.

Zipes DP, Libby P, Bonow RO, et al. eds. *Braunwald's heart disease: a textbook of cardiovascular medicine*, 7th ed. St. Louis, WB Saunders, 2005:76, 603.

A.12. What are the cardiovascular changes of pregnancy?

During the first trimester of pregnancy, the cardiac output increases to between 40% and 50% above normal and plateaus at approximately 28 weeks of gestation. It remains fairly stable until the stresses imposed by labor increase it further and may actually decline slightly in the final weeks of pregnancy. The increase in cardiac output is due to a 30% increase in stroke volume and a 15% increase in heart rate. Blood pressure, however, is not elevated because peripheral vascular resistance decreases.

During labor, cardiac output increases approximately 15% with uterine contractions during the latent phase, 30% in the active phase, and 45% in the expulsive phase when compared to prelabor values. The greatest increase in cardiac output occurs immediately postpartum when it increases an average of 80% above prelabor values. Cardiac output and heart rate decline to prelabor values within 1 hour of delivery and by approximately 24 hours, mean blood pressure and stroke volume return to their prelabor values. For the first 3 to 6 months after delivery, the cardiovascular changes of pregnancy resolve. It can take a year, however, for the residual effects of cardiovascular remodeling to subside.

Clark SL, Cotton DM, Lee LW, et al. Central hemodynamic assessment of normal term pregnancy. *Am J Obstet Gynecol* 1989;161(6):1439.

Datta S, ed. *Anesthetic and obstetric management of high-risk pregnancy*, 3rd ed. New York: Springer-Verlag, 2004:157.

Hughes SC, Levinson G, Rosen MA, eds. *Shnider and Levinson's anesthesia for obstetrics*, 4th ed. Philadelphia: Lippincott Williams & Wilkins, 2002:7.

Ueland K, Novy MJ, Peterson EN, et al. Maternal cardiovascular dynamics, IV: the influence of gestational age on the maternal cardiovascular response to posture and exercise. *Am J Obstet Gynecol* 1969;104:856–864.

Walters WAW, MacGregor WG, Hill M. Cardiac output at rest during pregnancy and the puerperium. *Clin Sci* 1966;30:1–11.

A.13. What changes may normally occur in heart sounds during pregnancy?

In a study of 50 normal pregnant women at varying stages in pregnancy, a phonocardiographic study found that the first heart sound might have an exaggerated split with increased loudness of both components. In up to 84% of pregnant patients, a third heart sound is also evident. Functional systolic murmurs, which disappear shortly after delivery, occur in more than 90% of pregnant women. Soft transient diastolic murmurs occur in 20% of these women, and 10% have continuous murmurs apparently arising from the breast vasculature. These murmurs alone, therefore, are not indicative of organic heart disease. Similarly, venous distention, tachycardia, edema, and breathlessness may be seen with pregnancy and not be a sign of heart disease.

Cutforth R, MacDonald CB. Heart sounds and murmurs in pregnancy. *Am Heart J* 1966; 71:741.

A.14. What are the normal electrocardiographic and echocardiographic changes seen during pregnancy?

During pregnancy, sinus tachycardia is common. Premature atrial and ventricular contractions can occur. The QRS axis may be deviated to the right or the left. In lead III, inverted P waves and small Q waves may be seen that disappear with inspiration. In leads V1 and V2, the R/S ratio is increased. Some ST-segment depression and flattening or inverting of the T waves may occur. Normal echocardiographic findings include approximately a 20% increase in right atrial and right ventricular sizes. The size of the left atrium increases approximately 15% whereas the left ventricular size increases approximately 10%. Left ventricular function is unchanged or slightly improved. The annuli of the pulmonary, tricuspid, and mitral valves dilate progressively, and some mild mitral regurgitation may be present. A small pericardial effusion may develop as well.

Carruth JE, Mivis SB, Brogan DR, et al. The electrocardiogram in normal pregnancy. *Am Heart J* 1981;102(6):1075.

Datta S, ed. *Anesthetic and obstetric management of high-risk pregnancy*, 3rd ed. New York: Springer-Verlag, 2004:157.

Zipes DP, Libby P, Bonow RO, et al. eds. *Braunwald's heart disease: a textbook of cardiovascular medicine*, 7th ed. St. Louis, WB Saunders, 2005:76, 1968.

A.15. What causes rheumatic heart disease?

Rheumatic heart disease may occur in patients who have had acute rheumatic fever. The diagnosis of acute rheumatic fever is a clinical one; there are no specific laboratory tests to confirm the diagnosis and the exact pathogenetic mechanism is unknown. The diagnosis is made using Jones criteria. In addition to the requirement of supporting evidence of an antecedent group A streptococcal tonsillopharyngitis infection, there are five major criteria: carditis, polyarthritis, Sydenham's chorea, erythema marginatum, and subcutaneous nodules. Several minor criteria exist. The presence of one major and two minor or two major criteria are needed for the diagnosis. Rheumatic fever usually first occurs in 6- to 15-year-old children. If carditis occurs, mitral insufficiency ensues and approximately 5 years later mitral stenosis can occur. Mitral stenosis is the most common valvular lesion (90%) in women with a history of rheumatic heart disease. Mitral valve insufficiency and aortic valve stenosis and insufficiency can also occur in these patients.

Hughes SC, Levinson G, Rosen MA, eds. *Shnider and Levinson's anesthesia for obstetrics*, 4th ed. Philadelphia: Lippincott Williams & Wilkins, 2002:456.

Mandell GL, Bennett JE, Dolan R. *Principles and practice of infectious diseases*, 6th ed. Philadelphia: Churchill Livingstone, 2005:2380.

A.16. What are the physiologic consequences of mitral stenosis?

The normal mitral valve orifice area is 4 to 6 cm^2. With mitral stenosis, the valve area is reduced. When the valve area reaches 2 cm^2, cardiovascular hemodynamics become impaired. As the area decreases further to 1 cm^2, left atrial pressure increases to approximately 25 mm Hg to maintain an adequate cardiac output. Left ventricular diastolic pressure is usually normal, and the diastolic atrioventricular pressure gradient is the hemodynamic hallmark of this condition. Pulmonary venous and capillary pressures increase, leading to exertional dyspnea. If pulmonary capillary pressure exceeds blood oncotic pressure, pulmonary edema can develop. Pulmonary hypertension can result from elevated left atrial pressure and pulmonary arteriolar constriction. If severe pulmonary hypertension develops, right-sided heart failure can occur. Factors that may increase pulmonary pressure include tachycardia, increased cardiac output, and atrial fibrillation.

Brady K, Duff P. Rheumatic heart disease in pregnancy. *Clin Obstet Gynecol* 1989;32:21.

Burrow GN, Duffy TP, eds. *Medical complications during pregnancy*, 5th ed. Philadelphia: WB Saunders, 1999:119–120.

Datta S, ed. *Anesthetic and obstetric management of high-risk pregnancy*, 3rd ed. New York: Springer-Verlag, 2004:180.

A.17. What are the ausculatory findings associated with mitral stenosis?

The first heart sound is increased. There may be an opening snap heard along the left sternal border. A diastolic rumbling murmur is present at the mitral area and may be best heard with the patient in the left lateral decubitus position.

Bickley LS, Hoekelman RA. *Bates' guide to physical examination and history taking*, 7th ed. Philadelphia: Lippincott Williams & Wilkins, 1999:331.

A.18. What may be seen on the electrocardiogram in patients with mitral stenosis?

There may be broadened diphasic P waves in lead V_1, which are indicative of left atrial enlargement. There may be signs of right-axis deviation and right ventricular hypertrophy. Atrial fibrillation may be present.

Dubin D. *Rapid interpretation of EKGs*, 5th ed. Tampa: Cover Publishing, 1996:159–162, 235–238.

A.19. What are the echocardiographic findings associated with mitral stenosis?

Two-dimensional (2D) echocardiography and Doppler ultrasonography are the mainstays of diagnosis and characterization of mitral stenosis. On 2D echo, the hallmark of mitral stenosis is thickening and restriction of motion of both mitral valve leaflets with the main process being fibrosis and fusion of the leaflets tips and proximal chordae. Early on due to inflammation and leaflet tip thickening which restricts tip but not leaflet motion, a characteristic "doming" of the valve occurs during diastole and the anterior leaflet has a "hockey stick" configuration (Fig. 42.1). As the stenosis progresses, the body of the leaflet may become involved and calcification can occur within the leaflets and on the subvalular apparatus including the chordae and papillary muscle tips. Left atrial enlargement can be seen. Pulmonary valve motion abnormalities and right ventricular enlargement may signify pulmonary hypertension. In addition to reduced excursion and thickening of the leaflets, M-mode echocardiography shows a decrease in the closure rate of the anterior mitral leaflet during early diastole; this results in a reduced E-F slope. M-mode and 2D echocardiography do not reliably predict the severity of mitral stenosis. In addition to determining the anatomic extent and severity of the lesion, Doppler echocardiography can assess the physiologic significance of the lesion. Doppler studies can provide an estimate of valve area that is within $\pm 0.4 \text{ cm}^2$ of those obtained by cardiac catheterization. During pregnancy, however,

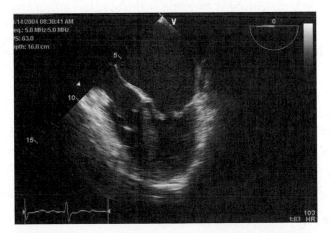

Figure 42.1 Two-dimensional echocardiography of the mitral valve showing severe mitral stenosis with the typical "hockey-stick" appearance.

mitral valve area calculations by Doppler may be inaccurate. Transesophageal echocardiography is helpful in assessing atrial thrombi.

Rokey R, Hsu HW, Moise KJ, et al. Inaccurate noninvasive mitral valve area calculation during pregnancy. *Obstet Gynecol* 1994;84:950.

Zipes DP, Libby P, Bonow RO, et al. eds. *Braunwald's heart disease:a textbook of cardiovascular medicine*, 7th ed. St. Louis: WB Saunders, 2005:212.

A.20. What is the effect of the physiologic changes of pregnancy on patients with mitral stenosis?

The increased physiologic cardiovascular load of pregnancy can cause patients to deteriorate and advance from one NYHA classification to another. With mild mitral stenosis, pregnancy is usually tolerated well. As the mitral valve area decreases to less than 1.5 cm^2, the pregnancy worsens the NYHA status by 1 to 2 classes.

Chestnut DH, ed. *Obstetric anesthesia: principles and practice*, 3rd ed. Philadelphia: Mosby, 2004:717.

A.21. If mitral stenosis is first recognized during pregnancy and symptoms develop, how would you treat the patient?

Heart rate reduction and a decreased left atrial pressure are the standard therapeutic goals for women with moderate to severe mitral stenosis. β-aderenergic receptor blockade is useful in preventing tachycardia. Atrial fibrillation of flutter should be treated aggressively; a rapid ventricular response compromises diastolic flow time and can lead to pulmonary edema. Emergency treatment includes digoxin, β-aderenergic receptor blockade and/or cardioversion if needed. Atrial fibrillation not only increases the risk of pulmonary edema but it also increases the likelihood of a thromboembolic event. Salt restriction and cautious use of diuretics can decrease left atrial pressure by decreasing blood volume. Avoidance of hypovolemia and decreased uteroplacental perfusion are essential.

If symptoms are uncontrolled by medical therapy, the mitral valve should be repaired or replaced. Percutaneous balloon valvuloplasty can be done using echocardiography or with appropriate radiation shielding of the fetus. For those with severe mitral stenosis, valve area less than 1 cm^2, surgical commissurotomy, or valve replacement has been done and is well tolerated by the mother, but fetal loss is high to greater than 30%.

Chambers CE, Clark SL. Cardiac surgery during pregnancy [Review]. *Clin Obstet Gynecol* 1994;37:316–323.

Datta S, ed. *Anesthetic and obstetric management of high-risk pregnancy*, 3rd ed. New York: Springer-Verlag, 2004:181.

Esteves CV, Auristela IOR, Braga SLN, et al. Effectiveness of percutaneous balloon mitral valvotomy during pregnancy. *Am J Cardiol* 1991;68:930–934.

A.22. What are the determinants of fetal oxygenation?

Fetal oxygenation is dependent on uteroplacental blood flow, oxygen-carrying capacity, oxygen affinity, arterial oxygen tension, placental diffusion capacity, placental vascular geometry, and placental oxygen consumption.

Hughes SC, Levinson G, Rosen MA, eds. *Shnider and Levinson's anesthesia for obstetrics*, 4th ed. Philadelphia: Lippincott Williams & Wilkins, 2002:24–25.

A.23. What are the determinants of uterine blood flow?

Uterine blood flow is derived from the Ohm's law, which states that pressure equals flow multiplied by resistance. Therefore, uterine blood flow is shown as follows:

$$\text{Uterine blood flow} = \frac{\text{uterine artery pressure} - \text{uterine venous pressure}}{\text{uterine artery resistance}}$$

Normally, 10% of maternal cardiac output goes to the uterus. Of this, the placenta receives 80%, and the myometrium receives the rest. Uterine blood flow is directly related to blood pressure; the uterine vessels do not autoregulate.

Hughes SC, Levinson G, Rosen MA, eds. *Shnider and Levinson's anesthesia for obstetrics*, 4th ed. Philadelphia: Lippincott Williams & Wilkins, 2002:22–23.

B. Preoperative Evaluation and Preparation

B.1. How is fetal well-being assessed during labor?

Fetal well-being is dependent on an intact uteroplacental unit. Simultaneous monitoring of fetal heart rate (FHR) and uterine contractions aids in the detection of fetal distress.

B.2. How are fetal heart rate (FHR) and maternal contractions monitored?

FHR can be monitored noninvasively using the Doppler technique or invasively using a fetal scalp electrode. Uterine contractions may be monitored noninvasively by a tocodynamometer, which measures the tightening of maternal abdominal muscles, or invasively by a transcervical pressure catheter hooked to a strain gauge.

Gabbe SG, Niebyl JR, Simpson JL, eds. *Obstetrics–normal and problem pregnancies*, 4th ed. New York: Churchill Livingstone, 2002:395–400.

B.3. What is the normal fetal heart rate (FHR) with beat-to-beat variability?

The normal FHR is 120 to 160 beats per minute with beat-to-beat variability. Abnormalities in FHR such as bradycardia, tachycardia, dysrhythmias, decreased or absent beat-to-beat variability, or transient decelerations can be a sign of fetal asphyxia.

Gabbe SG, Niebyl JR, Simpson JL, eds. *Obstetrics–normal and problem pregnancies*, 4th ed. New York: Churchill Livingstone, 2002:400–405.

B.4. What are transient or periodic decelerations?

Transient or periodic decelerations in FHR fall into the following three categories depending on their shape and timing with respect to maternal contractions (Fig. 42.2).

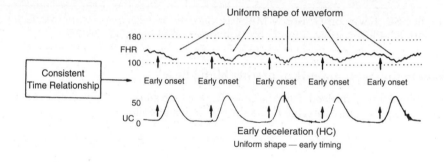

Early deceleration (HC)
Uniform shape — early timing

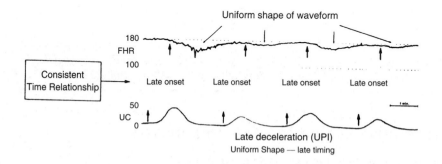

Late deceleration (UPI)
Uniform Shape — late timing

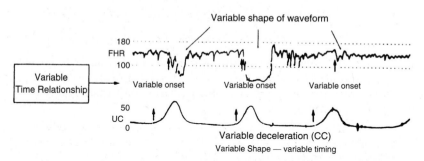

Variable deceleration (CC)
Variable Shape — variable timing

Figure 42.2 Fetal heart rate decelerations in relation to the time of onset of uterine contractions. (From Hon EH. *An atlas of fetal heart rate patterns.* New Haven: Harty Press, 1968, with permission.)

- Early, or type 1, decelerations are uniform FHR decreases that coincide with the onset, peak, and end of uterine contraction. This is a vagal response caused by fetal head compression and is usually not associated with fetal hypoxia.
- Late, or type 2, decelerations are a gradual decrease in FHR that begins after the onset of a contraction and lasts beyond the end of the contraction. They indicate uteroplacental insufficiency and require prompt evaluation and treatment.
- Variable, or type 3, decelerations occur variably and usually abruptly in relationship to contractions. They usually result from umbilical cord compression. Variable decelerations are further classified, depending on degree and duration, into mild, moderate, and severe categories.

Mild variable decelerations

- Usually insignificant
- FHR more than 80 beats per minute, or
- Any FHR deceleration lasting less than 30 seconds

Moderate variable decelerations

- May signify mild hypoxia
- FHR less than 70 beats per minute for 30 to 60 seconds
- FHR 70 to 80 beats per minute lasting more than 30 seconds

Severe variable decelerations

- Can indicate frank fetal acidosis
- FHR less than 70 beats per minute lasting more than 60 seconds

---

Cunningham FG, Leveno KJ, Bloom SL, et al. eds. *Williams Obstetrics*, 22nd ed. New York: McGraw-Hill, 2005:451–457.

Hughes SC, Levinson G, Rosen MA, eds. *Shnider and Levinson's anesthesia for obstetrics*, 4th ed. Philadelphia: Lippincott Williams & Wilkins, 2002:623–633.

B.5. How accurate is fetal heart rate (FHR) monitoring in predicting fetal well-being?

If the FHR tracing is normal, 99% of the time, the fetus is not depressed, as exhibited by a 5-minute Apgar score of more than 6. In contrast, however, if the FHR tracing is abnormal, in 50% of cases, the infants are normal and have no umbilical cord acidosis.

Uncertainty about diagnosing fetal distress from FHR patterns has given rise to the descriptions of these patterns as reassuring or nonreassuring. These fetal assessments are subjective clinical judgments. After more than 30 years of FHR pattern interpretation, there is finally some evidence emerging that certain combinations can be used meaningfully to identify normal and severely abnormal fetuses. True fetal distress patterns seem to be those where there is no beat-to-beat variability in conjunction with severe decelerations, persistent baseline rate changes, or both.

Cunningham FG, Leveno KJ, Bloom SL, et al. eds. *Williams Obstetrics*, 22nd ed. New York: McGraw-Hill, 2005:461.

Gabbe SG, Niebyl JR, Simpson JL, eds. *Obstetrics–normal and problem pregnancies*, 4th ed. New York: Churchill Livingstone, 2002:415–416.

Low JA, Mc Grath MJ, Marshall SJ, et al. The relationship between antepartum fetal heart rate, intrapartum fetal heart rate, and fetal acid-base status. *Am J Obstet Gynecol* 1986; 154(4):769–776.

Paul RH, Suidan AK, Yeh S-Y, et al. Clinical fetal monitoring, VII: the evaluation and significance of intra-partum baseline FHR variability. *Am J Obstet Gynceol* 1975;123(2): 206–210.

Schifrin BS, Dame L. Fetal heart rate patterns: prediction of Apgar score. *JAMA* 1972; 219(10):1322–1325.

B.6. In the fetus with a nonreassuring fetal heart rate (FHR) pattern, what other modalities can be used to assess whether hypoxia has led to acidosis? What are the normal values of fetal blood gases?

Fetal scalp capillary blood pH, FHR accelerations and fetal pulse oximetry are additional methods to assess fetal well-being. Significant fetal hypoxia leads to anaerobic metabolism and systemic fetal acidosis. There is a positive correlation of fetal scalp capillary blood pH with umbilical vein and artery pH. Fetal capillary blood pH values of 7.25 or more are normal, a pH value of 7.20 to 7.24 is classified as preacidotic, and a pH value less than 7.20 is considered acidotic, in which case delivery of the fetus should be performed immediately. Both pH and should be obtained to determine if the acidosis is metabolic or respiratory. Pco_2 determination is especially important when doing scalp sampling for variable decelerations because in this situation most acidosis is respiratory in origin. Fetal scalp capillary blood pH samples were obtained when FHR tracings were abnormal, because ominous FHR tracings are only associated with acidosis 48% of the time. Obviously, one must have access to the fetal scalp for fetal scalp sampling; therefore, this tool is not useful in abnormal presentations or placenta previa. In practice, fetal scalp sampling is being used less frequently because of the technical difficulties associated with it and the appreciation of the utility of FHR accelerations and beat-to-beat variability for predicting the presence or absence of acidosis.

In the fetus with a nonreassuring FHR tracing, any spontaneous or induced, that is, scalp or vibroacoustic stimulation, FHR accelerations indicate the absence of acidosis. The application of the interpretation of FHR accelerations should be restricted to the fetus with an otherwise nonreassuring FHR pattern.

Fetal pulse oximetry is a newer modality that is not widely used and has technical limitations. However, an oxygen saturation greater than 30% indicates that the fetus is not acidotic.

When the fetus has a persistently nonreassuring FHR pattern and backup methods do not provide reassurance, the delivery of the fetus should be immediate.

Normally, umbilical artery blood has the following characteristics:

- pH value, 7.28 ± 0.05
- Pco_2, 49.2 ± 8.4 mm Hg
- Po_2, 18.0 ± 6.2 mm Hg
- Bicarbonate, 22.3 ± 2.5 mEq per L

Umbilical vein blood has the following characteristics:

- pH, 7.35 ± 0.05
- Pco_2, 38.2 ± 5.6 mm Hg
- Po_2, 29.2 ± 5.9 mm Hg
- Bicarbonate, 20.4 ± 2.1 mEq per L

Bowe ET, Beard RW, Finster M, et al. Reliability of fetal blood sampling. Maternal fetal relationships. *Am J Obstet Gynecol* 1970;107:279–287.

Cunningham FG, Leveno KJ, Bloom SL, et al. eds. *Williams Obstetrics*, 22nd ed. New York: McGraw-Hill, 2005:457–460.

Gabbe SG, Niebyl JR, Simpson JL, eds. *Obstetrics–normal and problem pregnancies*, 4th ed. New York: Churchill Livingstone, 2002:419.

Goodwin TM, Milner-Masterson L, Paul RH. Elimination of fetal scalp blood sampling on a large clinical service. *Obstet Gynecol* 1994;83:971.

Low JA, Cox MJ, Karchmar EJ, et al. The prediction of intrapartum fetal metabolic acidosis by fetal heart rate monitoring. *Am J Obstet Gynecol* 1981;139(3):299–305.

Tejani N, Mann LI, Bhakthavathsalan A, et al. Correlation of fetal heart rate-uterine contraction patterns with fetal scalp blood pH. *Obstet Gynecol* 1975;46(4):392–396.

Yeoman ER, Hauth JC, Gilstrap LC III et al. Umbilical cord pH, Pco_2 and bicarbonate following uncomplicated term vaginal deliveries. *Am J Obstet Gynecol* 1985;151:798.

B.7. Can fetal scalp capillary blood pH sampling give false signals?

Yes. Sometimes depressed neonates can occur despite a normal fetal scalp capillary blood pH because of maternal alkalosis and/or drug effects. Conversely, with a low fetal scalp capillary blood pH, infants can be normal and well oxygenated if there is maternal acidosis or local scalp effects.

Bowen LW, Kochenour NK, Rehm NE, et al. Maternal-fetal pH difference and fetal scalp pH as predictors of neonatal outcome. *Obstet Gynecol* 1986;67(4):487–495.

Roversi GD, Canussio V, Spennacchio M. Recognition and significance of maternogenic fetal acidosis during intensive monitoring of labor. *J Perinat Med* 1975;3(1):53–67.

Seeds AE. Maternal-fetal acid-base relationships and fetal scalp-blood analysis. *Clin Obstet Gynecol* 1978;21(2):579–591.

B.8. What are the causes of acute fetal distress?

Uteroplacental dysfunction, umbilical cord compression, and uterine hypertonus are causes of acute fetal distress. Some causes of uteroplacental insufficiency include maternal hypotension, placental abruption, and pregnancy-induced hypertension. Umbilical cord compression can be secondary to umbilical cord prolapse and/or oligohydramnios. Uterine hypertonus or tetany may signify dehydration or hyperstimulation by parenteral oxytocin.

Cunningham FG, Leveno KJ, Bloom SL, et al, eds. *Williams Obstetrics*, 22nd ed. New York: McGraw-Hill, 2005:451–466.

Hughes SC, Levinson G, Rosen MA, eds. *Shnider and Levinson's anesthesia for obstetrics*, 4th ed. Philadelphia: Lippincott Williams & Wilkins, 2002:623–633.

B.9. What is the significance of meconium-stained amniotic fluid?

Although meconium staining occurs in 12% to 22% of all deliveries, most of the infants are not depressed; there is a high false-positive rate and low sensitivity for acidemia.

The physiology of meconium passage and its adverse sequelae are incompletely understood. Three theories have been suggested to explain the passage of meconium by the fetus, and the wide differences in the proposed theories may help explain the tenuous connection between meconium detection and infant mortality. The pathologic explanation proposes that in response to hypoxia the fetus passes meconium and that meconium, therefore, signals fetal compromise. Alternatively, *in utero* passage of meconium may indicate normal gastrointestinal tract maturation under neural control. A third alternative suggests that passage of meconium follows vagal stimulation from common but transient umbilical cord entrapment and resultant peristalsis.

Ramin et al. suggest that the high incidence of meconium in amniotic fluid during labor often represents a normal physiologic process. This meconium, however, becomes an environmental hazard when fetal acidemia occurs. Importantly, because acidemia occurs acutely, meconium aspiration is unpredicatable and likely, unpreventable. Greenwood et al. looked at women with clear amniotic fluid and emphasized that clear fluid is an unreliable sign of fetal well-being.

Evidence is accumulating that many infants with meconium aspiration syndrome have suffered hypoxia before birth. Blackwell et al. found that 60% of the infants with meconium aspiration syndrome had umbilical artery blood pH greater than or equal to 7.20; this suggests that this syndrome was unrelated to the neonates condition at delivery. Meconium aspiration syndrome is more likely when the meconium is thick, the pregnancy is postterm or the fetus is growth-restricted.

Blackwell SC, Moldenhauer J, Hassan SS, et al. Meconium aspiration syndrome in term neonates with normal acid-base status at delivery: is it different?. *Am J Obstet Gynecol* 2001;184:1422.

Cunningham FG, Leveno KJ, Bloom SL, et al. eds. *Williams Obstetrics*, 22nd ed. New York: McGraw-Hill, 2005:461, 675.

Greenwood C, Lalchandani S, MacQuillan K, et al. Meconium passed in labor: how reassuring is clear amniotic fluid?. *Obstet Gynecol* 2003;102:89.

Miller FC, Sacks DA, Yeh SY, et al. Significance of meconium during labor. *Am J Obstet Gynecol* 1975;122(5):573–580.

Ramin KD, Leveno KJ, Kelly MS, et al. Amniotic fluid meconium: a fetal environmental hazard. *Obstet Gynecol* 1996;87:181.

B.10. What is meconium aspiration syndrome?

Of the 10% to 15% of births with meconium-stained amniotic fluid, 5% of the infants develop meconium aspiration pneumonia. Of these infants, 30% require mechanical ventilation, and 3% to 5% may die.

Meconium is a combination of swallowed amniotic fluid, fetal hair, and gastrointestinal cells and secretions. Meconium aspiration syndrome is characterized by respiratory distress with a low lung compliance and a marked mismatch of ventilation to perfusion. Pneumothorax and/or pneumomediastinum are complications. With severe disease, pulmonary hypertension leading to persistent fetal circulation can occur.

Behrman RE, Kliegman RM, Jensen HB, eds. *Nelson textbook of pediatrics*, 17th ed. Philadelphia: WB Saunders, 2004:583.

B.11. What are the usual noninvasive tests used to evaluate the pregnant cardiac patient?

Physical examination, exercise tolerance test, chest roentgenograph using appropriate protective radiation sheilding, electrocardiogram (ECG), pulse oximeter oxygen saturation, Holter monitoring, and echocardiography with Doppler flow studies may all be useful in evaluating these patients. With less than 5 rads of radiation exposure, the risk of fetal anomalies is low; radiation exposure with a chest roentgenograph is approximately 20 millirads.

Zipes DP, Libby P, Bonow RO, et al. *Braunwald's heart disease:a textbook of cardiovascular medicine*, 7th ed. St. Louis: WB Saunders, 2005:1966.

B.12. What preoperative medications would you give this patient?

Recommendations for antibiotic prophylaxis against endocarditis are dependant on the cardiac lesion and the procedure being performed. As recommended by the American Heart Association, patients with acquired valvular dysfunction are at moderate risk for endocarditis, and endocarditis prophylaxis is not recommended for cesarean section or uncomplicated vaginal delivery in the moderate risk patient. If these patients were undergoing a procedure where antibiotic prophylaxis was recommended, such as dental extractions, the suggested prophylaxis is amoxicillin 2 g orally 1 hour before the procedure or ampicillin, 2 g intramuscularly (IM) or intravenously (IV), within 30 minutes of starting the procedure. For high-risk patients, such as those with a history of bacterial endocarditis, prosthetic cardiac valves, surgically constructed cardiac shunts, etc., the standard regimen is ampicillin, 2 g IV, and gentamicin, 1.5 mg per kg IV, given 60 minutes prior to starting the procedure followed 6 hours later by 1 g ampicillin IV or amoxicillin 1 g orally. Because of the difficulties in predicting complicated deliveries and the potentially devastating consequences of endocarditis, the need antibiotic prophylaxis should be individualized based on the above recommendations.

Pregnancy itself may not decrease gastric emptying, but during labor, gastric motility does decrease. Patients are considered at risk for aspiration pneumonitis if gastric volume exceeds 25 mL (0.4 mL/kg) and the pH level is less than 2.5. Gastric fluid volume and pH are not different in the pregnant patient versus their nonpregnant counterparts. Pregnant patients, however, are considered to be at an increased risk for aspiration of gastric contents. This is thought to be due to a decrease in lower esophageal sphincter tone, changes in the gastroesophageal junction angle and an increased risk of having difficulty with intubation. Although the exact time at which the risk increases is unclear, it seems prudent to consider the pregnant patient to have an increased risk for aspiration of gastric contents after 16 to 20 weeks' gestation. In this patient for emergency cesarean, an oral nonparticulate antacid such as 15 to 30 mL of 0.3 M sodium citrate given immediately before induction reduces the risk of developing aspiration pneumonitis. Ranitidine, cimetidine, and metoclopramide may also decrease this risk but require more time to be effective.

Chestnut DH, ed. *Obstetric anesthesia: principles and practice*, 3rd ed. Philadelphia: Mosby, 2004:256.

Dajani AS, Taubert KA, Wilson W, et al. Prevention of bacterial endocarditis: recommendations by the American Heart Association. *JAMA* 1997;277(22):1794.

Gabbe SG, Niebyl JR, Simpson JL, eds. *Obstetrics–normal and problem pregnancies*, 4th ed. New York: Churchill Livingstone, 2002:1010.

Goodman S. Anesthesia for nonobstetric surgery in the pregnant patient. *Semin Perinatol* 2002;26(2):136.

Kaplan EL, Bisplo A, Derrick W, et al. Prevention of rheumatic fever. *Circulation* 1977;55:1.

Hughes SC, Levinson G, Rosen MA, eds. *Shnider and Levinson's anesthesia for obstetrics*, 4th ed. Philadelphia: Lippincott Williams & Wilkins, 2002:391–393.

Zipes DP, Libby P, Bonow RO, et al. *Braunwald's heart disease:a textbook of cardiovascular medicine*, 7th ed. St. Louis, WB Saunders, 2005:1969.

C. Intraoperative Management

C.1. What monitors would you use in this functional New York Heart Association (NYHA) Class II patient during her cesarean section?

All pregnant cardiac patients should be monitored with an electrocardiogram (ECG), blood pressure monitoring, pulse oximetry, precordial or esophageal stethoscope, temperature monitor, Foley catheter, end-tidal carbon dioxide monitor (if general anesthesia), and neuromuscular blockage monitor (if general anesthesia).

C.2. When would you use invasive monitoring in a pregnant patient with cardiac disease?

New York Heart Association (NYHA) class I and II patients do not routinely require invasive hemodynamic monitoring. However, patients with class III and IV status are usually monitored with an intraarterial line for serial arterial blood gas determinations and continuous blood pressure monitoring. Additionally, central venous pressure (CVP) monitoring and pulmonary artery catheter placement are often used. Unlike CVP monitoring, the pulmonary artery catheter allows you to obtain added information on pulmonary artery pressure, pulmonary artery occlusion pressure, and thermodilution cardiac output.

Chestnut DH, ed. *Obstetric anesthesia: principles and practice*, 3rd ed. Philadelphia: Mosby, 2004:717.

Zipes DP, Libby P, Bonow RO, et al. eds. *Braunwald's heart disease: a textbook of cardiovascular medicine*, 7th ed. St. Louis, WB Saunders, 2005:1972.

C.3. What are the hemodynamic goals of intraoperative management of the pregnant patient with mitral stenosis?

- Avoid tachycardia.
- Maintain sinus rhythm.
- Avoid marked decreases in systemic vascular resistance.
- Avoid marked increases in central blood volume.
- Avoid increases in pulmonary vascular resistance.

Increased heart rates should be avoided because decreases in the amount of diastolic time for blood to flow across the stenotic mitral valve can lead to pulmonary edema and a decreased cardiac output. Atrial fibrillation with a rapid ventricular response similarly can result in cardiac decompensation, and the loss of atrial contraction is detrimental. Marked decreases in systemic vascular resistance should be avoided because compensatory increases in heart rate can result. Elevation of pulmonary vascular resistance, as can occur with hypercarbia, hypoxia, and acidosis, is also poorly tolerated by these patients.

Datta S, ed. *Anesthetic and obstetric management of high-risk pregnancy*, 3rd ed. New York: Springer-Verlag, 2004:181.

Hughes SC, Levinson G, Rosen MA, eds. *Shnider and Levinson's anesthesia for obstetrics*, 4th ed. Philadelphia: Lippincott Williams & Wilkins, 2002:456–460.

C.4. What anesthetic technique would you use for this emergency cesarean section?

The choices of anesthetic techniques for cesarean section are regional, spinal or epidural, or general anesthesia. In this case, a general anesthetic would be the anesthetic of choice. General anesthesia has a rapid onset, which is necessary because of fetal distress. In addition, if the patient has not been adequately hydrated with an intravenous crystalloid solution before a rapid regional anesthetic induction, the resulting decrease in systemic vascular resistance, hypotension, and reflex tachycardia can exacerbate fetal distress and lead to maternal cardiac decompensation in the patient with mitral stenosis. In the nonemergent setting, patients with mitral stenosis do well with epidural anesthesia for their vaginal delivery or cesarean section. Combined spinal-epidural analgesia has also been used successfully in these patients during vaginal delivery.

Chestnut DH, ed. *Obstetric anesthesia: principles and practice*, 3rd ed. Philadelphia: Mosby, 2004:718.

Hughes SC, Levinson G, Rosen MA, eds. *Shnider and Levinson's anesthesia for obstetrics*, 4th ed. Philadelphia: Lippincott Williams & Wilkins, 2002:460.

C.5. What technique could you use for this general anesthesia?

- Intravenous crystalloid solution through a large-bore cannula (if not already present) could be used.
- Place the patient on the table in the supine position with left lateral tilt to avoid aortocaval compression.
- Preoxygenate the mother and place monitors on her quickly. Preoxygenation may be accomplished by allowing her to breathe 100% oxygen by face mask for 3 to 5 minutes or to take four maximally deep inspirations if time is limited.
- After abdominal preparation and draping, perform a rapid sequence induction using thiopental sodium, 4 mg per kg, and succinylcholine, 1 mg per kg. Ketamine should be avoided because it can increase heart rate. Pregnant women do not experience severe fasciculations, so a defasciculatory dose of nondepolarizing muscle relaxant is not necessary to prevent a rise in intragastric pressure. Depending on the severity, mitral stenosis patients may benefit from a β-adrenergic receptor antagonist, such as esmolol, or a modest dose of opiod before or during induction of general anesthesia. Remember to inform the neonatologist in the delivery room about the medications that the mother has received.
- Endotracheal intubation: Mucosal swelling and capillary engorgement can make intubation more difficult. A smaller endotracheal tube, such as a 7-mm internal diameter (ID) tube, should be used. Cricoid pressure is maintained until the endotracheal tube cuff is inflated and the position checked. Cricoid pressure effectively prevents regurgitation with gastric pressures as high as 50 to 94 cm H_2O.
- Maintenance of anesthesia before the baby is delivered involves the following: N_2O with at least 50% oxygen, volatile anesthetic agent (e.g., 0.5% halothane or 1% sevoflurane), and muscle relaxant as needed (mivacurium, vecuronium, or cisatracurium). Isoflurane and desflurane probably should be avoided in this patient because they may cause tachycardia. Eucapnea should be maintained.
- Maintenance of anesthesia after the baby is delivered no longer requires fetal consideration. A narcotic technique can be implemented using, for instance, fentanyl, midazolam, muscle relaxant, nitrous oxide, and oxygen.
- After the delivery of newborn, be aware that bolus administration of either oxytocin, methylergonovine or 15-methyl prostaglandin F2-α can increase pulmonary vascular resistance.
- Extubation of the patient is done after her protective laryngeal reflexes have returned and the patient has regained conciousness.

Chestnut DH, ed. *Obstetric anesthesia: principles and practice*, 3rd ed. Philadelphia: Mosby, 2004:718.

Fanning GL. The efficacy of cricoid pressure in regurgitation of gastric contents. *Anesthesiology* 1970;32:553.

Hughes SC, Levinson G, Rosen MA, eds. *Shnider and Levinson's anesthesia for obstetrics*, 4th ed. Philadelphia: Lippincott Williams & Wilkins, 2002:223, 226.

Norris MC, Dewan DM. Preoxygenation for cesarean section. A comparison of two techniques. *Anesthesiology* 1985;62:827.

Thind GS, Bryson THL. Single dose suxamethonium and muscle pain in pregnancy. *Br J Anaesth* 1983;55:743.

C.6. If you had unexpectedly been unable to intubate this patient, how would you have managed the airway?

Figure 42.3 shows one way to deal with the failed intubation in the obstetric patient with an unrecognized difficult airway. However, other anesthetic techniques may be used. For instance,

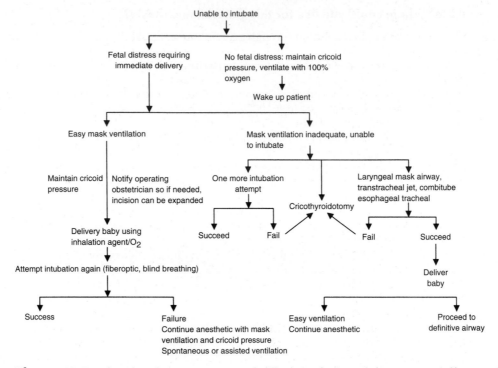

Figure 42.3 Algorithm for management of difficult intubation. If the surgeon infiltrates region with local anesthetic, it will decrease your general anesthetic requirement.

some would let the patient breathe spontaneously, and others would paralyze the patient while continuing mask ventilation. Remember that like face mask ventilation, the laryngeal mask airway does not prevent aspiration. The mother's life should not be endangered to deliver a distressed fetus. Calling for help when difficulties arise is wise.

Barker P, Langeton JA, Murphy PJ, et al. Regurgitation of gastric contents during general anesthesia using the laryngeal mask airway. *Br J Anaesth* 1992;69:314.

Benumof JL. The ASA difficult airway algorithm: new thoughts/considerations. In: *ASA refresher course lectures*. American Society of Anesthesiologists, 1995:253.

Benumof JL. Laryngeal mask airway and the ASA difficult airway algorithm. *Anesthesiology* 1996;84:686.

Green KS, Berger TH. Proper use of the combitube. *Anesthesiology* 1994;81:513.

C.7. Would this patient benefit from the use of β-blockade?

This patient is asymptomatic, and the β-blockade is unnecessary at this point. However, if compromising tachycardia should occur, β-blockade with drugs such as propanolol, atenolol, or esmolol may be useful, as may digoxin or cardioversion depending on her dysrhythmia.

In patients with mitral stenosis, it is important to prevent tachycardia. Al Kasab et al. have shown that pregnant patients with symptomatic mitral stenosis who receive β-blockade with propanolol or atenolol have a significant decrease in the incidence of pulmonary edema with no adverse neonatal side effects.

Al Kasab SM, Sabag T, Zaibag MA, et al. β-Adrenergic receptor blockage in the management of pregnant women with mitral stenosis. *Am J Obstet Gynecol* 1990;163:37.

C.8. What is the effect of the inhalation agents on uterine contractility?

If less than one minimum alveolar concentration of a potent volatile inhalation agent, such as isoflurane or sevoflurane, is used, there is no increase in blood loss or decrease in uterine contractility, because at these low concentrations, the uterus still responds to oxytocin. At higher concentrations, the uterine contractility is decreased and blood loss is increased.

Munson ES, Embro WJ. Enflurane, isoflurane and halothane and isolated human uterine muscle. *Anesthesiology* 1977;46:11.

Tjeuw MTB, Yao FS, Van Poznak A. Depressant effects of anesthetics on isolated human gravid and nongravid uterine muscle. *Chinese Med J* 1986;99(3):235–242.

Warren TM, Datta S, Ostheimer GW, et al. Comparison of the maternal and neonatal effects of halothane, enflurane and isoflurane for cesarean delivery. *Anesth Analg* 1983;62:516.

C.9. What is the Apgar scoring system?

The Apgar scoring system is used in the delivery to assess the neonate's condition at 1 minute and 5 minutes. Each of five categories is given a rating of 0 to 2, and the final score at each time is the sum of the individual category scores. Ten points is the best possible neonatal Apgar score (Table 42.1).

Apgar V. A proposal for a new method of evaluation of the newborn infant. *Curr Res Anesth Analg* 1953;32:260.

C.10. What is the significance of the Apgar scores?

Overall, Apgar scores qualitatively measure basic neurologic reflexes and correlate with generalized neonatal depression. They only loosely correlate with acidosis and asphyxia. Apgar scores aid in predicting mortality but poorly predict morbidity; the longer the Apgar score is low, the higher the neonatal mortality.

Table 42.1 Apgar Scoring System.

MNEMONIC	SIGN	SCORE		
		0	**1**	**2**
A	Appearance (color)	Blue, pale	Body pink, extremities blue	Pink
P	Pulse	Absent	< 100/ min	>100/ min
G	Grimace (reflex irritability; response to catheter in the nose)	Absent	Grimace	Cough, sneeze
A	Activity (muscle tone)	Limp	Some extremity flexion	Active motion
R	Respiratory effect	Absent	Slow, irregular	Good cry

Glodenberg RL, Huddelston JF, Nelson KG. Apgar scores and umbilical arterial pH in preterm newborn infants. *Am J Obstet Gynecol* 1984;149(6):651.

Low JA, Mc Grath MJ, Marshall SJ, et al. The relationship between antepartum fetal heart rate, intrapartum fetal heart rate, and fetal acid-base status. *Am J Obstet Gynecol* 1986;154(4):769.

Silverman F, Suidan J, Wasserman J, et al. The Apgar score: is it enough? *Obstet Gynecol* 1985;66(3):331.

C.11. At birth, what should be done to minimize the infant's risk of meconium aspiration syndrome?

It is agreed that the obstetrician should suction the mouth and nose of the newborn before the infant's first breath and the delivery of its shoulders. Depressed newborns and/or those with signs of airway obstruction should have endotracheal intubation and suctioning. Experts also recommend that vigorous newborns with meconium exposure not be intubated and suctioned.

Behrman RE, Kliegman RM, Jensen HB, eds. *Nelson textbook of pediatrics*, 17th ed. Philadelphia: WB Saunders, 2004:583.

Cunningham A, Lawson E, Martin E, et al. Tracheal suction and meconium: a proposed standard of care. *J Pediatr* 1990;116(1):153–154.

Linder N, Aranda JV, Tsur M, et al. Need for endotracheal intubation and suction in meconium-stained neonates. *J Pediatr* 1988;112:613.

Yoder BA. Meconium-stained amniotic fluid and respiratory complications: impact of selective tracheal suction. *Obstet Gynecol* 1994;83:77.

C.12. The Apgar score of the newborn was 3 at 1 minute. How would you treat the newborn?

In addition to minimizing heat loss and upper airway suctioning, this newborn is moderately depressed with the Apgar score of 3 or 4 and requires oxygen with positive pressure ventilation through face mask and nonrebreathing bag. If clinical improvement is not prompt, then endotracheal intubation should be undertaken. If ventilation with 100% oxygen does not lead to improvement, umbilical vessel catheterization and appropriate fluid and drug administration is required.

Levthner SR, Jansen RD, Hageman JR. Cardiopulmonary resuscitation of the newborn. *Pediatr Clin North America* 1994;41:893.

D. Postoperative Management

D.1. Immediately after the baby was delivered, the patient's oxygen saturation decreased. What is the differential diagnosis?

- Mechanical problems with the endotracheal tube
- Cardiac decompensation with pulmonary edema
- Pulmonary venous embolism: air, amniotic, thrombotic

Brady K, Dugg P. Rheumatic heart disease in pregnancy. *Clin Obstet Gynecol* 1989; 32:21.

Fong J, Gadalla R, Pierri MK, et al. Are Doppler-detected venous emboli during cesarean section air emboli? *Anesth Analg* 1990;71:254.

CHAPTER 43

Appendectomy for a Pregnant Patient

Farida Gadalla

A 25-YEAR-OLD WOMAN

at 32 weeks' gestation presented to the emergency room with vague right abdominal pain. She had lost her appetite and had two episodes of vomiting. Temperature was 37.5°C (99.5°F), pulse 100 beats per minute, hematocrit 34%, and white blood cell (WBC) count 15,000/μL.

A. Medical Disease and Differential Diagnosis

1. What is the differential diagnosis for this patient?
2. How would you attempt to make the diagnosis of acute appendicitis clinically?
3. What is the incidence of appendicitis during pregnancy?
4. Why is the incidence of gangrenous appendix higher in pregnant than in nonpregnant women?
5. What is Alders' sign?
6. What is the incidence of perforation of the appendix and in which trimester is it most likely to occur?
7. What is the incidence of surgery during pregnancy?
8. What are the main concerns associated with nonobstetric surgery in the pregnant patient?
9. What are the factors influencing teratogenicity in mammals? Discuss the teratogenicity of anesthetic agents.
10. Discuss the U.S. Food and Drug Administration (FDA) fetal risk categories for therapeutic agents and classify the most commonly used anesthetic agents.
11. How would you prevent intrauterine fetal asphyxia?
12. Although this patient presented with an acute abdomen, what is the major reason for nonobstetric surgical intervention in the pregnant patient?

B. Preoperative Evaluation and Preparation

1. What would you discuss with this patient preoperatively?
2. Is there a difference in the aim of anesthesia for delivery and for nonobstetric surgery in a pregnant patient?
3. How would you premedicate this patient?

C. Intraoperative Management

1. What factors would alter your anesthetic technique from that used for a nonpregnant patient?

2. Describe your technique and dosage if you choose epidural anesthesia.
3. If the patient is in need of supplemental medication, what would be your choice?
4. What vasopressor would you choose to improve uteroplacental perfusion?
5. When this patient arrived in the operating room, she was panic stricken and desired a general anesthetic. Describe your technique.
6. Does any controversy exist surrounding the use of nitrous oxide?
7. What is the incidence of fetal loss and what factors influence it?
8. If the patient was having surgery on her hand, what would you do differently?
9. What would you expect to see on the fetal monitor during an isoflurane-nitrous oxide-oxygen anesthetic?
10. The surgeon schedules the procedure as a laparoscopic one. Does this pose any problems?

D. Postoperative Management

1. When would you extubate this patient?
2. What monitors would you use postoperatively?
3. What other precautions would you take postoperatively?
4. What is the incidence of preterm delivery following nonobstetric surgery during pregnancy?
5. The next day the patient went into premature labor having "failed" tocolytic therapy. She now needed a cesarean section for prematurity and breech presentation. She required another general anesthetic. In what way would your technique differ from your previous anesthetic technique?

A. Medical Disease and Differential Diagnosis

A.1. What is the differential diagnosis for this patient?

The differential diagnosis includes the following:

Medical Conditions
- Sickle cell disease
- Porphyria
- Glomerulonephritis
- Pyelonephritis
- Pneumonia
- Withdrawal from drug addition

Obstetric Conditions
- Labor
- Abruptio placentae
- Chorioamnionitis

Gynecologic Conditions
- Salpingitis
- Degenerating myoma
- Ovarian cyst or tumor, either torted or ruptured
- Tubo-ovarian abscess

Surgical Conditions
- Appendicitis
- Cholecystitis
- Pancreatitis

- Mesenteric adenitis
- Intestinal obstruction

Baden JM, Brodsky JB, eds. *The pregnant surgical patient*. Mt. Kisco: Futura Publishing, 1985:165–166.

Chestnut DH, ed. *Obstetric anesthesia: principle and practice*, 3rd ed. Mosby, 2004:265.

Weinold AB. Appendicitis in pregnancy. *Clin Obstet Gynecol* 1983;26:801.

A.2. How would you attempt to make the diagnosis of acute appendicitis clinically?

Diagnosis is based on a detailed history and the following symptoms:

- Vague abdominal pain, variable in position because of the growing uterus
- Anorexia
- Vomiting

The signs are the following:

- Abdominal tenderness
- Rebound pain
- Abdominal guarding
- Rectal tenderness
- Mildly elevated temperature, 37°C to 38°C (98.6°F to 100.4°F)
- Mildly elevated pulse rate
- An increase in white blood cell (WBC), although this is not useful because of the already existing relative leukocytosis in pregnancy.

Baden JM, Brodsky JB, eds. *The pregnant surgical patient*. Mt. Kisco: Futura Publishing, 1985:150.

Chestnut DH, ed. *Obstetric anesthesia: principle and practice*, 3rd ed. Mosby, 2004:265.

Weingold AB. Appendicitis in pregnancy. *Clin Obstet Gynecol* 1983;26:801.

A.3. What is the incidence of appendicitis during pregnancy?

Appendicitis is the most common surgical emergency during pregnancy. Incidence varies from 1:350 to 1:10,000. Appendicitis is the reason for approximately two thirds of the laparotomies performed during pregnancy.

Babaknia A, Parsa H, Woodruff JD. Appendicitis during pregnancy. *Obstet Gynecol* 1977; 50:40.

Weingold AB. Appendicitis in pregnancy. *Clin Obstet Gynecol* 1983;26:801.

A.4. Why is the incidence of gangrenous appendix higher in pregnant than in nonpregnant women?

The incidence of gangrenous appendix is higher during pregnancy because the enlarging uterus pushes the appendix away from the abdominal wall (Fig. 43.1), thereby causing the diseased appendix to produce little pain. This will delay the diagnosis and allow the appendix time to become gangrenous. Another factor contributing to the delay in diagnosis of a nonobstetric

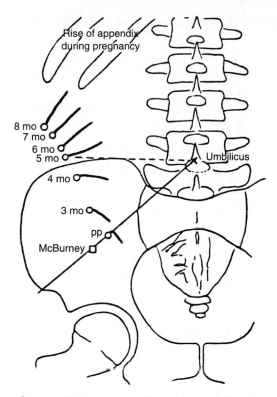

Figure 43.1 Changes in position and direction of the appendix during pregnancy. McBurney, McBurney's point; PP, prepregnancy. (From Baer JL, Reis RA, Arens RA. Appendicitis in pregnancy with changes in position and axis of normal appendix in pregnancy. *JAMA* 1932;98:1359, with permission.)

abdominal crisis is that useful diagnostic procedures such as radiography and laparoscopy are postponed because of concern for the fetus.

Baden JM, Brodsky JB, eds. *The pregnant surgical patient*. Mt. Kisco: Futura Publishing, 1985:150.

Weingold AB. Appendicitis in pregnancy. *Clin Obstet Gynecol* 1983;26:802.

A.5. What is Alders' sign?

Alders' sign is a clinical sign used to differentiate between uterine and appendiceal pain.

The pain is localized with the patient supine. The patient then lies on her left side. If the area of pain shifts to the left, it is presumed to be uterine.

Alders N. A sign for differentiating uterine from extrauterine complications of pregnancy. *Br Med J* 1951;2:1194.

A.6. What is the incidence of perforation of the appendix and in which trimester is it most likely to occur?

The incidence of perforation of the appendix is approximately 15%. Thirty percent of these occur in the first and second trimesters and 70% during the third trimester.

Weingold AB. Appendicitis in pregnancy. *Clin Obstet Gynecol* 1983;26:801.

A.7. What is the incidence of surgery during pregnancy?

The incidence of surgery is estimated at between 0.75% and 2.2%.

Baden JM, Brodsky JB, eds. *The pregnant surgical patient*. Mt. Kisco: Futura Publishing, 1985:223.

Mazze RI, Kallen B. Reproductive outcome after anesthesia and operations during pregnancy: a registry study of 5405 cases. *Am J Obstet Gynecol* 1989;16:1178–1185.

Shnider SM, Webster GM. Maternal and fetal hazards of surgery during pregnancy. *Am J Obstet Gynecol* 1965;92:891.

A.8. What are the main concerns associated with nonobstetric surgery in the pregnant patient?

The main concerns are maternal and fetal safety. To ensure maternal safety, awareness of the physiologic changes of the parturient is of great importance. Special care should be taken to prevent aspiration pneumonitis and supine hypotension syndrome. For fetal safety, it is essential to avoid teratogenic anesthetic agents and intrauterine fetal asphyxia.

Hawkins JL. Anesthesia for pregnant patient undergoing nonobstetric surgery. *ASA annual meeting refresher course lectures*. Park Ridge: American Society of Anesthesiologists, 2006:430.

Rosen MA. Management of anesthesia for the pregnant surgical patient. *Anesthesiology* 1999;91:1159–1163.

A.9. What are the factors influencing teratogenicity in mammals? Discuss the teratogenicity of anesthetic agents.

The factors influencing teratogenicity are genetic factors, nature, and dose of the anesthetic agent used, access of the agent to the fetus, and fetal developmental stage.

In this case, teratogenicity is unlikely because the most susceptible time in the human is that of organogenesis, between the 15th and the 30th day after conception; susceptibility declines thereafter to the 50th day. Almost all anesthetics are teratogenic in some animals. Before implantation of the ovum, teratogenicity leads to abortion. Later, malformation, functional deficiencies, and even death can occur. Large retrospective studies in the United States and United Kingdom suggest that female anesthesiologists and the wives of male anesthesiologists had significantly increased incidence of spontaneous abortion, and their children were more likely to have congenital anomalies than those of nonoperating room physicians. It has been suggested that chronic exposure to trace anesthetic gases was the causative factor. However, no documented reports are found of teratogenicity in humans ascribed to any anesthetic agent used during pregnancy. Nevertheless, we recommend that only time-tested anesthetics, instead of new agents, be used for the pregnant patient, especially in the first trimester of pregnancy.

Cohen EN, Bellville WJ, Brown BW Jr. Anesthesia, pregnancy, and miscarriage: a study of operating room nurses and anesthetists. *Anesthesiology* 1971;35:343.

Hawkins JL. Anesthesia for pregnant patient undergoing nonobstetric surgery. *ASA annual meeting refresher course lectures*. Park Ridge: American Society of Anesthesiologists, 2006:430.

Rosen MA. Management of anesthesia for the pregnant surgical patient. *Anesthesiology* 1999;91:1159–1163.

A.10. Discuss the U.S. Food and Drug Administration (FDA) fetal risk categories for therapeutic agents and classify the most commonly used anesthetic agents.

The FDA Fetal-risk Categories for Therapeutic Agents are the following:

- *Category A:* Controlled studies have shown no risk to the fetus during the first trimester and later trimesters as well. Risk is remote (e.g., water).
- *Category B:* Animal studies have demonstrated no fetal risk, but no controlled studies have been performed in humans. Animal studies have shown adverse fetal effects, but these results were not confirmed in controlled human studies. No risk is evident after the first trimester.
- *Category C:* Either studies have shown fetal risk in animals (teratogenic or embryocidal), but no controlled human studies have been performed, or there are no available data in humans or animals for an agent. Drugs of this class should be given only if the benefits outweigh the risks.
- *Category D:* Confirmed evidence exists for human fetal risk, but benefits are acceptable despite known risk (i.e., life or limb situations or serious disease for which no safer drugs exist [e.g., diazepam]).
- *Category X:* Agents of this class are contraindicated in pregnant patients for any reason because animal or human studies have displayed teratogenicity, or there is evidence of fetal risk from prior human experience. Fetal risk clearly outweighs any clinical benefit of their use in pregnancy (e.g., thalidomide).

The commonly used anesthetic agents are classified as follows:

Induction Agents
- Thiopental—C
- Methohexital—B
- Ketamine—C
- Etomidane—C
- Propofol—B

Inhalational Agents
- Halothane—C
- Enflurane—B
- Isoflurane—B
- Desflurane—B
- Sevoflurane—B
- Nitrous oxide (no classification)

Local Anesthetics
- 2-chloroprocaine—C
- Bupivacaine—C
- Lidocaine—B
- Ropivacaine—B

Narcotics
- Fentanyl—B
- Demerol—B
- Morphine—C
- Sufentanil—C

Fed Regist 1980;44:37434–37436.

A.11. How would you prevent intrauterine fetal asphyxia?

It is essential to maintain maternal homeostasis to ensure fetal well-being. Fetal oxygenation is directly dependent on maternal oxygen tension, oxygen saturation, hemoglobin content, oxygen affinity, and uteroplacental perfusion. Maternal hypoxia will result in fetal hypoxia and, if uncorrected, fetal abnormalities or death. Factors that decrease uterine blood flow must be avoided. Uterine blood flow is determined by uterine vascular resistance and uterine perfusion pressure. Uterine blood flow may be decreased by the following: maternal hypotension, stress (which releases maternal catecholamines), pain, anxiety, hypoxia, hypercarbia, hyperventilation, positive pressure ventilation, and pressor agents.

The following principles govern the administration of anesthesia to parturients:

- Delay elective surgery until after delivery.
- Try to avoid surgery during the first trimester.
- Use regional anesthesia when feasible.
- Attach greater importance to anesthetic management than to agents used.
- Change anesthetic management to conform to changes in maternal physiology.

No anesthetic technique is truly precluded for surgery in the pregnant patient. The avoidance of maternal hypoxia, hypotension, and hypovolemia is of greater importance than the choice of anesthetic technique.

Hawkins JL. Anesthesia for pregnant patient undergoing nonobstetric surgery. *ASA annual meeting refresher course lectures*. Park Ridge: American Society of Anesthesiologists, 2006:430.

Rosen MA. Management of anesthesia for the pregnant surgical patient. *Anesthesiology* 1999;91:1159–1163.

A.12. Although this patient presented with an acute abdomen, what is the major reason for nonobstetric surgical intervention in the pregnant patient?

Trauma occurs in 5% to 10% of all pregnancies and ranks first among nonobstetric causes of maternal death. Trauma, particularly blunt trauma to the abdomen, is the most common occasion for nonobstetric surgical intervention in the pregnant patient. Blunt trauma results in 61% of unsuccessful pregnancies. If admitted in shock, 80% of these patients miscarry. Uterine rupture can follow blunt trauma, particularly if the patient has had a previous cesarean section.

National Safety Council. *Accident facts*. National Safety Council, 1987.

Rothenberger D, Quattlebaum FW, Perry JF Jr, et al. Blunt maternal trauma. A view of 103 cases. *J Trauma* 1978;18:173.

B. Preoperative Evaluation and Preparation

B.1. What would you discuss with this patient preoperatively?

It is important to discuss her options concerning regional versus general anesthesia, emphasizing that statistically the fetal outcome is similar, but regional anesthesia is the technique of choice for the mother.

Shelley WC. Anesthetic considerations for nonobstetric surgery. *Clin Perinatol* 1982;9:149.

B.2. Is there a difference in the aim of anesthesia for delivery and for nonobstetric surgery in a pregnant patient?

Yes. The aim of obstetric anesthesia is to permit pain-free labor and delivery without interfering with the progress of labor, whereas the aim of surgical anesthesia is to provide maternal anesthesia without stimulating uterine activity and precipitating premature labor. Second, obstetric anesthesia should provide maternal analgesia without fetal neurologic depression and delayed neonatal breathing. Surgical anesthesia, on the other hand, is designed to maintain uteroplacental perfusion but without consideration for fetal neurologic or respiratory depression.

Diaz JH. Perioperative management of the pregnant patient undergoing non-obstetric surgery. *Anesth Rev* 1991;18:21–27, 27–34.

B.3. How would you premedicate this patient?

Premedication may be avoided by reassurance and support. If necessary, barbiturates can be given for sedation. Glycopyrrolate, which does not cross the placental barrier, can be used as a vagolytic and antisialagogue.

A nonparticulate antacid, such as 30 mL of 0.3 M sodium citrate, given about half an hour before surgery to prevent aspiration pneumonitis, and an H_2 receptor antagonist may also be given.

Chestnut DH, ed. *Obstetric anesthesia: principles and practice*, 3rd ed. Mosby, 2004:268.

Shelley WC. Anesthetic considerations for non-obstetric surgery. *Clin Perinatol* 1982;9:149.

C. Intraoperative Management

C.1. What factors would alter your anesthetic technique from that used for a nonpregnant patient?

The anatomic and physiologic changes of pregnancy alter the anesthetic technique in the following systems:

Cardiovascular System
- Increased blood volume (more increase in plasma than in red blood cell [RBC] count)
- Increased cardiac output (stroke volume and heart rate)
- Decreased peripheral resistance
- Decreased mean arterial blood pressure

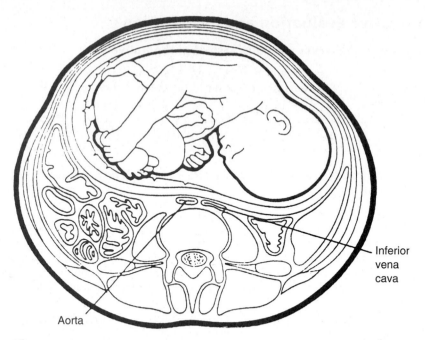

Figure 43.2 The pregnant uterus compressing the aorta and the inferior vena cava (aortocaval compression) in supine position. (From Ostheimer GW. *Regional anesthesia techniques in obstetrics.* New York: Breon Laboratories, 1980, with permission.)

- Vena caval and aortic compression in the supine position as shown in Fig. 43.2. (Therefore, the pregnant patient should be tilted by a wedge under her right hip.)

Respiratory System
- Increased minute ventilation
- Increased oxygen consumption
- Decreased functional residual capacity as shown in Fig. 43.3

Gastrointestinal System
- Decreased gastrointestinal motility and increased gastric emptying time
- Decreased volume of gastrointestinal secretions
- Increased gastric acidity
- Decreased lower esophageal tone because of increased progesterone levels (For these reasons, a pregnant patient beyond the first trimester should always be considered as having a full stomach and must be considered at risk for regurgitation and aspiration.)

Central Nervous System
- Decreased minimal alveolar capacity (MAC)
- Increased sensitivity to local anesthesia
- Decreased volume of epidural anesthetic required, because of engorgement of epidural veins and consequent decrease in size of epidural space

Skin and Mucous Membranes
- More friable mucous membranes and engorged mucosal capillaries (Therefore, avoid insertion of nasal airways, nasotracheal and nasogastric tubes.)

Metabolic
- Increase in oxygen consumption by 20%

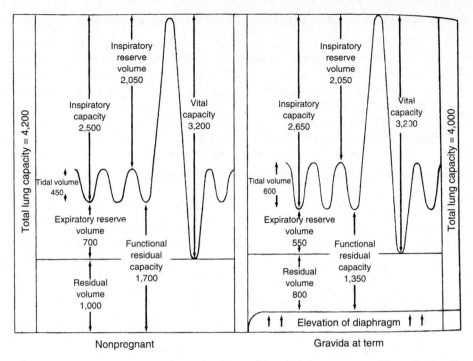

Figure 43.3 Pulmonary volumes and capacities during pregnancy. (From Bonica JJ. *Principles and practice of obstetric analgesia and anesthesia.* Philadelphia: FA Davis Co, 1967, with permission.)

Chestnut DH. *Obstetric anesthesia: principles and practice*, 3rd ed. Mosby, 2004:15–36.

C.2. Describe your technique and dosage if you choose epidural anesthesia.

The patient is placed in the left lateral decubitus position and is hydrated with 1,000 to 1,500 mL of crystalloid solution. She is then placed on her side or in the sitting position and prepared and draped. The epidural block is placed at L2-3 or L3-4 using the loss-of-resistance or hanging-drop technique. After testing for inadvertent spinal or intravascular placement, the local anesthetic is given in divided doses to attain a T4 level. This takes between one half and two thirds of the dose used for a nonpregnant patient (between 18- and 24-mL average volume). An inadvertent spinal injection is detected by the rapid onset of a solid motor block following a 2- to 5-mL test dose; and an intravascular injection is evidenced by signs of systemic toxicity (e.g., dizziness, tinnitus, or circumoral numbness).

The patient is once again placed in the left lateral decubitus position, oxygen is delivered by mask, and her blood pressure is monitored closely.

My choices of local anesthetics are either 2% lidocaine or 0.5% bupivacaine. These agents afford good analgesia with a degree of motor blockade that provides muscular relaxation.

Hughes SC, Levinson G, Rosen MA, eds. *Shnider and Levinson's anesthesia for obstetrics*, 4th ed. Philadelphia: Lippincott Williams & Wilkins, 2002:2249.

C.3. **If the patient is in need of supplemental medication, what would be your choice?**

It is best to use the narcotics that have been tried by time and appear to be safe, such as morphine and meperidine. Small doses of ketamine (0.25 mg/kg intravenously) may also be given.

Barion WM. Medical evaluation of the pregnant patient requiring non-obstetric surgery. *Clin Perinatol* 1985;12:488.

Hughes SC, Levinson G, Rosen MA, eds. *Shnider and Levinson's anesthesia for obstetrics*, 4th ed. Philadelphia: Lippincott Williams & Wilkins, 2002:249.

C.4. **What vasopressor would you choose to improve uteroplacental perfusion?**

Ephedrine was considered the safest vasopressor because it increases mean arterial pressure and uterine artery blood flow without a concomitant decrease in uteroplacental perfusion. The overall increase in cardiac output from the β-adrenergic stimulation of ephedrine will maintain uterine artery perfusion and compensate for its mild adrenergic vasoconstriction. Currently the ban on pure α agonists is much less rigid; as a number of current studies involving the use of both ephedrine and phenylephrine to treat maternal hypotension during spinal anesthesia for cesarean section, shows that phenylephrine did not adversely affect neonatal outcome and may even decrease the incidence of fetal acidosis.

Chestnut DH, ed. *Obstetric anesthesia: principles and practice*, 3rd ed. Mosby, 2004:425

Diaz JH. Perioperative management of the pregnant patient undergoing non-obstetric surgery. *Anesth Rev* 1991;18:21–27, 27–34.

Lee A, Ngan Kee WD, Gin T. A quantitative, systematic review of randomized controlled trials of ephedrine versus phenylephrine for the management of hypotension during spinal anesthesia for cesarean delivery. *Anesth Analg* 2002;94(4):920–926.

C.5. **When this patient arrived in the operating room she was panic stricken and desired a general anesthetic. Describe your technique.**

- Check the adequacy of the intravenous.
- Preoxygenate for at least 3 minutes to ensure denitrogenation and to avoid maternal and fetal hypoxemia during induction and intubation.
- Carry out induction using a rapid-sequence technique (precurarization, thiopental sodium, succinylcholine, cricoid pressure, and intubation using a cuffed endotracheal tube with a 7-mm internal diameter or less).
- Carry out maintenance using agents with a long history of safety, including morphine, meperidine, succinylcholine, nondepolarizing muscle relaxants, isoflurane, sevoflurane, and nitrous oxide-to-oxygen 50:50. (The inhalation anesthetics have the added advantage of relaxing the uterus in the hope of preventing premature labor.) Air/oxygen can also be used with the understanding that the omission of nitrous oxide can result in a drop in maternal blood pressure because of the need to use a higher concentration of volatile agents.
- Avoid hyperventilation and hypoventilation.
- Extubate when the patient is awake and has regained laryngeal reflexes.

Chestnut DH, ed. *Obstetric anesthesia: principles and practice*, 3rd ed. Mosby, 2004:268.

Pedersen H, Finster M. Anesthetic risk in the pregnant surgical patient. *Anesthesiology* 1979;51:439–451.

C.6. Does any controversy exist surrounding the use of nitrous oxide?

Yes, especially during early pregnancy. This is because nitrous oxide inhibits methionine synthetase potentially affecting DNA synthesis.

Nitrous oxide also increases adrenergic tone and decreases uterine blood flow. This, however, can be prevented by the addition of a volatile agent.

Nitrous oxide can cause teratogenic effects in animals during prolonged exposure at critical times. However, teratogenicity has not been demonstrated in humans.

Chestnut DH, ed. *Obstetric anesthesia: principles and practice*, 3rd ed. Mosby, 2004:260–261.

Hawkins JL. Anesthesia for the pregnant patient undergoing nonobstetric surgery. *ASA refresher courses in anesthesiology*, Vol. 25. Park Ridge: American Society of Anesthesiologists, 1997:100–105.

Rosen MA. Management of anesthesia for the pregnant surgical patient. *Anesthesiology* 1999;91:1159–1163.

C.7. What is the incidence of fetal loss and what factors influence it?

Prenatal loss may be caused by premature labor, but it also can be caused by generalized peritonitis and sepsis. Fetal loss is more related to the severity of the disease than to the surgical procedure or the anesthetic. The perinatal mortality rate in cases of prematurity because of generalized peritonitis is 200 to 350 per 1,000. The perinatal mortality rate for nonperforated appendicitis is approximately 50 per 1,000 women.

Duncan PG, Pope WDB, Cohen MM, et al. Fetal risk of anesthesia and surgery during pregnancy. *Anesthesiology* 1986;64:790–794.

Shnider SM, Webster GM. Maternal and fetal hazards of surgery during pregnancy. *Am J Obstet Gynecol* 1965;92:891.

Weingold AD. Appendicitis in pregnancy. *Clin Obstet Gynecol* 1983;26:801.

C.8. If the patient was having surgery on her hand, what would you do differently?

Initially, offer the patient the choice of a brachial plexus block or an intravenous regional technique. It is possible to monitor the fetal heart during surgery and to monitor for uterine contractions using a tocodynamometer. Continuous fetal heart monitoring using transabdominal Doppler is possible at approximately 18 weeks' gestation.

Biehl DR. Foetal monitoring during surgery unrelated to pregnancy. *Can Anaesth Soc J* 1985;32:455–459.

Hughes SC, Levinson G, Rosen MA, eds. *Shnider and Levinson's anesthesia for obstetrics*, 4th ed. Philadelphia:Lippincott Williams & Wilkins, 2002:249.

C.9. What would you expect to see on the fetal monitor during an isoflurane-nitrous oxide-oxygen anesthetic?

One would expect to see a decrease in beat-to-beat variability during anesthesia using inhalation agents.

Liu PL. Clinical reports: fetal monitoring in patients undergoing surgery unrelated to pregnancy. *Can Anaesth Soc J* 1985;32:525–532.

C.10. The surgeon schedules the procedure as a laparoscopic one. Does this pose any problems?

Laparoscopy has been performed during pregnancy both for diagnostic and procedural surgery. CO_2 pneumoperitoneum cause fetal respiratory acidosis. This leads to the recommendation of maintaining low intraabdominal pressure, limiting the duration of surgery, and using arterial blood gas analysis. However, a recent study concluded that capnography is adequate to guide ventilation during laparoscopic surgery. End-tidal CO_2 should be maintained approximately at 32 mm Hg.

Bhavani-Shankar K, Steinbrook RA, Brooks DC, et al. Arterial to end-tidal carbon dioxide pressure difference during laparoscopic surgery in pregnancy. *Anesthesiology* 2000;93:370–373.

Hawkins JL. Anesthesia for pregnant patient undergoing nonobstetric surgery. *ASA annual meeting refresher course lectures*. Park Ridge: American Society of Anesthesiologists, 2006:430.

D. Postoperative Management

D.1. When would you extubate this patient?

The patient can be extubated when she is fully awake and in command of her airway reflexes and able to avoid pulmonary aspiration.

Hughes SC, Levinson G, Rosen MA, eds. *Shnider and Levinson's anesthesia for obstetrics*, 4th ed. Philadelphia: Lippincott Williams & Wilkins, 2002:249.

D.2. What monitors would you use postoperatively?

- Electrocardiogram (ECG)
- Pulse oximeter
- Foley catheter
- Intermittent blood pressure and temperature monitoring
- Tocodynamometer to detect premature labor
- Fetal heart monitor to ensure fetal well-being

Shnider SM, Levinson G, eds. *Anesthesia for obstetrics*, 4th ed. Philadelphia: Lippincott Williams & Wilkins, 2002:262.

D.3. What other precautions would you take postoperatively?

- Provide adequate hydration.
- Continue left uterine displacement.
- Administer supplemental oxygen.

Many obstetricians use heavy sedation plus a course of β-agonist drugs to prevent premature labor. In our institution, all pregnant patients are observed on the obstetric floor for a minimum of 12 hours following nonobstetric surgery. Magnesium sulfate is given intravenously if labor occurs.

Hughes SC, Levinson G, Rosen MA, eds. *Shnider and Levinson's anesthesia for obstetrics*, 4th ed. Philadelphia: Lippincott Williams & Wilkins, 2002:249

D.4. What is the incidence of preterm delivery following nonobstetric surgery during pregnancy?

In a study of 778 women who underwent appendectomy while pregnant, 22% delivered during the following week if surgery occurred between 24 and 36 weeks' gestation.

Mazza RI, Källen B. Appendectomy during pregnancy. A Swedish registry study of 778 cases. *Obstet Gynecol* 1991;77:835–840.

D.5. The next day the patient went into premature labor having "failed" tocolytic therapy. She now needed a cesarean section for prematurity and breech presentation. She required another general anesthetic. In what way would your technique differ from your previous anesthetic technique?

- Do not precurarize the patient: magnesium sulfate prevents the muscle fasciculations that normally occur following the administration of succinylcholine.
- Use smaller doses of muscle relaxants: less is required because of the interaction between relaxants and magnesium.
- Avoid the use of narcotics until after delivery; then stop the inhalation agent and begin using a narcotic technique.

Hughes SC, Levinson G, Rosen MA, eds. *Shnider and Levinson's anesthesia for obstetrics*, 4th ed. Philadelphia: Lippincott Williams & Wilkins, 2002:249.

The Hematologic System

CHAPTER 44

Hemophilia and Coagulation Disorders

Jonathan Leff • Linda Shore-Lesserson • Robert E. Kelly

A 46-YEAR-OLD MAN

hemophiliac, human immunodeficiency virus (HIV) positive patient, was scheduled for elective elbow synovectomy with resection of the radial head due to limited, painful range of motion.

A. Medical Disease and Differential Diagnosis

1. What are the differences between hemophilia A, B, and C?
2. Describe the typical history and pathophysiology associated with von Willebrand's disease (vWD)?
3. What are the different components of factor VIII?
4. What is the difference between platelet adhesion and platelet aggregation?
5. Describe the physiologic events that occur following endothelial interruption in the blood vessel.
6. What prevents the extension of a clot beyond the site of injury?
7. Describe the procoagulant factors involved in the extrinsic, intrinsic, and common coagulation cascade.
8. Describe the levels of factor VIII necessary for hemostasis.
9. Describe the various laboratory tests that evaluate the coagulation cascade and the specific components measured by each.

10. Would there be any differences in preoperative factor replacement therapy between a patient with hemophilia A or hemophilia B?

B. Preoperative Evaluation and Preparation

1. What steps would you take to correct this patient's coagulation status before surgery?
2. What is meant by one unit of factor VIII clotting activity and how much does one unit of factor VIII clotting activity per kilogram of body weight increase factor VIII concentrations?
3. Would you administer factor VIII using a bolus or infusion technique?
4. Can a hemophiliac patient fail to mount an appropriate coagulation response following factor VIII infusion?
5. If a patient with hemophilia does not respond to a bolus injection of factor VIII, can an infusion technique be effective?
6. How much factor VIII activity is present in fresh frozen plasma (FFP)? What are the risks associated with administration of FFP?
7. What are the indications for the administration of FFP?
8. How is cryoprecipitate prepared? What are the components in cryoprecipitate? How much factor VIII activity is present in cryoprecipitate? What are the indications for cryoprecipitate?
9. Describe the advantages and disadvantages of the products that are available for transfusion of factor VIII activity.
10. What is the role of desmopressin (DDAVP) for hemostatic management in this patient?
11. What is the role of ε-aminocaproic acid (EACA) in the perioperative period for the hemophiliac patient?

C. Intraoperative Management

1. Is it safe to administer an intramuscular (IM) injection to this patient before surgery?
2. Would an axillary block be appropriate for this patient?
3. If general anesthesia is used as a technique, would it be safe to intubate the patient's trachea?
4. Would you use any special precautions for this patient who is positive for human immunodeficiency virus (HIV)?
5. What special considerations should be taken in choosing anesthetic drugs for this patient?
6. During the operative procedure, the surgeon indicated that significant blood loss had occurred. Would you transfuse this patient with packed red blood cells or whole blood?
7. During the transfusion of the first unit of whole blood, the patient's temperature rose from 36.8°C to 37.9°C (98.24°F to 100.22°F). What immediate steps should be taken by the anesthesiologist at this time?
8. Does giving blood intraoperatively increase the potential for the development of factor VIII inhibitors?
9. Can factor VIII be safely administered to patients who have developed circulating inhibitors?
10. The surgeon has requested the use of a tourniquet to minimize surgical bleeding. What are the physiologic and hemodynamic responses to tourniquet use?
11. Is it appropriate to suction the endotracheal tube and oropharynx of this patient before extubation?

D. Postoperative Management

    1. What special consideration should be given to postoperative pain management for this patient?

    2. What steps should be taken to enhance the coagulation status of this patient in the postoperative period while at home?

    3. Can this patient be treated with factor VIII supplements using home infusion?

A. Medical Disease and Differential Diagnosis

A.1. What are the differences between hemophilia A, B, and C?

Hemophilia, one of the oldest known genetic disorders, can be classified into type A, B, or C. Hemophilia A (factor VIII deficiency) is the most common form, accounting for 85% of all patients with hemophilia. It is an X-linked recessive disorder, and therefore occurs in men and homozygous women. Approximately 30% of patients have no family history; presumably their disease is caused by a new mutation. The disease results in a hemorrhagic tendency that, in its most severe form, can be life threatening. A screening test for hemophilia A is the partial thromboplastin time (PTT), which will be prolonged in all patients except those with mild disease. Measuring factor VIII activity will provide a definitive diagnosis.

Hemophilia B patients present with either deficient or defective factor IX, this entity represents 14% of hemophilia patients. This X-linked, genetic disorder has an inheritance pattern and clinical features that are similar to those of hemophilia A, but can be diagnosed by measuring both the concentration and function of factor IX.

The remaining 1% of hemophiliac patients suffers a deficiency in factor XI and is classified as hemophilia C, an autosomal disorder that is extremely rare except in Ashkenazi Jews. Hemophilia C can be distinguished from A and B by the absence of bleeding into joints and muscles. In addition, the degree of factor XI deficiency may not predict a patient's bleeding tendency in the postoperative period.

Barash PG, Cullen BF, Stoelting RK, eds. *Clinical anesthesia*, 5th ed. Philadelphia: Lippincott Williams & Wilkins, 2006:224–226.

Behrman RE, Kliegman RM, Jenson HB, eds. *Nelson textbook of pediatrics*, 16th ed. Philadelphia: WB Saunders, 2000:1508–1511.

Perkins JT, Vender JS. Transfusion therapy. In: Collins VJ, ed. *Physiologic and pharmacologic bases of anesthesia*. Baltimore: Williams & Wilkins, 1996:221.

Prasad M, Ted R. *Hemophilia C*. Montoya Hemophilia Center, Department of pediatrics, University of New Mexico. May 15, 2006

Stoelting RK, Dierdorf SF. *Anesthesia and co-existing diseases*, 4th ed. New York: Churchill Livingstone, 2002:490–492.

A.2. Describe the typical history and pathophysiology associated with von Willebrand's disease (vWD)?

vWD is the most common congenital bleeding disorder. The most common form of the disease is inherited as an autosomal dominant trait and has an incidence cited as high as 2% to 3%. Patients with vWD have a prolonged bleeding time, which clinically manifests as bruising, epistaxis, mucocutaneous bleeding, and menorrhagia in women. The diagnosis is suggested by the patient's history of a bleeding diathesis and the presence of a prolonged bleeding time, despite a normal platelet count. Laboratory analysis of vWD is useful for classifying the subtypes and to guide therapy. Type I vWD represents most afflicted patients and is marked by decreased levels of normal von Willebrand factor (vWF). First line treatment in type I disease is with desmopressin D-arginine vasopressin (DDAVP). Cryoprecipitate and fresh frozen plasma (FFP) also contain vWF and may be used in patients unresponsive to DDAVP. Type IIA vWD represents 15% to 30% of patients and is a qualitative defect in the platelet–vWF interaction. The number of vWF proteins can be normal, however, there is an absence of high and middle molecular weight vWF multimers. Type IIB vWD represents that subset of patients with enhanced platelet aggregation in the presence of ristocetin. Ristocetin is an antibiotic, formerly used to treat staphylococcus infection, which also initiates binding of vWF to platelet glycoprotein IB. In the absence of vWF no agglutination will occur with the ristocetin cofactor activity assay. A second assay was developed called the ristocetin induced platelet agglutination (RIPA), which utilizes the patients own platelets and plasma. This test is useful to distinguish a hyperaggregation tendency such as observed in type IIB vWD. In type IIN (Normandy) there is a decreased affinity of vWF to factor VIII and these patients are often misdiagnosed as having hemophilia A. The response to plasma can be helpful in distinguishing vWF deficiency from hemophilia. Hemophilia A patients will have a rapid rise of factor VIII levels following plasma or cryoprecipitate infusion but this is not sustained. The patients with vWD experience a similar initial rise in factor VIII, however, in contrast to hemophilia A, these patients are able to sustain the increase for over 48 hours. Types I and II vWD are inherited as autosomal dominant. Patients with type III vWF deficiency have little or no vWF multimers. DDAVP is not of benefit because these patients have no endogenous production of vWF. Type III vWD is inherited as an autosomal recessive trait. Types IIB and III are extremely rare. It is important to distinguish the subtypes of vWD because the use of DDAVP in types IIB and III may cause thrombocytopenia and increase platelet agglutination.

Barash PG, Cullen BF, Stoelting RK, eds. *Clinical anesthesia*, 5th ed. Philadelphia: Lippincott Williams & Wilkins, 2006:224–226.

Fischer GW, Shore-Lesserson L. Hematologic diseases. *In:* Fleisher L, ed. *Anesthesia and uncommon diseases*, 5th ed. Philadelphia: Elsevier Science, 2005:359–376.

Kovarik WD, O'Rourke PP. Pediatric and neonatal intensive care. In: Miller RD, ed. *Anesthesia*, 6th ed. Philadelphia: Churchill Livingstone, 2005:2481.

Stoelting RK, Dierdorf SF. *Anesthesia and co-existing diseases*, 4th ed. New York: Churchill Livingstone, 2002:490–492.

A.3. What are the different components of factor VIII?

Coagulant factor VIII is a plasma protein that has two components, factor VIII: von Willebrand factor (vWF) and factor VIII:c, each of which is under separate genetic control. The von Willebrand's component serves to adhere platelets to collagen in the subendothelial layer of blood vessels during primary hemostasis and to carry the factor VIII molecule. In hemophilia A, this factor VIII is deficient in quantity or quality.

Barash PG, Cullen BF, Stoelting RK, eds. *Clinical anesthesia*, 5th ed. Philadelphia: Lippincott Williams & Wilkins, 2006:224–226.

A.4. What is the difference between platelet adhesion and platelet aggregation.

Platelet adhesion is the affinity of platelets for nonplatelet surfaces, whereas platelet aggregation is the affinity of platelets for one another.

Barash PG, Cullen BF, Stoelting RK, eds. *Clinical anesthesia*, 5th ed. Philadelphia: Lippincott Williams & Wilkins, 2006:212–213.

A.5. Describe the physiologic events that occur following endothelial interruption in the blood vessel.

The small size of platelets relative to other blood components, such as red or white cells, results in slower transit in the blood vessel with resultant margination, the process in which the faster moving larger components push the platelets towards the walls of the blood vessel. As a result, platelets are in contact with the surface of the blood vessel and can immediately detect any break in the endothelium. Any endothelial break exposes platelets to subendothelial structures, including collagens and other activating proteins, which cause the glycoprotein receptors on the platelets to rapidly adhere to these substances. This adhesion begins the process of platelet activation, in which the shape of the platelet is changed and the contents of the cytoplasmic granule are released. These substances include factors such as adenosine diphosphate (ADP), which further stimulate platelet aggregation. The platelet plug that is formed in this process provides initial hemostasis, interaction with both fibrin and thrombin fuse the platelet plug for continued hemostasis. Activation of factor XIII produces crosspolymerization of the loose fibrin to produce a firm clot.

Barash PG, Cullen BF, Stoelting RK, eds. *Clinical anesthesia*, 5th ed. Philadelphia: Lippincott Williams & Wilkins, 2006:212–224.

Stoelting RK, Dierdorf SF. *Anesthesia and co-existing diseases*, 4th ed. New York: Churchill Livingstone, 2002:490–492.

A.6. What prevents the extension of a clot beyond the site of injury?

Localization of coagulation and control of primary hemostasis are controlled by many factors, including the dynamic tension between two prostaglandins, thromboxane A_2 and prostacyclin. Thromboxane A_2 is released at the site of vascular injury and stimulates vasoconstriction, adenosine diphosphate (ADP) release and platelet aggregation. In contrast, prostacyclin is produced by intact endothelial cells and prevents platelet aggregation and clot formation. In addition, clot localization is maintained by the dilution of procoagulants flowing in the blood, the removal of activated factors by the liver, the action of circulating procoagulant inhibitors such as antithrombin III and protein C and by the release of the serene protease tissue plasminogen activator (tPA). tPA digests fibrinogen as well as factors V and VIII, initiating the physiologic process of fibrinolysis and resulting in fibrin degradation (split) products, which are removed by the mononuclear phagocyte system.

Barash PG, Cullen BF, Stoelting RK, eds. *Clinical anesthesia*, 5th ed. Philadelphia: Lippincott Williams & Wilkins, 2006:212–214.

Stoelting RK, Dierdorf SF. *Anesthesia and co-existing diseases*, 4th ed. New York: Churchill Livingstone, 2002:490–492.

A.7. Describe the procoagulant factors involved in the extrinsic, intrinsic, and common coagulation cascade.

When normal blood is placed in a test tube, a clot will form without any added agents. The clotting factors involved in this reaction were originally classified as the "intrinsic" factors, because everything necessary for blood to clot was "intrinsic" to the test tube. The "extrinsic" path is another potent stimulus for thrombin formation and is initiated by exposure of tissue thromboplastin (tissue factor) to factor VII. The extrinsic and intrinsic pathways converge at factor X, to form the common pathway.

This classic separation of procoagulant factors into extrinsic, intrinsic and common coagulation cascades is not absolute due to the cross over of many factors. In fact, the current conception of coagulation uses a cell-based model and takes into account many *in vivo* pathways and the contribution of the endothelium itself. Although the classic intrinsic and extrinsic coagulation pathways does lead to the formation and activation of thrombin (and hence the amplification of coagulation), it fails to take into account the cellular components, which play a vital role in hemostasis.

The cell-based theory is thought to occur in three stages: initiation, amplification, and propagation. Each stage represents a different aspect of hemostasis at a cellular level with the end result being formation of thrombin and a stable clot. An appreciation of thrombin's role in the coagulation cascade is critical and the reason that all anticoagulation therapy is aimed at the inhibition of thrombin. In fact, the initiation phase of the cell based model is marked by the exposure of tissue factor to circulating factor VII. This activates the other two phases and serves as a potent catalyst for hemostasis. An understanding of this mechanism helps to illustrate how the drug Novoseven (activated factor VII) is such an effective hemostatic agent.

The common coagulation cascade is shown in Fig. 44.1.

Hoffman M, Monroe DM III. A cell-based model of hemostasis. *Thromb Haemost* 2001;85: 958–965.

Stoelting RK, Dierdorf SF. *Anesthesia and co-existing diseases*, 4th ed. New York: Churchill Livingstone, 2002:490–492.

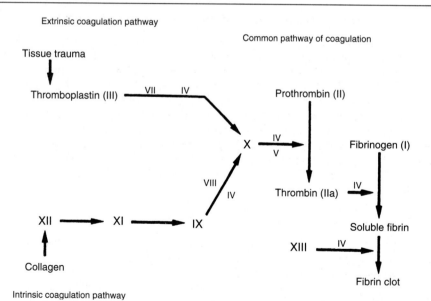

Figure 44.1 Schematic diagram of the procoagulant phase of coagulation depicting the cascade sequence in three steps, designated as the intrinsic, extrinsic, and common coagulation pathways. (From Stoelting RK, Dierdorf SF, McCammon RL, eds. Anesthesia and co-existing disease. 2nd ed. New York: Churchill Livingstone, 1988:577, with permission.)

Table 44.1 The Levels of Factor VIII Necessary for Hemostasis.

CLINICAL PRESENTATION	FACTOR VIII CONCENTRATION (% of normal)
Spontaneous hemorrhage	1–3
Moderate trauma	4–8
Hemarthrosis and deep skeletal muscle hemorrhage	10–15
Major surgery	>30

A.8. Describe the levels of factor VIII necessary for hemostasis.

The levels of factor VIII necessary for hemostasis are described in Table 44.1. When life-threatening airway or neurological bleeding has occurred, factor VIII levels of 100% should be achieved. Similarly, when major surgery is anticipated, correction to 100% factor VIII levels should be done preoperatively and maintained postoperatively (see section D.2).

Jamco RL, McClean WE, Terrin JM, et al. A prospective study of patterns of bleeding in boys with hemophilia. *Haemophilia* 1996;2:202–206.

Maxwell LB, Zuckerberg AL, Motoyama EK, et al. Systemic disorders in pediatric anesthesia. In: Motoyama EK, Davis PJ, eds. *Smith's anesthesia for infants and children*. St. Louis: Mosby 1996:857.

Stoelting RK, Dierdorf SF. *Anesthesia and co-existing diseases*, 4th ed. New York: Churchill Livingstone, 2002:490–492.

A.9. Describe the various laboratory tests that evaluate the coagulation cascade and the specific components measured by each.

There are numerous laboratory tests to evaluate specific components of the coagulation cascade. The standard skin bleeding time is one way to measure for platelet function; however, bleeding time may be prolonged due to factors other than platelet dysfunction such as anemia, low platelet count or patient movement. Moreover, no study has reported a correlation between an abnormal bleeding time and an increased risk of hemorrhage. More recent tests for analyzing platelet function include the Ultegra and the platelet function analyzer (PFA-100). Ultegra (Accumetrics, San Diego, CA), or "rapid platelet function assay" is a point-of-care monitor designed specifically to measure the platelet response to a thrombin receptor agonist peptide (TRAP). In whole blood, it measures TRAP activation-induced platelet agglutination of fibrinogen-coated beads using an optical detection system. Because of the importance of the GPIIb IIIa receptor in mediating fibrinogen-platelet interactions, the Ultegra has been especially useful in accurately measuring receptor inhibition in invasive cardiology patients receiving GPIIb IIIa inhibiting drugs. The platelet function analyzer, PFA-100 (Dade Behring, Miami, FL) is a monitor of platelet adhesive capacity that is valuable in its diagnostic abilities to identify drug-induced platelet abnormalities, Bernard Soulier syndrome, von Willebrand's disease (vWD), and other acquired and congenital platelet defects. The test is conducted as a modified *in vitro* bleeding time. Whole blood is drawn through a chamber by vacuum, and is perfused across an aperture in a collagen membrane coated with an agonist (epinephrine or adenosine diphosphate [ADP]). Platelet adhesion and formation of aggregates will seal the aperture, thereby indicating the "closure time" measured by the PFA-100. This test may be useful in detecting pharmacologic platelet dysfunction before cardiac surgery or may be able to accurately detect hypercoagulability after cardiopulmonary bypass (CPB).

Monitoring the coagulation cascade is usually performed with both the prothrombin time (PT) and the partial thromboplastin time (PTT). The PT is measured by adding tissue form thromboplastin (TF) to a blood specimen and measuring the time until clot formation. This test will detect abnormalities in factors VII, X, V, II, or I. A normal PT could occur with an abnormal fibrinogen level because the PT is only prolonged if the fibrinogen level is below 100 mg per dL. In order to standardize test results performed with different types of thromboplastin activating agents, standardization to the international sensitivity index has created the international normalized ratio (INR). The PTT is performed when partial thromboplastin is added to a test tube of blood and time is measured until clot forms, measuring factors XII, XI, IX, VIII, X, V, II, and I. This test can be modified by the addition of the surface activating factors XII and XI before the addition of the partial thromboplastin, creating the activated partial thromboplastin time (APTT). The APTT is a faster test than the PTT and is a standard test used in clinical practice. The activated clotting time (ACT) also is an accelerated version of the PTT and is activated by diatomaceous earth. This test is used most often to measure the efficiency of heparin use and is much less sensitive than the APTT to specific factor deficiencies. The thrombin time (TP) bypasses most of the coagulation cascade to measure the conversion of fibrinogen to fibrin, a useful test to determine both inadequate amounts of fibrinogen as well as inadequate fibrinogen molecules. The thromboelastogram (TEG) measures both the speed of clot formation as well as clot firmness. This monitor allows evaluation of a clot from early fibrin strand to fibrinolysis. The TEG tracing is made up of several parameters; reaction time (R value), coagulation time (K value), maximum amplitude (MA value), an α angle, and the amplitude 60 degrees after the maximal amplitude (A60). A deviation from a prototypical tracing represents a specific abnormality in the patient's coagulation cascade. An abnormal TEG tracing can correspond to conditions such as thrombocytopenia or factor deficiencies, allowing systematic analysis of intraoperative coagulation defects and a more directed approach to therapy (see Chapter 13, Section A.22).

Laboratory evaluation of the coagulation cascade can be defined as shown in Table 44.2.

Barash PG, Cullen BF, Stoelting RK, eds. *Clinical anesthesia*, 5th ed. Philadelphia: Lippincott Williams & Wilkins, 2006:219–224.

Fischer GW, Shore-Lesserson L. Hematologic diseases. *In:* Fleisher L, ed. *Anesthesia and uncommon diseases*, 5th edition. Philadelphia: Elsevier Science, 2005:359–376.

A.10. Would there be any differences in preoperative factor replacement therapy between a patient with hemophilia A or hemophilia B?

The patient with hemophilia A would need transfusion of factor VIII before surgery to correct factor VIII levels to approximately 100% of normal. Further supplementation should be repeated approximately every 1.5 hours. The patient with hemophilia B would need high initial doses of

---

Table 44.2 Specific Components Measured by Different Coagulation Tests.

LABORATORY TESTS	COMPONENTS MEASURED
Bleeding time	Platelet count, vascular integrity
Prothrombin time	I, II, V, VII, and X
Partial prothrombin time	I, II, V, VII, IX, X, XI, and XII
Thrombin time	I, II

factor IX due to a low recovery from the extensive distribution of factor IX both intravascularly and extravascularly. In addition, the longer half-life of factor IX (18 to 30 hours) requires less frequent dosing.

Lofqvist T, Nilsson I, Petersson C. Orthopaedic surgery in hemophilia. *Clin Ortho Rel Res* 1996;332:232–241.

Stoelting RK, Dierdorf SF. *Anesthesia and co-existing diseases*, 4th ed. New York: Churchill Livingstone, 2002:490–492.

B. Preoperative Evaluation and Preparation

B.1. What steps would you take to correct this patient's coagulation status before surgery?

Orthopedic surgical procedures requiring more factor replacement than might be expected are those in which a raw bone surface must heal, or those where a small amount of bleeding into or around a prosthetic joint could lead to infection and destruction of the surrounding tissue. In contrast, when the extremity or operative site can be held firm with plaster, or if good surgical apposition of tissues can be achieved with sutures, less factor replacement is required. Factor VIII levels of 30% of normal will usually provide adequate hemostasis; however, most clinicians will correct abnormal factor VIII levels to normal levels.

For a major orthopedic procedure, the factor VIII level should be corrected to 100% of normal approximately 1 to 2 hours before the procedure. A repeat dose should be given if the surgical procedure lasts more than 1.5 hours or if the measured factor VIII level falls below 40% of normal.

Lofqvist T, Nilsson I, Petersson C. Orthopaedic surgery in hemophilia. *Clin Ortho Rel Res* 1996;332:232–241.

B.2. What is meant by one unit of factor VIII clotting activity and how much does one unit of factor VIII clotting activity per kilogram of body weight increase factor VIII concentrations?

One unit of factor VIII clotting activity is defined as the amount present in one cc of fresh normal, pooled plasma. A single unit of factor VIII clotting activity per kilogram of body weight will increase plasma factor VIII levels approximately 2%. Therefore, to prescribe the factor VIII activity necessary to correct a 70-kg hemophilia patient with 5% factor VIII activity to 95% of normal, one would calculate as follows:

$$\frac{95\% - 5\%}{2\%} \times 70 \text{ kg} = 3,150 \text{ units of factor VIII}$$

Braunwald E, Fauci A, Kasper DL, et al. eds. *Harrison's principles of internal medicine*, 16th ed. New York: McGraw Hill, 2004:751–753.

Ellison N. Diagnosis and management of breeding disorders. *Anesthesiology* 1977;47:17–80.

Pisciotto PT, ed. *Blood transfusion therapy, a physician's handbook*, 3rd ed. Allenton: AABB, 1989.

B.3. Would you administer factor VIII using a bolus or infusion technique?

Factor VIII concentrates are very stable at room temperature after reconstitution and therefore are appropriate for infusion use. By titrating the infusion, the desired factor VIII level can be maintained, eliminating both the overshoot and the subtherapeutic levels seen with the bolus technique. While the infusion technique requires close observation, less total factor VIII is infused and therapeutic levels are maintained.

Schulman S, Gitel S, Martinowitz U. The stability of Factor VIII concentrates after reconstitution. *Am J Hematol* 1994;45:217–223.

Schulman S, Martinowitz U. Continuous infusion instead of bolus injections of factor concentrate? *Haemophilia* 1996;2:189–191.

B.4. Can a hemophiliac patient fail to mount an appropriate coagulation response following factor VIII infusion?

Approximately 10% to 20% of hemophiliacs will develop an antibody inhibitor against factor VIII and do not achieve the anticipated response following factor VIII infusion.

Stoelting RK, Dierdorf SF. *Anesthesia and co-existing diseases*, 4th ed. New York: Churchill Livingstone, 2002:490–492.

B.5. If a patient with hemophilia does not respond to a bolus injection of factor VIII, can an infusion technique be effective?

Some patients who do not respond well to bolus injections may have measurable low titers of inhibitors. A continuous infusion has proven to be effective in this situation to stop hemorrhage, because appropriate levels of the missing factor can be achieved relatively easily by the infusion method. Those patients with high titers and without measurable factor level during the infusion have also been known to stop bleeding with an infusion technique, likely due to the fact that complete inhibition of the factor only occurs after 1 to 2 hours. If the factor is continuously infused, there will always be some that is circulating, unneutralized and hemostatically active.

Gordon EM, Mungo R, Goldsmith JG. Lingual hemorrhage in a patient with hemophilia A complicated by a high titer inhibitor. *Am J Pediat Hematol Oncol* 1993;15:107–110.

Schulman S, Martinowitz U. Continuous infusion instead of bolus injections of factor concentrate? *Haemophilia* 1996;2:189–191.

B.6. How much factor VIII activity is present in fresh frozen plasma (FFP)? What are the risks associated with administration of FFP?

FFP is prepared from a single donor and contains all plasma proteins, including factor VIII. Factor VIII activity is between 0.7 and 0.9 units of clotting activity per mL of FFP. Following blood donation and plasma separation, approximately 200 mL of FFP are extracted.

The risks associated with the transfusion of FFP are similar to any other single donor blood product. These include associated blood proteins and infectious processes such as hepatitis B, hepatitis C, and human immunodeficiency virus (HIV). The incidence of transfusion-related infections have decreased over the years as screening procedures improved. Currently, the risk of transmitting hepatitis B infection following transfusion of FFP exceeds that of HIV and hepatitis C. The decrease in transfusion-related hepatitis C was secondary to nucleic acid testing which was initiated in 1999. Hepatitis B currently occurs at a frequency of 1/60,000 to 1/200,000 and hepatitis C occurs at 1/800,000 to 1/1,600,000. HIV infection currently occurs at 1 per 1.5 to 2 million-donor exposures. Current techniques for preparation of FFP including heat, detergent treatments and monoclonal antibody purifications can minimize or eliminate the risk of viral pathogen transmission. There are other risks associated with transfusion that are not related to transmission of infectious organisms. These include transfusion-related acute lung injury (TRALI) which occurs with in incidence of 1/5,000 units transfused and is more commonly seen after transfusion of FFP than other blood products. Other aspects of immune modulation are seen after transfusion and may increase the risk of infection and/or postoperative complications.

ASA Task Force. Practice guidelines for perioperative blood transfusions and adjuvant therapies: An updated report by the American Society of Anesthesiologists Task Force on Perioperative blood transfusions and adjuvant therapies. *Anesthesiology* 2006;105(1): 198–208.

Barash PG, Cullen BF, Stoelting RK, eds. *Clinical anesthesia*, 5th ed. Philadelphia: Lippincott Williams & Wilkins, 2006:209.

Goodnough LT. Risk of blood transfusion. *Anesthesiol Clin North Am* 2005;23:241–252.

Spahn DR, Casutt M. Eliminating blood transfusions. New aspects and perspectives. *Anesthesiology* 2000;93:244–255.

B.7. What are the indications for the administration of fresh frozen plasma (FFP)?

The National Institute of Health multidisciplinary consensus development panel determined that FFP was the most overused blood product for transfusion. Many clinicians have used FFP as a volume expander; however, indications for its use should be limited to documented evidence of isolated factor deficiency, reversal of antithrombin III deficiency, selected immunodeficiencies, thrombocytopenia purpura, or massive blood transfusion.

Barash PG, Cullen BF, Stoelting RK, eds. *Clinical anesthesia*, 5th ed. Philadelphia: Lippincott Williams & Wilkins, 2006:231–233.

B.8. How is cryoprecipitate prepared? What are the components in cryoprecipitate? How much factor VIII activity is present in cryoprecipitate? What are the indications for cryoprecipitate?

Cryoprecipitate is the fraction of plasma that precipitates when fresh frozen plasma (FFP) is thawed. In addition to factor VIII, this solution also contains significant levels of factor VIII: von Willebrand's factor (vWF), factor XIII and fibrinogen. This product contains high concentrations of factor VIII in a small volume, usually between 5 and 13 units of factor VIII clotting activity per mL.

Cryoprecipitate is indicated for patients with hemophilia, von Willebrand's disease (vWD), hypofibrinogenemia, as well as uremic platelet dysfunction. Small amounts of red cell fragments may be present in cryoprecipitate; therefore, it may sensitize Rh-negative individuals to the Rh antigens if the donor is Rh positive.

Barash PG, Cullen BF, Stoelting RK, eds. *Clinical anesthesia*, 5th ed. Philadelphia: Lippincott Williams & Wilkins, 2006:231–233.

Stoelting RK, Dierdorf SF. *Anesthesia and co-existing diseases*, 4th ed. New York: Churchill Livingstone, 2002:490–492.

Tetit CR, Klein HG. *Hemophilia, hemophiliacs and the health care delivery system*. Bethesda: Department of HEW Publication No. (NIH) 76–871, 1976:31.

B.9. Describe the advantages and disadvantages of the products that are available for transfusion of factor VIII activity.

The advantages and disadvantages of factor VIII products are shown in Table 44.3

Schulman S, Varon D, Keller N, et al. Monoclonal purified FVIII for continuous infusion: stability, microbiological safety, and clinical experience. *Thromb Haemostas* 1994;72: 403–407.

White GC, McMillan CW, Kindon HS. The use of recombinant antihemophilic factor in the treatment of two patients with classic hemophilia. *N Engl J Med* 1989;320:154.

B.10. What is the role of desmopressin (DDAVP) for hemostatic management in this patient?

This synthetic analog of the antidiuretic hormone is used to prepare mild and moderate hemophiliacs for minor surgery. Intravenous DDAVP will rapidly release preformed factor VIII complex, which leads to a two- to threefold increase in circulating factor VIII within 30 to 60 minutes of administration. In addition, factor VIII and von Willebrand's factor (vWF) are released from the endothelial cells. In a patient with mild or moderate hemophilia A or von Willebrand's disease (vWD), this influx of factor VIII may provide adequate hemostasis for minor elective surgical procedures. The half time of this released factor is approximately 12 hours and repeated administration of DDAVP will deplete the storage capacity in the endothelial cells.

Barash PG, Cullen BF, Stoelting RK, eds. *Clinical anesthesia*, 5th ed. Philadelphia: Lippincott Williams & Wilkins, 2006:224–226.

Stoelting RK, Dierdorf SF. *Anesthesia and co-existing diseases*, 4th ed. New York: Churchill Livingstone, 2002:490–493.

Table 44.3 The Advantages and Disadvantages of Factor VIII Products.

COMPONENT	ADVANTAGE	DISADVANTAGE
Cryoprecipitate	Readily available, long shelf life, relatively low risk of hepatitis and AIDS	Allergic reaction, hyperfibrinogenemia if large volumes are used
Factor VIII concentrates	Easily stored and reconstituted, long life, known potency	Multiple plasma product with high risk of infectious disease
Monoclonal purified factor VIII	Stability, biologic safety	Cost (?)

AIDS, acquired immunodeficiency syndrome.

B.11. What is the role of ε-aminocaproic acid (EACA) in the perioperative period for the hemophiliac patient?

EACA is an antifibrinolytic that has been used successfully in hemophiliac patients to prevent bleeding following minor surgical procedures. Its use in major surgical procedures has not been well documented. If DDAVP is to be used preoperatively, the release of plasminogen activator by DDAVP mandates the use of EACA as well.

Barash PG, Cullen BF, Stoelting RK, eds. *Clinical anesthesia*, 5th ed. Philadelphia: Lippincott Williams & Wilkins, 2006:232–233.

C. Intraoperative Management

C.1. Is it safe to administer an intramuscular (IM) injection to this patient before surgery?

IM injections can be safely administered to any patient with a factor VIII activity greater than 30%. Therefore, if appropriate factor VIII correction has occurred before surgery, an IM injection would be considered safe. However, it is unlikely that an IM injection would be necessary for this patient. If a sedative hypnotic or anticholinergic drug would be necessary before the induction of anesthesia, it would be prudent to use an intravenous route.

Sampson JF, Hamstra R, Aldrete JA. Management of hemophiliac patients undergoing surgical procedures. *Anesth Analg* 1979;58:133–135.

C.2. Would an axillary block be appropriate for this patient?

Regional anesthesia has long been considered contraindicated in patients with hemophilia due to the concern of hematoma formation at the regional site. With proper management of the coagulation status, regional techniques have been successfully performed in hemophiliac patients. As with any patient, the benefit of regional technique must be weighed against the potential risk associated with this technique. Certainly, in a patient with a full stomach, a regional technique might be more appropriate due to the relative risk of aspiration. For a completely elective procedure in the hemophiliac patient, a more prudent course might be general anesthesia.

Sampson JF, Hamstra R, Aldrete JA. Management of hemophiliac patients undergoing surgical procedures. *Anesth Analg* 1979;58:133–135.

C.3. If general anesthesia is used as a technique, would it be safe to intubate the patient's trachea?

Airway management of the hemophiliac patient presents a unique challenge for the anesthesiologist due to the risk of hemorrhage in the tongue or neck, which could completely compromise the upper airway of the patient. Therefore, manipulation of the airway during intubation should not be performed until appropriate replacement factors have been administered. Care should be used in placing the mask on the patient to avoid trauma to the lips, tongue, or face; elective laryngoscopy should only be attempted following preoperative factor correction and achievement of complete muscle relaxation. A smaller than predicted well-lubricated endotracheal tube should be used for intubation, nasal intubation with its propensity for epistaxis should be avoided.

Hyderally H, Stark DCC. Hemophilia: anesthetic implications. *Mt. Sinai J Med* 1977;44(3): 397–399.

C.4. Would you use any special precautions for this patient who is positive for human immunodeficiency virus (HIV)?

Standard precautions should be used for all patients regardless of their HIV status. Strict attention to aseptic technique throughout the surgical procedure should be emphasized (postoperative infections are more common in HIV positive patients undergoing orthopedic procedures such as these).

Thomason HC, Wilson FC, Lachiewiczpf, Kelley SS. Knee arthroplasty in hemophiliac arthropathy. *Clin Ortho* 1999;(360):169–173.

Stoelting RK, Dierdorf SF. *Anesthesia and co-existing diseases*, 4th ed. New York: Churchill Livingstone, 2002:566–570.

C.5. What special considerations should be taken in choosing anesthetic drugs for this patient?

Coexisting liver disease is a common complication in the hemophiliac patient due to hepatitis acquired from previous blood or factor transfusions. As a result, drugs that are metabolized by the liver should be used with caution in the hemophiliac patient. A balanced intravenous technique might be preferable to an inhaled anesthetic due to the reduced hepatic blood flow observed in an inhaled technique.

Stoelting RK, Dierdorf SF. *Anesthesia and co-existing diseases*, 4th ed. New York: Churchill Livingstone, 2002:490–492.

C.6. During the operative procedure, the surgeon indicated that significant blood loss had occurred. Would you transfuse this patient with packed red blood cells or whole blood?

In general, blood banks will fractionate donated blood into component parts, allowing individual transfusion of red cells, platelets, fresh frozen plasma (FFP) or cryoprecipitate. Following blood loss, oxygen carrying capacity and volume expansion are required, usually packed red blood cells and a salt solution are sufficient. In a hemophiliac patient, transfusion of packed red blood cells will further dilute already depressed circulating factor VIII levels; therefore, transfusion of whole blood in such a patient would be appropriate. With this technique, both oxygen carrying capacity and all components of coagulation will be replenished.

Miller RD, ed. *Miller's anesthesia*, 6th ed. Philadelphia: Churchill Livingstone, 2005:1821–1825.

C.7. During the transfusion of the first unit of whole blood, the patient's temperature rose from 36.8°C to 37.9°C (98.24°F to 100.22°F). What immediate steps should be taken by the anesthesiologist at this time?

Ruling out an acute hemolytic transfusion reaction should always be considered when a patient becomes febrile during a blood transfusion. The anesthesiologist should immediately discontinue the transfusion and blood should be drawn from the patient and sent to the blood bank with the questionable unit of blood to allow further cross matching. An additional tube of blood should be collected and allowed to sit undistributed for 5 to 10 minutes, allowing separation of red cells from plasma. The presence of free plasma hemoglobin in the serum is diagnostic of a hemolytic reaction. In the presence of an acute hemolytic blood transfusion reaction, profound hypotension requiring the use of vasopressors is likely. Fluid and diuretic therapy may be required to maintain renal function. A febrile reaction that is not due to an acute hemolytic transfusion reaction can occur with blood transfusion, these are usually self-limited. Once a transfusion reaction is ruled out, further investigation of the increase in temperature is warranted.

> Miller RD, ed. *Miller's anesthesia*, 6th ed. Philadelphia: Churchill Livingstone, 2005:1815–1817.

C.8. Does giving blood intraoperatively increase the potential for the development of factor VIII inhibitors?

Although 10% to 15% of all hemophiliac patients will develop a circulating inhibitor of factor VIII, there is no evidence that the development of such an inhibitor is related to the number of transfusions that the patient receives. As a result, the administration of blood products in this setting should not be withheld for fear of inducing an inhibitor response.

> Behrman RE, Kliegman RM, Jenson HB, eds. *Nelson textbook of pediatrics*, 16th ed. Philadelphia: WB Saunders, 2000:1508–1511.

C.9. Can factor VIII be safely administered to patients that have developed circulating inhibitors?

Occasionally patients with the most severe variance of hemophilia (factor levels <1%) develop immunoglobulin G (IgG) antibodies to the deficient factor. The inhibitors may be of low titer and transient, or of extremely higher titer and very persistent. The "Bethesda unit" of inhibition is defined as the amount of inhibitory activity in 1 mL of plasma that decreases the factor VIII level in 1 mL of normal plasma from 1 to 0.5 units. It is almost impossible to overpower a high-titer inhibitor, but, when life-threatening hemorrhage occurs, massive doses of factor VIII concentrates or plasmapheresis with replacement of factor VIII should be given and may be of temporary benefit. Replacement with large amounts of factor VIII concentrate may provide temporary hemostasis but will stimulate an increase in the antibody titer. Porcine factor VIII may provide hemostasis due to its distinct antigenicity, even in the presence of circulating inhibitor. Immunosuppressive therapy is of no value.

Alternative approaches to therapy of the hemophilic patient with inhibitors involve the use of other agents such as activated prothrombin complex concentrated (APCC), which contain activated vitamin K dependent enzymes as well as recombined factor VIIa. These activated coagulants enter the coagulation cascade distal to the level of factor VIII and therefore bypass the effects of the inhibitor. Thrombosis is a possible complication.

Porcine factor VIII is effective in hemophilia A patients with inhibitors. The porcine factor VIII provides adequate factor VIII activity in patients with less than 50 Bethesda units of inhibitor. The usual starting dose is 100 to 150 porcine units per kg.

> Behrman RE, Kliegman RM, Jenson HB, eds. *Nelson textbook of pediatrics*, 16th ed. Philadelphia: WB Saunders, 2000:1508–1511.
>
> DiMichele D. Hemophilia. *Pediatr Clin North Am* 1996;43:709.

Perkins JT, Vender JS. Transfusion therapy. In: Collins VJ, ed. *Physiologic and pharmacologic bases of anesthesia*. Baltimore: Williams & Wilkins, 1996:219–221.

C.10. The surgeon has requested the use of a tourniquet to minimize surgical bleeding? What are the physiological and hemodynamic responses to tourniquet use?

Although the tourniquet will provide optimal surgical conditions, the physiological and hemodynamic consequences are significant. Anaerobic metabolism distal to the tourniquet begins approximately 8 minutes following inflation, a decrease in nicotinamide adenine dinucleotide and creatine phosphate stores in muscle will occur over the next 30 to 60 minutes. As a result, cellular acidosis will cause the release of myoglobin, intracellular enzymes and potassium. In addition, the limb loses internal heat and may approach room temperature.

Hemodynamic changes are seen both when the tourniquet is inflated and deflated. Exsanguination of the limb and tourniquet inflation expands central venous blood volume, which may have significant hemodynamic consequences in a patient with limited cardiac reserve. Tourniquet deflation and reperfusion of the limb can be associated with profound decreases in central venous and arterial blood pressure, due to a decrease in vascular resistance with the washout of metabolites produced during the ischemic period. Prolonged inflation (>45 to 60 minutes) can result in systemic hypertension for reasons that are likely due to the presence of a critical level of ischemia in the muscle or nerve.

Miller RD, ed. *Miller's anesthesia*, 6th ed. Philadelphia: Churchill Livingstone, 2005:2423–2424.

C.11. Is it appropriate to suction the endotracheal tube and oropharynx of this patient before extubation?

Removal of secretions that might be aspirated is essential before the extubation of any patient; however, suctioning of the oropharynx of hemophiliac patient can trap mucosa in the suction catheter and result in the formation of an oral hematoma. In a hemophiliac patient, gentle oral suctioning under direct vision is appropriate to remove all secretions.

Hyderally H, Stark DCC. Hemophilia: anesthetic implications. *Mt. Sinai J Med* 1977;44(3): 397–399.

D. Postoperative Management

D.1. What special consideration should be given to postoperative pain management for this patient?

It is important to avoid any postoperative pain supplements that might produce a bleeding diathesis in the hemophiliac patient. Analgesics containing aspirin or nonsteriodal antiinflammatory drugs (NSAIDs) should obviously be avoided. Antihistamines and antitussives can inhibit platelet aggregation and prolong bleeding time. Narcotic analgesics or acetaminophen-based products should be appropriately titrated for postoperative pain management. If regional blockade with a catheter technique was used for anesthesia, postoperative analgesics should be administered through this route.

Hilgartner MW. *Factor replacement in hemophilia in the child and adult*. New York: Masson Publishers, 1983:78.

Miller RD, ed. *Miller's anesthesia*, 6th ed. Philadelphia: Churchill Livingstone, 2005:2732–2737.

D.2. What steps should be taken to enhance the coagulation status of this patient in the postoperative period while at home?

It is important that factor VIII levels are supplemented for at least 2 to 4 weeks following surgery. It has been shown that allowing factor VIII levels to fall to the levels normally associated with these patients can result in postoperative hemorrhage. Postoperatively many clinicians recommend maintaining levels at 80% of normal for the first 4 postoperative days, whereas others feel that levels of at least 40% of normal are adequate. There is a consensus that the factor VIII levels on postoperative days 5 to 8 should be maintained at 30% to 40% of normal, whereas levels of 10% to 20% of normal should be maintained for the following 2 to 4 weeks.

Hilgartner MW. *Factor replacement in hemophilia in the child and adult*. New York: Masson Publishers, 1983:76.

Inwood MJ, Meltzer DB. The female carrier of hemophilia: a problem for the anesthetist. *Can Anaesth Soc J* 1978;25(4):266–269.

Lofqvist T, Nilsson I, Petersson C. Orthopaedic surgery in hemophilia. *Clin Ortho Reh Res* 1996;332:232–241.

D.3. Can this patient be treated with factor VIII supplements using home infusion?

Administration of factor VIII concentrate by continuous infusion is routinely used at medical centers for postoperative inpatient hemophiliacs. In the transition of many surgical procedures to the outpatient arena, home infusion of factor VIII can provide the same level of hemostatic protection. Home infusion of purified factor VIII concentrate has been shown to be safe, efficacious and convenient for postoperative patients and should be used for this patient.

Carthaus RP, Novakova IRO. Total knee replacement in haemophilac arthropathy. *J Bone Joint Surg* 1988;70:382–385.

Varon D, Schulman S, Bashari D, Martinowitz U. Home therapy with continuous infusion of factor VIII after minor surgery or serious hemorrhage. *Hemophilia* 1996;2:207–210.

CHAPTER 45

Sickle Cell Disease

CHRIS R. EDMONDS • VINOD MALHOTRA

A 30-YEAR-OLD AFRICAN-AMERICAN WOMAN

with avascular necrosis of her right hip was admitted for a total hip arthroplasty. Her hematocrit was 22%, blood pressure was 130/90 mm Hg, and pulse was 107 beats per minute. She had a past medical history of recurrent joint and bone pain, jaundice, and abdominal pain requiring multiple hospitalizations for analgesia.

A. Medical Disease and Differential Diagnosis
1. What was the most likely medical problem in this patient?
2. What is sickle cell disease (SCD)?
3. What is sickle cell trait?
4. What are some of the other hemoglobinopathies and what are their clinical features?
5. What are the clinical features of SCD?
6. What is sickle cell crisis? Describe the different types of sickle cell crises?
7. Discuss the pathogenesis of sickle cell crisis.
8. What is acute chest syndrome (ACS)?

B. Preoperative Evaluation and Preparation
1. What preoperative evaluation would you perform on this patient before anesthesia?
2. How would you prepare this patient for general anesthesia/regional anesthesia?
3. Discuss preoperative exchange transfusion in this patient.
4. What are the indications for blood transfusion in SCD?

C. Intraoperative Management
1. Discuss the anesthetic management for this patient. Discuss both regional and general anesthesia considerations.
2. Discuss how the comorbidities associated with SCD can affect your anesthetic.
3. What precautions should one take to prevent sickling in this patient?

D. Postoperative Management
1. Discuss the postoperative management of this patient.
2. What complications might occur in this patient in the immediate postoperative period?
3. What is the treatment of sickle cell crisis?
4. What is the role of hyperbaric oxygen therapy in treatment of sickle cell crisis?

A. Medical Disease and Differential Diagnosis

A.1. What was the most likely medical problem in this patient?

For a young African-American patient presenting with a history of joint and bone pains, abdominal pain, and anemia, the most likely diagnosis is sickle cell disease (SCD). Other diagnoses to consider include other hemoglobinopathies, dermatomyositis, glucose-6-phosphate dehydrogenase (G6PD) deficiency, and porphyria. However, given the constellation of symptoms and the laboratory findings, SCD is the most likely diagnosis. A hemoglobin (Hb) electrophoresis will confirm the diagnosis and provide the percentage of abnormal HbS.

Barash PG, Cullen BF, Stoelting RK, eds. *Clinical anesthesia*, 5th ed. Philadelphia: Lippincott Williams & Wilkins, 2006:518–520.

A.2. What is sickle cell disease (SCD)?

SCD is a hereditary hemoglobinopathy resulting from inheritance of a *β-globin* gene mutation located on chromosome 11. The single-point mutation replaced adenosine with thymine. The mutant *β*-allele codes for production and assembly of a variant hemoglobin (*β*-S). The molecular basis of SCD has been demonstrated to be the substitution of valine for glutamic acid in the sixth position from the *N*-terminus of the *β* chains of hemoglobin (Hb). This substitution replaces a hydrophilic negative-charged amino acid with a hydrophobic nonpolar amino acid. This greatly destabilizes the structure of Hb. The mutation in *β*-S hemoglobin accelerates the denaturation of the Hb molecule and significantly decreases its solubility. Decreased oxygen tension causes conformational changes in the Hb molecule, allowing hydrophobic bonds to form between the BS-6 valine of one chain and the BS-85 phenylalanine and the BS-88 leucine of a second chain. This bond forms insoluble tetramers which bond with other tetramers to form long helical strands which subsequently polymerize, causing deformation of the red cell membrane into a sickle shape. The result is a red blood cell that is less able to transverse the capillaries of the microcirculation, disposing the end organ to hypoxia and ischemic damage when sickle cells are present in sufficient quantity. In the United States, the estimated prevalence of HbSS is 1:625 (0.2%) in people of African descent. Patients with sickle cell anemia have early mortality with median age of death in the late 40s to early 50s.

Bunn HF. Pathogenesis and treatment of sickle cell disease. *N Engl J Med* 1997;337:762.

Danzer BI, Birnbach DJ, Thys DM. Anesthesia for the parturient with sickle cell disease. *J Clin Anesth* 1996;8:598–602.

Firth PG, Head A. Sickle cell disease and anesthesia. *Anesthesiology* 2004;101:766–785.

Gregory GD, ed. *Pediatric anesthesia*, 4th ed. New York: Churchill Livingstone, 2002: 140–142.

Lane PA. Sickle cell disease. *Pediatr Clin North Am* 1996;43:639–664.

Roth EF, Elbaum D, Bookchin RM, et al. The conformational requirements for the mechanical precipitation of hemoglobin S and other mutants. *Blood* 1976;48:265–271.

Steinberg MH. Management of sickle cell disease. *N Engl J Med* 1999;340:1021.

Stoelting RK, Dierdorf SF. *Anesthesia and co-existing disease*, 4th ed. New York: Churchill Livingstone, 2002:478–482.

A.3. What is sickle cell trait?

Sickle cell trait is the heterozygous or carrier state of SCD. Sickle cell trait (HbAS) occurs in 8% to 10% of African Americans. HbAS cells begin to sickle only when oxygen saturation of hemoglobin (Hb) is less than 20%. No difference has been found between normal persons (HbAA) and those with HbAS regarding survival rates or incidence of severe disease, with one exception: patients with HbAS have a 50% increase risk of pulmonary infarctions. It has been suggested that sickle cell trait provides a survival advantage over hematologic normal individuals when infected by the malarial parasite *Plasmodium falciparum*. This may account for the high incidence of the mutation in the gene pool.

Allison AC. Protection afforded by sickle cell trait against subtertian malarial infection. *Br Med J* 1954;1:290–294.

Barash PG, Cullen BF, Stoelting RK, eds. *Clinical anesthesia*, 5th ed. Philadelphia: Lippincott Williams & Wilkins, 2006:518–520.

Firth PG, Head A. Sickle cell disease and anesthesia. *Anesthesiology* 2004;101:766–785.

A.4. What are some of the other hemoglobinopathies and what are their clinical features?

The most common hemoglobinopathies include thalassemia, hemoglobin C disease and sickle cell anemia. Thalassemia arises from alterations in one or more of the four genes that code for the α chain. The mildest form of thalassemia (loss of one α gene) presents as a mild form of anemia, whereas the most severe form (loss of all four genes) is incompatible with life. Hemoglobin C results from a mutation in the *β-globin* gene. Hemoglobin C disease is a relatively benign disease producing a mild hemolytic anemia and splenomegaly. However, when it is paired with a β-S mutation, the disease is more severe. Other rare hemoglobinopathies will not be discussed further.

Each hemoglobin gene mutation of the heterozygous form causes little or no clinical consequence, but when both genes of a heterozygote are abnormal, a disease state is evident. Heterozygous combinations such as HbS and HbC (HbSC disease), and β-thalassemia mutation (HbS-β-thalassemia) usually cause a milder clinical course than that of SCD.

Barash PG, Cullen BF, Stoelting RK, eds. *Clinical anesthesia*, 5th ed. Philadelphia: Lippincott Williams & Wilkins, 2006:518–520.

Bunn HF. Pathogenesis and treatment of sickle cell disease. *N Engl J Med* 1997;337:762.

Lane PA. Sickle cell disease. *Pediatr Clin North Am* 1996;43:639–664.

McGoldrick KE, ed. *Ambulatory anesthesiology: a problem-oriented approach*. Baltimore: Williams & Wilkins, 1995:68–69.

Steinberg MH. Management of sickle cell disease. *N Engl J Med* 1999;340:1021.

A.5. What are the clinical features of sickle cell disease (SCD)?

The clinical features of SCD are manifested through indolent end-organ damage with intermittent acute episode of severe pain and pulmonary complications. Although SCD is a disease of hemoglobin (Hb), it ultimately affects all organ systems. It is usually the acute problems that bring them to the attention of a physician. The clinical manifestations by organ systems are as follows:

Central Nervous System

- Cerebral vascular accidents
- Seizures and developmental retardation

- Chronic pain syndrome
- Proliferative retinopathy
- Peripheral neuropathy
- Poor school performance

Cardiac

- Cor pulmonale
- Left ventricular (LV) and right ventricular (RV) dysfunction
- Arrhythmias secondary to iron overload
- High output failure

Renal

- Chronic renal insufficiency
- Hyposthenuria
- Urinary tract infections
- Priapism
- Renal medulla infarctions
- Nephritic syndrome
- Inability to concentrate urine

Pulmonary

- Infarction, pulmonary fibrosis
- Restrictive lung disease
- Airway hyperactivity
- Acute chest syndrome

Gastrointestinal

- Liver disease
- Viral hepatitis secondary to transfusions
- Dyspepsia
- Cholelithiasis (gallstones)
- Sickle girdle syndrome (mesenteric ischemia)

Immunologic

- Auto infarction of the spleen
- Encapsulated organism infections
- Altered immune response predisposes them to overwhelming sepsis.

Orthopedic

- Avascular necrosis
- Infarction
- Osteomyelitis
- Dactylitis

Hemotologic

- Chronic anemia
- Difficulties in matching blood secondary to alloantibodies
- Hyperbilirubinemia
- Sequestration crises
- Aplastic crises
- Hemolytic crises

Vascular

- Leg ulcers

The progression and severity of SCD is variable. Many of the patients have an indolent course, whereas a smaller subset suffer from early end-organ failure and an early death. Pulmonary, neurologic, and renal disease are the leading causes of morbidity and mortality.

Barash PG, Cullen BF, Stoelting RK, eds. *Clinical anesthesia*, 5th ed. Philadelphia: Lippincott Williams & Wilkins, 2006:518–520.

Danzer BI, Birnbach DJ, Thys DM. Anesthesia for the parturient with sickle cell disease. *J Clin Anesth* 1996;8:598–602.

Firth PG, Head A. Sickle cell disease and anesthesia. *Anesthesiology* 2004;101:766–785.

Gregory GD, ed. *Pediatric anesthesia*, 4th ed. New York: Churchill Livingstone, 2002: 140–142.

Lane PA. Sickle cell disease. *Pediatr Clin North Am* 1996;43:639–664.

McMillan JA, De Angelis CD, Feigin RD, et al. eds. *Oski's pediatrics: principles and practice*, 3rd ed. Philadelphia: Lippincott Williams & Wilkins, 2006.

Steinberg MH. Management of sickle cell disease. *N Engl J Med* 1999;340:1021.

Stoelting RK, Dierdorf SF. *Anesthesia and co-existing disease*, 4th ed. New York: Churchill Livingstone, 2002:478–482.

A.6. What is sickle cell crisis?

Sickle cell crisis refers to the acute clinical picture generally caused by sickling of red blood cells *in the microcirculation.* Four main clinical types of crises have been described, as follows:

- Vascular occlusion crises with organ infarction and pain
- Hemolytic crises with hematologic features of sudden hemolysis (often associated with G6PD disease)
- Sequestration syndrome with sequestration of red blood cells in the liver and spleen causing their massive, sudden enlargement, and an acute fall in peripheral hematocrit
- Aplastic crises with bone marrow suppression

The most common crises in sickle cell disease (SCD) is vaso-occlusive crisis (VOC) which is characterized with intermittent, recurrent acute episodes of severe pain. It is generally felt that the central cause of pain is ongoing acute ischemia, vaso-occlusion, and infarction. The precise pathophysiology and nociceptive pathways have not been elucidated. Patients in VOC present with fever, anemia, spine pain, limb pain, and abdominal pain. They are tachypneic and may have an enlarged liver and spleen in addition to abdominal tenderness. Serjent et al. reported that in 118 patients having 183 painful crises, the location was noted to be in the lumbar spine (49%), abdomen (32%), femoral shaft (30%), and the knee (21%). There is usually no identifying triggering agent for most VOCs. The average rate of painful crises per patient year is 0.8%. There is a subset of patients (5.2%) that average 8 to 10 crises a year, which accounts for 33% of all hospitalizations. Mortality positively correlates with increased pain rate in adults.

Firth PG, Head A. Sickle cell disease and anesthesia. *Anesthesiology* 2004;101:766–785.

Lane PA. Sickle cell disease. *Pediatr Clin North Am* 1996;43:639–664.

Miller RD, ed. *Anesthesia*, 5th ed. New York: Churchill Livingstone, 2000:986–987.

Serjent GR, Ceulaer CD, Lethbridge R, et al. The painful crises of homozygous sickle cell disease: clinical features. *Br J Haematol* 1994;87:586–591.

Vijay V, Cavenagh JD, Yate P. The anaesthetist's role in acute sickle cell crisis. *Br J Anaesth* 1998;80:820–828.

A.7. Discuss the pathogenesis of sickle cell crisis.

The pathogenesis of sickle cell crises is precipitated by a triggering insult such as infection, surgical stress, or ischemia-reperfusion injury which catalyzes a complex interaction between sickled cells, endothelial regulation of flow, inflammatory cytokines, platelet aggregation factors, and vasoconstriction leading eventually to ischemia, infarction, and cell death. This cascade leads to a vicious cycle that eventually causes end-organ damage and dysfunction. End-organ damage that occurs in sickle cell states is attributable to three processes: the sickling of cells in blood vessels, which causes infarcts and consequent tissue destruction secondary to tissue ischemia; hemolytic crisis secondary to hemolysis; and aplastic crises that occur with bone marrow exhaustion, which can rapidly result in severe anemia. Factors associated with increased sickling include HbS more than 50% of the total hemoglobin (Hb), dehydration leading to increased blood viscosity, low oxygen tension, hypotension causing vascular stasis, hypothermia, and acidosis. Enhanced oxygen delivery by sickle Hgb causes a rightward shift of the oxyhemoglobin dissociation curve. Once deoxygenated, the HgbS molecule participates in polymerization more readily. Erythrocytes sickle at oxygen tension of 20 to 30 mmHg. The pathogenesis is shown in Fig. 45.1.

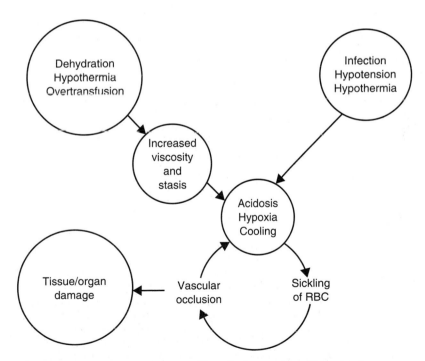

Figure 45.1 Pathogenesis of sickle cell crises. RBC, red blood cell.

Bunn HF. Pathogenesis and treatment of sickle cell disease. *N Engl J Med* 1997;337:762.

Firth PG, Head A. Sickle cell disease and anesthesia. *Anesthesiology* 2004;101:766–785.

Miller RD, ed. *Anesthesia*, 5th ed. New York: Churchill Livingstone, 2000:986–987.

Vijay V, Cavenagh JD, Yate P. The anaesthetist's role in acute sickle cell crisis. *Br J Anaesth* 1998;80:820–828.

A.8. What is acute chest syndrome (ACS)?

ACS is a term used to describe an acute pulmonary complication of SCD. It is defined by the finding of a new pulmonary infiltrate involving at least one complete lung segment on chest radiograph that is not due to atelectasis. It presents with a constellation of pulmonary symptoms and signs in a patient with SCD. These include fever (temperature 38.5°C [101.3°F]), wheezing, coughing, tachypnea, chest pain, and hypoxemia (<92% on room air). Pleural effusions (55%) are commonly seen on chest radiographs. ACS frequently follows vaso-occlusive crises (VOCs); therefore, vaso-occlusive pulmonary infarction may be a precipitating factor. Other causes include infection (viral, chlamydia, mycoplasma, and bacterial) and pulmonary fat embolism resulting from bone marrow necrosis. ACS is a common postoperative complication in SCD patients with a history of pulmonary disease following general anesthesia. ACS can be prevented by judicious hydration, incentive spirometry, effective analgesia, and avoidance of even mild hypothermia during the crises. ACS should be treated with bronchodilators, antibiotics, and exchange transfusion, when necessary.

Castro O, Brambilla DJ, Thorington B. The acute chest syndrome in sickle cell disease: incidence and risk factors. *Blood* 1994;84:643.

Emre U, Miller ST, Gutierez M, et al. Effect of transfusion in acute chest syndrome of sickle cell disease. *J Pediatr* 1995;125:901–904.

Stoelting RK, Dierdorf SF. *Anesthesia and co-existing disease*, 4th ed. New York: Churchill Livingstone, 2002:478–482.

Stuart MJ, Yamaja S. Sickle cell acute chest syndrome: pathogenesis and rationale for treatment. *Blood* 1999;94:1555.

Vichinsky EP, Haberkern CM, Neumayo L. A comparison of conservative and aggressive transfusion regimens in the perioperative management of sickle cell disease. *N Engl J Med* 1995;333:206–213.

B. Preoperative Evaluation and Preparation

B.1. What preoperative evaluation would you perform on this patient before anesthesia?

The aim of the preoperative assessment in a patient with sickle cell disease (SCD) is to determine the perioperative risk of this multisystemic disease and how the end-organ damage will affect the anesthetic management. A careful history and physical examination should be done and the cardiopulmonary status should be thoroughly investigated, in view of the increased incidence of cardiac and pulmonary morbidity in these patients. A history of frequent hospitalizations in the year before surgery significantly increases the likelihood of a vaso-occlusive crisis (VOC) in the perioperative period. Immunization status for Pneumovax and Haemophilus influenzae vaccine should be checked. Other characteristics that increase the perioperative risk are age, pregnancy, and infection. One should correct hypovolemia and treat infection appropriately preoperatively.

Laboratory investigation should include a complete blood count, blood urea nitrogen, serum creatinine, urinalysis, electrocardiogram, chest x-ray, pulse oximetry, and liver function tests. In addition, the following tests may be helpful:

- Arterial blood gas, if indicated
- Sickle cell preparation (if diagnosis is unclear)
- Hb electrophoresis to determine HbS, quantitatively
- Reticulocyte count
- Type and cross (alloimmunization may make this difficult)
- Pulmonary function test (if severe pathology or paroxysmal dyspnea)
- Neurologic imaging (if there are psychological or behavioral changes)

Barash PG, Cullen BF, Stoelting RK, eds. *Clinical anesthesia*, 5th ed. Philadelphia: Lippincott Williams & Wilkins, 2006:518–520.

Firth PG, Head A. Sickle cell disease and anesthesia. *Anesthesiology* 2004;101:766–785.

B.2. How would you prepare this patient for general anesthesia/regional anesthesia?

- Informed consent to explain the options, risk, and benefits for the different types of anesthetics used.
- Preoperative hydration to treat baseline volume deficit.
- Maintain euvolemia preoperatively (remembering that the patient is NPO and may have a urine concentration defect requiring volume replacement).
- Treat any infections preoperatively, if possible.
- Consider transfusion of red blood cells to maintain oxygen-carrying capacity. Transfusion guidelines should be based on comorbidities, surgical risk, and degree of anemia. Transfusions should be individualized and based on the patient's risk/benefit. Efforts should be made for leukocyte reduction techniques as with buffy coat poor red cells in order to reduce the incidence of leukocyte antigen alloimmunization. The goals of transfusion are to achieve an Hgb concentration of greater than 8 g per dL and to ensure that Hgb A represents more than 40% of the total Hgb present. Past practices of reducing Hgb S levels to <30% do not seem to improve outcome and increase transfusion-related complications.

Barash PG, Cullen BF, Stoelting RK, eds. *Clinical anesthesia*, 5th ed. Philadelphia: Lippincott Williams & Wilkins, 2006:518–520.

Lane PA. Sickle cell disease. *Pediatr Clin North Am* 1996;43:639–664.

Reed WF, Vichinsky EP. Transfusion practice for patients with sickle cell disease. *Curr Opin Hematol* 1999;6:432–436.

Schmalzer EA, Lee J, Brown AK, et al. Viscosity of mixtures of sickle and normal cells at varying hematocrit levels: implications for transfusion. *Transfusion* 1987;27:228–236.

Stoelting RK, Dierdorf SF. *Anesthesia and co-existing disease*, 4th ed. New York: Churchill Livingstone, 2002:478–482.

Vichinsky EP, Haberkern CM, Neumayer L, et al. A comparison of conservative and aggressive transfusion regimens in the perioperative management of sickle cell disease. *N Engl J Med* 1995;333:206–213.

B.3. Discuss preoperative exchange transfusion in this patient.

Controversy exists as to whether these patients benefit from preoperative exchange transfusion. For high-risk surgical procedures, the exchange transfusion should be performed with buffy coat–free packed red blood cells to reduce the HbS fraction to less than 40%. However, growing evidence indicates that most surgical procedures can be safely performed in patients with sickle cell disease (SCD) without aggressively transfusing. For example, for certain surgical procedures, it has been shown that a packed red blood cell transfusion done simply to increase the hemoglobin (Hb) level to 10 g per dL is as effective in decreasing perioperative morbidity as is exchange transfusions to reduce the HbS levels to less than 40%. Exchange transfusion is a therapy often used in patients with SCD complicated by acute chest syndrome (ACS). It is beneficial to keep the hematocrit lower than 35% with an exchange transfusion because an increased hematocrit will increase blood viscosity and stasis in the circulation.

Barash PG, Cullen BF, Stoelting RK, eds. *Clinical anesthesia*, 5th ed. Philadelphia: Lippincott Williams & Wilkins, 2006:518–520.

Koshy M, Weiner SJ, Miller ST, et al. Surgery and anesthesia in sickle cell disease. Cooperative study of sickle cell diseases. *Blood* 1995;86:3676–3684.

Stoelting RK, Dierdorf SF. *Anesthesia and co-existing disease*, 4th ed. New York: Churchill Livingstone, 2002:478–482.

Vichinsky EP, Haberkern CM, Neumayo L. A comparison of conservative and aggressive transfusion regimens in the perioperative management of sickle cell disease. *N Engl J Med* 1995;333:206–213.

B.4. What are the indications for blood transfusion in sickle cell disease (SCD)?

The indications for blood transfusion in SCD include the following:

Acute Conditions
- Vaso-occlusive crises (VOCs) with organ infarction and dysfunction
- Sequestration syndrome
- Acute hemolysis with exacerbation of anemia
- Aplastic crisis
- Acute chest syndrome (ACS)
- Acute multiorgan failure
- Severe unresponsive priapism
- Protracted painful crisis
- High-risk surgery (e.g., cardiovascular, thoracic)

Chronic Conditions
- Intractable leg ulcers
- Complicated pregnancy
- Stroke
- Recurrent painful syndrome
- Recurrent ACS

Embury SH, Hebbel RP, Mohandas N, eds. *Transfusion therapy in sickle cell disease: basic principles and clinical practice*. New York: Raven Press, 1994:781–798.

Reed WF, Vichinsky EP. Transfusion practice for patients with sickle cell disease. *Curr Opin Hematol* 1999;6:432–436.

C. Intraoperative Management

C.1. Discuss the anesthetic management for this patient. Discuss both regional and general anesthesia considerations.

The definitive anesthetic technique has not been established secondary to the wide clinical spectrum of sickle cell disease (SCD) and the different severities in the surgical procedures. Koshy et al. retrospectively reviewed 1,079 anesthetics and noted an apparent association between postoperative complications and the use of regional anesthesia. However, this study did not control for obstetric procedures and the tendency that clinicians often use regional anesthesia for sicker patients. Other studies did not find an adverse effect of regional anesthesia. Theoretically, regional anesthesia may produce a compensatory vasoconstriction in the nonblocked area but this has not been supported in the literature. Yaster et al. found that epidural analgesia markedly improved oxygenation in children in vaso-occlusive crises (VOCs) either through superior pain control or through opioid sparing effects. Therefore almost any anesthetic technique can be used provided the following principles are considered:

- Good intravenous access for maintenance of intravascular volume
- Adequate oxygenation
  Denitrogenation before induction of general anesthesia
- Endotracheal intubation for general anesthesia to ensure a controlled airway and adequate ventilation
- Maintenance of adequate oxygen-carrying capacity through judicious use of red cell transfusions
- Maintenance of normothermia
- Opioids for analgesia carefully titrated for perioperative and postoperative analgesia
- Avoidance of tourniquet use
- Consider regional analgesia
- Avoidance of hypotension and venous stasis to prevent sickling of red blood cells
- Avoidance of hypoventilation of lungs to prevent acidosis
- Possible increased inspired oxygen concentration to ensure maintenance of normal to increased PaO_2

Barash PG, Cullen BF, Stoelting RK, eds. *Clinical anesthesia*, 5th ed. Philadelphia: Lippincott Williams & Wilkins, 2006:518–520.

Garden MS, Grant RE, Jebraili S. Perioperative complications in patients with sickle cell disease. *Am J Orthop* 1996;25:353.

Gregory CGA, ed. *Pediatric anesthesia*, 4th ed. New York: Churchill Livingstone, 2002: 140–142.

Koshy M, Weiner SJ, Miller ST, et al. Surgery and anesthesia in sickle cell disease. Cooperative study of sickle cell diseases. *Blood* 1995;86:3676–3684.

Stoelting RK, Dierdorf SF. *Anesthesia and co-existing disease*, 4th ed. New York: Churchill Livingstone, 2002:478–482.

Yaster M, Tobin JR, Billett C, et al. Epidural analgesia in the management of severe vaso-occlusive sickle cell crises. *Pediatrics* 1994;93:310–315.

C.2. Discuss how the comorbidities associated with sickle cell disease (SCD) can affect your anesthetic.

Sickle cell anemia is a disease that can affect every end organ. Therefore evaluating the patient for end-organ dysfunction is paramount. This patient was anemic, tachycardic, and hypertensive.

She may have dyspepsia, a hyperreactive airway, chronic renal insufficiency, liver disease, and might be debilitated with cardiopulmonary complications. Patients with SCD often present with cardiomegaly, pulmonary hypertension, and heart failure. For this surgery, she will probably require transfusions and may be difficult to cross match. In the postoperative period, pulmonary infarcts and infection are common. All these problems, in addition to the potential for sickling crisis and/or sequestration syndrome, pose a greater risk than normal for perioperative morbidity and mortality. The patients at greater risk include those with a homozygous state SCD, sickle C disease (HbSC), and sickle thalassemia. In contrast, patients with sickle cell trait do not present an increased risk for intraoperative morbidity.

Covitz W, Espeland M, Gallagher D, et al. The heart in sickle cell anemia. The cooperative study of sickle cell disease. *Chest* 1995;108:1214–1219.

Gregory GD, ed. *Pediatric anesthesia*, 4th ed. New York: Churchill Livingstone, 2002: 140–142.

Koshy M, Weiner SJ, Miller ST, et al. Surgery and anesthesia in sickle cell disease. Cooperative study of sickle cell diseases. *Blood* 1995;86:3676–3684.

Stoelting RK, Dierdorf SF. *Anesthesia and co-existing disease*, 4th ed. New York: Churchill Livingstone, 2002:401–403.

C.3. What precautions should one take to prevent sickling in this patient?

Sickling of red blood cells is triggered by a variety of factors. One should avoid or correct factors that can precipitate sickling. Special precautions include the following:

- Avoid hypoxia by preoxygenating the patient and employing higher than usual concentrations of inspired oxygen.
- Prevent acidosis by maintaining adequate oxygenation, normovolemia, and cardiac output.
- Prevent respiratory acidosis by avoiding hypoventilation.
- Prevent stasis. This requires proper hydration and good regional blood flow. Blood viscosity should be maintained at a low level by limiting a rise in hematocrit to 35% and avoiding over transfusion.
- Avoid hypovolemia.
- Avoid hypothermia by using body warming and intravenous fluid warming devices perioperatively.
- Replace blood loss to prevent anemia.
- The use of tourniquets is controversial. Some advise against the use of tourniquets, although they have been used without ill effects by others. If a tourniquet is to be used, it should only be used when absolutely necessary and for as short a period as possible. Special attention should be paid to maintain adequate oxygenation and to prevent respiratory or metabolic acidosis at the time of tourniquet release.

Barash PG, Cullen BF, Stoelting RK, eds. *Clinical anesthesia*, 5th ed. Philadelphia: Lippincott Williams & Wilkins, 2006:518–520.

Gregory GD, ed. *Pediatric anesthesia*, 4th ed. New York: Churchill Livingstone, 2002: 140–142.

Stoelting RK, Dierdorf SF. *Anesthesia and co-existing disease*, 4th ed. New York: Churchill Livingstone, 2002:478–482.

D. Postoperative Management

D.1. Discuss the postoperative management of this patient.

The postoperative period is a crucial time with sickle cell disease (SCD). Surgical pain, hypoventilation, a high incidence of pulmonary infarction, and an expected decrease in PaO_2 will predispose these patients to the formation of sickle cells leading to the possibility of developing vaso-occlusive crisis (VOC) or acute chest syndrome (ACS). The mainstay of postoperative management is supportive and preventative care. Supplemental oxygen, maintenance of intravascular fluid volume, maintenance of normothermia, and adequate analgesia are important considerations. Supportive and preventative care should be continued in the extended postoperative period. Basic outline of routine postoperative care includes the following:

- Early mobilization
- Maintenance of normothermia
- Supplemental oxygenation
- Early effective analgesia or adjunctive analgesics—nonsteroidal antiinflammatory drug (NSAID), acetaminophen
- Maintain euvolemia
- Incentive spirometry
- Pulse oximetry
- Pulmonary monitoring
- Psychological support
- Consider regional analgesia

Barash PG, Cullen BF, Stoelting RK, eds. *Clinical anesthesia*, 5th ed. Philadelphia: Lippincott Williams & Wilkins, 2006:518–520.

Gregory GD, ed. *Pediatric anesthesia*, 4th ed. New York: Churchill Livingstone, 2002: 140–142.

Stoelting RK, Dierdorf SF, ed. *Anesthesia and co-existing disease*, 3rd ed. New York: Churchill Livingstone, 1993:401–403.

D.2. What complications might occur in this patient in the immediate postoperative period?

The postoperative complications most likely to occur in the sickle cell disease (SCD) patient include vaso-occlusive crisis (VOC), pulmonary infarction, acute chest syndrome (ACS), and infection. The incidence of postoperative respiratory infection is high and it is a leading cause of morbidity. Hypoxemic episodes are always a threat in that they might precipitate a sickling crisis. ACS is a potentially lethal postoperative complication in SCD patients who undergo general anesthesia for major surgery. Sequestration syndrome with shock is another potentially lethal complication, especially in the obstetric patient immediately postpartum. Patients with cardiomegaly and pulmonary hypertension are susceptible to heart failure. Renal and hepatic dysfunction may result in prolongation of the effects of certain medications.

Barash PG, Cullen BF, Stoelting RK, eds. *Clinical anesthesia*, 5th ed. Philadelphia: Lippincott Williams & Wilkins, 2006:518–520.

Stoelting RK, Dierdorf SF. *Anesthesia and co-existing disease*, 4th ed. New York: Churchill Livingstone, 2002:478–482.

Vichinsky EP, Haberkern CM, Neumayo L. A comparison of conservative and aggressive transfusion regimens in the perioperative management of sickle cell disease. *N Engl J Med* 1995;333:206–213.

D.3. What is the treatment of sickle cell crisis?

The treatment of sickle cell crisis is to break the vicious cycle of sickling, ischemia, infarction, pain, and end-organ failure. The principles of treatment of painful sickle cell crisis include the following:

- Bed rest
- Hydration
- Oxygen therapy
- Treatment of infection
- Analgesics (consider patient-controlled analgesia)
  - Consider regional analgesia
- Transfusion to reduce the HbS concentration
- Incentive spirometry
- Maintenance of normothermia

Barash PG, Cullen BF, Stoelting RK, eds. *Clinical anesthesia*, 5th ed. Philadelphia: Lippincott Williams & Wilkins, 2006:518–520.

Steinberg MH. Management of sickle cell disease. *N Engl J Med* 1999;340:1021.

Vijay V, Cavenagh JD, Yate P. The Anaesthetist's role in acute sickle cell crisis. *Br J Anaesth* 1998;80:820–828.

D.4. What is the role of hyperbaric oxygen therapy in treatment of sickle cell crisis?

Hyperbaric oxygen has been used empirically in some institutions for treatment of acute sickle cell crisis; however, it is not widely available. Although some published reports claim instant improvement of symptoms, others have failed to show beneficial effect. There is better evidence that therapy is useful in management of ischemic disorders of the anterior segment of the eye or in chronic leg ulcers. Studies have shown no apparent effects of hyperbaric oxygen on sickle cell morphology *in vitro*. It appears, then, that its reported benefit *in vivo* may be due to a decrease in the rate of sickling or improved tissue oxygenation by direct diffusion.

Mychaskiw G, Woodyard SA, Brunson CD, et al. *In vitro* effects of hyperbaric oxygen on sickle cell morphology. *J Clin Anesth* 2001;13:255–258.

Reynolds JD. Painful sickle cell crisis: successful treatment with hyperbaric oxygen therapy. *JAMA* 1971;216:1977–1978.

Wallyn CR, Jampl LM, Goldberg MF, et al. The use of hyperbaric oxygen in treatment of sickle cell hyphema. *Invest Ophthalmol Vis Sci* 1985;26:1155–1158.

Eye, Ear, Nose, and Throat

CHAPTER 46

Airway Trauma

RICHARD P. DUTTON

A 46-YEAR-OLD-MAN

was thrown from his motorcycle at a high rate of speed and impaled in the base of the neck by a tree branch. At presentation to the trauma center, he is awake and alert with heart rate (HR) = 122 beats per minute, blood pressure (BP) = 143/85 mm Hg, respiratory rate (RR) = 20 per minute, and oxygen saturation = 98% on 100% nonrebreathing mask. There is a 5-cm wide piece of wood protruding from his anterior lower neck at the sternal notch, without visible bleeding. The patient is neurologically intact but admits to consuming six beers in the hour before injury. His medical history is unremarkable.

A. Medical Disease and Differential Diagnosis

1. What variables mitigate injury from motorcycle collisions?
2. What other significant trauma may be present?
3. How is the initial assessment of a trauma patient organized?
4. How would you evaluate airway and breathing?
5. How would you evaluate the circulation?
6. How would you evaluate mental status and neurologic condition?
7. What diagnostic tests are indicated for this patient based on the mechanism of injury?
8. What are the zones of the neck and what is their clinical significance?
9. What immediate treatment is necessary before diagnostic studies?
10. When and where should the impaling object be removed?

B. Preoperative Evaluation and Preparation

1. What laboratory tests would you want?
2. What x-ray studies are most important to the anesthesiologist?
3. Is an electrocardiogram (ECG) necessary?
4. Should this patient be intubated before going for computed tomographic (CT) scanning?
5. When and where should this patient's airway be managed?
6. Are any prophylactic medications indicated?

C. Intraoperative Management

1. What monitors would you use? Is invasive monitoring necessary before definitive airway control?
2. What is the surgical approach to a Zone I neck injury?
3. Is the patient likely to require tube thoracostomy? Should this be placed before managing the airway?
4. What are the options for managing this patient's airway?
5. What are the risks of rapid-sequence induction in this patient?
6. What anesthetic agents would you use for a rapid-sequence induction?
7. How can you minimize the risk of exacerbating cervical spine trauma?
8. How can you minimize the risks of aspiration?
9. How would you anesthetize the airway for an awake intubation?
10. What are the risks of awake fiberoptic intubation?
11. If the patient cannot be ventilated, what options are available?
12. Would a laryngeal mask airway (LMA) or other pharyngeal airway be of assistance?
13. What surgical airway options are available in this case?
14. What maintenance anesthetics are indicated or contraindicated in this patient?
15. What complications will the surgical plan introduce?

D. Postoperative Management

1. What are the criteria for extubation?
2. What techniques may be used during extubation?
3. How does alcohol abuse and use of illicit drugs affect postoperative management?
4. What pain medication should be used?

A. Medical Disease and Differential Diagnosis

A.1. What variables mitigate injury from motorcycle collisions?

Trauma involving motorcycles accounts for 2% to 5% of all motor vehicle trauma but a higher proportion of death and serious injury is because of the relative exposure of the motorcycle rider to the environment. Factors such as youth, high speed, and intoxication contribute to motorcycle collisions just as they do for automobiles. Motorcycle riders are also much more susceptible to factors beyond their own control, such as lack of vigilance on the part of automobile and truck drivers, road conditions (oil or debris), and the weather.

Factors that can reduce the seriousness of motorcycle collisions when they do occur include helmets and protective clothing. Reenactment of a mandatory helmet law in the state of Washington in 1990 resulted in a decline in serious brain injury in motorcycle trauma victims from 20% to 9%, and a reduction in mortality from 10% to 6%. Full leather or synthetic "armor" reduces the risk of massive skin and soft tissue injuries in the event of a high-speed collision.

Mock CN, Maier RV, Boyle E, et al. Injury prevention strategies to promote helmet use decrease severe head injury at a level I trauma center. *J Trauma* 1995;39:29.

A.2. What other significant trauma may be present?

Motorcycle collisions are "high-energy" trauma that can result in injury to any organ system or region of the body. This patient will need a complete head-to-toe assessment and a number of diagnostic studies to establish the full extent of injury. Common injuries in motorcyclists include brain trauma from direct impact with the road and with other vehicles, pelvic fractures from impact with the frame of the bike, abdominal trauma from impact with the handlebars, and lower extremity orthopedic and soft tissue trauma from impact with the road.

A.3. How is the initial assessment of a trauma patient organized?

The initial management of trauma patients is best described by the tenets of the Advanced Trauma Life Support (ATLS) course, written by the American College of Surgeons Committee on Trauma. This course provides a unified philosophy and common language to organize practitioners from different specialties in the care of complex patients with the potential for multiple injuries. Assessment of the seriously injured patient begins with the ABCs: *A*irway, *B*reathing, and *C*irculation; followed by a brief neurologic examination and a catalogue of visible injuries. This "primary survey" is followed by diagnostic testing and a more detailed secondary survey, interrupted as necessary to provide life-saving resuscitative care.

Committee on Trauma, American College of Surgeons. *Advanced trauma life support program for doctors*. Chicago: American College of Surgeons, 1997.

A.4. How would you evaluate airway and breathing?

On first contact with the patient, the provider should attempt verbal communication: "How are you?" A patient who answers coherently in a normal voice has no immediate airway issue, adequate circulatory function, and no worse than minimal traumatic brain injury. In an unconscious patient, initial assessment is by looking, listening, and feeling for airflow. If airflow is absent, the airway should be opened by jaw thrust (*not* head tilt, as this may exacerbate a cervical spinal column injury), clearance of any visible foreign bodies or secretions, and placement of an oral or nasopharyngeal airway.

Breathing is assessed by observation of the chest wall and diaphragm once the airway is open, and by immediate placement of a pulse oximeter probe. Patients who are not breathing adequately should be assisted with bag-valve-mask ventilation while preparations are made for securing a definitive airway and instituting mechanical ventilation.

A.5. How would you evaluate the circulation?

Initial assessment for shock is by vital signs (heart rate, blood pressure, pulse oximetry) and physical examination (pallor, diaphoresis, peripheral circulation, visible or suspected hemorrhage). Mental status is also a useful sign: the patient in hemorrhagic shock will be first agitated and then lethargic. Young patients have significant compensatory reserves and will maintain a normal systolic blood pressure even in the face of hemorrhage as great as 40% of the blood volume. This state of compensated shock can be diagnosed by a narrowed pulse pressure (especially on automated sphygmomanometers), elevated heart rate, pallor, and abnormal lactate and base deficit. Shock in this patient could be the result of hemorrhage from chest or abdominal trauma (including a great vessel injury associated with the impalement) or tension pneumothorax in either side of the chest.

Committee on Trauma, American College of Surgeons. *Advanced trauma life support program for doctors*. Chicago: American College of Surgeons, 1997.

Dutton RP. Initial resuscitation of the hemorrhaging patient. In: Speiss B, Shander A, eds. *Perioperative transfusion medicine*. Philadelphia: Lippincott Williams & Wilkins, 2006:289–300.

A.6. How would you evaluate mental status and neurologic condition?

The quick neurologic examination consists of questions to determine alertness and orientation (assuming the patient is responsive) followed by gross motor examination of all extremities. In the less responsive patient, the Glasgow Coma Score (GCS) (Table 46.1) is used to stratify the degree of impairment: GCS 3 to 8 is a severe injury, GCS 9 to 13 is moderate traumatic brain injury, and GCS 14 to 15 is mild injury. Cranial nerve, spinal cord, and peripheral nervous system function is assessed by specific motor and sensory testing of each extremity during the secondary survey.

Teasdale G, Jennet B. Assessment of coma and impaired consciousness: a practical scale. *Lancet* 1974;2:81–84.

A.7. What diagnostic tests are indicated for this patient based on the mechanism of injury?

Because of the "high energy" mechanism of injury, this patient must be assessed from head to toe. Ultrasonography examination of the abdomen and chest is used to diagnose free peritoneal fluid, pneumothorax (in the hands of a skilled operator), and pericardial tamponade. Chest and pelvis plain-film radiography will reveal fractures, pneumothoraces, and hemothorax. Computed tomographic (CT) scanning should include the head, neck, chest, abdomen, and pelvis; newer technology will allow for 3D reconstructions of organs and vasculature with sensitivity and specificity equivalent to more traditional angiographic imaging.

This patient's obvious injury—to Zone III of the neck—will necessitate a focused assessment of the trachea, great vessels, esophagus, and bilateral pleural cavities. Traditionally this has been accomplished by a combination of plain-film radiography, angiography, bronchoscopy, and esophagoscopy. Increasing CT speed and resolution is leading to the increased use of this test at centers with experienced radiographers and traumatologists. The sequencing of diagnostic

Table 46.1 Glasgow Coma Score (GCS). The GCS is the sum of the best scores in each of three categories.

EYE-OPENING RESPONSE	VERBAL RESPONSE	MOTOR RESPONSE
4 = Spontaneous	5 = Oriented to name	6 = Follows commands
3 = To speech	4 = Confused	5 = Localizes to painful stimuli
2 = To pain	3 = Inappropriate speech	4 = Withdraws from painful stimuli
1 = None	2 = Incomprehensible sounds	3 = Abnormal flexion (decorticate posturing)
	1 = None	2 = Abnormal extension (decerebrate posturing)
		1 = None

studies will depend on the patient's stability. In this case, he is likely to require intubation and perhaps exploratory surgery first. A noninvasive study such as contrast-enhanced CT (with angiographic reconstructions) may help to guide the surgical approach to removal of the impaling object if the patient is calm and stable enough to tolerate the test.

Henry SM, Scalea TM. Assessment and initial management in the trauma patient. In: Prough DS, Fleisher L, eds. *Prob Anesth Trauma Care*, Vol. 13, no. 3, London: Lippincott Wiliams & Wilkins, 2002:271–278.

A.8. What are the zones of the neck and what is their clinical significance?

Zone I of the neck is the section superior to the angle of the mandible. Zone I vascular injuries pose a significant operative risk because distal control of an injured vessel cannot be achieved. Injuries in Zone I are therefore approached angiographically or as part of a more complex neurosurgical operation. Zone II is from the angle of the mandible down to the highest point of the clavicle. Injuries in Zone II are addressed through a lateral or transverse cervical incision, with the surgeon able to achieve both proximal and distal control of the carotid or jugular vessels before exploring the wound itself.

Zone III injuries, at the base of the neck, require the complex diagnostic workup described in the previous section, followed by a surgical approach that allows access to both the neck and chest. Partial or complete median sternotomy is often necessary to access an injured great vessel or to complete a tracheal or esophageal repair.

Britt LD, Peyser MB. Penetrating and blunt neck trauma. In: Mattox KL, Feliciano DV, Moore EE, eds. *Trauma*, 4th ed. New York: McGraw-Hill, 2000:437–439.

A.9. What immediate treatment is necessary before diagnostic studies?

The key to this case will be control of the patient's airway. Once hemodynamic stability is confirmed, the timing and sequence of diagnostic studies will be determined by the patient's degree of cooperation and ability to protect his own spontaneous ventilation. Although a computed tomographic (CT) scan before a controlled intubation in the operating room (OR) would be ideal, it is possible that the patient will decompensate before this can be accomplished. Preemptive airway control will allow for a more secure and safer diagnostic workup before the OR.

A.10. When and where should the impaling object be removed?

All things being equal, the impaling tree branch is best removed in the operating room (OR), in an anesthetized patient, with all of the personnel and equipment on hand to perform emergent median sternotomy and major vascular and/or tracheal surgery if necessary.

B. Preoperative Evaluation and Preparation

B.1. What laboratory tests would you want?

The patient should have a full set of laboratory studies, both to identify abnormalities and to establish a baseline for future changes. Hemoglobin and hematocrit will not indicate hemorrhage on the initial draw—the bleeding trauma patient is losing whole blood—but will drop with subsequent fluid resuscitation. Arterial blood gas and arterial or venous lactate measurement will be the most sensitive indicators of hypoperfusion and shock. Serum electrolytes will reveal baseline abnormalities, if any, and the effects of alcohol consumption and dehydration. Clotting studies are important to rule out congenital abnormalities or the effects of liver disease before what could be a major surgical procedure; coagulopathy at the time of trauma center admission is an indicator of substantial blood loss and severe hemorrhagic shock. Toxicology screening is indicated in every trauma patient and is important to rule out the use of drugs of abuse such as heroin or cocaine that have implications for the anesthesiologist.

Initial laboratory studies should also include a sample for the blood bank with the request for an urgent crossmatch of red cells and plasma. If there has been a major vascular injury, substantial blood loss is a possibility and should be treated with immediate transfusion of blood and coagulation factors.

Committee on Trauma, American College of Surgeons. *Advanced trauma life support program for doctors*. Chicago: American College of Surgeons, 1997.

Stein DM, Dutton RP, O'Connor J, et al. Determinants of futility of administration of recombinant factor VIIa in trauma. *J Trauma* 2005;59:609–615.

B.2. What x-ray studies are most important to the anesthesiologist?

Although all of the studies described in the preceding text will have some relevance, there are a few that have particular implications for the anesthesiologist. The chest radiograph and/or computed tomography (CT) scan will suggest the degree of tracheal involvement of the impaling object, the risk that there is a major vascular injury, or the presence of a pneumothorax. Plain radiographs or CT scan of the cervical spine will be useful in ruling out bony or ligamentous injury that might be exacerbated by manipulation of the neck during airway management.

B.3. Is an electrocardiogram (ECG) necessary?

In the absence of dysrhythmias on the cardiac monitor, the criteria for ordering a preoperative ECG are the same as in any other surgical candidate: a man aged 45 or older (or postmenopausal woman) or a patient presenting with symptoms or with a history suggestive of coronary artery disease. Dysrhythmias or visible injury to the precordium would be an indication for a baseline ECG and cardiac enzyme assay.

B.4. Should this patient be intubated before going for computed tomographic (CT) scanning?

The answer to this question involves an assessment of risks and benefits. If the patient is cooperative, if the vital signs are stable, if the CT scanner is close at hand, and if anesthesia personnel are available to accompany the patient, then an immediate CT scan would be indicated. If the patient is deteriorating in any way, if his degree of cooperation is in doubt, or if a CT scan would place the patient far from expert resources for an extended period of time, then it is wiser to secure the airway first. In this case, there is a possibility that successful airway management will precipitate patient deterioration (e.g., hemorrhage; conversion from simple to tension pneumothorax), which suggests that if airway management is attempted before CT, it should probably be done in the operating room (OR) with the surgical team on hand.

One approach to this kind of complex decision is to define an ideal course of care that provides the best information for each of the experts involved while minimizing risk to the patient and maximizing flexibility in dealing with changing circumstances. In this case, the surgeon and anesthesiologist might define a plan which includes transport to the OR; induction, intubation, and mechanical ventilation in this (safest possible) environment; transport to CT or angiography with the anesthesiologist in attendance for diagnostic studies; then return to the OR for definitive surgery.

B.5. When and where should this patient's airway be managed?

Because of the potential for rapid deterioration and the desire to examine the airway closely before and during the intubation process, the patient should be moved as rapidly as possible to the operating room (OR) before airway management is attempted. The surgical team should be on hand from the start and instruments should be available for video bronchoscopy, emergent tracheostomy, control of large vessel bleeding, and median sternotomy.

B.6. Are any prophylactic medications indicated?

Tetanus toxoid treatment is indicated for any trauma patient with an open wound who is more than 5 years removed from their last booster. Any patient with a significant open wound should receive prophylactic antibiotic therapy that covers gram-positive organisms for at least the first 24 hours following injury.

Prophylactic treatment to reduce the consequences of aspiration would be considered, but probably rejected in this case. Promotility agents such as metaclopramide and H_2 antagonists such as cimetidine will not have time to work before definitive airway control is achieved and the more immediate approach of administering oral bicitrate would be contraindicated because of the possibility of esophageal injury.

Because of the patient's history of intoxication, prophylactic intravenous administration of vitamins and thiamine is indicated. Prophylaxis against alcohol withdrawal and deep venous thrombosis are indicated in the immediate postoperative period.

C. Intraoperative Management

C.1. What monitors would you use? Is invasive monitoring necessary before definitive airway control?

Blood pressure, electrocardiography, capnography, and pulse oximetry should be employed as with any patient. A Foley catheter should be inserted, although urine output is not an accurate measure of intravascular volume status in a recently intoxicated patient. An arterial line is useful for moment-to-moment measurement of blood pressure and for easy access to blood for laboratory assay including arterial blood gases. A central venous catheter should be placed if there is need to monitor central venous intravascular volume, in anticipation of the need for rapid intravascular expansion (using a large-bore catheter such as a pulmonary artery introducer), and for the administration of vasoactive drugs. A pulmonary artery catheter is rarely indicated and seldom used acutely for resuscitation, although it may be helpful in selected patients with known coronary artery or valvular disease. Because of the potential for great vessel injury in this case, initial central access should be through the femoral vein.

Invasive monitoring lines are usually best placed after induction and intubation, when the patient is anesthetized and both surgeons and anesthesiologists can be working at the same time. Delaying surgical hemostasis in an unstable patient is unwise. In the case under discussion, it would be appropriate to place an arterial line in the operating room (OR) before airway management, as long as the patient remains cooperative and stable, and to place a femoral central line thereafter. Placing the arterial line on the right side will also allow for assessment of blood flow in the innominate artery during surgical exploration.

Duke J, Rosenberg SG. *Anesthesia secrets*. Philadelphia: Hanley & Belfas, 1996:219–222.

Karlin A. Hemodynamic monitoring of trauma patients during anesthesia. *Anesthesiol Clin North America* 1996;14:85–99.

C.2. What is the surgical approach to a Zone III neck injury?

In the present case, the surgery is likely to start with a collar incision through the impalement wound to allow for better visualization of the path of injury. If injury to the trachea or a great vessel is discovered, a partial or complete median sternotomy would be the next step. It is the uncertain nature of this patient's injuries that makes preoperative diagnostic information so valuable, which is why a computed tomographic (CT) scan before definitive surgery (but after airway management) is a strong consideration.

C.3. Is the patient likely to require tube thoracostomy? Should this be placed before managing the airway?

Pneumothorax and hemothorax are common in trauma patients and should be suspected and definitively ruled out following any "high energy" blunt trauma (motor vehicle collision, pedestrian struck, fall from a height) or any penetrating trauma to the neck, thorax, or upper abdomen. Immediate temporizing needle decompression and/or tube thoracostomy are indicated in any hemodynamically unstable patient with a suspicious injury, even before chest radiograph. Intubation and the change to positive pressure ventilation may precipitate decompensation in a patient with chest injury, due to either decreased preload in the setting of hemorrhage or increased intrathoracic pressure caused by conversion from simple to tension pneumothorax.

In this case, there is the possibility of pathology in either or both hemithoraces. A portable anterior–posterior chest radiograph should be obtained at the earliest moment, followed by computed tomography (CT) of the chest as outlined previously. If a simple pneumothorax is present, it is most prudent to prepare for chest tube placement (personnel, equipment) before airway management but to wait until the airway is secure before actually placing the chest tube.

C.4. What are the options for managing this patient's airway?

Choices for induction of anesthesia should be considered in concert with choices for securing the airway and transitioning to positive pressure ventilation. Airway management can occur with the patient awake under topical anesthesia or asleep, with either continued spontaneous ventilation (a "breathe down" induction with a volatile anesthetic) or an immediate transition to positive pressure, as in a rapid-sequence induction.

C.5. What are the risks of rapid-sequence induction in this patient?

Although most trauma patients are best managed with rapid-sequence induction and intubation, this case may represent an exception. Swelling or bleeding in the airway may make intubation physically difficult and the impaling object itself may prevent distal passage of an endotracheal tube. Further, dislodgement due to patient agitation or intubation attempts could precipitate hemorrhage or airway disruption. Finally, the transition from spontaneous to positive pressure ventilation could precipitate a tension pneumothorax.

C.6. What anesthetic agents would you use for a rapid-sequence induction?

Succinylcholine is the key component of a rapid-sequence intubation. No other relaxant provides as consistently good intubating conditions as quickly as succinylcholine. The usual dose for a trauma patient is 1.5 mg per kg—somewhat greater than normal to compensate for a potentially lower cardiac output in a hemorrhaging patient.

Because succinylcholine has no amnestic or analgesic properties, an induction sedative is also indicated in most patients. Any induction agent, including ketamine or etomidate, will precipitate hypotension in the hypovolemic patient with a high endogenous catecholamine level, so care with dosing is required. In young and previously healthy patients, sodium thiopental in a titrated dose from 1 to 5 mg per kg is effective and inexpensive. Etomidate (0.1–0.4 mg/kg) is a reasonable choice in elderly patients or in those with known cardiovascular disease.

Dutton RP, McCunn M. Anesthesia for trauma. In: Miller RD, ed. *Miller's anesthesia*, 6th ed. Philadelphia: Churchill Livingstone, 2005:2451–2495.

C.7. How can you minimize the risk of exacerbating cervical spine trauma?

Appropriate precautions must be taken to avoid worsening an occult spinal cord injury. In the worst case, fractures or ligamentous injury can leave the cervical spine so unstable that the normal manipulation of a direct laryngoscopy will injure the spinal cord. This is a low probability event but is of concern to the healthcare team because quadriplegia is a catastrophic complication.

Manual in-line cervical stabilization has been shown to be safe and effective in protecting the cervical spine over tens of thousands of direct laryngoscopies and is the common approach to urgent intubations in the trauma population. Another option commonly used only in patients with known cervical instability is an awake intubation over a fiberoptic bronchoscope. This approach allows for the least manipulation of the neck but requires a cooperative patient who can tolerate the time required for topical anesthesia of the airway and a slower intubation. Awake fiberoptic intubation may also increase the risk of aspiration in patients with a full stomach, especially if topical anesthesia of the pharynx and vocal cords is provided.

Other intubation devices may also decrease the need for manipulation of the neck. Good results have been achieved with the Bullard laryngoscope, lighted stylet intubations, and use of an intubating stylet with a less forceful laryngoscopy. Manual cervical stabilization is recommended with each of these approaches. In a difficult case such as the present one, the intubation technique chosen should be one that the anesthesiologist is experienced and comfortable with; this factor may be more relevant than the specific technology used.

Karlin A. Airway management of trauma victims. *Prob Anesth Trauma Care* 2002;13(3): 279–288.

Majernick TG, Bieniek R, Houston JB, et al. Cervical spine motion during orotracheal intubation. *Ann Emerg Med* 1986;15:417.

C.8. How can you minimize the risks of aspiration?

Because any significant injury is associated with decreased gastrointestinal motility, all trauma patients are considered to have full stomachs. The risk of aspiration is further increased by intoxication with drugs or alcohol, obesity, the use of analgesics, and injuries to the face, neck, or abdomen that may lead to bleeding within the gastrointestinal tract.

Minimization of risk is a function of how quickly the intubation must be accomplished. One component of prophylaxis is the normal use of rapid-sequence induction to minimize the time during which the airway is at risk. Another is the use of cricoid pressure (the Sellick maneuver) to obstruct the upper esophagus against passive reflux. Although recent magnetic resonance imaging research has shown significant variability in the relative anatomy of the cricoid ring and the esophagus, casting doubt on the efficacy of cricoid pressure, there is no reason not to do it in most cases. In the case under consideration, there would be a risk of dislodging the impaling object, making cricoid pressure inadvisable. It would be reasonable to administer an H_2 antagonist such as cimetidine and a promotility agent such as metaclopramide if time allowed, but these agents would require 1 to 2 hours to have any substantial effect. An oral antacid is contraindicated because of the potential injury to the esophagus.

Smith KJ, Dobranowski J, Yip G, et al. Cricoid pressure displaces the esophagus: an observational study using magnetic resonance imaging. *Anesthesiology* 2003;99(1): 60–64.

C.9. How would you anesthetize the airway for an awake intubation?

Innervation of the airway can be separated into three neural pathways. If nasal intubation is planned, some method of anesthetizing maxillary branches from the trigeminal nerve is required. Involvement of the posterior tongue will require blockade of the glossopharyngeal nerve. Structures more distal in the airway to the epiglottis will require blockade of vagal branches, with the superior laryngeal nerve supplying the pharyngeal apparatus and the recurrent laryngeal nerve supplying the vocal cord and the tracheal mucosa.

The trigeminal nerve, which supplies sensory innervation to the nasal mucosa, can be anesthetized by inserting a nasal airway lubricated with lidocaine jelly into the patent naris. Mixing the lidocaine jelly with oxymetazoline 0.05%, phenylephrine 10 mg, or 4% cocaine may help vasoconstrict the nasal blood vessels and diminish bleeding from the nasal mucosa. The liquid local anesthetic and vasoconstrictor may also be applied in droplet form from a syringe.

The glossopharyngeal nerves of interest are the tonsillar nerves, which provide sensation to the mucosa overlying the palatine tonsil and continuous parts of the soft palate, and the sensory branches to the posterior one third of the tongue. First, one must provide topical intraoral anesthesia with local anesthetic spray or nebulized lidocaine. Following topical anesthesia of the tongue, the mouth is opened wide and the posterior tonsillar pillar (palatopharyngeal fold) is identified. Then, a 22-gauge needle can be inserted at the caudad portion of the tonsillar pillar. The needle tip is inserted submucosally and following careful aspiration for blood 5 mL of 0.5% lidocaine is injected. The block is then repeated on the contralateral side. A similar block can be performed with direct application of anesthetic soaked cotton to the bilateral tonsillar fossae.

The vagus nerve supplies innervation to the mucosa of the airway from the level of the epiglottis to the distal airways through both the superior and recurrent laryngeal nerves. A superior laryngeal nerve block and a translaryngeal block can be useful in anesthetizing these pathways. With the patient lying supine, a 22-gauge needle attached to a syringe is directed at the most posterior palpable part of the hyoid bone, near the greater cornu, and anterior to the carotid sheath. The needle must be parallel to the table and never directed posteriorly for fear of penetrating the carotid sheath. When the needle strikes the hyoid, it is carefully walked caudad until it just slips off the hyoid, and then advanced a short distance through the hyothyroid membrane. Aspiration should produce nothing. Then 2 mL of 2% lidocaine is injected and the block repeated on the opposite side.

The translaryngeal block is performed with a 20- or 22-gauge needle attached to a syringe. The needle is inserted through the cricothyroid membrane in the midline and air is aspirated. The patient is asked to inhale deeply and then to exhale fully. At the end of expiration, 4 mL of 2% to 4% lidocaine is injected rapidly and the needle is quickly removed. The resultant coughing will ensure a wide distribution of local anesthetic droplets throughout the airway. If stability of the cervical spine is in doubt, then in-line stabilization should be held while the block is performed and coughing occurs.

Brown DL. *Atlas of regional anesthesia*. Philadelphia: WB Saunders, 1992:181–200.

Gotta AW, Sullivan CA. Anesthesia of the upper airway using topical anesthetic and laryngeal nerve block. *Br J Anaesth* 1981;53:1055–1058.

C.10. What are the risks of awake fiberoptic intubation?

The greatest risk of awake fiberoptic intubation is deterioration of the patient's airway or mental status (or both) during the procedure. Ineffective topical anesthesia can lead to agitation and combativeness, which in turn leads to increased use of intravenous sedatives. Blood and secretions in the airway can cause coughing, laryngospasm, or aspiration. Oversedation causes respiratory depression and desaturation, which can pressure the anesthesia providers and lead to hasty decisions. More uncommon complications include injury to nerves or vessels during local nerve blocks, toxicity from local anesthesia ingestion, and direct injury to the laryngeal or pharyngeal mucosa.

This particular case also includes the possibility of inadvertent dislodgement of the impaling tree branch during sedation and topicalization or during the intubation effort itself. Bleeding from a loss of tamponade or open disruption of the airway could necessitate a sudden change in anesthetic and surgical plans. Although awake fiberoptic intubation in the operating room is a reasonable starting point for this case, the anesthesiologists and surgeons involved must be prepared for other eventualities. These would include both rapid-sequence intubation and emergency surgical airway access.

C.11. If the patient cannot be ventilated, what options are available?

Failure of awake fiberoptic intubation in this case should be followed by an immediate attempt at rapid-sequence intubation. If repetitive strain injuries (RSIs) are not possible and the patient cannot be ventilated by mask or laryngeal mask airway (LMA), then a surgical airway may be required. An alternate technique involves placing a 14-gauge catheter over a needle through the cricothyroid membrane, removing the needle and using the catheter for jet ventilation. This technique provides a temporary route for oxygenation, as a bridge to a surgical airway, but is recognized as highly tenuous. Kinking or dislodgement of the jet catheter are common complications, with tension pneumothorax a possibility if the catheter tip is displaced into the paratracheal tissues.

Benumof JL, Scheller MS. The importance of transtracheal jet ventilation in the management of the difficult airway. *Anesthesiology* 1989;71:769 778.

C.12. Would a laryngeal mask airway (LMA) or other pharyngeal airway be of assistance?

Although an LMA or other supraglottic airway support device is often a great help in the difficult airway algorithm, this case may represent an exception. Establishing an efficient mask airway is beneficial if the cause of patient distress is neurologic (diminished respiratory drive due to anesthesia or traumatic brain injury) or related to pharyngeal anatomy (obstruction after muscle relaxation). Supraglottic ventilation will not help with more distal causes of airway obstruction, such as laryngospasm, tracheal disruption, or massive aspiration. Although an LMA or equivalent device should be on hand when this patient is brought to the operating room (OR), it is relatively less likely to be of use.

C.13. What surgical airway options are available in this case?

As with the laryngeal mask airway (LMA), surgical airway access is beneficial when the cause of airway obstruction is proximal to the intervention. Cricothyroidotomy—the fastest and most readily performed surgical airway procedure—is therefore of benefit in patients who cannot be intubated and have airway obstruction involving the pharynx or larynx. This procedure may be accomplished by surgical opening of the cricothyroid membrane and placing an endotracheal tube into the trachea. Operative cricothyrotomy can be performed more rapidly than conventional tracheostomy; however, it is more traumatic to the larynx and the cricothyrotomy tube should be removed after 24 hours. If the patient cannot be decannulated at this time a conventional tracheostomy should replace the cricothyrotomy.

Tracheostomy, performed lower in the airway, requires more extensive surgical dissection, takes longer, and carries a greater risk of hemorrhage secondary to thyroid tissue trauma. Surgical access to the lower trachea might be necessary in the present case if the impaling object has transected or significantly disrupted the airway. This would be accomplished essentially through the wound itself but would require a partial or complete median sternotomy and the full resources of the operating room (OR).

Britt LD, Peyser MB. Penetrating and blunt neck trauma. In: Mattox KL, Feliciano DV, Moore EE, eds. *Trauma*, 4th ed. New York: McGraw-Hill, 2000:437–439.

C.14. What maintenance anesthetics are indicated or contraindicated in this patient?

If initial awake fiberoptic examination of the trachea (at the time of intubation) rules out an airway injury, then muscle relaxation to facilitate surgical exploration would be appropriate for the duration of the case. Any of the commonly used intermediate acting nondepolarizing relaxants could be used. If an airway injury is present, then management of the patient using inhalational anesthesia alone, with continued spontaneous ventilation, offers additional security in the event of airway discontinuity during the course of surgical repair. Sevoflurane, because of its greater palatability, is the easiest volatile anesthetic to administer without interrupting the patient's ventilation. Care must be taken to ensure adequate fluid volume replacement during a pure inhalational anesthetic as hemodynamic instability is possible. Nitrous oxide is contraindicated when the potential for pneumothorax exists or when airway continuity is in doubt.

Narcotics will certainly be required for postoperative analgesia and may offer some intraoperative advantages as well. Once airway patency is assured, a narcotic-based anesthetic provides for the lowest level of circulating catecholamines, making it easier to assess and manage fluid resuscitation. The usual concern with delayed emergence in a patient receiving a large dose of narcotics is not relevant in this case as the patient will most likely require postoperative mechanical ventilation. The only caveat to intraoperative narcotics is the potential need to sustain spontaneous ventilation while the airway is assessed; narcotic administration should, therefore, be delayed until the anesthetic and surgical plans have become clear.

C.15. What complications will the surgical plan introduce?

Maintenance of homeostasis in the face of surgical provocations is the theme of many anesthetics and the present case is no exception. At some point—ideally after anesthetic induction, successful airway management, and placement of lines and monitors—the impaling object is going to be removed from the patient's neck. Blunt object impalements in patients seen alive in the trauma center may produce less organ-specific damage than predicted from the location and course of the injury due to the ability of mobile anatomic structures to deform away from low-speed penetrations. Even so, it is entirely possible that this object has injured one of the great vessels or the trachea and that removing it might lead to torrential bleeding or significant disruption of the airway. The anesthesia team must be prepared to change course rapidly from a spontaneous breathing inhalational approach (assuming that airway continuity is the initial concern) to a hemodynamically friendly narcotic-based approach if blood loss and hemorrhagic shock become the major issue. An open discussion of both surgical and anesthetic plans, including likely contingencies, is highly recommended before beginning definitive treatment.

D. Postoperative Management

D.1. What are the criteria for extubation?

Assuming that the case goes well and the patient's anatomic injuries are successfully repaired, it is appropriate to consider emergence and extubation when the following criteria are satisfied:

- Hemodynamic stability with complete cessation of bleeding and normal systemic coagulation.
- Adequate respiratory drive and reserve including complete return of neuromuscular function.
- Acceptable mental status. The patient should be calm, cooperative, comfortable, and able to follow commands.
- Evidence of airway patency. Edema at the site of injury will not be an issue with an endotracheal tube in place but might obstruct the airway quickly following extubation. Although not 100% predictive, the presence of an air leak around the endotracheal tube when the cuff is deflated is very reassuring.
- Completion of the diagnostic workup for "high-energy" trauma, including indicated computed tomographic (CT) scans and laboratory studies. It would be poor judgment to extubate the patient only to have the orthopedic surgeons schedule him for urgent pelvic surgery.

Dutton RP, McCunn M. Anesthesia for trauma. In: Miller RD, ed. *Miller's anesthesia*, 6th ed. Philadelphia: Churchill Livingstone, 2005:2451–2495.

D.2. What techniques may be used during extubation?

The best results from extubation will be achieved when the patient is most calm and comfortable and when the extubation itself is as nonstimulating. The appropriate level of sedation and analgesia is a complicated, controversial, and a very important question. Sedative agents such as benzodiazepines and propofol will diminish the patient's respiratory drive, cooperation, and ability to protect the airway, and should be minimized. The right level of narcotics, on the other hand, will allow for a comfortable patient with diminished airway reactivity, who can open their eyes and follow commands but is not otherwise distressed by the endotracheal tube or ventilator. The endotracheal tube should be suctioned ahead of time, and extubation deferred if there are copious secretions. Enough time should be allowed after suctioning for the stimulation to pass and the patient to relax. The posterior pharynx is then suctioned, the patient is asked to inhale deeply, the cuff is deflated, and the endotracheal tube is removed in one swift motion as the patient exhales.

The airway is in jeopardy immediately after extubation because edema and secretions may compromise respiratory function. Continuous pulse oximetry in a monitored setting is required and humidified oxygen should be administered for at least 24 hours postoperatively.

D.3. How does alcohol abuse affect postoperative management?

Symptomatic withdrawal from alcohol usually occurs within 24 hours and manifests as agitation, tachycardia, and hypertension. Delirium tremens (DTs) can occur thereafter if prophylactic therapy is not initiated. Prophylaxis should consist of a small basal dose of benzodiazepines or a low-dose intravenous alcohol infusion, with frequent assessment of mental status and the willingness to provide supplemental short-acting benzodiazepines if symptoms develop. The plan for DT prophylaxis should be coordinated with the pain management plan, ideally under the direction of a single individual, to provide for overall consistency and to avoid oversedation and respiratory arrest secondary to polypharmaceutical administration.

D.4. What pain medication should be used?

Postoperative analgesia in this case will depend on the extent of the surgical procedure and on the individual tolerance of the patient. Soft tissue exploration of the neck, including surgery on the trachea or major vessels, requires relatively little postoperative analgesia. Titrated intravenous narcotics can be used in the first 24 hours with a rapid transition to an oral narcotic/acetaminophen preparation thereafter. Median sternotomy or other significant extension of the surgery into the chest will necessitate more intensive postoperative analgesia including continuous narcotic infusion although the patient remains intubated, followed by intravenous patient-controlled analgesia after emergence and extubation. Nonsteroidal antiinflammatory drugs (NSAIDs) are an appropriate adjuvant therapy once the risk of traumatic hemorrhage is past.

CHAPTER 47

Open-Eye Injury

Theresa T. Kudlak

A 28-YEAR-OLD OTHERWISE HEALTHY MAN
presented to the emergency room with a fishhook embedded in his eye. He had eaten a full meal just before the fishing accident.

A. Medical Disease and Differential Diagnosis

1. Why is this patient a particular challenge to the anesthesiologist?
2. What are the determinants of intraocular pressure (IOP) under normal circumstances? What is the normal range? What was the IOP in this patient's injured eye?
3. How is aqueous humor formed and eliminated?
4. How is IOP affected by arterial P_{CO_2}, systemic blood pressure, coughing and vomiting, deep inspiration, and hypoxemia?
5. What is the role of the central nervous system (CNS) on IOP?
6. What is glaucoma?
7. Is atropine premedication contraindicated in patients with glaucoma?
8. How do carbonic anhydrase inhibitors work to decrease IOP? By what mechanism may osmotic agents decrease IOP?
9. Are carbonic anhydrase inhibitors or osmotic diuretics indicated in open-globe injuries?
10. Are topically applied ophthalmic medications absorbed systemically? How can this absorption be reduced? Which eyedrops may have effects that are of concern to the anesthesiologist?

B. Preoperative Evaluation and Preparation

1. Is an open-globe injury always a surgical emergency?
2. What preoperative evaluation would you require?
3. The patient had eaten shortly before the accident. Would you attempt to pass a nasogastric tube or to administer emetics to empty the stomach?
4. Could this case be done with topical anesthesia or a retrobulbar block?
5. How would you premedicate this patient?

C. Intraoperative Management

1. What are some factors that may increase the risk of vitreous herniation during induction and maintenance of anesthesia?
2. Will you intubate this patient? Would you consider a laryngeal mask airway? How does intubation affect IOP? How can this effect be minimized?
3. Would you consider an awake intubation?

4. Is succinylcholine contraindicated in open-globe injuries? How does succinylcholine affect IOP?

5. Does pretreatment with nondepolarizing muscle relaxants prevent the succinylcholine-induced elevation in IOP?

6. How do nondepolarizing muscle relaxants affect IOP?

7. How will you perform a rapid-sequence induction and intubation without using succinylcholine?

8. What are the effects of ketamine on the eye?

9. Would you consider the use of etomidate as an induction agent? What about propofol?

10. How do inhalation agents affect IOP and by what mechanism?

11. During the procedure, the patient's pulse suddenly dropped to 40 beats per minute. What do you think was happening? What is the oculocardiac reflex (OCR)?

12. What are the afferent and efferent pathways of the OCR?

13. What factors contribute to the incidence of the OCR?

14. How do you diagnose and treat the OCR?

15. Is atropine useful?

16. Can retrobulbar block prevent the OCR? Is it appropriate in this patient?

D. Postoperative Management

1. Would you reverse the neuromuscular blockade in this patient?

2. Do reversal doses of atropine affect IOP?

3. What would you do before extubating this patient?

4. When would you extubate this patient?

5. The patient awakened in the recovery room and complained of pain and tearing in the opposite eye. The conjunctiva was inflamed. What was the likely cause?

6. Will taping the eyes shut or applying ointment prevent corneal abrasions? Are there any contributing factors?

7. What should you do when you suspect that your patient might have a corneal abrasion?

8. A month after the surgical repair, the patient complained of impaired vision in the operative eye. He was examined and found to have a detached retina. As part of the surgical treatment, the ophthalmologist injected a gas bubble into the patient's posterior chamber. Why is this important to an anesthesiologist?

A. Medical Disease and Differential Diagnosis

A.1. Why is this patient a particular challenge to the anesthesiologist?

The combination of a full stomach and an open-globe injury presents a unique challenge to the anesthesiologist. In addition to the increased risk of aspiration of gastric contents, any drug or maneuver that raises intraocular pressure (IOP) in the injured, open eye may cause extrusion of the vitreous humor and loss of vision when the globe is opened.

Cunningham AJ, Barry P. Intraocular pressure: physiology and implications for anesthetic management. *Can Anaesth Soc J* 1986;33:195.

Holloway KB. Control of the eye during general anaesthesia for intraocular surgery. *Br J Anaesth* 1980;52:671.

Miller RD, ed. *Miller's anesthesia*, 6th ed. New York: Churchill Livingstone, 2005:2533–2534.

A.2. What are the determinants of intraocular pressure (IOP) under normal circumstances? What is the normal range? What was the IOP in this patient's injured eye?

IOP is determined by the balance between production and drainage of aqueous humor, by changes in choroidal blood volume, and by vitreous volume and extraocular muscle tone. Resistance to outflow of aqueous humor in the trabecular tissue is probably the factor that maintains IOP within physiologic range, but the mechanism of homeostasis is unknown.

Normal IOP is 12 to 16 torr in the upright posture and increases by 2 to 4 torr in the supine position.

When the globe is open, the IOP is lowered, and may be as low as ambient pressure. Our concern in this case is for the relative volume of choroid and vitreous humor within the eye. If this volume should increase while the eye is opened, the vitreous humor may be lost. Any deformation of the eye by external pressure in the globe may cause an increase in IOP.

Cunningham AJ, Barry P. Intraocular pressure: physiology and implications for anaesthetic management. *Can Anaesth Soc J* 1986;33:195–208.

Jay JL. Functional organization of the human eye. *Br J Anaesth* 1980;52:649.

Kumar C, Dodds C, Fanning G, eds. *Ophthalmic anaesthesia*. Lisse, The Netherlands: Swets and Zeitlinger BV, 2002:23–25.

LeMay M. Aspects of measurement in ophthalmology. *Br J Anaesth* 1980;52:655.

Smith GB. *Ophthalmic anaesthesia*. Baltimore: University Park Press, 1983:1–13.

A.3. How is aqueous humor formed and eliminated?

Aqueous humor is a clear fluid that occupies the anterior and posterior chambers of the eye. Its total volume is 0.3 mL. Aqueous humor is produced primarily by an active secretory process from the ciliary body in the posterior chambers at an equilibrium rate of 2 μL per minute. The aqueous then circulates through the pupil to the anterior chamber, passes through the trabeculated Fontana's spaces, and enters Schlemm's canal. From here, the fluid drains into the episcleral veins and finally into the cavernous sinus or jugular venous systems (Fig. 47.1).

Cunningham AJ, Barry P. Intraocular pressure: physiology and implications for anaesthetic management. *Can Anaesth Soc J* 1986;33:195–208.

Jay JL. Functional organization of the human eye. *Br J Anaesth* 1980;52:649.

LeMay M. Aspects of measurement in ophthalmology. *Br J Anaesth* 1980;52:655.

McGoldrick K, ed. *Anesthesia for ophthalmic and otolaryngologic surgery*. Philadelphia: WB Saunders, 1992:180–182.

A.4. How is intraocular pressure (IOP) affected by arterial P_{CO_2}, systemic blood pressure, coughing and vomiting, deep inspiration, and hypoxemia?

The choroidal arterioles vasodilate in response to hypercapnia and constrict during hypocapnia, thereby changing intraocular volume and pressure. However, the effect is minimal within the normal physiologic range of P_{CO_2}.

Minor fluctuations in arterial blood pressure also have minimal effects on IOP, although IOP may be seen to increase when hypertension is sustained and can fall significantly with induced hypotension. Changes in venous pressure, on the other hand, have a major impact on IOP. Vomiting, coughing, and bucking on the endotracheal tube cause a dramatic increase in IOP by

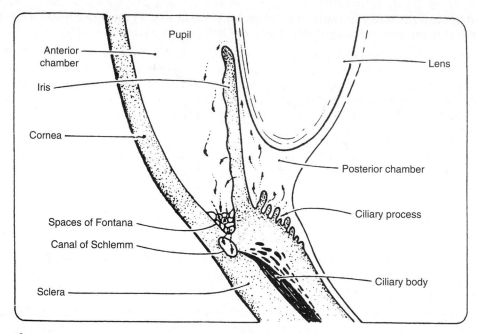

Figure 47.1 Sites of formation, circulation, and drainage of aqueous humor. (From Cunningham AJ, Barry B. Intraocular pressure: physiology and implications for anesthetic management. *Can Anaesth Soc J* 1986;33:197, with permission.)

30 to 40 torr. These actions, and also Valsalva's maneuver, cause congestion in the venous system, which impedes outflow of aqueous humor and increases the volume of choroidal blood.

A deep inspiration may reduce IOP by 5 torr. Hypoxemia may increase IOP through choroidal vasodilatation.

Calobrisi BL, Lebowitz P. Muscle relaxants and the open globe. *Int Anesthesiol Clin* 1990;28(2):83–88.

Cunningham AJ, Barry P. Intraocular pressure: physiology and implications for anaesthetic management. *Can Anaesth Soc J* 1986;33:195.

Miller RD, ed. *Anesthesia*, 6th ed. New York: Churchill Livingstone, 2005:2531–2533.

Murphy DF. Anesthesia and intraocular pressure. *Anesth Analg* 1985;64:520.

Smith RB, Aass AA, Nemoto EM. Intraocular and intracranial pressure during respiratory alkalosis and acidosis. *Br J Anaesth* 1981;53:967.

A.5. What is the role of the central nervous system (CNS) on intraocular pressure (IOP)?

The CNS influences IOP through alterations in extraocular muscle tone or, indirectly, by hormonal or hemodynamic changes.

Cunningham AJ, Barry P. Intraocular pressure: physiology and implications for anaesthetic management. *Can Anaesth Soc J* 1986;33:195.

Miller RD, ed. *Miller's anesthesia*, 6th ed. New York: Churchill Livingstone, 2005:2531–2533.

A.6. What is glaucoma?

Glaucoma is a pathologic elevation of intraocular pressure (IOP) caused by increased resistance to outflow of aqueous humor from the anterior chamber of the eye. It is classified as either open- or closed-angle glaucoma, depending on the anatomy and pathophysiology. Chronic elevation of IOP interferes with the intraocular blood supply and normal metabolism of the cornea. It can result in corneal opacities or decreased retinal blood flow.

The pathophysiology in glaucoma involves increased resistance to the flow of aqueous humor through Fontana's spaces as a result of scarring of the trabecular network or thickening of the endothelial covering of these channels. In closed-angle glaucoma the iris bulges forward, blocking the access of aqueous humor to the trabecular network. This may occur with pupillary dilation or an acutely swollen lens.

Johnson DH, Brubaker RF. Glaucoma: an overview. *Mayo Clin Proc* 1986;61:59.

LeMay M. Aspects of measurement in ophthalmology. *Br J Anaesth* 1980;52:655.

A.7. Is atropine premedication contraindicated in patients with glaucoma?

It was previously thought by some clinicians that atropine was contraindicated in patients with glaucoma, especially narrow-angle glaucoma. However, this claim is true only when atropine is given intravenously (IV) or topically to the eye and causes pupillary dilation (mydriasis). Atropine in a standard premedication dose of 0.4 mg intramuscularly (IM) causes no increase in IOP in either open- or closed-angle glaucoma because only approximately 0.0001 mg is absorbed by the eye. Therefore, intramuscular atropine for premedication is acceptable. However, scopolamine has a greater mydriatic effect than atropine. Therefore, scopolamine is not recommended for premedication in patients with known or suspected narrow-angle glaucoma.

Adams AK, Jones RM. Anaesthesia for eye surgery: general considerations. *Br J Anaesth* 1980;52:663.

Barash PG, Cullen BF, Stoelting RK, eds. *Clinical anesthesia*, 5th ed. Philadelphia: Lippincott Williams & Wilkins, 2006:977–978.

Miller RD, ed. *Anesthesia*, 6th ed. New York: Churchill Livingstone, 2005:2532.

Rosen DA. Anesthesia in ophthalmology. *Can Anaesth Soc J* 1962;9:545.

Schwartz H, deRoeth A, Papper EM. Preanesthetic use of atropine in patients with glaucoma. *JAMA* 1957;165:144.

A.8. How do carbonic anhydrase inhibitors work to decrease intraocular pressure (IOP)? By what mechanism may osmotic agents decrease IOP?

Carbonic anhydrase inhibitors, such as acetazolamide, interfere with the sodium-pump mechanism necessary for secretion of aqueous humor. An intravenous dose acts in 5 minutes, with maximal effect in 20 to 30 minutes. Chronic acetazolamide therapy may result in potassium depletion.

Osmotic agents, such as mannitol, increase plasma oncotic pressure relative to that of aqueous humor and produce an acute, transient drop in IOP. The maximum reduction in IOP occurs after 30 to 45 minutes and the effect lasts 5 to 6 hours.

Barash PG, Cullen BF, Stoelting RK, eds. *Clinical anesthesia*, 5th ed. Philadelphia: Lippincott Williams & Wilkins, 2006:978–979.

McGoldrick KE. Ocular drugs and anesthesia. *Int Anesthesiol Clin* 1990;28(2): 72–77.

A.9. Are carbonic anhydrase inhibitors or osmotic diuretics indicated in open-globe injuries?

No. If the globe is open, the intraocular pressure (IOP) is low, and these agents are not useful. In addition, they may cause transient choroidal congestion, which could lead to loss of ocular contents.

Smith GB. *Ophthalmic anaesthesia*. Baltimore: University Park Press, 1983.

A.10. Are topically applied ophthalmic medications absorbed systemically? How can this absorption be reduced? Which eyedrops may have effects that are of concern to the anesthesiologist?

Topical ophthalmic drugs may be absorbed through the conjunctiva or may drain through the nasolacrimal duct and be absorbed through the nasal mucosa. Absorption is increased when the eye is instrumented, diseased, or traumatized. Finger pressure on the inner canthus for a few minutes after instillation of eyedrops will impede absorption by occluding the nasolacrimal duct.

Usage of the following topical medications may have implications for the anesthesiologist.

Atropine

Atropine is used to produce mydriasis and cycloplegia. The 1% solution contains 0.2 mg to 0.5 mg of atropine per drop. Systemic reactions, seen primarily in children and older adults, include tachycardia, flushing, thirst, dry skin, and agitation. Atropine is contraindicated in closed-angle glaucoma.

Scopolamine

One drop of the 0.5% solution has 0.2 mg of scopolamine. Central nervous system (CNS) excitement can be treated with physostigmine, 0.015 mg per kg intravenously (IV), repeated one or two times in a 15-minute period. Scopolamine is contraindicated in closed-angle glaucoma.

Cyclopentolate (cyclogel)

Cyclopentolate, a short-acting mydriatic and cycloplegic, may cause transient neurotoxic effects, such as incoherence, visual hallucinations, slurred speech, ataxia, and seizures. It is contraindicated in closed-angle glaucoma.

Tropicamide (mydriacyl)

Tropicamide is used to produce mydriasis for refraction or funduscopic examination. It may have CNS effects and can elevate intraocular pressure (IOP) in closed-angle glaucoma.

Phenylephrine hydrochloride (neosynephrine)

Phenylephrine hydrochloride is used to produce capillary decongestion and pupillary dilatation. Applied to the cornea, phenylephrine hydrochloride can cause palpitations, nervousness, tachycardia, headache, nausea and vomiting, severe hypertension, reflex bradycardia, and subarachnoid hemorrhage. Solutions of 2.5%, 5%, and 10% (6.25-mg phenylephrine per drop) are available. The dose is 1 drop per eye per hour of the 2.5% solution (children) or the 5% solution (adults).

Epinephrine

Topical 2% epinephrine will decrease aqueous secretion, improve outflow, and lower IOP in open-angle glaucoma. Side effects include hypertension, palpitations, fainting, pallor, and tachycardia. The effects last approximately 15 minutes. One drop of 2% solution contains 0.5 to 1 mg of epinephrine. Epinephrine 1:200,000 in a balanced salt solution is sometimes continuously infused into the anterior chamber during cataract surgery. Systemic effects may occur.

Timolol maleate (timoptic)

Timolol Maleate is a β-blocker used in the treatment of chronic glaucoma. Side effects include light-headedness, fatigue, disorientation, depressed CNS function, and exacerbation of asthma. Bradycardia and bronchospasm may occur as well as potentiation of systemic β-blockers.

Betaxolol HCl (betoptic)

Betaxolol HCl is a cardioselective (β-1) blocking agent used to treat glaucoma. It may be hazardous in patients with sinus bradycardia, heart block, or heart failure.

Acetylcholine

Acetylcholine may be injected intraoperatively into the anterior chamber to produce miosis. Side effects are due to its parasympathetic action and include hypotension, bradycardia, and bronchospasm. Intravenous atropine is an effective treatment.

Echothiophate iodide (phospholine iodide)

Echothiophate iodide, a cholinesterase inhibitor, is used as a miotic agent. It may prolong the effect of both succinylcholine and ester-type local anesthetics. Levels of pseudocholinesterase decrease by 80% after 2 weeks on the drug. It takes 3 to 6 weeks for return to normal pseudocholinesterase activity after stopping the drug (4 weeks for return to 75% activity). Succinylcholine and ester-type local anesthetics should be avoided. Demecarium is another such cholinesterase inhibitor.

Cocaine

Cocaine is used to produce vasoconstriction and to shrink mucous membranes during dacryocystorhinostomy. One drop of 4% solution contains approximately 1.5 mg of cocaine, and the maximum dose is approximately 3 mg per kg. Systemic effects may be seen with a dose as low as 20 mg and involve the CNS, respiratory, and cardiovascular systems.

Ballin N, Becker B, Goldman ML. Systemic effects of epinephrine applied topically to the eye. *Invest Ophthalmol* 1966;5:125.

Barash PG, Cullen BF, Stoelting RK, eds. *Clinical anesthesia*, 5th ed. Philadelphia: Lippincott Williams & Wilkins, 2001:980–982.

Fraundfelder FT, Scafidi AF. Possible adverse effects from topical ocular 10 percent phenylephrine. *Am J Ophthalmol* 1978;84:447.

Johnson DH. Glaucoma: an overview. *Mayo Clin Proc* 1986;61:59.

Lansche RK. Systemic reactions to topical epinephrine and phenylephrine. *Am J Ophthalmol* 1966;49:95.

McGoldrick KE. Ocular drugs and anesthesia. *Int Anesthesiol Clin* 1990;28(2):72–77.

Miller RD, ed. *Miller's anesthesia*, 6th ed. New York: Churchill Livingstone, 2005:2536–2537.

deRoeth A, Bettbar WD, Rosenberg P. Effect of phospholine iodine on blood cholinesterase levels. *Am J Ophthalmol* 1963;49:586.

B. Preoperative Evaluation and Preparation

B.1. Is an open-globe injury always a surgical emergency?

No. In most cases surgery is not required immediately, and some time may be spent in adequately preparing the patient for anesthesia and surgery. However, the surgery should probably be performed within 12 hours to minimize the possibility of infection and other complications. Delaying surgery for gastric emptying to occur is not reliable as gastric emptying may be prolonged in this stressful situation.

Arthur DS, Dewar KMS. Anaesthesia for eye surgery in children. *Br J Anaesth* 1980;52:681.

Miller RD, ed. *Miller's anesthesia*, 6th ed. New York: Churchill Livingstone, 2005:2533–2534.

Smith GB. *Ophthalmic anaesthesia*. Baltimore: University Park Press, 1983:44–49.

B.2. What preoperative evaluation would you require?

An accurate, thorough history, and physical examination are the best means of evaluating this patient preoperatively and should reveal any existing medical problems that will guide your selection of preoperative laboratory tests.

In this otherwise healthy young patient, no routine laboratory tests are indicated, unless they are required by the institution in which you are practicing. In cases in which more extensive trauma is suspected, other injuries must also be addressed, such as fractures to the skull and orbit, intracranial hemorrhage, and other injuries as suggested by the history and physical examination.

Barash PG, Cullen BF, Stoelting RK, eds. *Clinical anesthesia*, 5th ed. Philadelphia: Lippincott Williams & Wilkins, 2006:982–983.

Miller RD, ed. *Miller's anesthesia*, 6th ed. New York: Churchill Livingstone, 2005:982–983.

B.3. The patient had eaten shortly before the accident. Would you attempt to pass a nasogastric tube or to administer emetics to empty the stomach?

Absolutely not. These procedures are contraindicated when there has been a perforation of the eye. Gagging, vomiting, and straining could cause a potentially disastrous increase in intraocular pressure (IOP). A cough can increase central venous pressure and choroidal blood volume and may raise IOP by 34 to 40 torr.

Adams AK, Jones RM. Anaesthesia for eye surgery: general considerations. *Br J Anaesth* 1980;52:663.

Arthur DS, Dewar KMS. Anaesthesia for eye surgery in children. *Br J Anaesth* 1980;52:681.

Cunningham AJ, Barry P. Intraocular pressure: physiology and implications for anaesthetic management. *Can Anaesth Soc J* 1986;33:195.

B.4. Could this case be done with topical anesthesia or a retrobulbar block?

General anesthesia is the preferred technique for open-globe injuries: the patient is fully immobile and there is no time limit for the procedure. In this case where the patient is not NPO, an endotracheal tube will guard against aspiration.

A retrobulbar or peribulbar injection has the potential to increase intraocular pressure (IOP) because of the volume of local anesthetic used and the likelihood of the patient squeezing his eyes during the injection. However, there have been reports of successful use of blocks for repair of open-globe injuries. Topical anesthesia with intravenous (IV) sedation has also been used to repair the globe in select patients with limited injury when general anesthesia is contraindicated.

Boscia F, Tegola MG, Columbo G, et al. Combined topical anesthesia and sedation for open-globe injuries in selected patients. *Ophthalmology* 2003;110:1555–1559.

Lo MW, Chalfin S. Retrobulbar anesthesia for repair of ruptured globes. *AM J Ophthalmol* 1997;123:820–831.

Scott IU, McCabe CM, Flynn HW. Local anesthesia with intravenuous sedation for surgical repair of selected open globe injuries. *Am J Ophthalmol* 2002;134:707–711.

B.5. How would you premedicate this patient?

Premedications should be given parenterally because gastrointestinal absorption is unreliable. Sedatives and anxiolytics may be given as necessary. Metoclopramide (0.15 mg/kg intramuscularly [IM] or intravenously [IV]) may be used to facilitate gastric emptying and to increase the tone of the cardiac sphincter. Narcotics should be used cautiously because they may cause nausea and vomiting. Nonparticulate antacids and H_2-receptor antagonists (cimetidine 2 mg/kg IM) should be considered to reduce the risk of aspiration pneumonitis. Intravenous droperidol (0.01 mg/kg) or ondansetron (0.1 mg/kg) can be given for antiemesis.

Atropine or glycopyrrolate will be useful to reduce secretions and gastric acidity, and they may also inhibit the oculocardiac reflex (OCR).

Barash PG, Cullen BF, Stoelting RK, eds. *Clinical anesthesia*, 5th ed. Philadelphia: Lippincott Williams & Wilkins, 2006:988.

Cunningham AJ, Barry P. Intraocular pressure: physiology and implications for anaesthetic management. *Can Anaesth Soc J* 1986;33:195.

Smith GB. *Ophthalmic anaesthesia*. Baltimore: University Park Press, 1983:44–49.

C. Intraoperative Management

C.1. What are some factors that may increase the risk of vitreous herniation during induction and maintenance of anesthesia?

- Face mask pressing on the eyeball
- Increased pressure from coughing, straining, bucking, and head-down position
- Extraocular muscle spasm induced by depolarizing muscle relaxants or surgical stimulation during light anesthesia
- Poorly applied cricoid pressure, which blocks venous drainage from the eye
- Choroidal congestion from hypercarbia, hypoxia, osmotic diuretics, intubation, or increases in blood pressure

Cunningham AJ, Barry P. Intraocular pressure: physiology and implications for anaesthetic management. *Can Anaesth Soc J* 1986;33:195–208.

Holloway KB. Control of the eye during general anaesthesia for intraocular surgery. *Br J Anaesth* 1980;52:671.

Libonati MM, Leahy JJ, Ellison N. The use of succinylcholine in open-eye surgery. *Anesthesiology* 1985;62:637–640.

C.2. Will you intubate this patient? Would you consider a laryngeal mask airway? How does intubation affect intraocular pressure (IOP)? How can this effect be minimized?

It is imperative that this patient be intubated not only to maintain the airway, which is close to the surgical field, but also to avoid pressure by a face mask on the eyeball and to minimize the risk of aspiration. Although the laryngeal mask airway has been used successfully in ophthalmologic anesthesia, it is not appropriate in this case because it does not protect the airway from aspiration. Many studies have demonstrated a significant increase in IOP caused by laryngoscopy and intubation under varying states of anesthetic depth and muscle relaxation. IOP may be increased even when there is no visible reaction to intubation. This increase in IOP can be attenuated by topical laryngeal anesthesia and by increased depth of anesthesia to reduce coughing, straining, and increases in blood pressure. The cardiovascular response to intubation can also be reduced by intravenous lidocaine (1.5 mg/kg), β-blockers, α_2 agonists or calcium channel blockers. Topical anesthesia of the larynx is not recommended in a full-stomach situation because of the increased risk of aspiration.

Akhtar TM, McMurray P, Kerr WJ, et al. A comparison of laryngeal mask airway with tracheal tube for intra-ocular ophthalmic surgery. *Anaesthesia* 1992;47:668–671.

Barash PG, Cullen BF, Stoelting RK, eds. *Clinical anesthesia*, 5th ed. Philadelphia: Lippincott Williams & Wilkins, 2006:988–989.

Cook JH. The effect of suxamethonium on intraocular pressure. *Anaesthesia* 1981;36:359.

Gefke K, Anderson LW, Friesel H. Intravenous lidocaine as a suppressant of cough and laryngospasm with extubation after tonsillectomy. *Acta Anaesthesiol Scand* 1983;27:112.

Libonati MM, Leahy JJ, Ellison N. The use of succinylcholine in open-eye surgery. *Anesthesiology* 1985;62:637–640.

Miller RD, ed. *Miller's anesthesia*, 6th ed. New York: Churchill Livingstone, 2005:2532–2533.

Smith RB, Aass AA, Nernoto EM. Intraocular and intracranial pressure during respiratory alkalosis and acidosis. *Br J Anaesth* 1981;53:967.

C.3. Would you consider an awake intubation?

Awake intubation is frequently accompanied by coughing and bucking and is risky in an open-globe injury when other safe methods of intubation are available. However, when dealing with a possible compromised airway or difficult intubation, an awake fiberoptic intubation expertly done under careful sedation may be indicated to safely secure the airway.

Calobrisi BL, Lebowitz P. Muscle relaxants and the open globe. *Int Anesthesiol Clin* 1990;28(2):83–88.

C.4. Is succinylcholine contraindicated in open-globe injuries? How does succinylcholine affect intraocular pressure (IOP)?

The use of succinylcholine in open-globe injuries is controversial. In the intact eye, following thiopental induction, succinylcholine has been shown to increase IOP by 6 to 8 torr between

1 and 4 minutes after administration. Tracheal intubation further increases IOP. IOP returns to baseline in 5 to 7 minutes. In open-globe injuries, succinylcholine use has been associated with loss of ocular contents. The increase in IOP may be mediated by prolonged tonic contraction of the extraocular muscles, although IOP has been shown to rise after succinylcholine even when the extraocular muscles have been severed. Other factors that may be contributory include choroidal blood flow, increased central venous pressure, and increased resistance to outflow of aqueous humor resulting from the cycloplegic effects of succinylcholine.

The hemodynamic response to laryngoscopy or intubation may have a much more significant effect on IOP than succinylcholine alone. Simply blinking will raise the IOP in a normal eye by 10 to 15 torr, similar to the effect of succinylcholine. Pretreating with nifedipine or lidocaine, which deepens the anesthesia, may attenuate the increase in IOP following succinylcholine and intubation.

Calobrisi BL, Lebowitz P. Muscle relaxants and the open globe. *Int Anesthesiol Clin* 1990;
    38(2):83–88.

Cook JH. The effect of suxamethonium on intraocular pressure. *Anaesthesia* 1981;36:359.

Cunningham AJ, Barry P. Intraocular pressure: physiology and implications for anaesthetic
    management. *Can Anaesth Soc J* 1986;33:195–208.

Holloway KG. Control of the eye during general anaesthesia for intraocular surgery. *Br J
    Anaesth* 1980;52:671.

Kelly RE, Dinner M, Turner LS, et al. Succinylcholine increases intraocular pressure in the
    human eye with the extraocular muscles detached. *Anesthesiology* 1993;79:948–952.

Lincoff HA. The effect of succinylcholine on intraocular pressure. *Am J Ophthalmol*
    1955;40:501.

Moreno RJ, Kloess P, Carlson DW. Effect of succinylcholine on the intraocular contents of
    open globes. *Ophthalmology* 1991;98:636–638.

Murphy DS, Davis MJ. Succinylcholine use in emergency eye operation. *Can J Anaesth*
    1987;34:101.

Smith RB, Babinski M, Leano N. The effect of lidocaine on succinylcholine-induced rise in
    intraocular pressure. *Can Anaesth Soc J* 1979;26:482.

C.5. Does pretreatment with nondepolarizing muscle relaxants prevent the succinylcholine-induced elevation in intraocular pressure (IOP)?

Available data are contradictory on this question, probably reflecting different methods of IOP measurement under varying depths of anesthesia with a variety of anesthetic adjuvant agents. Many techniques have been tried to prevent succinylcholine-induced elevation of IOP, and none has been consistently effective. However, there is no published report of loss of ocular contents when succinylcholine use has been preceded by pretreatment with a nondepolarizing relaxant and barbiturate for induction, and many anesthesiologists feel this is a safe combination for rapid-sequence induction in the open-eye, full-stomach situation.

Bourke DL. Open-eye injuries. *Anesthesiology* 1985;63:727.

Calobrisi BL, Lebowitz P. Muscle relaxants and the open globe. *Int Anesthesiol Clin* 1990;
    28(2):83–88.

Cunningham AJ, Barry P. Intraocular pressure: physiology and implications for anaesthetic
    management. *Can Anaesth Soc J* 1986;33:195–208.

Hartman GS, Fiamengo SA, Riker WF Jr. Succinylcholine: mechanism of fasciculations and their prevention by d-tubocurarine or diphenylhydantoin. *Anesthesiology* 1986;65: 405.

Holloway KB. Control of the eye during general anaesthesia for intraocular surgery. *Br J Anaesth* 1980;52:671.

Konchigeri HN, Lee YE, Venugopal K. Effect of pancuronium on intraocular pressure changes induced by succinylcholine. *Can Anaesth Soc J* 1979;26:479.

Libonati MM, Leahy JJ, Ellison N. The use of succinylcholine in open-eye surgery. *Anesthesiology* 1985;62:637–640.

McGoldrick KE. The open globe: is an alternative to succinylcholine necessary? *J Clin Anesth* 1993;5:1.

Meyers EF, Krupin T, Johnson M, et al. Failure of nondepolarizing neuromuscular blockers to inhibit succinylcholine-induced increased intraocular pressure: a controlled study. *Anesthesiology* 1978;48:149.

Miller RD, Way WL, Hickey RF. Inhibition of succinylcholine-induced increased intraocular pressure by nondepolarizing muscle relaxants. *Anesthesiology* 1968;29:123.

Murphy DF. Anesthesia and intraocular pressure. *Anesth Analg* 1985;64:520.

C.6. How do nondepolarizing muscle relaxants affect intraocular pressure (IOP)?

Nondepolarizing muscle relaxants either decrease or have no effect on IOP.

Abbott MA. The control of intraocular pressure during the induction of anaesthesia for emergency eye surgery. A high-dose vecuronium technique. *Anaesthesia* 1987;42: 1008.

Agarwal LP, Mathur SP. Curare in ocular surgery. *Br J Ophthalmol* 1952;36:603.

Calobrisi BL, Lebowitz P. Muscle relaxants and the open globe. *Int Anesthesiol Clin* 1990; 28(2):83–88.

Cunningham AJ, Kelly CP, Farmer J, et al. The effect of metocurine and pancuronium combination in intraocular pressure. *Can Anaesth Soc J* 1982;29:617.

Litwiller RW, Di Fazio CA, Rushia EL. Pancuronium and intraocular pressure. *Anesthesiology* 1975;42:750.

Maharaj RJ, Humphrey D, Kaplan N, et al. Effects of atracurium on intraocular pressure. *Br J Anaesth* 1984;56:459.

Miller RD, ed. *Miller's anesthesia*, 6th ed. New York: Churchill Livingstone, 2005:2532–2533.

Schneider MJ, Stirt JA, Finholt DA. Atracurium, vecuronium, and intraocular pressure in humans. *Anesth Analg* 1986;65:877.

C.7. How will you perform a rapid-sequence induction and intubation without using succinylcholine?

The safety of the patient must always be the primary concern; the preservation of the injured eye is secondary. Measures must be taken to guarantee adequate anesthetic depth and to blunt the hemodynamic responses to laryngoscopy and endotracheal intubation. Pretreatment measures such as narcotics, β-blockers, calcium channel blockers, lidocaine, or midazolam should be considered. Before induction, the patient should breathe 100% oxygen for several minutes, administered by a gently applied face mask. Anesthesia can then be induced using carefully applied cricoid pressure with intravenous sodium thiopental (5 mg/kg) or propofol (2 to 3 mg/kg) and a nondepolarizing muscle relaxant. Several options exist:

- Pancuronium (0.15 to 0.2 mg/kg) will provide intubation condition in 90 seconds. Tachycardia and prolonged muscle relaxation may be a problem.
- Atracurium (0.5 mg/kg) will allow safe intubation in 3 minutes. A larger bolus (1.5 mg/kg) will allow intubation in 60 to 90 seconds, but may cause hypotension, tachycardia, and histamine release.
- Cisatracurium—because of its intermediate onset of action, cisatracurium (0.10 to 0.15 mg/kg) is not recommended for rapid-sequence endotracheal intubations. Cisatracurium (0.4 mg/kg) 8× ED95 will allow intubation in 90 seconds without histamine release, but duration of action may exceed 60 minutes.
- Vecuronium (0.2 mg/kg) should provide adequate intubating conditions after 90 seconds.
- Rocuronium (0.8 to 1.0 mg/kg) gives excellent intubating conditions at 60 to 70 seconds. Time to recovery is variable and may take 45 to 60 minutes.
- An alternative is to pretreat the patient with a small dose of the nondepolarizing relaxant several minutes before induction, which may shorten the onset of action and lessen the dose required of subsequently administered relaxant. This has been referred to as a *priming* dose. Its use is controversial in that it may lead to diplopia, muscle weakness, respiratory distress, and aspiration while offering no definite advantage over the use of larger initial doses of nondepolarizing muscle relaxants. The doses for rapid tracheal intubation with succinylcholine or various nondepolarizing relaxants are listed in Chapter 19, Section C.4, Table 19.4.

Whatever technique is selected, it is essential to monitor the degree of muscle relaxation with a neuromuscular blockade monitor. It is also possible to intubate the patient without any muscle relaxant at all after a deep level of anesthesia has been reached, but this is not a recommended technique. Not only is the airway unprotected for a long period of time but also prevention of bucking cannot be guaranteed and positive pressure ventilation by face mask may exert pressure on the eye.

Abbott MA. The control of intraocular pressure during the induction of anaesthesia for emergency eye surgery. A high-dose vecuronium technique. *Anaesthesia* 1987;42:1008.

Barash PG, Cullen BF, Stoelting RK, eds. *Clinical anesthesia*, 5th ed. Philadelphia: Lippincott Williams & Wilkins, 2006:988–989.

Brown EM, Krishnaprasad D, Smiller BG. Pancuronium for rapid-induction technique for tracheal intubation. *Can Anaesth Soc J* 1979;26:489.

Foldes F. Rapid tracheal intubation with nondepolarizing neuromuscular blocking drugs. The priming principle. *Br J Anaesth* 1984;56:663.

Lennon RL, Olson RA, Gronert GA. Atracurium or vecuronium for rapid sequence endotracheal intubation. *Anesthesiology* 1986;64:510.

Mehta MP, Choi WW, Geris SD, et al. Facilitation of rapid endotracheal intubations with divided doses of nondepolarizing neuromuscular blocking drugs. *Anesthesiology* 1985;62:392.

Musich J, Walts LF. Pulmonary aspiration after a priming dose of vecuronium. *Anesthesiology* 1986;64:517.

Rich AL, Witherspoon CD, Morris RE, et al. Use of nondepolarizing anesthetic agents in penetrating ocular injuries. *Anesthesiology* 1986;65:108.

Schneider MJ, Stirt JA, Finholt DA. Atracurium, vecuronium, and intraocular pressure in humans. *Anesth Analg* 1986;65:87.

Sosis MB. On use of priming with vecuronium in a patient with an open globe and a full stomach. *Anesth Analg* 1990;70:336.

C.8. What are the effects of ketamine on the eye?

Ketamine may cause nystagmus and blepharospasm and is, therefore, not suitable for ophthalmic surgery. Studies with respect to the effect of ketamine on intraocular pressure (IOP) have shown both increased and decreased IOP in children and no change in IOP in adults premedicated with diazepam and meperidine. This may depend on whether ketamine is administered through the intramuscular (IM) or intravenous (IV) route.

Antal M. Ketamine anesthesia and intraocular pressure. *Ann Ophthalmol* 1978;10:1281.

Ausinch E, Rayborn RL, Munsen ES, et al. Ketamine and intraocular pressure in children. *Anesth Analg* 1976;55:73.

Cunningham AJ, Barry P. Intraocular pressure: physiology and implication for anaesthetic management. *Can Anaesth Soc J* 1986;33:195.

Peuler M, Glass DD, Arens JF. Ketamine and intraocular pressure. *Anesthesiology* 1975;5:575.

Yoshikawa K, Murai Y. The effect of ketamine on intraocular pressure in children. *Anesth Analg* 1971;50:199.

C.9. Would you consider the use of etomidate as an induction agent? What about propofol?

Although etomidate has been associated with a decrease in intraocular pressure (IOP) when used as an induction agent, the unpredictable incidence of generalized myoclonus seen with etomidate use and resultant elevation of IOP may preclude its use in open-globe injuries, unless rapid and complete prior muscle relaxation can be guaranteed. Propofol, with its antiemetic properties and ability to decrease IOP, would be an excellent choice for induction.

Berry JM, Merin RG. Etomidate myoclonus and the open globe. *Anesth Analg* 1989;69:256–259.

Calla S, Gupta A, Sen N, et al. Comparison of the effects of etomidate and thiopentone on intraocular pressure. *Br J Anaesth* 1987;59:437.

Ferrari LR, Donlon JV. A comparison of propofol, midazolam and methohexital for sedation during retrobulbar and peribulbar block. *J Clin Anesth* 1992;4:93.

C.10. How do inhalation agents affect intraocular pressure (IOP) and by what mechanism?

Inhalation agents cause dose-related decreases in IOP as a consequence of the following:

- Reduced aqueous humor production
- Depression of the central nervous system (CNS) control center
- Facilitation of aqueous humor outflow
- Decreased extraocular muscle tension
- Lowered arterial blood pressure

The degree of IOP reduction is proportional to the depth of anesthesia.

Cunningham AJ, Barry P. Intraocular pressure: physiology and implications for anaesthetic management. *Can Anaesth Soc J* 1986;33:195.

Miller RD, ed. *Miller's anesthesia*, 6th ed. New York: Churchill Livingstone, 2000:2532–2533.

C.11. During the procedure, the patient's pulse suddenly dropped to 40 beats per minute. What do you think was happening? What is the oculocardiac reflex (OCR)?

The OCR may be manifested by bradycardia, bigeminy, ectopy, nodal rhythms, atrioventricular block, and cardiac arrest. It is caused by traction on the extraocular muscles (especially medial rectus), ocular manipulation, or manual pressure on the globe. The OCR is commonly seen during eye muscle surgery, detached retina repair, or enucleation or whenever there is extensive traction or rotation of the eyeball.

Barash PG, Cullen BF, Stoelting RK, eds. *Clinical anesthesia*, 4th ed. Philadelphia: Lippincott Williams & Wilkins, 2001:973.

Miller RD, ed. *Miller's anesthesia*, 6th ed. New York: Churchill Livingstone, 2005:2529–2530.

C.12. What are the afferent and efferent pathways of the oculocardiac reflex (OCR)?

The OCR is trigeminovagal. The afferent pathway is by way of the ciliary ganglion to the ophthalmic division of the trigeminal nerve and through the gasserian ganglion to the main sensory nucleus in the fourth ventricle. The efferent pathway is the vagus nerve.

Adams AK, Jones RM. Anaesthesia for eye surgery: general considerations. *Br J Anaesth* 1980;52:663.

Barash PG, Cullen BF, Stoelting RK, eds. *Clinical anesthesia*, 5th ed. Philadelphia: Lippincott Williams & Wilkins, 2006:980.

Smith GB. *Ophthalmic anesthesia*. Baltimore: University Park Press, 1983:66–72.

C.13. What factors contribute to the incidence of the oculocardiac reflex (OCR)?

Preoperative anxiety, light general anesthesia, hypoxia, hypercarbia, and increased vagal tone because of age or drugs. The reported incidence of cardiac rhythm changes during eye muscle surgery is 32% to 82%. The incidence is higher in children.

Miller RD, ed. *Miller's anesthesia*, 6th ed. New York: Churchill Livingstone, 2005:2530.

Smith GB. *Ophthalmic anesthesia*. Baltimore: University Park Press, 1983:66–72.

C.14. How do you diagnose and treat the oculocardiac reflex (OCR)?

- Monitor the electrocardiogram intraoperatively and during any eye manipulation.
- Stop the surgical stimulus immediately.
- Ensure that ventilation is adequate.
- Ensure sufficient anesthetic depth.

The OCR may fatigue with repeated stimulation.

Miller RD, ed. *Miller's anesthesia*, 6th ed. New York: Churchill Livingstone, 2005:2530.

Smith GB. *Ophthalmic anesthesia*. Baltimore: University Park Press, 1983:66–72.

C.15. Is atropine useful for the oculocardiac reflex (OCR)?

Atropine use is controversial. Atropine, 0.4 mg intramuscularly (IM), as a premedicant has no vagolytic effect after 60 minutes and is of no value in preventing or treating the OCR. Atropine, 0.4 mg intravenously (IV), is effective for 30 minutes in preventing bradycardia associated with the OCR. Doses greater than 0.5 mg IV can cause tachycardia, which may be detrimental in certain patients with heart disease. At least 2 to 3 mg is required to ensure a total vagal block.

Blanc VF. Anticholinergic premedication for infants and children on the oculocardiac reflex [Letter]. *Can Anaesth Soc J* 1983;30:683.

Miller RD, ed. *Miller's anesthesia*, 6th ed. New York: Churchill Livingstone, 2005:2530.

Steward DJ. Anticholinergic premedication in infants and children on the oculocardiac reflex [Reply]. *Can Anaesth Soc J* 1983;30:684.

C.16. Can retrobulbar block prevent the oculocardiac reflex (OCR)? Is it appropriate in this patient?

Retrobulbar block injection is not only unreliable in preventing the OCR but may, during the injection, cause OCR, cardiac arrest, or retrobulbar hemorrhage.

Local infiltration of the recti muscles and a delicate operating technique may decrease the incidence of OCR. In this patient, retrobulbar block is relatively contraindicated because it may increase intraocular pressure (IOP).

Allen ED, Elkington AR. Local anesthesia and the eye. *Br J Anaesth* 1980;52:689.

McGoldrick KE. Complications of regional anesthesia for ophthalmic surgery. *Yale J Biol Med* 1993;66:443.

Miller RD, ed. *Miller's anesthesia*, 6th ed. New York: Churchill Livingstone, 2005:2530.

D. Postoperative Management

D.1. Would you reverse the neuromuscular blockade in this patient?

There is no contraindication to reversal, provided that efforts are made to minimize coughing or bucking on the tube.

D.2. Do reversal doses of atropine affect intraocular pressure (IOP)?

Reversal doses of atropine, when given in conjunction with neostigmine, do not significantly alter IOP and this combination may be safely used, even in patients with glaucoma.

Barash PG, Cullen BF, Stoelting RK, eds. *Clinical anesthesia*, 5th ed. Philadelphia: Lippincott Williams & Wilkins, 2006:991.

Cunningham AJ, Barry P. Intraocular pressure: physiology and implications for anaesthetic management. *Can Anaesth Soc J* 1986;33:195.

D.3. What would you do before extubating this patient?

- Empty the stomach with an orogastric tube while the patient is still paralyzed.
- Suction the pharynx with the patient still paralyzed or deeply anesthetized.
- Give an antiemetic, such as droperidol 0.01 mg per kg intravenously (IV) or ondansetron 0.1 mg per kg IV, 20 to 30 minutes before the end of surgery.
- Give lidocaine 1.5 mg per kg IV or remifentanil 0.5 to 0.8 μg per kg IV to prevent coughing during emergence.

Gefke K, Anderson LW, Friesel E. Intravenous lidocaine as a suppressant of cough and laryngospasm with extubation after tonsillectomy. *Acta Anaesthesiol Scand* 1983;27:112.

Miller RD, ed. *Miller's anesthesia*, 6th ed. New York: Churchill Livingstone, 2005:2534.

D.4. When would you extubate this patient?

There may be a conflict between the desire to extubate awake because of the full stomach and the desire to extubate deep to prevent coughing and bucking. Because modern techniques of eye repair involve minimal risk of suture disruption with coughing, one may extubate awake, thereby protecting the airway.

D.5. The patient awakened in the recovery room and complained of pain and tearing in the opposite eye. The conjunctiva was inflamed. What was the likely cause?

General anesthesia decreases tear production and reduces normal mechanical eyelid closure. Corneal abrasions are the most common perioperative ocular injury, and this patient's complaints are consistent with that diagnosis.

Barash PG, Cullen BF, Stoelting RK, eds. *Clinical anesthesia*, 5th ed. Philadelphia: Lippincott Williams & Wilkins, 2006:991–992.

Miller RD, ed. *Miller's anesthesia*, 6th ed. New York: Churchill Livingstone, 2005:2537.

D.6. Will taping the eyes shut or applying ointment prevent corneal abrasions? Are there any contributing factors?

There is no guarantee that an eye that has been taped shut or lubricated will not sustain a corneal abrasion. Most anesthesiologists protect the eyes in some way; however, abrasions still occur. Corneal abrasions represent the most common ophthalmic complication associated with general anesthesia. The incidence may be as high as 44% when no preventative measures have been taken and the cornea is exposed. The mechanism is thought to be drying of or direct trauma to exposed cornea. Possible contributing factors may be mask anesthesia, prone position, or having the patient's face in the surgical field.

Barash PG, Cullen BF, Stoelting RK, eds. *Clinical anesthesia*, 5th ed. Philadelphia: Lippincott Williams & Wilkins, 2006:991–992.

Bronheim D, Abel M, Neustein S. Corneal abrasions following non-ophthalmic surgery: a retrospective view of 35,253 general anesthetics. *Anesthesiology* 1995;83:A1071.

Gild WM, Posner KL, Caplan RA, et al. Eye injuries associated with anesthesia. *Anesthesiology* 1992;76:204–208.

D.7. What should you do when you suspect your patient might have a corneal abrasion?

Prompt consultation with an ophthalmologist should be solicited for precise diagnosis and treatment. The patient should be reassured that corneal abrasions usually heal and that relief of pain occurs within 24 to 48 hours. Possible treatments include eye patching and topical administration of antibiotics, short-acting cycloplegics, or antiinflammatory agents. The use of eye patches is controversial.

A topical anesthetic for the cornea should never be given to a patient for self-administration. Misuse may cause delayed wound healing and keratopathy.

Hulbert MFG. Efficacy of eye pad in corneal healing after corneal foreign body removal. *Lancet* 1991;337:643.

Jampal HD. Patching for corneal abrasions. *JAMA* 1995;274:1504.

Kaiser PK. The Corneal Abrasion Patching Study Group. A comparison of pressure patching versus no patching for corneal abrasions sue to trauma or foreign body removal. *Ophthalmology* 1995;102:1936–1942.

D.8. A month after the surgical repair, the patient complained of impaired vision in the operative eye. He was examined and found to have a detached retina. As part of the surgical treatment, the ophthalmologist injected a gas bubble into the patient's posterior chamber. Why is this important to an anesthesiologist?

If a patient with intraocular gas needs to undergo general anesthesia before the gas bubble resorbs, nitrous oxide must be avoided because the gas will expand thereby increasing intraocular pressure (IOP). The effects on the eye may be disastrous. Various types of gasses may be injected, with different durations. Patients are usually given bracelets to inform anesthesiologists that they have gas in their eye and nitrous oxide must be avoided.

Fu AD, McDonald HR, Eliott D, et al. Complications of general anesthesia using nitrous oxide in eyes with preexisting gas bubbles. *Retina* 2002;22(5):569–574.

Hart RH, Vote BJ, Borthwick JH, et al. Loss of vision caused by expansion of Intraocular perfluoropropane ($C_3 F_8$) gas during nitrous oxide anesthesia. *Am J Ophthalmol* 2002;134(5):761–763.

CHAPTER 48

Laser Treatment for Laryngeal Lesions

Marcus Gutzler • Matthew C. Gomillion

A 7-YEAR-OLD GIRL

with a past history of recurrent respiratory papillomatosis (RRP) is scheduled for direct laryngoscopy and possible reexcision. The patient has had 10 papilloma reexcisions over the course of the previous 2 years. Currently, she is undergoing adjuvant treatment with α-interferon, but now presents again with slowly progressive hoarseness.

A. Medical Disease and Differential Diagnosis

1. What is the cause of recurrent respiratory papillomatosis (RRP)?
2. Does delivery through cesarean section prevent infection of the neonate with human papilloma virus (HPV)?
3. Is this an unusual presentation for RRP?
4. What are the available treatment options for RRP?
5. What are common adverse effects of α-interferon therapy?
6. What is the differential diagnosis of hoarseness in this child?

B. Preoperative Evaluation and Preparation

1. What are the key points of the preanesthetic history and physical examination in this patient?
2. What preoperative laboratory tests are necessary?
3. How should this child be premedicated before coming to the operating room?
4. What are the special considerations for anesthetic setup in this case?

C. Intraoperative Management

1. What is a laser and how does it work?
2. What are the characteristics of laser radiation?
3. Discuss some advantages associated with the use of lasers for laryngeal surgery?
4. What are some disadvantages of lasers compared with microdebriders?
5. How would you protect the external surface of a conventional endotracheal tube for use during laser microlaryngoscopy?
6. What are the disadvantages of foil-wrapped tubes?
7. What special endotracheal tubes are available for laser surgery?
8. How would you manage an airway fire?

9. What is the Venturi effect?
10. What is Venturi jet ventilation?
11. How would you institute and conduct manual jet ventilation?
12. How is anesthesia maintained during jet ventilation?
13. What are the complications of jet ventilation?
14. Are there contraindications for the use of jet ventilation?
15. Discuss airway management options during laryngeal papilloma resection?
16. How would you plan to monitor this patient?
17. How would you induce anesthesia for an intermittent apnea technique?

D. Postoperative Management

1. After uneventful laser microlaryngeal resection using jet ventilation, the patient was extubated in the operating room and then transferred to the recovery room. What are the common postoperative complications?

A. Medical Disease and Differential Diagnosis

A.1. What is the cause of recurrent respiratory papillomatosis (RRP)?

RRP, a disease of the respiratory mucosa characterized by benign nonkeratinizing squamous papillomata, is caused by the human papilloma virus (HPV). On the basis of shared genetic code homologies, HPV are grouped and numbered. Although there are approximately 100 different HPV types identified to date, with respect to RRP, two types stand out: HPV 6 and 11. They are not only the causative agents for RRP but are also responsible for 90% of genital warts (Condylomata accuminata).

Derkay CS, Faust RA. Recurrent respiratory papillomatosis. In: Cummings C, Haughey B, Thomas JR, et al. eds. *otolaryngology: head and neck surgery*, 4th ed. New York: Mosby, 2005:4370–4383.

A.2. Does delivery through cesarean section prevent infection of the neonate with human papilloma virus (HPV)?

HPV has been estimated to be present in the genital tract of as many as 25% of all women of childbearing age worldwide. Although recurrent respiratory papillomatosis (RRP) is the most common benign neoplasm of the larynx in children, its true incidence and prevalence are uncertain. It is estimated that each year 1,500 to 2,500 new cases of childhood-onset RRP occur in the United States. Therefore, only a minority of children of virus-carrying mothers will become symptomatic, which is not to say, that the number of virus-carrying children is not much higher. Even in parturients with an active genital condyloma lesion, the child's risk for contracting the disease when normal spontaneous vaginal delivery (NSVD) is chosen is only approximately 1 in 400.

The route of transmission (i.e., transplacental, perinatal, or postnatal) is not completely understood, as is the preventive value of cesarean sections in parturients known to carry the virus. Cesarean section with the sole intention of preventing the disease in the newborn is therefore not recommended. It may have a role in preventing excessive maternal bleeding likely to result from NSVD or in circumventing pelvic outlet obstruction secondary to excessive lesions.

Centers for Disease Control and Prevention. *Sexually transmitted disease guidelines*. http://www.cdc.gov/STD/treatment/6-2002 TG.htm. 2002.

Derkay CS, Faust RA. Recurrent respiratory papillomatosis. In: Cummings C, Haughey B, Thomas JR, et al. eds. *otolaryngology: head and neck surgery*, 4th ed. New York: Mosby, 2005:4370–4383.

A.3. Is this an unusual presentation for recurrent respiratory papillomatosis (RRP)?

Recurrence of voice changes despite repeated surgical interventions is unfortunately not that rare in patients with respiratory papillomatosis. Hoarseness, stridor—and if severe enough—the development of respiratory distress from airway obstruction are the most consistent signs and symptoms of patients with RRP. Oral, tracheobronchial, and pulmonary involvements are also known to occur.

At present, there is no cure for RRP and no modality that would lead to eradication of the virus from the respiratory mucosa. Local recurrences are therefore to be expected.

Derkay CS, Faust RA. Recurrent respiratory papillomatosis. In: Cummings C, Haughey B, Thomas JR, et al. eds. *otolaryngology: head and neck surgery*, 4th ed. New York: Mosby, 2005:4370–4383.

A.4. What are the available treatment options for recurrent respiratory papillomatosis (RRP)?

As stated in the preceding text, there is no cure but only disease control for relentless and recurrent papillomatosis. The current standard of care is surgical therapy with the goal of complete removal of papillomata and preservation of normal structures as much as possible.

As scarring from overaggressive laryngeal resections may lead to precisely the adverse clinical effects that surgical therapy seeks to avoid or minimize (dysphonia, airway compromise), most experienced surgeons will accept incomplete papilloma resection, especially when near delicate structures such as the anterior laryngeal commissure. Even with the removal of all clinically evident papilloma, latent virus remains in adjacent tissue.

With respect to surgical technique, the CO_2 laser used to be the mainstay of therapy since the 1970s. According to a recent survey by the American Society of Pediatric Otolaryngology (ASPO), this has changed. Most members participating in this survey now rely on the use of the microdebrider as the preferred surgical therapy. The microdebrider is considered to be just as precise a surgical tool as the CO_2 laser, while at the same time being easier to use.

In addition, there seems to be an increasing role for adjuvant medical therapy (α-interferon and various antiviral agents) for severe cases, with the number of patients on adjuvant treatment doubled since the early 1990s (22% in the recent survey mentioned earlier).

Derkay CS, Faust RA. Recurrent respiratory papillomatosis. In: Cummings C, Haughey B, Thomas JR, et al. eds. *otolaryngology: head and neck surgery*, 4th ed. New York: Mosby, 2005:4370–4383. In;

Schraff S, Derkay CS, Burke B, et al. American Society of Pediatric Otolaryngology members' experience with recurrent respiratory papillomatosis and the use of adjuvant therapy. *Arch Otolaryngol Head Neck Surg* 2004;130:1039–1042.

A.5. What are common adverse effects of α-interferon therapy?

Interferons (IFNs) are potent cytokines that possess antiviral, immunomodulating, and antiproliferative activities. Of the three known major classes of IFNs (α, β and γ) only α-interferon is clinically used in recurrent respiratory papillomatosis (RRP). Therapy is initiated at 5 million units per m^2 body surface area administered by subcutaneous injection on a daily basis for 28 days, then

3 days per week for at least a 6-month trial. After 6 months in children with excellent responses and no severe side effects, the dosage can be decreased to 3 million units per m² for 3 days a week with further slow weaning as tolerated. Common adverse effects associated with systemic application are an acute, relatively benign influenza-like syndrome, characterized by fever, chills, headache, myalgia, arthralgia, nausea, vomiting, and diarrhea, as well as more serious dose-limiting comorbidities, namely myelosuppression and neurotoxicity. Neurotoxicity is characterized by somnolence, confusion, behavioral disturbance, and rarely, seizures, debilitating neurasthenia, and depression. Alopecia and personality change are common in IFN-treated children. Cardiovascular toxicity (hypotension and tachycardia) and hepatotoxicity seem to be more rare.

Derkay CS, Faust RA. Recurrent respiratory papillomatosis. In: Cummings C, Haughey B, Thomas JR, et al. eds. *otolaryngology: head and neck surgery*, 4th ed. New York: Mosby, 2005:4370–4383.

Hayden FG. Chemotherapy of microbial diseases: antiviral agents (Nonretroviral). In: Brunton L, Lazo J, Parker K, et al. eds. *Goodman and Gilman's the pharmacological basis of therapeutics*, 11th ed. New York: McGraw Hill, 2005:1243–1273.

A.6. What is the differential diagnosis of hoarseness in this child?

Hoarseness always indicates some abnormality of laryngeal structure or function. Given the patient's previous history local papilloma recurrence and/or postoperative scarring of laryngeal structures seem likely causes in this patient. A broader differential diagnosis for hoarseness in children would be as follows:

- Anatomic and Congenital Causes
  - Cystic lesions (laryngocele, thyroglossal cyst)
  - Vocal fold nodules
  - Glottic webs
- Neoplastic Causes
  - Squamous cell carcinoma
  - Recurrent respiratory papillomatosis (RRP)
- Neurologic Causes
  - Central (e.g., intracerebral hemorrhage, hydrocephalus)
  - Peripheral neuropathies
- Inflammatory
  - Gastroesophageal reflux
  - Rheumatoid arthritis
  - Angioneurotic edema
- Infectious
  - Croup syndrome
  - Laryngotracheobronchitis
  - Epiglottitis

McMurray JS. Disorders of phonation in children. *Pediatr Clin North Am* 2003;50:363–380.

B. Preoperative Evaluation and Preparation

B.1. What are the key points of the preanesthetic history and physical examination in this patient?

Of obvious concern in these patients is to quickly detect and address any serious respiratory compromise; in the absence of severe respiratory distress, a detailed history should be obtained.

A review of previous anesthetic experiences with particular emphasis on problems pertaining to airway management would be a good starting point. Weight, general health, associated comorbidities, recent respiratory infections, allergies, medications and nothing by mouth (NPO) status are all of obvious importance. A search for serious adverse effects as a result of the interferon (IFN) therapy should be done.

With respect to the voice changes, a more indepth investigation may offer some clues as to the suspected location: A low-pitched, coarse, fluttering voice suggests a subglottic lesion, whereas a high-pitched, cracking voice, aphonia or breathy voice suggests a glottic lesion. Associated high-pitched stridor also suggests a glottic or subglottic lesion. Because of the precision of laryngeal mechanics, hoarseness may result from a remarkably small lesion. On the other hand, if the origin of the lesion is remote from the vocal cords, hoarseness may result from a significantly larger lesion.

The concern here is to recognize the lesion that could potentially result in complete airway obstruction once anesthesia has been induced. When in doubt, a flexible nasopharyngoscopy—if not already done before arrival in the operating room (OR)—should be considered immediately preoperatively.

Derkay CS. Recurrent respiratory papillomatosis. *Laryngoscope* 2001;111:57–69.

B.2. What preoperative laboratory tests are necessary?

In recent years, the value of routine preoperative laboratory screening has been questioned. For a surgical procedure not associated with significant intraoperative blood loss in a child who is not at increased risk for severe and physiologic important anemia, no laboratory tests are required.

This patient may however no longer fall into this latter category. After all, α-interferon is associated with serious side effects, such as neurotoxicity and myelosuppression. Because effects of myelosuppression may not be easily diagnosed by history and physical examination, one might argue that at least obtaining a hematocrit would be in order in this particular patient.

Steward DJ. Preoperative evaluation and preparation for surgery. In: Gregory GA, ed. *Principles of pediatric anesthesia*, 4th ed. New York: Churchill Livingstone, 2002:184.

B.3. How should this child be premedicated before coming to the operating room (OR)?

Children with recurrent respiratory papillomatosis (RRP) are often quite anxious and apprehensive coming back to the OR for yet another reexcision. A reassuring preoperative visit by the anesthesiologist should help allay fears. Sedative premedication should be used very carefully, especially in the child with significant respiratory distress. It should not be administered without close monitoring and the immediate availability of oxygen, suction and positive pressure ventilation. Anticholinergic premedication may be used to dry up oral secretions.

Brett CM, Zwass MS. Eyes, ears, nose, throat and dental surgery. In: Gregory GA, ed. *Principles of pediatric anesthesia*, 4th ed. New York: Churchill Livingstone, 2002:687–688.

B.4. What are the special considerations for anesthetic setup in this case?

Before the initiation of anesthesia, the anesthesiologist should discuss the case with the surgeon. The anesthesiologist should seek a thorough understanding of the surgical plan and must keep in close communication with the surgeon throughout the procedure. A strategy for maintaining oxygenation and ventilation during the case, while at the same time working around surgical needs, must be devised. Special equipment (e.g., laser, jet ventilator, bronchoscopes, etc.) must be present and in good working condition.

Preparations for successfully dealing with the difficult pediatric airway should be made by both the anesthesia (difficult airway cart, senior pediatric anesthesiologist) and the surgical team (open tracheotomy set and experienced otolaryngologist on standby).

Whether a laser will be used or not greatly impacts on airway management. The biggest concern here is prevention of an airway fire. Also, a plan to effectively deal with such a disaster, should it occur, needs to be firmly established beforehand. Aside from that, all operating room (OR) staff must wear protective eye gear and laser masks when working around the laser.

Derkay CS. Recurrent respiratory papillomatosis. *Laryngoscope* 2001;111:57–69.

C. Intraoperative Management

C.1. What is a laser and how does it work?

Electromagnetic radiation consists of photons, and photons have properties consistent with both particles and waves. Like radio waves and Roentgen waves, visible light is another form of electromagnetic radiation.

The characteristic features of these different forms of radiation are their respective wavelengths. Visual light is electromagnetic radiation with wavelengths in the range from 385 to 760 nm, shorter wavelengths are ultraviolet, and longer wavelengths are infrared.

Laser is an acronym for light amplification by stimulated emission of radiation. What makes laser distinctive is the high energy density that it provides, and the ability to transfer large quantities of energy rapidly to remote locations.

Several concepts are important for a basic understanding of the phenomenon of laser:

- *The photoelectric effect.* Light of a certain wavelength (e.g., blue) causes metal to eject electrons at a rate proportional to the brightness of the light, whereas intense light at other colors (e.g., red, orange, yellow) cannot.
- *The orbital model.* Electrons circling the nuclei of atoms are constrained to a few specific orbital patterns and radii. Each orbital is associated with a specific energy level. The energy differences between electron orbitals are specific to different atoms. The only way an electron can move from one orbital to another of higher or lower energy is to absorb or emit, respectively, an amount of energy exactly equal to the difference in energy between the two orbitals.
- *Stimulated absorption.* The process by which a photon's energy is captured by an electron, thereby lifting the electron into a higher energy orbital (the electrons get excited).
- *Spontaneous emission.* The converse process by which an electron drops to lower orbital, in the process sending out a photon to carry away the excess energy.
- *Population inversion.* Many (as opposed to one single) electrons achieve a higher energy level (higher orbital). Once a photon comes along, it starts a chain reaction (i.e., amplification) of stimulated emission.

The essential components of a laser system include a laser medium (gaseous or solid) containing the atoms whose electrons create the laser light, resonating mirrors to boost laser efficiency, and an energy source to excite the atoms of the laser medium into producing laser light. The energy pump actually provides the means for obtaining a population inversion of orbital electrons of the laser medium. A pair of axial mirrors permits repeated passes of collimated photons through the medium, allowing maximum amplification by stimulated emission. One of the mirrors is partially transmitting, finally allowing the laser beam to emerge.

Rampil IJ. Anesthesia for laser surgery. In: Miller RD, ed. *Miller's anesthesia*, 6th ed. Philadelphia: Churchill Livingstone, 2005:2573–2588.

C.2. What are the characteristics of laser radiation?

The high energy density of laser is the result of three characteristics:

- There is a high degree of monochromaticity; that is, other than with ordinary light the range of wavelengths is very limited.
- Electromagnetic fields of all photons in the laser beam oscillate synchronously in identical phase, a phenomenon called *coherence*, again distinct from ordinary light where the electromagnetic fields are phased randomly.
- Whereas ordinary light beams spread out in all directions from a point source, laser light remains in a narrow collimated beam.

These characteristics allow for a very concentrated energy delivery, often producing heating at a rate of many thousand degrees per second with lasers in current clinical application.

Rampil IJ. Anesthesia for laser surgery. In: Miller RD, ed. *Miller's anesthesia*, 6th ed. Philadelphia: Churchill Livingstone, 2005:2573–2588.

C.3. Discuss some advantages associated with the use of lasers for laryngeal surgery?

With laser light, tissue penetration is mostly a function of wavelength. Long-wavelength laser light, such as that from CO_2 (operating at 10,600 nm), is completely absorbed by water in the first few layers of cells. The thermal effect is therefore largely limited to the point of entry into the target tissue. This results in explosive vaporization of the surface tissue of the target with surprisingly little damage to underlying cells. When coupled to an operating microscope, the laser vaporizes the lesions with precision, causing minimal bleeding and edema, an obvious advantage, especially in small pediatric airways.

Derkay CS. Recurrent respiratory papillomatosis. *Laryngoscope* 2001;111:57–69.

Rampil IJ. Anesthesia for laser surgery. In: Miller RD, ed. *Miller's anesthesia*, 6th ed. Philadelphia: Churchill Livingstone, 2005:2573–2588.

C.4. What are some disadvantages of lasers compared with microdebriders?

There are significant risks associated with the use of laser for laryngeal surgery.

Special eye protection for both patient and staff are indispensable, as the powerful laser beam may otherwise cause serious ocular injury. Other body parts need also to be carefully protected from inadvertent laser exposure in order to prevent tissue injury. Inappropriate and aggressive use of the laser may also cause injury to mucosa primarily not affected by disease and create an environment suitable for implantation of viral particles and thereby may actually promote spread of the disease. Laser-induced pneumothorax has been reported after a laryngeal procedure. Although the thermal effect is largely limited to the point of entry into the target tissue, if not used judiciously especially near delicate structures such as the anterior or posterior laryngeal commissure, laser may cause unacceptable scarring and subsequent abnormal vocal fold function.

Laser smoke contains water vapor and destroyed tissue material. It has been found to contain active viral DNA, a potential source of infection for operating room (OR) personnel. Smoke may also obstruct the surgeon's view during the resection.

The biggest concern with laser use however revolves around the generation of an airway fire through ignition of the endotracheal tube (ETT) by inadvertent laser strike, a potentially fatal complication if not effectively dealt with quickly.

When comparing the microdebrider and the CO_2 laser, there is evidence suggesting that removing papillomas using the microdebrider is associated with better short-term improvement in voice quality, and shorter procedure time, which may ultimately translate to reduced operative cost. Heat-induced scarring of nearby tissues is not a concern, there is no need for circumstantial protection from inadvertent laser strike, and the risk for an airway fire should be no higher than in a standard case.

Derkay CS, Faust RA. Recurrent respiratory papillomatosis. In: Cummings C, Haughey B, Thomas JR, et al. eds. *otolaryngology: head and neck surgery*, 4th ed. Chapter 196. New York: Mosby, 2005:4370–4383.

Pasquale K, Wiatrak B, Woolley A, et al. Microdebrider versus CO2 laser removal of recurrent respiratory papillomas: a prospective analysis. *Laryngoscope* 2003;113(1):139–143.

Rampil IJ. Anesthesia for laser surgery. In: Miller RD, ed. *Miller's anesthesia*, 6th ed. Philadelphia: Churchill Livingstone, 2005:2573–2588.

Werkhaven JA. Microlaryngoscopy-airway management with anaesthetic techniques for CO2 laser. *Pediatr Anesth* 2004;14:90–94.

C.5. How would you protect the external surface of a conventional endotracheal tube (ETT) for use during laser microlaryngoscopy?

Inadvertent laser strike can ignite and burn any hydrocarbon material in the airway, including ETTs. Because of their close proximity to the operative field, ETTs pose a serious fire hazard during laser use, especially in the oxygen-enriched environment of a general anesthetic.

All commonly used ETTs are potentially flammable, but to some degree flammability is a function of the material used to manufacture the tube. Unfortunately, the now commonplace clear polyvinylchloride (PVC) plastic tubes seem to catch fire much more easily than older red rubber tubes. Also, red rubber tubes seem to lead to less toxic combustion products once ignited.

In addition to limiting the amount of oxygen used to ventilate the patient to as low as tolerated, one strategy to make the use of conventional PVC tubes safer, is to guard it with reflective tape. Conventional aluminum or copper tape is an inexpensive (although not U.S. Food and Drug Administration [FDA]-approved) way to offer some protection against brief laser strike. FDA-approved tape is also available (Merocel Laser Guard, Medtronic USA).

Should a cuffed tube be used, the cuff in itself cannot unfortunately be protected from laser strike in this manner. Cuff breakage increases the fire hazard, as it will allow access of oxygen-enriched gas mixtures to the hypopharynx. One strategy here to reduce risk is to fill the cuff with an indicator dye (e.g., methylene blue in normal saline) to detect a break early. The cuff should also be covered with wet gauze or neurosurgical sponges to retard heating.

To wrap a PVC tube with tape, the tube should be clean and fat free, thereby facilitating tape adhesion. The tube diameter should be chosen 1 to 2 mm smaller than usual. Mastisol will further enhance the stickiness to the ETT. Wrapping should start at the distal end or just proximal to the cuff and be continued up to the level of the uvula. The distal end of the tape should be cut at a 60-degree angle, and the tube should then be wrapped in a spiral with approximately 30% overlap, avoiding sharp edges and leaving no PVC exposed.

Rampil IJ. Anesthesia for laser surgery. In: Miller RD, ed. *Miller's anesthesia*, 6th ed. Philadelphia: Churchill Livingstone, 2005:2573–2588.

C.6. What are the disadvantages of foil-wrapped tubes?

Disadvantages of metallic foil-wrapped tubes include risk of trauma to pharyngeal and laryngeal tissues by sharp edges. The tube will lose elasticity and be more prone to kink. If foil becomes detached, the protective effect is lost and aspirated foil may lead to airway obstruction. The reflective surface enhances the risk of inadvertent laser strike of surrounding tissues.

Brett CM, Zwass MS. Eyes, ears, nose, throat and dental surgery. In: Gregory GA, ed. *Principles of pediatric anesthesia*, 4th ed. New York: Churchill Livingstone, 2002:687–688.

C.7. What special endotracheal tubes (ETTs) are available for laser surgery?

The U.S. Food and Drug Administration (FDA)-approved specialized tubes for laser surgery are commercially available. In essence, there are metal- and silicone-based tubes.

The Xomed Laser Shield and Laser Shield II (Medtronic, USA) are silicone-based tubes with laser-reflective aluminum containing coating or reflective aluminum wrap with smooth fluoroplastic overwrap on the outside (in the case of the Laser Shield II). Although these tubes may withstand laser strikes longer then conventional tubes, they will ignite as well with longer exposure.

Two FDA-approved metal tube models are commercially available for use with CO_2 laser. First, there is the Laser Flex tube (Mallinckrodt, USA), an airtight stainless steel spiral tube with two distal polyvinylchloride (PVC) cuffs. If one ruptures, the second unruptured cuff will still limit egress of oxygen-rich gas. Second, the Bivona Fome-Cuf (Bivona, USA) is an aluminum spiral tube with an outer silicone coating. This tube has a specially designed self-inflating foam sponge-filled cuff, which will remain expanded even after laser puncture. Not surprisingly, the rigidity and bulkiness of these tubes are practical disadvantages that discourage from their routine use, especially in pediatric patients. Even with these metal tubes, fire hazard is still a concern.

Green JM, Gonzalez RM, Sonbolian N, et al. The resistance to carbon dioxide laser ignition of a new endotracheal tube: Xomed Laser-Shield II. *J Clin Anesth* 1992;4(2):89–92.

Rampil IJ. Anesthesia for laser surgery. In: Miller RD, ed. *Miller's anesthesia*, 6th ed. Philadelphia: Churchill Livingstone, 2005:2573–2588.

C.8. How would you manage an airway fire?

In case of an airway fire rapid and effective action is required. The "4 E's"–mnemonic may help to stay focused, when suddenly faced with this frightening situation:

- *E*xtract
- *E*liminate
- *E*xtinguish
- *E*valuate

All combustible material (endotracheal tube [ETT], pledgets) must be *e*xtracted from the airway at once. Oxygen supply through the tube must be quickly *e*liminated by disconnection from the circuit. Continued flow through a burning tube would lead to a blowtorch effect. Any residual fires need to be *e*xtinguished with normal saline. Ventilation with 100% oxygen should then be provided by mask, and anesthesia should be continued. *E*valuation of the injury is then in order and should be done with direct laryngoscopy and rigid bronchoscopy, thereby assessing the upper and lower airway. Any apparent airway damage makes reintubation the most prudent approach. For severe injury a low tracheotomy may be indicated.

Rampil IJ. Anesthesia for laser surgery. In: Miller RD, ed. *Miller's anesthesia*, 6th ed. Philadelphia: Churchill Livingstone, 2005:2573–2588.

Werkhaven JA. Microlaryngoscopy-airway management with anaesthetic techniques for CO2 laser. *Pediatr Anesth* 2004;14:90–94.

C.9. What is the Venturi effect?

The Venturi effect originally describes the impact of constricted channels on fluid flow. As fluid passes through a constriction of a Venturi tube (a tube with two open ends and a narrowing in its midsection), it must speed up. At the same time, its hydrostatic pressure drops. This pressure drop is proportional to flow, and can for example be used to measure flow in pipes without interfering with flow.

Ihra G, Aloy A. On the use of Venturi's principle to describe entrainment during jet ventilation. *J Clin Anesth* 2000;12:417–419.

C.10. What is Venturi jet ventilation?

The jet injector technique of ventilation for upper airway surgery was introduced by Sanders in 1967.

A high-pressure gas source is connected to a stiff, narrow cannula, positioned at the inlet of the laryngoscope. With a manual switch, gas boluses are delivered. In the lumen of the laryngoscope, the high-velocity stream of gas encounters stationary gas, which it pushes forward. Each jet bolus entrains ambient air through the open laryngoscope entrance, substantially augmenting the volume of the bolus and diluting the oxygen fraction of the jet.

Whether or not truly based on the phenomenon known as the *Venturi effect*, the jet injector provides a simple approach to deliver physiologic tidal volumes in a nongas tight delivery system. Venturi ventilation has become synonymous with jet ventilation in the medical literature.

Ihra G, Aloy A. On the use of Venturi's principle to describe entrainment during jet ventilation. *J Clin Anesth* 2000;12:417–419.

McRae K. Anesthesia for airway surgery. *Anesthesiol Clin North America* 2001;19(3):497–541.

C.11. How would you institute and conduct manual jet ventilation?

Before effective jet ventilation can begin, the operating laryngoscope must be inserted, the larynx adequately exposed and evaluated for appropriateness for jet ventilation, the suspension system installed, and the jet injector needle attached to the laryngoscope and properly aligned with the axis of the trachea. All of this takes time in an anesthetized apneic patient. Therefore, it is our preference at the New York Presbyterian Hospital-Weill-Cornell Medical Center to begin with laryngoscopy and intubation using a standard polyvinylchloride (PVC) endotracheal tube (ETT) if the airway appears appropriate for jet ventilation. Uninterrupted ventilation can now be performed while the operating laryngoscope and jet injector are positioned. When ready, the ETT is removed and jet ventilation begun. Alternatively, following anesthesia induction and demonstration of an adequate mask airway, the patient is paralyzed and the operating laryngoscope and jet injector are inserted and positioned while the patient is apneic.

Ventilation begins with a jet pressure of 5 to 10 *psi* in infants and children and 15 to 20 *psi* in adults. The jet pressure is gradually increased until adequate chest excursions are noted.

Jet ventilation should produce good clinical expansion of the chest at a rate appropriate for the patient's age. The inspiratory-to-expiratory (I:E) ratio should allow for complete passive exhalation in between jet applications. Monitoring of peripheral arterial saturation is mandatory as is monitoring ventilation both by auscultation and palpation.

Derkay CS, Faust RA. Recurrent respiratory papillomatosis. In: Cummings C, Haughey B, Thomas JR, et al. eds. *otolaryngology: head and neck surgery*, 4th ed. New York: Mosby, 2005:4370–4383.

Rampil IJ. Anesthesia for laser surgery. In: Miller RD, ed. *Miller's anesthesia*, 6th ed. Philadelphia: Churchill Livingstone, 2005:2573–2588.

C.12. How is anesthesia maintained during jet ventilation?

As delivery of inhalational anesthetics is impractical with jet ventilation (operating room pollution, inability to precisely regulate their concentrations), most authors favor a total intravenous technique. Combining a hypnotic agent such as propofol with a short-acting opioid (ideally remifentanil), hypnosis, amnesia and analgesia can all be achieved although at the same time allowing for a rapid recovery of the patient at the end of the procedure. Temporary muscle relaxation can be achieved with either a short-acting or intermediate-duration muscle relaxants.

Donlon JV, Doyle DJ, Feldman MA. Anesthesia for eye, ear, nose, and throat surgery. In: Miller RD, ed. *Miller's anesthesia*, 6th ed. Philadelphia: Churchill Livingstone, 2005: 2527–2556.

C.13. What are the complications of jet ventilation?

Complications associated with jet ventilation include dehydration of the mucosa, inadequate oxygenation and ventilation, gastric distension, regurgitation and even rupture. Pneumomediastinum and pneumothorax have been reported, and seem to occur mostly when applying jet ventilation with a (partially) obstructed airway occurring for example during partial closure of the vocal cords. This is best avoided by using muscle relaxation during jet ventilation.

Borland LM. Airway management for CO_2 laser surgery on the larynx: venturi jet ventilation and alternatives. *Int Anesthesiol Clin* 1997;35:99–106.

Jaquet Y, Monnier P, Van Melle G, et al. Complications of different ventilation strategies in endoscopic laryngeal surgery. A 10 year review. *Anesthesiology* 2006;104:52–59.

C.14. Are there contraindications for the use of jet ventilation?

Jet ventilation is most suited for patients with normal, unobstructed airways and normal lung and chest wall compliance.

The ability to fully exhale in between jet applications is crucial. If this is not possible (glottic lesion, significant interarytenoid scarring, laryngospasm) jet ventilation may not be appropriate. Decreased chest wall compliance such as in obese patients may lead to inadvertent gastric distension, further worsening respiratory compliance. Advanced chronic obstructive disease with its inherent prolonged exhalation phase may again make jet ventilation unpractical and in the presence of pulmonary bullae even hazardous. Significant overbite especially when combined with retrognathia makes orolaryngotracheal alignment challenging and accidental gastric hyperinflation likely.

Borland LM. Airway management for CO_2 laser surgery on the larynx: venturi jet ventilation and alternatives. *Int Anesthesiol Clin* 1997;35:99–106.

Jaquet Y, Monnier P, Van Melle G, et al. Complications of different ventilation strategies in endoscopic laryngeal surgery. A 10 year review. *Anesthesiology* 2006;104:52–59.

C.15. Discuss airway management options during laryngeal papilloma resection?

In addition to Venturi jet ventilation, there are three different widely accepted methods for managing the airway during papilloma resection—controlled mechanical ventilation through a small endotracheal tube (ETT), spontaneous ventilation, and apneic anesthesia with intermittent ventilation.

Except for the first option, all methods require an at least temporarily unsecured, unprotected airway during parts of the surgical resection. As reassuring as a secured airway may feel to the anesthesiologist, using an ETT during airway laser surgery entails the above-mentioned risk of an airway fire. Also, surgical exposure is often suboptimal in the presence of an ETT, as the tube limits access to parts of the larynx. In a recent web-based survey, use of an ETT seems now to be the least favored management technique among participating otolaryngologists.

Access to all parts of the laryngeal mucosa using spontaneous ventilation without an additional airway device (e.g., tube, laryngeal mask airway) is excellent. For obvious reasons, muscle relaxation is not an option, and the moving surgical field is a drawback of this technique, potentially making the surgical resection more demanding.

Intermittent apnea offers a solution to this problem. During apnea with intermittent ventilation, the patient is repeatedly ventilated using a standard ETT. Use of 100% oxygen will extend the tolerable apnea time to follow, although inadvertent movement is best avoided using muscle relaxants. The tube is then removed periodically and the surgeon allowed operating for brief periods of time, although the peripheral saturation is closely monitored. The patient is reintubated and reoxygenated before desaturation sets in, and thereby readied for another period of apnea to follow, allowing for further resection as needed. Spreading the virus to more distal parts of the airway by repeated reintubations is a concern with this technique.

Along with spontaneous ventilation, intermittent apnea techniques seem to be favored by most members of the American Society of Pediatric Otolaryngology (ASPO) participating in the above-mentioned survey.

Derkay CS, Faust RA. Recurrent respiratory papillomatosis. In: Cummings C, Haughey B, Thomas JR, et al. eds. *otolaryngology: head and neck surgery*, 4th ed. New York: Mosby, 2005:4370–4383.

Jaquet Y, Monnier P, Van Melle G, et al. Complications of different ventilation strategies in endoscopic laryngeal surgery. A 10 year review. *Anesthesiology* 2006;104:52–59.

Schraff S, Derkay CS, Burke B, et al. American society of pediatric otolaryngology members' experience with recurrent respiratory papillomatosis and the use of adjuvant therapy. *Arch Otolaryngol Head Neck Surg* 2004;130:1039–1042.

C.16. How would you plan to monitor this patient?

Routine monitors include a pulse oximeter, noninvasive blood pressure measurements, an electrocardiogram (EKG), a precordial stethoscope, a temperature probe, an oxygen analyzer, a CO_2 detector and a neuromuscular blockade monitor. In this otherwise healthy patient scheduled for relatively minor surgery without the potential for significant blood loss or fluid shifts, no additional monitoring is necessary.

http://www.asahq.org/publicationsAndServices/standards/02.pdf

C.17. How would you induce anesthesia for an intermittent apnea technique?

The choice of anesthetic induction is critically dependent upon the presence of signs and symptoms, suggesting possible airway compromise on induction. If those are present, the logical choice in an adult patient is an awake fiberoptic intubation, thereby not only allowing to secure the airway but also enabling evaluation of the subglottic airway before tube placement.

In children and uncooperative adults an inhalation induction using sevoflurane is the most reasonable approach. Maintenance of spontaneous ventilation is again critical. In this scenario, muscle relaxants are unsafe, until it is clear that the patient can be ventilated and/or intubated. If severe compromise is present, an awake tracheotomy under local anesthesia may be the safest means of managing the airway.

Blind techniques (lightwand, blind oral or nasal intubation) cannot be recommended in this setting, as they carry the risk of bleeding and loss of the airway with an obstructing lesion.

A word of caution here: papillomas are dynamic lesions in a sense that they may grow rapidly thereby questioning the validity of any but the most recent endoscopic airway examinations. Also, the absence of suggestive signs and symptoms does not truly guarantee a patent airway, once anesthesia has been induced. Hence the extreme caution in managing these patients is essential.

If the patient has truly no airway compromise, any routine induction technique (intravenous or inhalational) can be used safely.

Donlon JV, Doyle DJ, Feldman MA. Anesthesia for eye, ear, nose, and throat surgery. In: Miller RD, ed. *Miller's anesthesia*, 6th ed. Philadelphia: Churchill Livingstone, 2005: 2527–2556.

D. Postoperative Management

D.1. After uneventful laser microlaryngeal resection using jet ventilation, the patient was extubated in the operating room and then transferred to the recovery room. What are the common postoperative complications?

Laryngeal edema can occur early in the postoperative period and is usually manifested by retractions and inspiratory stridor in the recovery room. After microlaryngeal surgery, patients may benefit from humidified oxygen, intravenous steroids (e.g., dexamethasone), and racemic epinephrine inhalation. Laryngospasm may develop because of laryngeal hyperactivity. To reduce the incidence of laryngospasm, topical anesthesia to the larynx may be used. If laryngospasm develops postoperatively, it is treated initially with positive pressure ventilation with 100% oxygen. More severe forms of laryngospasm may require the use of small doses of succinylcholine (1/10 of a normal induction dose, i.e., 0.1 mg/kg intravenously). The occurrence of barotrauma with jet ventilation has been described and should be kept in mind. Pulmonary complications as a result of retained secretions and subsequent atelectasis have been reported.

Donlon JV, Doyle DJ, Feldman MA. Anesthesia for eye, ear, nose, and throat surgery. In: Miller RD, ed. *Miller's anesthesia*, 6th ed. Philadelphia: Churchill Livingstone, 2005: 2527–2556.

Jaquet Y, Monnier P, Van Melle G, et al. Complications of different ventilation strategies in endoscopic laryngeal surgery. A 10 year review. *Anesthesiology* 2006;104:52–59.

CHAPTER 49

Airway Obstruction in Childhood: Stridor and Croup Syndromes

MILES DINNER

A 3-YEAR-OLD BOY

was brought to the emergency room because of respiratory distress. He was noted to be stridulous with substernal retractions and excessive drooling. He complained of a sore throat and had a fever of 39.5°C (103.1°F).

A. Medical Disease and Differential Diagnosis

1. What is stridor?
2. How does stridor correlate with anatomic location?
3. Define croup. What is the clinical presentation of laryngotracheitis?
4. What is the differential diagnosis of acute upper airway obstruction in the pediatric population?
5. How is the severity of croup assessed?
6. What is the medical management of croup? Does this have applications for the anesthesiologist?
7. What is epiglottitis? What are its common causes? What is the incidence?
8. What are the clinical manifestations of epiglottitis?
9. How is the diagnosis of epiglottitis made?
10. What is postextubation croup? How is it managed?
11. What are the nonacute causes of partial airway obstruction in children?

B. Preoperative Evaluation and Preparation

1. Is intubation always required in children with epiglottitis?
2. Why is general anesthesia administered to a child with epiglottitis?
3. How would you prepare the patient for anesthesia?

C. Intraoperative Management

1. How is the airway of the child with epiglottitis best secured?
2. How would you induce anesthesia?
3. Should a child with epiglottitis undergo a rapid-sequence induction?
4. Is awake intubation a practical alternative to secure the patient's airway?

5. What would you do if the airway cannot be secured with intubation?
6. Should this patient have a nasotracheal or orotracheal tube placed?
7. Shortly after intubation, frothy secretions were obtained on suctioning the endotracheal tube. What is the reason for this? How can this be treated?

D. Postoperative Management

1. How long should this patient remain intubated? What criteria determine extubation time?
2. How would you make this patient comfortable during the course of being intubated?
3. What outcome can one expect for the child with acute epiglottitis?

A. Medical Disease and Differential Diagnosis

A.1. What is stridor?

Stridor is the high-pitched adventitious sound produced in the respiratory cycle by the turbulent flow of respiratory gases through a segmental narrowing in the airway. It can be biphasic, inspiratory or expiratory depending on the anatomic location.

A.2. How does stridor correlate with anatomic location?

Inspiratory stridor is characteristic of laryngeal or supraglottic obstruction. Such conditions as laryngeal papillomatosis, laryngeal web, laryngomalacia and vocal cord paresis produce inspiratory stridor. Expiratory stridor is usually typical of intrathoracic processes such as extrinsic tracheal compression by a vascular ring or mass, tracheomalacia or bronchotracheitis. Biphasic stridor is indicative of lesions or infections involving both the larynx and subglottis such as the croup syndrome, subglottic stenosis or intralaryngeal masses.

A.3. Define croup. What is the clinical presentation of laryngotracheitis?

Croup is a generalized term referring to infections of the upper respiratory tract with a characteristic cough, inspiratory stridor, and possible respiratory distress. Other terms namely, *laryngotracheobronchitis, spasmodic croup,* and *bacterial tracheitis* are interwoven within the croup syndrome but have specialized meanings. For instance, spasmodic croup suggests a noninfectious inflammatory process as opposed to the viral etiology of laryngotracheobronchitis. Most cases occur during the colder months. There is a 2:1 man to woman prevalence. Also known as *laryngotracheobronchitis* because of the structures involved, croup is usually caused by the *Haemophilus parainfluenzae* virus type 1, although type 2 and 3 may cause disease. It affects children between 1 and 3 years of age, with a median age of 18 months. It manifests subacutely as an exacerbation of cold symptoms with low fever, barking cough, and hoarseness. Exudative inflammation of the upper airway may cause dyspnea and in extreme cases can lead to exhaustion and frank hypoxia. In most cases, it is self-limited and benign.

Behrman RE, Kliegman RM, Jensen HB, eds. *Nelson textbook of pediatrics*, 17th ed. Philadelphia: WB Saunders, 2004:1405–1409.

Cherry JD. Croup (laryngitis, laryngotracheitis, spasmodic croup, laryngotracheobronchitis, bacterial tracheitis, and laryngotracheobronchopneumonitis). In: Fein RD, Cherry JD, Demmler GJ, et al. eds. *Textbook of pediatric infectious diseases*, 5th ed. Philadelphia: WB Saunders, 2004:252.

A.4. What is the differential diagnosis of acute upper airway obstruction in the pediatric population?

A full differential for this condition involves a host of infectious causes. Among the most important are bacterial tracheitis, diphtheria, retropharyngeal abscess, peritonsillar abscess, measles, and Ebstein-Barr (EB) viral infection. Other cause to be considered are thermal burns, foreign body aspiration, laryngeal fractures, angioneurotic edema, vocal cord paralysis, and uvulitis. Anatomic anomalies include hemangiomas, laryngeal papillomas and congenital subglottic stenosis, which may exist silently until an underlying infection causes exacerbation and manifests with obstructive symptomatology.

Castro-Rodriguez JA, Holberg CJ, Morgan WJ, et al. Relation of two different subtypes of croup before age three to wheezing, atopy, and pulmonary function during childhood: a prospective study. *Pediatrics* 2001;107:512.

Gorelick MH, Baker MD. Epiglottitis in children: 1979 through 1992. *Arch Pediatr Adolesc Med* 1994;148:47.

A.5. How is the severity of croup assessed?

One evaluates the following parameters in assessing severity of the illness: (a) work of breathing—is there tachypnea and or retractions? (b) Chest wall motion—is the tidal volume adequate with inspiration, (c) overall appearance—is the child cyanotic, obtunded, comfortable? (d) Vocal quality—is there stridor, diminished voice or cry? Severe croup unresponsive to the medical therapy may require intubation. Once the diagnosis of croup has been established, the child is given a croup score, which helps determine therapy (Table 49.1).

Westley CR, Cotton EK, Brooks JG. Nebulized racemic epinephrine by IPPB for the treatment of croup: a double-blind study. *Am J Dis Child* 1978;132:484.

A.6. What is the medical management of croup? Does this have applications for the anesthesiologist?

Mild croup is treated with inspired gas humidification, hydration, and oxygen to improve the attendant hypoxemia. Croup tents, croupettes, and blow by oxygen are helpful. Steroids and racemic epinephrine are the prime modalities of therapy. If the patient has moderate retractions

Table 49.1 The Westley Croup Score.

	0	1	2	3	4	5
Cyanosis	None				With agitation	At rest
Level of Consciousness	Normal, including sleep					Disoriented
Stridor	None	With agitation	At rest			
Air Entry	Normal	Decreased	Markedly decreased			
Retractions	None	Mild	Moderate	Severe		

Mild croup has a score <2, moderate is between 3 and 7, and severe has a score >8.

and appears dyspneic, 0.5 mL of a 2.25% racemic epinephrine solution in 2.5 mL of normal saline can be administered through a nebulizer.

Airway resistance can be high with the reactive transudation and resultant intraluminal narrowing. By vasoconstricting the arterioles of the mucosal vasculature, racemic epinephrine relieves edema. The epinephrine is prepared as a mixture of the L and D isomers to limit cardiac stimulation. Patients improve markedly, but the clinician should be cautioned that the relief may be short lived and rebound airway compromise may occur after the epinephrine wears off. The β_2 activity will cause bronchial smooth muscle relaxation. Avoid racemic epinephrine in children with glaucoma and ventricular outflow obstruction.

Dexamethasone and budesonide when given early in viral croup can be beneficial in reducing inflammation and alleviating symptoms. This takes time to work however requiring hours for effective onset. The pediatric dose of dexamethasone is 0.6 mg per kg orally or intramuscularly. Clinical evaluation of topical steroids such as budesonide has shown effective improvement especially with laryngeal edema. Nebulized budesonide has been shown to be as effective as dexamethasone in treatment.

Behrman RE, Kliegman RM, Jensen HB, eds. *Nelson textbook of pediatrics*, 17th ed. Philadelphia: WB Saunders, 2004:1405–1409.

Cetinkaya F, Tufekci BS, Kutluk G. A comparison of nebulized budesonide, and intramuscular, and oral dexamethasone for treatment of croup. *Int J Pediatr Otorhinolaryngol* 2004;68:453.

Westley CR, Cotton EK, Brooks JG. Nebulized racemic epinephrine by IPPB for the treatment of croup: a double-blind study. *Am J Dis Child* 1978;132:484.

A.7. What is epiglottitis? What are its common causes? What is the incidence?

Epiglottitis is an inflammation of the epiglottis usually secondary to an infectious process. It was first described in the latter 19th century. It can involve other supraglottic structures such as the arytenoid, false cords, and posterior tongue leading to obstruction of the airway. Progression of swelling can rapidly lead to complete airway occlusion and death. Table 49.2 contrasts epiglottitis with croup. Epiglottitis is most often bacterial in origin. The causative agent is usually *Haemophilus influenzae* type B. *Streptococcus pneumoniae* has also been infrequently associated with epiglottitis, and recently group A β-hemolytic streptococci have been on the increase. Burn injury, neoplastic infiltration, caustic ingestion, lymphoproliferative disease and angioneurotic edema are also causes of this process. The incidence has declined to 1.8 per 10,000 admissions

Table 49.2 Characteristics of Croup and Epiglottitis.

	CROUP	EPIGLOTTITIS
Etiology	Parainfluenza virus	*Haemophilus influenzae*
Age	Infancy 4 mo to 2 y	2–5 y
Onset	Subacute exacerbation of preexistent URI	Acute
Temperature	Low-grade fever	High fever
Course	Usually mild, stridor may worsen at night	Rapid progress of symptoms
Symptoms	Barky cough, stridor	Dysphagia, sore throat Dysphonia, respiratory distress

URI, upper respiratory infection.

at the Children's Hospital of Philadelphia after the haemophilus influenzae B (Hib) vaccine. The median age has increased from 3 years to 6½ years over the past decade, and currently the prevalence is higher in adults than children. In one study, five cases of epiglottitis occurred amongst children who had been immunized.

Behrman RE, Kliegman RM, Jensen HB, eds. *Nelson textbook of pediatrics*, 17th ed. Philadelphia: WB Saunders, 2004:1405–1409.

Shah RK, Roberson DW, Jones DT. Epiglottitis in the haemophilus influenzae type B vaccine era: changing trends. *Laryngoscope* 2004;114:557.

A.8. What are the clinical manifestations of epiglottitis?

This illness presents acutely in the otherwise healthy child between 2 and 5 years of age with fever as high as 40°C (104°F). Within a few hours the epiglottic inflammation progresses and the child becomes dyspneic. The child sits forward to use the accessory muscles of respiration and complains of a fullness and pain in the throat. Speech sounds muffled known as a *hot potato voice*. Salivation is often characteristic and swallowing is difficult. The child appearing anxious and toxic concentrates only on breathing. The older child will assume a tripod posture with the neck extended to maximize air entry. As the child fatigues, cyanosis leading to complete asphyxia may ensue without intervention. Inspiratory effort is maximal with severe airway compromise, and negative pressure pulmonary edema can occur. Chest auscultation may reveal decreased breath sounds.

Behrman RE, Kliegman RM, Jensen HB, eds. *Nelson textbook of pediatrics*, 17th ed. Philadelphia: WB Saunders, 2004:1405–1409.

Cressman WR, Myer CM. Diagnosis and management of croup and epiglottitis. *Pediatr Clin North Am* 1994;41:265–276.

A.9. How is the diagnosis of epiglottitis made?

Acute epiglottitis is a dire emergency and any child whose clinical presentation warrants the diagnosis of epiglottitis must be evaluated promptly in a hospital. Pharyngoscopy to visualize an inflamed epiglottitis should not be attempted in an office setting, because this can stimulate upper airway reflexes and lead to increasing dyspnea. All medical centers should have in place a management protocol that standardizes the approach to this rapidly progressive and fatal disease and that involves a team of physicians and nurses from the specialties of pediatrics, otolaryngology, and anesthesiology. A logical approach is as follows:

- The child is kept calm with a parent in attendance at all times. Supplementary oxygen, maintenance of a sitting position, and reassurance are essential.
- If the patient clinically conforms to a classical presentation of epiglottitis, the operating room is alerted and the child is taken there immediately for intubation.
- With other diagnostic considerations, such as a foreign body in the upper airway, retropharyngeal abscess, congenital anomalies, and croup, the child may be escorted to radiology. The time taken for the x-ray examination should obviously be avoided in the critically ill child. A physician skilled in airway management should accompany the child with all necessary resuscitation equipment available.
- The classic thumb sign on a lateral x-ray film is an aptly named shape seen with epiglottic enlargement. However, the absence of this sign does not eliminate the diagnosis of epiglottitis. Croup is distinguished by the steeple sign representing a uniform narrowing of the subglottic

airway by inflammation. Recently, magnetic resonance imaging has demonstrated the standard measurements for the hypopharyngeal space in various age groups, and it has correlated this measurement with the change produced by epiglottic inflammation. This may be a useful tool in the future to assess the severity of airway involvement.

- Laboratory evidence is nonspecific, although a high white count with bands and polymorphonuclear leukocytes is more suggestive of epiglottitis than of croup.
- Fiberoptic pharyngoscopy can be most effective if performed gently by a skilled examiner; it immediately confirms or eliminates the diagnosis. Do not perform a laryngoscopy if anxiety is increased by the procedure and hence exacerbates airway obstruction.

Davis HW, Gartner JC, Galvis AG, et al. Acute upper airway obstruction: croup and epiglottitis. *Pediatr Clin North Am* 1981;28:859.

Diaz JH. Croup and epiglottitis in children: the anesthesiologist as diagnostician. *Anesth Anal* 1985;64:621.

Shorten GD, Opie NJ, Graziotti P, et al. Assessment of upper airway anatomy in awake, sedated and anaesthetized patients using magnetic resonance imaging. *Anaesth Intensive Care* 1994;22:165.

A.10. What is postextubation croup? How is it managed?

Anesthesiologists are often in the position of treating patients with postextubation airway edema, which resembles croup in its symptomatology.

Pediatric patients undergoing general endotracheal anesthesia can and may mimic many of the physical signs of the croup syndrome following extubation. The tracheal and subglottal mucosa have become irritated by the plastic tube, which initiates an inflammatory response causing airway luminal narrowing. Because airway resistance is inversely proportional to the fourth power of the tracheal radius (with turbulent flow, this increases to the fifth power), the pediatric airway is especially compromised by edema. Halving the lumen will increase laminar airflow resistance 16 times.

Postextubation croup may manifest more frequently in a patient who has received large quantities of fluid or transfusions; maintained unusual or strained lateral head positioning; has a history of smoke inhalation, restrictive congenital anomalies such as a tracheoesophageal fistula, or acquired subglottic stenosis secondary to prolonged intubation as a neonate; has a coexistent upper respiratory infection, especially bronchitis; or has a cuffed endotracheal tube under high pressure.

Management involves reducing airway constriction by administering nebulized racemic epinephrine, steroids, and humidifications of inspired gases. On occasion, reintubating with a soft endotracheal tube one half to one size smaller than previously used is necessary until the inflammation subsides. Note that topical lidocaine ointment can have vasodilatory actions and should not be used in patients with postextubation croup.

Davis HW, Gartner JC, Galvis AG, et al. Acute upper airway obstruction: croup and epiglottitis. *Pediatr Clin North Am* 1981;28:859.

Ferrari LR. Anesthesia for pediatric ear, nose and throat surgery. *In: Barash PG, ed. ASA refresher courses in anesthesiology*, Vol. 24. Park Ridge: American Society of Anesthesiology, 1996:66.

A.11. What are the nonacute causes of partial airway obstruction in children?

Several congenital anomalies are associated with respiratory difficulties. These can be subdivided into intrinsic and extrinsic pathologies as follows.

Extrinsic pathologies

- Cystic hygroma—a proliferation or expansion of lymphatic channels, usually in the cervical region, which can compress the airway and lead to enlargement of the tongue.
- Vascular anomalies—abnormalities of the aortic arch usually caused by aberrant vessels leads to compression of the airway. This is often position dependent and may be responsible for coughing and wheezing when the patient is supine.
- Neoplastic compression of the trachea by lymphoma, hemangioma, neurofibromatosis, rhabdomyosarcoma, and other neural tumors in the mediastinum may occur and enlarge or compress airway structures.

Intrinsic pathologies

- Subglottic stenosis—especially as acquired in previously intubated neonates. This form of airway narrowing occurs below the vocal cords, and it can lead to marked airway obstruction with respiratory infections. The congenital form may not be appreciated until an upper respiratory infection is present, when stridor may occur.
- Vocal cord paralysis—considered the second most common laryngeal anomaly in children, it is associated with the Arnold-Chiari malformation.
- Laryngeal structural anomalies—webs, laryngoceles, and cysts.

Perry H. Stridor. In: Fleisher GR, Ludwig S, Henretig FM, eds. *Textbook of pediatric emergency medicine*, 5th ed. Philadelphia: Lippincott Williams & Wilkins, 2006:1632–1634.

B. Preoperative Evaluation and Preparation

B.1. Is intubation always required in children with epiglottitis?

Selected patients may even be managed under very vigilant circumstances without intubation provided that there is no impending obstructive danger. However, contemporary practice warrants the establishing of an airway with an endotracheal tube. Nasotracheal intubation is most often used for ease of maintaining the child's comfort and safety. Endoscopic evaluation using appropriate fiberoptic airway endoscopy is a major advance in the management of epiglottitis.

Damm M, Eckel HE, Jungehulsing M, et al. Airway endoscopy in the interdisciplinary management of acute epiglottitis. *Int J Pediatr Otorhinolaryngol* 1996;38:41.

B.2. Why is general anesthesia administered to a child with epiglottitis?

General anesthesia facilitates several activities. It gives the examiner a thorough look at the supraglottic area, which would be impossible and dangerous in the awake child. In addition, endotracheal intubation can be accomplished under controlled, relaxed conditions without trauma and laryngospasm. Intubation can be difficult because of the swelling and deformation of the paraepiglottic tissues. Clinicians who have no experience with this unusual appearance will find it easier to visualize landmarks and secure the airway when the patient is in a surgical plane of anesthesia.

Diaz JH. Croup and epiglottitis in children. *Anesthesiology* 1985;64:628.

B.3. How would you prepare the patient for anesthesia?

Expedience is crucial. Once the diagnosis is made and the operating room alerted, the child is transported accompanied by his or her parents and a physician with supportive equipment. It is not necessary to place an intravenous line, because this can be done more easily under anesthesia without upsetting the child. Any maneuver that causes the child to cry will potentially interfere with breathing. The child should, therefore, be kept calm and constantly reassured. Nasal prong or face tent oxygen should be provided and portable pulse oximetry should be used.

Equipment, which is prepared in the operating room, includes a suitable mask and endotracheal tube, sized two gauges (1-mm diameter) smaller than normally expected. Lidocaine, succinylcholine, atropine, and ketamine in convenient dilutions should be readily available. A cricothyrotomy tray should be available as a precaution.

The parent is dressed in operating room attire to accompany the child into the operating room. Before induction, the parent is instructed on his or her role in comforting the child, encouraging complicity with mask breathing, and gently holding the child when the inhalation induction commences. The parent should also be told that as the child begins to fall asleep he or she will be asked to leave the room. For anesthesiologists unaccustomed to the presence of parents in the operating room, the extra anxiety created by parental presence can be attenuated by having them depart just as the patient begins to get sleepy. When parents can provide their assistance in an emotionally controlled, supportive way, a smooth, safe anesthetic induction can usually be well facilitated.

Berry FA. Management of the pediatric patient with croup or epiglottitis. *ASA annual meeting refresher course lectures*. Park Ridge: American Society of Anesthesiologists, 1990:261.

C. Intraoperative Management

C.1. How is the airway of the child with epiglottitis best secured?

Little debate occurs over the safety and efficacy of endotracheal intubation provided that supportive staff is readily available. The endotracheal tube should be sized down 0.5 or 1.0 mm due to the inherent swelling and to protect against postextubation complications. Thick, copious secretions must be cleared frequently to prevent obstruction, and the child must be sedated properly to prevent the tube from dislodging and to allow for its toleration. In the smaller hospital without a pediatric intensive care facility or experienced personnel, a tracheotomy may be the safest route.

C.2. How would you induce anesthesia?

Verbal assurance is constantly given. The child is seated on the parent's lap in the operating room and is preoxygenated. Sevoflurane is a good choice of induction agent as it is less pungent than other irritative gases such as desflurane and is usually well tolerated without a high incidence of laryngospasm, coughing or other irritative reflexes. Halothane is also well tolerated and, due to its greater solubility than sevoflurane, may have the added advantage of providing for a longer sustained level of surgical anesthesia. This may be of value during laryngoscopy. In either case, the inhalational agent should be initiated slowly and increased in concentration as tolerated. A flavored mask with a pleasant scent may be helpful to enlist the child's cooperation. As the child tires, the supine position is assumed. If there are any considerations of gastric contents regurgitation either due to a recent meal or antecedent history of reflux, cricoid pressure is applied as a safeguard against aspiration. The patient may undergo a brief period of excitement during which care is taken not to be overly zealous with ventilatory assistance. Spontaneous, unassisted ventilation continues and an intravenous line is started. Glycopyrrolate 0.01 mg per kg is given intravenously as an antisialagogue. Ventilatory assistance but not control is provided to limit hypercarbia. End-tidal gas analysis is continually monitored and the airway is adjusted to provide maximal tidal exchange. Sevoflurane is augmented as tolerated to 8% provided cardiovascular stability is maintained to allow the child to pass into a plane of surgical anesthesia. If halothane is used, 3% to 4% concentration is used. If there is airway obstruction, anesthetic uptake may be delayed. Therefore, a much prolonged induction time may be necessary to achieve a deeply anesthetized patient with a slow inhalation induction. When the patient is in a deep plane of surgical anesthesia (remember that the minimal alveolar concentrations [MACs] of halothane and sevoflurane in children are higher than those in adults), a careful laryngoscopy is carried out. Paralysis is unnecessary in this deep plane of anesthesia. However, if several attempts are required with the possibility of the patient becoming light and reactive, cisatracurium (0.5 mg/kg) or mivacurium (0.2 mg/kg) will serve to maintain stable intubating conditions. This should be given only after it has been shown that the patient can be ventilated with a bag and mask.

DeSoto H. Anesthesia for pediatric ENT surgery—routine and emergent. *ASA annual meeting refresher course lectures*. Park Ridge: American Society of Anesthesiologists, 2000:252.

Hall SC. The child with a difficult airway: recognition and management. *ASA annual meeting refresher course lectures*. Park Ridge: American Society of Anesthesiologists, 2006:412.

Spalding MB, Ala-Kokko TI. The use of inhaled sevoflurane for endotracheal intubation in epiglottitis. *Anesthesiology* 1998;89:1025.

C.3. Should a child with epiglottitis undergo a rapid-sequence induction?

In the child with a full stomach, a mask induction leaves the airway unprotected from aspiration of gastric contents. However, a rapid-sequence induction may predispose the patient to severe hypoxia and hypoventilation should the clinician not be able to intubate expediently. Because the supraglottic landmarks are distorted by erythema and edema, recognition of the glottic inlet is obscured. In the spontaneously breathing patient, small air movements and the resultant secretional bubbling may highlight the glottic opening. In addition, paralysis in no way secures ventilatability.

If the patient must be manually ventilated, it is possible to meet with complete obstruction secondary to invagination of the swollen supraglottic tissues into the laryngeal introitus. In such a case, positive end-expiratory pressure (PEEP) or the jaw-thrust maneuver may fail to correct the airway obstruction.

Should the child be too agitated to cooperate with an inhalational induction, an intramuscular dose of ketamine (2 to 3 mg/kg) will accomplish sedation and preserve ventilation. However, it may accentuate airway reflexes, and the clinician should be wary of laryngospasm.

DeSoto H. Anesthesia for pediatric ENT surgery—routine and emergent. *ASA annual meeting refresher course lectures*. Park Ridge: American Society of Anesthesiologists, 2000:252.

Hall SC. The child with a difficult airway: recognition and management. *ASA annual meeting refresher course lectures*. Park Ridge: American Society of Anesthesiologists, 2006:412.

C.4. Is awake intubation a practical alternative to secure the patient's airway?

Some authors suggest awake intubation with topical anesthesia. In such cases the anesthesiologist should be alerted to the possibility of adenoidal bleeding, difficult visualization, agitation, trauma, and compromised ventilation. Unless one has acquired great skill at awake pediatric intubation in the child with a normal airway, this technique should be avoided in these patients.

Diaz JH. Croup and epiglottitis in children. *Anesthesiology* 1985;64:628.

C.5. What would you do if the airway cannot be secured with intubation?

Percutaneous transtracheal ventilation can be performed. This involves inserting a needle through the cricothyroid membrane as follows. Localize the cricothyroid membrane and topically cleanse the area with antiseptic. Anesthetize the skin with lidocaine and then insert a 16-gauge catheter (attached to needle) in the inferior portion of the midline cricothyroid membrane. Keep the angle of the needle directed caudally and attach a 3-mL syringe to the needle barrel applying negative pressure. If the syringe contains a few milliliters of saline, air bubbles will be apparent when the trachea is entered. Following entry, advance the catheter into the trachea. Depending on the hub size, a 3.0-mm or 3.5-mm endotracheal tube adapter can be inserted into the catheter to interface with an Ambu bag. Alternatively, a 6.5-mm or 7.0-mm endotracheal tube adapter can be inserted into a 3-mL syringe without the plunger to interface with an Ambu bag or anesthesia circuit. Jet ventilation can also be applied with high-pressure tubing keeping careful observation of respiratory dynamics and saturation.

Delaney WA, Kaiser RE. Percutaneous transtracheal jet ventilation made easy. *Anesthesiology* 1991;74:952.

C.6. Should this patient have a nasotracheal or orotracheal tube placed?

The patient will better tolerate a nasal tube for prolonged intubation. Oropharyngeal toilet is also easier. However, because the intubation can be difficult with epiglottitis and may predispose the patient to the problems listed in section C.4, the orotracheal route is easier and thus safer. Once the airway is secured orally, a nasotracheal tube can be inserted with laryngoscopic guidance. The Magill forceps may be necessary to facilitate insertion of the nasal tube.

C.7. Shortly after intubation, frothy secretions were obtained on suctioning the endotracheal tube. What is the reason for this? How can this be treated?

Davis et al. describes 7% of these patients as having pulmonary edema after intubation. This phenomenon relates to the transudation into the alveoli during periods of increased transpulmonary pressure. This occurs especially during obstructed inspiration. If the obstruction is complete, it is referred to as the *Müller* maneuver. The high negative pressures are buffered by the decreased venous return during exhalation. However, relief of the airway obstruction facilitates the extravasation of fluid for an increased venous return.

Treatment of this negative pressure pulmonary edema requires positive end-expiratory pressure (PEEP). Diuretics and fluid restriction are not required because this condition is generally self-correcting.

Davis HW, Gartener JC, Galvis AG, et al. Acute upper airway obstruction: croup and epiglottitis. *Pediatr Clin North Am* 1981;28:859.

D. Postoperative Management

D.1. How long should this patient remain intubated? What criteria determine extubation time?

Earlier studies have shown a mean intubation duration of 36 hours in 23 patients with a range of 19 to 67 hours. These patients were treated with ampicillin or chloramphenicol and the epiglottis was visualized before extubation. The current antibiotic regimen is cefazolin 75 to 100 mg/kg/day in three divided doses or clindamycin 30 to 40 mg/kg/day in three divided doses with the addition of a third generation cephalosporin such as cefotaxime or ceftriaxone.

Criteria for extubation include an increased air leak around the endotracheal tube as well as decreased erythema and edema. Vernon and Sarnaik, however, feel that instrumentation and examination of the child is unnecessary and extubation at 36 to 48 hours can easily be accomplished in all patients. Hopkins recommended that the flexible fiberoptic laryngoscope be used to visualize the epiglottis and determine extubation time.

Damm M, Eckel HE, Jungehulsing M, et al. Airway endoscopy in the interdisciplinary management of acute epiglottitis. *Int J Pediatr Otorhinolaryngol* 1996;38:41.

Hopkins RL. Extubation in epiglottitis. *Anesth Analg* 1984;63:468.

Rothstein P, Lister G. Epiglottitis: duration of intubation and fever. *Anesth Analg* 1983;62: 785.

Vernon DD, Sarnaik AP. Extubation in epiglottitis. *Anesth Analg* 1984;63:469.

D.2. How would you make this patient comfortable during the course of being intubated?

The child must be kept sedated to minimize movement, to prevent deliberate extubation, and to provide anxiolysis. Midazolam (0.075 mg/kg) as a starting dose titrated upward to effect followed by a continuous infusion of 0.04 mg/kg/hour will be effective in this regard. If necessary a fentanyl infusion (1 to 2 μg/kg/hour)) can be supplemented. A bilateral superior laryngeal nerve block in experienced hands allows for better endotracheal tube toleration.

Of course respiratory care, humidification, suctioning, and secretion mobilization must receive attention.

Davis HW, Gartner JC, Galvis AG, et al. Acute upper airway obstruction: croup and epiglottitis. *Pediatr Clin North Am* 1981;28:859.

D.3. What outcome can one expect for the child with acute epiglottitis?

Residual airway problems are unusual in most children. Most children who are diagnosed in time and intubated go on to a full recovery without sequela. Complications include associated pneumonia, respiratory failure, hypoxia, and cardiac arrest.

CHAPTER 50

Cleft Palate

AARTI SHARMA

A 3-MONTH-OLD MALE INFANT

was scheduled for repair of a cleft lip and a cleft palate. According to his pediatrician, the infant was born at full term and had no other medical problems.

A. Medical Disease and Differential Diagnosis

1. Describe the anatomic concept of a cleft palate and a cleft lip.
2. What is the cause of a cleft lip and a cleft palate?
3. What is the incidence of a cleft lip and a cleft palate?
4. Discuss the pathophysiology of a cleft lip and palate in the neonate and the older child (e.g., age >5 years).
5. What other conditions are associated with a cleft lip and a cleft palate?
6. What is Pierre Robin syndrome?
7. What is Treacher Collins syndrome?
8. What kind of specialized team care would these patients need?
9. Discuss indications and timing of closure of a cleft lip and palate.
10. What is velopharyngeal incompetence and how can it be diagnosed?
11. What is the relation of tonsillectomy and adenoidectomy to velopharyngeal incompetence?

B. Preoperative Evaluation and Preparation

1. What information do you need before closure of a cleft lip and palate?
2. What preoperative orders are needed?

C. Intraoperative Management

1. What monitors will you need for cheiloplasty and palatoplasty?
2. Discuss the induction and the anesthetic management for cleft lip and palate.
3. What positioning is recommended for cleft palate repair surgery?
4. What are the reported complications of this type of surgery and anesthesia?
5. Briefly describe the surgical techniques used to repair cleft defects.
6. How does a pharyngeal flap affect anesthetic management or any subsequent anesthetic administered to this patient?
7. What is an Abbe flap? What are its anesthetic implications?
8. What is the crucial problem of anesthesia for cleft palate? Enumerate the consequences of failure.
9. What is laryngospasm? How would you make a diagnosis of laryngospasm?
10. How would you manage the patient with laryngospasm?

D. Postoperative Management

1. What complications of cleft lip and cleft palate surgery may be seen in the recovery room?

2. How do you protect the airway postoperatively?

3. How would you control postoperative pain in patients following a cleft lip and a cleft palate repair?

A. Medical Disease and Differential Diagnosis

A.1. Describe the anatomic concept of a cleft palate and a cleft lip.

Congenital clefts of upper lip occur because of failure of fusion of the maxillary and the medial and the lateral nasal processes. They vary from notch in the upper lip to a cleft through the lip and the floor of the nose involving the alveolar ridge, or they may be complete cleft of the lip and the palate.

The cleft palate is divided into prepalatal and postpalatal clefts. The incisive foramen marks the boundary between the two. They both have different embryologic development. Prepalatal cleft involves anterior palate, alveolus, lip, nostril floor, and ala nasi. Postpalatal clefts may extend anywhere from soft and hard palate to the incisive foramen. The third type is a submucosal cleft in which a bone defect exists without a mucosal defect. The most common cleft of the palate is a left complete cleft of the prepalatal and palatal structures. The second most common is a midline cleft of all the soft palate and part of the hard palate without a cleft in the prepalatal area. Various degrees of the cleft palate and lip are shown in Fig. 50.1.

Aston SJ, Beasley RW, Thorne CHM, eds. *Grabb and Smith's plastic surgery*, 5th ed. Philadelphia: Lippincott-Raven, 1997:245–263.

Gregory GA, ed. *Pediatric anesthesia*, 4th ed. New York: Churchill Livingstone, 2002:731.

A.2. What is the cause of a cleft lip or a cleft palate?

Major components of face develop between 4 and 7 weeks of fetal life. There are three mesodermal islands, one central and two lateral. Prepalatal clefts are caused by the failure of these mesodermal elements to develop and fuse. Palatal clefts are caused when the palatal ridges fail to migrate medially, contact, and fuse (Fig. 50.1).

Aston SJ, Beasley RW, Thorne CHM, eds. *Grabb and Smith's plastic surgery*, 5th ed. Philadelphia: Lippincott-Raven, 1997:230–234.

A.3. What is the incidence of a cleft lip and a cleft palate?

Cleft lip and cleft palate may occur together or separately. A cleft lip with or without a cleft palate occurs in 1:1,000 births. A cleft palate alone occurs in approximately 1:2,500 births. A cleft lip with or without a cleft palate is more common in boys, whereas isolated cleft palate is more common in girls.

The highest incidence of a cleft lip and a cleft palate occurs among Asians (1.61:1,000 births), whereas the lowest incidence is in African Americans (0.3:1,000 births). The incidence in whites is intermediate (0.9:1,000 births).

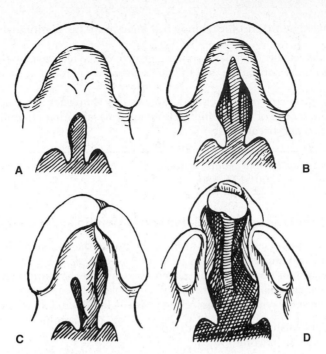

Figure 50.1 Various degrees of cleft palate and lip. **A:** Cleft of the soft palate only. **B:** Cleft of the soft and hard palate as far forward as the incisive foramen. **C:** Complete unilateral alveolar cleft, usually involving the lip. **D:** Complete bilateral alveolar cleft, usually associated with bilateral clefts of the lip. (From McCarthy JG, ed. Cleft lip and palate and craniofacial abnormalities. In: *Plastic surgery,* Vol 4. Philadelphia: WB Saunders, 1990, with permission.)

Aston SJ, Beasley RW, Thorne CIIM, eds. *Grabb and Smith's plastic surgery,* 5th ed. Philadelphia: Lippincott-Raven, 1997:245–255.

A.4. Discuss the pathophysiology of a cleft lip and palate in the neonate and the older child (e.g., age >5 years).

Cleft palate is responsible for some major physiologic disorders. The pharynx communicates more extensively with the nasal fossae and the oral cavity. The complex mechanisms of swallowing, breathing, hearing (through the eustachian tube), and speech are, therefore, impaired.

The presence of a cleft lip and palate in a neonate results in feeding difficulties. The neonate cannot suck because the cleft makes the creation of a negative pressure difficult. Breast-feeding is improbable and bottle-feeding is difficult.

Essentially all children with a cleft palate have middle ear disease because abnormal anatomy of the nasopharynx adversely affects eustachian tube function. Chronic middle ear effusion produces varying degree of conductive hearing loss. Nasal septation between food and air is absent, creating a nonphysiologic mixing chamber in the nasopharynx. Not infrequent this is associated with chronic rhinorrhea that must be distinguished preoperatively from infection.

Secondary defects of tooth development, growth of the ala nasi, and velopharyngeal function (contact between the soft palate and the posterior pharynx for speech and swallowing) can also occur.

Psychologic problems may be considerable as this youngster approaches school age and peer association. The speech of these children is typically nasal with an inability to sound the so-called plosives (*p/k/d/t*) and fricatives (*s/f*).

Malek R, ed. *Cleft lip and palate, lesions, pathophysiology and primary treatment.* London: Martin Dunitz, 2001:124–130.

A.5. What other conditions are associated with a cleft lip and a cleft palate?

Associated anomalies occur 30 times more frequently in the patient with isolated cleft palate than in the noncleft population.

The most common nonsyndrome-related abnormalities are umbilical hernias, clubfoot, and limb and ear deformities.

The most common syndromes associated with a cleft lip and a cleft palate are

- Velocardiofacial (Shprintzen's) syndrome
- Van der Woude's syndrome
- Stickler's syndrome
- Pierre Robin syndrome
- Fetal alcohol syndrome
- Goldenhar's syndrome (facio-auriculo-vertebral syndrome or hemifacial microsomia)
- Treacher Collins syndrome
- Nager syndrome
- Down syndrome

Sumner E, Hatch D, eds. *Pediatric anesthesia*, 2nd ed. London: Arnold, 2000:383–384.

A.6. What is Pierre Robin syndrome?

This syndrome is characterized by retrognathia or micrognathia, glossoptosis, and airway obstruction. For facial cleft surgeons, Pierre Robin syndrome is defined by a triad of clinical criteria:

- Retrognathia
- Severe respiratory and/or digestive disorders in early infancy
- Cleft palate

An incomplete cleft of the palate is associated with the syndrome in approximately 50% of these patients. In patients with micrognathia (small jaw) or retrognathia, the chin is posteriorly displaced causing the tongue to fall backward toward the posterior pharyngeal wall. This results in obstruction of the airway on inspiration. Crying or straining by these children can often keep the airway open. However, when the child relaxes or sleeps, airway obstruction occurs. Because of these respiratory problems, feeding may become very difficult. This can lead to a sequence of events: glossoptosis, airway obstruction, crying or straining with increased energy expenditure, and decreased oral intake. This vicious cycle of events if untreated can led to exhaustion, cardiac failure, and ultimately death.

Jones KL, ed. *Smith's recognizable patterns of human malformation*, 7th ed. Philadelphia: WB Saunders, 2006:262.

A.7. What is Treacher Collins syndrome?

It is highly complex disease process consisting of

- Hypoplastic cheeks, zygomatic arches, and mandible
- Microtia with possible hearing loss
- High arched or cleft palate
- Macrostomia (abnormally large mouth)
- Antimongoloid slant to the eyes
- Colobomas (notching of the outer portion of the lower eyelid)
- Increased anterior facial height
- Malocclusion (anterior open bite)
- Small oral cavity and airway with normal-sized tongue
- Pointed nasal prominence

Jones KL, ed. *Smith's recognizable patterns of human malformation*, 7th ed. Philadelphia: WB Saunders, 2006:280–281.

A.8. What kind of specialized team care would these patients need?

These patients need a pediatrician to maintain their overall health and a surgeon and an anesthesiologist to accomplish the various surgeries. They would need a speech therapist to prevent or overcome the speech deficiencies and an orthodontist for early orthodontic intervention to develop and maintain relatively normal bite and dentition. The care team also includes geneticist, pediatric dentist, prosthodontist, psychologist, medical social worker, and public health nurse.

Nelson WE, Behrman RE, et al. eds. *Nelson textbook of pediatrics*, 17th ed. Philadelphia: WB Saunders, 2004:1207–1208.

A.9. Discuss indications and timing of closure of cleft lip and palate.

Functional goals of cleft palate surgery are normal speech, hearing, and maxillofacial growth. It is thought that speech and hearing are improved by early cleft palate repair (before 24 months of age) and that the delayed closure (after 4 years) is associated with less retardation of midfacial growth. An early two-stage palate repair is advocated in management of these patients. The recommended sequence involves closure of the soft palate at 3 to 6 months of age with secondary closure of the residual hard palate at 15 to 18 months of age. This sequence takes advantage of the early physiology and growth that occurs in the soft palate, which is vital in the development of speech. Furthermore, it avoids the potential pitfalls of the growth disturbance related to early periosteal undermining of palatal and vomerine tissue. This repair sequence also provides total palatal closure before speech evolves. If soft palate is repaired at the time of lip repair, an additional anesthetic is avoided.

Malek R, ed. *Cleft lip and palate, lesions, pathophysiology and primary treatment*. London: Martin Dunitz, 2001:197–205.

A.10. What is velopharyngeal incompetence and how can it be diagnosed?

Velopharyngeal incompetence is inability of soft palate in fulfilling its role in closing the nasopharynx, thereby affecting the phonation seriously.

To produce plosive sounds, *p/k/t/d*, or the sibilants, *s/sh*, the soft palate must touch the posterior pharyngeal wall to close the nose. Failure of closure results in the typical hypernasal speech. The most common cause of this is the cleft palate, but patients with congenitally short palates and no cleft can also have this typical speech. Treatment consists of surgical lengthening of the palate by the pushback operation with or without pharyngeal flap. The diagnosis of velopharyngeal incompetence can be suggested by the child's speech. More objective diagnosis can be obtained by direct vision of the soft palate while the child is pronouncing certain keywords (*kah, kah*), by the fogging of the hand mirror placed under the nose during speech, and from cinefluorographic x-ray films.

In patients with velopharyngeal incompetence, videofluoroscopy and nasopharyngoscopy can provide information that will help select the appropriate procedure, either pharyngoplasty or posterior pharyngeal flap.

Dudas JR, Deleyiannis FW, Ford MD, et al. Diagnosis and treatment of velopharyngeal insufficiency: clinical utility of speech evaluation and videofluoroscopy. *Ann Plast Surg* 2006;56(5):511–517.

A.11. What is the relation of tonsillectomy and adenoidectomy to velopharyngeal incompetence?

There is often a considerable mass of tonsillar and adenoidal tissue at the age when surgery is usually performed, and, in addition to the latent danger of infection, the flap used in pharyngoplasty creates an obstruction that seriously complicates their subsequent removal. Furthermore, bulky tonsils may hinder retrodisplacement of the soft palate or block the air flow by obstructing cavum, which has already been reduced in volume by the retrodisplacement and the presence of the flap. It is, therefore, preferable to remove the tonsils and adenoids a few months before pharyngoplasty. The parents may wonder why this decision has been made, because they have been repeatedly told that the adenoids should not be removed in case of cleft palate because this might create or aggravate velar insufficiency. However, once velar inadequacy is confirmed, the parents are in a position to understand that these precautions are no longer justified and that the adenoids can represent a source of problems if not treated with radical measures. During tonsillectomy it is important to leave the tonsillar pillars absolutely intact, because their muscle structure has a vital physiologic role.

Malek R, ed. *Cleft lip and palate, lesions, pathophysiology and primary treatment*. London: Martin Dunitz, 2001:146.

B. Preoperative Evaluation and Preparation

B.1. What information do you need before closure of a cleft lip and palate?

Preoperative anesthetic evaluation is invaluable and includes the history and physical examination and suitable laboratory data. It gives a picture of the patient's general health. Hemoglobin level, which is often low in very young infants, should be obtained. If Treacher Collins or Pierre Robin syndrome is suspected, an x-ray film of the mandible may be helpful. Examination of the mouth may indicate potential intubation problems. The examination also offers a good opportunity to appraise the family environment, because parental cooperation is essential for proper postoperative care.

Most surgeons repair a cleft lip when the baby is 6 to 10 weeks old and repair a cleft palate at 6 to 12 months of age. The exact age of repair will depend on the size and health of the child and the surgeon's preference.

Because periosteoplasty and lip adhesions are carried out as soon as the segments are in alignment and the surgery is less extensive, the rule of 10 can be used with moderate license:

- *Weight.* Approximately £10
- *Hemoglobin.* 10 g or more
- *White blood cell count.* Less than 10,000 per μL
- *Age.* Can be less than 10 weeks

With open cleft palate, however, it is common to have crusting and low-grade infection of the nasopharynx because of food and fluid regurgitation through the cleft. It is nearly impossible to eliminate this completely. Unless an acute inflammation process is present, this does not lead to complications.

Barrett BM Jr, ed. *Patient care in plastic surgery.* St. Louis: Mosby, 1996:343–344.

B.2. What preoperative orders are needed?

Preoperative fasting has been a prerequisite for elective surgery. An issue of particular importance to the pediatric patient is the wonderful changes that have taken place regarding preoperative fasting. Recent work has shown that prolonged fasting does not reduce the risk of aspiration pneumonitis during anesthesia. This has led to reduction in the fasting times. Reduced fasting increases patient comfort and there may be less potential for intraoperative hypoglycemia. Fasting guidelines for infants and children are shown in Table 50.1.

Because multiple operations may be required, the emotional trauma of each hospital experience must be minimized. The most common premedication used at Cornell Medical center in pediatric patients is oral midazolam. Dose can range from 0.25 to 0.5 mg per kg orally. Children younger than 8 months rarely require premedication. Children with anticipated difficulty in airway management and those with propensity toward airway obstruction are better off without premedication.

Special orders include antibiotics if the infant or child has associated congenital heart disease and the typing and crossmatching of a unit of blood for palatal surgery.

Cote CJ. Preparation, premedication and induction of anesthesia in children. *ASA annual meeting refresher course lectures.* Park Ridge: American Society of Anesthesiologists, 2001;243.

Table 50.1 Minimum Fasting Period (Hours) for Pediatric Patients.

	CLEAR FLUIDS	BREAST MILK	FORMULA OR COW'S MILK	SOLIDS
Children	2	—	6	6
3–12 mo	2	4	6	6
<3 mo	2	4	4	6

C. Intraoperative Management

C.1. What monitors will you need for cheiloplasty and palatoplasty?

Heart rate, respiration, blood pressure, temperature, and oxygen saturation are monitored at all times. An electrocardiogram provides visual and audible evidence of the electrical activity of the heart. A precordial stethoscope monitors both heart and respiratory sounds. It is particularly important in this patient because once the surgery has begun, the anesthesiologist no longer has easy direct access to the airway. The use of pulse oximetry and an end-tidal CO_2 monitor is indispensable. Temperature should be monitored per rectum or axilla. A warming blanket should be used in these patients to avoid hypothermia. Blood loss determination should be made by a calibrated catchment trap in the suction line and by weighing sponges. Blood loss rarely exceeds 10% of circulating blood volume; however, properly crossmatched and screened blood should be available but used only if absolutely necessary.

C.2. Discuss the induction and the anesthetic management for cleft lip and palate.

After suitable monitors are attached, the infant is induced with oxygen, nitrous oxide, and either sevoflurane or halothane. Because cardiac depressant effects of sevoflurane are less pronounced than that of halothane, we prefer to use sevoflurane for induction. In addition, myocardium is more sensitive to exogenous epinephrine with use of halothane. Recommended maximal dose of lidocaine for palate or lip surgery is 5 mg per kg and of epinephrine 10 μg per kg. This epinephrine dose is for hypocarbic or normocarbic patients.

Once the patient is asleep, an intravenous line is established and appropriate intravenous fluids are started. Intubation can be facilitated with nondepolarizing muscle relaxants such as vecuronium 0.1 mg per kg. Muscle relaxants should be withheld if any possibility of difficulty in intubation exists.

Laryngoscopy in patient with a cleft lip is generally straightforward, but the cleft palate has the capability to trap and immobilize a straight blade. Should this occur, the anesthesiologist must first recognize the problem and then consider inserting a gauze pack or a dental roll in the cleft before laryngoscopy.

To achieve a cosmetic repair, symmetry is essential, so the tube should exit the mouth in the midline without facial distortion from either the tube or the securing tape. Some surgeons prefer to suture the tube to the lower gum.

An orogastric tube should be passed to empty the stomach of gas and secretions, and it should be removed before preparation of the surgical field.

A pharyngeal pack of moistened ribbon gauze is inserted for a cleft lip repairs; as for a cleft palate repair the surgeon inserts the gag before insertion of the pharyngeal pack. Following the gag and pack insertion, ventilation should be reassessed, because tube compression may have occurred. To avert eye injury, an ocular lubricant is placed in the eyes, and the upper eyelids are splinted shut with tape.

During the surgery it is necessary to have good communication and cooperation between the surgeon and the anesthesiologist because the surgeon's tools and hands and the anesthesiologist's endotracheal tube and apparatus all occupy the same very small space.

Gregory GA, ed. *Pediatric anesthesia*, 4th ed. New York: Churchill Livingstone, 2002:731.

C.3. What positioning is recommended for cleft palate repair surgery?

Correct positioning of the child is important for the plastic surgeon, who sits at the head of the operating table. Head extension must be maximal for cleft palate surgery. The entire body is raised with a thick foam mat or folded blanket, allowing the head to drop back hyperextended into a stockinette head support. Not only does this position provide good exposure but it also allows blood to flow away from larynx and toward the nasopharynx allowing it to be removed by suction.

C.4. What are the reported complications of this type of surgery and anesthesia?

Anesthetic complications include obstruction of the endotracheal tube, inadvertent extubation during the procedure, and cardiac arrest. Postanesthetic complications include airway obstruction, bleeding with or without aspiration, and pneumonia. Complications not related to anesthetic management are wound healing, diarrhea, and otitis media. The mortality rate has been reported to be less than 0.5%.

Gregory GA, ed. *Pediatric anesthesia*, 4th ed. New York: Churchill Livingstone, 2002:731–732.

C.5. Briefly describe the surgical techniques used to repair cleft defects.

The Furlow procedure is the most common technique for cleft palate closure. It involves opposing z-plasties of the mucosa and the musculature of the soft palate. The goal is to separate the nonfunctioning attachments to the posterior border of the hard palate and to displace the mucosa and the musculature posteriorly.

Other basic surgical techniques include: von Langenbeck technique, Schweckendiek technique, two-flap technique, three flap/V-Y technique.

Although most of the repairs do not involve repairing the muscular sling, doing so allows better palatal and Eustachian tube function.

Sadove AM, van Aalst JA, Culp JA. Cleft palate repair: art and issues. *Clin Plast Surg* 2004; 31(2):231–241.

C.6. How does pharyngeal flap affect anesthetic management or any subsequent anesthetic administered to this patient?

The presence of this flap prohibits nasoendotracheal intubation and makes many nasal techniques difficult (e.g., insertion of nasogastric tube). The degree of obstruction is related to the width of the flap. Traumatic rupture of this flap secondary to attempted nasotracheal intubation could produce bleeding, aspiration, and laryngospasm.

Traumatic rupture of soft palate can occur from placement of laryngeal mask airway.

Knowledge of prior surgery is essential to good anesthetic management. Following the pushback and pharyngeal flap operation (pharyngoplasty) significant airway obstruction has been noted in the early postoperative period. Sleeping pulse oximetry has demonstrated obstruction and desaturation in the first 48 to 72 hours.

Dearlove O, Perkins RJ, Briggs G. Anaesthesia after cleft palate repair. *Anaesthesia* 2004; 59(10):1032.

Somerville NS, Fenlon S, Boorman J, et al. Disruption of cleft palate repair following the use of the laryngeal mask airway. *Anaesthesia* 2004;59(4):401–403.

C.7. What is an Abbe flap? What are its anesthetic implications?

An Abbe flap is a full-thickness pedicle flap taken from the lower lip and swung on its own artery to a position in the upper lip to replace a tissue deficit resulting from any cause, such as surgical excision of malignancy or loss of tissue in a bilateral cleft lip. The lips must remain closed until the flap "takes," and then it can be detached from its blood supply. Usually this operation is performed in children of an older age under local anesthesia, but it occasionally requires general anesthesia if the patient is young. All the problems of a closed mouth, such as the possibility of vomiting and aspiration, are encountered in addition to those associated with preservation of the flap.

Furlow LT Jr. Flaps for cleft lip and palate surgery. *Clin Plast Surg* 1990;17:633–644.

C.8. What is the crucial problem of anesthesia for cleft palate? Enumerate the consequences of failure.

The establishment, maintenance, and protection of the airway comprise the crucial problem of anesthesia for palate surgery. Failure to establish, maintain, and protect the airway results in tachypnea, CO_2 retention, hypoxemia, increased bleeding, hypovolemia, arrhythmia, cardiac arrest, and death. The major cause of cardiac arrest in infants and children is hypoxia. The fear of retinopathy of prematurity (ROP) should not cloud judgment in the operating room.

Cote CJ, Ryan JF, Todres ID, et al. eds. *A practice of anesthesia for infants and children*, 3rd ed. Philadelphia: WB Saunders, 2001:116–117, 212, 225–241.

C.9. What is laryngospasm? How would you make a diagnosis of laryngospasm?

This is defined as glottic closure resulting from a reflex constriction of the laryngeal muscles. It is much more common in pediatric anesthesia than in adults. Incidence is twice that of adults in older children and three times that of adults in younger children. Airway complications are further increased in children with upper respiratory tract infections. In the pediatric patient, the oxygen consumption is greater and so the consequences of laryngospasm in children are more serious. The oxygen consumption is highest in the youngest patients.

Laryngospasm seems to occur during anesthesia for two reasons: first, a lack of inhibition of glottic reflexes because of central nervous system depression and second, increased number of stimuli—such as manipulation of the airway, secretions or blood irritating the cords, and stimulation of visceral nerve endings at an inadequate depth of anesthesia.

Sumner E, Hatch DJ, eds. *Pediatric anesthesia*, 2nd ed. London: Arnold, 2000:205–206.

C.10. How would you manage the patient with laryngospasm?

Laryngospasm may be partial or complete. Partial spasm will be diagnosed by a characteristic stridulous noise and a mismatch between the patient's respiratory effort and the disappointingly small movements of the reservoir bag. Methods of overcoming laryngospasm include applying positive pressure to the airway, deepening anesthesia, and administering muscle relaxants or a bolus of propofol. Recently, it was found that a bolus of propofol works extremely quickly, without the side effects of succinylcholine. The exact mechanism of action of propofol is not clear, but it could be due to increasing the depth of anesthesia or direct effect on the glottis. When there is complete laryngospasm there will be silence with regards to air movement. The application of positive pressure may not be helpful in these circumstances and indeed may make the situation worse by forcing the false cords against the tightly closed true cords. It is much better to relax the cords before the hypoxia is severe. Succinylcholine can be given intramuscular or intravenous.

Sumner E, Hatch DJ, eds. *Pediatric anesthesia*, 2nd ed. London: Arnold, 2000:205–206.

D. Postoperative Management

D.1. What complications of cleft lip and cleft palate surgery may be seen in the recovery room?

Complications include airway obstruction, bleeding, and hypothermia. Airway obstruction is the result of closure of the cleft structures plus some edema secondary to trauma. In case of pushback procedure with or without a pharyngeal flap, the obstruction is due to the new posterior position of the palate and the pharyngeal flap.

Combination of a closed palate, a small mandible pushing the tongue into a small pharynx, edema, blood, and the residual effects of anesthesia make postextubation airway obstruction more likely. There could also be swelling of the tongue due to mouth gag placement during surgery.

Anesthesiologist must be aware of the potential problems such as subglottic edema, flap edema, increased oral secretions, posterior displacement of tongue, mucosal swelling of hypopharynx, overlooked throat pack.

Blood loss is not an anesthetic complication but its replacement is an anesthesiologist's responsibility, as is prevention of aspiration.

Hypothermia delays emergence and produces metabolic acidosis and respiratory and myocardial depression. The most important problem for the anesthesiologist is maintenance of airway.

Motoyama EK, Davis PS, eds. *Smith's anesthesia for infants and children*, 7th ed. St. Louis: Mosby, 2006:733–735.

D.2. How do you protect the airway postoperatively?

Following palatoplasty, the pharynx and nasopharynx are suctioned before extubation. Some anesthesiologists advocate that this be done with the aid of the laryngoscope to ensure removal of any mucus, blood, or clots. If suctioning is done before removing the Dingman gag, the laryngoscope may not be necessary. The infant should be as awake as possible. A long traction suture is placed through the tongue and tied loosely. Traction on the suture stimulates respiration and clears the airway. Neither an oral nor a nasal airway should be inserted unless absolutely necessary; either one could disrupt the sutures and undo all the surgical work. The traction suture is removed when the infant leaves the recovery room.

Following palate surgery, the infant is placed in prone or lateral position with the head dependent, turned to the side, and hyperextended. This position can be achieved with a jack placed under the foot of the crib or by placing a bulky bath blanket under the hips of the infant. Any blood or mucus will accumulate in the dependent cheek or roll out of the mouth.

Following cleft lip surgery, a Logan bow is frequently used to take the tension off the newly sutured lip. The infant can still be placed in the lateral position. Elbow restraints are essential, and they are placed on the infant or the child before leaving the operating room. A high-humidity atmosphere is recommended postoperatively to reduce the incidence of tracheitis, but others have failed to show any correlation between the use of humidity and the incidence of tracheitis.

Aston SJ, Beasley RW, Thorne CHM, eds. *Grabb and Smith's plastic surgery*, 5th ed. Philadelphia: Lippincott-Raven, 1997:247.

Table 50.2 Opioid Analgesics for Pediatric Patients.

DRUGS	DOSAGE	FORM
Fentanyl	1 μg/kg	IV
Morphine	0.05–0.1 mg/kg	IV
Meperidine	1 mg/kg	IV
Codeine	1.5 mg/kg q4h	PO: 15-mg, 30-mg, 60-mg tablets; syrup 15 mg/mL
Oxycodone	0.15 mg/kg	PO: 5-mg tablets; syrup 5 mg/mL

IV, intravenous; PO, by mouth.

Motoyama EK, Davis PS, eds. *Smith's anesthesia for infants and children*, 7th ed. St. Louis: Mosby, 2006:733–735.

D.3. How would you control postoperative pain in patients following a cleft lip and cleft palate repair?

The continuum of pain management continues through to the recovery room, the pediatric intensive care unit, or to an inpatient bed in patients with cleft lip or cleft palate repair. No child should be discharged from recovery room with uncontrolled pain.

Local anesthetic infiltration by surgeon can provide some amount of postoperative pain relief. Infraorbital nerve block can be used for pain control after cleft lip repair. Nasopalatine and palatine nerve block will provide palatal hard and soft tissue anesthesia.

Opioid analgesics that can be used postoperatively are shown in Table 50.2.

Nonopioid analgesics that can be used postoperatively are shown in Table 50.3.

Badgwell JM, ed. *Clinical pediatric anesthesia.* Philadelphia: Lippincott-Raven, 1997:229–235.

Sumner E, Hatch DJ, eds. *Pediatric anesthesia*, 2nd ed. London: Arnold, 2000:272–278.

Table 50.3 Nonopioid Analgesics for Pediatric Patients.

DRUG	DOSAGE	FORMS AVAILABLE
Acetaminophen (Tylenol)	10–15 mg/kg PO maximum 2,600 mg/d	Tablets: 80 mg Syrup: 325 mg/5 mL Suppositories: 120, 325, 650 mg
Ibuprofen (Motrin)	10–20 mg/kg PO q6h	Tablets: 300, 400 mg Syrup: 100 mg/5 mL
Ketorolac (Toradol)	0.5 mg/kg IV to load (maximum dose 30 mg) 0.5 mg/kg q8h intramuscularly or intravenously (limit use to 48 hr)	Parenteral form used intramuscularly/intravenously

IV, intravenous; PO, by mouth.

CHAPTER 51

Congenital Heart Disease with a Cervical Mass in Infancy

MILES DINNER

A 1-WEEK-OLD MALE INFANT

was diagnosed shortly after birth with an interrupted aortic arch (IAA). The workup revealed the child to have a 22q11 deletion syndrome (formerly known as *DiGeorge syndrome*). An enlarging cervical mass was noted and the child was brought to the operating room for exploration.

A. Medical Disease and Differential Diagnosis

1. What is the 22q11 deletion syndrome?
2. What are the associated cardiovascular defects in 22q11 deletion syndrome?
3. What are the endocrinologic consequences of 22q11 deletion syndrome and the attendant manifestations?
4. What are the immunologic findings in DiGeorge syndrome?
5. What is the differential diagnosis of cervical masses in infancy?
6. What is a cystic hygroma? What are the complications? What is the treatment?
7. What is the interrupted aortic arch (IAA) anomaly?
8. What is the pathophysiology of the IAA syndrome?
9. How is ductal patency maintained?
10. What are the side effects of prostaglandin infusion?
11. What is the hyperoxia test?

B. Preoperative Evaluation and Preparation

1. What preoperative studies should be obtained to evaluate the neck mass?
2. How would you categorize the difficult airway in children?
3. What features of the difficult airway can be noted on physical examination?
4. How would you optimize preoperatively the ability to secure the airway in the operating room?
5. What laboratory studies are necessary before surgery?
6. What are the causes of congestive heart failure (CHF) in the infant? How would you assess this infant on your preoperative evaluation for signs of CHF?

7. How would you optimize the preoperative treatment of CHF?
8. How would you premedicate this infant?
9. When is premedication useful in infants and children?
10. Before the planned surgery, the infant is scheduled for a magnetic resonance imaging (MRI) scan. You are asked to ensure that the baby remains immobile for a period of 20 minutes to perform the scan adequately. How would you accomplish this?

C. Intraoperative Management

1. What anesthesia equipment, circuit, and monitors would you use?
2. Describe techniques other than direct laryngoscopy that would be useful for securing the airway in this baby.
3. How would you monitor blood loss in this patient?
4. What anesthetic technique should be used in a patient who may experience severe loss of blood intraoperatively?
5. How would you induce anesthesia in this infant?
6. Would you use nitrous oxide?
7. Intraoperatively, the surgeon must dissect the tumor in the anterior mediastinum and needs to have a quiet surgical field. How would you accomplish this in the infant?

D. Postoperative Management

1. How would you manage this patient postoperatively?

A. Medical Disease and Differential Diagnosis

A.1. What is the 22q11 deletion syndrome?

Formerly known as *DiGeorge syndrome*, this constellation of abnormalities results from an embryogenic disruption in the formation of the third and fourth aortic arches. It occurs in approximately 1 in 4,000 births. The velocardiofacial syndrome (VCFS) with features of facial, palatal, developmental, and cardiac abnormalities is distinct from the DiGeorge syndrome but has the same 22q11 deletion.

The common clinical features are hypocalcemia, immunodeficiency, dysmorphic facial features, palatal and velopharyngeal dysfunction, renal anomalies, and congenital heart disease (CHD). A significant number of patients with tetralogy of Fallot, and interrupted aortic arch (IAA), have a 22q11 deletion.

The DiGeorge anomaly is characterized by thymic and parathyroid aplasia or hypoplasia, cardiovascular defects, and dysmorphic facies. It arises as a consequence of a developmental defect in the embryology of the third and fourth pharyngeal pouches. It is currently thought to be caused by inadequate neural crest migration into the pharyngeal pouches with the subsequent limitation in growth of the derivative structures. The condition arises either from Mendelian disorders, teratogen exposure, or cytogenetic abnormalities. A chromosome 22q11 microdeletion is a constant finding.

Goldmuntz E. DiGeorge syndrome: new insights. *Clin Perinatol* 2005;32:963–978.

A.2. What are the associated cardiovascular defects in 22q11 deletion syndrome?

Congenital heart defects are found in 75% of patients with this syndrome. Approximately 50% of patients with the 22q11 deletion syndrome have an aortic arch anomaly. Most patients with the DiGeorge syndrome have associated anatomic cardiovascular anomalies involving the aortic arch system. Of these, the most common abnormality is an interrupted aortic arch (IAA) seen in approximately half the number of neonates with this condition. Persistent truncus arteriosus is seen in approximately one third and the remainder have tetralogy of Fallot or an isolated ventricular septal defect (VSD). These defects arise during the crucial developmental stages of the truncoconal parts of the heart from the pharyngeal pouch derivatives. Cardiac magnetic resonance imaging (MRIs) are invaluable in defining the aortic arch anatomy in detail

Marino B, Digilo MC, Toscano A, et al. Congenital heart defects in patients with DiGeorge syndrome. *Genet Couns* 1999;10:25.

McElhinney DB, Driscoll DA, Levin ER, et al. Chromosome 22q11 deletion in patients with ventricular septal defect: frequency and associated cardiovascular anomalies. *Pediatrics* 2003;112:472–476.

A.3. What are the endocrinologic consequences of the 22q11 deletion syndrome and the attendant manifestations?

Aplasia of the thymus occurs in approximately 60% of patients with the 22q11 syndrome. These patients fail to make parathyroid hormone, or they are severely deficient in its production. Subsequently, hypocalcemia occurs. Hypocalcemia in the neonate is often difficult to detect clinically, but it can lead to irritability, jitteriness, twitching or frank seizure activity, failure to thrive, tachycardia, and hypotension. Stridor, syncope, and carpopedal spasm may occur. Trousseau's sign (carpopedal spasm elicited by an inflated blood pressure cuff) and Chvostek's sign (twitching of facial muscles after tapping the facial nerve) can be seen. Growth hormone and thyroid hormone deficiency have been reported.

Brauner R, Le Harivel De Gonneville A, Kindermans C, et al. Parathyroid function and growth in 22q11.2 deletion syndrome. *J Pediatr* 2003;142:504–508.

Lynch BJ, Rust RS. Natural history and outcome of neonatal hypocalcemia and hypomagnesemia. *Pediatr Neurol* 1994;11:23.

A.4. What are the immunologic findings in DiGeorge syndrome?

Patients with DiGeorge syndrome demonstrate marked variability in the degree of involvement of the immune system. Total lymphocyte counts, percent of T cells, and T-lymphocyte function ranges from normal to severely depressed. The most consistent abnormality is a decrease in total T cells. Spontaneous resolution of immunodeficiency occurs in some patients, but progressive loss of function can be seen in others. Patients with the partial DiGeorge anomalad can be immunized and generate good antibody responses; therefore, humoral immunity is often intact as is functional cellular immunity.

Markert ML, Alexieff MJ, Li J, et al. Complete DiGeorge syndrome: development of rash, lymphadenopathy, and oligoclonal T cells in 5 cases. *J Allergy Clin Immunol* 2004;113(4): 734–741.

Martin-Matros MA, Perez Duemas BP, et al. Clinical and immunological spectrum of partial DiGeorge syndrome. *J Investig Allergol Clin Immunol* 2000;10:352.

A.5. What is the differential diagnosis of cervical masses in infancy?

Neck masses can originate from a congenital anatomic anomaly, neoplasm, or infection. In the first category are branchial cysts, thyroglossal duct cysts, and failed thymic descent. Branchial cysts arise in the embryo from the thymic stalk or the pharyngeal pouch. They may be present at birth or arise later. They lie beneath the sternomastoid muscle and may bulge out from the anterior border. They can become infected and, thereby, enlarge with pus. When this occurs, the airway or upper esophagus may be compressed. Thyroglossal duct cysts are spherical, midline masses that may extend back to the base of the tongue, and may represent all the thyroid tissue that the baby has. The thymus gland arises high in the neck and must descend in the embryo to the anterior mediastinum. If this caudad movement becomes arrested, the thymus can appear as a soft, compressible mass along the anterior border of the sternocleidomastoid muscle.

Infectious masses can be due to tuberculosis, Kawasaki's disease, Ebstein-Barr (EB) viral infection, Ludwig's angina, and cat-scratch disease. Neoplastic masses in the cervical region can be teratomas, hemangiomas, neurofibromas, lymphomas, goiters, or cystic hygromas. Teratomas are firm, midline masses arising adjacent to the thyroid isthmus. Hemangiomas may be extensive and compress vital structures. Neurofibromas may arise individually, or as a consequence of neurofibromatosis (von Recklinghausen's syndrome), and they can be very large. A goiter represents an enlarged thyroid gland, which may be hypothyroid, hyperthyroid, or euthyroid.

Long AA. *Principles and practice of pediatric infectious diseases*, 2nd ed. Orlando: WB Saunders, 2003:170–171.

Ungkamont V, Yellan RF, Weissman JL. Head and neck space infections in infants and children. *Otolaryngol Head Neck Surg* 1995;11:375.

A.6. What is a cystic hygroma? What are the complications? What is the treatment?

Cystic hygroma is a developmental malformation of the lymphatic system that is found most often in the posterior triangle of the neck and axilla of children. They are divided into suprahyoid and subhyoid masses. They are compressible masses that are most often found in infants younger than 1 year, and they intermittently enlarge. Suprahyoid masses can be extremely difficult to manage because of the obstructive symptoms and feeding difficulties, and they may become infected, producing rapid compromise of breathing.

Complete surgical removal of these masses is often impossible and repeat debulking is sometimes the only treatment. Facial paresis may be a consequence of resection. The mortality of obstructing cystic hygroma diagnosed prenatally exceeds 20% following delivery. Intubation of the neonate during delivery under uninterrupted maternal–fetal circulation has been performed to prevent the fatal consequences of immediate postpartum airway obstruction. Bleomycin has also been used as a sclerosing agent with favorable results.

Burezq H, Williams B, Chitte SA. Management of cystic hygromas: 30 year experience. *J Craniofac Surg* 2006;17(4):815–818.

Descamps P, Jourdain O, Paillet C, et al. Etiology, prognosis and management of nuchal cystic hygroma. *Eur J Obstet Gynecol Reprod Biol* 1997;71:3–10.

A.7. What is the interrupted aortic arch (IAA) anomaly?

IAA is a group of three anatomic abnormalities in which the aorta has a complete atresia at a site somewhere along the arch. If untreated, it is uniformly lethal within 1 week of life as a consequence of closure of the ductus arteriosus. In type A, which accounts for 43%, the aorta is interrupted between the left subclavian artery and the aortic isthmus. Type B, the most common (53%) has the lack of continuity between the left carotid and the left subclavian arteries. The defect in type C (4%) is between the right and left carotid arteries. A ventricular septal defect (VSD) is present in most patients with this anomaly. Approximately 50% of patients with IAA have DiGeorge syndrome. IAA can also coexist with a single ventricle and atrioventricular (AV) canal.

Brown JW, Ruzmetov M, Okada Y, et al. Outcomes in patients with interrupted aortic arch and associated anomalies: a 20-year experience. *Eur J Cardiothorac Surg* 2006;29(5): 666–673.

Goldmunte E, Clark BJ, Mitchell LE. Frequency of 22q11 deletions in patients with conotruncal defects. *J Am Coll Cardiol* 1998;32:492.

A.8. What is the pathophysiology of the interrupted aortic arch (IAA) syndrome?

Because of the discontinuity between the descending aorta and the arch, no blood can flow to the descending aorta unless a patent ductus arteriosus exists. If the ductus is inadequate to provide perfusion to the lower body because of its closure, severe metabolic acidosis, and renal insufficiency develops. With a ventricular septal defect (VSD), most of the cardiac output will be directed into the pulmonary vascular bed (PVB) as the ductus closes. Patients are at risk for a profound low output syndrome. Unless ductal patency can be maintained, death will occur. Symptoms will include tachypnea, lethargy, and poor feeding. Two-dimensional echocardiography is diagnostic.

Chin AJ, Jacobs ML. Morphology of the VSD in two types of interrupted aortic arch. *J Am Soc Echocardiogr* 1996;9:199.

A.9. How is ductal patency maintained?

Ductal patency is maintained by the infusion of prostaglandin E_1 (PGE_1). Both PGE_1 and prostaglandin E_2 (PGE_2) are produced endogenously in the ductus, metabolized in the lungs, and achieve high levels in the fetus relative to adults. Among the endogenous prostaglandins, PGE_2 is the most important. Postnatally, the levels fall associated with increased metabolism resulting from the increase in pulmonary blood flow. An infusion of prostaglandin will delay the natural closure of the ductus and improve systemic arterial oxygenation. In the case of an interrupted aortic arch (IAA), circulation to the lower body is totally dependent on the patency of the ductus, and, therefore, continual infusion of PGE_1 is critical to keep the infant alive. The infusion is titrated at a rate of 0.05 to 0.1 μg/kg/minute. Because of its relatively long half-life, discontinuation of the drip will not acutely cause ductal closure in the event of inadvertent stoppage.

Freed MD, Heymann MA, Lewis AB, et al. Prostaglandin E_1 in infants with ductus arteriosus-dependent congenital heart disease. *Circulation* 1981;64:1889.

Hermes-DeSantis ER, Clyman RI. Patent ductus arteriosus: pathophysiology and management. *J Perinatol* 2006;26(Suppl):14–18.

A.10. What are the side effects of prostaglandin infusion?

Prostaglandin infusion has a variety of side effects ranging from fever to hypotension, seizures, flushing, and edema. Platelet aggregation may be reduced. Apnea is noted in premature infants and those weighing less than 2 kg. Therefore, infants are intubated prophylactically and mechanical ventilation may be necessary in these babies. A separate intravenous line must be used.

Lake CL, Booker PD, eds. *Pediatric cardiac anesthesia*, 4th ed. Philadelphia: Lippincott, Williams & Wilkins 2005:110.

A.11. What is the hyperoxia test?

This test is performed to distinguish pulmonary cause of cyanosis from cardiac ones. In this test, arterial O_2 tension is taken in the right arm representing preductal blood with the patient breathing 100% O_2 for 10 minutes. Supplemental oxygen in patients with pulmonary disease usually significantly augments systemic oxygenation, whereas this is not the case in cyanotic congenital heart defects. Of course in severe pulmonary conditions, there may be a failure to raise the oxygen tension meaningfully but the chest x-ray would be valuable in affirming the diagnosis of lung pathology. Similarly, in some congenital heart lesions with mixing such as truncus arteriosus, the supplemental O_2 decreases pulmonary vascular resistance (PVR) resulting in an increase in oxygen tension but rarely more than 150 mm Hg.

Tingelstad J. Consultation with the specialist: nonrespiratory cyanosis. *Pediatr Rev* 1999;20: 350–352.

B. Preoperative Evaluation and Preparation

B.1. What preoperative studies should be obtained to evaluate the neck mass?

Because of the extremely variable nature, invasiveness, and potential for airway compression, magnetic resonance imaging (MRI) studies and a sonogram should be obtained before surgery. These studies will better define the nature of the cystic hygroma and highlight the region of airway compression. These cysts are known to invade the anterior mediastinum and can, therefore, cause extrinsic distortion of the lower airway anywhere from the cricoid ring to the carina. Cyst fluid can be aspirated under sonography to reduce the size of the mass and potentially relieve compressive symptoms. On rare occasions, there may be ingrowth of the pericardium and displacement of the lung. For suprahyoid masses, radiologic studies will define the scope of laryngeal compression and retropharyngeal involvement, which will obviously affect the ability to intubate the trachea. A flexible neonatal bronchoscopic examination can define extrinsic compressive deformations of the airway.

B.2. How would you categorize the difficult airway in children?

Children with difficult airways can be grouped into four main groups. The first group includes children who have congenital anomalies affecting the airway such as vascular rings, laryngomalacia, micrognathia, and neurofibromatosis. Second would be children with an acute acquired obstruction such as injury or foreign body. The third group includes infectious causes such as retropharyngeal abscess, croup, diphtheria, and peritonsillar abscess. In the last group are those children who prove to be difficult to visualize on intubation and who do not have known congenital abnormalities.

Hall SC. The child with a difficult airway: recognition and management. *ASA annual meeting refresher course lectures*. Park Ridge: American Society of Anesthesiologists, 2006; 412.

B.3. What features of the difficult airway can be noted on physical examination?

Starting at the mouth and working caudally, we can examine a host of physical features that can challenge the clinician. Many anatomic abnormalities can be discerned before direct laryngoscopy. Conditions that result in a constricted oral opening, such as scleroderma, epidermolysis bullosa, burn cicatrization, or congenital microstomia, prevent insertion of the laryngoscope. A small lower jaw and maxillary protrusion often accompany the anterior larynx, making laryngeal inlet exposure during laryngoscopy impossible. This is seen in children with syndromes such as Pierre Robin, Apert's, Crouzon's, Treacher Collins, and many other craniofacial syndromes.

Macroglossia as a consequence of certain metabolic storage diseases, cystic abnormalities, and hamartomatous tumors of the tongue (Goltz syndrome) can make effective laryngoscopy impossible.

Temporomandibular ankylosis, as seen in patients with juvenile rheumatoid arthritis and other rheumatic processes, may prevent mouth opening. A narrow, high-arched palate may suggest a problematic intubation. Neck extension problems may accompany some neuromuscular disorders, trauma, arthritis, or Goldenhar's syndrome.

Berry FA, ed. *Anesthetic management of difficult and routine pediatric patients*. New York: Churchill Livingstone, 1986:167.

Wetmore RF, Muntz HR, McGill TJ. *Pediatric otolaryngology: principles and practical pathways*. New York: Thieme Medical, 2000:775.

B.4. How would you optimize preoperatively the ability to secure the airway in the operating room?

Because of the risk inherent in inducing anesthesia in this infant, plan for a fiberoptic laryngoscopy. The infant bronchoscope is of such small diameter that it does not have a suction port and visualization is especially impaired because of secretions. An antisialagogue is a must to permit proper anatomic recognition through the fiberoptic scope. Glycopyrrolate (0.01 mg/kg) given half an hour before anesthesia will limit secretions without the excessive tachycardia that may occur with atropine. In this infant with cardiac compromise, any unnecessary stress on the heart should be avoided. An appropriate laryngeal mask airway (LMA), in this case a no.1, should be readied as should equipment trays for emergency cricothyrotomy. Adjunctive devices such as a rigid infant bronchoscope with video imaging can be tremendously useful should fiberoptic or classical laryngoscopy prove too difficult. An appropriate-sized rigid scope can serve to visualize the laryngeal inlet and can serve to hold the endotracheal tube as an introducing stylet to facilitate intubation.

American Society of Anesthesiologists Task Force on Management of Difficult Airway. Practice guidelines for management of the difficult airway. *Anesthesiology* 1993;78:597.

DeLeo A. Pediatric upper airway endoscopy. *ORL Head Neck Nurs* 2005;23:29.

B.5. What laboratory studies are necessary before surgery?

Because of the strong association of 22q11 deletion syndrome with hypocalcemia, serum calcium should be measured. In addition, because of the inherent dysphagia with a cystic hygroma, the infant will not have been feeding. To ensure that adequate parenteral nutrition and hydration were provided, serum glucose and sodium levels should be noted. Because of the potential for severe metabolic acidosis secondary to underperfusion of the lower body through the interrupted descending aorta, a serum pH and bicarbonate concentrations must be obtained. A $PaCO_2$ will indicate the adequacy of ventilation in the face of a potentially obstructing mass and a baseline PaO_2 will serve as a guideline to the infant's degree of congestive heart failure (CHF), pulmonary insufficiency, and central shunting.

Because the surgery can be extensive with a significant loss of blood, a baseline complete blood count with hematocrit should be obtained. In addition, the prothrombin time (PT) and partial thromboplastin time (PTT) should be obtained before surgery of this magnitude because of the possibility of baseline immaturity in coagulation factor production and the inherent bleeding potential from the large dissection that will be done. Specific gravity of the urine will suggest the diagnosis of dehydration, although urinary concentrating ability does not mature until the infant is 3 months of age. A chest x-ray film will define the state of the lungs and indicate whether there is tracheal deviation.

B.6. What are the causes of congestive heart failure (CHF) in the infant? How would you assess this infant on your preoperative evaluation for signs of CHF?

The causes of CHF can be divided into five major areas:

- Cardiac rhythm disturbances (heart block and supraventricular tachycardia)
- Volume overload (anemia, sepsis, and ventricular septal defect [VSD])
- Systolic ventricular dysfunction (myocarditis, malnutrition, and dilated cardiomyopathy)
- Pressure overload (aortic stenosis and coarctation)
- Diastolic ventricular dysfunction (pericardial tamponade and restrictive cardiomyopathy)

CHF occurs either in response to an excessive volume or pressure load, or as a consequence of myocardial muscle impairment. Volume overload is due to factors causing a large increase in cardiac output (e.g., large VSD or ductus arteriosus). In these circumstances, there must be a sufficiently large enough left-to-right shunt to cause a severe strain on the heart. In the normal newborn, these lesions do not usually produce heart failure until 1 to 2 months of age because it takes longer than usual for the pulmonary vascular resistance (PVR) to fall. The elevated PVR protects the left ventricle from the stress of overcirculation. This is not true in premature infants who do not manifest the same degree of pulmonary arteriolar constriction. Therefore, they are susceptible to large left-to-right shunts early and show CHF more easily.

Regurgitant valvular lesions can lead to CHF. In complex congenital heart disease (CHD) such as truncus arteriosus or tricuspid atresia with transposition, the additional stress of hypoxemia or univentricular overload may herald the early onset of CHF. Large arteriovenous malformations may occur intracranially and cause CHF. Excessive pressure loads are seen in obstruction to cardiac output from aortic stenosis, aortic coarctation, and aortic interruption. In the immediate newborn period, right-sided CHF is seen with greater frequency because of severe pulmonary hypertension. Pulmonary hypertension has many causes: intrinsic lung parenchymal insufficiency or pathology as in diaphragmatic hernia, meconium aspiration or hyaline membrane disease, chronic hypoxemia, hypervolemia, and polycythemia.

Primary myocardial failure is unusual in the newborn; it occurs with endocardial fibroelastosis, or anomalous coronary circulation. However, the myocardium in the infant is susceptible to depression from metabolic derangements such as hypoglycemia, hypocalcemia, or birth asphyxia. Certainly, severe anemia with the associated decrease in systemic and myocardial oxygen supply forces an increase in myocardial work that can lead to CHF.

Infants are different from adults in their manifestations of CHF. Because of possible coexisting lung disease in many premature infants, signs of cardiac dilation may be absent because of the decreased systemic venous return from elevated intrathoracic pressure. Although immature, the carotid baroreceptors still initiate an increase in sympathetic outflow in response to reduced perfusion. The increased α-adrenergic stimulation impairs blood flow to the systemic arteriolar beds, resulting in cold, underperfused extremities, and diminished splanchnic perfusion. Fatigue, loss of appetite, and failure to thrive follow. Tachycardia from β-receptor stimulation occurs. Generalized sweating results from sympathetic cholinergic fiber stimulation. Extracellular water increases because of decreased renal excretion of sodium from a lowered glomerular filtration rate. Peripheral pitting edema is much less common in infants than older children and adults. The venous system in infants is extremely distensible and, therefore, raised right atrial pressure may not show large jugular venous engorgement. The most prominent manifestation of CHF in the infant is tachypnea. As pulmonary venous pressure is elevated from left ventricular failure, the lung compliance falls because of the augmented interstitial fluid. Breathing becomes rapid and shallow and the resultant increase in oxygen requirement causes a cyclic dependency to maintain both tachycardia and tachypnea. Subcostal retractions are seen because of the increase in respiratory effort.

Infants have a greater lymphatic drainage capacity than adults and, therefore, can clear interstitial accumulations more readily. Therefore, rales are not as frequent a manifestation of CHF in infants as in adults. The bronchial mucosa may be swollen because of the engorgement of the bronchial venous system. The lumen of the airway is narrowed, resulting in wheezing that is often seen in infantile CHF. Hepatomegaly is a cardinal sign of right ventricular failure in infants.

Behrman RE, Kliegman RM, Jensen HB, eds. *Nelson textbook of pediatrics*, 17th ed. Philadelphia: WB Saunders, 2004:1582–1586.

B.7.   How would you optimize the preoperative treatment of congestive heart failure (CHF)?

The typical manifestations of CHF in infants, namely tachycardia, tachypnea, subcostal retractions, and rhonchi, are also cardinal signs of pulmonary infection in this age-group. They are hard to distinguish. Often, they coexist and treatment must address both conditions. In this patient, the structural abnormality, the interrupted aortic arch (IAA), needs surgical correction; however, correction must be deferred until the neck mass is resected. In this infant, the CHF is caused by pressure overload from the IAA and the hypocalcemia is due to parathyroid hormone insufficiency. Calcium must be normalized by intravenous infusion. If glucose is low as would be expected in undernourishment, glycogen depletion from the stress of illness, or increased utilization, it should be supplemented by slow intravenous administration. Myocardial work is compromised by the presence of metabolic acidosis, which occurs as a consequence of the increased lactic acid production during anaerobic metabolism. The pH should be normalized with sodium bicarbonate. Because of the attendant sodium load, tromethamine (THAM) may be an alternative.

Myocardial function should be optimized with digitalis in most infants with CHF. However, in the IAA syndrome, there may be decreased renal perfusion. As a consequence, the digoxin levels may rise and toxicity may occur. Catecholamine (e.g., dopamine or dobutamine) should be infused to boost contractility. Pulmonary symptoms should be treated with antibiotics and positive pressure ventilation with oxygen carefully adjusted to arterial blood gas measurements. Intubation and mechanical ventilation may be necessary in many infants with CHF. Diuresis with furosemide will promote restoration of pulmonary compliance by decreasing lung water in conjunction with fluid restriction

Balaguru D, Artman M, Auslander M. Management of heart failure in children. *Curr Probl Pediatr* 2000;30:5–30.

Kambam J. *Cardiac anesthesia for infants and children*. St. Louis: Mosby, 1994:117–118.

B.8. How would you premedicate this infant?

Infants younger than 2 years do not routinely require preoperative anxiolytics or narcotics. Premedicants such as midazolam have no place in this scenario. An infant with a compromised airway and circulation cannot tolerate any degree of respiratory depression. Therefore, no sedatives should be given at all. As mentioned, because a fiberoptic intubation is planned, glycopyrrolate should be given for its antisecretory activity.

B.9. When is premedication useful in infants and children?

Patients with dynamically responsive cyanotic congenital heart disease (CHD) (e.g., tetralogy of Fallot) benefit from premedication before coming to the operating room. In these children, the inherent anxiety of transfer to unfamiliar surroundings, change in temperature, and parental separation may trigger infundibular spasm and reduce pulmonary blood flow thereby leading to a blue spell. Acute hypoxemia is not an optimal state in which to initiate an anesthetic induction. Therefore, sedation with oral midazolam or rectal pentobarbital is useful to allay the child's impending state of panic and reduce the risk of provoking a hypoxemic spell. Of course premedication is always helpful to make the overall experience of the operating room less imposing to the young child. In producing variable degrees of amnesia and reducing the potential for physical agitation, premedication offers a real benefit for those children who are intensely frightened of the operating room.

B.10. Before the planned surgery, the infant is scheduled for a magnetic resonance imaging (MRI) scan. You are asked to ensure that the baby remains immobile for a period of 20 minutes to perform the scan adequately. How would you accomplish this?

Given this infant's extreme risk of complete airway occlusion, there is no safe method other than endotracheal intubation, which will guarantee immobility on demand and ensure a patent airway. The routine method of sedating an infant for a MRI scan, namely chloral hydrate, oral midazolam, should not be used here. Establishing an airway emergently in this infant may be impossible even with a laryngeal mask airway (LMA), and, therefore, sedation can proceed only after the trachea is intubated. Section C.2 shows details on fiberoptic intubation in infants. Of course if the infant has demonstrated a postprandial sleep cycle and can take PO fluids, it may be well worth the attempt at an MRI by using nothing at all except the inherent feeling of wellness from a full stomach.

C. Intraoperative Management

C.1. What anesthesia equipment, circuit, and monitors would you use?

Because of the depressed cellular immunity, this patient is susceptible to infection. Therefore, particularly strict attention must be paid to sterile technique during line placement and instrumentation of the patient. The anesthesiologist must wear gowns and gloves to protect the infant. Sterility of the disposable circle system, mask, endotracheal tube, fiberoptic bronchoscope, and laryngoscope should be ensured. Routine monitors for all surgery on infants include a precordial stethoscope, rectal temperature probe, electrocardiogram, blood pressure, capnograph, and spirometer. Multiple pulse oximeters should be used to offer flexibility in the event of dysfunction. In this case, the interrupted aortic arch (IAA) prevents saturation data from the lower body and left arm. End-tidal expired gas concentrations should be recorded of anesthetic gases, nitrogen, and oxygen. Accurate capnography in small infants may be hampered by side-arm gas sampling resulting from the relatively high gas flows relative to the expired gas flow from the infant.

In this procedure, an arterial line should be inserted in the right radial site, because the aortic arch interruption will not allow for pressure determination on the left side. Because of the potential for significant blood loss, a central line should be placed either through the femoral vein or subclavian vein if possible. Keep in mind the distorted anatomy and the potential for difficulty in cannulation with the subclavian site. If the subclavian site is elected, before proceeding with this complicated case, a chest x-ray film should be obtained to document the absence of a pneumothorax and good line position. The femoral vein may be chosen as an alternate site. Catheter length is important, and it is easy in an infant to inadvertently place the central line across the tricuspid valve, in which case misleading values of the right ventricular pressure would be obtained. Remember in setting the transducer height that small variances in the alignment of the zero point can result in relatively large central venous pressure (CVP) value discrepancies. Therefore, the transducer should be placed with great care to approximate the right atrial level and be moved accordingly as the table height is changed.

The neuromuscular junction should be monitored with electrodes on a readily visible extremity.

Schreiber C, Eicken A, Vogt M, et al. Repair of interrupted aortic arch: results after more than 20 years. *Ann Thorac Cardiovasc Surg* 2000;70:1896.

C.2. Describe techniques other than direct laryngoscopy that would be useful for securing the airway in this baby.

It is highly unlikely that laryngeal visualization could be accomplished in this infant with direct visualization. On the computed tomography (CT) scan the mass is seen to elevate the tongue and deviate the larynx to the side. Because of this limitation in direct visualization, the clinician should be well acquainted with alternative methods before emergently instituting them. The following techniques can be useful when laryngoscopy cannot be accomplished easily.

Retrograde cricothyroid wire

Although technically difficult, the retrograde cricothyroid wire technique can be successful, and it is best for oral intubation. A guidewire is inserted through a large-gauge needle used to puncture the cricothyroid membrane and is threaded cephalad to be retrieved out through the mouth. This wire then serves as a stent for placement of the endotracheal tube.

Blind nasal intubation

Although very successful in the adult patient, the blind nasal intubation technique can be difficult in infants or small children. Certainly, performing an awake, sedated intubation in this manner mandates giving adequate topical anesthesia to a less than cooperative infant. In addition, the smaller endotracheal tubes used in pediatrics are far more compliant than others, especially when warmed with nasopharyngeal respiratory gases, which makes it difficult to maintain the anterior curve on the tube to enter the larynx. Styletted nasal tubes should be used only by clinicians skilled in this specialized technique.

Nasal intubation with laryngoscope and magill forceps

If the larynx cannot be visualized by laryngoscopy, an anesthetized spontaneously breathing nasal intubation with laryngoscopic assistance can be carried out in some patients. In this case, great care is taken to ensure that the patient maintains adequate ventilatory exchange during the inhalational induction. Halothane or sevoflurane is initiated, because either is less pungent and more easily tolerated than the other halogenated ethers, and the anesthesiologist should be ever mindful that total obstruction is possible in some of these infants because of their airway abnormalities. If spontaneous breathing can be maintained, the intubation should be attempted after a surgical plane of anesthesia is achieved. The laryngoscope is used to visualize the epiglottis, and the tip of the endotracheal tube is aligned with the help of a Magill forceps and then advanced in the subepiglottic region. Capnographic monitoring during this maneuver can help verify the direction of the endotracheal tube tip.

Fiberoptic intubation

Fiberoptic intubation is most successful when carried out as the initial maneuver. It may be impossible to use after several unsuccessful attempts with conventional laryngoscopy because the upper airway is then often traumatized and hypersecretory. Fiberoptic technology is still not widely disseminated to the infant population. Most centers do not have the smallest, "ultrathin" bronchoscopes, which come as small as 2.2 mm in diameter. Limitations are found in their use because of the size and lack of a suction port. The endotracheal tube requires good lubrication before threading over the scope.

In older patients, three specialized fiberoptic methods are available that may be useful in intubating difficult infants. First, the clinician can pass a guidewire through the suction port of the larger instrument to serve as a stylet for the endotracheal tube. Second, the scope can be used to visualize and guide a nasal endotracheal tube inserted into the opposite nostril. Finally, a 4.5-mm tube can be placed at the laryngeal orifice to be used as a stent for inserting a small guidewire, which can in turn be used to place a smaller endotracheal tube.

Another useful technique is the application of a laryngeal mask airway (LMA) as a guide for the endotracheal tube.

Transtracheal jet ventilation can be used when applicable. In this technique, a 16-gauge intravenous catheter is placed through the cricothyroid membrane and jet ventilation with 100% oxygen is provided. A second intravenous catheter is placed through the cricothyroid membrane and a guidewire (0.021 in. diameter J-tip) is introduced with cephalad angulation. Jet ventilation continues as the guidewire is threaded through the nose and connected to the working part of a fiberoptic scope. The scope is then advanced through the laryngeal inlet and a tube is now threaded over the scope when the guidewire is removed. Sedation can be provided with a remifentanil drip (0.1 to 0.2 μg/k/minute). Of course, safety is the foremost consideration in any technique for inserting an artificial airway. If the anesthesiologist cannot perform a cricothyrotomy, personnel capable of an accurate and quick cricothyrotomy should be on hand in case of a life-threatening loss of airway control. In an emergency cricothyrotomy, a longitudinal incision is made in the skin and fascia above the cricothyroid membrane, after which the cricothyroid membrane is punctured and entered with a small endotracheal tube. Another technique uses a 14-gauge angiocatheter, which is inserted into the cricothyroid membrane. Intratracheal location is verified by the loss of resistance with an attached syringe and the aspiration of air. The catheter is attached to a 3-mL syringe (without plunger), which is then connected to the Y-piece of the anesthesia circuit by an adapter from a 7.0-mm internal diameter (ID) endotracheal tube.

Auden SM. Additional techniques for managing the difficult pediatric airway. *Anesth Analg* 2000;90:878.

Hall SC. The child with a difficult airway, recognition and management. *ASA annual meeting refresher course lectures*. Park Ridge: American Society of Anesthesiologists, 2006; 412.

C.3. How would you monitor blood loss in this patient?

In many of these procedures, blood loss can be significant, often exceeding the patient's calculated blood volume. Often, much of this loss is not measurable because blood is either lost under the drapes or irrigated away. Certainly meticulous weighing of sponges and observation of suction canisters are important, but blood loss can be continuous from the time of skin incision and be seemingly relentless for an inexperienced clinician. Absolute changes in the central venous pressure (CVP) are a relative guide to the volume in the central compartment, but no one isolated value correlates with a known blood volume. A falling CVP in association with a downward trend in blood pressure during periods of surgical intervention known to produce significant bleeding should be treated aggressively with brisk transfusion. If blood loss is allowed to continue, severe hypotension can rapidly ensue.

C.4. What anesthetic technique should be used in a patient who may experience severe loss of blood intraoperatively?

Blood loss should be replaced milliliter for milliliter to prevent falling behind in volume. It is wise to choose an anesthetic technique that produces a relatively stable blood pressure throughout the surgery, so that new downward trends in blood pressure can be attributable to blood loss and not to pharmacologic action. For instance, if a steady level of isoflurane and nitrous oxide anesthesia is given at 1.25 minimal alveolar concentration (MAC) with a resultant mean arterial pressure (MAP) 15% lower than awake, further dips in MAP during surgical intervention can be taken as intravascular volume depletion secondary to bleeding and replaced accordingly. This interpretation would be obscured if there were frequent anesthetic interventions associated with MAP changes (e.g., intermittent narcotization, pancuronium bolusing, droperidol or other α-blockade administration) or up and down titration of hypotension-inducing agents.

An important clue to the blood volume loss of the patient is the blood pressure at a MAC of anesthesia. If a stable pressure is established at a given MAC of inhalational agent, a lower than expected blood pressure at this MAC is almost always indicative of hypovolemia and, therefore, calls for fluid or blood replacement. Frequent hematocrit determinations drawn with the arterial blood gases are important. Remember it is most unusual in an otherwise healthy infant to produce hypotension with intravascular overload.

C.5. How would you induce anesthesia in this infant?

After securing the airway with fiberoptic intubation or awake tracheotomy and checking for bilateral breath sounds, narcotic titration with fentanyl should be given in repeated doses of 2 μg per kg. Remember, this infant may behave sensitively to any anesthetic agent because of the cardiovascular anomalies. Therefore, beat-to-beat monitoring of the blood pressure with an arterial line, as the fentanyl is administered, ensures inadvertent drops in pressure. Because this patient is not going to be extubated, fentanyl can be given in the range of 50 μg per kg or higher to allow for dense analgesia. Because this will be a long procedure, pancuronium can be administered slowly to mitigate against the tachycardia. If tolerated, small concentrations of approximately 0.5% to 4% desflurane or sevoflurane 0.25% to 1.5% can be administered to synergize with the narcotic and assist with amnesia and unconsciousness. The prostaglandin infusion should be maintained throughout the entire surgery.

C.6. Would you use nitrous oxide?

The adult experience suggests that nitrous oxide may have augmenting effects on pulmonary vascular resistance (PVR), especially in patients with already elevated PVR. It may also decrease cardiac index in conjunction with narcotics. In infants, however, little consequence is seen in administering nitrous oxide unless there is a profound myocardial disturbance. It is avoided by some anesthesiologists because of the potential of expanding intravascular air bubbles.

Kambam J. *Cardiac anesthesia for infants and children*. St. Louis: Mosby, 1994:130.

C.7. **Intraoperatively, the surgeon must dissect the tumor in the anterior mediastinum and needs to have a quiet surgical field. How would you accomplish this in the infant?**

Double-lumen tubes are not used in the neonatal age-group because of the exceedingly small lumen and the technical difficulties of securing both lungs. Instead, a single-lumen endotracheal tube can be advanced to the right or left main stem bronchus to allow for one-lung ventilation. This may be fraught with consequences in this infant with interrupted aortic arch (IAA), but it can still be attempted. Keep in mind that hypoxic pulmonary vasoconstriction may not occur readily in the neonate and excessive shunting may be in evidence. In addition, having an infant on one-lung ventilation may lead to an elevated $PaCO_2$ from pulmonary insufficiency. During thoracotomies in infants for pulmonary banding or Blalock-Taussig shunts it is not uncommon to see extremely elevated $PaCO_2$ values from retraction of the lung, especially the right side, which has almost 60% of the total lung surface area.

Lew YS. Pediatric one lung anesthesia by selective bronchial intubation. *Singapore Med J* 2000;51:398.

McGahren ED, Kern DA, Rodgers BM. Anesthetic technique for pediatric thoracoscopy. *Ann Thorac Surg* 1995;60:927–930.

D. Postoperative Management

D.1. How would you manage this patient postoperatively?

This procedure, involving extensive dissection around the neck and upper thorax, warrants that the patient stay intubated or have a tracheostomy placed. A tremendous amount of upper airway and neck edema will surely ensue, which would make extubation life threatening. To facilitate care over the next day, the patient should be well narcotized and paralyzed if necessary to coordinate effective mechanical ventilation. Artificial ventilation and oxygen supplementation should be titrated to arterial blood gas determinations. In addition, the prostaglandin drip must be continued to ensure ductal patency. Generous narcotic supplementation will ensure that the pulmonary vascular resistance (PVR) stays in a state of relative quiescence. If an endotracheal tube is maintained, fiberoptic visualization of the laryngeal inlet after 24 hours will enable a more educated decision on the suitability of extubation. Anatomic airway factors aside, the interrupted aortic arch (IAA) and associated congestive heart failure (CHF) will make extubation of this baby more challenging. Assuming all other factors are under control, the following ventilatory parameters should be met before extubation: normal arterial blood gases with satisfactory oxygenation of 28% O_2, spontaneous tidal volume greater than 5 mL per kg, and inspiratory force greater than 12 cm H_2O. One should always be on the alert for airway obstruction and ready to intercede with reintubation or tracheostomy if prompt deterioration occurs.

SECTION XI

Miscellaneous

CHAPTER 52

Myasthenia Gravis

Cephas P. Swamidoss • Cynthia A. Lien

A 25-YEAR-OLD FEMALE

G3P2 with a 24-week intrauterine fetal demise, presents for dilation and evacuation, in the setting of a history of increasing diplopia and dysphagia. She has a known history of myasthenia gravis (MG), diagnosed 10 years previously and underwent a thymectomy for thymoma during the first trimester of her second pregnancy 2 years ago. Since then she has been in remission and on no medications. Her vital signs were as follows: pulse rate, 60 beats per minute; blood pressure, 150/80 mm Hg; and respiratory rate 20 breaths per minute. Her arterial oxygen saturation was 98% on room air. She is 155 cm tall and weighs 65 kg.

A. Medical Disease and Differential Diagnosis

1. What is the clinical course of myasthenia gravis (MG)?
2. What is the cause of MG and how is the diagnosis made?
3. What should be included in this patient's differential diagnosis?
4. What is the difference between MG and Lambert–Eaton syndrome?
5. What is the incidence of MG?
6. Describe the clinical classification of MG.
7. How is myasthenia classified in the pediatric age-group?
8. What treatment regimens are available for patients with MG?
9. What are the electrical and humoral events that take place during normal neuromuscular transmission? How are these altered in patients with MG?
10. What is the role of surgery in the treatment of MG?

    11. What is the effect of pregnancy on the course of MG?

    12. What is the effect of MG on pregnancy?

B. Preoperative Evaluation and Preparation

    1. How should you assess these patients preoperatively?

    2. What preoperative laboratory data are required?

    3. Should this patient be premedicated?

C. Intraoperative Management

    1. How should this patient be monitored intraoperatively?

    2. What anesthetic regimen would you choose for this patient?

    3. Can neuromuscular blocking agents be used in patients with MG?

D. Postoperative Management

    1. Would you anticipate that this patient will require prolonged postoperative ventilatory support?

    2. How should this patient's postoperative pain be treated?

    3. This patient was extubated in the operating room without difficulty, and 40 minutes later, she complained of feeling weak and unable to breathe. Why?

A. Medical Disease and Differential Diagnosis

A.1. What is the clinical course of myasthenia gravis (MG)?

The hallmark of the symptoms of MG is fluctuating muscle weakness that worsens with exertion and improves after a period of rest. Patients with MG are strongest after resting and therefore feel energized immediately after waking from sleep. Their weakness worsens as the day progresses.

The presentation of MG is usually insidious, occurring over months to years. The initial symptoms are commonly ocular and consist of ptosis and diplopia. Ptosis can be unilateral or bilateral, symmetric or asymmetric, and typically alternates between eyes. The diplopia is usually intermittent. Extraocular muscle involvement can vary from single muscle paresis to total ophthalmoplegia. Muscle fatigue can result in nystagmus. The pupil is usually spared in MG. Ocular symptoms usually progress to more generalized ones in 80% to 85% of patients with MG. The prognosis is better if the symptoms remain confined to those associated with ocular disturbances for more than 2 years.

Involvement of the bulbar muscles produces dysarthria, dysphagia, and difficulty chewing. Weight loss may occur as a result of decreased oral intake and nasal regurgitation, and a nasal twang in the voice can indicate palatal weakness. Involvement of the facial muscles, particularly the elevators of the angles of the mouth (levator labii superioris and levator anguli oris), results in the characteristic myasthenia "snarl."

Although limb muscle weakness occurs in only 15% to 20% of myasthenics, it can manifest as the inability to do simple everyday tasks like pulling, reaching, or lifting. Proximal muscles are more commonly involved than distal muscles. Rarely, weakness of the neck extensor muscles (rectus capitis posterior major, rectus capitis posterior minor) may occur. Patients affected in this way are unable to keep their heads upright.

Respiratory muscle weakness presents as dyspnea, particularly in the supine position. If the diaphragm is involved, there is a decreased forcefulness of cough and an inability to project the voice.

Many factors may exacerbate the symptoms of MG. These include physical and emotional stress, infection, exposure to bright sunlight, and particularly in case of predominantly ocular symptoms, any increase in temperature associated with infection and hyperthyroidism. Medications including quinidine, procainamide, aminoglycosides, penicillamine, and calcium channel blockers can also worsen symptoms. An infection treated with an offending antibiotic may be enough to exacerbate severe respiratory compromise and may necessitate mechanical ventilation.

Drachman DB. Myasthenia gravis. *N Engl J Med* 1994;330(25):1797–1810.

Grob D, Arsura EL, Brunner NG, et al. Part IV. Diagnosis and treatment of myasthenia gravis. The course of myasthenia gravis and therapies affecting outcome. *Ann N Y Acad Sci* 1987;505:472–499.

Kennedy FS, Moersch FP. Myasthenia gravis—a clinical review of 87 cases observed between 1915 and the early part of 1932. *Can Med Assoc J* 1937;37:216.

Rakel RE, ed. *Conn's current therapy*, Philadelphia: WB Saunders, 2006:1134–1141.

Scherer K, Bedlack RS, Simel DL. Does this patient have Myasthenia Gravis? *JAMA* 2005; 293:1906–1914.

Schwendimann RN, Burton E, Minagar A. Management of Myasthenia Gravis. *Am J Ther* 2005;12:262–268.

Snell R, Katz J, eds. *Clinical anatomy for anesthesiologists*. Norwalk: Appleton & Lange, 1998.

Yanoff M, Duker JS, eds. *Ophthalmology*. London: Mosby, 1999.

A.2. What is the cause of myasthenia gravis (MG) and how is the diagnosis made?

MG is an autoimmune disease caused by an antibody to and T-cell attack on the nicotinic acetylcholine receptor (AChR) of the motor endplate. Antibodies are detected in 80% of patients with generalized weakness and 50% of patients with ocular disease only. T-cell stimulation is theorized to occur after sensitization within the thymus to a protein similar or identical to the embryonic AChR. In approximately 85% of MG patients, pathologic alterations of the thymus gland are found—10% tumors, 75% hyperplasia of lymphoid follicles within the medullas of the thymus. Blockade of AChR results in abnormally decreased membrane moor endplate potential owing to a reduction in the number of functional AChR at the neuromuscular junction. This lowered neurotransmission at the neuromuscular junction (NMJ) causes the clinical symptoms of muscle fatigue in myasthenic patients.

A diagnosis of MG is usually made by history and clinical examination. It is then confirmed with several diagnostic tests. Clinical tests of stress endurance include monitoring a prolonged upward gaze, holding an outstretched hand in abduction, and determination of vital capacity. These tests provide objective information about fatigability. Other tests that confirm a diagnosis of MG include the following:

- Electrophysiologic tests
- Pharmacologic tests
- Serologic tests

Electrophysiologic testing involves stimulation of a peripheral nerve with a supramaximal stimulus of 2 Hz four times over 2 seconds in a train-of-four pattern. A decrease in twitch response of more than 10%, when the fourth response is compared with the first, is diagnostic of MG. Myasthenic patients also show less posttetanic facilitation than their healthy counterparts. The sensitivity of this stimulation test is 50% to 70%.

Single-fiber electromyography is a more sensitive electrophysiologic test. It evaluates the time interval between two muscle fiber action potentials in the same motor unit. As the same nerve innervates both muscle fibers, the time variation between their action potentials, known as *jitter*, is a manifestation of neuromuscular junction transmission. In patients with MG, the "jitter" is increased. The sensitivity of this test is higher than 90%, although it is not specific for MG.

Pharmacologic testing involves the administration of the anticholinesterase edrophonium. For this diagnostic test, the patient is fatigued with a task that can be easily assessed, such as slurred speech or vital capacity, and then is given edrophonium. Patients with myasthenia show dramatic improvement within 2 minutes with intravenous administration of 2.5 to 9 mg of edrophonium.

The curare test may also be used to demonstrate that impulse transmission can be markedly reduced at the neuromuscular junction in patients with MG. This test is rarely used because of the morbidity and mortality that is associated with it. Because myasthenic patients can have up to 70% of their AChRs blocked, their margin of safety of impulse transmission is greatly reduced. Therefore, they can develop profound neuromuscular blockade and respiratory arrest after the administration of even a small dose of parenteral D-tubocurarine. The test can be done as either a regional or a systemic test. With the regional test, a tourniquet is applied to each arm and inflated. In one arm, a dose of 0.2 mg of D-tubocurarine in 20 mL of normal saline is given intravenously. In the other arm, 20 mL of normal saline is given intravenously. Muscle function is tested before, during, and every few minutes with electromyography until 16 minutes after administration of D-tubocurarine on normal saline. In MG, a marked decrease in muscle response is seen in the arm receiving the D-tubocurarine. During a systemic test, 0.5- to 1-mg increments of D-tubocurarine to a maximum dose of 0.03 mg per kg are administered intravenously to exacerbate myasthenic symptoms. In myasthenic patients, marked weakness is seen with less than 10% of the normal curarizing dose. Muscle function is assessed 5 minutes after each dose. The test is stopped as soon as exacerbation of weakness is observed. Because the regional curare test examines only select muscle groups, the systemic curare test is more sensitive than the regional one. The regional curare test, however, is the safer of the tests because of decreased potential for respiratory compromise. It is based on the principle that patients with MG can have even as many as 70% of their AChR blocked and can therefore develop severe weakness even if as little as 10% of the normal dose of D-tubocurarine is administered intravenously. A test is positive when any exacerbation of weakness is observed.

Serologic testing involves identification of AChR antibodies. Antibodies to AChR are a serum marker for the diagnosis of MG and are detected in 80% of patients with generalized MG and 50% of patients with only ocular symptoms. Antibodies to striated muscle are also detected in patients with MG, and their presence in high titers is usually associated with thymoma. Although the antibody level does not correlate with the severity of the disease or the patient's prognosis, the antibody tests are still more specific than any other test for MG.

Other tests that have helped to corroborate the diagnosis of myasthenia include nystagraphy and stapedius reflexometry.

Davies DW, Steward DJ. Myasthenia gravis in children and anesthetic management for thymectomy. *Can Anaesth Soc J* 1973;20:253.

Drachman DB. Myasthenia gravis. *N Engl J Med* 1994;330(25):1797–1810.

Foldes FF, Klonymus DH, Maisel W, et al. A new curare test for the diagnosis of myasthenia gravis. *JAMA* 1968;203:649.

Goetz CJ, Pappert EJ, eds. *Textbook of clinical neurology*. Philadelphia: WB Saunders, 2003: 1024–1026.

Rakel RE, ed. *Conn's current therapy*. Philadelphia: WB Saunders, 2006:1134–1141.

Samaha FJ. Electrodiagnostic studies in neuromuscular disease. *N Engl J Med* 1971; 285:1244.

Schwendimann RN, Burton E, Minagar A. Management of myasthenia gravis. *Am J Ther* 2005;12:262–268.

Viets HR, ed. *Myasthenia gravis*. Springfield: Charles C Thomas Publisher, 1961:411–434.

Yanoff M, Duker JS, eds. *Ophthalmology*. London: Mosby, 1999.

A.3. What should be included in this patient's differential diagnosis?

Although this patient's diagnosis is consistent with myasthenia gravis (MG), a number of disorders mimic MG and should be included in the initial differential diagnosis. Botulism and Lambert–Eaton syndrome (LES) can cause both weakness and ophthalmoplegia. Botulism affects cranial nerves early. A change in pupillary light response and an increased response on repetitive nerve stimulation can differentiate it from MG.

LES causes a distal muscle weakness that improves after exercise. It is associated with oat cell tumor of the lung in 50% of cases. It is also associated with a defect in the autonomic nervous system, which manifests as dry mouth, orthostatic hypotension, and urinary retention.

Thyrotoxicosis can present with generalized weakness and abnormal thyroid function. Neurasthenic patients characteristically have weakness, which disappears when individual muscle groups are tested. Progressive external ophthalmoplegia, restricted cardiomyopathies, muscular dystrophies, brain tumors, amyotrophic lateral sclerosis, myasthenic polymyopathy with hypersensitivity to neostigmine, and drugs like D-penicillamine, D-tubocurarine, aminoglycosides, quinine, procainamide, and calcium channel blockers can also cause myasthenia-like symptoms.

Drachman DB. Myasthenia gravis. *N Engl J Med* 1994;330(25):1797–1810.

Eisenkraft JB. Anesthetic considerations in patients with myasthenia gravis. *Cardiothorac Vasc Anesth Update* 1990;1:1.

Fleisher LA, ed. *Anesthesia and uncommon disease*, 5th ed. Philadelphia: WB Saunders, 2006: 320–322.

Goetz CJ, Pappert EJ, eds. *Textbook of clinical neurology*. Philadelphia: WB Saunders, 2003: 1024–1026.

Green DM. Weakness in the ICU. *Neurologist* 2005;11(6):338–347.

A.4. What is the difference between myasthenia gravis (MG) and Lambert–Eaton syndrome (LES)?

Characteristics of MG and LES are presented in Table 52.1.

Book WJ, Abel M, Eisencraft JB. Anesthesia and neuromuscular diseases. *Anesthesiol Clin North America* 1996;14:3.

Fleisher AL, ed. *Anesthesia and uncommon disease*, 5th ed. Philadelphia: WB Saunders, 2006:320–322.

Healy T, Cohen P, eds. *Wylie and Churchill-Davidson's a practice of anesthesia*, 6th ed. London: Edward Arnold, 1995:143.

Yanoff M, Duker JS, eds. *Ophthalmology*. London: Mosby, 1999.

A.5. What is the incidence of myasthenia gravis (MG)?

MG is relatively rare and has an incidence of approximately 1 of 30,000 people. One and a half times more women than men develop the disease. Men who have this disease have a higher

Table 52.1 Characteristics of Myasthenia Gravis and Lambert—Eaton Syndrome.

CHARACTERISTICS	MYASTHENIA GRAVIS	LAMBERT—EATON SYNDROME
Gender most commonly affected	Female	Male
Age at onset	20–40 y	50–70 y
Presenting signs	Weakness of ocular, bulbar, and facial muscles; fatigue with activity; muscle pains are uncommon; normal tendon reflexes	Weakness and fatigability of the proximal muscles; transient increase in strength on activity; muscle pains common; tendon reflexes reduced or absent
Pathology	Thymus gland most often abnormal, with 15%–20% of patients having thymoma	Small cell carcinoma of the lung usually present
Electromyographic response	Voltage decrement to repeated stimulation, with a good response to anticholinesterases	Voltage increment to repeated stimulation and a poor response to anticholinesterases
Response to muscle relaxants	Increased sensitivity to nondepolarizing neuromuscular blocking agents and a variable response to succinylcholine	Sensitivity to nondepolarizing neuromuscular blocking agents and a normal to increased response to succinylcholine
Presence of antibodies	Antibodies to the acetylcholine receptor present	Antibodies to calcium channel—associated protein synaptogamin are present
Abnormality of autonomic nervous system	Not present	Present
Treatment	Steroids, plasmapheresis, azathioprine, and thymectomy	Steroids, plasmapheresis, azathioprine, and 3,4-diaminopyridine

incidence of thymoma. There is a bimodal pattern of incidence that varies with the gender of the patient. Among women, it occurs within the second and third decade of life—the primary reproductive decades of life. In men, it is seen more commonly in the fifth and sixth decade. Patients younger than 16 years account for less than 10% of cases of myasthenia.

Patients with MG tend to have a higher incidence of autoimmune diseases. These include autoimmune thyroid disease, rheumatoid arthritis, systemic lupus erythematosus, and diabetes mellitus, suggesting a partial genetic predisposition for myasthenia.

Drachman DB. Myasthenia gravis. *N Engl J Med* 1994;330(25):1797–1810.

Ferrero S, Pretta S, Nicoletti A, et al. Myasthenia gravis: management issues during pregnancy. *Eur J Obstet Gynecol Reprod Biol* 2005;121:129–138.

Goetz CJ, Pappert EJ, eds. *Textbook of clinical neurology*. Philadelphia: WB Saunders, 2003:1024–1026.

Gurjar M, Jagia M. Successful management of pregnancy-aggravated maystenic crisis after complete remission of the disease. *Aust N Z J Obstet Gynaecol* 2005;45:331–332.

Rakel RE, ed. *Conn's current therapy*. 54th ed. Philadelphia: WB Saunders, 2006:1134–1141.

Sthoeger Z, Nieman A, Elbirt D, et al. High prevalence of systemic lupus erythematosus in 8 myasthenia gravis patients: a clinical and serological study. *Am J Med Sci* 2006; 331(1):4–9.

A.6. Describe the clinical classification of myasthenia gravis (MG)?

The clinical classification by Osserman and Genkins groups patients with myasthenia on the basis of their symptomatology are as follows:

- *Class 1:* ocular symptoms only
- *Class 1A:* ocular symptoms with electromyographic evidence of peripheral muscle involvement
- *Class 2A:* mild generalized symptoms
- *Class 2B:* more severe and rapidly progressive symptoms
- *Class 3:* acute and presenting in weeks to months with severe bulbar symptoms
- *Class 4:* late in the course of disease with severe bulbar symptoms and marked generalized weakness

Andreoli T, Carpenter C, Griggs R, et al. eds. *Cecil essentials of medicine*, 6th ed. Philadelphia: WB Saunders, 2004:921–922.

Osserman KE, Genkins G. Studies in myasthenia gravis: review of a 20 year experience in over 1200 patients. *Mt Sinai J Med* 1971;38:497–538.

A.7. How is myasthenia classified in the pediatric age-group?

In pediatric patients, myasthenia gravis (MG) is classified as neonatal transient, neonatal persistent, or juvenile.

Neonatal transient myasthenia is the classification assigned to infants born to mothers with MG. Most of these infants have circulating acetylcholine receptor (AChR) antibodies that have been passively transferred from mother to baby. The antibodies are transient. Only 12% of these infants have myasthenic symptoms. The symptoms with which they present include a feeble cry, poor feeding effort, respiratory difficulty, general or facial weakness, and ptosis. These symptoms last an average 18 days.

Neonatal persistent MG is very rare. Onset is at 2 to 3 months of age. These patients have no detectable antibodies to AChR.

Juvenile myasthenia is very similar to the MG with which adults present.

Andreoli T, Carpenter C, Griggs R, et al. eds. *Cecil essentials of medicine*, 6th ed. Philadelphia: WB Saunders, 2004:921–922.

Ferrero S, Pretta S, Nicoletti A, et al. Myasthenia gravis: management issues during pregnancy. *Eur J Obstet Gynecol Reprod Biol* 2005;121:129–138.

Fleisher L, ed. *Anesthesia and uncommon disease*, 5th ed. Philadelphia: WB Saunders, 2006: 320–322.

A.8. What treatment regimens are available for patients with myasthenia gravis (MG)?

A number of different forms of treatment for MG are available. They can be broadly classified as follows:

- Pharmacologic
- Surgical
- Plasmapheresis

Pharmacologic treatment with anticholinesterases and immunosuppressants is aimed at manipulation of acetylcholine (ACh) levels and the immune system.

Anticholinesterases have been used as the initial therapy for symptoms of MG since 1934. By inhibiting the enzymatic metabolism of ACh, these drugs prolong the duration of ACh at the postsynaptic membrane of the neuromuscular junction. Because patient response to these agents is variable, varying from patient to patient and within a patient over the course of a day, patient education and their involvement in their medical care are required for optimal use of anticholinesterases.

The most common side effects of anticholinesterases are due to the muscarinic effects of ACh and include bradycardia, gastrointestinal cramps, bronchospasm, and an increase in oral and respiratory secretions. The increase in oral secretions can be problematic, particularly for those patients who have bulbar symptoms with already compromised swallowing and in those patients with respiratory muscle involvement.

Excessive therapy with anticholinergic agents can result in a cholinergic crisis. This will manifest as profound weakness and is due to excess ACh at the neuromuscular junction, which produces a persistent depolarization of the muscle fiber. These symptoms may start a vicious cycle of treating the weakness as myasthenic weakness with anticholinesterases, and further exacerbating the cholinergic crisis. In distinguishing clinically between the two, pupillary size may offer some clue to the etiology of the weakness. Hypercarbia in myasthenic patients causes sympathetic stimulation and dilation of pupils. In a cholinergic crisis, ACh causes constriction of the pupils. It should be noted that patients with primarily ocular symptoms often respond poorly to cholinesterase inhibitors.

Pyridostigmine (Mestinon) is the most commonly used drug for treatment of myasthenia because it causes fewer muscarinic side effects than neostigmine. Its onset of action is 15 to 30 minutes after oral administration, the peak effect is within 1 to 2 hours, and the duration of action is 3 to 4 hours. It is available in three doses 10, 30, and 60 mg, and the typical daily doses range between 30 and 120 mg divided into three to six doses over 24 hours. A long-acting, 180 mg slow-release preparation can be used overnight. A long-acting form of pyridostigmine is also available. Unless the patient has profound morning weakness or nocturnal respiratory distress, it is not commonly used. There is an increased risk of overdosage with the long-acting form of this anticholinesterase.

Edrophonium (Tensilon), 5 to 10 mg intravenously, has been used between regularly scheduled doses of anticholinesterases to determine whether the patient is receiving too much or too little medication.

Anticholinesterases do not have an impact on the primary pathology, which is immunologic, and are rarely used alone.

Corticosteroids are used to complement, rather than replace, anticholinesterase therapy. Seventy percent to 80% of patients have complete remission of their disease within weeks to months of treatment with adequate doses of prednisone. Clinical improvement after initiation of steroid therapy is slow and may take weeks. Starting with small doses of steroids can minimize an initial deterioration in a patient's condition. Corticosteroids exert their immunosuppressive effects at many levels of the immune system. They reduce the amount of acetylcholine receptor (AChR) antibodies and diminish the anti-AChR reactivity of the peripheral blood lymphocytes.

A number of different dosing regimens have been suggested. An alternate-day regimen lessens the degree of side effects. The common side effects seen with high-dose steroids are generalized immunosuppression, infection, cataracts, myopathy, osteoporosis, diabetes, and peptic ulcer disease. Most patients require approximately 40 to 60 mg of prednisone per day.

Cytotoxic drugs like azathioprine and cyclosporine are used in conjunction with steroids and anticholinesterases to reduce the total dose of steroids. Azathioprine acts predominantly on T cells. It is useful in patients in whom corticosteroids are contraindicated. Although it is well tolerated by patients, many months to a year may be required to see its maximal therapeutic effect. Cyclosporine inhibits the production of interleukin-2 by helper T cells. Its efficacy is similar to that of azathioprine, but its maximal therapeutic effect is seen within 1 to 2 months. Its side effects include nephrotoxicity and hypertension.

Adrenocorticotropic hormone (ACTH; corticotropin) has been used in the treatment of severe MG and is often useful when previous therapy with steroids has failed. This form of treatment, however, is being replaced with plasmapheresis.

Plasmapheresis has been found to effectively remove circulating antibodies and is typically reserved to stabilize patients undergoing myasthenic crisis or preoperatively in patients with severe weakness. After therapy, a patient's condition improves rapidly, but the effects are short lived. When plasmapheresis is used in conjunction with pooled intravenous immunoglobulins in doses of 400 mg/kg/day for 5 days on alternate days, there is a rapid improvement, which can last for several weeks.

With an increasing understanding of the immune system, there are some novel potential treatments for MG such as targeting the specific T and B cells, and a nonselective removal of helper T cells, which are responsible for producing the antibodies to AChR. Induction of tolerance to self-antigens by their ingestion has been shown to prevent MG in animal models.

Andreoli T, Carpenter C, Griggs R, et al. eds. *Cecil's essentials of medicine*, 6th ed. Philadelphia: WB Saunders, 2004:921–922.

Atlee JL, ed. *Complications in anesthesia*. 2nd ed. Philadelphia: WB Saunders, 2006:484–486.

Goetz CJ, Pappert EJ, eds. *Textbook of clinical neurology*. Philadelphia: WB Saunders, 2003: 1024–1026.

Rakel RE, ed. *Conn's current therapy*. 54th ed. Philadelphia: WB Saunders, 2006:1134–1141.

Schwendimann RN, Burton E, Minagar A. Management of myasthenia gravis. *Am J Ther* 2005;12:262–268.

Tackenber B, Hemmer B, Oertel WH, et al. Immunosuppresive treatment of ocular myasthenia gravis. *BioDrugs* 2001;15:369–378.

A.9. What are the electrical and humoral events that take place during normal transmission? How are these altered in patients with myasthenia gravis (MG)?

Normally, the charge inside a cell is negative relative to the extracellular environment. The potential difference is 70 to 90 mV. During an action potential, the ionic fluxes that occur cause the interior of the cell to become positive by approximately 40 mV. The nerve action potentials cause the release of quanta of acetylcholine (ACh) from nerve terminals. The ACh crosses the synaptic cleft and attaches to the receptor site on the sarcolemma, causing depolarization. This depolarization is called the *endplate potential*. If the threshold for excitation is exceeded by the summation of many endplate potentials, an action potential invades the muscle cell membrane and spreads along its surface, causing muscle contraction.

In MG, the amount of ACh released from the presynaptic sites is normal or even increased. There are, however, histologic alterations found at the neuromuscular junctions to which alterations in transmission of impulses can be attributed. These consist of a widening of the synaptic space at the neuromuscular junction and a degeneration of the junctional folds. Most importantly, the concentration of the functional acetylcholine receptors (AChRs) on the postsynaptic membrane is often reduced by more than 70%. Antibodies to the AChR are responsible for this decrement. These AChR antibodies are directed against various epitopes on the postsynaptic receptor. They decrease the amount of functioning ACh by a number of mechanisms, which include direct blockade, complement-mediated lysis, and increased receptor-degradation rate.

Atlee JL, eds. *Complications in anesthesia*, 2nd ed. Philadelphia: WB Saunders, 2006:484–486.

Drachman DB. Myasthenia gravis. *N Engl J Med* 1994;330(25):1797–1810.

Harvard CWH, Scadding GK. Myasthenia gravis: pathogenesis and current concepts in management. *Drugs* 1983;26:174.

A.10. What is the role of surgery in the treatment of myasthenia gravis (MG)?

Although the efficacy of thymectomy is based on retrospective data, it is a widly accepted therapy for myasthenic patients, particularly those with thymoma and early-onset generalized MG. Thymectomy has been used as a treatment for MG since 1939, when the removal of a cyst from the thymus of a patient with MG, described by Blalock, resulted in remission of the disease. The goal of thymectomy as a treatment for MG is to induce remission, permitting a reduction in the immunosuppressive medication. Fifty percent to 80% of patients undergoing thymectomy will demonstrate clinical improvement after thymectomy, and 21% to 38% of patients will go into clinical remission (compared with the 13% of medically treated patients).

The exact role of the thymus in the pathogenesis of MG is likely the T-cell–mediated production of acetylcholine receptor (AChR) antibodies. Thymic epithelial cells and AChRs share similar epitopes. A thymoma is seen in 15% of patients with MG, and thymic hyperplasia is seen in 80% of patients. The clinical improvement frequently seen after thymectomy is further evidence of an association of the thymus in MG. Therefore, thymectomy may be a logical choice for most patients with MG. It is not, however, done in prepubertal children and in those patients with predominantly ocular symptoms. Furthermore, if the symptoms of the disease respond to medical management, patients are not candidates for surgery.

The surgical approach to thymectomy for MG can be either transsternal or transcervical. The transsternal approach allows for better surgical exposure and a more thorough excision. The main advantage of the transcervical approach is that it is minimally invasive. Mortality with this approach is close to 0% versus 9% with the transsternal approach. Furthermore, the incidence of requiring postoperative ventilation is 10% after transcervical thymectomy, compared with 50% after the transsternal approach. The rates of remission with the two surgical approaches are comparable. Thymectomy may induce perioperative myasthenic crises. Optimizing medical therapy preoperatively may minimize this risk.

Atlee JL, ed. *Complications in anesthesia*, 2nd ed. Philadelphia: WB Saunders, 2006:484–486.

Buchinghan JM, Howard FM, Bernaty PE, et al. The value of thymectomy in myasthenia gravis. *Ann Surg* 1976;184:453.

Drachman DB. Myasthenia gravis. *N Engl J Med* 1994;330(25):1797–1810.

Kissel JT, Franklin GM. Treatment of myasthenia gravis. *Neurology* 2000;55(1):3–4.

Papasetas AE, Genkins G, Kornfield P, et al. Comparison of the results of transcervical and transsternal thymectomy in myasthenia gravis. *Ann N Y Acad Sci* 1981;377:766.

Schwendimann RN, Burton E, Minagar A. Management of myasthenia gravis. *Am J Ther* 2005;12:262–268.

A.11. What is the effect of pregnancy on the course of myasthenia gravis (MG)?

The course of MG during pregnancy is unpredictable at best—control at the beginning of the pregnancy does not predict exacerbations or remissions. Worsening symptoms occur in one third of pregnant women. Although these exacerbations can occur at any time, they are more likely to occur during the first trimester *or* the first month postpartum. Twenty percent to 40% of women experience an improvement in symptoms during the second and third trimesters. Peurperal complications, such as infections, seem to increase the risk of exacerbation of MG symptoms and should be promptly recognized and treated. MG mother mortality risk is inversely correlated to the duration of the disease, the highest risk being in the first year and the minimal risk 7 years after the onset of the disease.

Batocchi AP, Majolini L, Evoli A, et al. Course and treatment of myasthenia gravis during pregnancy. *Neurology* 1999;52:447–452.

Djelmis J, Sostarko M, Mayer D, et al. Myasthenia gravis in pregnancy: report on 69 cases. *Eur J Obstet Gynecol Reprod Biol* 2002;104:21–25.

Ellison J, Thompson AJ, Walker ID, et al. Thrombocytopenia and leucopenia precipitated by pregnancy in a woman with myasthenia gravis. *Br J Obstet Gynaecol* 2000;107: 1052–1054.

Ferraro S, Pretta S, Noicoletti A, et al. Myasthenia gravis: management issues during pregnancy. *Eur J Obstet Gynecol Reprod Biol* 2005;121:129–138.

Hoff JM, Dalveit AK, Gilhus NE. Myasthenia gravis: consequences for pregnancy, delivery and the newborn. *Neurology* 2003;61:1362–1366.

Scott JS. Immunologicla disease in pregnancy. *Prog Allergy* 1977;23:321–366.

A.12. What is the effect of myasthenia gravis (MG) on pregnancy?

The effect of MG on pregnancy is relatively small. There is no increase in the rate of spontaneous abortion or low birth weight children. Although MG does not increase the rate of premature birth, there is some suggestion of an increased rate of premature rupture of membranes among women with MG. This etiology is unclear, but some think it is related to the course of medications taken by the mother with MG. There are case reports of preeclampsia in the setting of MG but no study has proved an increased risk due to MG. It is recommended that pregnant patients with MG have frequent follow-up with their obstetricians, every 2 weeks in the first and second trimesters and every week in the third trimester. Ultrasound evaluations are necessary during pregnancy to detect signs of fetal akinesia. Fetal monitoring for signs of hypoxia is also very important during myasthenic exacerbations.

Ellison J, Thompson AJ, Walker ID, et al. Thrombocytopenia and leucopenia precipitated by pregnancy in a woman with myasthenia gravis. *Br J Obstet Gynaecol* 2000;107: 1052–1054.

Ferraro S, Pretta S, Noicoletti A, et al. Myasthenia gravis: management issues during pregnancy. *Eur J Obstet Gynecol Reprod Biol* 2005;121:129–138.

Hoff JM, Dalveit AK, Gilhus NE. Myasthenia gravis: consequences for pregnancy, delivery and the newborn. *Neurology* 2003;61:1362–1366.

B. Preoperative Evaluation and Preparation

B.1. How should you assess these patients preoperatively?

The preoperative interview should be used to identify factors that may be predictive of the need for postoperative ventilation. These factors include duration and severity of the disease and the total daily requirement of pyridostigmine or other medications. This information can guide the anesthesiologist in formulating the anesthetic plan, choosing preoperative medications and appropriately arranging for postoperative care. Myasthenic patients are usually knowledgeable about their medication; they are often able to adjust their own regimen on the basis of their clinical status.

Whether to alter a patient's anticholinesterase medication preoperatively is still much debated. In patients with mild symptoms, discontinuation of anticholinesterase would seem to be preferable as its continued use can complicate anesthesia by rendering patients more susceptible to vagal arrhythmias. Furthermore, anticholinesterase inhibits plasma cholinesterase and acetylcholinesterase. Because of this, the metabolism of ester local anesthetics, succinylcholine, and mivacurium may be slowed. Certainly, patients who are dependent on their medication should continue it. In this case, however, the anesthesiologist needs to be aware that postoperative requirements may be markedly reduced. Whether the patient is taking or has taken steroids in the past year should also be determined.

Because other autoimmune diseases occur with increased frequency in myasthenic patients and can have their own anesthetic implications, evidence of hypothyroidism, pernicious anemia, systemic lupus erythematosus, and rheumatoid arthritis should be sought.

Book WJ, Abel M, Eisencraft JB. Anesthesia and neuromuscular diseases. *Anesthesiol Clin North America* 1996;14:3.

Fleisher L, ed. *Anesthesia and uncommon disease*, 5th ed. Philadelphia: WB Saunders, 2006: 320–322.

Stoelting RK, Dierdorf SF, eds. *Anesthesia and coexisting disease*, 4th ed. New York: Churchill Livingstone, 2002:522–527.

B.2. What preoperative laboratory data are required?

The need for laboratory studies should be tailored to the patient's history. In addition to routine preoperative laboratory data, myasthenic patients should have electrolyte abnormalities ruled out, particularly hypokalemia, which can exacerbate weakness. Because many of these patients are on steroids, blood glucose levels should be determined. Cyclosporine blood levels should be obtained to adjust dosing and avoid toxic levels. Blood counts and hepatic and renal function should also be checked.

If the patient will require a general anesthetic for their surgical procedure, a preoperative arterial blood gas analysis and pulmonary function tests would serve as baseline for extubation, particularly if it is anticipated that the patient will be mechanically ventilated postoperatively. By definition, patients with thymomas have an anterior mediastinal mass that should be evaluated for tracheal compression and deviation. This may affect the ease of endotracheal intubation. Myasthenic patients can have intrathoracic airway or vascular obstruction on anesthetic induction. Flow–volume loops preoperatively can indicate whether the obstruction is intrathoracic or extrathoracic.

B.3. Should this patient be premedicated?

A preoperative visit should include explanation of the anesthetic procedure and the possibility of postoperative mechanical ventilation. Often, these measures serve to allay anxiety and decrease the need for preoperative sedation. Medications that cause respiratory depression should be avoided. Glycopyrrolate can be given to reduce the increased secretions resulting from treatment with anticholinesterases. Stress-dose steroids should be given in the perioperative period for patients who are taking steroids preoperatively.

Barash PG, Cullen BF, Stoelting RK, eds. *Clinical anesthesia*, 5th ed. Philadelphia: Lippincott Williams & Wilkins, 2006:507–509.

Stoelting RK, Dierdorf SF, eds. *Anesthesia and coexisting disease*, 4th ed. New York: Churchill Livingstone, 2002:522–527.

C. Intraoperative Management

C.1. How should this patient be monitored intraoperatively?

These patients should be monitored with an electrocardiogram, blood pressure cuff, pulse oximeter, esophageal temperature, and end-tidal capnography. Depending on the nature of the procedure and the severity of the patient's myasthenia, an arterial line may be warranted to monitor arterial blood gases during the processes of weaning from mechanical ventilation and extubation of the trachea.

A nerve stimulator should be used to monitor muscle strength even if muscle relaxants are not used intraoperatively. Inhalational anesthetics have been shown to cause depression of the twitch response in the absence of a muscle relaxant in patients with myasthenia gravis (MG). They are extremely sensitive to the neuromuscular junction (NMJ)—depressing properties of volatile anesthetics.

Wahlin A, Havermark KG. Enflurane (Ethrane) anesthesia on patients with myasthenia gravis. *Acta Anaesthesiol Belg* 1974;2:215.

C.2. What anesthetic regimen would you choose for this patient?

There are a number of options for anesthetizing this patient ranging from a general endotracheal tube anesthetic to a *Proseal* LMA to regional anesthesia and even monitored anesthesia care. The decision as to what is right for this patient in this situation depends on weighing the risks of pregnancy induced aspiration with the anesthetic risks associated with myasthenia gravis (MG), particularly in the postoperative period. The most conservative anesthesia providers would place the risks of aspiration above those of MG and proceed with a general endotracheal anesthetic. Others would weigh the aspiration risks with those of the difficult airway in a pregnant woman *or* those of postoperative complications due to MG and plan for a regional or monitored care anesthetic. There is no correct answer. Whatever the chosen course, the anesthetic regimen for this patient should be planned to provide the least and briefest interference with ventilatory and neuromuscular function.

In the setting of a general anesthetic, the patient should be preoxygenated before induction of anesthesia with agents like thiopental, propofol, or etomidate. Opioids should be used cautiously because these patients are very sensitive to their respiratory depressant effects. Ventilation with 100% oxygen should be assisted and then controlled as necessary. Once an adequate airway is established, a volatile anesthetic can be added to the oxygen. Muscle relaxants are rarely required for laryngoscopy and intubation, if the patient is deeply enough anesthetized. Four percent topical lidocaine may be sprayed to vocal cords before intubation. Ventilation should be controlled to ensure adequate gas exchange and anesthesia should be maintained with oxygen, nitrous oxide, and a volatile anesthetic with or without a continuous infusion of a short-acting intravenous anesthetic. Desflurane and an intermediate-acting muscle relaxant have been reported as an effective combination. Dexmetetomidine or propofol may be considered for total intravenous anesthesia (TIVA)-based techniques. Remifentanil, with its short duration of action, may be an appropriate choice of opioid in these patients. As surgery is completed, the anesthesia is tapered to allow for prompt emergence. The patient should not be extubated until awake and responsive, strong, and able to generate a negative inspiratory force of at least -30 cm H_2O. Additionally, the patient should be able to maintain normal oxygenation and normocapnia before extubation of his trachea.

If a regional anesthetic is chosen, either an epidural or a spinal anesthetic, depending on the dermatomal level achieved, preservation of the thoracic muscles may be desirable in preserving the greatest amount of ventilatory function.

Ferrero S, Pretta S, Nicoletti A, et al. Myasthenia gravis: management issues during pregnancy. *Eur J Obstet Gynecol Reprod Biol* 2005;121:129–138.

Fleisher L, ed. *Anesthesia and uncommon disease*, 5th ed. Philadelphia: WB Saunders, 2006: 320–322.

Gurjar M, Jagia M. Successful management of pregnancy-aggravated maystenic crisis after complete remission of the disease. *Aust N Z J Obstet Gynaecol* 2005;45:331–332.

Stoelting RK, Dierdorf SF, eds. *Anesthesia and coexisting disease*, 4th ed. New York: Churchill Livingstone, 2002:522–527.

C.3. Can neuromuscular blocking agents be used in patients with myasthenia gravis (MG)?

The myasthenic patient's response to muscle relaxants is altered because of the inherent disease process and because of treatment with anticholinesterase agents. The depolarizing muscle relaxant succinylcholine has been used to facilitate endotracheal intubation. However, myasthenic patients have a variable response to succinylcholine, which depends on their medical treatment. In patients not receiving anticholinesterases, the decreased number of functional receptors makes the endplates "resistant" to the effects of succinylcholine. The dose therefore needs to be increased to reliably facilitate intubation. In patients treated with anticholinesterases, plasma cholinesterase activity is decreased. Therefore, more succinylcholine reaches the motor endplate. As succinylcholine metabolism is decreased in these patients, the neuromuscular block can be prolonged from 4 to 87 minutes. Formation of a phase II block has been reported to occur after a single intubating dose of 0.5 mg per kg of succinylcholine. Although the use of succinylcholine is not contraindicated in patients with MG, some clinicians prefer not to use it because of the risk of prolonged neuromuscular block.

In contrast to what is seen after the administration of succinylcholine, the response of the patient with MG to nondepolarizing drugs is extremely predictable. They are exquisitely sensitive to the nondepolarizing drugs and frequently demonstrate a profound weakness after administration of a precurarizing dose of muscle relaxant. This sensitivity is due to the fact that the number of acetylcholine receptor (AChR) is decreased by up to 70% in these patients. The number of available receptors is just sufficient to produce endplate potentials that are above the threshold required for neuromuscular transmission and muscle contraction. This reduced receptor concentration reduces the dose of relaxant required for muscle relaxation. Blockade of 70% of receptors, or an effective decrease in the number of receptors by this same amount, will cause a fade in the mechanomyographic response to a train-of-four stimuli in patients without MG.

Despite this increased sensitivity to nondepolarizing muscle relaxants, they can be safely used in patients with MG. Markedly decreased doses, however, should be used. Pancuronium has been reported to cause 95% neuromuscular blockade with only one fourth of the usual dose used for maintenance of neuromuscular block (0.005–0.01 mg/kg). The intermediate-acting muscle relaxants may be more suitable for patients with MG because of their shorter duration of action. Doses ranging from 10% to 50% of those required in patients without myasthenia were used, and prompt extubation was accomplished after either spontaneous recovery or antagonism of the residual neuromuscular block. Because of the metabolism of mivacurium by plasma cholinesterase, it may not be well suited for patients with MG.

Barash PG, Cullen BF, Stoelting RK, eds. *Clinical anesthesia*, 5th ed. Philadelphia: Lippincott Williams & Wilkins, 2006:507–509.

Blitt CD, Wright WA, Peat J. Pancuronium and the patient with myasthenia gravis. *Anesthesiology* 1975;42:624.

Buzello W, Noeldge G, Krieg N, et al. Vecuronium for muscle relaxation in patients with myasthenia gravis. *Anesthesiology* 1986;64:507.

Fleisher L, ed. *Anesthesia and uncommon disease*, 5th ed. Philadelphia: WB Saunders, 2006: 320–322.

Foldes FF, McNall PG. Myasthenia gravis: a guide for anesthesiologists. *Anesthesiology* 1962;23:837.

Lake CL. Curare sensitivity in steroid related myasthenia gravis: a case report. *Anesth Analg* 1978;57:132.

Nilsson E, Meretoja OA. Vecuronium dose response and maintenance requirements in patients with myasthenia gravis. *Anesthesiology* 1990;73:28.

Vacanti CA, Ali HH, Schweiss JF, et al. The response of myasthenia gravis to atracurium. *Anesthesiology* 1985;62:692.

D. Postoperative Management

D.1. Would you anticipate that this patient will require prolonged postoperative ventilatory support?

A number of predictive criteria for the need for prolonged postoperative ventilatory support have been proposed. Leventhal, Orkin, and Hirsch assigned a scoring system to four factors as follows:

Duration of more than 6 years: 12 points
History of chronic obstructive pulmonary disease: 10 points
Pyridostigmine, more than 750 mg per day: 8 points
Vital capacity less than 2.9 L: 4 points

Patients scoring less than 10 points in their series could be extubated immediately after surgery; those scoring more than 12 points required postoperative ventilatory support. This system of predicting whether a patient will require prolonged intubation and ventilation is not universally applicable. Patients undergoing transsternal thymectomy require postoperative ventilation more frequently than those undergoing transcervical thymectomy, perhaps because the less invasive procedure has less of an effect on respiratory function.

Similarly, myasthenic patients undergoing an upper abdominal operation are more likely to require postoperative ventilation than patients undergoing a more peripheral procedure. Obviously, each patient must be considered individually when assessing the need for postoperative ventilatory support.

Barash PG, Cullen BF, Stoelting RK, eds. *Clinical anesthesia*, 5th ed. Philadelphia: Lippincott Williams & Wilkins, 2006:507–509.

Eisencraft JB, Papasetas AE, Kahn CH, et al. Predicting the need for postoperative mechanical ventilation in myasthenia gravis. *Anesthesiology* 1986;65:79.

Eisencraft JB, Papasetas AE, Posner JN, et al. Prediction of ventilatory failure following transcervical thymectomy in myasthenia gravis. *Ann N Y Acad Sci* 1987;505: 888.

Grant RP, Jenkins LC. Prediction of the need for postoperative mechanical ventilation in myasthenia gravis. A dose response study. *Anesthesiology* 1988;69:760.

Leventhal SR, Orkin FK, Hirsch RA. Prediction of the need for post operative ventilation in myasthenia gravis. *Anesthesiology* 1980;53:26.

Stoelting RK, Dierdorf SF, eds. *Anesthesia and coexisting disease*, 4th ed. New York: Churchill Livingstone, 2002:522–527.

D.2. How should this patient's postoperative pain be treated?

The patient's postoperative analgesic regimen should be designed to avoid any respiratory compromise. Because these patients are exquisitely sensitive to the respiratory depressant effects of parenteral narcotics, these should be used sparingly. Epidural administration of opioids is an alternative to parenteral administration. They may provide better pain relief with smaller doses of medication and therefore cause less ventilatory depression.

Barash PG, Cullen BF, Stoelting RK, eds. *Clinical anesthesia*, 5th ed. Philadelphia: Lippincott Williams & Wilkins, 2006:507–509.

Smith CA. Postoperative management after thymectomy. *Br Med J* 1975;1:309.

D.3. This patient was extubated in the operating room without difficulty, and 40 minutes later, she complained of feeling weak and unable to breathe. Why?

The anesthesiologist needs to determine whether this exacerbation of weakness is due to a cholinergic crisis or a myasthenic crisis. During myasthenic crisis, patients have a decreased response to anticholinesterases. A cholinergic crisis is caused by an overdose of anticholinesterases. Either can be suspected in the immediate postoperative period, when the stress of surgery can cause an exacerbation of myasthenic weakness and when anticholinergic requirements may be altered. In either case, increased muscle weakness may require ventilatory support.

With either myasthenic or cholinergic crisis, increases in muscle weakness, salivation, and sweating occur. It has been recommended that the two crises be differentiated from each other on the basis of the patient's response to an intravenously administered dose of 10 mg of edrophonium. The patient in a myasthenic crisis should show some improvement in muscle strength. The patient in cholinergic crisis will show either no increase in muscle strength or a worsening of respiratory distress.

Fleisher L, ed. *Anesthesia and uncommon disease*, 5th ed. Philadelphia: WB Saunders, 2006: 320–322.

CHAPTER 53

Malignant Hyperthermia

HENRY ROSENBERG • VINOD MALHOTRA • DANA LYNN GURVITCH

A 7-YEAR-OLD BOY

with kyphoscoliosis was scheduled for ambulatory surgery for repair of strabismus under general anesthesia. Previous anesthetic history included an uneventful sevoflurane and nitrous oxide anesthesia for bilateral myringotomy. However, the mother was very nervous because a first cousin of the boy had died under anesthesia in Wisconsin the previous year.

A. Medical Disease and Differential Diagnosis

1. What was the problem of concern in this case?
2. What is malignant hyperthermia (MH)?
3. What are the clinical features of a susceptible patient?
4. Does the history of previous uneventful sevoflurane anesthesia reasonably exclude the patient's susceptibility to MH?
5. What are the clinical features of the syndrome?
6. What are the laboratory findings during an acute crisis of MH?
7. What is the incidence of this syndrome?
8. What is the mode of inheritance of the disease?
9. What genetic disorder results in MH susceptibility?
10. What is the pathophysiology of the syndrome?
11. What laboratory tests can further substantiate the susceptibility of the patient to MH?
12. What is neuroleptic malignant syndrome (NMS)?

B. Preoperative Evaluation and Preparation

1. How would you prepare this patient for anesthesia and surgery?
2. Is dantrolene prophylaxis indicated?
3. What laboratory tests would you obtain before surgery?
4. Is outpatient surgery appropriate for this patient?
5. In anticipation of general anesthesia, what preparations would you make?

C. Intraoperative Management

1. What anesthetic techniques and agents would you employ?
2. What anesthetic agents are contraindicated?
3. If the surgeon wants to use local anesthesia for a procedure, what agents will you recommend?
4. What is the significance of masseter muscle spasm occurring after succinylcholine administration?

5. Twenty minutes into the procedure, the patient developed increasing tachycardia with ventricular premature beats and mottled skin. What emergency measures would you take?

6. What modalities would you monitor closely during management of the crisis?

D. Postoperative Management

1. What complications may follow this syndrome?

2. What would be your follow-up in this case?

3. What would you advise the patient and the family?

A. Medical Disease and Differential Diagnosis

A.1. What was the problem of concern in this case?

The patient was a 7-year-old boy with kyphoscoliosis and strabismus and a history of an anesthetic-related death in the family in Wisconsin. Therefore, in addition to the respiratory problems associated with kyphoscoliosis, he presented a likelihood of susceptibility to malignant hyperthermia (MH) syndrome. The supporting factors for strong suspicion were the family history, kyphoscoliosis and the geographic location. There is a high density of MH susceptible families in the state of Wisconsin.

Gronert GA, Pessah IN, Muldoon S, et al. Malignant hyperthermia. In: Miller RD, ed. *Miller's Anesthesia*. 6th ed. New York: Elsevier Science Churchill Livingstone, 2005:1169–1190.

Strazis KP, Fox AW. Malignant hyperthermia: a review of published cases. *Anesth Analg* 1993;77(2):297–304.

Wedel DJ. Malignant hyperthermia and neuromuscular disease. *Neuromuscul Disord* 1992;2(3):157–164.

A.2. What is malignant hyperthermia (MH)?

MH, first described by Denborough and Lovell in 1960, is a clinical syndrome of a markedly accelerated metabolic state characterized by elevated core temperature, tachycardia, tachypnea, hypercarbia, rigidity, acidosis, and hyperkalemia. Death is likely if untreated. In almost every instance, the clinical syndrome occurs in a susceptible patient when a "triggering" anesthetic agent is employed. However, not all signs appear in all cases. In rare situations an MH crisis has appeared in humans in the absence of anesthetic drugs.

Denborough MA, Lovell RRH. Anesthetic deaths in a family. *Lancet* 1960;2:45.

Rosenberg H, Brandom BW, Sambuughin NK, et al. Malignant hyperthermia and other pharmacogenetic disorders. In: Barash P, Cullen B, Stoelting R, eds. *Clinical anesthesia*, 5th ed. Philadelphia: Lippincott Williams & Wilkins, 2006:529–556.

A.3. What are the clinical features of a susceptible patient?

A family history, if present, particularly in a first-degree relative, is a strong indicator of malignant hyperthermia (MH) susceptibility. Nonspecific signs such a kyphoscoliosis have been linked to MH but without firm scientific evidence. There are however a few myopathic disorders that are known to be associated with MH susceptibility. They include central core disease, King-Denborough

Table 53.1 ASSOCIATED MUSCULOSKELETAL DISORDERS IN PATIENTS SUSCEPTIBLE TO MALIGNANT HYPERTHERMIA.

Kyphoscoliosis
Hypotonia
Exercise-induced rhabdomyolysis
Central core disease
Multiminicore disease
King syndrome

syndrome, and multiminicore disease (Table 53.1). Most patients susceptible to MH do not have obvious musculoskeletal disorders or a positive family history.

McCarthy TV, Quane KA, Lynch PJ. Ryanodine receptor mutations in malignant hyperthermia and central core disease. *Hum Mutat* 2000;15:410–417.

Rosenberg H, Dirksen RA. *Malignant Hyperthermia*. Genetests web site. www.genetests.org, 2006.

Rosenberg H, Brandom BW, Sambuughin NK, et al. Malignant hyperthermia and other pharmacogenetic disorders. In: Barash P, Cullen B, Stoelting R, eds. *Clinical anesthesia*, 5th ed. Philadelphia: Lippincott Williams & Wilkins, 2006:529–556.

Strazis KP, Fox AW. Malignant hyperthermia: a review of published cases. *Anesth Analg* 1993;77(2):297–304.

A.4. Does the history of previous uneventful sevoflurane anesthesia reasonably exclude the patient's susceptibility to malignant hyperthermia (MH)?

No, it does not. Cases may occur during a second or subsequent anesthetic course.

Bendixen D, Skovgaard LT, Ording H. Analysis of anaesthesia in patients suspected to be susceptible to malignant hyperthermia before diagnostic *in vitro* contracture test. *Acta Anaesthesiol Scand* 1997;41(4):480–484.

A.5. What are the clinical features of the syndrome?

The clinical features of malignant hyperthermia (MH) are the result of an uncontrolled, exaggerated, hypermetabolic state triggered by the use of potent inhalation anesthetic agents and succinylcholine. In humans, only a few cases of MH have been thought to occur as a result of environmental factors other than anesthetic agents. Common manifestations include the following:

Specific for malignant hyperthermia

- Increase in end-tidal CO_2 during constant ventilation (the most sensitive and specific sign)
- Generalized rigidity (extremely high specificity)
- Masseter muscle rigidity (MMR)
- Increased temperature (not uncommonly higher than 40°C [104°F])

Nonspecific

- Tachycardia (the earliest and most consistent clinical sign however not specific)
- Tachypnea

- Arrhythmias
- Skin mottling
- Profuse sweating
- Altered blood pressure

Hyperkalemic cardiac arrest

Sudden hyperkalemic cardiac arrest has been reported after the administration of MH trigger agents in children with undiagnosed myopathy, especially Duchenne's or Becker's muscular dystrophy. This response is not a result of similar pathophysiologic changes typical for MH, but rather muscle membrane destruction leading to hyperkalemia.

The treatment is similar to treatment for hyperkalemia, that is, glucose and insulin, calcium chloride or gluconate, hyperventilation.

Kleopa K, Rosenberg H, Heiman-Patterson T. Malignant hyperthermia-like episode in Becker muscle dystrophy. *Anesthesiology* 2000;93:1535–1557.

Larach MG, Localio AR, Allen GC, et al. A clinical grading scale to predict malignant hyperthermia susceptibility. *Anesthesiology* 1994;80(4):771–779.

Larach MG, Rosenberg H, Gronert GA, et al. Hyperkalemic cardiac arrest during anesthetics in infants and children with occult myopathies. *Clin Pediatr* 1997;36:9–18.

A.6. What are the laboratory findings during an acute crisis of malignant hyperthermia (MH)?

The laboratory values once again reflect changes of a hypermetabolic state and muscle tissue damage (Table 53.2).

Table 53.2   THE LABORATORY FINDINGS OF ACUTE MALIGNANT HYPERTHERMIA.

Metabolic and respiratory acidosis
Arterial blood gases
    $\downarrow\downarrow$ pH
    $\uparrow\uparrow\uparrow$ P_{CO_2}
    Mild decreases in P_{O_2}
Electrolytes
    $\uparrow$ K
    $\uparrow$ Ca or decreased
    $\uparrow$ Mg
Serum
    $\uparrow$ Lactate
    $\uparrow$ Pyruvate
    $\uparrow$ Creatine kinase
    $\uparrow$ Lactate dehydrogenase
    $\uparrow$ Aldolase
    $\uparrow$ Myoglobin
    Increased INR, increased FSP, increased PT/PTT

$\uparrow$, mild to moderate increase; $\uparrow\uparrow$, moderate to major increase; $\uparrow\uparrow\uparrow$, extreme change; INR, international normalized ratio; FSP, fibroblast secretory protein; PT, prothrombin time; PTT, partial thromboplastin time.

Ali SZ, Taguchi A, Rosenberg H. Malignant hyperthermia. *Best Pract Res Clin Anesth* 2003;17: 519–533.

A.7. What is the incidence of this syndrome?

The incidence of clinical malignant hyperthermia (MH) is difficult to measure as many clinical syndromes resemble MH and often the anesthetic management is altered when initial signs suggesting MH are detected. The incidence also depends on the prevalence in a population of genetic mutations causal for MH as well as the prevalence of use of MH trigger agents.

One of the earliest epidemiologic studies of MH was conducted in Denmark where an estimate of the incidence of fulminant MH was noted to be 1 in 260,000 general anesthetics and 1 in 60,000 anesthetics where succinylcholine was used. The incidence was even higher, that is, 1 in 5,000 anesthetics, when such signs as masseter muscle rigidity (MMR), unexplained tachycardia and unexplained fever were included.

In a particular province of Quebec, Canada, the prevalence of MH was calculated as 0.2% of the population based on a detailed genealogic study of families with MH susceptibility.

More recently, genetic studies have suggested that the prevalence of mutations that are causal for MH is 1 in 3,000 in France and in Japan.

The incidence of clinical MH appears to be higher in children and in men.

Bachand M, Vachon N, Boisvert M, et al. Clinical reassessment of malignant hyperthermia in Abitibi-Temiscamingue. *Can J Anaesth* 1997;44(7):696–701.

Monnier N, Krivosic-Horber R, Payen JF, et al. Presence of two different genetic traits in malignant hyperthermia families: implication for genetic analysis, diagnosis, and incidence of malignant hyperthermia susceptibility. *Anesthesiology* 2002; 97:1067–1074.

Ording H. Incidence of malignant hyperthermia in Denmark. *Anesth Analg* 1985;64:700–704.

A.8. What is the mode of inheritance of the disease?

Malignant hyperthermia (MH) is inherited in humans in an autosomal dominant manner with reduced penetrance and variable expressivity. MH is heterogenetic with up to seven gene loci implicated.

More than 50% of MH cases are linked to the ryanodine receptor gene located on chromosome 19. More than 100 mutations have been found in that gene with up to 30 documented to be causal for the syndrome.

In MH susceptible pigs, the inheritance is autosomal recessive with only one DNA change noted to account for all cases.

Litman RS, Rosenberg H. Malignant hyperthermia. Update on susceptibility testing. *JAMA* 2005;239:2918–2924.

McCarthy TV, Sandra Healey JM, Jeffron JA, et al. Localization of the malignant hyperthermia susceptibility locus to human chromosome 19q12-13.2. *Nature* 1990;343: 562–563.

A.9. What genetic disorder results in malignant hyperthermia (MH) susceptibility?

In almost all cases, the MH-susceptible patient has a defective calcium channel located in the membrane of the sarcoplasmic reticulum (SR) of skeletal muscle. This channel is termed the *ryanodine receptor* (RYR) because it binds the plant alkaloid ryanodine. The channel is closely associated with other proteins and structures, such as the dihydropyridine calcium channel that mediates transfer of voltage change to the RYR-1 receptor. Other proteins associated with the ryanodine receptor include triadin, and FK 506–binding protein. However, mutations associated with MH susceptibility are found mainly in the gene for the ryanodine receptor. As many as 30% of families susceptible to MH harbor one of approximately 30 causal mutations for MH, with approximately 60 other mutations that are yet to be characterized.

The dihydropyridine receptor (DHPR) gene, also involved in intracellular calcium control, has been associated with MH susceptibility in a few families.

There are probably other genes that may lead to MH susceptibility but are much less common than those associated with the *RYR-1* and the *DHPR* genes.

Of interest is the observation that the genetic mutations associated with central core disease that also predisposes to MH, are located on the *RYR-1* gene as well. It is hypothesized that in this disorder there is a constant leak of calcium from the SR, thereby depleting the reserves of calcium and leading to inadequate activation of actin and myosin and hence muscle weakness.

Recently a mouse model of MH has been created by artificially incorporating one of the causal MH mutations into the mouse genome. The mouse displays signs typical of MH during exposure to MH trigger agents and also on exposure to raised environmental temperature.

Chelu MG, Goonasekera SA, Durham WJ, et al. Heat- and anesthesia-induced malignant hyperthermia in an RyR1 knock-in mouse. *FASEB J* 2006;20(2):329–330.

Monnier N, Krivosic-Horber R, Payen JF, et al. Presence of two different genetic traits in malignant hyperthermia families: implication for genetic analysis, diagnosis, and incidence of malignant hyperthermia susceptibility. *Anesthesiology* 2002;97:1067–1074.

Robinson RL, Hopkins PM. A breakthrough in the genetic diagnosis of malignant hyperthermia. *Br J Anesth* 2001;86:166–168.

Sambuughin N, Holley H, Muldoon S, et al. Screening of the entire ryanodine receptor type 1 coding region for sequence variants associated with malignant hyperthermia susceptibility in the North American population. *Anesthesiology* 2005;102:515–521.

A.10. What is the pathophysiology of the syndrome?

The malignant hyperthermia (MH) clinical syndrome results from an abnormal and uncontrolled elevation of intracellular calcium levels in skeletal muscle. The pathophysiology is as follows: The process of calcium release from the sarcoplasmic reticulum (SR) normally begins with depolarization of the sarcolemma which is transmitted through the t-tubules to the dihydropyridine receptor which in turn activates the calcium channel termed the *ryanodine receptor* to release calcium.

The elevated calcium removes the inhibition of actin and myosin interaction that leads to mechanical force generation. The calcium release occurs through a channel within the SR called the *ryanodine* receptor. Reuptake of calcium returns the intracellular cytoplasmic concentration of calcium to normal and muscle relaxation takes place. Reuptake is mediated through a calcium adenosine triphosphate (ATP)ase pump mechanism.

There are a variety of intermediate proteins that also regulate the intrasarcoplasmic reticulum concentration of calcium such as calsequestrin and intracellular proteins as well.

The control of calcium release is highly regulated because, when muscle contraction takes place, a variety of energy-consuming steps are required resulting in ATP breakdown and heat production.

In an MH episode, the ryanodine receptor calcium channel is locked in an open position leading to an uncontrolled release of calcium with elevation of intracytoplasmic calcium levels and continuous muscle activation as well as ATP breakdown. The SR calcium pump is unable to resequester the calcium. ATP breakdown during this process aggravates heat production further.

Energy-consuming processes take place through glycolysis as well as oxidative phosphorylation. Eventually ATP levels are insufficient to maintain sarcolemmal integrity and potassium leaks from the cell resulting in hyperkalemia. Myoglobinemia occurs for the same reason as does an increase of a number of enzymes, including creatine kinase.

Gronert GA, Pessah IN, Muldoon S, et al. Malignant hyperthermia. In: Miller RD, ed. *Anesthesia*. 6th ed. New York: Elsevier Science Churchill Livingstone, 2005:1169–1190.

A.11. What laboratory tests can further substantiate the susceptibility of the patient to malignant hyperthermia (MH)?

The most accurate diagnostic test for MH is the exposure of biopsied skeletal muscle to halothane, caffeine, and, more recently ryanodine or chlorocresol. In this test, approximately 2 g of muscle is harvested from the thigh under regional, or in the case of a child, general anesthesia. Strips or fascicles of muscle weighing 100 to 200 mg are suspended in a water bath at 37°C (98.6°F), and exposure is made to either halothane, caffeine, ryanodine, or chlorocresol in specific graded concentrations. The isometric contracture, not contraction, response to muscle is measured through strain gauge following specific guidelines. The threshold and height of the contracture is measured and a diagnosis of MH is made based on the contracture threshold and strength exceeding specific values.

The test is highly sensitive, close to 100%, but there are false positives, up to 20% of positives may be false positives. Nevertheless the value of the test resides in ruling out MH susceptibility with certainty.

Because the test is invasive and costly and requires strict adherence to specific requirements there are only approximately 10 testing centers in North America. There are more than 20 in Europe.

The patient and his/her history are carefully evaluated by the biopsy center before recommending the test.

Molecular genetic testing for malignant hyperthermia susceptibility

The era of DNA testing for MH susceptibility began in 1990 when a mutation in the *RYR-1* gene was shown to be causal for MH in pigs. In humans several genes have been associated with MH, however the *RYR-1* gene is probably responsible for most cases of MH. At present 28 mutations in the *RYR-1* gene have been found in humans that are causal for MH. Unfortunately no mutation accounts for more than a small percent of all patients with MH susceptibility. The chief advantage of genetic testing is all that is required is a blood sample and the specimen may be shipped to the laboratory. The main limitation of genetic testing is the sensitivity of approximately 25% even testing for presence of the 28 mutations. The sensitivity will improve as more mutations are identified.

Patients should consider genetic testing if: (a) they have had a positive contracture test; (b) a family member has had a positive contracture test; (c) they have suffered a very likely MH episode but have not had a contracture test; (d) a family member has been found to have a causal mutation.

In those patients who are tested and a causal mutation identified, those with the mutation are MH susceptible (high specificity) but those without the mutation *cannot* be considered MH negative as they may harbor another mutation.

At present there are two clinical testing laboratories for diagnosing MH susceptibility: PreventionGenetics (www.preventiongenetics.com) and the DNA diagnostic laboratory at the University of Pittsburgh (http://path.upmc.edu/divisions/mdx/diagnostics.html).

The decision to undergo genetic testing is complex because the test, although requiring only a blood sample, costs approximately $800 for the search for the 23 mutations. However once a mutation is found, the cost for screening family members is $200 each.

The pros and cons of testing should be discussed with either an MH expert or a genetic counselor.

Allen GC, Rosenberg H, Fletcher J. Safety of general anesthesia in patients tested negative for malignant hyperthermia susceptibility. *Anesthesiology* 1990;72:619–622.

Iaizzo PA, Wedel DJ, Gallagher WJ. *In vitro* contracture testing for determination of susceptibility to malignant hyperthermia: a methodological update. *Mayo Clin Proc* 1991;66:998–1001.

Rosenberg H, Antognini JF, Muldoon S. Testing for malignant hyperthermia. *Anesthesiology* 2002;96:232–237.

A.12. What is neuroleptic malignant syndrome (NMS)?

The NMS is also a hypermetabolic syndrome characterized by hyperthermia, rigidity, rhabdomyolysis, acidosis, and tachycardia, features that mimic malignant hyperthermia (MH). However, NMS is precipitated by a variety of neuroleptic drugs including haloperidol, the atypical antipsychotics, phenothiazines, and other centrally acting drugs.

This syndrome differs from MH in that central dopamine depletion is responsible for the clinical picture. The mainstays of treatment are benzodiazepines and a dopamine agonist such as bromocriptine. Patients also respond symptomatically to dantrolene therapy.

A variety of drug-induced hyperthermic syndromes resemble MH such as the serotonin syndrome. The most common situation for the serotonin syndrome is the administration of meperidine in a patient on monoamine oxidase (MAO) inhibitor drugs.

Ecstasy and other methylenedioxymethamphetamine (MDMA) agonists also produce hyperthermia. Again the signs may resemble MH, but the pathophysiology is very different.

Anesthesiologists may encounter NMS in patients who are sedated with haloperidol in the intensive care unit (ICU) and on infrequent occasions when patients are given dopamine agonist agents such as metoclopramide, and promethazine.

Caroff SN, Mann SC. Neuroleptic malignant syndrome. *Med Clin North Am* 1993;77(1): 185–202. *www.nmsis.org*.

B. Preoperative Evaluation and Preparation

B.1. How would you prepare this patient for anesthesia and surgery?

Preoperative preparation should include a detailed medical history, assessment of the patient's physical status, evaluation of laboratory findings including creatinine kinase (CK), and specific investigations to determine the susceptibility of the patient to malignant hyperthermia (MH). Three possible scenarios are as follows:

- The halothane caffeine contracture test result is normal. The patient should be considered not susceptible to MH and the anesthetic should be nonrestrictive.
- The halothane caffeine contracture test is abnormal, implying MH susceptibility. Or a mutation associated with MH is identified. In this case, trigger-free anesthetic agents should be employed and all preparations should be made to quickly treat the syndrome if it develops.

- The halothane caffeine contracture test is not available. This is very frequently the case because this test is done in only a few centers in the country. In such situations, the patient should be treated as malignant hyperthermia syndrome (MHS) and all appropriate steps should be followed.

Allen GC, Rosenberg H, Fletcher J. Safety of general anesthesia in patients tested negative for malignant hyperthermia susceptibility. *Anesthesiology* 1990;72:619–622.

Rosenberg H, Brandom BW, Sambuughin NK, Fletcher JE. Malignant hyperthermia and other pharmacogenetic disorders. In: Barash P, Cullen B, Stoelting R, eds. *Clinical anesthesia*, 5th ed. Philadelphia: Lippincott Williams & Wilkins, 2006:529–556.

B.2. Is dantrolene prophylaxis indicated?

If a nontriggering anesthetic is administered with appropriate monitoring to a malignant hyperthermia (MH)-susceptible patient, dantrolene prophylaxis is not necessary.

With the judicious use of trigger-free anesthetics, the incidence of MH is extremely unlikely. Dantrolene can cause side effects, such as nausea, vomiting, pain at the injection site, and depression of the twitch response, which can predispose the patient to respiratory insufficiency in the postoperative period.

Carr AS, Lehman J, Cunliffe M, et al. Incidence of malignant hyperthermia reactions in 2,214 patients undergoing muscle biopsy. *Can J Anaesth* 1995;42(4):281–286.

B.3. What laboratory tests would you obtain before surgery?

Chest radiograph and electrocardiogram (ECG) should be ordered if dictated by his kyphoscoliosis or other associated medical illness. Otherwise, there is no routine laboratory testing indicated for strabismus surgery in this child. Serum creatinine kinase (CK) is of value as a baseline test and should be obtained.

B.4. Is outpatient surgery appropriate for this patient?

With the use of trigger-free anesthetics and appropriate monitoring, surgery normally performed as an outpatient can be performed safely. Postoperative admission to the hospital solely on the basis of malignant hyperthermia (MH) susceptibility is not warranted. When MH occurs, it is usually in the immediate postoperative period and usually not beyond 2 hours postoperatively. Therefore, it is prudent to keep the patient longer than usual in the postanesthesia care unit (PACU) in monitored setting and a little longer in the ambulatory discharge area.

Allen GC, Rosenberg H, Fletcher J. Safety of general anesthesia in patients tested negative for malignant hyperthermia susceptibility. *Anesthesiology* 1990;72:619–622.

Pollock N, Langton E, McDonnell N, et al. Malignant hyperthermia and day stay surgery. *Anaesth Intensive Care* 2006;34(1):40–45.

Yentis SM, Levine MF, Hartley EJ. Should all children with suspected or confirmed malignant hyperthermia susceptibility be admitted after surgery? A 10-year review. *Anesth Analg* 1992;75(3):345–350.

B.5. In anticipation of general anesthesia, what preparations would you make?

A satisfactory preparation for administering anesthesia to this patient should include measures to prevent and treat an acute crisis of malignant hyperthermia (MH). The following should be available:

Equipment

- Drain, remove or disable vaporizers.
- Fresh circuit, reservoir bag, and soda lime.
- Flush machine and ventilator by flowing 10 L oxygen per minute for 10 minutes.
- Routine American Society of Anesthesiologists (ASA) monitors including:
  - Pulse oximeter
  - Capnometer
  - Core Temperature monitor
  - Electrocardiogram (ECG) and BP monitors

Items to have available:

Cooling aids

- Hypothermia blanket
- Crushed ice
- Cold saline for irrigation and intravenous infusion
- Nasogastric tube and Foley catheter for cavity cooling

Drugs

- Sodium bicarbonate, mannitol, furosemide, dantrolene (intravenous), sterile water, antiarrhythmics, insulin, 50% dextrose, and calcium chloride
- *Avoid* calcium channel blockers because of interaction with dantrolene, possibly resulting in cardiac arrest.

Ali SZ, Taguchi A, Rosenberg H. Malignant hyperthermia. *Best Pract Res Clin Anesth* 2003; 17:519–533.

Malignant Hyperthermia Association of the United States (MHAUS). *Clinical update 2005: managing malignant hyperthermia*. Sherburne: MHAUS, 2005.

San Juan AC Jr, Wong KC, Port JD. Hyperkalemia after dantrolene and verapamil-dantrolene administration in dogs. *Anesth Analg* 1998;67(8):759–762.

C. Intraoperative Management

C.1. What anesthetic techniques and agents would you employ?

The main approach is avoidance of potent inhalation agents and succinylcholine. If possible, local or regional anesthesia is preferred. Anesthesia may be induced with a barbiturate, benzodiazepine, or hypnotic, and the patient should be ventilated with 100% oxygen. Fentanyl or other opioid may be added to ensure adequate depth of anesthesia. Topical anesthesia of the larynx and vocal cords may be achieved with a local anesthetic spray. The trachea is intubated with or without the use of a short-acting or intermediate-acting nondepolarizing muscle relaxant. Anesthetic maintenance is achieved using oxygen and nitrous oxide, a narcotic, and a nondepolarizing relaxant as required. Total intravenous anesthesia (TIVA) is a good choice for anesthesia as well.

Vital signs are monitored with very close attention to capnography.

C.2. What anesthetic agents are contraindicated?

In general, the anesthetic agents to be avoided include potent inhalation agents and depolarizing muscle relaxant. Of the agents commonly employed currently, the following have been implicated in triggering malignant hyperthermia (MH):

- *Inhalation agents*—halothane enflurane, isoflurane, desflurane, and sevoflurane
- *Muscle relaxants*—succinylcholine

Fu ES, Scharf JE, Mangar D, et al. Malignant hyperthermia involving the administration of desflurane. *Can J Anaesth* 1996;43(7):687–690.

Otsuka H, Komura Y, Mayumi T, et al. Malignant hyperthermia during sevoflurane anesthesia in a child with central core disease. *Anesthesiology* 1991;75(4):699–701.

C.3. If the surgeon wants to use local anesthesia for a procedure, what agents will you recommend?

Both ester and amide local anesthetics are now considered safe for use in malignant hyperthermia syndrome (MHS) patients.

Harrison GG, Morrell DF. Response of MHS swine to intravenous infusion of lignocaine and bupivacaine. *Br J Anesth* 1980;52:385–387.

Maccani RM, Wedel DJ, Melton A, et al. Femoral and lateral femoral cutaneous nerve block for muscle biopsies in children. *Paediatr Anaesth* 1995;5(4):223–227.

C.4. What is the significance of masseter muscle spasm occurring after succinylcholine administration?

Rigidity of the jaw muscles after administration of succinylcholine is referred to as *masseter muscle rigidity* (MMR). MMR presages clinical malignant hyperthermia (MH) in up to 30% of cases. Even in the absence of clinical MH, myoglobinuria in individuals with MMR is common postoperatively. MMR probably occurs in individuals of all ages regardless of malignant hyperthermia syndrome (MHS) status; however, MMR is more common in children, particularly following gas anesthesia induction

MMR has been reported in 1% of children after halothane/succinylcholine induction and in adults after succinylcholine administration. Should MMR occur, elective surgery should be postponed, the patient observed in an intensive care unit (ICU) setting for 24 hours seeking myoglobinuria specifically.

In the case of an emergency surgical procedure, the anesthetic should be converted to a "nontrigger" technique and the patient observed for early signs of MH. Dantrolene and other MH treatment procedures should be made ready.

The patient and/or family should be advised to be evaluated for MH susceptibility.

The incidence of MMR and MH episodes in children have recently decreased as a result of recommendations that the use of succinylcholine in children be reserved for emergency situations.

Gronert GA, Rosenberg H. Management of patients in whom trismus occurs following succinylcholine. *Anesthesiology* 1988;68:653–655.

Kaplan RF. *Malignant hyperthermia: ASA refresher courses.* Philadelphia: JB Lippincott, 1994:169–180.

O'Flynn RP, Schutak JG, Rosenberg H. Masseter muscle rigidity and malignant hyperthermia susceptibility in pediatric patients. An update on management and diagnosis. *Anesthesiology* 1994;80(6):1228–1233.

Rosenberg H, Fletcher JE. Masseter muscle rigidity and malignant hyperthermia susceptibility. *Anesth Analg* 1985;65:161–164.

Schwartz L, Rockoff MA, Koka BV. Masseter spasm with anesthesia incidence and implications. *Anesthesiology* 1984;61:722–775.

C.5. Twenty minutes into the procedure with sevoflurane anesthesia, the patient developed increasing tachycardia with ventricular premature beats and mottled skin. What emergency measures would you take?

Although tachycardia may arise from other more common causes, such as a light plane of anesthesia and/or hypovolemia, its association with dysrhythmia in this patient—who has malignant hyperthermia syndrome (MHS)—is the first key to the onset of the syndrome. End-expiratory CO_2 should be monitored, and if rising despite increasing minute ventilation the diagnosis of malignant hyperthermia (MH) should be strongly considered. As time is of the essence, the following steps should be taken; this constitutes a critical emergency.

- Stop all anesthetics and surgery (if possible).
- Hyperventilate the patient with 100% oxygen.
- Obtain help and assistance through the MH hotline of the Malignant Hyperthermia Association of the United States (MHAUS): 1-800-MH-HYPER.
- Administer specific drug therapy—start dantrolene sodium early while muscle perfusion is still present. An initial intravenous dose of 2.5 mg per kg should be followed by repeated doses of 1 to 2 mg per kg to a total of 10 mg per kg depending on the patient's response. More dantrolene may be administered if clinically indicated.
- Initiate aggressive cooling immediately for rapidly increasing temperatures and for those higher than 40°C (104°F)—methods for cooling include the following: surface cooling with the patient on a cooling blanket and packed in ice; gastric, rectal, or peritoneal lavage with iced saline; and iced intravenous fluids (saline). Cooling should be stopped when the patient's temperature falls to lower than 38°C (100.4°F), to prevent inadvertent hypothermia.
- Treat acidosis with sodium bicarbonate (2 mEq/kg initial dose and titrate as necessary).
- Treat hyperkalemia with sodium bicarbonate, insulin, and 50% dextrose.
- Treat arrhythmias with standard antiarrhythmics, and avoid calcium channel blockers if dantrolene has been given.
- Arterial line, Foley catheter should be inserted in all cases of MH. Central venous catheterization should be considered for unstable patients or where aggressive therapy is needed.
- Maintain urine output with mannitol or furosemide.
- Follow creatinine kinase (CK) levels every 12 hours.
- Check electrolytes and coagulation parameters.
- Register the patient and the event with the North American MH Registry.
- Forms may be obtained through MHAUS. The web site for the North American MH registry is www.mhreg.org

Ali SZ, Taguchi A, Rosenberg H. Malignant hyperthermia. *Best Pract Res Clin Anesth* 2003; 17:519–533.

C.6. What modalities would you monitor closely during management of the crisis?

The modalities that should be monitored closely include the following:

- End-tidal carbon dioxide
- Arterial blood gases/electrolytes/coagulation
- Core temperature
- Creatinine kinase (CK) levels
- Myoglobin levels
- Urine output

D. Postoperative Management

D.1. What complications may follow this syndrome?

Disseminated intravascular coagulation syndrome is a major complication of malignant hyperthermia (MH) especially when the patient's temperature exceeds 41°C (105.8°F). Other complications include renal failure, hyperkalemia, and compartment syndrome. As a result of massive muscle breakdown, the patient may be weak for days and also complain of muscle cramps and pain.

Rosenberg H, Brandom BW, Sambuughin NK, et al. Malignant hyperthermia and other pharmacogenetic disorders. In: Barash P, Cullen B, Stoelting R, eds. *Clinical anesthesia*, 5th ed. Philadelphia: Lippincott Williams & Wilkins, 2006:529–556.

D.2. What would be your follow-up in this case?

The vigorous therapy started in the operating room should be continued in the immediate postoperative period into the postanesthesia care unit (PACU) or the intensive care unit (ICU). Dantrolene administration should be continued for at least 36 hours after an episode is controlled at a dose of 1 mg per kg every 4 to 6 hours titrated to signs of malignant hyperthermia (MH). Serum creatinine kinase (CK) should be followed until normalized.

Other laboratory values that should be followed until normalized include:

- Arterial blood gases
- Electrolytes
- Coagulation profile

Body temperature should be monitored along with other vital signs. Recrudescence of MH occurs in approximately 25% of treated cases and therefore the patient should be watched in an ICU setting for at least 36 hours following an episode.

Rosenberg H, Brandom BW, Sambuughin NK, et al. Malignant hyperthermia and other pharmacogenetic disorders. In: Barash P, Cullen B, Stoelting R, eds. *Clinical anesthesia*, 5th ed. Philadelphia: Lippincott Williams & Wilkins, 2006:529–556.

D.3. What would you advise the patient and the family?

The patient and his family should be warned of the dangerous nature of this syndrome and should be advised to carry an identification band at all times. The pedigree of the family should be prepared and the members should be investigated for susceptibility to this syndrome and issued medical identification bracelets or pendants accordingly.

The Malignant Hyperthermia Association of the United States (MHAUS) has been active since 1981 and offers current information and advice on patient management as well as identification bracelets and a variety of material for health care professionals. The following is some useful contact information:

Emergency hotline: 1-800-MH-HYPER
Address: MHAUS, 39 East State Street, P.O. Box 1609, Sherburne, NY 13815
Phone: 1-800-98-MHAUS
Internet: www.mhaus.org

In addition, the patient and his family should consult with one of the malignant hyperthermia diagnostic centers to discuss further evaluation. A complete listing is available through MHAUS.

The patient should be registered with the North American MH Registry.
Forms may be obtained through MHAUS.
The web site for the North American MH Registry is www.mhreg.org
The phone number is (888) 274–7899
The Registry is located at the Children's Hospital of the University of Pittsburgh. The director is Dr. Barbara Brandom.

Suggested Resources

Web sites of the MH Association of the US: www.mhaus.org
www.nmsis.org
    Web site of the European MH Group: www.emhg.org
Website of the North American MH Registry: www.MHReg.org

Latest reviews
orphanet.org
genetests.org

CHAPTER 54

Prolonged Postoperative Apnea

PETER SAVARD • MATTHEW R. BELMONT

A YOUNG WOMAN

experienced severe lower abdominal pain and vaginal bleeding after eating a large meal. Upon examination in the emergency room, a pelvic mass was found and emergency laparotomy was proposed for presumed ruptured ectopic pregnancy.

Anesthesia was induced with a rapid sequence technique including succinylcholine. The patient remained apneic, not only throughout the procedure but also in the recovery room. Her husband arrived and stated that several other members of her family had had similar difficulty.

A. Medical Disease and Differential Diagnosis

1. Describe the humoral events in normal neuromuscular transmission.
2. What is acetylcholinesterase?
3. What is serum cholinesterase?
4. How does succinylcholine resemble acetylcholine (ACh)?
5. How does succinylcholine differ from ACh?
6. What is the incidence of atypical cholinesterase activity?
7. What is the significance of the dibucaine number?
8. Discuss possible cardiovascular effects of succinylcholine. What patients are especially at risk?
9. What are some factors that can lower pseudocholinesterase levels?
10. Should succinylcholine be routinely used in pediatric anesthesia?
11. Can mivacurium be used in patients with abnormal pseudocholinesterase?

B. Preoperative Preparation

C. Intraoperative Management

1. When should the first dose of nondepolarizing muscle relaxant be given?
2. How is the choice among muscle relaxants made?
3. What is "train-of-four (TOF)?"
4. When is it safe to reverse muscle relaxants? What factors affect reversal?
5. What is adequate neuromuscular recovery, and are clinical signs of reversal useful? Is TOF a reliable measure?

6. What percentage of postjunctional receptors must be blocked before transmission is diminished?

D. Postoperative Management

1. What is the differential diagnosis for postoperative apnea? How would you treat it?

A. Medical Disease and Differential Diagnosis

A.1. Describe the humoral events in normal neuromuscular transmission.

It is generally accepted that the synthesis and release of acetylcholine (ACh) involves a cycle of events. ACh is first formed in the cytoplasm of the nerve terminal from acetyl coenzyme A and choline in a reaction catalyzed by the soluble enzyme choline acetyltransferase. An energy-dependent transporter then accumulates ACh within vesicles containing 5,000 to 10,000 molecules of ACh. The ACh contained in a single vesicle is often referred to as a *quantum* of transmitter. Release of ACh is a Ca^{2+}-dependent process and is triggered by an increase in the concentration of free Ca^{2+} within the nerve terminal. This results from the opening of voltage-gated Ca^{2+} channels by the depolarization of the nerve impulse. This Ca^{2+} signal triggers the fusion of synaptic vesicles with the presynaptic membrane and subsequently exocytosis, resulting in the release of a "quantum" of several thousand ACh molecules into the synaptic cleft. The released ACh binds to α subunits of the acetylcholine receptors (AChRs). These ligand-gated cation channels allow sodium to enter and depolarize the muscle cell membrane at synaptic sites. This local depolarization leads to the activation of nearby voltage-gated sodium channels, which amplify and propagate action potentials across the surface of the muscle fiber and into the transverse tubules where Ca^{2+} channels are present at high density, releasing large amounts of Ca^{2+} from the sarcoplasmic reticulum and resulting in muscle contraction. The translation of electrical signaling at the surface membrane into intracellular Ca^{2+} release from the sarcoplasmic reticulum is known as *excitation–contraction coupling*.

Naguib M. Advances in neurobiology of the neuromuscular junction: implications for the anesthesiologist. *Anesthesiology* 2002;96(1):202–231.

A.2. What is acetylcholinesterase?

Acetylcholinesterase is a relatively specific enzyme that hydrolyzes acetylcholine (ACh) faster than it does other choline esters. It is found in red blood cells, the central nervous system, and the neuromuscular junction. It is responsible for hydrolyzing and inactivating the ACh produced during normal neuromuscular transmission. It does not hydrolyze succinylcholine and is inhibited by the drug.

Miller RD, ed. *Miller's anesthesia*, 6th ed. Philadelphia: Elsevier Science, 2005:642.

Taylor P, Schumacher M, MacPhee-Quingley K, et al. The structure of acetylcholinesterase: relationship to its function and cellular disposition. *Trends Neurosci* 1987;10:93.

A.3. What is serum cholinesterase?

This enzyme, also called *cholinesterase, pseudocholinesterase, butyrylcholinesterase,* and *nonspecific cholinesterase,* hydrolyzes many choline esters, including succinylcholine. It is found in many human tissues, but not in the red blood cell. It is synthesized in the liver. Its physiologic function is unknown, but it may hydrolyze choline esters, such as propionylcholine and butyrylcholine, which may be formed by bacterial action in the gut and by the enzyme systems responsible for the formation of acetylcholine (ACh).

Massoulie J, Bon S. Molecular forms of cholinesterase and acetylcholinesterase in vertebrates. *Annu Rev Neurosci* 1982;5:57.

Miller RD, cd. *Miller's anesthesia*, 6th ed. Philadelphia: Elsevier Science, 2005:642.

Pantuck EJ. Plasma cholinesterase: gene and variations. *Anesth Analg* 1993;77:380–386.

A.4. How does succinylcholine resemble acetylcholine (ACh)?

Succinylcholine causes depolarization of the postsynaptic membrane by opening channels in the same manner as ACh.

Brunton L, ed. *Goodman and Gilman's the pharmacological basis of therapeutics*, 11th ed. New York: McGraw-Hill, 2006:223.

Durant MW, Katz RI. Suxamethonium. *Br J Anaesth* 1982;54:195.

A.5. How does succinylcholine differ from acetylcholine (ACh)?

Succinylcholine persists for a longer duration at the neuromuscular junction, primarily because of its resistance to acetylcholinesterase. The depolarization is longer lasting, resulting in a period of repetitive excitation, eliciting muscle fasciculations followed by a flaccid paralysis.

Albuquerque EX, Akaike A, Shaw KP, et al. The interaction of anticholinesterase agents with the acetylcholine receptor–ionic channel complex. *Fundam Appl Toxicol* 1984;14:S27.

Brunton L, ed. *Goodman and Gilman's the pharmacological basis of therapeutics*, 11th ed. New York: McGraw-Hill, 2006:223.

Viby-Mogensen J. Correlation of succinylcholine duration of action with plasma cholinesterase activity in subjects with the genotypically normal enzyme. *Anesthesiology* 1980;53:517.

A.6. What is the incidence of atypical cholinesterase activity?

The incidence of atypical cholinesterase activity varies with the population studied, but it is approximately 1 of 2,800 in the general population of the United States, with a 1:1 male/female ratio.

Kalow W, Genest K. A method for detection of atypical forms of human serum cholinesterase: determination of dibucaine numbers. *Can J Biochem* 1957;35:339.

Maddineni VR, Mirakhur RK. Prolonged neuromuscular block following mivacurium. *Anesthesiology* 1993;78:1181–1184.

A.7. What is the significance of the dibucaine number?

The dibucaine number is used to identify the heterozygote. Dibucaine in 10^{-5} mol per L concentration produces the maximum difference in inhibition between the usual and the atypical forms of serum cholinesterase. The term *dibucaine number* has been applied to the

Table 54.1 RELATION BETWEEN DIBUCAINE NUMBER AND DURATION OF SUCCINYLCHOLINE NEUROMUSCULAR BLOCKADE.

TYPE OF PSEUDOCHOLINESTERASE	GENOTYPE	FREQUENCY	DIBUCAINE NUMBER[a]	RESPONSE TO SUCCINYLCHOLINE OR MIVACURIUM
Homozygous typical	EuEu	Normal	70–80	Normal
Heterozygous	EuEa	1/480	50–60	Slightly prolonged
Homozygous atypical	EaEa	1/3,200	20–30	Markedly prolonged

[a]The dibucaine number indicates the percentage of enzyme inhibited.

percentage of inhibition of serum cholinesterase. The usual homozygote has a dibucaine number of approximately 80, the atypical homozygote has a value less than 30, and the heterozygote has a value between 45 and 69. The relation between the dibucaine number and the duration of succinylcholine neuromuscular blockade is shown in Table 54.1.

Kalow W, Genest K. A method of detection of atypical forms of human serum cholinesterase: determination of dibucaine numbers. *Can J Biochem* 1957;35:339–353.

Miller RD, ed. *Miller's anesthesia*, 6th ed. Philadelphia: Elsevier Science, 2005:488–489.

A.8. Discuss possible cardiovascular effects of succinylcholine. What patients are especially at risk?

Succinylcholine stimulates all cholinergic autonomic receptors, including nicotinic receptors in both sympathetic and parasympathetic ganglia as well as muscarinic receptors in the sinus node of the heart. Cardiac arrhythmias may easily arise as a result of this generalized autonomic stimulation. These arrhythmias include sinus bradycardia, nodal (junctional) rhythms, and ventricular arrhythmias. Individuals especially at risk are those with predominantly vagal tone, such as children who have not received atropine. Sinus bradycardia has also been noted in adults and appears more commonly when a second dose of the drug is given approximately 5 minutes after the first. The bradycardia may be prevented by thiopental, atropine, ganglion-blocking drugs, and nondepolarizing neuromuscular blockers.

Belmont MR. Succinylcholine. *Curr Opin Anesth* 1995;8:362–366.

Leiman BC, Katz J, Butler BD. Mechanisms of succinylcholine-induced arrhythmias in hypoxic or hypoxic/hypercarbic dogs. *Anesth Analg* 1987;66:1292.

Miller RD, ed. *Miller's anesthesia*, 6th ed. Philadelphia: Elsevier Science, 2005:489.

A.9. What are some factors that can lower pseudocholinesterase levels?

These include liver disease, advanced age, malnutrition, pregnancy, burns, oral contraceptives, monoamine oxidase inhibitors, echothiophate, cytotoxic drugs, neoplastic disease, anticholinesterase drugs, tetrahydroaminacrine, hexafluorenium, and metoclopramide.

Miller RD, ed. *Miller's anesthesia*, 6th ed. Philadelphia: Elsevier Science, 2005:487–488.

A.10. Should succinylcholine be routinely used in pediatric anesthesia?

No, unless there is urgent need to secure the airway rapidly. An increasing number of reports of adverse cardiovascular reactions, hyperkalemic cardiac arrests, and the possibility of malignant hyperthermia argue against routine use. The introduction of new shorter acting nondepolarizing muscle relaxants has decreased the need for the use of succinylcholine and caused a modification of the package insert as advocated by the U.S. Food and Drug Administration (FDA).

Belmont MR. Succinylcholine. *Curr Opin Anesth* 1995;8:362–366.

Miller RD, ed. *Miller's anesthesia*, 6th ed. Philadelphia: Elsevier Science, 2005:2378–2379.

Rosenberg H, Gronert GA. Intractable cardiac arrest in children given succinylcholine. *Anesthesiology* 1992;77:1054.

Schulte-Sasse VU, Eberlein HJ, Schumucker I, et al. Should the use of succinylcholine during pediatric anesthesia be reevaluated? *Anesthesiol Reanim* 1993;18:13.

A.11. Can mivacurium be used in patients with abnormal pseudocholinesterase?

The duration of action of mivacurium is directly related to the plasma cholinesterase activity of the patient. As with succinylcholine, the neuromuscular blocking effect of mivacurium is prolonged in patients with atypical plasma cholinesterase. In patients homozygous for the atypical enzyme, mivacurium acts as a very potent, long-acting nondepolarizer with a duration that can last for several hours depending on dose. When mivacurium is given to those who are heterozygous for the atypical gene, effects of the drug last 8 to 20 minutes longer than in healthy subjects.

Belmont MR, Rubin L, Lien C, et al. Mivacurium. *Anaesth Pharmacol Rev* 1995;3:1–12.

Ostergaard D, Jensen F, Jensen E, et al. Influence of plasma cholinesterase activity on recovery from mivacurium induced neuromuscular blockade in phenotypically normal patients. *Acta Anaesthesiol Scand* 1992;36:702–706.

Ostergaard D, Jensen F, Jensen E, et al. Mivacurium-induced neuromuscular blockade in patients with atypical plasma cholinesterase. *Acta Anaesthesiol Scand* 1993;37:314–318.

B. Preoperative Preparation

In this emergency situation, there was no opportunity to be aware of the atypical cholinesterase variant.

C. Intraoperative Management

C.1. When should the first dose of nondepolarizing muscle relaxant be given?

Recovery from the intubating dose of succinylcholine must be demonstrated before proceeding with paralysis with any of the nondepolarizers.

C.2. How is the choice among muscle relaxants made?

A muscle relaxant can be chosen based on onset characteristics, duration of action, and method of metabolism (Table 54.2). Muscle relaxants can be characterized as short, intermediate, and long duration. Metabolism may or may not be dependent on liver and kidney function.

Table 54.2 CHARACTERISTICS OF COMMONLY USED MUSCLE RELAXANTS.

DRUG	ED_{95} UNDER N_2O/O_2 (mg/kg)	DOSE FOR INTUBATION (mg/kg)	INTUBATION TIME (s)	CLINICAL DURATION (min)	METABOLISM (%)	ELIMINATION KIDNEY (%)	ELIMINATION LIVER (%)
Ultrashort acting							
Succinylcholine	0.5	1.0	60	5–10	Plasma cholinesterase (98–99)	<2	0
Short acting							
Mivacurium	0.08	0.2–0.25	120	12–15	Plasma cholinesterase (95–99)	<5	0
Intermediate acting							
Vecuronium	0.05	0.1–0.2	120	45–60	Liver (30–40)	40–50	50–60
Rocuronium	0.3	0.6–1.0	90	45–55	None	<10	>70
Cisatracurium	0.05	0.15–0.2	120	45–60	Hofmann elimination (77)	16	—
Long acting							
α-Tubocurarine	0.5	0.5–0.6	150	100–120	None	80	20
Pancuronium	0.07	0.08–0.12	150	100–120	Liver (10–20)	85	15
Pipecuronium	0.05	0.08–0.10	180	100–120	10	>90	<10
Doxacurium	0.025	0.05–0.08	240	120–150	None	>90	<10

Kaplan J, ed. *Cardiac anesthesia*, 5th ed. Philadelphia: WB Saunders, 2006:615–616.

Miller RD, ed. *Miller's anesthesia*, 6th ed. Philadelphia: Elsevier Science, 2005:2379–2380.

C.3. What is "train-of-four (TOF)?"

TOF is a method of assessing a neuromuscular block that consists of four indirect stimuli given at a rate of 2 Hz. As described by Ali, Utting, and Grey and Lee, the count of TOF can quantify the degree of block between 75% and 100%. During recovery, the reappearance of individual twitches may vary among patients. Satisfactory reversibility can be assured with one twitch of TOF corresponding to approximately 25% recovery. This information adds significantly to the practitioner's ability to judge the timing of reversal, recovery, and ultimately to safe extubation.

Ali HH, Utting J, Grey T. Quantitative assessment of residual antidepolarizing block. *Br J Anaesth* 1971;43:478.

Lee C. Train-of-4 quantitation of competitive neuromuscular block. *Anesth Analg* 1975;54: 649–653.

C.4. When is it safe to reverse muscle relaxants? What factors affect reversal?

It is safest to have some degree of spontaneous recovery before anticholinesterases are given, because their effectiveness depends on the degree of recovery present when they are given. More intense blocks require a longer recovery time and neostigmine is more effective than edrophonium in antagonizing intense blockade. Increasing the dose of reversal can help shorten the recovery time but there is no benefit in administering neostigmine at more than 70 μg per kg. The rate of recovery of the underlying relaxant affects the recovery after reversal as well. Short-acting neuromuscular blockers are reversed faster than intermediates, which recover faster than long-acting relaxants.

Donati F, Smith CE, Bevan DR. Dose response relationships for edrophonium and neostigmine as antagonists of moderate and profound atracurium blockade. *Anesth Analg* 1989;68:13.

Gencarelli PJ, Miller RD. Antagonism of ORG NC45 (vecuronium) and pancuronium neuromuscular blockade by neostigmine. *Br J Anaesth* 1982;54:53.

Miller RD, ed. *Miller's anesthesia*, 6th ed. Philadelphia: Elsevier Science, 2005:518–523.

Rupp SM, McChristian JW, Miller RD, et al. Neostigmine and edrophonium antagonism of varying intensity neuromuscular blockade induced by atracurium, pancuronium, or vecuronium. *Anesthesiology* 1986;64:711.

Smith CE, Donati F, Bevan DR, et al. Dose–response relationships for edrophonium and neostigmine as antagonists of atracurium and vecuronium neuromuscular blockade. *Anesthesiology* 1989;71:37.

C.5. What is adequate neuromuscular recovery and are clinical signs of recovery useful? Is train-of-four (TOF) a reliable measure?

Once the TOF ratio returns to more than 70%, sustained eye opening and head lift are possible. In awake volunteers, vital capacity, inspiratory force, and peak expiratory flow rates are at clinically acceptable values. Although a TOF at this ratio may provide some assurance of respiratory adequacy, it is not a guarantee that the muscles of airway protection are functional or that the patient is comfortable. Heavy eyelids, blurred vision, difficulty swallowing, and general discomfort can be observed even with a TOF ratio at 90%. Subjective assessment of the TOF fade is not reliable. Even when experienced observers evaluated responses, the presence of fade was frequently missed despite ratios as low as 50%. Because of this, the TOF count should be used intraoperatively to predict the extent of neuromuscular block and the ease with which residual block can be antagonized.

Kopman AF. Tactile evaluation of train-of-four count as an indicator of reliability of antagonism from vecuronium or atracurium-induced neuromuscular blockade. *Anesthesiology* 1991;75:588–593.

Pavlin EG, Holle RH, Schoene RB. Recovery of airway protection compared with ventilation in humans after paralysis with curare. *Anesthesiology* 1989;70:381–385.

Viby-Mogensen J, Jensen NH, Engbaek J, et al. Tactile and visual evaluation of the response to train-of-four stimulation. *Anesthesiology* 1985;63:440–442.

C.6. What percentage of postjunctional receptors must be blocked before transmission is diminished?

It remains important to remember that 75% of the receptors must be blocked before neuromuscular transmission is affected. After 75% of the receptors are occupied, there is an abrupt decline in transmission and surgical relaxation; that is, a TOF count between 1 and 2 corresponds to approximately 85% to 95% receptor blockade. This fact combined with the inherent lack of precision in TOF assessment underscores the need for adequate reversal at the end of a case.

Partridge B. Basic pharmacology of neuromuscular blocking agents. *Anesthesiol Clin North America* 1993;11(2):222–225.

D. Postoperative Management

D.1. What is the differential diagnosis for postoperative apnea? How would you treat it?

The differential diagnosis for postoperative apnea includes the following:

- Residual anesthetic agent
- Residual narcotic
- Residual muscle relaxant
- Hypocarbia
- Occurrence of some medical complication during anesthesia, such as stroke or embolism

Treatment of the patient would include discontinuance of anesthetics, checking the depth of narcosis and considering a titrated reversal of narcotics with naloxone, reversal of nondepolarizing relaxants with atropine and neostigmine, and determination of arterial blood gases and appropriate adjustment of ventilation. Ventilatory and circulatory support should be continued while arrangements are made for determination of cholinesterase unitage. Should these indicate an atypical cholinesterase, sedation and mechanical ventilation should continue until spontaneous recovery of neuromuscular function returns. Postoperatively, the patient and family should be informed. The patient should also be given a letter to be transmitted to any anesthesiologist who might provide future care for the patient.

Miller RD, ed. *Miller's anesthesia*, 6th ed. Philadelphia: Elsevier Science, 2005:2717–2718.

CHAPTER 55

Burns

Michael Tjeuw

A 45-YEAR-OLD MAN

who was smoking in bed sustained 40% second- and third-degree burns over his face, neck, chest, and upper extremities. He had a history of hypertension, angina, and angioplasty of the right coronary artery 1 year ago. He has smoked three packs of cigarettes per day for 20 years and he drinks alcohol daily. He is scheduled for tangential excision of eschar on the third day. Blood pressure, 190/100 mm Hg; heart rate, 120 beats per minute; and weight, 110 kg.

A. Medical Disease and Differential Diagnosis

1. How do you classify the burn injury?
2. How do you express the extent of the burn injury?
3. Should the "rule of nines" be used in children?
4. What is the definition of a major burn according to the American Burn Association?
5. What functions does the skin perform?
6. What pathophysiologic changes accompany major thermal injury?
7. Name some of the known mediators released with thermal injury. What are the responses to those mediators?
8. What is the prognosis for this patient? What major factors affect his prognosis?
9. What are the most common causes of death?
10. Does this patient have a smoke inhalation burn? How do you make the diagnosis?
11. Could you name some of the chemical products of combustion?
12. What is carbon monoxide poisoning? How do you treat carbon monoxide poisoning?
13. What resuscitative measure would you institute immediately in this patient with 40% burns?
14. What fluid formula would you use?
15. What cardiovascular changes typify the burn injury?
16. Is the immune system affected in burn injury? How?
17. What hematologic changes occur in burn injury?
18. What changes occur in liver function? What are the anesthetic implications of such changes?
19. What are Curling ulcers? How can they be prevented?
20. What complications are associated with electrical burns?

B. Preoperative Evaluation and Preparation

1. What preoperative preparations would you order? What are particular concerns in this patient?

2. What are the various operative and management options available for severely burned patients?

3. What is tangential excision split-thickness skin graft? What are the principles of this grafting technique?

4. What are the advantages and disadvantages of early tangential excision split-thickness skin graft?

5. What is this patient's mean arterial blood pressure? How do you calculate it?

6. Are you concerned about this patient's blood pressure? What treatment would you institute?

7. How do α_2-adrenergic agonists work?

8. This patient was ventilated with respirator settings of tidal volume 1,200 mL; respiratory rate, 20 breaths per minute; FIO_2, 60%; and positive end-expiratory pressure, 10 cm H_2O. Arterial blood gas analyses showed the following: pH, 7.25; PO_2, 56 mm Hg; PCO_2, 60 mm Hg; and O_2 saturation, 80%. How would you interpret these arterial blood gas analysis results? What are the possible causes of high PCO_2 and low PO_2?

9. How do you calculate oxygen content and oxygen delivery? What factors govern the oxygen delivery to the tissues? What are the causes of tissue hypoxia?

10. What are the symptoms and signs of alcohol withdrawal? Are you concerned that this patient could develop delirium tremens?

11. How would you prevent the adverse effects of alcohol withdrawal?

C. Intraoperative Management

1. What monitors would you use in the operating room?

2. What information can be obtained from an arterial line and a pulmonary artery catheter? How are these calculations performed?

3. If the patient had not been intubated, how would you proceed with the anesthetic induction?

4. Why is awake intubation considered the safest?

5. What anesthetic agents would you use? Discuss inhalation versus intravenous agents.

6. Why are you concerned about the patient's body temperature? What is normothermia for a burned patient?

7. How is temperature best maintained?

8. What derangements occur with hypothermia?

9. What muscle relaxant would you use?

10. Why is succinylcholine contraindicated in burned patients? For how long should it be avoided?

11. What other adverse effects are associated with succinylcholine?

12. How are the doses of nondepolarizing muscle relaxants affected by burn injury?

13. How are muscle relaxants such as curare, pancuronium, cisatracurium, vecuronium, doxacurium, rocuronium, and pipecuronium metabolized and eliminated? Which of them has significant histamine release?

14. What is the difference between metabolism and elimination of drugs?

15. What complications are associated with electrical burns?

D. Postoperative Management

1. How would you monitor this patient during transport?
2. What is meant by diffusion hypoxia? How do you prevent it?
3. Why do patients often shiver in the recovery room on emergence from anesthesia?
4. Discuss the causes of oliguria in the recovery room.

A. Medical Disease and Differential Diagnosis

A.1. How do you classify the burn injury?

Burns are classified as first, second, or third degree. First-degree, or superficial, burns are characterized by simple erythema of the skin, with only microscopic destruction of superficial layers of the epidermis. Second-degree, or partial-thickness, burns extend through the epidermis into the dermis. Even when most of the epithelium is destroyed, regeneration may occur from epithelial cells surrounding hair follicles or sweat glands. Third-degree, or full-thickness, burns are characterized by total, irreversible destruction of all the skin, dermal appendages, and epithelial elements. Spontaneous regeneration of epithelium is not possible and the burns are described as full-thickness burns. Such burns require the application of skin grafts if the development of scar tissue is to be avoided. Fourth-degree burns refer to deep thermal injuries involving fascia, muscle, or bone (Table 55.1).

Brunicardi FC, Anderson DK, eds. *Schwartz's principles of surgery*, 8th ed. New York: McGraw-Hill, 2005:189–216.

MacLennan N, Heimbach DM, Cullen BF. Anaesthesia for major thermal injury. *Anesthesiology* 1998;89:749–770.

A.2. How do you express the extent of the burn injury?

The extent of the burn injury is expressed as a percentage of the total body surface area (TBSA) displaying either second- or third-degree burns. It is most commonly estimated by the "rule of

---

Table 55.1 Classification of Burn Depth.

CLASSIFICATION	BURN DEPTH	OUTCOME
Superficial		
First degree	Confined to epidermis	Heals spontaneously
Partial thickness		
Second degree		
Superficial dermal burn	Epidermis and upper dermis	Heals spontaneously
Deep dermal burn	Epidermis and deep dermis	Requires excision and grafting for rapid return of function
Full thickness		
Third-degree burn	Destruction of epidermis and dermis	Wound excision and grafting required Some limitation of function and scar formation
Fourth-degree burn	Muscle, fascia, bone	Complete excision required, limited function

(From MacLennan N, Heimbach DM, Cullen BF. Anesthesia for major thermal injury. *Anesthesiology* 1998;89:749–779, with permission.)

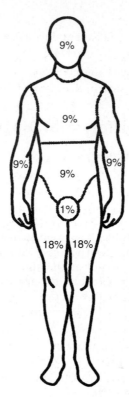

Figure 55.1 The rule of nines for determining the percentage of body surface area burned in adults. (From MacLennan N, Heimbach DM, Cullen BF. Anesthesia for major thermal injury. *Anesthesiology* 1998;89:749–770, with permission.)

nines" (Fig. 55.1). The major anatomic portions of the adult may be divided into multiples of 9% of the body surface area. The proportion of each of these areas is estimated and the sum represents the percentage of the TBSA burn. The percentages of body surface are as follows:

- Head and neck   9%
- Right upper extremity   9%
- Left upper extremity   9%
- Right lower extremity   18%
- Left lower extremity   18%
- Anterior trunk   18%
- Posterior trunk   18%
- Perineum   1%

Brunicardi FC, Anderson DK, eds. *Schwartz's principles of surgery*, 8th ed. New York: McGraw-Hill, 2005:189–216.

MacLennan N, Heimbach DM, Cullen BF. Anesthesia for major thermal injury. *Anesthesiology* 1998;89:749–770.

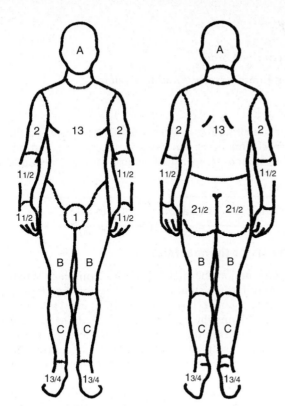

Relative percentages of areas affected by growth

AREA	AGE IN YEARS					
	0	1	5	10	15	Adult
A: half of head	9½	8½	6½	5½	4½	3½
B: half of thigh	2¾	3¼	4	4¼	4½	4¾
C: half of leg	2½	2½	2¾	3	3¼	3½

Figure 55.2 Diagram and table for determining the percentage of body surface area burned in children. (From MacLennan N, Heimbach DM, Cullen BF. Anesthesia for major thermal injury. *Anesthesiology* 1998;89:749–770, with permission.)

A.3. Should the "rule of nines" be used in children?

The "rule of nines" may not be used to estimate total body surface area (TBSA) burns in children because the surface area of the head and neck in children is significantly larger than 9%, and that of the lower extremities is smaller. More precise methods, such as the Lund and Browder chart, may be used to provide greater accuracy by taking into account the changing proportions of the body from infancy to adulthood (Fig. 55.2).

Brunicardi FC, Anderson DK, eds. *Schwartz's principles of surgery*, 8th ed, New York: McGraw-Hill, 2005:189–216.

MacLennan N, Heimbach DM, Cullen BF. Anesthesia for major thermal injury. *Anesthesiology* 1998;89:749–770.

A.4. What is the definition of a major burn according to the American Burn Association?

The American Burn Association defines a major burn as follows:

- Full-thickness burns more than 10% total body surface area (TBSA)
- Partial-thickness burns more than 25% in adults or 20% at extremes of age

- Burns involving face, hands, feet, or perineum
- Inhalation, chemical, or electrical burns
- Burns in patients with serious preexisting medical disorders

Adapted from the American Burn Association Injury Severity Grading System.

A.5. What functions does the skin perform?

The skin is the largest organ of the body, with surface area ranging from 1.5 to 2.0 m^2 in the adult. It protects the invasion of microorganisms. It performs other functions in thermal regulation, fluid and electrolytes homeostasis, and sensation (touch, temperature, pain). The skin also has metabolic functions including vitamin D metabolism.

Herndon DN, ed. *Total burn care*, 2nd ed. Philadelphia: WB Saunders, 2002:184–185.

A.6. What pathophysiologic changes accompany major thermal injury?

The pathophysiologic alterations that accompany major thermal injury are complex. When destroyed, skin, which is the largest organ of the body, has a systemic impact. Thermal regulation, fluid and electrolyte homeostasis, and protection against bacterial infection are affected. Immediately after a burn injury, mediators released from the burn wound contribute to local inflammation and edema. A large amount of fluid is lost from the vascular compartment into the burn wound. Sequestration in the extravascular space results in significant hemoconcentration. Increased secretion of antidiuretic hormone (ADH) may decrease or even completely inhibit urinary output. It has been shown that during the first 4 days after a burn, an amount of albumin equal to twice the total plasma albumin content is lost through the wound. Half of this fluid remains sequestered in the extravascular space for 3 weeks or more before returning to the intravascular compartment.

The metabolic rate is markedly increased after the burn injury. Depending on the size of the burn, the increase in metabolic rate can be doubled or tripled with a proportionate increase in oxygen consumption and carbon dioxide production. This hypermetabolic state will continue for weeks or months until full skin coverage is achieved and the tissue repair processes are complete. Cardiac output is often decreased in patients with major burns. This decrease is not entirely explained by the rapid reduction in circulating blood volume. It has been shown that a circulating myocardial-depressant factor exists in both humans and laboratory animals.

Changes in vascular integrity occur in other areas remote from the injury site. The entire vascular compartment in the body becomes permeable to circulating macromolecules, such as dextran. This capillary leak syndrome is manifested as edema. In the lung, severe pulmonary edema can be life threatening.

Pulmonary function decreases markedly. Functional residual capacity is reduced. Both lung compliance and chest wall compliance decrease markedly. The alveolar-arterial ($PAO_2–PaO_2$) oxygen gradient increases. Minute ventilation is increased; it can be as high as 40 L per minute (normal, 6 L per minute).

Brunicardi FC, Anderson DK, eds. *Schwartz's principles of surgery*, 8th ed. New York: McGraw-Hill, 2005:189–216.

Herndon DN, ed. *Total burn care*, 2nd ed. Philadelphia: WB Saunders, 2002:79–85.

MacLennan N, Heimbach DM, Cullen BF. Anesthesia for major thermal injury. *Anesthesiology* 1998;89:749–770.

A.7. Name some of the known mediators released with thermal injury? What are the responses to those mediators?

After a thermal injury, mediators released from the burn wound contribute to local inflammation and edema. Local mediators include histamine, prostaglandins, bradykinin, nitric oxide, serotonin, and substance P.

In minor burns, the inflammatory process is limited to the wound itself. In major burns, local injury triggers the release of circulating (systemic) mediators, resulting in a systemic response. This is characterized by hypermetabolism, immune suppression, and the systemic inflammatory response syndrome (protein catabolism, sepsis, multiple organ failures).

The systemic mediators are cytokines (interleukins), endotoxin, and nitric oxide (Fig. 55.3).

Brunicardi FC, Anderson DK, eds. *Schwartz's principles of surgery*, 8th ed. New York: McGraw-Hill, 2005:189–216.

Herndon DN, ed. *Total burn care*, 2nd ed. Philadelphia: WB Saunders, 2002:81–83.

MacLennan N, Heimbach DM, Cullen BF. Anesthesia for major thermal injury. *Anesthesiology* 1998;89:749–770.

A.8. What is the prognosis for this patient? What major factors affect his prognosis?

The prognosis for this patient is very poor. Statistical survival based on total body surface area (TBSA) alone would predict a less than 50% chance of survival. Other factors that affect

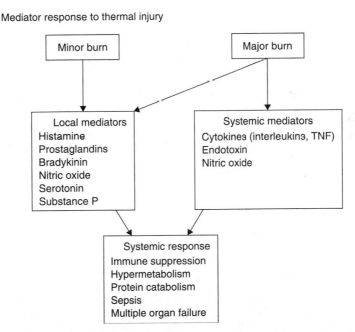

Figure 55.3 Mediators released with thermal injury and the response to their release. TNF, tumor necrosis factor. (From MacLennan N, Heimbach DM, Cullen BF. Anesthesia for major thermal injury. *Anesthesiology* 1998;89:749–770, with permission.)

his prognosis are age, size and depth of burn, associated pulmonary injury, and preexisting medical disease. In view of this patient, who had angioplasty for coronary artery disease and hypertension and who is a heavy smoker and obese, the risk of myocardial infarction is greatly increased.

A.9. What are the most common causes of death?

With the understanding of vigorous early fluid resuscitation, hypovolemic shock is not common in United States. The major early cause of death is asphyxia. The most common cause of long-term mortality is septic complications.

A.10. Does this patient have a smoke inhalation burn? How do you make the diagnosis?

The patient probably sustained a smoke inhalation burn. Smoke inhalation should be highly suspected in patients who were burned in an enclosed space, received burns of the face, were burned while under the influence of alcohol or drugs, or lost consciousness at the time of the accident.

A patient with smoke inhalation often exhibits no physical signs or symptoms during the first 24 hours after the burn. Diagnosis is dependent on a high index of suspicion and careful physical and laboratory examination. The early symptoms and signs of respiratory tract injury include singed nasal hair; burned nasal mucosa, lips, and mouth; hoarseness; wheezing; and brassy cough with soot in the sputum. The posterior pharynx may appear red and the larynx may appear edematous. Radiographic findings are usually negative immediately after injury; this is the "clear or lucid period." Laboratory tests include blood gas analysis, carboxyhemoglobin concentration, xenon scans, and fiberoptic bronchoscopy.

Brunicardi FC, Anderson DK, eds. *Schwartz's principles of surgery*, 8th ed. New York: McGraw-Hill, 2005:189–216.

Herndon DN, ed. *Total burn care*, 2nd ed. Philadelphia: WB Saunders, 2002:233–234.

MacLennan N, Heimbach DM, Cullen BF. Anesthesia for major thermal injury. *Anesthesiology* 1998;89:749–770.

A.11. Could you name some of the chemical products of combustion?

Carbon monoxide is produced by incomplete combustion of carbon-containing compounds such as wood, coal, and gasoline. Other chemical products of combustion include ammonia, nitrogen dioxide, sulfur dioxide, and chlorine. These chemicals combine with water to produce strong acids and alkalines.

MacLennan N, Heimbach DM, Cullen BF. Anesthesia for major thermal injury. *Anesthesiology* 1998;89:749–770.

A.12. What is carbon monoxide poisoning? How do you treat carbon monoxide poisoning?

Carbon monoxide is the leading cause of hypoxia in survivors of burn injuries. Carbon monoxide has a 200 times greater affinity for hemoglobin than oxygen and therefore displaces oxygen from its hemoglobin-binding sites. Fortunately, this reaction is a competitive, reversible one, so oxygen therapy should be instituted immediately. The half-life for carbon monoxide elimination from hemoglobin can be shortened from 4 hours to 45 minutes with an inspired oxygen concentration of 100%. Although the PaO_2 may be normal, the actual content of oxygen in the blood is markedly reduced.

Brunicardi FC, Anderson DK, eds. *Schwartz's principles of surgery*, 8th ed. New York: McGraw-Hill, 2005:189–216.

Fein A, Leff A, Hopewell PC. Pathophysiology and management of the complications resulting from fire and the inhaled products of combustion: review of the literature. *Crit Care Med* 1980;94:98.

Herndon DN, ed. *Total burn care*, 2nd ed. Philadelphia: WB Saunders, 2002:235.

A.13. What resuscitative measure would you institute immediately in this patient with 40% burns?

Vigorous fluid resuscitation should be instituted immediately to combat the danger of hypovolemia from translocation of intravascular volume into the burn edema, which acts as a "third space." Fluid must be administered adequately to ensure good tissue perfusion and adequate urine output. The airway should be maintained to ensure adequate ventilation. If an upper airway burn is involved, endotracheal intubation is indicated.

A.14. What fluid formula would you use?

Over the last 30 years, many fluid formulas have been developed as guides to initial resuscitation in hypovolemic shock after burn injury. Most use various combinations of crystalloid and colloid solutions, but they differ widely in the colloid/crystalloid ratio and in the rate of fluid administration. Although much controversy still surrounds the use of "the solution" for resuscitation in burn shock, scientific investigation supports the need for both crystalloid and colloid solutions (Table 55.2). Which formula is used to begin such therapy matters little, as long as it is modified according to the patient's changing requirements. The Parkland formula, popularized by Baxter, has been adopted in most burn centers because of its simplicity, reduced cost, and equivalent outcome and is currently the standard against which new formulas must be compared.

Parkland formula

First 24 Hours

- *Electrolyte solution (lactated Ringer's).* 4 mL/kg/percentage of body area with second- and third-degree burn

Table 55.2 Fluid Resuscitation for Adults with Major Burns.

Crystalloid Regimens		
Parkland	Lactated Ringer's	4 mL/kg/% burn
Modified Brooke	Lactated Ringer's	2 mL/kg/% burn
Colloid regimens		
Evans	Normal saline	1 mL/kg/% burn
	Colloid	1 mL/kg/% burn
	5% Dextrose	2,000 mL/24 hr
Brooke	Lactated Ringer's	1.5 mL/kg/% burn
	Colloid	0.5 mL/kg/% burn
	5% Dextrose	2,000 mL/24 hr

(From MacLennan N, Heimbach DM, Cullen BF. Anesthesia for major thermal injury. *Anesthesiology* 1998;89:749–770, with permission.)

- *Administration rate.* Half the solution given in the first 8 hours, one quarter in the second 8 hours, one quarter in the third 8 hours
- *Urine output.* Maintain at 0.5 to 1.0 mL/kg/hour

Second 24 Hours

- *Glucose in water.* To replace evaporated water loss and maintain serum sodium concentration of 140 mEq per L
- *Colloid solutions (e.g., albumin).* Amount proportional to burn
  - *30% to 50% burn:* 0.3 mL/kg/percentage of burn
  - *50% to 70% burn:* 0.4 mL/kg/percentage of burn
  - *Larger than 70% burn:* 0.5 mL/kg/percentage of burn
- *Urine output.* Maintain at 0.5 to 1.0 mL/kg/hour

Brunicardi FC, Anderson DK, eds. *Schwartz's principles of surgery*, 8th ed. New York: McGraw-Hill, 2005:189–216.

Herndon DN, ed. *Total burn care*, 2nd ed. Philadelphia: WB Saunders, 2002:90–94.

MacLennan N, Heimbach DM, Cullen BF. Anesthesia for major thermal injury. *Anesthesiology* 1998;89:749–770.

A.15. What cardiovascular changes typify the burn injury?

Cardiovascular changes develop in several phases. Acutely, fluid sequestration in the burned area and from capillary leak is caused by direct thermal destruction of the capillary membranes. This results in a massive shift of fluids and proteins from the intravascular compartment to the interstitial spaces. This shift of fluid accounts for the marked decrease in circulating blood volume, resulting in hypotension or the initial burn shock. Decreased blood volume and decreased cardiac output would trigger catecholamine release, resulting in severe vasoconstriction, which may further compromise forward flow and tissue perfusion. Release of myocardial-depressant factors may further depress cardiac output through its direct action on myocardial contractility.

Brunicardi FC, Anderson DK, eds. *Schwartz's principles of surgery*, 8th ed. New York: McGraw-Hill, 2005:189–216.

Hendon DN, ed. *Total burn care*, 2nd ed. Philadelphia: WB Saunders, 2002:83–85.

Sugi K, Theissen J, Traber LD, et al. Impact of carbon monoxide on cardiopulmonary dysfunction after smoke inhalation injury. *Circ Res* 1990;66:69–75.

A.16. Is the immune system affected in burn injury? How?

Both the cellular and the humoral components of the immune system are impaired. The presence of devitalized tissue greatly increases the risk of wound infection and systemic sepsis. Endotoxins cause changes in cellular function. Macrophage activity in the alveolar is impaired. Changes in phagocytic and chemotactic properties of neutrophils have been demonstrated. Strict antiseptic precautions must be observed in these patients.

Brunicardi FC, Anderson DK, eds. *Schwartz's principles of surgery*, 8th ed. New York: McGraw-Hill, 2005:189–216.

Herndon DN, ed. *Total burn care*, 2nd ed. Philadelphia: WB Saunders, 2002:334–335,350–351.

A.17. What hematologic changes occur in burn injury?

Hematologic changes can be seen in erythrocytes (red blood cells [RBCs]), platelets, and the coagulation mechanism.

Erythrocytes (RBCs). Immediately after injury, the hematocrit level increases as noncellular fluid translocates into the interstitium. Anemia is more often the case after fluid resuscitation because of RBC damage and hemolysis during the heating injury. There is shortened RBC half-life and reduction of production due to circulating inhibitory factors.

Platelets. The platelet count usually decreases because of dilutional and consumption by formation of microaggregates in the skin and smoke damaged lung. The platelet level returns to normal by the end of the first week unless sepsis or multiple system organ failure occurs.

Coagulation. Both the thrombotic and the fibrinolytic mechanisms are activated, and clotting factors decrease. Disseminated intravascular coagulopathy is rare but can occur, particularly in fourth-degree burns involving structures deep to the skin.

Brunicardi FC, Anderson DK, eds. *Schwartz's principles of surgery*, 8th ed. New York: McGraw-Hill, 2005:189–216.

MacLennan N, Heimbach DM, Cullen BF. Anesthesia for major thermal injury. *Anesthesiology* 1998;89:749–770.

A.18. What changes occur in liver function? What are the anesthetic implications of such changes?

Hypoperfusion during burn shock can result in decreased hepatic function, severely depressing the detoxification capacity of the liver. Decreased levels of albumin may result in greater free fractions of bound drugs such as benzodiazepines and phenytoin. In contrast, the injury-stimulated rise in the acute-phase reactant α_1-acid-glycoprotein increases the binding of basic drugs such as muscle relaxants, lidocaine, and propranolol.

Brunicardi FC, Anderson DK, eds. *Schwartz's principles of surgery*, 8th ed. New York: McGraw-Hill, 2005:189–216.

Herndon DN, ed. *Total burn care*, 2nd ed. Philadelphia: WB Saunders, 2002:190.

Martyn JAJ. The use of neuromuscular relaxants in burn patients. In: Rupp SM, ed. *Problems in anesthesia*. Philadelphia: JB Lippincott, 1989:482.

A.19. What are Curling ulcers? How can they be prevented?

Curling ulcer is a stress ulcer of the duodenum commonly found after a severe burn. Gastric ulceration may occur also. Without treatment, the incidence is as high as 80%. The frequency and severity correlate with the size of the burn. They may present with gastric bleeding. They can be prevented with prophylactic antacids, H_2-antagonists, and early enteral feeding.

Brunicardi FC, Anderson DK, eds. *Schwartz's principles of surgery*, 8th ed. New York: McGraw-Hill, 2005:189–216.

MacLennan N, Heimbach DM, Cullen BF. Anesthesia for major thermal injury. *Anesthesiology* 1998;89:749–770.

A.20. What complications are associated with electrical burns?

The burn from electrical current results from the conversion of electrical energy to thermal energy. The damages may vary and are determined by the area of contact, the resistances of the tissues, and the duration of current flow. Often, only the surface entrance and exit sites on the skin show visible injury because of the high current concentrations at these points. Deep tissues such as muscles, tendons, blood vessels, and nerves can be severely injured. Vascular complications such as thrombosis can be late complications. The heart is particularly susceptible to electrical damage. Ectopy and congestive heart failure can be signs of electrical injury.

B. Preoperative Evaluation and Preparation

B.1. What preoperative preparations would you order? What are particular concerns in this patient?

Preoperative preparations should include a medical history, physical examination, and the usual concerns regarding cardiac disease, pulmonary disease, renal function, liver function, anesthetic history, and family history. Of particular concern in this patient are hypertension, ischemic heart disease, angioplasty of left main coronary artery, and the history of heavy smoking and heavy alcohol consumption.

The adequacy of fluid volume resuscitation should be assessed.
Hemodynamic stability should have been achieved.

Laboratory tests should include complete blood cell count, platelet count, electrolytes, blood urea nitrogen, creatinine, coagulation studies, urinalysis, liver function test, electrocardiogram (ECG), chest radiograph, and arterial and venous blood gases.

Other data that may be helpful include central venous pressure (CVP), pulmonary capillary wedge pressure (PCWP), cardiac output, and cardiac index (CI).

In view of this patient's left main coronary artery disease, cardiac enzymes studies in conjunction with cardiologist involvement would be beneficial.

B.2. What are the various operative and management options available for severely burned patients?

Deep partial-thickness and full-thickness burns will not heal spontaneously and require excision and skin graft. The burned skin or eschar is a good culture medium for bacterial growth. Although topical antibiotic creams such as silver sulfadiazine can be applied to control the infection, the definitive treatment is excision of eschar.

The timing and extent of burn wound excision are still debatable; there has been a shift toward earlier excision and grafting. The most widely used approach involves an initial 48-hour period of stabilization, followed by tangential excision split-thickness skin graft (TE/STSG). The extent of excision is limited to 20%. These procedures are repeated every 2 days until the eschar excision is complete. Some favor very early excision (<24 hours from the time of burn).

Brunicardi FC, Anderson DK, eds. *Schwartz's principles of surgery*, 8th ed. New York: McGraw-Hill, 2005:189–216.

Herndon DN, ed. *Total burn care*, 2nd ed. Philadelphia: WB Saunders, 2002:170–180.

MacLennan N, Heimbach DM, Cullen BF. Anesthesia for major thermal injury. *Anesthesiology* 1998;89:749–770.

B.3. What is tangential excision split-thickness skin graft (TE/STSG)? What are the principles of this grafting technique?

TE/STSG is a procedure to debride the dead skin and graft on new layers. The burn eschar is sharply excised from the underlying subcutaneous tissue. Brisk capillary bleeding signifies that adequate excision has been achieved and viable tissue uncovered. Skin grafts may be either full thickness or split (partial) thickness. Full-thickness grafts include all layers of epidermis and dermis in their sample. Therefore, the donor site must be closed primarily. Suitable donor sites are the skinfolds of the axilla and groin. A tissue expander is commonly used to increase the available donor skin. Full-thickness grafts have the advantage of better cosmesis and durability, and they are useful when tissue bulk is desired. More commonly, STSGs are used. These grafts are obtained by slicing the superficial layers of the skin through the level of the dermal pegs. Because maturation of skin cells occurs as they migrate superficially, the graft has many viable layers of dermal cells. When placed on a viable bed of subcutaneous tissue, ingrowth of vessels occurs and the graft remains viable. In addition, because the excision of donor skin is through the dermis, the deep basement membrane and skin appendages remain intact. Hence, the donor site will heal on its own, architecturally normal, usually with only mild discoloration.

Brunicardi FC, Anderson DK, eds. *Schwartz's principles of surgery*, 8th ed. New York: McGraw-Hill, 2005:189–216.

Herndon DN, ed. *Total burn care*, 2nd ed. Philadelphia: WB Saunders, 2002:172–177.

B.4. What are the advantages and disadvantages of early tangential excision split-thickness skin graft?

By excising the burn eschar early (within 7 to 10 days), one can remove the bacterial load quickly and achieve prompt skin coverage with resultant lessening of septic complications; the hospital and recovery phases are therefore shortened. Very early excision (within 24 hours), however, has the disadvantage of the patient undergoing a major operation during the resuscitative phase of the injury. The patient is not optimally stabilized, and there is an increase in anesthetic risk.

Cultured epithelial autografts are an exacting new technique that can be of great use in patients with large total body surface area (TBSA) burns in which donor sites are few in number.

Brunicardi FC, Anderson DK, eds. *Schwartz's principles of surgery*, 8th ed. New York: McGraw-Hill, 2005:189–216.

Herndon DN, ed. *Total burn care*, 2nd ed. Philadelphia: WB Saunders, 2002:170–180.

Herndon DN, Barrow RE, Rutan TC, et al. A comparison of conservative versus early excision. *Ann Surg* 1989;209(5):547–553.

Munster AM, Weiner SH, Spence RJ. Cultured epidermis for the coverage of massive burn wounds: a single center experience. *Ann Surg* 1990;211:676–680.

B.5. What is this patient's mean arterial blood pressure? How do you calculate it?

The patient's blood pressure is 190/100 mm Hg; therefore, his mean arterial blood pressure is 130 mm Hg (mean arterial pressure = diastolic pressure + one third of pulse pressure, which is the difference between systolic and diastolic pressure).

B.6. Are you concerned about this patient's blood pressure? What treatment would you institute?

The blood pressure is quite high (190/100 mm Hg). Knowing that this patient has a history of ischemic heart disease with symptoms of angina that required angioplasty of the left main coronary artery 1 year ago, I am very concerned about his hypertension and would like to control the blood pressure to the normal range.

The following intravenous vasodilators may be used:

- Nitroprusside
- Nitroglycerine α_2-agonist such as clonidine

In view of his tachycardia (heart rate, 120 beats per minute), I would prefer an α_2-agonist. Increased afterload and tachycardia would increase oxygen demand on the heart and increase the risk of myocardial infarction.

Adequate volume resuscitation should be assessed, so obtaining pulmonary capillary wedge pressure (PCWP), cardiac output (CO), cardiac index (CI), and systemic vascular resistance would be helpful in instituting treatment.

B.7. How do α_2-adrenergic agonists work?

α_2-Agonists such as clonidine stimulate the presynaptic α_2-receptors centrally in the medulla of the brainstem and inhibit the release of norepinephrine, thereby decreasing sympathetic outflow from the vasopressor centers in the brainstem. Decreased sympathetic outflow results in vasodilation, decreased blood pressure, and bradycardia.

Katzung BG, ed. *Basic and clinical pharmacology*, 8th ed. New York: McGraw-Hill, 2001: 160–162.

B.8. This patient was ventilated with respirator settings of tidal volume, 1,200 mL; respiratory rate, 20 breaths per minute; FIO_2, 60%; and positive end-expiratory pressure, 10 cm H_2O. Arterial blood gas analyses showed the following: pH, 7.25; PO_2, 56 mm Hg; PCO_2, 60 mm Hg; and O_2 saturation, 80%. How would you interpret these arterial blood gas analysis results? What are the possible causes of high PCO_2 and low PO_2?

Arterial blood gas analysis results are abnormal. This patient was hypoventilated with high PCO_2 of 60 mm Hg (normal PCO_2 is 35 to 45 mm Hg), although the minute volume was 24 L (1,200 mL × 20), the increase in minute volume might not have compensated for his hypermetabolic state with marked increase in CO_2 production.

Ventilation/perfusion mismatch is the most common cause of hypoxemia. Causes of ventilation/perfusion mismatches range from dead space to shunt. The common causes are atelectasis, pneumonia, and pulmonary edema.

This patient had respiratory acidosis and probably mild metabolic acidosis.

Malposition of endotracheal tube with single-lung ventilation is a possible cause that should be ruled out.

B.9. How do you calculate oxygen content and oxygen delivery? What factors govern the oxygen delivery to the tissues? What are the causes of tissue hypoxia?

Oxygen content consists of oxygen in combination with hemoglobin and oxygen dissolved in plasma and can be expressed as:

Oxygen content (mL/dL) $= 1.31 \times$ hemoglobin (g/dL) $\times O_2$, saturation (%) $+ 0.003 \times PO_2$
Normal $CaO_2 = 20.73$ mL per 100 mL
Normal $C_vO_2 = 15.76$ mL per 100 mL

Oxygen delivery is the product of cardiac output (CO) and arterial oxygen content.

$DO_2 = CO \times CaO_2$
$= CO \times ([1.31 \times$ hemoglobin $\times O_2$, saturation$] + 0.003 \times PO_2)$

Three main factors govern the oxygen delivery: cardiac output, hemoglobin, and arterial oxygen saturation.

Tissue hypoxia may be due to the following:

- Inadequate cardiac output: "stagnant anoxia"
- Inadequate arterial oxygen saturation: "anoxic anoxia"
- Reduction of hemoglobin concentration: "anemic anoxia"

Lumb AB. *Nunn's applied respiratory physiology*, 6th ed. Philadelphia: Butterworth-Heinemann, 2005:188.

B.10. What are the symptoms and signs of alcohol withdrawal? Are you concerned that this patient could develop delirium tremens?

Minor withdrawal symptoms are anorexia, insomnia, tremors, mild disorientation, hallucination, and convulsion. These symptoms usually peak within 10 to 30 hours of cessation of drinking. Major withdrawal symptoms occur later and are characterized by severe autonomic hyperactivity, which includes anxiety, tachycardia, diaphoresis, tremors, fever, hallucination, and global convulsion. These major symptoms are also known as *delirium tremens*. There is a real concern that this patient could develop withdrawal syndrome. Early treatment should be instituted.

B.11. How would you prevent the adverse effects of alcohol withdrawal?

Sedatives, such as benzodiazepines, are effective in preventing the withdrawal symptoms. If autonomic hyperactivity symptoms occur, β-blockers are helpful to attenuate the symptoms, especially tachycardia and dysrhythmias.

C. Intraoperative Management

C.1. What monitors would you use in the operating room?

The routinely used monitors, such as electrocardiogram (ECG), blood pressure, temperature, inspired oxygen, pulse oximetry, and capnography, should be used in this patient. A urinary catheter is essential to assess urine output. An indwelling arterial line is helpful, because a standard blood pressure cuff would be difficult to apply over the areas to be grafted and harvested. A pulmonary artery catheter or central venous pressure (CVP) catheter is recommended for the severely burned patient, especially a patient with ischemic heart disease.

C.2. What information can be obtained from an arterial line and a pulmonary artery catheter? How are these calculations performed?

The arterial line can display direct continuous blood pressure, thereby providing continuous real-time monitoring of blood pressure. This is most useful in fluctuating hypotensive or hypertensive situations. In conditions such as atrial fibrillation or ventricular tachycardia, variations in ventricular response or blood pressure can be recognized instantly. In addition, it serves as ready vascular access for blood sampling—for example, arterial blood gas analyses, electrolytes, hematocrit, and blood sugar levels.

Pulmonary artery catheter allows measurement of pulmonary capillary wedge pressure (PCWP). The PCWP parallels left atrial pressures. Left atrial pressure reflects left ventricular end-diastolic pressure, which is helpful in assessing the preload status of the left ventricle. Central venous pressure (CVP), although useful as a rough estimate of preload, does not correlate with left ventricular end-diastolic pressure when either isolated right-sided or left-sided cardiac dysfunction occurs.

The multilumen pulmonary artery catheters are capable of measuring CVP and cardiac output (CO) through the thermodilution method. It also permits sampling of mixed venous blood. These measurements permit calculation of many hemodynamic variables.

$$\text{Cardiac index (CI)} = \frac{CO}{\text{Body surface area}} \quad \text{(normal 2.8 to 4.2 L/min/m}^2)$$

$$\text{Stroke volume(SV)} = \frac{CO}{\text{Heart rate}} \quad \text{(normal 60–80 mL/beat)}$$

$$\text{Stroke index(SI)} = \frac{CI}{\text{Heart rate}} \quad \text{(normal 40–65 mL/beat/m}^2)$$

$$\text{Systemic vascular resistance(SVR)} = \frac{\text{Mean BP} - \text{CVP}}{CO} \times 80$$

$$\text{(normal 900–1,400 dynes/sec/cm}^5)$$

$$\text{Pulmonary vascular resistance(PVR)} = \frac{\text{Mean PAP} - \text{PCWP}}{CO} \times 80$$

$$\text{(normal 150–250 dynes/sec/cm}^5)$$

Mixed venous blood samples are needed for shunt calculations:

$$\frac{O_s}{Q_t} = \frac{Cco_2 - Cao_2}{Cco_2 - C\overline{v}o_2}$$

Cco_2 = pulmonary capillary oxygen content
Cao_2 = artery oxygen content
$C\overline{v}o_2$ = mixed venous oxygen content

A low mixed venous oxygen level (<30 mm Hg) is suggestive of inadequate tissue perfusion.

Miller RD, ed. *Miller's anesthesia*, 6th ed. Philadelphia: Elsevier: Churchill Livingstone, 2005:1325–1333.

C.3. If the patient had not been intubated, how would you proceed with the anesthetic induction?

One should anticipate a difficult intubation because this patient has burns over his face and neck. Burns on the face may cause severe edema of the face, pharynx, and larynx, so careful assessment of the mouth opening, pharynx, and larynx should be performed. The safest way to secure the airway is to do an awake intubation with topical anesthesia and mild sedation; it can be achieved with either direct or fiberoptic-guided intubation. If prolonged postoperative intubation is anticipated, the nasotracheal route should be considered. A nasotracheal tube is more easily secured in place, is better tolerated by the patient, and permits better oral hygienic care. Vasoconstriction of the nasal mucosa may be achieved with phenylephrine drops.

C.4. Why is awake intubation considered the safest?

Awake intubation is considered the safest way to secure an airway because when the patient is awake and breathing spontaneously, the patient is less likely to obstruct the upper airway by the tongue and is less likely to have oxygen desaturation. The anesthesiologist does not have to ventilate using a mask and is therefore less likely to distend the stomach.

If the patient is breathing spontaneously and has adequate oxygenation, the anesthesiologist has more time to do a proper laryngoscopy or manipulation of the endotracheal tube. Identifying the passage of air from the glottis may be helpful in blind intubation.

C.5. What anesthetic agents would you use? Discuss inhalation versus intravenous agents.

For the severely burned patient, once the airway is secured, high-dose narcotic-muscle relaxant technique would be preferred, because this technique offers good intraoperative hemodynamic stability in critically ill patients, coupled with excellent postoperative analgesia.

The narcotics such as morphine, meperidine (Demerol), fentanyl, or sufentanil can be used because they do not depress myocardial contractility, whereas inhalation agents depress the myocardium. If inhalation agents are chosen, the concentration should be carefully titrated to prevent loss of cardiovascular compensation.

C.6. Why are you concerned about the patient's body temperature? What is normothermia for a burned patient?

Massively burned patients with loss of skin have constant evaporation from open surfaces. They tend to develop severe intraoperative hypothermia. The tendency is exaggerated by the effects of general anesthesia on the temperature-regulating centers, by vasodilation and by the cool relatively dry environment of the operating room. The infusion of a large amount of intravenous fluids at room temperature also contributes to the development of hypothermia.

Normothermia for a burned patient is approximately 38.5°C because the burned patient develops a resetting of the centrally mediated thermostat.

Brunicardi FC, Anderson DK, eds. *Schwartz's principles of surgery*, 8th ed. New York: McGraw-Hill, 2005:189–216.

Herndon DN, ed. *Total burn care*, 2nd ed. Philadelphia: WB Saunders, 2002:175.

C.7. How is temperature best maintained?

Hypothermia is an ever-present problem. Burned patients have lost their natural insulation of the skin. Heat loss can occur through convection, conduction, and evaporation. Methods to maintain normothermia should involve active warming and prevention of heat loss. We administer all fluids and blood transfusions through the blood- and/or fluid-warming device. A thermal mattress is placed under a single-layer sterile sheet on the operating table and is prewarmed, although this method is not very effective. Warming the operating room to temperatures between 24°C (75.2°F) and 27°C (80.6°F) with a relative humidity higher than 50% is particularly effective. The areas of the patient's body not immediately involved in the surgery must be covered. Heated, humidified circuits are most effective in minimizing the heat loss from ventilation with cold anesthetic gases.

C.8. What derangements occur with hypothermia?

Hypothermia causes many physiologic changes. Hypothermia decreases metabolism, heart rate, cardiac output, and blood pressure. At temperatures less than 28°C (82.4°F), atrial pacing becomes irregular and ventricular ectopic increases. Ventricular fibrillation occurs between 25°C (77°F) and 30°C (86°F) in the human adult.

Decreasing the rate of metabolism can prolong the duration of many anesthetic drugs. Decreased hepatic blood flow could slow the delivery of drugs to the site of metabolism.

Hypothermia shifts the oxygen dissociation curve to the left, resulting in a reduced release of oxygen by hemoglobin. However, the shift to the left is compensated by two factors, namely an increase in dissolved oxygen in the plasma and an increase in dissolved carbon dioxide, which increases acidity and tends to shift the curve to the right.

Miller RD, ed. *Miller's anesthesia*, 6th ed. New York: Churchill Livingstone, 2005:1581–1582.

C.9. What muscle relaxant would you use?

A nondepolarizing muscle relaxant should be used. Depolarizing relaxant should be avoided. In general, the choice of muscle relaxant should be based on the duration of the operation and the presence of any coexisting diseases that might affect the elimination of the drug. Muscle relaxants without histamine release would be preferred, such as vecuronium, rocuronium, pipecuronium, and doxacurium.

C.10. Why is succinylcholine contraindicated in burned patients? For how long should it be avoided?

Succinylcholine is contraindicated in burned patients because injection of succinylcholine may cause a significant transient increase in serum potassium levels as high as 13 mEq per L, resulting in ventricular tachycardia, fibrillation, and cardiac arrest. This hyperkalemic response begins approximately 5 to 15 days after the burn and persists for 2 to 3 months or longer, irrespective of degree and size of burn injury.

The exact mechanism responsible for this response is not known. Gronert and Theye postulated that the abrupt release of potassium is from the hypersensitive muscle membranes. Apparently, extrajunctional acetylcholine receptors are found on the muscle membranes of burned patients. Stimulation of these receptors may mediate the potentially lethal efflux of potassium.

The exact time period for this hypersensitivity is unclear. Most authors recommend the avoidance of succinylcholine from 24 to 48 hours after the burn injury and extension of succinylcholine well until complete healing has occurred. A hyperkalemic response has been reported in a patient after 480 days. The recommended limit now is extended to approximately 2 years after the burned skin has healed.

Gronert GA, Theye RA. Pathophysiology of hyperkalemia induced by succinylcholine. *Anesthesiology* 1975;43:89–99.

Miller RD, ed. *Miller's anesthesia*, 6th ed. New York: Churchill Livingstone, 2005:530.

Schaner PJ, Brown RL, Kirksey TD, et al. Succinylcholine-induced hyperkalemia in burned patients. *Anesth Analg* 1969;48:764–770.

Tolmie JD, Joyce TH, Mitchell GD. Succinylcholine danger in the burned patient. *Anesthesiology* 1967;28:467–470.

C.11. What other adverse effects are associated with succinylcholine?

Adverse effects of succinylcholine are many. Its side effects are as follows:

- Hyperkalemia, particularly following burns, spinal cord injuries and generalized major trauma: a single case report of a marked hyperkalemic response to succinylcholine in a patient with a closed head injury without peripheral paralysis
- Increased intracranial and intraocular pressures: the practical importance of which is controversial
- Increased intragastric pressure: counterbalanced by the increase in lower esophageal pressure, which reduces or eliminates the increased risk of regurgitation
- Muscle pains: more likely to concern the patient with minor injuries who ambulates soon after surgery

- Prolonged paralysis in patients with atypical pseudocholinesterase
- Cardiac arrhythmias, particularly bradycardia after repeated doses
- Trigger for malignant hyperthermia

Miller RD, ed. *Miller's anesthesia*, 6th ed. Philadelphia: Elsevier: Churchill Livingstone, 2005:489–492.

C.12. How are the doses of nondepolarizing muscle relaxants affected by burn injury?

In general, burn patients show great resistance to the nondepolarizing relaxants. Martyn et al. first reported that burn patients required a five times higher plasma concentration of d-tubocurarine to attain a given percentage of twitch depression compared with healthy subjects. The dose of pancuronium is increased by 2.5 times.

Although these patients have altered pharmacokinetics and increased plasma protein binding of the relaxants, most of the increased requirement appears to be due to alterations in the number and affinity of the junctional receptors. This alteration is quite variable.

Martyn JAJ, Liu LMP, Szyfelbein SK, et al. The neuromuscular effects of pancuronium in burned children. *Anesthesiology* 1983;59:561–564.

Martyn JAJ, Szyfelbein SK, Ali HH, et al. Increased D-tubocurarine requirement following major thermal injury. *Anesthesiology* 1980;52:352–355.

Miller RD, ed. *Miller's anesthesia*, 6th ed. Philadelphia: Elsevier: Churchill Livingstone, 2005:530.

C.13. How are the muscle relaxants such as curare, pancuronium, cisatracurium, vecuronium, doxacurium, rocuronium, and pipecuronium metabolized and eliminated? Which of them has significant histamine release?

See Table 55.3.

C.14. What is the difference between metabolism and elimination of drugs?

Drug metabolism is the chemical modification of a substance. There are two phases: Phase I metabolism involves chemical reactions of oxidation, reduction, and hydrolysis. Many of these involve catalysis by the cytochrome P450 system in the liver. Phase II metabolism involves *conjugations*, or the combining of endogenous substances with drugs. This is also known as *the synthetic mode of biotransformation*.

Table 55.3   The Metabolism, Elimination, and Histamine Release of Muscle Relaxants.

RELAXANT	HEPATIC ELIMINATION (%)	RENAL ELIMINATION (%)	PLASMA METABOLISM (%)	HISTAMINE RELEASE
Curare	20	80	None	Moderate
Pancuronium	15–40	60–85	None	None
Cisatracurium	None	16	Hoffmann elimination 77	None
Vecuronium	60	40	None	None
Pipecuronium	<10	>90	None	None

Source: From Miller RD, ed. *Anesthesia,* 5th ed, New York: Churchill Livingstone, 2000:435–440, with permission.

Drug elimination involves all processes, which include metabolism, renal and hepatobiliary excretion, and pulmonary excretion such as CO_2 and anesthetic gases.

Miller RD, ed. *Miller's anesthesia*, 6th ed. Philadelphia: Elsevier: Churchill Livingstone, 2005:70.

D. Postoperative Management

D.1. How would you monitor this patient during transport?

This patient was most likely intubated, paralyzed, apneic, and still under the influence of general anesthetic. Monitoring should be directed toward respiration, oxygenation, and hemodynamics. These can be achieved by a transport monitor capable of monitoring electrocardiogram (ECG), blood pressure, central venous pressure (CVP), and pulse oximeter. Ventilation should be controlled with an Ambu bag with supplemental oxygen during transport.

D.2. What is meant by diffusion hypoxia? How do you prevent it?

Fink et al. in 1954 first reported diffusion hypoxia during recovery from nitrous oxide-oxygen anesthesia. A mild degree of hypoxia may develop for more than 10 minutes when nitrous oxide-oxygen anesthesia is concluded and the patient is allowed to breathe room air. The arterial oxygen saturation may fall 5% to 10% and often reaches values less than 90% (Pao_2 <60 mm Hg). This occurs at the time when nitrous oxide is eliminated rapidly through the lungs. Nitrous oxide is 35 times more soluble in blood than nitrogen. Therefore, the amount of nitrous oxide diffused from blood to alveoli is much more than the amount of nitrogen diffused from alveoli to blood. Hence, alveolar oxygen is diluted by nitrous oxide. Diffusion hypoxia can be prevented by the inhalation of high concentrations of oxygen for several minutes before the patient is allowed to breathe room air.

Fink R. Diffusion anoxia. *Anesthesiology* 1955;16:511–519.

Fink R, Carpenter SL, Holiday DA, et al. Diffusion anoxia during recovery from nitrous oxide-oxygen anesthesia. *Fed Proc* 1954;13:354.

D.3. Why do patients often shiver in the recovery room on emergence from anesthesia?

Postanesthetic shivering is commonly observed in the recovery room. It is more commonly seen after receiving inhalational general anesthetics. It is thought that inhalation agents inhibit the temperature-regulating centers in the hypothalamus, and shivering is a thermoregulatory response to intraoperative hypothermia (the operating room is always cold). Shivering is a mechanism to produce heat to maintain normothermia. However, the precise mechanism of shivering is not fully explained because many patients who shiver are normothermic. It is postulated that the tremor pattern results from anesthetic-induced disinhibition of normal descending control over spinal reflexes. Similar nonthermoregulatory tremor has been seen in women during labor.

Miller RD, ed. *Miller's anesthesia*, 6th ed. Philadelphia: Elsevier: Churchill Livingstone, 2005:1582.

D.4. Discuss the causes of oliguria in the recovery room.

Oliguria is defined arbitrarily as the production of less than 400 mL of urine in 24 hours. When oliguria occurs, it is a functional manifestation of various clinical entities referred to as *acute renal failure* (ARF). The syndrome of ARF may be classified into the following three groups:

- *Prerenal ARF (hypovolemic).* There is no structural damage to the kidney. The reduction in renal blood flow results in a reduced filtration rate and a decrease in urinary flow. It is reversible with volume expansion. However, if untreated, it can progress to the ischemic form of acute tubular necrosis.
- *Renal ARF (acute tubular necrosis).* There is structural damage to the renal tubules. The damage may be due to ischemia or nephrotoxic substances.
- *Postrenal ARF (obstruction of urinary outflow).* Pus, tubular debris, clots of blood, and crystalluria can cause bilateral obstruction of the ureters. The flow of urine is completely suppressed in contrast to the low flows found in prerenal and renal disease.

One must determine the cause of the oliguria because the management can vary greatly. To identify the cause of oliguria, one must make a careful assessment of the urinary sediment. Presence of renal tubular cells, renal tubular cell casts, and pigmented granular casts is strong evidence for the diagnosis of acute tubular necrosis. A normal urinary sediment supports a diagnosis of hypovolemic renal failure. Other data, such as central venous pressure (CVP), pulmonary artery diastolic pressure, and pulmonary capillary wedge pressure (PCWP) can give valuable information about the state of hydration.

CHAPTER 56

Trauma

RALPH L. SLEPIAN • JAIDEEP K. MALHOTRA

A 31-YEAR-OLD MAN

sustained a multiple stab wounds to the left upper quadrant of his abdomen and in the left hemithorax. Vital signs were as follows: blood pressure, 85/60 mm Hg; heart rate, 130 beats per minute; respiratory rate, 32 breaths per minute; temperature, 34.5°C (94.1°F). Hematocrit was 27%. He was emergently brought to the operating room for an exploratory laparotomy and possible thoracotomy.

A. Medical Disease and Differential Diagnosis

1. How is trauma classified?
2. What are the injuries associated with thoracic trauma?
3. What are the injuries associated with cardiac trauma?
4. How is the initial assessment and management of the trauma patient performed?
5. What constitutes a primary survey and what is its objective?
6. What constitutes a secondary survey and what is its objective?
7. What are the signs and symptoms of a hemothorax? What is the definition of massive hemothorax?
8. What are the indications for a thoracotomy to treat a hemothorax?
9. How are pneumothoraces categorized?
10. What are the most commonly injured organs in blunt abdominal trauma?
11. What is a Focused Abdominal Sonography for Trauma (FAST) examination?
12. What is diagnostic peritoneal lavage (DPL)?
13. Why was diagnostic peritoneal lavage (DPL) not performed for this patient?
14. Define shock.
15. What are the four types of shock?
16. List the signs and symptoms of shock.
17. What is the pathophysiology of hypovolemic shock?
18. How would you classify hemorrhage?
19. What is the initial treatment of hemorrhagic shock?
20. Would you choose crystalloid or colloid therapy to treat hypovolemic shock?
21. Is there a place for dextran or hetastarch (Hespan) in treating hypovolemic shock?
22. Is there a place for hypertonic saline (HTS) in the treatment of hypovolemic shock?

B. Preoperative Evaluation and Preparation

1. What premedication would you order?
2. What preoperative testing would you order?

C. Intraoperative Management

1. How would you monitor this patient?
2. How would you induce anesthesia?
3. What technique could you use if one-lung ventilation was indicated?
4. What agents would you choose to maintain anesthesia?
5. What muscle relaxant would you choose?
6. What can be done to decrease the incidence of intraoperative awareness?
7. Five minutes after intubation, the peak airway pressure increased from 30 to 50 cm H_2O. What are the possible causes?
8. How would you make a diagnosis of tension pneumothorax?
9. What is the treatment of tension pneumothorax?
10. The patient's blood loss was continuing and the hematocrit was 18%. What type of blood would you give if the type and cross-match are not completed?
11. What precautions should be taken if more than 2 units of type O Rh-negative un-cross-matched whole blood is given?
12. What are the complications associated with any blood transfusion?
13. What is considered a massive transfusion?
14. What are the complications associated with a massive transfusion?
15. Can the shift of the oxygen-hemoglobin dissociation curve be quantitated?
16. How is hypothermia defined?
17. What are the adverse effects of hypothermia?
18. What is the treatment of hypothermia?
19. What are the effects of blood transfusion on the immune system?
20. What are the guidelines for transfusion of blood products?
21. If the patient were a member of the Jehovah's Witness religious sect, would you give a blood transfusion?
22. If a child is a Jehovah's Witness and suffered from hemorrhagic shock, what would you do?
23. Are there artificial blood substitutes available?

D. Postoperative Management

1. What is acute respiratory distress syndrome [ARDS])?
2. How is ARDS treated?
3. In the recovery room, you are called to see this patient because of oliguria. How would you evaluate and treat this patient?

A. Medical Disease and Differential Diagnosis

A.1. How is trauma classified?

Trauma is usually separated into two distinct categories: penetrating and blunt trauma. Both can cause havoc on the body's vascular, visceral, musculoskeletal, and nervous systems.

A.2. What are the injuries associated with thoracic trauma?

Penetrating injuries associated with thoracic trauma are typically associated with stabbings and gunshot wounds, the latter being causing far more destruction as a result of the much greater amount of kinetic energy being transferred to the thoracic cavity from the impact of the bullet. As a result, gunshot wounds to the thorax are diffuse and much more likely to be fatal as compared to stabbings.

Blunt injuries to the chest are far more common than penetrating injuries. The most common causes of blunt injuries are deceleration injuries (as a result of motor vehicle accidents) and crush injuries. These can range from relatively minor injuries such as rib fractures to more severe ones such as lung contusion, tracheobronchial tears, flail chest, pneumothorax, hemothorax, injuries to the great vessels, and traumatic ruptures of the esophagus and/or diaphragm.

Kaplan JA, Slinger PD. *Thoracic anesthesia*, 3rd ed. New York: Churchill Livingstone, 2003: 315–326.

A.3.   What are the injuries associated with cardiac trauma?

Penetrating cardiac injuries often lead to immediate cardiovascular collapse and patients rarely survive to reach the operating room. Blunt cardiac trauma injuries include cardiac contusion (most common), pericardial ruptures, rupture of a chamber, valvular tears, coronary artery injuries, and ventricular aneurysms.

Kaplan JA, Slinger PD. *Thoracic anesthesia*, 3rd ed. New York: Churchill Livingstone, 2003: 315–326.

A.4.   How is the initial assessment and management of the trauma patient performed?

A systematic and organized approach to the assessment and management of the trauma patient has been developed by the American College of Surgeons and is taught as Advanced Trauma Life Support (ATLS). Initial evaluation and management as stated by ATLS consists of five components:

- The primary survey
- Resuscitation
- The secondary survey
- Continued monitoring and reevaluation
- Definitive care

Kaplan JA, Slinger PD. *Thoracic anesthesia*, 3rd ed. New York: Churchill Livingstone, 2003: 315–326.

A.5.   What constitutes a primary survey and what is its objective?

The assessment of the trauma patient consists of the primary and secondary survey. The function of the primary survey is to identify and treat immediately life-threatening injuries. The life-threatening injuries associated with chest trauma are:

- Lost airway
- Tension pneumothorax
- Massive hemothorax
- Open pneumothorax
- Cardiac tamponade
- Flail chest

Kaplan JA, Slinger PD. *Thoracic anesthesia*, 3rd ed. New York: Churchill Livingstone, 2003: 315–326.

Thoracic trauma: chest trauma initial evaluation. www.trauma.org/thoracic, 2007.

A.6. What constitutes a secondary survey and what is its objective?

The secondary survey is a more detailed examination aimed at identifying other non–life-threatening injuries and planning further laboratory and radiographic studies and forming a workable differential diagnosis. Examples of chest injuries identified on secondary survey are the following:

- Simple pneumo/hemothorax
- Rib fractures
- Pulmonary contusion
- Non–life-threatening blunt myocardial injury

Kaplan JA, Slinger PD. *Thoracic anesthesia*, 3rd ed. New York: Churchill Livingstone, 2003: 315–326.

Thoracic trauma: chest trauma initial evaluation. www.trauma.org/thoracic, 2007.

A.7. What are the signs and symptoms of a hemothorax? What is the definition of a massive hemothorax?

The signs and symptoms of a hemothorax include diminished breath sounds on the affected side, hemorrhagic shock, and mediastinal shift. A massive hemothorax is defined as a rapid accumulation of greater than 1,500 mL of blood in the thoracic cavity.

Reed AP, Yudkowitz FS. *Clinical cases in anesthesia*, 3rd ed. New York: Churchill Livingstone, 2005:481–493.

A.8. What are the indications for a thoracotomy to treat a hemothorax?

Hemothorax, if severe enough, can lead to hemmorhagic shock. Therefore, timely diagnosis and treatment is of utmost importance. After a chest tube is placed, if drainage of blood is greater than 1,200 mL, or if drainage is greater than 200 mL per hour for over 4 hours, then a thoracotomy is indicated. Alternatively, if the patient is older than 60 years, then if drainage is greater than 100 mL per hour for over 4 hours, a thoracotomy is also indicated. However, if the patient does not meet these criteria but is still hemodynamically unstable or if ventilation is difficult, then emergent surgery should be performed.

Reed AP, Yudkowitz FS. *Clinical cases in anesthesia*, 3rd ed. New York: Churchill Livingstone, 2005:481–493.

A.9. How are pneumothoraces categorized?

Pneumothoraces are categorized into three broad categories: open, closed, and tension pneumothorax. Pneumothoraces, like hemothoraces, can cause severe hypoxemia, impair venous return, and cause a severe mediastinal shift.

Open pneumothoraces are a result of penetrating wounds and allow intrathoracic pressure to equalize with atmospheric pressure. The result is introduction of outside air every time the patient takes a breath. Definitive treatment is to close the wound and placement of a chest tube.

Closed pneumothoraces can result from both blunt and penetrating trauma to the chest. It is defined as the presence of air in the pleural space. Diagnosis can be made radiographically, but the patients' condition precludes obtaining a chest radiograph in many trauma situations. In such cases, diagnosis can be made by physical examination, that is, by percussion or by diminished or absent breath sounds. Treatment is placement of a chest tube if the patient is unstable or if the pneumothorax is greater than 10% of the pleural cavity.

Tension pneumothorax is the progressive build up of air within the pleural space that cannot escape. Essentially, it is a "one-way valve" which is exacerbated by positive pressure ventilation. This progressive build up of air can cause a mediastinal shift, acute rise in airway pressures and obstruction of venous return. All of these factors can result in a sudden and dramatic cardiovascular collapse.

Kaplan JA, Slinger PD. *Thoracic anesthesia*, 3rd ed. New York: Churchill Livingstone, 2003: 315–326.

Thoracic Trauma: Chest Trauma—Pneumothorax. www.trauma.org/thoracic, 2007.

A.10. What are the most commonly injured organs in blunt abdominal trauma?

In blunt abdominal trauma, the most commonly injured organs are the spleen, liver, kidneys, and bowel. Generally, blunt abdominal trauma leads to higher mortality rates than penetrating trauma. The reason is multifactorial and includes greater difficulty in diagnosis and frequent association with other injuries, such as head injury, chest trauma, and fractures.

A.11. What is a Focused Abdominal Sonography for Trauma (FAST) examination?

FAST is a rapid ultrasonography examination performed in the trauma resuscitation room looking specifically for fluid (blood) in the peritoneum, pericardium, or thorax. Currently, FAST is indicated for all hemodynamically unstable blunt trauma patients. It may also have a role in some patients with penetrating trauma.

Trauma ultrasonography—the FAST and beyond. www.trauma.org/radiology/FASTintro .html, 2007.

A.12. What is diagnostic peritoneal lavage (DPL)?

Peritoneal lavage is a procedure performed in the emergency room to help determine whether a patient has internal bleeding that requires an exploratory laparotomy. It is done by performing a mini-laparotomy under local anesthesia. A catheter is then placed into the abdomen and is aspirated for gross blood. Aspiration of 10 mL of blood is considered a positive finding. A grossly bloody aspirate is indicative of solid or vascular injury. If less than 10 mL of blood is aspirated, then 1 L of lactated Ringer's solution or normal saline (NS) is allowed to drain into the abdomen. The lavage fluid is then allowed to return by gravity, and it is sent to the laboratory for analysis. Criteria for a positive peritoneal lavage are an erythrocyte count of 100,000 per mm^3, a white blood cell (WBC) count of 500 per mm^3, the presence of bile or food particles, and a fluid amylase concentration of 175 U per dL. WBC level itself should not determine the need for laparotomy. The level of WBCs also does not rise initially, but its rise requires several hours. Alkaline phosphatase and amylase are contained in the small bowel and spill into the abdominal cavity after injury. These levels tend to rise early in injury. Amylase in lavage fluid has been seen as a more accurate marker than alkaline phosphatase. If the peritoneal lavage meets one or more of these criteria, then the patient comes to the operating room for an exploratory laparotomy.

Roberts JR, ed. *Clinical procedures in emergency medicine*. 4th ed. Philadelphia: WB Saunders, 2004:853.

A.13. Why was diagnostic peritoneal lavage (DPL) not performed for this patient?

Peritoneal lavage was not done for two reasons. First, it is felt that all penetrating wounds to the abdomen need to be surgically explored. Second, this patient was exhibiting signs of shock and obviously needed to be sent to the operating room without delay.

Before computed tomography (CT) and ultrasonography (US) technologies, DPL was the only mechanism to rapidly evaluate the abdomen for injury. CT now allows for evaluation of all intraperitoneal organs and the retroperitoneum (an area inaccessible to DPL). US has been used for detecting fluid in pouches and gutters and is effective in determining injury to solid viscera. If patients are stable, US and CT should be used unless other injuries take priority and the patient needs to go to the operating room before any objective abdominal examination can be completed.

In penetrating trauma, DPL allows for rapid establishment of a hemoperitoneum and for discovery of intraperitoneal injury.

A.14. Define shock.

Shock is defined as the circumstance of insufficient oxygen delivery to sustain aerobic metabolism in vital cells of essential organs. Shock of all forms appears to be invariably related to inadequate tissue perfusion. The low-flow state in vital organs seems to be the final common denominator in all forms of shock.

Townsend CM, ed. *Sabiston textbook of surgery*. 17th ed. Philadelphia: WB Saunders, 2004:67.

A.15. What are the four types of shock?

For a working classification of shock, the following classification offered by Blalock in 1934 is still useful and functional:

- *Hematogenic (hypovolemic, hemorrhagic) shock*—characterized by a loss of circulatory blood volume.
- *Cardiogenic shock*—characterized by an inability of the myocardium to pump blood.
- *Vasogenic (septic) shock*—characterized by an infection that causes a decrease in peripheral vascular resistance.
- *Neurogenic shock*—characterized by an impairment of the central nervous system-mediated control of vascular tone.

Townsend CM, ed. *Sabiston textbook of surgery*. 17th ed. Philadelphia: WB Saunders, 2004:67–109.

A.16. List the signs and symptoms of shock.

Tachycardia, hypotension, cool extremities, pallor, oliguria, tachypnea, decreased capillary refill, anxiety, restlessness, and loss of consciousness are signs and symptoms of shock.

A.17. What is the pathophysiology of hypovolemic shock?

Cardiovascular derangement

An acute decrease in circulating blood volume leads to an increase in sympathetic activity with an outpouring of epinephrine and norepinephrine from the adrenal gland. The α-adrenergic response causes vasoconstriction, which shunts blood from the skin, viscera, and muscle, thereby preserving the coronary and cerebral circulation. With constriction of both precapillary and postcapillary sphincters, a reduction occurs in hydrostatic pressure of the capillary bed, which allows the osmotic pressure to draw fluid back into the vascular space from the interstitial space. This process of hemodilution tends to expand the patient's blood volume. In addition to the vasoconstriction and hemodilution, a tachycardic response may be noted.

Myocardial-depressant factor is a peptide thought to be released from the pancreas during low-flow states. This peptide is thought to be responsible for some of the decreased cardiac performance seen in trauma patients. Pancreatectomy and various myocardial-depressant factor antagonists demonstrate protective myocardial effects during shock in animals.

Acid–base disturbance

Metabolic acidosis is almost always seen in association with a shock state. As a result of decreased blood flow or a low rate of perfusion, oxygen delivery to vital organs is reduced and consequently a mandatory change occurs from aerobic to anaerobic metabolism. This shift will lead to the production of lactic acid instead of carbon dioxide as the end product of metabolism. The increase in lactic acid leads to a metabolic acidosis.

Marx JA, ed. *Rosen's emergency medicine: concepts and clinical practice*, 5th ed. St. Louis: Mosby, 2002:93.

Townsend CM, ed. *Sabiston textbook of surgery*. 17th ed. Philadelphia: WB Saunders, 2004: 77–78.

A.18. How would you classify hemorrhage?

Classification of hemorrhage based on blood loss is as follows:

Class I: Blood loss of up to 15% of the blood volume: normal pulse and blood pressure
Class II: Blood loss of up to 30% of the blood volume: tachycardia, decreased urine output, and anxiety
Class III: Blood loss of up to 40% of the blood volume: marked tachycardia, hypotension, tachypnea, oliguria, and anxiety
Class IV: Blood loss of more than 40% of the blood volume: tachycardia and hypotension, tachypnea, anuria, confusion, and lethargy

Crystalloid therapy can be used to treat blood losses of up to 30%. The lower limit of human tolerance to acute normovolemic anemia has not been established; oxygen delivery is believed to be adequate when a hemoglobin level is as low as 7 g per dL.

American College of Physicians. Practice strategies for elective red blood cell transfusion. *Ann Intern Med* 1992;116:403–406.

Committee on Trauma, American College of Surgeons. *Advanced trauma life support: program for physicians*. Chicago: American College of Surgeons, 1993.

Dutton RP. Shock and trauma anesthesia. *Anesthesiol Clin North America* 1999;17: 83–95.

Stehling LC, Doherty DC, Faust RJ, et al. Practice guidelines for blood component therapy: a report by the ASA Task Force on Blood Component Therapy. *Anesthesiology* 1996;84:732–747.

A.19. What is the initial treatment of hemorrhagic shock?

The initial treatment of hemorrhagic shock is to attempt to stabilize hemodynamics by administering fluids and blood products as required to maintain tissue perfusion and oxygen delivery.

Kruskall MS, Mintz PD, Bergin JJ, et al. Transfusion therapy I emergency room medicine. *Ann Emerg Med* 1988;17:327–335.

A.20. Would you choose crystalloid or colloid therapy to treat hypovolemic shock?

Crystalloid solutions can sustain hemodynamics and deliver adequate oxygenation in healthy patients who have lost as much as 30% of their total blood volume. There continues to be some controversy about the use of crystalloid versus colloid therapy.

Proponents of crystalloid therapy believe that both intravascular and interstitial fluid losses occur in hypovolemic shock, and that these can be readily replaced with crystalloids. Another benefit of crystalloids is the decrease in blood viscosity, which may enhance perfusion. A particular advantage to lactated Ringer's solution is that lactate is metabolized to bicarbonate, which may help to buffer the patient's acidosis. Finally, in this age of medical economics, the cost of crystalloid is much less than that of colloid. Because crystalloid leaves the intravascular space and enters the interstitial space, large quantities are needed and some fear that these quantities may lead to both pulmonary and peripheral edema, although studies have not confirmed this fear.

Proponents of colloid therapy believe that much less volume of fluid is needed to counteract hypovolemic shock. Colloids maintain the oncotic pressure and hold the interstitial fluids in the intravascular space, which is felt to possibly prevent pulmonary edema. However, if leaky alveolar capillary membranes are seen within the lung, colloids may worsen pulmonary edema.

Choi P, Yip G, Quinonez L, et al. Crystalloids vs. colloids in fluid resuscitation: a systematic review. *Crit Care Med* 1999;27:200–209.

Miller RD, ed. *Miller's anesthesia*, 6th ed. Philadelphia: Elsevier: Churchill Livingstone, 2005:1786.

Orlinsky M, Shoemaker W, Reis E, et al. Current controversies in shock and resuscitation. *Surg Clin North Am* 2001;81:6.

A.21. Is there a place for dextran or hetastarch (Hespan) in treating hypovolemic shock?

Dextran and hetastarch are synthetic polysaccharide solutions with varying mean molecular weights. Dextran 40, dextran 70, and hetastarch have all been used as volume expanders. Dextrans are relatively inexpensive, increase effective blood volume, and decrease blood viscosity. However, their negative aspects are considerable. They impair coagulation by coating platelets, and they impair typing and cross-matching by coating red blood cells (RBCs). In addition, anaphylactic reactions have been reported.

A.22. Is there a place for hypertonic saline (HTS) in the treatment of hypovolemic shock?

HTS is now being used for resuscitation at some major centers. Its effects tend to be of short duration, so it is not used alone. HTS is under investigation as a resuscitative agent, particularly in the prehospital setting, because small volumes may have beneficial cardiovascular effects. However, if one combines HTS and dextran, the effective resuscitation will be prolonged. HTS is usually supplied as 7.5% NaCl, often combined with a colloid, 6% dextran 70. The optimal dose is thought to be 4 mL per kg.

The potential advantage is that the greater the sodium concentration, the less total volume will be required for resuscitation. A serious potential danger exists in that patients may become hypernatremic, which can lead to brain dehydration. In patients with high intracranial pressure (ICP), this brain dehydration may have a potential benefit in lowering ICP.

HTS solutions have been used successfully in hemorrhagic shock resuscitation in animals and humans. This type of fluid resuscitation offers the advantage of requiring smaller volumes for a similar effect (4 to 5 mL/kg), making it especially attractive for use during prehospital resuscitation. HTS has been shown to elevate mean arterial pressure and cardiac output and increase renal, mesenteric, total splanchnic, and coronary blood flow. HTS causes a small and transient rise in circulating volume by transcapillary refill. These beneficial effects after controlled hemorrhage have been established. Its hypertonic nature and small volume usage are particular advantages in traumatic brain injury. HTS promotes redistribution of fluid into the vascular compartment and decreases ICP. HTS also seems to offer similar advantages to improvement in microcirculatory flow of the spinal cord. Use of these products during uncontrolled hemorrhage, however, has been strongly questioned.

Henry S, Scalea T. Resuscitation in the new millennium. *Surg Clin North Am* 1999;79:6.

Marx JA, ed. *Rosen's emergency medicine: concepts and clinical practice*, 5th ed. St. Louis: Mosby, 2002:353.

McCunn M, Karlin A. Nonblood fluid resuscitation: more questions than answers. *Anesthesiol Clin North America* 1999;17:1.

Orlinsky M, Shoemaker W, Reis E, et al. Current controversies in shock and resuscitation. *Surg Clin North Am* 2001;81:6.

B. Preoperative Evaluation and Preparation

B.1. What premedication would you order?

None. This is a critically ill patient who is coming to the operating room for emergency surgery. Narcotics and sedatives would be contraindicated because they could worsen his already tenuous hemodynamic state.

B.2. What preoperative tests would you order?

Because of the emergent nature of the trauma setting, preoperative tests and imaging studies are frequently limited. If the patient is hemodynamically unstable, any preoperative evaluation is often impossible. However, if the patient is stable, a portable chest x-ray, arterial blood gas, complete blood count, and Focused Abdominal Sonography for Trauma (FAST) can be obtained in a relatively short period of time in the emergency department or operating room before surgery. Often these tests can be obtained while the patient is being prepared for emergency surgery. This information can be combined with other monitoring adjuncts such as oxygen saturation, invasive blood pressure and electrocardiogram (ECG) to evaluate the patient and formulate an appropriate management strategy.

C. Intraoperative Management

C.1. How would you monitor this patient?

Routine noninvasive monitor would include electrocardiogram (ECG), blood pressure cuff, O_2 monitor, pulse oximeter, end-tidal CO_2, esophageal stethoscope, temperature probe, and Foley catheter.

Invasive monitors for this patient would include an arterial line and a central venous catheter. An arterial line is useful for blood sampling and direct blood pressure monitoring. The central venous line is helpful for determining the patient's volume status. A pulmonary artery catheter may be indicated if the patient shows signs of heart failure.

C.2. How would you induce anesthesia?

Because all trauma patients are considered to have a full stomach, the best way to protect the patient's airway is to perform an awake intubation. For an uncooperative patient, one could do a rapid sequence induction. First, the patient should be preoxygenated for 3 to 5 minutes, if hemodynamics will allow. Then, one could give a defasciculation dose of a nondepolarizing muscle relaxant. Next, ketamine, 1.0 to 2.5 mg per kg, might be given, followed by succinylcholine, 1.5 mg per kg, while maintaining cricoid pressure. Ketamine was chosen in this case because of its cardiovascular-stimulating effects and the patient's unstable hemodynamics. If the patient was adequately resuscitated in the emergency room, then one could possibly use a small dose of thiopental or midazolam/fentanyl for induction.

If the patient is comatose, in severe shock, or in full arrest on admission to the resuscitation room, no drug other than oxygen and possibly a neuromuscular blocking drug is required until the patient's blood pressure and heart rate sufficiently rebound so anesthetics can be titrated. In awake traumatized patients who are thought to be hypovolemic, etomidate is best tolerated.

Wilson WC, Patel N, Hoyt DB, et al. Perioperative anesthetic management of patients with abdominal trauma. *Anesthesiol Clin North America* 1999;17(1):211–236.

C.3. What technique could you use if one-lung ventilation was indicated?

If the patient does not already have a secure airway, the airway should be secured in the manner described in the previous question. One-lung ventilation is indicated in this situation if the patient is bleeding from one lung and protection of the other lung is required, or to improve the surgical field (lower priority). Once the airway is secured, there are several ways to obtain one-lung ventilation. The easiest and safest technique would be to attach a bronchoscopy adapter to the endotracheal tube (ETT) and to pass an embolectomy catheter (bronchial blocker) through the bronchoscopy adapter and ETT. The bronchial blocker position can be confirmed by fiber-optic bronchoscopy. The point at which the bronchial blocker enters the bronchoscopy adapter can then be sealed with pliable "bone wax" (a pliable form of sterile bees wax which is soft and kneadable).

Another method of obtaining one-lung ventilation would be to change the ETT to a double-lumen tube through a Cook exchange catheter. The major risks of this option are losing a previously secured airway and aspiration while attempting to change the tube.

Other options would be to use a Univent tube while initially securing the airway or using an Arndt endotracheal blocker if available.

C.4. What agents would you choose to maintain anesthesia?

As the patient stabilizes and the hemodynamics improve, other anesthetic agents can be carefully titrated to prevent hypotension, as follows:

- Sedatives or amnestics should be added to the anesthetic as soon as tolerated. Remember to start with small doses and to check the patient's reaction to the drugs between doses.
- Narcotics should be titrated to control the hemodynamic response to surgery.
- Nitrous oxide must be carefully considered, because it has the capacity to accumulate in closed airspaces.
- Inhalational anesthetics may be used in low concentrations so the patient's hemodynamics are not compromised.

C.5. What muscle relaxant would you choose?

Vecuronium, rocuronium, and cisatracurium are free of cardiovascular side effects and have an intermediate duration of action. They are acceptable choices. Pancuronium is a long-acting muscle relaxant with vagolytic properties that may be deleterious to the patient.

Curare, metocurine, atracurium, and mivacurium all have the potential to cause hypotension and therefore would not be chosen for this patient.

C.6. What can be done to decrease the incidence of intraoperative awareness?

The incidence of intraoperative awareness is commonly cited as approximately 0.2%. This is probably an overestimation. In other sources, the incidence of traumatic intraoperative recall associated with pain is less that 0.03%. The American Society of Anesthesiologists Closed Claims database states that claims associated to recall during anesthesia constitute 1.5%. An increased relative risk of recall is seen in certain types of surgery, including cardiac surgery, cesarean sections, and trauma surgery. This most likely represents intentional light anesthesia associated with higher levels of stimulation. Recently, the Bispectral Index (BIS) by Aspect Medical Systems (Natick, MA) and the PSA 4000 by Physiometrix (Billerica, MA) have been used as monitors of intraoperative awareness. It has been shown that patients with a BIS value of 50 were able to respond to verbal commands less than 10% of the time. Although this information may be potentially useful, the application of these monitors during a trauma resuscitation may not be easily accomplished.

Kerssens C, Klein J, vander Woerd A, et al. Auditory information processing during adequate propofol anesthesia monitored by electroencephalogram Bispectral Index. *Anesth Analg* 2001;92:1210–1214.

Lubke GH, Kerssens C, Gershon RY, et al. Memory function droning general anesthesia for emergency cesarean sections. *Anesthesiology* 2001;92:1029–1034.

O'Connor MF, Daves SM, Tung A, et al. BIS monitoring to prevent awareness during general anesthesia. *Anesthesiology* 2001;94:520–522.

Rampil I. Monitoring depth of anesthesia. *Curr Opin Anesthesiol* 2001;14:649–653.

C.7. Five minutes after intubation, the peak airway pressure increased from 20 to 40 cm H_2O. What were the possible causes?

- Tension pneumothorax
- Bronchospasm
- Endobronchial intubation

- Pulmonary edema
- Secretions
- Kink in the anesthesia circuit or endotracheal tube (ETT)

C.8. How would you make a diagnosis of tension pneumothorax?

A tension pneumothorax can be defined by the absence of breath sounds on the affected side. The chest movement may be asymmetric. Neck veins will be full, and systemic hypotension can occur if the tension pneumothorax is severe. Any patient who deteriorates under anesthesia and has wounds to the upper abdomen, lower neck, or ribs should be assumed to have a tension pneumothorax until proven otherwise.

Marx JA, ed. *Rosen's emergency medicine: concepts and clinical practice*, 5th ed. St. Louis: Mosby, 2002:1513.

C.9. What is the treatment of tension pneumothorax?

Immediate decompression of the chest is mandatory for tension pneumothorax because a patient's hemodynamics will deteriorate. Diagnosis is made clinically not by radiograph. An 18-gauge Angiocath is placed into the second intercostal space at the midclavicular plane. After the air escapes, confirming your diagnosis, and the lung is decompressed, a chest tube should be placed.

Marx JA, ed. *Rosen's emergency medicine: concepts and clinical practice*, 5th ed. St. Louis: Mosby, 2002:1513.

C.10. The patient's blood loss was continuing and the hematocrit was 18%. What type of blood would you give if the type and cross-match are not completed?

This patient should have blood transfused as soon as possible. Type O Rh-negative packed cells are the universal donor. This should be started while type-specific blood is being made available. Whenever the type-specific blood is ready, one can switch to it. However, if the transfusion begins with type O Rh-negative *whole blood* and more than 2 units has been infused, only type O Rh-negative blood should continue to be used. Usually, by the time a patient reaches the operating room from the emergency room, a partial cross-match can be done. This usually takes 5 to 10 minutes, after which time type-specific blood can be transfused.

Miller RD, ed. *Miller's anesthesia*, 6th ed. Philadelphia: Elsevier: Churchill Livingstone, 2005:1804.

Roberts JR, ed. *Clinical procedures in emergency medicine*, 4th ed. Philadelphia: WB Saunders, 2004:513.

C.11. What precautions should be taken if more than 2 units of type O Rh-negative un-cross-matched whole blood is given?

The plasma from type O Rh-negative *whole blood* contains anti-A and anti-B antibodies, which can cause hemolytic reactions with type A and type B blood cells if given in significant quantities. Therefore, only type O Rh-negative blood should continue to be transfused, although this will lead to minor hemolytic of the patient's own red blood cells (RBCs). The patient should not receive his type-specific blood until the blood bank determines that the transfused anti-A and anti-B antibody levels have fallen sufficiently low to permit safe transfusion of type-specific blood. This usually requires a 2-week waiting period.

However, packed red blood cells (PRBCs) have smaller volumes of plasma and are virtually free of anti-A and anti-B antibodies. Therefore, whenever type-specific blood is not yet available, type O Rh-negative un–cross-matched PRBCs should be used in preference to type O Rh-negative *whole blood*. Once type-specific blood is available, it can be used safely.

Cain JG. Current practices in fluid and blood component therapy in trauma. *Semin Anesth* 2001;20(1):28–35.

Miller RD, ed. *Miller's anesthesia*. 6th ed. Philadelphia: Elsevier: Churchill Livingstone, 2005:1804.

C.12. What are the complications associated with any blood transfusion?

Transfusion reactions

- Febrile reactions occur in approximately 1% of all transfusions. In an awake patient, this is usually no more than an annoyance that requires decreasing the infusion rate.
- Allergic reactions to properly cross-matched blood will manifest as an increase in temperature, pruritus, and urticaria. This may be difficult to diagnose in the anesthetized patient. Treatment consists of administration of antihistamines and discontinuation of the transfusion.
- Hemolytic reactions occur when incompatible blood is administered. Caused by activation of the complement system, they can be life threatening. In the awake patient, fever, chills, dyspnea, substernal, and lumbar pain are seen in addition to hypotension. Under general anesthesia, the only sign that is not masked is hypotension. Also, if free hemoglobin can be documented in the plasma or urine, this too would be indicative of a transfusion reaction. Substances released by the hemolyzed cells can lead to disseminated intravascular coagulation (DIC) and acute renal failure (ARF). Treatment consists of immediate discontinuation of the transfusion. Hypotension should be treated with hydration, vasopressors, and inotropic agents if needed. Urinary output must be maintained by adequate hydration. Although its value is uncertain, sodium bicarbonate has been used to alkalinize the urine to improve the solubility of the hemoglobin-degradation products. The risk of an ABO-incompatible transfusion is 1:33,500 red blood cell (RBC) transfusions. Mortality associated with this remains high, at approximately 40%.

Transmission of disease

- Transmission of disease can be a serious problem. Human immunodeficiency virus (HIV), hepatitis B virus, hepatitis C virus, and cytomegalovirus can all be transmitted by transfusion. Because the risk of disease transmission increases with each unit of blood or its components given, they must be carefully scrutinized before they are administered. The incidence of posttransfusion HIV infection is 1:493,000 (1:200,000 to 1:2,000,000) per transfused unit of blood. The risk of hepatitis B transmission is approximately 1 per 63,000 units. The risk of hepatitis C transmission is 1:103,000 (1:30,000 to 1:150,000) per unit transfused. Cytomegalovirus is the most common viral agent transmitted by blood transfusion; however, it produces clinically important infections only in immunodepressed patients. Malaria, syphilis, Lyme disease, Chagas' disease, and other diseases may also be transmitted through transfusion of blood and blood products. The aggregate infection risk is approximately 1 per 34,000. As new nonhemoglobin solutions appear on the market, less blood will be transfused and disease transmission will diminish.

Microembolization

- Microembolization can occur from the transfusion of blood or its components. Stored blood forms microaggregates that are too small to be removed by the standard 170-micron blood filters. Smaller filters have been developed to remove these particles. However, when using blood filters of the 20- to 40-micron range, the rate of transfusion is dramatically decreased because of the increased resistance of the filters. Some early reports suggested that these microaggregates may lead to pulmonary dysfunction, but this has never been proven.

Goldman L, Bennett JC, ed. *Cecil textbook of medicine*, 22nd ed. Philadelphia: WB Saunders, 2004:997.

Kruskall MS, Mintz PD, Bergin JJ, et al. Transfusion therapy in emergency room medicine. *Ann Emerg Med* 1988;17:329–331.

Landers DF, Dullye KK. Vascular access and fluid resuscitation in trauma: issues of blood and blood products. *Anesthesiol Clin North America* 1999;17(1):125–135.

Lee GR, ed. *Wintrobe's clinical hematology*, 11th ed. Baltimore: Lippincott Williams & Wilkins, 2003:859–873.

Miller RD, ed. *Miller's anesthesia*, 6th ed. New York: Churchill Livingstone, 2005:1799.

Schreiber GB, Busch MP, Kleinman SH, et al. The risk of transfusion-transmitted viral infections. *N Engl J Med* 1996;334:1685.

Spahn DR, Casutt M. Eliminating blood transfusions: new aspects and perspectives. *Anesthesiology* 2000;83:242–255.

C.13. What is considered a massive transfusion?

A massive transfusion is defined as the replacement of the patient's total blood volume in a 24-hour period. This is usually between 8 and 10 units of packed red blood cells (PRBCs). Many trauma cases far exceed this amount and may require other blood components in addition to the RBCs.

Miller RD, ed. *Miller's anesthesia*, 6th ed. Philadelphia: Elsevier: Churchill Livingstone, 2005:1807–1808.

C.14. What are the complications associated with a massive transfusion?

Complications of a massive transfusion include dilutional coagulopathy, disseminated intravascular coagulation (DIC), fibrinolysis, citrate toxicity, hyperkalemia, hypokalemia, acid–base imbalance, impaired hemoglobin function, and hypothermia.

- Dilutional coagulopathy usually becomes a problem during massive transfusions. Both platelets and coagulation factors are markedly decreased and must be replaced. They should be administered after laboratory documentation of the deficiency. It is no longer accepted practice to give fresh frozen plasma (FFP) routinely after 5 units of packed red blood cell (PRBC), and it is not proper to give platelets after 10 units of PRBC. At present, dilutional coagulopathies appear to be rare, even with the transfusion of one blood volume. Approximately 40% of the coagulation factors remain after one blood volume replacement, and this should be sufficient to allow normal coagulation. Platelets can be reduced to 30% to 40% of normal after one blood volume transfusion. This decrease will usually represent a platelet count less than 100,000 per μL and may lead to a prolonged bleeding time.
- DIC and fibrinolysis may occur after massive transfusions. An important triggering event of DIC and fibrinolysis is shock, with its accompanying tissue ischemia, acidemia, and waste product accumulation. Therefore, early and prompt treatment of hypoperfusion is mandatory.
- Citrate toxicity is frequently discussed, but it is rarely a problem. However, in the pediatric population, citrate toxicity is much more of a problem and should be considered in any child

who does not respond to rapid volume administration of blood products. Citrate is added to stored blood to bind calcium and therefore prevent clotting. The citrate anticoagulant stays with the plasma, and obviously FFP would contain much more citrate that PRBCs. Citrate binds calcium and decreases the patient's ionized calcium level. Hypocalcemia may present as a prolongation of the QT interval with little effect of cardiac performance. In some cases, ventricular performance may be compromised. However, cardiac performance may also be decreased by acidemia, hyperkalemia, and hypothermia, which all accompany the shock state. Therefore, the routine administration of supplemental calcium is not indicated. A point worth noting is that citrate is metabolized to bicarbonate, and it can contribute to posttransfusion metabolic alkalosis.

- Hyperkalemia can be a rare occurrence in the massively transfused patient. Plasma potassium levels of stored whole blood range between 12 and 32 mEq per L. The potassium level increases approximately 1 mEq/L/day in stored blood. A unit of whole blood would contain between 4 and 8 mEq of potassium, which is hardly enough to cause hyperkalemia. A unit of PRBC contains insignificant amounts of potassium because most plasma is removed. However, in the shock state with hypoperfusion and acidemia, hyperkalemia may become evident.
- Hypokalemia is also a possibility after a massive transfusion. Citrate is metabolized to bicarbonate, resulting in a metabolic alkalosis that can cause hypokalemia. In addition, the transfused RBCs take up potassium, which can also result in hypokalemia.
- Acid–base imbalance is a problem after massive transfusion. Banked blood with a pH level of 6.8 is acidotic and may worsen the acidosis that accompanies shock. However, this acidosis is easily reversible with the restoration of normal perfusion. No need is seen to give supplemental bicarbonate based on an arbitrary number of units transfused. However, if a metabolic acidosis persists, then sodium bicarbonate is warranted. As stated, citrate from stored blood and lactate from lactated Ringer's solution are metabolized to bicarbonate, and this can cause a metabolic alkalosis.
- Impaired hemoglobin function is a theoretic possibility after massive transfusion. The 2,3-diphosphoglycerate (2,3-DPG) level is decreased in banked blood. This will shift the oxygen–hemoglobin dissociation curve to the left, and oxygen will be held more tightly by the hemoglobin molecule. However, no studies have documented any adverse effects from this.
- Hypothermia is an obvious consequence of infusing cold banked blood. Therefore, it is recommended that the blood be reconstituted with warm normal saline (NS). In addition, all fluids should pass through a warming device to help prevent hypothermia.

Drummond JC, Petrovitch CT. The massively bleeding patient. *Anesthesiol Clin North America* 2001;19(4):633–649.

Goskowicz R. The complications of massive blood transfusion. *Anesthesiol Clin North America* 1999;17(4):959–978.

Miller RD, ed. *Miller's anesthesia*, 6th ed. Philadelphia: Elsevier: Churchill Livingstone, 2005:1799–1830.

C.15. Can the shift of the oxygen-hemoglobin dissociation curve be quantitated?

Yes, the shift of the oxygen-hemoglobin dissociation curve is quantified by means of the P_{50} values (i.e., the partial pressure of oxygen at which hemoglobin is 50% saturated with oxygen). A leftward shift of the curve indicates a low P_{50} value. The normal P_{50} value of blood is 27 mm Hg and the normal level of 2,3-diphosphoglycerate (2,3-DPG) is 4.8 mmol per mL of erythrocytes.

Lumb AB. *Nunn's applied respiratory physiology*, 6th ed. Philadelphia: Butterworth-Heinemann, 2005:177–179.

C.16. How is hypothermia defined?

Hypothermia is defined as a core body temperature of less than 35°C (95°F). A trauma patient brought to the emergency room may already be hypothermic. Prolonged exposure to a cold operating room, evaporative heat loss from the respiratory tract, infusions of cold fluids, and loss of heat production secondary to shock cause decreased core temperature in most patients.

All skin surfaces not in the surgical field should be covered to reduce convective and radiant heat loss. Humidification of inspired gases reduces evaporative heat loss from the lung. All intravenous fluids should be warmed.

Warming the operating room may also lessen heat loss, as will the use of warming blankets.

Miller RD, ed. *Miller's anesthesia*, 6th ed. Philadelphia: Elsevier: Churchill Livingstone, 2005:1579.

Roberts JR, ed. *Clinical procedures in emergency medicine*, 4th ed. Philadelphia: WB Saunders, 2004:514–515.

C.17. What are the adverse effects of hypothermia?

- Shivering-induced increase in O_2 consumption by as much as 400%
- A leftward shift in the oxygen-hemoglobin dissociation curve
- Decreased coagulation of blood
- Increased epinephrine and norepinephrine levels, causing vasoconstriction
- As hypothermia becomes severe, possible decreases in both heart rate and blood pressure
- Cardiac irritability, leading to ventricular fibrillation

Miller RD, ed. *Miller's anesthesia*, 6th ed. Philadelphia: Elsevier: Churchill Livingstone, 2005:1581–1583.

Tanaka M, Nagasaki G, Nishikawa T. Moderate hypothermia depresses arterial baroreflex control of heart rate during, and delays its recovery after general anesthesia in humans. *Anesthesiology* 2001;95:1.

C.18. What is the treatment of hypothermia?

The normal response to hypothermia is shivering, which is blocked by general anesthesia. Therefore, it is of utmost importance to prevent and treat hypothermia. Recommendations include the following:

- Increase the temperature of the operating room.
- Use a warming blanket.
- Preheat intravenous fluids.
- Pass all fluids through a warming device.
- Use low-flow anesthesia.
- Use a heat moisture exchanger in the anesthesia circuit.

C.19. What are the effects of blood transfusion on the immune system?

Blood transfusion will result in immunologic changes that can be harmful in some patients and helpful in others. This immunomodulation occurs from immune suppression. The blood components crucial to these changes are thought to be the white blood cells (WBCs) or plasma.

An example of a beneficial effect is the increased survival of the renal allograft in patients who had received a prior transfusion. In patients who have cancer, a possible harmful effect of immunosuppression is the increased cancer recurrence rate seen in patients who have had prior transfusion. Finally, a number of clinical studies have demonstrated that perioperative transfusion is associated with an increased incidence of infection and sepsis.

Landers DF. Blood transfusion-induced immunomodulation. *Anesth Analg* 1996;82(1):187–204.

Lee GR, ed. *Wintrobe's clinical hematology*, 11th ed. Baltimore: Lippincott Williams & Wilkins, 2003:859–873.

C.20. What are the guidelines for transfusion of blood products?

The New York Presbyterian Hospital Guidelines for blood product usage are as follows:

Red blood cell transfusion criteria

- Hemoglobin (Hb) level less than 8 g per dL and mean red cell volume within normal limit (81 to 100 fL, 70 to 125 fL for patients aged 14 years)
- Hb level less than 8 g per dL and high risk/acute bleed[1]
- Hb level less than 11 g per dL and clinically symptomatic[2]
- Hb level less than 11 g per dL and bleed more than 1 U per 24 hours
- Any Hb level and high risk[1] and acute bleed
- Any Hb level and symptomatic[2] and acute bleed
- Any Hb level and bleed more than 2 U per 24 hours, or more than 15% of blood volume per 24 hours

Platelet transfusion criteria

- Platelet count less than 20,000 per μL without thrombotic thrombocytopenic purpura (TTP), idiopathic thrombocytopenic purpura, posttransfusion purpura, or hemolytic-uremic syndrome
- Platelet count less than 50,000 per μL with minor bleed, preoperative for a minor procedure or prematurity
- Platelet count less than 90,000 per μL with bleed requiring RBC transfusion or preoperative for a major procedure
- Massive RBC transfusion (>8 U/24 hours)
- Bleeding time longer than 10 minutes
- Open heart surgery transfusion of more than mean number of RBC units (6 units/case)

Fresh frozen plasma transfusion criteria

- Massive transfusion more than 8 units of RBC per 24 hours (>1 blood volume infants/children)
- Abnormal coagulation test results prothrombin time more than 15 seconds or partial thromboplastin time more than 45 seconds during prior 24 hours or known congenital coagulation factor disorder and bleeding or prophylaxis for major procedures
- Clinical evidence of abnormal bleeding from venipuncture sites or generalized oozing
- Patients with diagnosis of thrombotic thrombocytopenic purpura (TTP)
- Open heart surgery transfusion of more than mean number of RBC units (6 units/case)

Cryoprecipitate transfusion criteria

- Massive transfusion more than 8 units of RBCs per 24 hours
- Open heart surgery transfusion of more than mean number of RBC units (6 units/case)

---

[1]High risk includes patients with coronary artery disease, chronic pulmonary disease, cerebrovascular disease, or congenital or acquired anemia.

[2]Symptomatic includes patients with signs or symptoms of anemia, such as tachycardia, angina, electrocardiographic changes or of neonatal respiratory distress, known hemoglobinopathy, and so forth.

- Bleeding or invasive procedure with hypofibrinogemia or disseminated intravascular coagulation (DIC)
- Deficient factor VIII of von Willebrand factor or abnormal fibrinogen and presurgical or bleed

New York Presbyterian Hospital. *Weill/Cornell Medical Center Protocols*. 2006.

Stehling LC, Doherty DC, Faust RJ, et al. Practice guidelines for blood component therapy: a report by the ASA Task Force of Blood Components Therapy. *Anesthesiology* 1996;84:732–747.

C.21. If a patient were a member of the Jehovah's Witness religious sect, would you give a blood transfusion?

Jehovah's Witnesses are best known for refusing the transfusion of blood and blood products. This belief is based on the Bible (Acts 15:28–29). In the awake and otherwise competent adult, courts have ruled that physicians cannot be held liable if they comply with a patient's directive and withhold life-saving blood administration after specific and detailed informed consent of the consequences of such an omission of treatment. The issue becomes clouded when patients are incompetent, unconscious (most Jehovah's Witnesses carry cards informing medical personnel of their religious beliefs), or minors. They believe all hope of eternal life is forfeited if they accept a transfusion. Therefore, a blood transfusion is considered a physical violation. The right of a Jehovah's Witness to refuse a blood transfusion is absolute. The courts have upheld their rights to refuse a blood transfusion. Most witnesses take adequate legal steps to relieve the liability of the medical personnel. Most carry a medical alert card that states their wishes and they usually have made arrangements for proxy or surrogate decision makers. In addition, an open and honest avenue of communication must exist between the patient, surgeon, and anesthesiologist.

They will refuse transfusion of whole blood, packed red blood cells (PRBCs), white blood cells (WBCs), plasma, and platelets. However, they will allow the use of cardiopulmonary bypass, dialysis, or similar equipment, as well as intraoperative blood salvage where the extracorporeal circulation is uninterrupted. Their religious understanding does not absolutely prohibit albumin, immune globulins, or hemophiliac preparations; those products must be decided on an individual basis. They accept all nonblood replacements, including nonblood colloids, crystalloids, dextrans, or oxygen-carrying blood substitutes.

An anesthesiologist may refuse to care for any patient when a procedure is elective. In an emergency situation, legal and ethical requirements apply. Conversely, any competent adult also has the right to refuse any therapy, and to treat such a patient against that person's will is to commit battery.

Dasen KR, Niswander DG, Schlenker RE. Autologous and allogenic blood products for unanticipated massive blood loss in a Jehovah's Witness. *Anesth Analg* 2000;90:553–555.

Roberts JR, ed. *Clinical procedures in emergency medicine*, 4th ed. Philadelphia: WB Saunders, 2003:520–521.

Waters JH, Potter PS, Booke M. Cell salvage in the Jehovah's Witness patient. *Anesth Analg* 2000;90:229.

C.22. If a child is a Jehovah's Witness and suffered from hemorrhagic shock, what would you do?

Care of minors presents the greatest concern and often leads to legal action against the parents under child-neglect status. Such actions are questioned by Jehovah's Witnesses who do seek good medical care for their children, while claiming that consideration be given to their families' religious beliefs. Doctors can appeal to the court for permission to transfuse blood to children of this sect who are underage. In an unforeseeable emergency, generally, blood may be given without consulting a court.

C.23. Are there artificial blood substitutes available?

Three types of artificial blood are being investigated: hemoglobin solutions, liposome-encapsulated hemoglobin, and perfluorocarbons.

Hemoglobin solutions

Hemoglobin can now be prepared from outdated human blood. Intravascular free hemoglobin has a high affinity for oxygen and is quickly excreted. Hemoglobin can now be modified and dissolved in an isotonic medium that will decrease renal filtration, prolong intravascular life, and restore a normal P_{50} of oxygen. Hemoglobin solutions can restore circulating blood volume and provide adequate tissue oxygenation in animal models. Detrimental effects include renal toxicity and increased systemic and pulmonary vascular pressures.

Liposome-encapsulated hemoglobin

Hemoglobin can be membrane encapsulated for modification. It is then possible to add 2,3-diphosphoglycerate (2,3-DPG), or inositol hexaphosphate to the membrane, thereby adjusting the P_{50} to match the RBCs. In theory, the encapsulated hemoglobin will have a longer intravascular duration and greater oxygen-carrying capacity. The membrane is being further modified to try to decrease the deposition in the reticuloendothelial system, thereby further increasing the intravascular duration.

Perfluorocarbons

Perfluorocarbons are synthetic substances that have a capacity for dissolved oxygen. It is unlikely these will be useful because a high PaO_2 is needed to allow the perfluorocarbon to carry even small amounts of dissolved oxygen. Initial studies of stromafree hemoglobin have shown potential harm in renal function, and stromafree hemoglobin is not approved for clinical use.

Human studies have been disappointing because of unacceptable side effects, such as renal failure, platelet dysfunction, and vasoconstriction. No product has been approved for use in trauma patients, although phase III trials are under way in centers throughout the United States using hemoglobin-based oxygen carriers. Currently, artificial blood substitute use is not indicated.

Lee GR, ed. *Wintrobe's clinical hematology*, 11h ed. Baltimore: Lippincott Williams & Wilkins, 2003:859–873.

Miller RD, ed. *Miller's anesthesia*, 6th ed. Philadelphia: Elsevier: Churchill Livingstone, 2005:1804.

Townsend CM, ed. *Sabiston textbook of surgery*, 17th ed. Philadelphia: WB Saunders, 2004: 134.

D. Postoperative Management

D.1. What is acute respiratory distress syndrome (ARDS)?

ARDS is an acute respiratory failure seen in patients with healthy lungs after being exposed to shock, trauma, sepsis, aspiration, transfusion, burns, or toxic inhalation. Initially, when this lung injury was thought to be related to the shock state and its resuscitation, names such as "shock lung" and "traumatic wet lung" were applied to acute respiratory insufficiently following injury. It is now recognized that many types of lung insults will result in damage to the alveolar capillary membrane, resulting in leakage of proteinaceous fluid from the intravascular space into the interstitium and subsequently into the alveolar spaces. This injury with its resulting interstitial and alveolar edema produces a clinical picture ranging from mild to severe pulmonary dysfunction that can actually be fatal.

Acute lung injury (ALI) is characterized by impaired oxygenation, defined as a ratio of PaO_2/FIO_2 of 300 or less; bilateral pulmonary infiltrates on the frontal chest radiograph; and a pulmonary artery occlusion of 18 mm Hg or more. ARDS is defined as ALI with a PaO_2/FIO_2 ratio of 200 or less. ARDS is characterized by the following:

- Hypoxemia—is relatively unresponsive to increasing inspired oxygen concentration
- Decreased pulmonary compliance—clinically appears as stiff lungs
- Initially normal chest radiograph progressing to diffuse infiltrates or even to areas of complete consolidation
- Decrease in resting lung volumes, specifically functional residual capacity

---

Amato MB, Barbas CS, Medeiros DM, et al. Effect of a protective-ventilation strategy on mortality in the acute respiratory distress syndrome. *N Engl J Med* 1998;338:345–354.

Rakel RE, ed. *Conn's current therapy*, 57th ed. Philadelphia: WB Saunders, 2005:251–253.

D.2. How is acute respiratory distress syndrome (ARDS) treated?

The treatment of ARDS is primarily supportive. Currently, mechanical ventilation is the mainstay of supportive therapy for ARDS. The principal goal of mechanical ventilation is to minimize the deleterious effects on gas exchange. Unfortunately, mechanical ventilation has also been associated with further lung injury. Excessive alveolar volumes (volutrauma), high mean and peak airway pressures (barotrauma), and shearing forces caused by frequent collapse and opening of alveolar units are responsible for this further lung injury. Positive end-expiratory pressure (PEEP) is used to increase oxygenation at a fixed FIO_2.

Investigators have looked at lung protection in patients with ARDS. Strategies were used to prevent ventilator-associated lung injury. Amato et al. used a strategy to limit peak inspiratory pressures by using low tidal volumes (<6 mL/kg) and the institution of PEEP. Their strategy was associated with a lower 28-day mortality (38% vs. 71%), higher weaning rate (66% vs. 29%), and lower barotrauma rate (7% vs. 42%).

The National Heart, Lung, and Blood Institute ARDS network reported improved survival in patients using a low tidal volume strategy (6 mL/kg vs. 12 mL/kg). These investigators found a decrease in mortality of approximately 25% in the intervention group compared with the control group.

Amato MB, Barbas CS, Medeiros DM, et al. Effect of a protective-ventilation strategy on mortality in the acute respiratory distress syndrome. *N Engl J Med* 1998;338:345–354.

Brower R, Ware L, Berthiaume Y, et al. Treatment of ARDS. *Chest* 2001;120:4.

National Institutes of Health. *National Heart, Lung, and Blood Institute ARDS Network.* 2000.

Rakel RE, ed. *Conn's current therapy*, 57th ed. Philadelphia: WB Saunders, 2005:251–253.

D.3. **In the recovery room, you are called to see this patient because of oliguria. How would you evaluate and treat this patient?**

Oliguria is a decrease in urinary output to less than 0.5 mL/kg/hour.

Acute renal failure (ARF) is a syndrome characterized by a rapid (hours to weeks) decline in glomerular filtration rate and retention of nitrogenous waste products such as blood urea nitrogen (BUN) and creatinine. The kidney is remarkable in its ability to recover from almost complete loss of function. Most ARF is reversible. ARF is associated with major in-hospital morbidity and mortality. The diagnosis of ARF usually hinges on serial analysis of BUN and serum creatinine.

Renal failure can be divided into three categories.

Prerenal

Prerenal failure is the most common cause of ARF and is an appropriate physiologic response to renal hypoperfusion. It is usually caused by a low cardiac output due to hypovolemia or cardiac failure. It can be evaluated by checking the patient's heart rate, blood pressure, central venous pressure, pulmonary capillary wedge pressure, and cardiac output. If hypovolemia is the cause, then treatment would consist of a fluid bolus. If the patient is in cardiac failure, then inotropic support and diuretics could be administered. Severe renal hypoperfusion may cause ischemic acute tubular necrosis (ATN). Therefore, prerenal azotemia and ischemic ATN are part of a spectrum of manifestations of renal hypoperfusion.

Renal

Intrinsic renal failure is generally due to toxic injury or ischemia. Ischemic injury is caused by a decrease in perfusion pressure that can lead to renal cellular dysfunction. Substances that affect renal tubular function in addition to renal blood flow can cause toxic injury. Ischemic ATN, unlike prerenal azotemia, is associated with injury to renal parenchyma and does not resolve immediately on restoration of renal perfusion. In its more extreme form, renal hypoperfusion may result in bilateral renal cortical necrosis and irreversible renal failure. Urinalysis may show cells and/or casts that are indicative of ARF. Intrinsic renal failure can be minor and short lived, or it can progress to chronic renal failure, depending on the severity of the insult. In the absence of congestive heart failure, use of diuretics should generally be avoided as they can exacerbate ATN. In particular, loop diuretics increase oxygen and adenosine triphosphate (ATP) consumption at the level of the tubules.

Postrenal

Urinary tract obstruction accounts for less than 5% of cases of ARF. Urinary tract obstruction must be sought and corrected to treat possible causes of postrenal oliguria. This usually requires irrigation and/or changing of the Foley catheter. Consider the possibility of and intraoperative mishap causing postrenal obstruction.

Brenner BM, ed. *Brenner and rector's the kidney*, 7th ed. Philadelphia: WB Saunders, 2004:1215–1230.

CHAPTER 57

Scoliosis

Victor M. Zayas

A 14-YEAR-OLD GIRL

with scoliosis is scheduled for posterior spine fusion with segmental instrumentation. She has been told that her scoliosis is idiopathic. Her past medical history is unremarkable but her mother states that she appears to get short of breath more easily than her friends when she plays basketball.

A. Medical Disease and Differential Diagnosis

  1. What is scoliosis?
  2. What is the most common type of scoliosis?
  3. What are other types of scoliosis?
  4. How is the severity of scoliosis assessed and why is the severity important?
  5. What abnormalities in pulmonary function tests are most commonly seen in scoliosis? What is the cause of these abnormalities?
  6. What is the most common arterial blood gas abnormality seen in scoliosis? What are possible causes for this abnormality?
  7. What abnormalities of ventilatory drive may be associated with scoliosis?
  8. How may the cardiovascular system be affected in patients with scoliosis?
  9. What is the relation between scoliosis and malignant hyperthermia?

B. Preoperative Evaluation and Preparation

  1. What should the anesthesiologist know about the nature of the spinal curve?
  2. What aspects of the history are most important?
  3. What aspects of the physical examination are most important?
  4. Why is a preoperative neurologic assessment important?
  5. What tests would you order preoperatively?
  6. What preparation should the patient have preoperatively?
  7. What should you consider in ordering preoperative medications?

C. Intraoperative management

  1. What monitoring would you use?
  2. What is the incidence of neurologic complications in scoliosis surgery and which patients are at highest risk?
  3. What monitoring techniques are used to minimize neurologic complication?
  4. What are somatosensory evoked potentials (SSEPs) and how are they used?
  5. How reliable are SSEPs for predicting spinal injury?

6. What are motor evoked responses (MEPs) and how are they used?

7. How is spinal cord monitoring affected by anesthetic agents? What other factors affect spinal cord monitoring?

8. What should be done if the SSEPs or MEPs become abnormal during surgery?

9. How is the wake-up test performed? What complications can occur during a wake-up test?

10. Four hours into the surgical procedure, the surgeon reports some bubbling in the thoracic portion of the wound. Shortly thereafter, end-tidal CO_2 decreases abruptly from 35 to 18 mm Hg, heart rate increases from 80 to 120 beats per minute (bpm), blood pressure begins to fall, and arterial saturation decreases to 90%. On auscultation through esophageal stethoscope, you hear a loud gurgling murmur. What is your diagnosis?

11. How common is significant air embolism during scoliosis surgery?

12. What should be done if air embolism is suspected?

13. What is the optimal anesthetic technique for scoliosis surgery?

14. What complications occur related to positioning the patient?

15. How will the surgical procedure influence estimated blood loss and fluid requirements?

16. What is transfusion-related lung injury (TRALI)?

17. What techniques can be used to minimize transfusion requirements?

18. What techniques would you use to produce deliberate hypotension during scoliosis surgery? What is the major concern of using this technique?

D. Postoperative Management

1. When would you extubate the patient?

2. What should be done to optimize pulmonary status?

3. What laboratory tests should be ordered postoperatively?

4. What fluid therapy would you use postoperatively?

5. What complications may occur following scoliosis surgery?

A. Medical Disease and Differential Diagnosis

A.1. What is scoliosis?

The spine normally curves posteriorly in the thoracic region and anteriorly in the lumbar region. These physiologic curves are the thoracic kyphosis and the lumbar lordosis, respectively. The spine is not normally curved when viewed from the front or back. Scoliosis refers to a lateral curvature of the spine. Curves are classified as structural or nonstructural. A nonstructural curve, such as lumbar scoliosis from a leg length discrepancy, will resolve when the patient is supine or uses a shoe lift and does not require surgical correction. In contrast, structural scoliosis lacks normal flexibility and does not correct with bending or lying supine. In addition to the lateral curvature of the spine, the vertebrae are rotated and the rib cage may be markedly deformed (Fig. 57.1). As demonstrated in the computed tomography (CT) scan image in Fig. 57.2, this thoracic deformity may lead to a significant decrease in total lung volume. Particularly note the decrease in left lung volume relative to the right.

A.2. What is the most common type of scoliosis?

Idiopathic scoliosis is the most common type of scoliosis (70% of all cases) and occurs in an infantile, a juvenile, or an adolescent form. As the name implies, the cause is unknown but

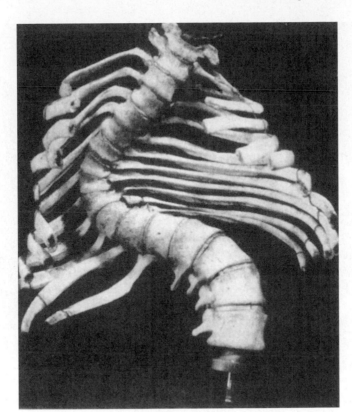

Figure 57.1 In addition to producing a lateral deformity of the spine, scoliosis also results in rotation of the vertebral bodies and significant rib cage deformity.

appears to be multifactorial, including abnormalities of collagen, brainstem function, equilibrium, hormones, and growth. Genetic factors are important in its development as evidenced by an increased incidence of scoliosis in relatives of affected patients. Recent evidence suggests that pronounced forms of scoliosis (curve >11 degrees) occur only in the carriers of a mutant allele with incomplete penetrance (30% of men, 50% of women).

The prevalence of idiopathic scoliosis in large screening studies depends upon the definition of scoliosis and the population screened. The prevalence of spinal curves greater than 10 degrees is 1.5% to 3%, greater than 20 degrees it is 0.3% to 0.5%, and greater than 30 degrees it is 0.2% to 0.3%. The adolescent form of idiopathic scoliosis is by far the most common in the United States. The prevalence was 1.2% in a large screening study of one and one quarter million students aged 10 to 16 years. The male to female prevalence ratio depends in part on the age of the patient, but scoliosis requiring surgical correction is more common in women.

Axenovich TI, Zaidman AM, Zorkoltscva IV, et al. Segregation analysis if idiopathic scoliosis: demonstration of a major gene defect. *Am J Med Genet* 1999;86:389–394.

Lonstein JE. Adolescent idiopathic scoliosis. *Lancet* 1994;344(8934):1407–1412.

Lonstein JE, Bjorklund S, Wanniger MH, et al. Voluntary school screening for scoliosis in Minnesota. *J Bone Joint Surg* 1982;64A:481–488.

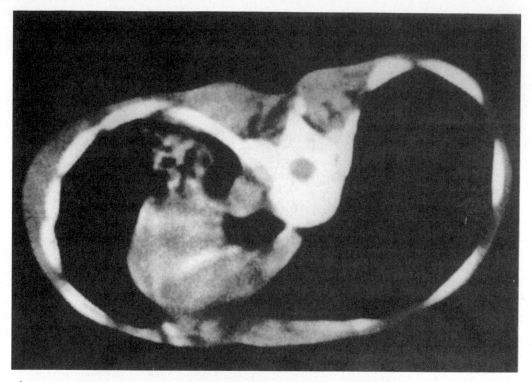

Figure 57.2 A computed tomography (CT) scan of the thorax demonstrating significant loss of lung volume due to the rib cage deformity.

Weinstein SL, ed. *The pediatric spine: principles and practice*. New York: Raven Press, 1994: 445–462.

Yawn BP, Yawn RA. A population-based study of school scoliosis screening. *JAMA* 1999; 282(15):1427–1432.

A.3. What are other types of scoliosis?

There are many etiologic classifications of structural scoliosis. Neuromuscular scoliosis (paralytic scoliosis) may occur as a result of diseases such as cerebral palsy, muscular dystrophy, poliomyelitis, familial dysautonomia and so on. This type of scoliosis is associated with significantly increased intraoperative blood loss compared with idiopathic scoliosis. Congenital scoliosis is the result of congenital anomalies such as hemivertebrae and fused vertebrae or ribs. Neurofibromatosis and Marfan's syndrome are also associated with scoliosis. These underlying conditions may have a major impact on the anesthetic plan. The classification of structural scoliosis is as follows:

Idiopathic

- Infantile
- Juvenile
- Adolescent

Neuromuscular (Paralytic)

- Neuropathic
  - Upper motor neuron (e.g., cerebral palsy, spinal cord injury)
  - Lower motor neuron (e.g., poliomyelitis, meningomyelocoele)
  - Familial dysautonomia
- Myopathic
  - Muscular dystrophy
  - Myotonic dystrophy

Congenital

- Hemivertebrae
- Congenitally fused ribs

Neurofibromatosis
Mesenchymal disorders

- Marfan's syndrome
- Ehlers–Danlos syndrome

Trauma

- Vertebral fracture or surgery
- Postthoracoplasty
- Postradiation

Bradford DS, Lonstein JE, Ogilvie JW, et al. eds. *Moe's textbook of scoliosis and other spinal deformities*. Philadelphia: WB Saunders, 1987:41–45.

Sethna NF, Zurakowski D, Brustowicz RM, et al. Tranexamic acid reduces intraoperative blood loss in pediatric patients undergoing scoliosis surgery. *Anesthesiology* 2005;102: 727–732.

A.4. How is the severity of scoliosis assessed and why is the severity important?

In 1966, the Scoliosis Research Society standardized the method for assessing the severity of scoliosis. The most common measure of severity is Cobb's angle. Fig. 57.3 illustrates how Cobb's angle is measured on a roentgenogram of the spine. A perpendicular *(2)* is constructed from the bottom of the lowest vertebrae *(1)* whose bottom tilts towards the concavity of the curve, and another perpendicular *(4)* from the top of the highest vertebrae *(3)* whose top tilts towards the concavity. The angle *(5)* at which these perpendiculars intersect is Cobb's angle. Numerous studies have documented that the more severe the thoracic curve (greater Cobb's angle), the more profound the disturbance in pulmonary function. Surgical treatment is usually recommended for curves greater than 45 to 50 degrees. Curves greater than 60 degrees are usually associated with decreases in pulmonary function.

In a recent series of 79 patients with thoracic scoliosis, the mean Cobb's angle was 45 degrees and vital capacity was decreased by an average of 22%. Figure 57.4 demonstrates that forced vital capacity (FVC) and forced expiratory volume (FEV_1) decrease with increasing thoracic curve severity.

Scoliosis severity and impairment of pulmonary function also increase with greater number of vertebrae involved, more cephalad location of the curve, and loss of the normal thoracic kyphosis. Severe curves have a worse prognosis because they tend to progress and if long standing can

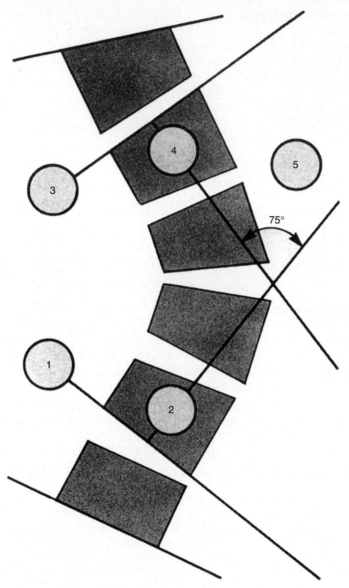

Figure 57.3 Measurement of the curve in scoliosis using Cobb's angle. (Reprinted with permission from Levine DB. Scoliosis. *Curr Opin Rheumatol* 1987;2:191.)

cause permanent damage of the lung parenchyma, respiratory failure, cor pulmonale, and death. It is important to note that patients with neuromuscular types of scoliosis may have a much more profound decrease in pulmonary function for any given curve severity.

Bradford DS, Lonstein JE, Ogilvie JW, et al. eds. *Moe's textbook of scoliosis and other spinal deformities*. Philadelphia: WB Saunders, 1987:586–587.

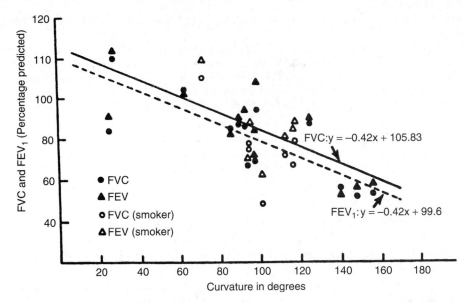

Figure 57.4 Relation between forced vital capacity (FVC), and forced expiratory volume in one second (FEV₁), and size of the curve in 20 patients with thoracic scoliosis. (Reproduced with permission from Weinstein SL, Zaval DC, Ponseti IV, et al. Idiopathis scoliosis. Long-term follow-up and prognosis in untreated patients. *J Bone Joint Surg* 1981;63:702.)

Kearon C, Viviani GR, Kirkley A, et al. Factors determining pulmonary function in adolescent idiopathic thoracic scoliosis. *Am Rev Respir Dis* 1993;148(2):288–294.

Levine DB. Scoliosis. *Curr Opin Rheumatol* 1990;2:190–195.

Weinstein SL, ed. *The pediatric spine: principles and practice.* New York : Raven Press, 1994: 463–477.

Weinstein SL, Zaval DC, Ponseti IV, et al. Idiopathis scoliosis. Long-term follow-up and prognosis in untreated patients. *J Bone Joint Surg Am* 1981;63:702–712.

A.5. What abnormalities in pulmonary function tests are most commonly seen in scoliosis? What is the cause of these abnormalities?

A decrease in lung volumes, a restrictive pattern, is most commonly seen in thoracic scoliosis. The greatest reduction occurs in the vital capacity, which is typically reduced to 60% to 80% of predicted. Total lung capacity, functional residual capacity (FRC), inspiratory capacity, and expiratory reserve volume are also decreased. An increase in residual volume has been reported in patients with congenital scoliosis and in patients with idiopathic scoliosis 3 years following corrective spine fusion.

During exercise, ventilation is adequate but tidal volume is reduced and respiratory rate is increased. Maximal work capacity may also be decreased. Unless there is coexisting obstructive airway disease, the ratio of the forced expiratory volume in 1 second to the forced vital capacity (FEV₁/FVC) is normal. Impaired respiratory muscle function also occurs in scoliosis as evidenced by a decrease in inspiratory force to 70% of normal values. The decrease in inspiratory force is probably due to the inspiratory muscles working at a mechanical disadvantage due to the chest wall deformity.

These abnormalities in pulmonary function are usually the result of abnormal thoracic cage geometry producing a marked decrease in chest wall compliance rather than any abnormality in the lungs or respiratory muscles themselves. These changes in chest wall compliance can be mimicked in normal volunteers by chest strapping. Exceptions include congenital and infantile scoliosis in which growth of the lungs may be impaired early in development by the thoracic deformity.

Bradford DS, Lonstein JE, Ogilvie JW, et al. eds. *Moe's textbook of scoliosis and other spinal deformities*. Philadelphia: WB Saunders, 1987:585–592.

Cooper DM, Rojas JV, Mellins RB, et al. Respiratory mechanics in adolescents with idiopathic scoliosis. *Am Rev Respir Dis* 1984;130:16–22.

Day GA, Upadhyay SS, Ho EKW, et al. Pulmonary functions in congenital scoliosis. *Spine* 1993;19(9):1027–1031.

Jones RS, Kennedy JD, Hasham F, et al. Mechanical inefficiency of the thoracic cage in scoliosis. *Thorax* 1981;36:456–461.

Kearon C, Viviani GR, Killian KJ. Factors influencing work capacity in adolescent idiopathic thoracic scoliosis. *Am Rev Respir Dis* 1993;148(2):295–303.

Weinstein SL, Zavala DC, Ponseti IV. Idiopathic scoliosis: long term follow up and prognosis in untreated patients. *J Bone Joint Surg* 1981;63:702–712.

A.6. What is the most common arterial blood gas abnormality seen in scoliosis? What are possible causes for this abnormality?

It has been documented that patients with thoracic scoliosis have arterial oxygen desaturation compared to normal controls. Both arterial P_{CO_2} and pH are usually normal. Several studies have failed to show a correlation between the severity of the spinal curve and the amount of arterial oxygen desaturation.

Arterial hypoxemia is probably caused by ventilation/perfusion ($\dot{V}/\dot{Q}$) inequalities. Decreased diffusing capacity and alveolar hypoventilation may also play a role. However, the diffusing capacity is not decreased sufficiently to be the sole cause of the hypoxemia. Similarly, alveolar ventilation at rest and during exercise is usually normal; therefore, arterial P_{CO_2} is usually normal. It has been reported that some patients have a closing capacity higher than functional residual capacity (FRC), resulting in premature airway closure during normal tidal breathing. Other studies have failed to demonstrate this finding. Some authors have reported an increase in the ratio of dead space to tidal volume (V_D/V_T), while other recent series have found V_D/V_T to be normal. This discrepancy may be related to the patient population studied, the severity of the scoliosis or both. Severe and/or long-standing scoliosis can produce severe $\dot{V}/\dot{Q}$ abnormalities, alveolar hypoventilation, CO_2 retention, and more severe hypoxemia. If not surgically treated, severe scoliosis increases the risk of premature death from respiratory failure after 40 years of age. A survey of patients with respiratory failure in Sweden found that a vital capacity less than 50% of predicted and a Cobb's angle greater than 100 degrees indicated an increased risk of respiratory failure.

Bergofsky EH. Respiratory failure in disorders of the thoracic cage. *Am Rev Respir Dis* 1979;119:643–669.

Kafer ER. Respiratory and cardiovascular functions in scoliosis and the principles of anesthetic management. *Anesthesiology* 1980;32:339–351.

Pehrsson K, Nachemson A, Olofson J, et al. Respiratory failure in scoliosis and other thoracic deformities. *Spine* 1992;17:714–718.

Weber W, Smith JP, Briscoe WA, et al. Pulmonary function in asymptomatic adolescents with idiopathic scoliosis. *Am Rev Respir Dis* 1975;111:389–397.

A.7. What abnormalities of ventilatory drive may be associated with scoliosis?

The slope of the ventilatory response to CO_2 may be decreased in patients with scoliosis. This is probably not specific to scoliosis as this response is known to be reduced in situations in which the work of breathing is increased even in the absence of a chest wall deformity. Patients with mild scoliosis have been reported to exhibit abnormal ventilatory patterns in response to hypoxemia and hypercarbia. This pattern tends to minimize the work of breathing, a higher respiratory rate, and lower tidal volume.

It has also been demonstrated that during maximal exercise, patients with mild to moderate scoliosis exhibit a significantly decreased ventilatory capacity, reduced exercise tolerance and oxygen consumption despite normal pulmonary function testing at rest.

Barrios C, Perez-Encinas C, Maruenda JI, et al. Significant ventilatory restriction in adolescents with mild or moderate scoliosis during maximal exercise tolerance test. *Spine* 2005;30(14):1610–1615.

Kafer ER. Respiratory and cardiovascular functions in scoliosis and the principles of anesthetic management. *Anesthesiology* 1980;32:339–351.

Smyth RJ, Chapman KR, Wright TA, et al. Ventilatory patterns during hypoxia, hypercapnia, and exercise in adolescents with mild scoliosis. *Pediatrics* 1986;77(5):692–697.

Weber W, Smith JP, Briscoe WA, et al. Pulmonary function in asymptomatic adolescents with idiopathic scoliosis. *Am Rev Respir Dis* 1975;111:389–397.

A.8. How may the cardiovascular system be affected in patients with scoliosis?

Patients with scoliosis may develop elevated pulmonary vascular resistance and pulmonary hypertension. This may result in right ventricular hypertrophy and, eventually, right ventricular failure. A 50-year study of untreated scoliosis demonstrated that the mortality rate of these patients was twice that of the general population and respiratory failure or right heart failure accounted for 60% of the deaths.

The increase in pulmonary vascular resistance is probably due to several factors. Hypoxemia produces pulmonary vasoconstriction, an increase in pulmonary vascular resistance, and hence an increase in pulmonary arterial pressure. Chronic hypoxemia will produce hypertensive vascular changes and pulmonary hypertension may become irreversible. It has also been proposed that the chest wall deformity compresses some lung regions, increasing vascular resistance in those regions. Finally, if scoliosis develops in the first 6 years of life, the growth of the pulmonary vascular bed may be impaired by the chest wall deformity. Supporting this concept are reports of a decrease in the number of vascular units per lung volume in patients with scoliosis.

The most common cardiovascular abnormality in patients with scoliosis is mitral valve prolapse. Antibiotic prophylaxis should be administered before catheterization of the bladder or laryngoscopy in these patients.

Some conditions that are associated with scoliosis also affect the cardiovascular system. Patients with Duchenne's muscular dystrophy develop a cardiomyopathy in the second decade of life that may not be appreciated on the basis of clinical symptoms as these patients are unable to exercise. The electrocardiogram may reveal tachycardia, prolonged PR and QRS intervals,

ST abnormalities, bundle branch block, Q waves in the left precordial leads and tall R waves in the right precordial leads. Ejection fraction may be decreased on echocardiogram.

Patients with Marfan's syndrome may have mitral and aortic insufficiency, aneurysm of the proximal ascending aorta, and abnormalities of the conduction system.

The association of scoliosis and congenital heart disease has been well established. While no specific cardiac lesion has been identified, some series have suggested that scoliosis is more common in patients with cyanotic heart disease.

Bradford DS, Lonstein JE, Ogilvie JW, et al. eds. *Moe's textbook of scoliosis and other spinal deformities*. Philadelphia: WB Saunders, 1987:609–611.

Kafer ER. Respiratory and cardiovascular functions in scoliosis and the principles of anesthetic management. *Anesthesiology* 1980;32:339–351.

Kawakami N, Mimatsu K, Deguchi M, et al. Scoliosis and congenital heart disease. *Spine* 1995;20(11):1252–1255.

A.9. What is the relation between scoliosis and malignant hyperthermia?

In 1970, a statistical, retrospective review of 89 patients who developed malignant hyperthermia reported that 6 of these patients had "idiopathic kyphoscoliosis." While this report suggests an association between idiopathic scoliosis and malignant hyperthermia, data are not yet available regarding the incidence of this disorder in scoliosis patients. Certainly some scoliosis patients do have an increased risk of malignant hyperthermia due to their underlying disease. For example, patients with certain muscle disorders such as central core muscular dystrophy are at increased risk of developing malignant hyperthermia and also develop scoliosis (also see Chapter 53).

Britt BA, Kalow W. Malignant hyperthermia: a statistical review. *Can Anaesth Soc J* 1970;17: 293–315.

Brownell AKW. Malignant hyperthermia: relationship to other diseases. *Br J Anaesth* 1988; 60:303–308.

B. Preoperative Evaluation and Preparation

B.1. What should the anesthesiologist know about the nature of the spinal curve?

It is important to identify the location of the curve, the age of onset, its severity, the direction of the curve, and the etiology of the scoliosis. The location of the curve is important because thoracic scoliosis is associated with pulmonary function abnormalities. Cervical scoliosis may cause difficulties in airway management and may be associated with other congenital anomalies.

The age of onset of scoliosis is of critical importance because the lung continues to grow and develop from birth until 8 years of age. The number of alveoli increases from approximately 20 million at birth to 250 million at 4 years of age. The development of significant thoracic scoliosis during this phase of rapid growth impairs lung development. A significant reduction in alveolar number has been demonstrated in patients with early-onset thoracic scoliosis, predisposing these patients to impaired gas exchange and pulmonary hypertension.

The severity of the curve is important because thoracic curves greater than 60 degrees generally produce significant decreases in pulmonary function. Curves greater than 100 degrees may be associated with significant impairment in gas exchange. Most curves in adolescent idiopathic scoliosis are convex to the right just as most people are right handed. A left thoracic convexity should raise your index of suspicion to look for other underlying conditions and congenital anomalies. Finally, an understanding of the etiology of the scoliosis is important because underlying conditions such as muscular dystrophy or cerebral palsy will influence anesthetic management.

Bradford DS, Lonstein JE, Ogilvie JW, et al. eds. *Moe's textbook of scoliosis and other spinal deformities*. Philadelphia: WB Saunders, 1987:585–592.

Weinstein SL, ed. *The pediatric spine: principles and practice*. New York: Raven Press, 1994: 421–429.

B.2. What aspects of the history are most important?

Cardiopulmonary reserve should be assessed by questioning the patient about shortness of breath, dyspnea on exertion, exercise tolerance and so on. As a general rule, patients who can exercise normally and "keep up with friends" in vigorous activities will have good cardiopulmonary function. Pulmonary symptoms such as episodes of wheezing or cough may indicate parenchymal lung disease and alter perioperative management. Patients with muscular dystrophy, Marfan's syndrome and neurofibromatosis should be questioned about symptoms suggestive of cardiac conduction abnormalities such as palpitations or syncope.

Weinstein SL, ed. *The pediatric spine: principles and practice*. New York: Raven Press, 1994: 421–429.

B.3. What aspects of the physical examination are most important?

Particular emphasis in the physical examination should be directed towards the heart and lungs. Auscultation of the lungs may reveal wheezing or rales suggesting obstructive airway disease or parenchymal lung disease. On examination of the heart, in addition to auscultating for murmurs and gallops, signs of pulmonary hypertension and right ventricular hypertrophy should be sought. Pulmonary hypertension causes accentuation of the pulmonic component of the second heart sound and a right ventricular lift indicates right ventricular enlargement. Signs of right ventricular failure include engorged neck veins, an enlarged liver due to passive liver congestion, and lower extremity edema. If neurofibromatosis is suspected, the skin should be examined for the presence of *cafe au lait spots* or cutaneous neurofibroma. The airway should be evaluated closely for abnormalities such as cervical scoliosis, neurofibroma, or high arched palate associated with Marfan's syndrome that may make endotracheal intubation difficult.

Weinstein SL, ed. *The pediatric spine: principles and practice*. New York: Raven Press, 1994: 421–429.

B.4. Why is a preoperative neurologic assessment important?

A preoperative neurologic assessment is important because patients who have preexisting neurologic deficits are at increased risk for developing spinal cord injury during scoliosis surgery. Furthermore, it is important to document preoperative neurologic function in order to avoid confusion about postoperative neurologic complications.

B.5. What tests would you order preoperatively?

It is probably best to tailor diagnostic testing based on the severity of the scoliosis and underlying conditions rather than ordering a standard battery of diagnostic tests. In the current climate emphasizing medical cost containment, each institution needs to critically reassess preoperative testing. This healthy 14-year-old may only need a complete blood count before surgery. If the history or physical examination suggests that pulmonary reserve is decreased, then standard pulmonary function testing should be considered. If vital capacity is significantly diminished, an arterial blood gas is indicated. If routine pulmonary function testing reveals evidence of obstructive airway disease (a decrease in the ratio of the forced expiratory volume in 1 second to the forced vital capacity (FEV_1/FVC) or a decrease in forced expiratory flow ($FEF_{25\%-75\%}$), then a bronchodilator should be administered to determine if the airway obstruction is reversible.

Patients with onset of scoliosis in the first 8 years of life should have pulmonary function testing, arterial blood gas analysis, and an electrocardiogram. If the electrocardiogram reveals abnormalities such as right ventricular hypertrophy (large R in V_1 and V_2), right atrial enlargement ($P_{wave} > 2.5$ mm) or evidence of a cardiomyopathy, an echocardiogram, or even cardiac catheterization may be indicated, particularly if pulmonary hypertension is suspected.

Kafer ER. Respiratory and cardiovascular functions in scoliosis and the principles of anesthetic management. *Anesthesiology* 1980;32:339–351.

B.6. What preparation should the patient have preoperatively?

The patient should be prepared both physiologically and psychologically for surgery. First, preoperative teaching of coughing and incentive spirometry should be emphasized. Patients with evidence of parenchymal lung disease, or obstructive airway disease should have aggressive pulmonary toilet and/or bronchodilator therapy preoperatively. Finally, if an intraoperative wake-up test is planned (see subsequent text), the patient should be informed and reassured that he or she will feel no pain or discomfort. It is helpful to rehearse the wake-up test during the preoperative visit.

B.7. What should you consider in ordering preoperative medications?

Heavy premedication and narcotics are probably best avoided in patients with neuromuscular disease, evidence of pulmonary hypertension, impaired gas exchange, or markedly decreased pulmonary function. Use of an antisialagogue may be desirable as many of these surgical procedures are performed in the prone position and copious secretions may wet the tape securing the endotracheal tube and cause it to slip.

C. Intraoperative management

C.1. What monitoring would you use?

Minimal monitoring for posterior spine fusion should include blood pressure, electrocardiogram, pulse oximetry, end-tidal CO_2, esophageal stethoscope, core temperature, and spinal cord monitoring. A radial artery catheter is used for continuous monitoring of blood pressure, particularly if deliberate hypotension is planned to reduce blood loss. This will also facilitate obtaining blood samples for blood gas and hematocrit determination. All patients should have a urinary catheter placed to document urine output during and particularly after the surgical procedure. Monitoring of central filling pressures may be indicated if the expected blood loss is large, or cardiovascular disease is present or suspected. A pulmonary artery catheter may be useful in patients with cardiomyopathy from Duchenne's muscular dystrophy, and patients with pulmonary hypertension or right ventricular failure in order to optimize volume replacement therapy. When placing pulmonary artery catheters in patients with pulmonary hypertension it must be considered that the risk of pulmonary artery rupture, a complication with a mortality rate of 50%, is increased in patients with pulmonary hypertension. Neuromuscular blockade should be monitored if a balanced anesthetic technique is used.

C.2. What is the incidence of neurologic complications in scoliosis surgery and which patients are at highest risk?

In the 1987 morbidity report of the Scoliosis Research Society, the rate of complete or partial paraplegia was 0.26%. A recent study of 6,334 patients undergoing anterior, posterior, or combined anterior/posterior spinal fusion reported an overall rate of spinal injury of 0.28%. Of note, combined anterior/posterior procedures had a significantly higher rate of spinal cord injuries (1.12%) compared to either anterior (0.0%) or posterior (0.21%) procedures.

It has been proposed that distraction of the cord and straightening of the deformity compresses the spinal cord and disrupts the arterial blood supply of the cord. The spinal cord and nerve roots may also be injured directly by hooks or instrumentation.

Prevention of neurologic complications begins with identification of the high-risk group. Patients are at increased risk for developing paraplegia if they have a severe rigid deformity (>120 degrees), kyphosis, neurofibromatosis, congenital or postinfectious scoliosis, a preexisting neurologic deficit, or more invasive instrumentation. Congenital scoliosis is associated with intraspinal anomalies including lipomas, tethered cord, cysts, and teratomas that also increase the risk of postoperative neurologic complications. A preoperative myelogram or magnetic resonance imaging (MRI) is indicated in these patients. Preoperative prophylaxis with high-dose corticosteroids should be considered for patients with a preexisting neurologic deficit.

Cole JD, Arlet V, Donaldson W, et al. Complications in spinal fusion for adolescent idiopathic scoliosis in the millennium. A report of the scoliosis society morbidity and mortality committee. *Spine* 2006;31(3):291–298.

C.3. What monitoring techniques are used to minimize neurologic complication?

The two monitoring techniques most commonly used in the United States to monitor spinal cord function during scoliosis surgery are somatosensory evoked potentials (SSEPs) and the intraoperative wake-up test. More recently, motor evoked potentials (MEPs) are being used to assess the integrity of the spinal motor pathways. In many centers, MEP monitoring has replaced the routine use of the wake-up test.

Bernard J, Pereon Y, Fayet G, et al. Effects of isoflurane and desflurane on neurogenic motor and somatosensory-evoked potential monitoring for scoliosis surgery. *Anesthesiology* 1996;85(5):1013–1019.

Bradford DS, Lonstein JE, Ogilvie JW, et al. eds. *Moe's textbook of scoliosis and other spinal deformities*, Philadelphia: WB Saunders, 1987:471–472.

Lonstein JE. Adolescent idiopathic scoliosis. *Lancet* 1994;344:1407–1412.

Weinstein SL, ed. *The pediatric spine: principles and practice*. New York: Raven Press, 1994:1764–1765.

C.4. What are somatosensory evoked potentials (SSEPs) and how are they used?

Sensory information from the periphery passes through the posterior columns of the spinal cord on its way to the cerebral cortex. The functional integrity of this pathway can be continually

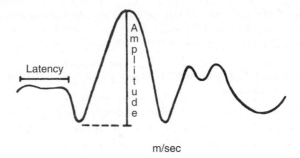

m/sec

Figure 57.5 Typical somatosensory evoked potential trace. (Reprinted with permission from Cunningham JN Jr, Laschinger JC, Merkin HA, et al. Measurement of spinal cord ischemia during operations on the thoracic aorta: initial clinical experience. *Ann Surg* 1982;196:285–296.)

assessed by monitoring SSEPs. This technique involves applying repeated electrical stimuli to a peripheral nerve (e.g., posterior tibial nerve) and measuring the evoked response over the cerebral cortex and subcortical regions using standard electroencephalogram (EEG) scalp electrodes. As these evoked potentials are of very low amplitude, computer averaging or summation must be used to distinguish these potentials from background noise and the patient's EEG. A typical evoked potential waveform is shown in Fig.57.5. The time interval between electrical stimulation of peripheral nerve to recording the evoked response over the cortex is defined as the latency. An increase in the latency (slower conduction), a decrease in the amplitude, or a complete loss of the evoked potential should be considered indicative of surgical injury or ischemia until proved otherwise. It is difficult to define standard values for latency and amplitude because of the differences in recording technique among laboratories and therefore it is important to be familiar with the normal limits for the system that is in use. In general, an increase in latency of 10%–15% or more, and a decrease in amplitude of greater than 50% should be cause for concern.

Miller RD, eds. *Miller's anesthesia*, 6th ed. Philadelphia: Elsevier: Churchill Livingstone, 2005:1511–1550.

Nash CL, Brown RH. Current concepts review-spinal cord monitoring. *J Bone Joint Surg* 1989;71A(4):627–630.

C.5. How reliable are somatosensory evoked potentials (SSEPs) for predicting spinal injury?

Normal intraoperative SSEPs are good predictors of normal postoperative sensory function. Although posterior (sensory) and anterior (motor) spinal injuries tend to occur together during spine surgery or spinal trauma, there have been reports of postoperative paraplegia with normal intraoperative SSEPs. This probably represents selective ischemia in the distribution of the anterior spinal artery. Sensory function and SSEPs are preserved because the posterior columns receive their blood supply from the posterior spinal arteries. For this reason, it is probably best not to rely exclusively on SSEPs to monitor spinal cord function during scoliosis surgery.

In a recent survey of 173 orthopedic spinal surgeons, it was found that experienced SSEP monitoring teams had fewer neurologic complications per 100 cases than teams with less experience. Neurologic defects with normal SSEPs (false negative) occurred in only 0.063% of cases.

Lesser RP, Raudzens P, Luders H, et al. Postoperative neurological deficits may occur despite unchanged intraoperative somatosensory evoked potentials. *Ann Neurol* 1986;19:22–25.

Nash CL, Brown RH. Current concepts review-spinal cord monitoring. *J Bone Joint Surg* 1989;71A(4):627–630.

Nuwer MR, Dawson EG, Carlson LG, et al. SSEP spinal cord monitoring reduces neurologic deficits after scoliosis surgery: results of a large multicenter study. *Electroencephalogr Clin Neurophysiol* 1995;96:6–11.

Spielholz NI, Benjamin NV, Engler GL, et al. Somatosensory evoked potentials during decompression and stabilization of the spine: methods and findings. *Spine* 1979;4:500.

C.6. What are motor evoked responses (MEPs) and how are they used?

MEPs assess the integrity of the spinal motor pathways (anterior columns). MEPs are elicited by transosseous electrical stimulation of the motor cortex using scalp electrodes, or by stimulation of the anterior columns using epidural electrodes. Conduction of these stimuli through the motor pathways is monitored as peripheral nerve impulses, electromyographic signals, or actual limb movements.

C.7. How is spinal cord monitoring affected by anesthetic agents? What other factors affect spinal cord monitoring?

All anesthetic agents may affect spinal monitoring to a varying degree. This has been documented for potent inhalation agents, propofol, nitrous oxide, benzodiazepines, droperidol, etomidate, ketamine, barbiturates, and even narcotics. Narcotics probably have the least effect on somatosensory evoked potentials (SSEPs) of all these agents. Cortical SSEPs and motor evoked potentials (MEPs) are very sensitive to nitrous oxide and potent inhalational agents, while subcortical SSEPs are more resistant. The addition of nitrous oxide to isoflurane has been shown to have a profound effect on MEPs. MEPs are also profoundly affected by benzodiazepines and thiopental, while ketamine may enhance MEPs.

Nitrous oxide produces a decrease in amplitude in SSEPs without an increase in latency. Isoflurane, sevoflurane, halothane and so on have similar effects on SSEPs: a dose-dependent increase in latency and decrease in amplitude. The addition of nitrous oxide appears to produce a larger decrease in amplitude than addition of 1% isoflurane or enflurane to a fentanyl-based anesthetic.

Muscle relaxants have no effect on SSEPs or MEP impulses monitored from peripheral nerves. However, muscle relaxants will affect the intensity of the motor response, which may lead to confusion interpreting MEPs.

While it is important to realize that anesthetic agents can affect spinal cord monitoring, excellent results can be obtained if anesthetic depth is stable. For example, it is preferable to administer narcotics by continuous infusion rather than by intermittent doses. It is most important to maintain a stable anesthetic before and during periods when monitoring is critical, that is, during spine distraction or instrumentation.

A decrease in arterial pressure below levels of cerebral autoregulation, hypothermia, hematocrits below 15% and hypoxia will affect both SSEPs and MEPs.

Miller RD, eds. *Miller's anesthesia*, 6th ed. Philadelphia: Elsevier: Churchill Livingstone, 2005:1511–1550.

C.8. What should be done if the somatosensory evoked potentials (SSEPs) or motor evoked potentials (MEPs) become abnormal during surgery?

If spinal cord monitoring becomes abnormal, the anesthesiologist should ensure that oxygen delivery and spinal cord perfusion are adequate. Hypovolemia and anemia should be corrected. Arterial oxygen tension should be optimized and arterial Pco_2 should be normalized if the patient is being hyperventilated. It has been reported that normalizing arterial pressure if deliberate hypotension is being used, or raising arterial pressure above normal may improve spinal cord perfusion and restore SSEPs to normal. The surgeon should seek a surgical cause such as too much distraction or surgical trespass with instrumentation and correct the problem as quickly as possible. If the abnormality persists despite corrective action, a wake-up test should be performed to determine if the instrumentation should be adjusted or removed. There is evidence that the shorter the interval between detection of injury and removal of instrumentation, the better the neurologic outcome.

Grundy BL, Nash CL, Brown CR. Arterial pressure manipulation alters spinal cord function during correction of scoliosis. *Anesthesiology* 1981;54:249–253.

C.9. How is the "wake-up" test performed? What complications can occur during this test?

The wake-up test is used to assess the integrity of the spinal motor pathways and is performed by "lightening" the depth of anesthesia sufficiently to allow the patient to follow commands. This is usually done as soon as all instrumentation is in place, or if an abnormality has been detected with spinal cord monitoring. The patient is first instructed to squeeze the anesthesiologist's hand, confirming that he is responsive, and then asked to move his feet and toes. If the patient is able to squeeze his hands but unable to move his feet, the amount of spine distraction must be reduced until a safe degree of correction is achieved. When the patient moves his feet, anesthesia is quickly deepened with small doses of propofol (0.5 mg/kg) and a muscle relaxant. Recall of intraoperative events is very unusual with this technique.

The anesthesiologist should have one or two assistants available in the event the patient moves excessively during the wake-up test. Although this occurs rarely when an adequate amount of narcotic has been administered, it is best to be prepared. The author does not recommend use of narcotic antagonists because of the potential for the patient to experience pain and become agitated in the prone position. If naloxone is deemed necessary to arouse the patient, a small dose (0.3–0.5 μg/kg) should be administered and repeated every 2 to 3 minutes until the respiratory depression of the narcotic is reversed. It is not typically necessary to reverse neuromuscular blockade if at least three twitches are present on train-of-four stimulation.

Complications of this technique include extubation in the prone position, recall of intraoperative events, myocardial ischemia, self-injury, and dislodgment of instrumentation. Air embolus from open venous sinuses may occur if the patient is breathing spontaneously and inhales vigorously.

C.10. Four hours into the surgical procedure, the surgeon reports some bubbling in the thoracic portion of the wound. Shortly thereafter, end-tidal CO_2 decreases abruptly from 35 to 18 mm Hg, heart rate increases from 80 to 120 beats per minute (bpm), blood pressure begins to fall, and arterial saturation decreases to 90%. On auscultation through esophageal stethoscope, you hear a loud gurgling murmur. What is your diagnosis?

This constellation of symptoms strongly suggests venous air embolism. There are at least two reports indicating that air bubbling in the wound may be the first clinical sign of an air embolus before cardiovascular collapse. This is thought to occur as a result of retrograde flow of blood containing entrained air through the valve-less venous system due to an increase in central venous pressure. Central venous pressure rises as a result of an air lock in the right heart. Positive pressure ventilation and pressure on the spine during placement of hardware may also produce bubbling of entrained air.

Adornato DC, Gildenberg PL, Ferrario CM, et al. Pathophysiology of intravenous air embolism in dogs. *Anesthesiology* 1978;49(2):120–127.

Will J, Schwend RM, Albin MS, et al. Intraoperative visible bubbling of air may be the first sign of venous air embolism during posterior surgery for scoliosis. *Spine* 2005; 30(20):629–635.

C.11. How common is significant air embolism during scoliosis surgery?

Fortunately, clinically significant air embolism is probably uncommon. However, a number of cases of fatal air embolism have been reported during scoliosis surgery in children. Most, but not all cases, involve extensive surgical dissection with excessive bleeding. The mortality rate in the reported cases may be 50%.

C.12. What should be done if air embolus is suspected?

If an air embolus is suspected, the surgical field should be immediately flooded with saline, ventilation begun with 100% oxygen, and intravascular fluid administered to increase central venous pressure. Air is most likely entrained from open epidural and paravertebral veins and venous sinuses in decorticated bone. Flooding the field with saline prevents air entrainment. Ventilation with 100% oxygen reduces the volume of the air embolus, particularly if nitrous oxide was administered. Hypovolemia and low central venous pressure favor air entrainment by increasing the pressure gradient between open veins and the right atrium.

If the patient requires cardiopulmonary resuscitation, placing the patient in the left lateral decubitus position during external cardiac massage may improve blood flow by breaking the air lock of the pulmonary outflow tract. Removing air through either a central catheter or by direct intracardiac aspiration has also been advocated.

McCarthy RE, Lonstein JE, Mertz JD, et al. Air embolism in spinal surgery. *J Spinal Disord* 1990;3:1–5.

Sutherland RW, Winter RJ. Two cases of fatal air embolism in children undergoing scoliosis surgery. *Acta Anaesthesiol Scand* 1997;41(9):1073–1076.

C.13. What is the optimal anesthetic technique for scoliosis surgery?

There is no simple answer for the optimal anesthetic technique. Most patients with idiopathic scoliosis are healthy adolescents who tolerate anesthesia and surgery well, and a wide variety of techniques have been used successfully. The primary concern is the ability to provide an anesthetic that is suitable for spinal cord monitoring. Before the use of MEP monitoring, anesthetic techniques were tailored to facilitate the wake-up test. Monitoring of MEPs has now replaced routine use of the wake-up test in many centers. Although cortical somatosensory evoked potentials (SSEPs) and motor evoked potentials (MEPs) may be measurable in most healthy adults receiving 50% to 70% nitrous oxide and 0.5 minimal alveolar concentration (MAC) isoflurane, this combination is not suitable in small children or those with preexisting neurologic deficits. Furthermore, MEPs may be more sensitive to the combination of nitrous oxide and potent inhalational agents than cortical SSEPs.

Therefore, a typical anesthetic is a combination of a low-dose potent agent (e.g., isoflurane 0.4%) in 50% oxygen per air mixture, with a propofol/narcotic-based intravenous anesthetic. Infusion of ketamine at a low dose (0.1–0.2 mg/kg/hour) may improve MEP monitoring. Muscle relaxants, if used, should be administered by continuous infusion and titrated to a constant train-of-four as the neuromuscular blockade will affect the intensity of the motor response.

Succinylcholine should be avoided in patients with muscle disorders. Its administration in patients with Duchenne's muscular dystrophy may produce hyperkalemia, cardiac arrhythmias, myoglobinuria, or precipitate malignant hyperthermia. Patients with myotonic muscular dystrophy may exhibit sustained skeletal muscle contractions in response to succinylcholine. This may produce difficulty in ventilation and intubation.

C.14. What complications occur related to positioning the patient?

If the head is not positioned carefully, pressure on the eyes may cause thrombosis of the central retinal artery producing loss of vision or blindness. The horseshoe-type head rest (Fig. 57.6) has been implicated in a number of reports of unilateral eye blindness and should be used with great caution if at all. The head should be positioned without excessive flexion or extension and in such a way that the face and eyes can be inspected easily. The position of the head and neck will move during surgical manipulation of the spine and should be inspected frequently during the procedure. Patients with Marfan's syndrome and neurofibromatosis may have abnormalities of the cervical spine and must be turned and positioned with great caution.

The upper extremities should be positioned at no more than 90 degrees of abduction to the trunk as illustrated in Fig. 57.7A. Figure 57.7B demonstrates improper arm positioning because the arms are abducted above the head. This stretches the brachial plexus and may result in a brachial plexus palsy. Both axillae should be inspected to ensure that the frame does not compress the axillary sheath. Figure 57.8B demonstrates improper positioning on the frame resulting in pressure on the axilla. Proper positioning is shown in Figure 57.8A. Note that there is ample space between the thoracic bolster of the frame and the axilla. Care should be taken to pad the ulnar nerves at the elbow. Impairment of ventilation and increased bleeding from increased venous pressure may occur if the abdomen is compressed by the operating frame.

C.15. How will the surgical procedure influence estimated blood loss and fluid requirements?

A variety of surgical procedures are commonly performed for posterior spine fusion. The blood lost during these procedures may be considerable and varies according to the procedure, the operative time, the number of segments fused, whether deliberate hypotension is used, and other factors. Even when deliberate hypotension is used, blood loss in the range of 15 to 25 mL per kg is not uncommon during uncomplicated spine fusion with Harrington rods or Cotrel-Dubousset instrumentation. This represents a blood loss of 1 to 2 L for a 70-kg patient. Postoperative bleeding may equal or exceed this, emphasizing the need for continued monitoring of these patients in the postoperative period. More extensive procedures such as combined anterior-posterior spine fusion, instrumentation into the pelvis, or especially osteotomy of the spine to correct rigid deformities may be associated with blood loss exceeding the patient's own blood volume (75 mL/kg). Patients who require these more extensive procedures are frequently those with neuromuscular scoliosis (Duchenne's muscular dystrophy, cerebral palsy) who may already have diminished reserves.

Moderate third-space losses of intravascular fluid occur during scoliosis surgery. These should be replaced with balanced salt solution at a rate of 5 to 7 mL/kg/hour. This is in addition to

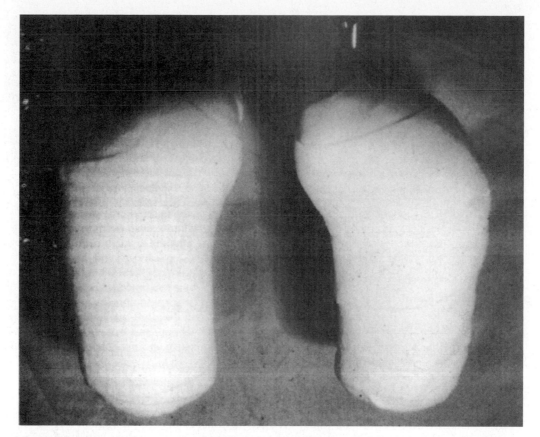

Figure 57.6 This horseshoe-type headrest has been associated with unilateral eye blindness due to pressure on the eye during surgery. The forehead rests on the upper portion with the chin free in the wider, open portion.

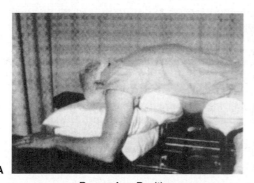

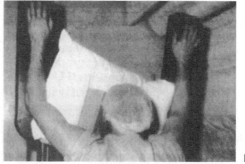

A   B

Proper Arm Position   Improper Arm Position

Figure 57.7 Proper arm position and improper arm position during scoliosis surgery. **A:** Degrees of abduction (relative to the trunk). **B:** Improper arm positioning with the arms abducted above the head. This results in stretching of the brachial plexus.

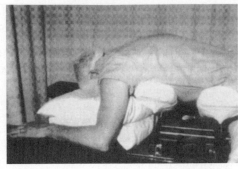
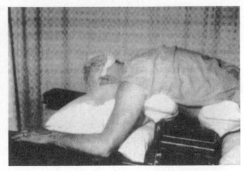

A   Proper Frame Position   Improper Frame Position   B

Figure 57.8 Proper and improper positioning on the four poster frame during spine surgery. **A:** Proper positioning on the frame with ample space between the axilla and the thoracic bolster of the frame. **B:** Improper positioning on the frame resulting in compression of the axillary sheath by the thoracic bolster of the frame.

any deficit or maintenance requirements. Procedures that are more extensive may require higher infusion rates.

Guay J, Haig M, Lortie L, et al. Predicting blood loss in surgery for idiopathic scoliosis. *Can J Anaesth* 1994;41(9):775–781.

C.16. What is transfusion-related acute lung injury (TRALI)?

Transfusion-related acute lung injury (TRALI) is noncardiogenic pulmonary edema occurring within 1 to 6 hours of transfusion of a plasma-containing blood product. In intubated patients it presents as copious, pink, frothy pulmonary edema fluid in the endotracheal tube. While clinically indistinguishable from adult respiratory distress syndrome (ARDS), TRALI is associated with a much lower mortality rate (5%–10%). Typically, the chest x-ray and arterial oxygen saturation return to baseline within 72 hours. The exact mechanism of TRALI is unknown, but evidence points to pathologic antibodies in donor plasma causing agglutination of white blood cells on pulmonary endothelial cells. Platelet transfusions have been most commonly implicated. Therapy is supportive, similar to that for ARDS.

Popovsky MA, Davenport RD. Transfusion-related acute lung injury: femme fatale? *Transfusion* 2001;41:312–315.

Silliman CC. Transfusion-related acute lung injury. *Transfus Med Rev* 1999;13(3):177–186.

C.17. What techniques can be used to minimize transfusion requirements?

There are several techniques to minimize homologous blood transfusion requirements. A simple and important way to minimize bleeding is to minimize intraabdominal pressure, as any increase in abdominal pressure is transmitted to the vertebral venous plexus, increasing venous bleeding. Careful positioning will avoid external pressure on the abdomen, and muscle relaxants or deeper levels of anesthesia have been used to prevent a rise in abdominal wall tension.

Isovolemic hemodilution may also be used to minimize red cell loss during surgery. Before incision the hematocrit is lowered 20% to 25% by removing blood aseptically and storing it in anticoagulated bags. Intravascular volume is maintained by replacing the blood with three times the volume of a balanced saline solution, or an equal volume of colloid. Intraoperatively, the previously withdrawn blood is replaced as needed. Obviously this technique requires careful monitoring of intravascular volume status and hemoglobin level. Some patients who are Jehovah's Witnesses and will not accept blood transfusions may accept this type of blood conservation method because the blood can be kept in continuity with the circulation.

Salvaging of blood during the surgical procedure can play an important role as an adjunct to an autologous blood program. In our experience, 50% to 60% of the red blood cells lost can be recovered, concentrated, washed, and return to the patient using commercially available autotransfusion devices. These red cells are obviously lacking in platelets and plasma. Some Jehovah's Witness patients may also accept this technique if the autotransfusion device is kept in continuity with the circulation.

The use of an antifibrinolytic agent such as tranexamic acid has been shown to decrease blood loss in pediatric patients undergoing scoliosis surgery. These agents may be of particular benefit in patients with neuromuscular scoliosis such as Duchenne's muscular dystrophy. These patients have significantly greater intraoperative blood loss compared with idiopathic scoliosis. The antifibrinolytic agent is administered as a loading dose followed by a continuous infusion before the activation of the fibrinolytic system, which occurs with surgical incision.

Deliberate hypotension has been used widely to decrease blood loss and improve operating conditions during spine fusion surgery. It has been shown to decrease blood loss 30% to 50% when mean arterial pressure is maintained at 50 to 60 mm Hg.

Fontana JL, Welborn L, Mongan P, et al. Oxygen consumption and cardiovascular function in children during profound intraoperative hemodilution. *Anesth Analg* 1995; 80:219–225.

Miller RD, eds. *Miller's anesthesia*, 6th ed. Philadelphia: Elsevier: Churchill Livingstone, 2005:2418–2420.

Sethna NF, Zurakowski D, Brustowicz RM, et al. Tranexamic acid reduces intraoperative blood loss in pediatric patients undergoing scoliosis surgery. *Anesthesiology* 2005;102: 727–732.

C.18. What techniques would you use to produce deliberate hypotension during scoliosis surgery? What is the major concern of using this technique?

Many techniques have been used to produce deliberate hypotension. These include using high doses of potent inhalation anesthetic agents, vasodilators (sodium nitroprusside, nitroglycerin, adenosine), ganglionic blocking agents (trimethaphan), β-adrenergic blocking agents (propranolol, esmolol), angiotensin-converting enzyme inhibitors (captopril), and combinations of these agents. As high doses of potent anesthetics interfere with spinal cord monitoring and make it more difficult to perform an intraoperative wake-up test, this technique is not commonly used to produce deliberate hypotension during scoliosis surgery. Animal experiments have suggested that deliberate hypotension with trimethaphan may be associated with a decrease in spinal cord blood flow compared with sodium nitroprusside or nitroglycerin. A commonly utilized technique employs a short acting vasodilator such as sodium nitroprusside and a short-acting β-adrenergic blocker such as esmolol. Mean arterial pressure can be rapidly stabilized at 50 to 65 torr and will return to normal within minutes of discontinuing these agents.

The major concern of using deliberate hypotension during scoliosis surgery is the potential for spinal cord blood flow to be compromised with resultant spinal cord injury. This is of particular concern when the spine is distracted because levels of hypotension that are considered safe under normal conditions may compromise spinal cord blood flow after spine distraction. A study in dogs demonstrated that spinal cord blood flow decreases with deliberate hypotension but returns to baseline levels after approximately 35 minutes. Therefore, it has been recommended that the spine should not be distracted for 35 minutes after the start of deliberate hypotension.

In patients at high risk for development of neurologic injury (see section 2), it is important to balance the potential benefits of deliberate hypotension with the potential risks, and if deliberate hypotension is utilized, it is probably prudent to maintain mean arterial pressure no lower than 60 or 65 torr.

Grundy BL, Nash CL, Brown CR. Arterial pressure manipulation alters spinal cord function during correction of scoliosis. *Anesthesiology* 1981;54:249–253.

Kling TF, Ferguson NV, Leach AB, et al. The influence of induced hypotension and spine distraction on canine spinal cord blood flow. *Spine* 1985;10:878–883.

Miller RD, eds. *Miller's Anesthesia*. 6th ed. Philadelphia: Elsevier: Churchill Livingstone, 2005:2418–2420.

D. Postoperative Management

D.1. When would you extubate the patient?

The decision to continue mechanical ventilation in the postoperative period is usually made preoperatively. Most patients with adolescent idiopathic scoliosis have mild to moderate pulmonary function abnormalities and may be extubated in the operating room. Mechanical ventilation should be continued in patients with severe restrictive lung defects (vital capacity less than 30% of predicted) or severe gas exchange abnormalities such as CO_2 retention. Postoperative mechanical ventilation should be considered for patients with Duchenne's muscular dystrophy, familial dysautonomia, or severe cerebral palsy.

The parameters for extubation given below are the same as for other respiratory disorders:

- Vital capacity >10 mL per kg
- Tidal volume >3 mL per kg
- Spontaneous respiratory rate <30 per minute
- Negative inspiratory force >−30 cm H_2O

Bradford DS, Lonstein JE, Ogilvie JW, et al. eds. *Moe's textbook of scoliosis and other spinal deformities*. Philadelphia: WB Saunders, 1987:590.

D.2. What should be done to optimize pulmonary status?

Incentive spirometry should be taught preoperatively and should be used aggressively in the postoperative period. Coughing and deep breathing should be encouraged. Patients with obstructive or reactive airway disease will benefit from bronchodilators. Narcotics should be used judiciously with the goal of providing adequate analgesia to allow coughing and incentive spirometry without excessive respiratory depression.

D.3. What laboratory tests should be ordered postoperatively?

Upon arrival in the recovery room, blood should be sent for analysis of arterial blood gases, hematocrit, electrolytes, blood urea nitrogen (BUN), creatinine, and if blood loss has been large, platelet count, prothrombin, and partial thromboplastin time. Determination of arterial blood gases should be repeated if clinically indicated. Hyponatremia with high urinary sodium excretion has been reported following scoliosis surgery and has been attributed to the syndrome of inappropriate antidiuretic hormone secretion (SIADH). These patients produce small amounts of concentrated urine and excrete large amounts of urinary sodium. Efforts to increase urine output by administration of fluid are unsuccessful and worsen the hyponatremia. Therefore, serum electrolyte concentrations should be measured at least every 12 hours for the first 24 hours, and then daily for the first 2 days. Rapid decreases in serum sodium concentration or sodium concentrations less than 125 mEq per L may produce swelling of brain cells (intracellular "edema") and convulsions.

Brenner BM, Rector FC, eds. *The kidney*. Philadelphia: WB Saunders, 1986:418.

Burrows FA, Shutack JG, Crone RK. Inappropriate secretion of antidiuretic hormone in a postsurgical pediatric population. *Crit Care Med* 1983;11(7):527–531.

D.4. What fluid therapy would you use postoperatively?

Significant losses of intravascular fluid continue to occur in the postoperative period. These should be replaced with balanced salt solution such as lactated Ringer's to maintain urine output at a minimum of 0.5 to 1 mL/kg/hour. Hypotonic fluids should be avoided in the first 24 to 36 hours postoperatively. The risk of postoperative hyponatremia is increased if fluid replacement is excessive or if hypotonic fluid is administered. Some authors recommend the use of colloid replacement solutions as serum albumin is often decreased following scoliosis surgery.

Brenner BM, Rector FC, eds. *The kidney*. Philadelphia: WB Saunders, 1986:418.

Burrows FA, Shutack JG, Crone RK. Inappropriate secretion of antidiuretic hormone in a postsurgical pediatric population. *Crit Care Med* 1983;11(7):527–531.

D.5. What complications may occur following scoliosis surgery?

Complications that have been reported in the postoperative period include pneumothorax, atelectasis, pleural effusion, hemothorax, thoracic duct injury, and neurologic injury. Pneumothorax may occur due to both anterior and posterior surgical dissections, as well as secondary to central venous line placement. A chest x-ray should be obtained upon arrival in the postanesthesia care unit. Atelectasis may occur due to prolonged supine positioning and the use of narcotics. Anterior spine fusion by thoracotomy poses the greatest risk of pulmonary complications. Almost 100% of patients undergoing these procedures will develop some degree of atelectasis. Incentive spirometry and deep breathing should be emphasized and may require specialized nursing care.

In addition to intraoperative neurologic complications during instrumentation or distraction of the spine, there have been a number of reports of delayed paraplegia in the first few days postoperatively. This emphasizes the need for continued monitoring of neurologic status postoperatively.

In the first few postoperative days, adynamic ileus occurs commonly and some authors recommend placement of nasogastric tubes in all patients. Less commonly, superior mesenteric artery syndrome has been reported to occur in 0.5% of patients. This presents with nausea, vomiting, and abdominal pain after a mean time of 7.2 days. This is probably due to compression of the distal third of the duodenum by the superior mesenteric artery as a result of anatomic changes related to straightening of the spine.

Altiok H, Lubicky JP, DeWald CJ, et al. The superior mesenteric artery syndrome in patients with spinal deformity. *Spine* 2005;30(19):2164–2170.

Kahanowitz N, Levine DB. Iatrogenic complications of spinal surgery. *Contemp Orthop* 1984;9(2):23–39.

Stockl B, Wimmer C, Innerhofer P, et al. Delayed anterior spinal artery syndrome following posterior scoliosis correction. *Eur Spine J* 2005;14:906–909

Weinstein SL, ed. *The pediatric spine: principles and practice*. New York: Raven Press, 1994: 1761–1784.

CHAPTER 58

Hypoxia and Equipment Failure

JAMES B. EISENKRAFT • ANDREW B. LEIBOWITZ

A 70-YEAR-OLD MAN

is to undergo cystoscopy and transurethral resection of a bladder tumor under general anesthesia through a laryngeal mask airway. He gave a history of mild asthma and used an albuterol inhaler when necessary. Breathing room air ($FIO_2 = 0.21$), his pulse oximeter saturation reading (SpO_2) was 94%.

A. Medical Disease and Differential Diagnosis

1. What is hypoxia and what is hypoxemia?
2. Is PaO_2 related to age?
3. Was this patient hypoxemic?
4. What is a pulse oximeter and what is a hemoximeter?
5. How does a pulse oximeter work?
6. How is a pulse oximeter calibrated?
7. What may affect the accuracy of a pulse oximeter?
8. How do methemoglobin and carboxyhemoglobin affect SpO_2 readings?
9. What is capnometry and what is capnography? Of what value are they in patient monitoring?
10. What is meant by the term *end-tidal CO_2 ($PETCO_2$) concentration*?
11. What is the appearance of a normal capnogram and what is its significance?
12. What are mainstream and sidestream gas analyzers?
13. Show some common capnograms and provide a differential diagnosis of each event.
14. What is the arterial–alveolar difference in CO_2?
15. What are some of the important safety features of the contemporary anesthesia workstation?
16. What are common sites for gas leakage?
17. How can the anesthesia machine be checked for leaks?

B. Preoperative Evaluations and Preparation

1. What should be included in the equipment checkout in preparation for anesthesia?
2. What emergency equipment should be readily available to the anesthesiologist?
3. How should this patient be premedicated?

C. Intraoperative Management

1. How should this patient be monitored?

2. After uneventful inhalation mask induction, cystoscopy was begun and the SpO_2 was noted to decrease to 81% with the patient breathing O_2 at 2 L per minute and N_2O at 3 L per minute. The patient developed respiratory distress. The laryngeal mask airway was easily maintained and no gross secretions were noted. What acute diagnostic and therapeutic interventions would you perform?

3. The patient was tracheally intubated. Squeezing the reservoir bag in the circle system failed to ventilate the lungs and a leak was noted. What are the common sites for gas leaks?

D. Postoperative Management

1. What criteria would you use to establish readiness for tracheal extubation?
2. What are the causes of postoperative hypoxemia?
3. What is the difference between shunt, ventilation/perfusion mismatch, and dead space?
4. What is the differential diagnosis of pulmonary edema?
5. How should the ventilator be set if mechanical ventilation is required postoperatively?
6. What other changes in routine therapy should be considered?
7. What methods of oxygen administration may be used postoperatively?

A. Medical Disease and Differential Diagnosis

A.1. What is hypoxia and what is hypoxemia?

Hypoxia is defined as reduction of oxygen supply to tissue below physiologic levels. Hypoxemia is defined as deficient oxygenation of the blood. From the anesthesiologist's perspective, hypoxia is usually considered to be decreased oxygen tension (Po_2) inside the body at the tissue level or outside the body (e.g., hypoxic gas mixture), and hypoxemia is decreased oxygen tension in the arterial blood (Pao_2).

Dorland WAN. *Dorland's illustrated medical dictionary*, 28th ed. Philadelphia: WB Saunders, 1994:812.

Wilson W. Perioperative hypoxia. In: Atlee JL, ed. *Complications in anesthesia*. Philadelphia: WB Saunders, 1999:175.

A.2. Is Pao_2 related to age?

Yes. There is an age-dependent decrease in the Pao_2. In 1972, Marshall and Whyche suggested the following relationship in subjects breathing room air:

$$\text{mean } Pao_2 \text{ in mm Hg} = 102 - 0.33 \text{ (age in years) mm Hg}$$

About this regression line, there are 95% confidence limits (2 standard deviations [SDs]) of 10 mm Hg.

Sorbini et al. found that mean Pao_2 decreased from 95 ± 2 mm Hg (SD) at age 20 years, to 73 ± 5 at age 75 years. In both men and women, the decrease in Pao_2 was 4 to 5 mm Hg per decade.

Marshall BE, Whyche MQ. Hypoxemia during and after anesthesia. *Anesthesiology* 1972;37: 178.

Sorbini CA, Grassi V, Salinas E, et al. Arterial oxygen tension in relation to age in healthy subjects. *Respiration* 1968;25:3–13.

A.3. Was this patient hypoxemic?

No. A hemoglobin oxygen saturation reading of 94% does not signify hypoxemia. This patient is five decades older than a 20-year-old subject; therefore, his mean PaO_2 should be 5×5 mm Hg per decade, which is 25 mm Hg less than that (95 mm Hg) expected in a 20-year-old (see section A.2, Sorbini et al.).

$$95 - 25 = 70 \text{ mm Hg}$$

or, using the Marshall and Whyche equation (see section A.2),

$$102 - 0.33(70) = 79 \text{ mm Hg}$$

Assuming normal adult hemoglobin, temperature, and pH, this PaO_2 corresponds to a hemoglobin oxygen saturation of approximately 94% on the normal hemoglobin oxygen saturation versus PO_2 curve.

Although the definitions of hypoxemia given in sections A.1 and A.2 must take age into consideration, from a practical point of view, hypoxemia (in the absence of anemia) is generally considered to exist when the PaO_2 is less than 60 mm Hg, which is equivalent to a hemoglobin oxygen saturation of 90%.

Forbes RB, Layman AJ. Anticipating common intraoperative problems. In: Longnecker DE, Tinker JH, Morgan GE Jr, eds. *Principles and practice of anesthesiology*, 2nd ed. St. Louis: Mosby–Year Book, 1998:108.

Lumb AB. *Nunn's applied respiratory physiology*, 6th ed. Philadelphia: Elsevier Science, 2005:166.

A.4. What is a pulse oximeter and what is a hemoximeter?

The pulse oximeter is a noninvasive device that provides an estimate (designated the SpO_2%) of the arterial hemoglobin saturation with oxygen. It is a transmissive oximeter in which the patient's fingertip (or other probe site; e.g., earlobe) serves as an *in vivo* cuvette through which light at two different wavelengths is transmitted.

If one requires an accurate determination of the arterial hemoglobin saturation with oxygen, an arterial blood sample must be drawn and analyzed using a laboratory cooximeter, sometimes called a *hemoximeter*. The laboratory cooximeter is a transmissive oximeter that uses six or more different wavelengths of light to measure total hemoglobin ($HbTOT$), oxygenated hemoglobin (HbO_2), deoxygenated ("reduced") hemoglobin (RHb), methemoglobin (metHb), carboxyhemoglobin (HbCO), and other dyshemoglobins such as sulfhemoglobin. Because each species of hemoglobin has a characteristic absorbance spectrum (i.e., absorbance vs. wavelength), examination of a sample of blood using these six or eight wavelengths permits identification and quantification of each hemoglobin species. Conventional pulse oximeters use only two wavelengths of light, therefore they are unable to determine all of the different hemoglobin species. Fractional saturation (HbO_2%) is defined as $HbO_2/(HbO_2 + RHb + HbCO + metHb)$—that is, HbO_2 per total Hb. Functional saturation (SaO_2) is defined as $HbO_2/(HbO_2 + RHb)$. Note that dyshemoglobins are absent from the denominator in the definition of SaO_2.

Barker SJ, Tremper KK. Pulse oximetry. In: Ehrenwerth J, Eisenkraft JB, eds. *Anesthesia equipment: principles and applications*. St. Louis: Mosby–Year Book, 1993:249–263.

A.5. How does a pulse oximeter work?

The pulse oximeter combines the technologies of spectrophotometry and optical plethysmography. In the pulse oximeter probe, light-emitting diodes transmit red light at wavelengths 660 nm and infrared light at 960 nm through the fingertip or other probe site. Light that passes through the probe site is sensed by a single photodetector and expressed as absorbance at each wavelength. The ratio of absorbances, 660/990 nm, is related to the hemoglobin saturation with oxygen. This is spectrophotometry. Detection of pulsatile flow is by optical plethysmography. With each pulse of arterial blood, the probe site (e.g., fingertip) increases in volume, the path length of light increases, and the absorbance of light at 660 nm and 940 nm increases. This *pulse-added* absorbance is considered to be due to the pulsatile flow of arterial blood at the probe site, so that the ratio of pulse-added absorbances, 660/990 nm, can be used to provide an estimate of hemoglobin oxygen saturation in arterial blood.

Pologe JA. Pulse oximetry: technical aspects of machine design. *Int Anesthesiol Clin* 1987; 25:137–153.

A.6. How is a two-wavelength pulse oximeter calibrated by the manufacturer?

Each pulse oximeter manufacturer creates an empiric calibration algorithm, that is, one that is based on observations in human volunteers. The algorithm relates the average ratio of pulse-added absorbances, 660/990 nm, to the actual hemoglobin oxygen saturation in arterial blood samples drawn simultaneously and analyzed in a laboratory hemoximeter. Observations are made with the volunteers breathing varying FiO_2 values so data for saturations as low as 70% are obtained. The calibration algorithm that is created relates the ratio (R) of pulse-added absorbances, 660/990 nm, to the laboratory cooximeter readings of HbO_2 or SaO_2%, depending on the pulse oximeter manufacturer. The calibration algorithm is then stored in the software of the pulse oximeter as a "lookup" table. Therefore the pulse oximeter merely measures R, consults its "lookup" table, and displays the corresponding saturation reading as SpO_2. The pulse oximeter does not actually measure saturation; it infers it from the ratio (R) and therefore it predicts what the laboratory hemoximeter would read if an arterial sample drawn at that moment were analyzed.

A high value for R corresponds to a low SpO_2 reading; R = 1 corresponds to an SpO_2 reading of 85%; and a low value for R corresponds to a high SpO_2 reading. Whenever the SpO_2 reading is approximately 85%, one should consider the possibility of a spurious reading due to the "R = 1" phenomenon.

The pulse oximeter (SpO_2) reading is usually specified to have a standard deviation (SD) of 2%. Therefore, if the SpO_2 is 96%, there is a 68% likelihood that the true saturation (as measured by a hemoximeter) is 96 ± 2% (i.e., ±1 SD) and a 95% likelihood that the true saturation is 96 ± 4% (i.e., ±2 SD).

Kelleher JF, Ruff RH. The penumbra effect-vasomotion–dependent pulse oximeter artifact due to probe malposition. *Anesthesiology* 1989;71:787–791.

Pologe JA. Pulse oximetry: technical aspects of machine design. *Int Anesthesiol Clin* 1987; 25:137–153.

A.7. What may affect the accuracy of a two-wavelength pulse oximeter?

The two-wavelength pulse oximeter is most accurate when the conditions of its clinical use most closely resemble those of its calibration. Spurious readings or failure may occur during patient movement (e.g., shivering, peripheral nerve stimulation, and "twitching"), presence of intense ambient light (low signal/noise ratio), electrocautery use, administration of intravenous dyes with absorbance peaks at 660 nm (e.g., methylene blue), presence of dyshemoglobins (e.g., methemoglobin, carboxyhemoglobin, and sulfhemoglobin), nail polish, poor pulsatile flow at the probe site (e.g., hypotension, vasoconstriction, Raynaud's disease), and venous pulsations (e.g., tricuspid regurgitation).

Recent improvements in pulse oximetry technology include paradigms to increase the signal/noise ratio, thereby permitting motion artifact reduction and increased sensitivity to pulsatile flow. Such pulse oximeters have significantly lower failure rates during patient movement (such as in the postanesthesia care unit) and during conditions of low flow (e.g., hypothermia).

Barker SJ. "Motion-resistant" pulse oximetry: a comparison of new and old models. *Anesth Analg* 2002;95:967–972.

Eisenkraft JB, Barker SJ. Monitoring oxygenation and ventilation. In: Youngberg JA, Lake CL, Roizen MF, et al, eds. *Cardiac, thoracic and vascular anesthesia.* New York: Churchill Livingstone, 2000:307–327.

A.8. How do the methemoglobin (met HB) and carboxyhemoglobin (HbCO) affect SpO$_2$ readings?

In methemoglobin, iron in the heme moiety is oxidized (such as by dapsone, benzocaine, nitric oxide, prilocaine) to the Fe^{3+} state rather than being in the normal Fe^{2+} state. Methemoglobin cannot carry oxygen and creates a physiologic anemia. The absorbance spectrum for metHb shows it to have similar absorbances at 660 and 940 nm. Therefore, the more metHb that is present, the more R tends toward 1 and the SpO$_2$ reading toward 85%. In the presence of metHb, the SpO$_2$ reading overestimates the fractional saturation and underestimates the functional saturation.

In carbon monoxide (CO) poisoning, CO combines with Hb to create a physiologic hypoxemia. HbCO has a similar absorbance to HbO$_2$ at 660 nm, but a very low absorbance at 940 nm. In the presence of HbCO, the SpO$_2$ overestimates fractional saturation and underestimates functional saturation. Although blood that is poisoned with carbon monoxide appears "cherry red" in color to the naked eye, and therefore may look like it is fully saturated with oxygen, it is important to recognize that the ratio of absorbances 660/940 nm suggest blood with a hemoglobin oxygen saturation in the 90s. In a subject breathing FIO$_2$ of 1 (when functional saturation is 100%), as the level of HbCO increases, SpO$_2$ decreases from close to 100% down to approximately 91%.

If the presence of dyshemoglobins is suspected, arterial blood must be drawn and analyzed in a hemoximeter to obtain accurate readings of saturation.

Pulse oximetry technology continues to improve. Very recently, the Masimo Company (Irvine, CA) has announced the introduction of a pulse oximeter that uses eight wavelengths of light (Masimo Rainbow SET Pulse CO-Oximetry), similar to the hemoximeter. This will offer the unique ability to accurately measure carbon monoxide (SpCO), methemoglobin (SpMet) and potentially other future parameters like fractional arterial oxygen saturation (SpaO2) and total hemoglobin (SpHbt), all noninvasively.

Barker SJ, Tremper KK. The effect of carbon monoxide inhalation on pulse oximetry and transcutaneous PO$_2$. *Anesthesiology* 1987;66:677–679.

Barker SJ, Curry J, Redford D, et al. Measurement of carboxyhemoglobin and methemglobin by pulse oximetry: a human volunteer study. *Anesthesiology* 2006;105:892–897.

Barker SJ, Tremper KK, Hyatt J. Effects of methemoglobin on pulse oximetry and mixed venous oximetry. *Anesthesiology* 1989;70:112–117.

A.9. What is a capnometer and what is capnography? Of what value are they in patient monitoring?

A capnometer is a device that measures the tension (millimeters of mercury) or concentration (volumes %) of carbon dioxide in the gas near the patient's airway during ventilation. Capnography is the graphic display of the CO_2 concentration on the y-axis against time on the x-axis.

Capnometry may be achieved using different technologies that can monitor CO_2. Most capnometers now use infrared spectroscopy to measure the P_{CO_2} (i.e., CO_2 partial pressure in millimeters of mercury). A built-in barometer measures barometric pressure (P_B) so that CO_2 can also be displayed as a percentage ($P_{CO_2} \times 100/P_B = \%CO_2$).

Capnography is one of the American Society of Anesthesiologists' standards for basic anesthetic monitoring. ("Continual monitoring for the presence of expired carbon dioxide shall be performed unless invalidated by the nature of the patient, procedure or equipment.") It is the "gold standard" for establishing presence of ventilation.

ASA standards for basic anesthetic monitoring (approved October 21, 1986 and last amended October 25, 2005). Park Ridge: American Society of Anesthesiologists, 2005.

Eisenkraft JB, Raemer DB. Monitoring gases in the anesthesia delivery system. In: Ehrenwerth J, Eisenkraft JB, eds. *Anesthesia equipment: principles and applications.* St. Louis: Mosby–Year Book, 1993:201–220.

A.10. What is meant by the term "end-tidal CO_2 (P_{ETCO_2}) concentration?"

End-tidal CO_2 (P_{ETCO_2}) is the tension of CO_2 in the exhaled gas at the end of an exhalation. Because this gas originates from the alveoli, it is considered to represent the CO_2 tension in the alveolar gas (P_{ACO_2}). The P_{ACO_2} results from the combination of gases coming from ideal alveoli, where ventilation and perfusion are perfectly matched and the CO_2 concentration is the same as arterial (P_{ACO_2}), and alveolar dead space (alveoli that are ventilated but not perfused) where CO_2 concentration is the same as inspired (P_{ICO_2}) and is normally zero.

The presence of a normal capnogram and P_{ETCO_2} depends on (a) production of CO_2 by the tissues, (b) cardiac output and pulmonary blood flow to carry CO_2 to the lungs, and (c) ventilation. Monitoring of P_{ETCO_2} can be used to adjust the setting of a mechanical ventilator and monitor ventilation, as well as detect ventilator malfunctions and breathing system problems such as leaks, incompetent unidirectional valves, exhausted CO_2 absorbent, metabolic problems (e.g., malignant hyperthermia), and gas embolism.

Lumb AB. *Nunn's applied respiratory physiology,* 6th ed. Philadelphia: Elsevier Science, 2005: 157–158.

A.11. What is the appearance of a normal capnogram and what is its significance?

A typical normal capnogram (P_{CO_2} vs. time) is shown in Fig. 58.1. Four phases have been described.

Phase I. This is the expiratory baseline. During exhalation, CO_2-free gas from the mechanical dead space (e.g., flexible or "goose-neck" connector) and anatomic dead space (large conducting airways) flows past the CO_2 sampling port.

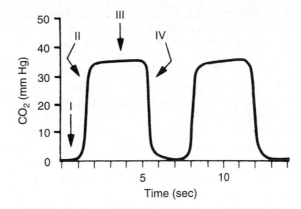

Figure 58.1 Phases of the normal capnogram. *(Phase I)* Inspiratory baseline; *(Phase II)* expiratory upstroke; *(Phase III)* expiratory plateau; and *(Phase IV)* inspiratory downstroke. (From Good ML. Capnography: uses, interpretation, and pitfalls. In: *ASA refresher courses in anesthesiology.* American Society of Anesthesiologists, 1990:179, with permission.)

Phase II. This is the expiratory upstroke. It is due to CO_2 from alveoli mixed with dead space gas arriving at the sensor and is usually a steep upslope.

Phase III. This is the expiratory or alveolar plateau and is due to alveolar CO_2.

In patients with healthy lungs, it is nearly horizontal, but in patients with obstructive airways disease, there is a more pronounced upward slope. The maximum expired CO_2 is usually considered as the end-tidal CO_2 (P_{ETCO_2}).

The angle between the upstroke of phase II and the plateau of phase III is referred to as the *α angle*. The angle between phase III and IV is the *β angle*. An increase in the *α* angle and slope of phase III is seen commonly in acute bronchospasm. The angle usually decreases with treatment of the bronchospasm.

Phase IV. This is the inspiratory downstroke. During the commencement of inspiration, fresh (i.e., CO_2-free) gas is inhaled past the sensor and the capnogram falls sharply to baseline.

Lumb AB. *Nunn's applied respiratory physiology,* 6th ed. Philadelphia: Elsevier Science, 2005: 162.

A.12. What are mainstream and sidestream gas analyzers?

In a mainstream or nondiverting type of analyzer, the gas analyzer sensor is brought to the airway itself and no gas is removed from the breathing system. A cuvette with a quartz window is placed between the breathing system and the tracheal tube connector. As respired gases flow past the window in the cuvette, a beam of infrared radiation (wavelength 4.3 μm) is directed through the window. Absorbance of infrared radiation at 4.3 μm is used to measure P_{CO_2}. At present, only CO_2 is measured using mainstream analysis. Advantages of the nondiverting analyzer are rapid response time, accurate waveform, and no need to scavenge gases. Disadvantages are that this additional device in the airway can be a site for a disconnect and needs sterilization between cases, limitation to CO_2 analysis only, need for heating because water vapor condensing on the window causes error, and blocking of the window by secretions or blood.

A sidestream or diverting gas analyzer aspirates gas from the breathing circuit through a sampling adapter placed by the airway. The sampled gas passes down a sampling catheter (usually 6–10 feet in length) to reach the gas analyzer. Advantages of diverting analyzers are that the breathing circuit adapter is disposable. The analyzer, being remote from the airway, can be more versatile and incorporate several technologies in one "box" to analyze gases (e.g., infrared for CO_2, N_2O, anesthetic agents; paramagnetic sensor or fuel cell for O_2; or Raman scattering for CO_2, O_2, agents, N_2O, and N_2). Disadvantages of sidestream sampling analysis are slower response times, possibility of sampling leaks, errors due to length of the gas sampling tube, need to scavenge gases from the analyzer after analysis, and susceptibility of the sampling tube to becoming clogged by water or secretions. Because of their versatility in regard to gas monitoring, most anesthetizing locations now use sidestream sampling analyzers.

Eisenkraft JB, Raemer DB. Monitoring gases in the anesthesia delivery system. In: Ehrenwerth J, Eisenkraft JB, eds. *Anesthesia equipment: principles and applications.* St. Louis: Mosby–Year Book, 1993:201–220.

A.13. Show some common capnograms and provide a differential diagnosis of each event.

Elevated baseline = the amount of CO_2 present in inspired gas (Fig. 58.2A).

- Capnometer not properly calibrated to zero
- Delivery of CO_2 to breathing system through fresh gas inflow
- Incompetent unidirectional valves
- Failure of CO_2 absorber (channeling, exhaustion, bypass)

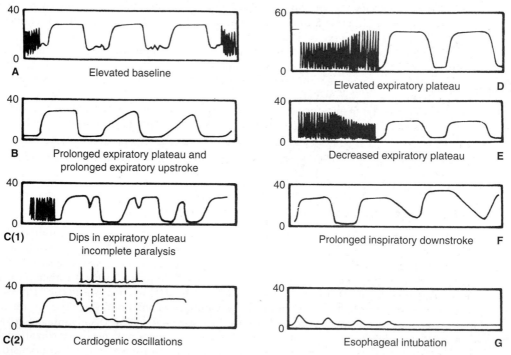

Figure 58.2 Abnormal capnograms.

Prolonged expiratory plateau and expiratory upstroke (Fig. 58.2B)

- Mechanical obstruction to exhalation
- Chronic obstructive pulmonary disease
- Bronchospasm

Dips in expiratory plateau (Fig. 58.2C[1])

- Patient making spontaneous inspiratory effort
- "Curare cleft"

Cardiogenic oscillations if synchronized with electrocardiogram (Fig. 58.2C[2])

- Ventilator pressure relief valve perturbations

Elevated expiratory plateau (Fig. 58.2D)

- Incorrect calibration
- Increased CO_2 production/delivery versus laparoscopic CO_2 gas insufflation
- Decreased CO_2 removal
- Hypoventilation
- Leak

Decreased expiratory plateau (Fig. 58.2E)

- Incorrect calibration
- Air leak into gas sampling system
- Hyperventilation
- Decreased CO_2 production (hypothermia)
- Increased arterial–alveolar CO_2 gradient (ventilation/perfusion mismatch pulmonary embolus)

Prolonged inspiratory downstroke and raised baseline (Fig. 58.2F)

- Incompetent or missing inspiratory unidirectional valve
- Inspiratory obstruction to gas flow (e.g., kinked tube)

Esophageal intubation (Fig. 58.2G)

As CO_2 that has been insufflated into the stomach during bag-mask ventilation, or CO_2 produced as a result of ingestion of a carbonated beverage, is washed out during esophageal ventilation, the CO_2 waveform disappears within a few breaths.

Good ML, Gravenstein N. Capnography. In: Ehrenwerth J, Eisenkraft JB, eds. *Anesthesia equipment: principles and applications.* St. Louis: Mosby–Year Book, 1993:237–248.

A.14. What is the arterial–alveolar difference in CO_2?

The arterial–alveolar difference in CO_2 is usually expressed as the difference between the arterial and end-tidal CO_2 tensions. In an ideal alveolus, the P_{ACO_2} equals P_{aCO_2} and the "P_{aCO_2}–P_{ACO_2}" difference is zero. Ventilation of unperfused alveoli, however, leads to alveolar dead space or wasted alveolar ventilation. Because the end-tidal CO_2 (P_{ETCO_2}) comprises gas from both ideal and dead space alveoli, the "P_{aCO_2}–P_{ACO_2}" difference is a measure of alveolar dead space ventilation.

$$\text{Tidal volume} = 500 \text{ mL, anatomic dead space} = 150 \text{ mL}$$

$$P_{aCO_2} = 40 \text{ mm Hg}; P_{ETCO_2} = 36 \text{ mm Hg}$$

$$\text{Alveolar tidal volume} = (500 - 150) = 350 \text{ mL}$$

$$\text{Ratio of } \frac{\text{Alveolar dead space}}{\text{Alveolar tidal volume}} = \frac{P_{aCO_2} - P_{ETCO_2}}{P_{aCO_2}} = \frac{40 - 36}{40} = 10\%$$

Therefore, 350 mL × 10% = 35 mL wasted ventilation from each alveolar tidal volume

$$\text{Ideal alveolar ventilation} = (350 - 35) = 315 \text{ mL per breath}$$

In this example, physiologic dead space = anatomic + alveolar

$$= 150 + 35 = 185 \text{ mL per breath.}$$

$$\frac{\text{Physiologic dead space}}{\text{Tidal volume}} = \frac{185}{500} = 37\%$$

Therefore, $Paco_2$–$Paco_2$ measures alveolar dead space ventilation as a percentage of total alveolar ventilation. The alveolar dead space is increased by ventilation in excess of perfusion, or a decrease in perfusion, such as occurs with pulmonary embolism. Shunt has minimal effect on $Paco_2$–$Paco_2$.

$Paco_2$–$Paco_2$ is normally 3 to 5 mm Hg in the patient under general anesthesia, but it is not constant. Therefore, although one commonly uses $Petco_2$ to noninvasively estimate $Paco_2$, only an arterial blood sample can provide an accurate measure of $Paco_2$, and this should be measured when critical, such as during neurosurgical anesthesia.

Lumb AB. *Nunn's applied respiratory physiology*, 6th ed. Philadelphia: Elsevier Science, 2005: 120.

A.15. What are some of the important safety features of the contemporary anesthesia workstation?

Because most problems with anesthesia machines are due to use error, safety design of the contemporary workstation is at four levels.

Features intended to prevent human error

The medical gas pin index and diameter index safety systems ensure that medical gas connections are made correctly. Therefore, one cannot hang an N_2O cylinder in an O_2 hanger yoke, or connect an N_2O hose to the O_2 pipeline inlet of the machine.

The "fail-safe" valve is a pressure-sensitive device that interrupts flow of all hypoxic gases on the machine to their flow control valves if the supply pressure of O_2 in the high-pressure system (i.e., components upstream of the O_2 flow control needle valve) falls below a threshold (20 psig in Datex-Ohmeda machines; 12 psig in Dräger Narkomed machines).

When the pressure of O_2 in the high-pressure system falls below 30 psig, an oxygen supply pressure failure alarm is annunciated. The oxygen flow control knob is "touch coded"; that is, it is fluted and larger in diameter than the other gas flow control knobs and is located on the right of all other gas flow control valves.

Key-fill systems for anesthesia vaporizers are safety features that also decrease the likelihood of atmospheric contamination during vaporizer filling. The most important of such systems is the Saf-T-Fill system used on desflurane (Suprane) bottles and desflurane vaporizers because the filling with desflurane of a vaporizer specific for another agent could result in a lethal overdose of desflurane.

A pressure relief valve built into the machine common gas outlet, breathing system, or ventilator provides some protection against positive pressure barotrauma.

Features to correct for use error

Gas flow proportioning systems ensure a minimum O_2 concentration of 25% when N_2O and O_2 are being used. Therefore, if the anesthesiologist were to accidentally attempt to increase the flow of N_2O, either the O_2 flow would be increased automatically (Datex-Ohmeda) system or the flow of N_2O would be limited according to the flow of O_2 that was set.

On older machines, during use of the anesthesia ventilator, changes in fresh gas flow, I:E ratio, or respiratory rate cause changes in delivered tidal volume (V_T) that might result in overventilation, underventilation, or even barotrauma. On modern systems (e.g., Datex-Ohmeda S5ADU and Aisys workstations that incorporate a 7900 series ventilator that has the Smart Vent feature; Dräger Narkomed 6000 series, Fabius GS and Apollo workstations), once the ventilation parameters have been set, they are maintained because the ventilator automatically compensates for changes in gas flow settings. In the Datex-Ohmeda workstations V_T is monitored continually by a computer. If measured V_T changes from that set to be delivered, the computer adjusts the volume delivered by the ventilator bellows. Drager and Datascope workstations use fresh gas decoupling to maintain a constant V_T. In this system, during the inspiratory phase, a decoupling valve closes so that fresh gas entering the breathing system is directed into the reservoir bag and only gas from the ventilator is delivered to the patient. During exhalation the ventilator chamber refills from the fresh gas flow and the fresh gas that was collected in the reservoir bag during the previous inspiration.

A vaporizer interlock system prevents the simultaneous use of more than one vaporizer.

Monitoring systems

A monitor of O_2 in the gas delivered to the patient is mandated to be enabled and the low O_2 concentration alarm activated whenever the workstation is capable of delivering an anesthetic gas mixture from the common gas outlet.

Other monitors in the anesthesia workstation include pressure, volume, flow, and gas composition. Some also incorporate airway gas flow monitoring. The breathing system low-pressure monitor alarm is automatically enabled when the ventilator is turned on.

Alarm systems

Contemporary workstations incorporate a prioritized alarm system with high-, medium-, and low-priority alarms that have visible and audible alerts when set parameter limits are exceeded.

An important safety feature of all modern machines is the preuse checkout, or an approved departmental adaptation of the U.S. Food and Drug Administration's (FDA) 1993 checklist. The machine must be checked out by an educated user. Item no. 1 on the FDA checklist is that an alternative means to ventilate the patient's lungs be present and functioning. Therefore, if a problem arises with the machine, the patient's lungs can be ventilated using a self-inflating resuscitation bag. If a machine problem arises and the cause/remedy is not immediately obvious, one should instinctively reach for the resuscitation bag and call for help.

Brockwell RC, Andrews JJ. Delivery systems for inhaled anesthetics. In: Barash PG, Cullen BF, Stoelting RK. *Clinical anesthesia*, 5th ed. Philadelphia: Lippincott Williams & Wilkins, 2006:557.

Eisenkraft JB. Anesthesia delivery system. In: Longnecker DE, Tinker JH, Morgan GE Jr, eds. *Principles and practice of anesthesiology*, 2nd ed. St. Louis: Mosby–Year Book, 1998:1011–1063.

Eisenkraft JB. Complications of anesthesia delivery systems. In: *ASA refresher courses in anesthesiology*. American Society of Anesthesiologists, 2005;33:65–78.

Standard specification for particular requirements for anesthesia workstations and their components. West Conshohocken: American Society for Testing and Materials, 2000. No. F1850-00.

A.16. What are common sites for gas leakage?

Because gas can leak from numerous points in the workstation and breathing system, the anesthesiologist must be able to trace the flow of gases from their supply and storage sources, through the system components. Most commonly, leaks occur in the breathing system and/or low-pressure parts of the machine (i.e., components downstream of the gas flow control valves). For the breathing system, trace the flow of gas from the common gas outlet, through the antidisconnect fitting and hose, to the breathing circuit fresh gas inlet. Trace the flow of gas past the inspiratory valve, inspiratory limb, gas sampling connector, elbow, to the tracheal tube or airway device. Common sites for leaks include a partially deflated tracheal tube cuff or a disconnection of the sidestream sampling gas analyzer sampling line. Check flow back down the expiratory limb, spirometer, expiratory valve, absorber, pressure gauge, pressure sampling lines, and any user-added components such as filters, humidifiers, and positive end-expiratory pressure (PEEP) valves. Check both the bag and the ventilator circuits for gas leaks.

Leaks in the machine low-pressure system can occur as a result of cracked rotameter flow tubes, incorrectly mounted vaporizers, vaporizer leak around agent filling device, or fracture in the gas piping. Leaks in the high-pressure system usually result from defective valves, connectors, and hanger yokes.

Eisenkraft JB, Sommer RM. Equipment failures. In: Benumof JL, Saidman LJ, eds. *Anesthesia and perioperative complications,* 2nd ed. St. Louis: Mosby–Year Book, 1999: 112–160.

A.17. How can the machine be checked for leaks?

Leaks in the machine low-pressure system should be tested for according to the manufacturer's specific recommendations for that particular brand and model.

In general, Dräger Narkomed machines (Narkomed 2B, Narkomed 2C, Narkomed 3, and Narkomed 4) are tested using a positive pressure leak check. In principle, the inspiratory and expiratory connections on the absorber are connected by a short length of 22-mm-diameter tubing (i.e., the circle breathing system tubing is removed). The reservoir bag (usually 3 liters) is removed and a test terminal is connected to the bag mount. A short piece of plastic tubing and a sphygmomanometer bulb are connected to the test terminal. With no gases flowing and with the pop-off valve closed, the system is pressurized to 50 cm H_2O by squeezing the sphygmomanometer bulb. Pressure should not decrease by more than 20 cm H_2O in 30 seconds. In this test, the pressure is applied to all of the rigid components of the breathing system and through the fresh gas hose into the machine low-pressure system all the way back to the flow control valves. This test is then repeated with each vaporizer turned on in turn to test for leaks in each vaporizer.

Some anesthesia machines (e.g., Datex-Ohmeda Modulus I, Modulus II, Excel) have a one-way "outlet check valve" at the common gas outlet. Other models (e.g., Modulus II Plus, Modulus CD) have no outlet check valve. The presence of an outlet check valve precludes the application of a positive pressure leak check. Whether or not such a valve is present, a negative pressure leak test can be used to check the low-pressure system. In this test, a suction bulb (negative pressure leak-check device) is connected to the common gas outlet. With all gases off and vaporizers off, the bulb is squeezed empty and then connected to the common gas outlet of the workstation. Reexpansion of the bulb should not occur in less than 30 seconds. The test is repeated with each vaporizer turned on in turn to check for leaks in the vaporizers.

The U.S. Food and Drug Administration (FDA) 1993 preuse checkout recommendations describe the use of the negative pressure (bulb) leak-check device and state that the bulb should not refill within 10 seconds. The anesthesiologist must understand how to perform a low-pressure system leak check and must have the means (i.e., appropriate leak-check device) to check his or her own particular machine.

The newer electronic anesthesia workstations incorporate an automated checkout to test for leaks. The user of the workstations must understand what the automated checkout is designed to do, and more importantly, what it does not do. Even with an automated preuse checkout, there are steps that must be performed manually as prompted and directed by the checkout screen.

Brockwell RC, Andrews JJ. Delivery syaytems for inhaled anesthetics. In: Barash PG, Cullen Bf, Stoelting RK. *Clinical anesthesia*, 5th ed. Philadelphia: Lippincott Williams & Wilkins, 2006:557.

Food and Drug Administration. *Anesthesia apparatus checkout recommendations*. 1993. Available at: www.fda.gov/cdrh/humfac/anesckot.html.

Myers JA, Good ML, Andrews JJ. Comparison of tests for detecting leaks in the low pressure system of anesthesia gas machines. *Anesth Analg* 1997;84:179–184.

B. Preoperative Evaluation and Preparation

B.1. What should be included in the equipment checkout in preparation for anesthesia?

In 1993 the U.S. Food and Drug Administration (FDA) published its *14-Step Anesthesia Apparatus Checkout Recommendations,* as follows:

This checkout, or a reasonable equivalent, should be conducted before administration of anesthesia. These recommendations are only valid for an anesthesia system that conforms to current and relevant standards and includes an ascending bellows ventilator and at least the following monitors: capnograph, pulse oximeter, oxygen analyzer, respiratory volume monitor (spirometer), and breathing system pressure monitor with high- and low-pressure alarms. This is a guideline that users are encouraged to modify to accommodate differences in equipment design and variations in local clinical practice. Such local modifications should have appropriate peer review. Users should refer to the operator's manual for the manufacturer's specific procedures and precautions, especially the manufacturer's low-pressure leak test (step no.5).

Emergency ventilation equipment

Step 1. Verify backup ventilation equipment is available and functioning.

High-pressure system

Step 2. Check oxygen cylinder supply.

- Open O_2 cylinder and verify at least half full (~1,000 psi).
- Close cylinder.

Step 3. Check central pipeline supplies.

- Check that hoses are connected and pipeline gauges read approximately 50 psi.

Low-pressure systems

Step 4. Check initial status of low-pressure system.

- Close flow control valves and turn vaporizers off.
- Check fill level and tighten vaporizers' filler caps.

Step 5. Perform leak check of machine low-pressure system.

- Verify that the machine master switch and flow control valves are off.
- Attach "suction bulb" to common fresh gas outlet.
- Squeeze the bulb repeatedly until it is fully collapsed.
- Verify that the bulb stays fully collapsed for at least 10 seconds.

- Open one vaporizer at a time and repeat the tests as discussed earlier.
- Remove suction bulb, and reconnect fresh gas hose.

Step 6. Turn on machine master switch and all other necessary electrical equipment.
Step 7. Test flowmeters.

- Adjust flow of all gases through their full range, checking for smooth operation of floats and undamaged flow tubes.
- Attempt to create a hypoxic O_2/N_2O mixture and verify correct changes in flow and/or alarm.

Scavenging system

Step 8. Adjust and check scavenging system.

- Ensure proper connections between the scavenging system and both the adjustable-pressure limit (APL, or "pop-off") valve and ventilator relief valve.
- Adjust waste gas vacuum (if possible).
- Fully open APL valve and occlude Y-piece.
- With minimum O_2 flush activated, allow the scavenger reservoir bag to distend fully and then verify that the absorber pressure gauge reads less than 10 cm H_2O.

Breathing system

Step 9. Calibrate O_2 monitor.

- Ensure monitor reads 21% in room air.
- Verify low O_2 alarm is enabled and functioning.
- Reinstall sensor in circuit and flush breathing system with O_2.
- Verify that monitor now reads more than 90%.

Step 10. Check initial status of breathing system[1]

- Set selector switch to "bag" mode.
- Check that breathing circuit is complete, undamaged, and unobstructed.
- Verify that CO_2 absorbent is adequate.
- Install breathing circuit accessory equipment (e.g., humidifier, PEEP valve) to be used during the case.

Step 11. Perform leak check of the breathing system.

- Set all gas flows to zero (or minimum).
- Close APL (pop-off) valve and occlude Y-piece.
- Pressurize breathing system to approximately 30 cm H_2O with O_2 flush.
- Ensure that pressure remains fixed for at least 10 seconds.
- Open APL (pop-off) valve and ensure that pressure decreases.

Manual and automatic ventilation systems

Step 12. Test ventilation systems and unidirectional valves.

- Place a second breathing bag on the Y-piece.
- Set appropriate ventilator parameters for the next patient.
- Switch to automatic ventilation ("ventilator") mode.
- Fill bellows and breathing bag with O_2 flush and then turn the ventilator on.

---

[1]In step no. 10, checking adequacy of the CO_2 absorbent should include changing or hydrating it if there is any possibility that it may have become desiccated. This is because desiccated soda lime can react with desflurane, enflurane, and isoflurane to produce high levels of carbon monoxide in the breathing system. Baralyme is no longer available for use as an absorbent.

- Set O_2 flow to minimum, and other gas flows to zero.
- Verify that during inspiration bellows deliver appropriate TV and that during expiration bellows fills completely.
- Set fresh gas flow to approximately 5 L per minute.
- Verify that the ventilator bellows and simulated lungs fill and empty appropriately without sustained pressure at end expiration.
- Check for proper action of unidirectional valves.
- Exercise breathing circuit accessories to ensure proper function.
- Turn ventilator off and switch to manual ventilation ("bag/APL") mode.
- Ventilate manually and ensure inflation and deflation of artificial lungs and appropriate feel of system resistance and compliance.
- Remove second breathing bag from the Y-piece.

Monitors

Step 13. Check, calibrate, and/or set alarm limits of all monitors.

- Capnometer
- Pulse oximeter
- Oxygen analyzer
- Respiratory volume monitor (spirometer)
- Pressure monitor
- High- and low-airway alarms

Final position

Step 14. Check final status of machine.

- Vaporizers off
- APL valve open
- Selector switch to "bag"
- All flowmeters to zero
- Patient suction level adequate
- Breathing system ready to use

Berry PD, Sessler DI, Larson MI. Severe carbon monoxide poisoning during desflurane anesthesia. *Anesthesiology* 1999;90:613–616.

B.2. What emergency equipment should be easily available to the anesthesiologist?

In checking the anesthesia machine, step no. 1 on the U.S. Food and Drug Administration (FDA) checklist is to verify that backup ventilation equipment is available and functioning. This means a self-inflating resuscitation bag appropriate for patient size (adult vs. pediatric) is present and tested. Emergency airway management equipment must be available. The latter may be stored in a "difficult airway cart."

It is also important to have available a means to perform an emergency cricothyrotomy for the "cannot intubate, cannot ventilate" scenario and a means to ventilate/oxygenate through the cricothyroid catheter, once placed. A suitable device is the Sanders injector system.

Other emergency equipment includes a working flashlight, a backup battery for any electricity-dependent workstation, an O_2 tank and regulator, a malignant hyperthermia cart, a "code" cart/defibrillator, a difficult airway cart, a fire extinguisher, knowledge of appropriate response to a fire, and an evacuation plan.

B.3. How should this patient be premedicated?

The goal of premedication must be established preoperatively. Commonly considered objectives listed in order of most to least common are as follows:

- Anxiolysis
- Minimization of gastric volume and acidity when "full stomach" is of concern
- Antibiotic prophylaxis (commonly administered intravenously in the operating room) before surgical incision
- Antisialagogue effect

This patient may require anxiolysis. Premedication for anxiolysis in an ambulatory patient must consider the patient's need to arrive from home and ambulate, as well as the desire for rapid return of clear mental status postoperatively. Most commonly, therefore, no agent is administered preoperatively. Alternatively, for the highly anxious patient, a small dose of a short-acting agent (e.g., lorazepam, 1 to 2 mg orally) may be administered with a few sips of water 30 to 60 minutes preoperatively.

Porter BP, Gomez MN. Premedication. In: Longnecker DE, Tinker JH, Morgan GE Jr, eds. *Principles and practice of anesthesiology*, 2nd ed. St. Louis: Mosby–Year Book, 1998: 52–72.

C. Intraoperative Management

C.1. How should this patient be monitored?

The "Standards for Basic Anesthetic Monitoring" are established by the American Society of Anesthesiologists and were last amended in October 2005. In summary, they are as follows:

- *Standard I:* Qualified anesthesia personnel shall be present in the room throughout the conduct of all general anesthetics, regional anesthetics, and monitored anesthesia care.
- *Standard II:* During all anesthetics, the patient's oxygenation, ventilation, circulation, and temperature shall be continually evaluated.

Oxygenation

- *Inspired gas:* During every administration of general anesthesia using an anesthesia machine, the concentration of oxygen in the patient breathing system shall be measured by an oxygen analyzer with a low oxygen concentration limit alarm in use.*
- *Blood oxygenation:* During all anesthetics, a quantitative method of assessing oxygenation such as pulse oximetry shall be employed.* When the pulse oximeter is utilized, the variable pitch pulse tone and the low threshold alarm shall be audible to the anesthesiologist or the anesthesia care team personnel.* Adequate illumination and exposure of the patient are necessary to assess color.*

Ventilation

- Every patient receiving general anesthesia shall have the adequacy of ventilation continually evaluated. Qualitative clinical signs such as chest excursion, observation of the reservoir breathing bag and auscultation of breath sounds are useful. Continual monitoring for the presence of expired carbon dioxide shall be performed unless invalidated by the nature of the patient, procedure or equipment. Quantitative monitoring of the volume of expired gas is strongly encouraged.*
- When an endotracheal tube or laryngeal mask is inserted, its correct positioning must be verified by clinical assessment and by identification of carbon dioxide in the expired

gas. Continual end-tidal carbon dioxide analysis, in use from the time of endotracheal tube/laryngeal mask placement, until extubation/removal or initiating transfer to a postoperative care location, shall be performed using a quantitative method such as capnography, capnometry or mass spectroscopy.* When capnography or capnometry is utilized, the end-tidal CO_2 alarm shall be audible to the anesthesiologist or the anesthesia care team personnel.*

- When ventilation is controlled by a mechanical ventilator, there shall be in continuous use a device that is capable of detecting disconnection of components of the breathing system. The device must give an audible signal when its alarm threshold is exceeded.
- During regional anesthesia and monitored anesthesia care, the adequacy of ventilation shall be evaluated by continual observation of qualitative clinical signs and/or monitoring for the presence of exhaled carbon dioxide.

Circulation

- Every patient receiving anesthesia shall have the electrocardiogram continuously displayed from the beginning of anesthesia until preparing to leave the anesthetizing location.*
- Every patient receiving anesthesia shall have arterial blood pressure and heart rate determined and evaluated at least every 5 minutes.*
- Every patient receiving general anesthesia shall have, in addition to the above, circulatory function continually evaluated by at least one of the following: palpation of a pulse, auscultation of heart sounds, monitoring of a tracing of intraarterial pressure, ultrasound peripheral pulse monitoring, or pulse plethysmography or oximetry.

Body temperature

- Every patient receiving anesthesia shall have temperature monitored when clinically significant changes in body temperature are intended, anticipated or suspected.

Under extenuating circumstances, the responsible anesthesiologist may waive the requirements marked with an asterisk (*); it is recommended that when this is done, it should be so stated (including the reasons) in a note in the patient's medical record.

The reader should visit the ASA website for the most recent version of the standards http://www.asahq.org/publicationsAndServices/standards/02.pdf

---

Eichhorn JH. Standards for patient monitoring. In: Longnecker DE, Tinker JH, Morgan GE Jr, eds. *Principles and practice of anesthesiology,* 2nd ed. St. Louis: Mosby–Year Book, 1998:791–801.

C.2. **After uneventful inhalation mask induction, cystoscopy was begun and the SpO$_2$ was noted to decrease to 81% with the patient breathing O$_2$ at 2 L per minute and N$_2$O at 3 L per minute. The patient developed respiratory distress. The laryngeal mask airway was easily maintained and no gross secretions were noted. What acute diagnostic and therapeutic interventions would you perform?**

Immediately the patient should be examined for airway obstruction, bilateral breath sounds and the quality of the breath sounds. The FIO_2, end-tidal CO_2, heart rate, blood pressure, and SpO_2 should also be checked. The bladder irrigation fluid intake and output, as well as the intravenous fluid intake, should be reviewed.

Therapeutically the FIO_2 should be increased immediately to 1 and a change to manually assisted ventilation should be considered. If the SpO_2 does not increase rapidly in response to these interventions, then tracheal intubation and initiation of positive pressure ventilation should be performed.

Dorotta I, Basali A, Ritchey M, et al. Transurethral resection syndrome after bladder peforation. *Anesth Analg* 2003;97:1536.

C.3. The patient was tracheally intubated. Squeezing the reservoir bag in the circle system failed to inflate the lungs and a leak was noted. What are the common sites for gas leaks?

A leak can occur anywhere in the gas circuit. One might logically check for a leak in the circuit starting from the tip of the tracheal tube and working backward toward the gas delivery system, recognizing the following common potential sites:

- Incomplete seal between the tracheal tube cuff and the trachea
- Connection between the tracheal tube and the gas hose (e.g., the elbow adapter)
- Spirometric and end-tidal monitoring connections at both the patient end (near the connection between the gas hose and endotracheal tube) and the monitoring end
- Connection between inspiratory and expiratory gas hoses and the machine
- Within the low-pressure system including the unidirectional valves, adjustable-pressure limit (APL) valve, reservoir bag/bellows housing, absorber, vaporizers, flowmeters, and scavenging system

Equipment checking and maintenance. In: Dorsch JA, Dorsch SE. *Understanding anesthesia equipment*, 4th ed. Baltimore: Williams & Wilkins, 1998:949–956.

D. Postoperative Management

D.1. What criteria would you use for tracheal extubation?

In the operating room, traditional extubation criteria fall into two categories: global and respiratory. Global criteria include return of consciousness, demonstration of ability to protect the airway, adequate reversal of residual neuromuscular blockade, absence of hypothermia, and presence of a normal metabolic milieu (e.g., no significant anemia, acidosis, and electrolyte abnormality). Commonly applied respiratory criteria are a vital capacity more than 15 mL per kg, a negative inspiratory force of more than -20 cm H_2O, and an SpO_2 more than 90% while breathing an FIO_2 less than 0.40.

Patients with a respiratory insult and the need for postoperative mechanical ventilation in the postanesthesia care unit or intensive care unit may be assessed using additional criteria. The ratio of respiratory rate to tidal volume is now widely used. This is also called the *rapid shallow breathing index* (RSBI). The idea is that slow deep breathing during minimal respiratory support predicts successful extubation and that rapid shallow breathing predicts probable failure. To determine this ratio, the patient is observed breathing from a T-bar, or a low level of pressure support (PS) (e.g., <10 cm H_2O) and the following is calculated:

$$RSBI = \text{respiratory rate (breaths per minute)/tidal volume (in liters)}$$

When the RSBI is more than 100, the implication is that the patient is exhibiting rapid shallow breathing and will predictably fail an extubation attempt. When the RSBI is less than 100, it is assumed that the patient can breathe at a rate and tidal volume that can be easily maintained after extubation and will be adequate to maintain a normal PaO_2 and $PaCO_2$. If during the period of observation while breathing from a T-bar or on PS, the patient develops signs of distress such as diaphoresis, agitation, tachycardia, bradycardia, hypertension, or hypotension, the trial is abandoned and the patient is said to have had a weaning failure.

Yang KL, Tobin MJ. A prospective study of indexes predicting the outcome of trials of weaning from mechanical ventilation. *N Engl J Med* 1991;324:1445–1450.

D.2. What are the causes of postoperative hypoxemia?

The etiology of hypoxemia can be classified physiologically or pathologically.

Physiologically, all instances of hypoxemia have only four potential causes:

- Low F_{IO_2}
- Hypoventilation (which will also be associated with an increased $Paco_2$)
- Ventilation/perfusion mismatch
- Shunt

Pathologically, common etiologies likely to present postoperatively include airway obstruction, atelectasis (especially with upper abdominal retraction and Trendelenburg positioning), right mainstem intubation, aspiration, pulmonary edema, and pulmonary embolus.

Feeley TW, Macario A. The post anesthesia care unit. In: Miller RD. *Anesthesia*, 6th ed. New York, Churchill-Livingstone, 2005:2710–2714.

D.3. What is the difference between shunt, ventilation/perfusion mismatch, and dead space?

The relative quantity of perfusion and ventilation defines these terms. A normal lung has a small portion in which perfusion and ventilation are perfectly matched. Two extreme conditions may exist at either end of the spectrum of perfectly matched perfusion and ventilation; those extremes are shunt and dead space ventilation.

In a shunt, the alveolus is perfused, but it is not ventilated. The physiologic result is hypoxemia. This is characterized by a failure of the Pao_2 to rise despite an increase in the F_{IO_2}. Hypoxemia caused by small amounts of shunted blood (i.e., less than 20% of cardiac output) is easily overcome by increasing the F_{IO_2}. This is because the blood that is not shunted will contain enough "extra" dissolved oxygen to make up for the deficit that the shunted blood contributes to the combined total of blood oxygen content. Once the shunt fraction approaches 0.3 (30%), increasing the F_{IO_2} even to 1 will not be effective in preventing hypoxemia. The term *venous admixture* is often used synonymously for shunt.

In dead space, the alveolus is ventilated, but it is not perfused; hence, the alveolar space is essentially "dead." The physiologic result is hypercarbia. This is characterized by a failure to maintain a normal $Paco_2$ despite an increase in minute ventilation (i.e., tidal volume × respiratory rate).

Ventilation/perfusion mismatch is the term applied to any condition that is not a perfect match—that is, shunt or dead space. The physiologic result is a variable combination of hypoxemia and hypercarbia. The resultant degree of hypoxemia and hypercarbia depends on the relative contribution of partial shunt and dead space.

Benatar SR, Hewlett AM, Nunn JF. The use of iso-shunt lines for the control of oxygen therapy. *Br J Anaesth* 1973;45:711–718.

Lumb AB. *Nunn's applied respiratory physiology,* 6th ed. Philadelphia: Elsevier Science, 2005: 122–126.

Petros AJ, Doré CJ, Nunn JF. Modification of the iso-shunt lines for low inspired oxygen concentrations. *Br J Anaesth* 1994;72:515–522.

D.4. What is the differential diagnosis of pulmonary edema?

Pulmonary edema is usually thought to be either cardiac or noncardiac in etiology. The differential diagnosis of pulmonary edema is shown in Table 58.1.

Conditions that physiologically result from an increase in the pressure within the vessel that cause transudation of fluid from inside the vessel to outside the vessel are traditionally termed *congestive heart failure* (CHF). CHF will be associated with a diminution of cardiac function and an increase in the left ventricular end-diastolic pressure.

A decrease in the pressure outside of the vessel may also result in the net movement of fluid from inside to outside. The classic example of this would be negative pressure pulmonary edema, a condition seen in young patients who are inspiring against a closed glottis.

A change in the permeability of the vessel wall is the major cause of pulmonary edema seen in acute lung injury (ALI) and acute respiratory distress syndrome (ARDS). These conditions require a history of exposure to a risk factor, the development of bilateral infiltrates on chest radiography, and documentation of the absence of heart failure either by echocardiogram or pulmonary artery catheterization. Risk factors for ALI and ARDS include aspiration, long bone fracture, massive transfusion related acute lung injury (TRALI), pancreatitis, inhalational injury, and sepsis (Table 58.1).

In this patient, acute fluid overload from absorption of bladder irrigation fluid should be considered. Physiologically, this picture resembles CHF and will respond to treatment with diuretics.

Dorotta I, Basali A, Ritchey M, et al. Transurethral resection syndrome after bladder perforation. *Anesth Analg* 2003;97:1536.

Geer RT. Pulmonary complications of anesthesia. In: Longnecker DE, Tinker JH, Morgan GE Jr, eds. *Principles and practice of anesthesiology*, 2nd ed. St. Louis: Mosby–Year Book, 1998:2356–2357.

D.5. How should the ventilator be set if mechanical ventilation is required postoperatively?

Parameters that must be set include the mode, respiratory rate, tidal volume, positive end-expiratory pressure (PEEP), and F_{IO_2}.

Patients with an acute need for mechanical ventilation should be given full support with the mode set as volume control (VC), with which all breaths are delivered by the ventilator. Other modes to be considered as the patient improves include synchronized intermittent mandatory ventilation (SIMV), pressure support (PS), and combinations of SIMV and PS.

Tidal volume has traditionally been set at 10 mL per kg. Normally, during spontaneous ventilation, the respiratory rate is 12 to 16 breaths per minute and the tidal volume is 6 mL per kg.

Table 58.1 Differential Diagnosis of Pulmonary Edema.

CONDITION	PATHOPHYSIOLOGY	SAMPLE CAUSE
Congestive heart failure	↑ Filling pressure, ↓ cardiac output	Myocardial infarction
Negative pressure pulmonary edema	↑ Outside–inside pressure gradient	Laryngospasm
Acute lung injury and acute respiratory distress syndrome	↑ Permeability	Sepsis, aspiration

However, during spontaneous ventilation, there are yawns and sighs that prevent atelectasis. Yawns and sighs are not administered during routine mechanical ventilation. Therefore, standard mechanical ventilation settings use a lower respiratory rate and higher tidal volume than spontaneous values, resulting in the same minute ventilation and no need for sigh (150% of tidal volume) breaths.

Traditional mechanical ventilation has been recognized as a potential cause of morbidity and mortality when applied to injured lungs. The excessive tidal volume is thought to cause alveolar injury and worsen lung damage (i.e., volutrauma). This should be distinguished from the more easily recognized concern of pneumothorax, resulting from ventilation of stiff lungs with high inflation pressures, commonly referred to as *barotrauma*. Hence, the current recommendation in acute lung injury (ALI) and acute respiratory distress syndrome (ARDS) is that the tidal volume be set at 6 mL per kg of premorbid weight. Additionally, the peak inspiratory pressure should ideally be less than 35 cm H_2O. This may result in CO_2 retention, but if the pH is more than 7.25, no intervention is necessary. If CO_2 retention is severe and the pH is less than 7.25 after increasing the respiratory rate to as high as 20 breaths per minute, then administration of sodium bicarbonate should be considered.

To maximize oxygenation and limit exposure to potentially toxic concentrations of oxygen (i.e., $FIO_2 = 1$), usually an end-expiratory pressure of 10 cm H_2O is set.

In addition to standard monitoring, prolonged mechanical ventilation in ALI and ARDS will require arterial line placement to facilitate frequent arterial blood gas determinations. Further, a daily chest radiograph will be required.

The Acute Respiratory Distress Syndrome network. Ventilation with lower tidal volumes as compared with traditional tidal volumes for acute lung injury and the acute respiratory distress syndrome. *N Engl J Med* 2000;342:1301–1308.

D.6. If this patient had acute lung injury (ALI) secondary to aspiration, besides low tidal volume ventilation, what other changes in routine therapy should be considered?

The newest "proven" management strategy noted to improve lung function and shorten the duration of mechanical ventilation and intensive care of patients with ALI is conservative administration of intravenous fluids. Although the protocol employed in the National Institutes of Health (NIH)-sponsored study is too lengthy to expound on in this chapter, suffice it to say the excessive administration of fluid is harmful whereas minimizing intravenous fluids appears to be safe and not associated with other organ insufficiency or failure.

Wiedemann HP, Wheeler AP, Bernard GR, et al. National Heart, Lung, and Blood Institute Acute Respiratory Distress Syndrome (ARDS) Clinical Trials Network. Comparison of two fluid-management strategies in acute lung injury. *N Engl J Med* 2006;354: 2564–2575.

D.7. What methods of oxygen administration may be used postoperatively?

Most postoperative patients who are prone to develop hypoxemia may be managed with a nasal cannula or face mask. Nasal cannulas are cheap and comfortable, but regardless of flow rates, they cannot achieve an FIO_2 of more than 0.30. Face masks have the capability of delivering a wide range of precise FIO_2 levels of up to 1.

Occasionally, a patient may require more aggressive oxygenation than nasal cannula or face mask can provide, but less invasive than tracheal intubation and mechanical ventilation. Noninvasive positive pressure ventilation should be considered. Continuous positive airway pressure and bilevel positive airway pressure (BiPAP) may be applied. These modes may be used in patients who either have previously used these devices at home or who are on the verge of requiring tracheal intubation and mechanical ventilation but have conditions thought to be rapidly resolving (e.g., congestive heart failure [CHF] and chronic obstructive pulmonary disease exacerbation). These patients usually do not require an arterial catheter but need frequent assessment of their respiratory effort, particularly their respiratory rate and use of accessory muscles, as well as continuous SpO_2 monitoring.

Antonelli M, Conti G, Rocco M, et al. A comparison of noninvasive positive pressure ventilation and conventional mechanical ventilation in patients with acute respiratory failure. *N Engl J Med* 1998;339:429–435.

CHAPTER 59

Electroconvulsive Therapy

PATRICIA FOGARTY MACK

A 72-YEAR-OLD MAN

with major depressive disorder is scheduled for electroconvulsive therapy (ECT). His past medical history reveals significant coronary artery disease status after three-vessel coronary bypass surgery 5 years ago. He also has chronic atrial fibrillation. He had a transient ischemic attack (TIA) 2 years previously after which he underwent left carotid endarterectomy. In addition, he has sleep apnea and gastroesophageal reflux disease (GERD). The patient weighs 115 kg and is 5 ft 3 in. tall and had a Mallampati class 2 airway. Medications include warfarin, atenolol, and esomeprazole (Nexium).

A. Medical Disease and Differential Diagnosis

    1. What are the indications for electroconvulsive therapy (ECT)?

    2. Are there any contraindications to ECT?

    3. What is the mechanism of action of ECT?

B. Preoperative Evaluation and Preparation

    1. How would you assess the cardiac status of this patient?

    2. How should his anticoagulation be managed during ECT therapy?

    3. What implications do his history of sleep apnea have on management of ECT?

    4. How does his history of transient ischemic attack (TIA) and carotid endarterctomy impact your preoperative evaluation?

    5. Is ECT contraindicated in a patient with a permanent pacemaker or implantable cardiovertor-defibrillator?

C. Intraoperative Management

    1. Describe the hemodynamic response to ECT in a typical patient?

    2. Is an arterial line warranted in this patient?

    3. By what means would you attempt to maximize hemodynamic stability?

    4. Describe the cerebral hemodynamic effects of ECT.

    5. How would you proceed with an anesthetic induction for this procedure?

    6. How do you intend to manage his airway during each treatment?

D. Postoperative Management

    1. The patient is extremely agitated upon emergence. Discuss the risk factors for postictal agitation (PIA) as well as the therapeutic options?

    2. After three consecutive uneventful inpatient treatments, the psychiatrist asks if the patient may undergo ECT as an outpatient. Would you agree to this plan?

A. Medical Disease and Differential Diagnosis

A.1. What are the indications for electroconvulsive therapy (ECT)?

For centuries it had been noted that psychosis did not tend to occur in those people with epilepsy. Since the 16th century patients with severe mental illness were treated with various agents, such as camphor, to induce seizures (pharmacoconvulsive therapy). ECT was first instituted in the late 1930s and gained acceptance in providing a better-controlled seizure. The addition of curare, followed in 1951 by succinylcholine greatly diminished incidence of fracture due to the convulsions. Finally, the advent of methohexital, which ensured unconsciousness without significantly diminishing the seizure, led to its acceptance as an efficacious and safe treatment.

From the mid-1970s through the 1980s many new drug treatments for psychiatric illness were developed and found to be efficacious. ECT fell into disfavor as a barbaric treatment, when compared to pharmacotherapy.

In the past 15 years the pendulum has again swung back in favor of ECT as a safe and effective treatment for drug-resistant major depressive disorder and bipolar disorder.

Specific indications for ECT include, but are not limited to major depressive disorder and bipolar disorder, nonchronic schizophrenia (especially with affective or catatonic symptoms) and schizoaffective disorder. Although usually reserved as a second-line therapy for those who are resistant to pharmacologic treatment, ECT has in some circumstances been recommended as a first-line therapy, especially if a rapid response is urgently required as in patients with severe suicidal potential, malnutrition/dehydration and catatonia. Finally, ECT has been recommended in patients who are unable to tolerate pharmacotherapeutic agents for any reason, including during pregnancy.

American Psychiatric Association. *The practice of electroconvulsive therapy, a task force report of American Psychiatric Association*, 2nd ed. Washington, DC: American Psychiatric Association, 2001:5–26.

A.2. Are there any contraindications to electroconvulsive therapy (ECT)?

In the past the only absolute contraindication was an intracranial mass lesion or vascular malformation; however, ECT has been performed successfully in patients with these diseases. There is considered to be significantly increased risk in patients with intracranial space occupying lesions, any condition associate with intracranial hypertension, recent myocardial infarction with diminished ventricular function, severe hypertension especially associated with pheochromocytoma, evolving stroke, retinal detachment and any American Society of Anesthesiologists (ASA) physical status 4 or 5 patient.

American Psychiatric Association. *The practice of electroconvulsive therapy, a task force report of American Psychiatric Association*, 2nd ed. Washington, DC: American Psychiatric Association, 2001:27–30.

A.3. What is the mechanism of action of electroconvulsive therapy (ECT)?

The mechanism of ECT is unknown. There are many neurochemical, neuroendocrine, electrophysiologic and neuropsychological theories regarding the mechanism of ECT. See Table 59.1.

In addition, although it has been long assumed that a generalized seizure of adequate duration is sufficient for effective treatment, recent research shows that barely suprathreshold stimulation, especially with unilateral ECT is not as efficacious. Current research suggests that something

Table 59.1 Mechanism of Action of Electroconvulsive Therapy—Physiological Theories.

Neurophysiological
Anticonvulsant (changes in seizure threshold)
Cerebral blood flow and metabolic rate changes
Increased slow-wave EEG activity
Antidelerium/sleep theories

Neuroendocrinologic
Prolactin release
Neuropeptide release
Melatonin

Neurochemical
Stimulation of β receptors
Monoamine release
Modulation of serotonin

EEG, electroencephalography.

about the process of seizure generalization may be more important than the duration of the seizure.

B. Preoperative Evaluation and Preparation

B.1. How would you assess the cardiac status of this patient?

The cardiac status of the patient needs to be assessed as it would for any other general anesthetic. As there can be periods of significant tachycardia and hypertension following seizure induction, it would be useful to ensure that there is no longer significant myocardium at risk for ischemia and that systolic function is not compromised. If this information cannot be obtained from patient history and assessment of his functional status, it may be useful to obtain a stress test and echocardiogram. Bear in mind that it may be difficult to get an accurate history of functional status from patients who are psychotic or severely depressed.

American Psychiatric Association. *The practice of electroconvulsive therapy, a task force report of American Psychiatric Association*, 2nd ed. Washington, DC: American Psychiatric Association, 2001:77–80.

B.2. How should his anticoagulation be managed during electroconvulsive therapy (ECT) therapy?

The anticoagulation for his atrial fibrillation should be continued throughout his course of therapy, maintaining an international normalized ratio (INR) between 2.0 and 3.0. Although intracerebral hemorrhage is a theoretic concern, a retrospective study from the Mayo clinic suggests that ECT can be safely performed in patients on warfarin therapy.

American Psychiatric Association. *The practice of electroconvulsive therapy, a task force report of American Psychiatric Association*, 2nd ed. Washington, DC: American Psychiatric Association, 2001:40–41.

Mehta V, Mueller PS, Gonzalez-Arriaza HL, et al. Safety of electroconvulsive therapy in patients receiving long-term warfarin therapy. *Mayo Clin Proc* 2004;79:1396–1401.

B.3. What implications do his history of sleep apnea have on management of electroconvulsive therapy (ECT)?

His history of sleep apnea is important because suboptimal management of respiratory function may reduce efficacy of treatment and increase complications. Hypocarbia is sometimes required to ensure adequate seizure duration. Additionally, after onset of seizure activity, oxygen consumption is increased dramatically as is CO_2 production. Hypercarbia can exacerbate the tachycardia and hypertensive responses to seizure. Therefore, adequate mask ventilation is required to ensure optimal respiratory status. The use of a laryngeal mask airway (LMA) may be required to ensure adequate ventilation in this patient.

Finally, if the patient uses continuous positive airway pressure (CPAP) or bilevel positive airway pressure (BIPAP) at home it may be useful to have that machine available to the patient in the postprocedure period when postanesthetic and postictal somnolence may compromise his ability to maintain a patent airway.

Saito S. Anesthesia management for electroconvulsive therapy: hemodynamic and respiratory management. *J Anesth* 2005;19:142–149.

B.4. How does his history of transient ischemic attack (TIA) and carotid endarterectomy impact your preoperative evaluation?

In many instances where there has been a TIA or stroke, the patient will undergo a head computed tomography (CT) before their first course of electroconvulsive therapy (ECT). At Weill Cornell Medical Center, the practice is for most patients to receive a head CT before initiation of ECT to rule out an organic cause for depression. Although a comprehensive neurologic examination is routinely recommended by the American Psychiatric Association before ECT, it may be that in this patient more sophisticated neuropsychological testing would be useful in documenting subtle deficits and establishing a true baseline. Finally, if the patient has not had follow up carotid Doppler examination, it may be useful to ensure that there has not been restenosis or that no new plaques have formed. This is particularly important in view of the fact that the rate pressure product may be increased by as much as 400% in the sympathetic phase of the cardiac response.

American Psychiatric Association. *The practice of electroconvulsive therapy, a task force report of American Psychiatric Association*, 2nd ed. Washington, DC: American Psychiatric Association, 2001:77–80.

B.5. Is electroconvulsive therapy (ECT) contraindicated in a patient with a permanent pacemaker or implantable cardiovertor-defibrillator?

See Chapter 9, section C.11.

C. Intraoperative Management

C.1. Describe the hemodynamic response to electroconvulsive therapy (ECT) in a typical patient?

First, a parasympathetic discharge occurs within a few seconds of application of the electrical stimulus. This may result in bradycardia, which may be profound and even progress to asystole.

Because many patients are volume depleted due to poor oral intake or mildly hypotensive secondary to their psychotropic medications, they can be susceptible to further hypotension due to anesthetic induction. Within 1 minute, sympathetic activation due to the seizure results in a tachycardia and at times dysrhythmias as well as hypertension to up to 150% of baseline values. This hypertension usually lasts for between 2 and 5 minutes. If the patient is not adequately ventilated, hypercarbia may add to the hypertension. During the first ECT treatment the electrical stimulus may often be titrated upward in succession until a generalized seizure occurs. When a generalized seizure does not follow the electrical stimulation, the parasympathetic response predominates and the patient may experience a sustained bradycardia.

With such a dramatic increase in heart rate and blood pressure, the rate pressure product, an indicator of myocardial oxygen demand, is significantly elevated. This can lead to electrocardiographic ischemia as well as regional wall motion abnormalities on echocardiography.

Bready LL, Tyler DS. Electroconvulsive therapy. In: MauriceS Albin, ed. *Textbook of neuroanesthesia with neurosurgical and neuroscience perspectives*. New York: McGraw-Hill, 1997:707–734.

Messina AG, Paranicas M, Katz B, et al. Effect of electroconvulsive therapy on the electrocardiogram and the echocardiogram. *Anesth Analg* 1992;75:511–514.

Saito S. Anesthesia management for electroconvulsive therapy: hemodynamic and respiratory management. *J Anesth* 2005;19:142–149.

C.2. Is an arterial line warranted in this patient?

No, in spite of the potential dramatic perturbations in heart rate and blood pressure, these responses are fairy predictable and can be attenuated by judicious use of anticholinergics and antihypertensives. Atropine (0.4 mg) or glycopyrrolate (0.2 mg) are used to prevent the bradycardia associated with the parasympathetic discharge. The tachycardia and hypertension seen as part of the sympathetic response can be prevented with short acting β-blockade, nitroglycerin, or even remifentanil, administered just at the beginning of the sympathetic stimulation.

Severe cardiac complications during electroconvulsive therapy (ECT) are very rare.

Bready LL, Tyler DS. Electroconvulsive therapy. In: MauriceS Albin, ed. *Textbook of neuroanesthesia with neurosurgical and neuroscience perspectives*. New York: McGraw-Hill, 1997:707–734.

Saito S. Anesthesia management for electroconvulsive therapy: hemodynamic and respiratory management. *J Anesth* 2005;19:142–149.

C.3. By what means would you attempt to maximize hemodynamic stability?

First, one should continue antihypertensive medication on the evening before and the morning of the procedure. Second, a small dose of atropine (0.4 mg) or glycopyrrolate (0.2 mg) may be given several minutes before the electrical stimulation in order to prevent the subsequent bradycardia. At Weill Cornell Medical Center we are more likely to use glycopyrrolate as it is a quaternary compound, which will not cross an intact blood–brain barrier. In addition, the tachycardic response from the seizure is not as pronounced when glycopyrrolate is used as compared with atropine. Anticholinergic pretreatment is most important on the first treatment when the electrical stimulation is being titrated and it is likely not to progress into a generalized seizure on the first or second stimulus. If the pretreatment with an anticholinergic leaves a fragile patient with an undesirable tachycardia, we may omit it during subsequent treatments as long as the bradycardia is not too severe or prolonged.

Similarly, medications to attenuate the sympathetic response are typically not administered until it is certain that the seizure will generalize. This results in a requirement for very fast-acting drugs to control heart rate and blood pressure. The drug of choice at Cornell Medical Center is esmolol (0.5 to 1.0 mg/kg) or labetalol (5 to 20 mg). If there is a contraindication to β-blockade, diltiazem, nicardipine, or sodium nitroprusside may be substituted. Nitroglycerin may be particularly useful in patients with ischemic cardiac disease.

Saito S. Anesthesia management for electroconvulsive therapy: hemodynamic and respiratory management. *J Anesth* 2005;19:142–149.

C.4. Describe the cerebral hemodynamic effects of electroconvulsive therapy (ECT).

Electrically induced seizures lead to cerebral hyperemia (increase in cerebral blood flow) as documented by transcranial Doppler and near-infrared spectroscopy. This response occurs even if the seizure does not generalize, suggesting that they are a result of the electric stimulation itself. The increase in cerebral blood flow has been shown to be related to the degree of systemic hypertension and occurs whether bilateral or unilateral stimulus is applied. Although there is a correlation with systemic hypertension, the systemic antihypertensives do not fully ameliorate the increase in cerebral blood flow. This is due to the fact that these drugs have differing effects on the cerebral and systemic circulations.

Saito S. Anesthesia management for electroconvulsive therapy: hemodynamic and respiratory management. *J Anesth* 2005;19:142–149.

C.5. How would you proceed with an anesthetic induction for this procedure?

Anesthetic induction may be accomplished with any one of a number of medications. Traditionally methohexital (0.5 to 1.0 mg/kg) has been the induction agent of choice because it has very little effect on seizure duration and has a rapid onset and recovery profile. Unfortunately, methohexital is no longer available in many areas. At Weill Cornell Medical Center we now use etomidate (0.2 to 0.3 mg/kg). In research studies etomidate provides for longer seizure duration when compared to methohexital and propofol; however, postictal hypertension is more severe and myoclonic contractions may be undesirable. Although adrenal suppression has been reported in patients on continuous infusions of etomidate, there are no reports of adrenal suppression in patients receiving multiple bolus doses of etomodate as part of a course of ECT. In patients in whom etomidate is not well tolerated, propofol or thiopental may be used. Studies concur that propofol and thiopental reduce seizure duration; however, there is controversy as to how this reduction in seizure duration impacts the efficacy of therapy.

Muscle relaxation is usually achieved with succinylcholine (0.5 to 1.0 mg/kg) unless there is a contraindication. In that case an appropriate nondepolarizing muscle relaxant may be substituted.

Bready LL, Tyler DS. Electroconvulsive therapy. In: MauriceS Albin, ed. *Textbook of neuroanesthesia with neurosurgical and neuroscience perspectives*. New York: McGraw-Hill, 1997:707–734.

Saito S. Anesthesia management for electroconvulsive therapy: hemodynamic and respiratory management. *J Anesth* 2005;19:142–149.

C.6. How do you intend to manage his airway during each treatment?

The diagnosis of sleep apnea and the patient's body habitus raise concerns regarding the ease and effectiveness of mask ventilation. In spite of these concerns, I would proceed with a plan for mask ventilation with a backup plan of laryngeal mask airway (LMA) or intubation. As electroconvulsive therapy (ECT) is usually administered three times a week, repeated intubations may lead to airway trauma and edema. Gastroesophageal reflux disease (GERD) may also be of concern; however, we do not intubate patients for ECT solely because of GERD. Our plan would include continuation of medication to reduce stomach acid and promote gastric emptying, as well as a dose of preinduction sodium bicitrate.

Effective mask ventilation is important for several reasons. First, hypocapnea may lower seizure threshold and promote more effective therapy. Second, avoidance of hypercapnea postseizure is necessary as hypercapnea will exacerbate hypertension and tachycardia.

In anticipation of potential difficult ventilation during ECT, we proceed with preoxygenation for 3 to 5 minutes. As soon as induction is accomplished both an oral and a well-lubricated nasal airway will be placed. A second person ideally is available in case two-person ventilation is required. We find that Jackson-Reese circuits are advantageous for ventilation during ECT. First they allow you to adjust the amount of positive pressure administered; second, the weight of an Ambu-bag can sometimes make maintenance of ideal mask placement difficult; finally, as the patient regains spontaneous ventilation, he or she may breathe comfortably and effectively through the Jackson-Reese circuit. If mask ventilation were not effective, I would place an appropriately sized LMA.

If necessary for adequate ventilation, intubation may be considered. Unfortunately, repeated intubations over several days and weeks may lead to glottic edema and trauma.

Saito S. Anesthesia management for electroconvulsive therapy: hemodynamic and respiratory management. *J Anesth* 2005;19:142–149.

D. Postoperative Management

D.1. The patient is extremely agitated upon emergence. Discuss the risk factors for postictal agitation (PIA) as well as the therapeutic options?

PIA manifests as disorientation, inability to consistently follow commands, and motor agitation. Risk factors for PIA include prolonged seizure duration, bilateral versus unilateral electroconvulsive therapy (ECT), and concomitant lithium therapy. In addition, low doses of induction agent as well as very low doses of succinylcholine are considered risk factors. The etiology of low-dose succinylcholine may be related to excess lactate production in those patients who have greater manifestation of clinical seizure activity. Increased lactate levels were noted in patients who experienced PIA versus those who did not.

It is of critical importance to rule out nonconvulsive status epilepticus as an etiology for the PIA. Nonconvulsive status may present as agitation or conversely as mutism.

Treatment of PIA usually consists of benzodiazepene, such as midazolam 1 to 2 mg. If this is not effective, haloperidol may be added. In some circumstances, propofol as a bolus or an infusion have been effective.

Augoustides JG, Greenblatt E, Abbas MA, et al. Clinical approach to agitation after electroconvulsive therapy: a case report and literature review. *J ECT* 2002;18(4):213–217.

D.2. After three consecutive uneventful inpatient treatments, the psychiatrist asks if the patient may undergo electroconvulsive therapy (ECT) as an outpatient. Would you agree to this plan?

Outpatient ECT has become an acceptable therapeutic option in our institution for many patients. Primarily, it is used for maintenance therapy. It may also be used to complete an initial course of ECT provided that the first several treatments are uneventful medically, i.e., no respiratory or cardiovascular problems, and that the patient is demonstrating improvement in psychiatric status. In addition, because psychiatric patients may be unreliable in following preoperative instructions, such as nothing by mouth (NPO) status, they must have another adult who assumes responsibility for ensuring that those instructions are followed. Of course they must also have an escort to bring them home.

Finally, there needs to be close communication between the treating psychiatrist and the ECT psychiatrist to keep abreast of any change in psychiatric status or in any medical condition.

CHAPTER 60

Ambulatory Surgery

KATHRYN E. MCGOLDRICK • MATTHEW C. GOMILLION

A 40-YEAR-OLD WOMAN

desiring permanent sterility was scheduled for bilateral laparoscopic tubal ligation in the ambulatory surgical suite. Her preoperative outpatient questionnaire indicated a history of glaucoma. Additionally, she had surgery 3 weeks ago under general anesthesia for a detached retina, and her postoperative course was complicated by severe postoperative nausea and vomiting (PONV). She is 5 ft 3 in. tall, weighs 190 pounds, and complains of chronic fatigue. Her only medications consist of "eye drops."

A. Medical Disease and Differential Diagnosis

1. What are the anesthetic implications of glaucoma?
2. What side effects and important anesthetic interactions are associated with eye drops used to treat glaucoma?
3. Should glaucoma medications be discontinued before elective surgery?
4. Is this patient morbidly obese?
5. What medical conditions may be associated with obesity and morbid obesity?

B. Preoperative Evaluation and Preparation

1. What advantages does outpatient surgery offer?
2. What are the goals of the preoperative evaluation of the surgical outpatient?
3. In order to thoroughly screen for disease, should one put all outpatients through a full battery of laboratory testing?
4. What preoperative laboratory testing is necessary for the surgical outpatient?
5. Which outpatients should receive a preoperative chest roentgenogram?
6. In which patients is an electrocardiogram (ECG) necessary before outpatient anesthesia and surgery?
7. Would a patient's age or physical status influence the decision to perform outpatient surgery?
8. What patients would be considered inappropriate for ambulatory surgery?
9. What questions are critically important to ask this woman when obtaining her medical history?
10. How would you premedicate this patient?
11. Should every outpatient receive prophylaxis against acid aspiration pneumonitis?
12. Is an overnight fast justified for all outpatients?

C. Intraoperative Management

1. What are the important considerations in choosing an anesthetic technique for outpatient surgery?
2. What are the anesthetic implications of recent retinal detachment surgery?
3. How would you monitor this patient?
4. What is the Bispectral Index (BIS) monitor and what information does it convey?
5. What benefits might be derived from using a BIS monitor?
6. Is BIS monitoring applicable to children?
7. What are the major limitations of BIS monitoring?
8. What does a BIS reading of 56 mean?
9. What are the anesthetic options for laparoscopy?
10. What anesthetic agents would you use to induce and maintain general anesthesia in this patient?
11. Would you avoid the use of nitrous oxide in this ambulatory patient?
12. Discuss the physiologic changes induced by laparoscopy.
13. In addition to the physiologic changes described in the preceding text, what other intraoperative complications are associated with laparoscopy?
14. Why is carbon dioxide the insufflation agent of choice for laparoscopy?
15. What are some alternatives to carbon dioxide for laparoscopy?

D. Postoperative Management

1. What are the common causes of nausea and vomiting in outpatients?
2. How would you pharmacologically prevent postoperative nausea and vomiting (PONV) in the susceptible ambulatory patient?
3. How is postoperative pain treated?
4. If the patient complained of eye pain postoperatively, how would you manage the situation?
5. What criteria would you use to establish that a patient can be safely discharged after ambulatory surgery?
6. How would you decide when to discharge a patient after regional anesthesia?
7. What instructions should be given to an ambulatory surgical patient upon discharge?

A. Medical Disease and Differential Diagnosis

A.1. What are the anesthetic implications of glaucoma?

With open-angle glaucoma, elevated intraocular pressure (IOP) exists in conjunction with an anatomically patent anterior chamber angle. It is thought that sclerosis of trabecular tissue produces impaired aqueous filtration and drainage. Treatment consists of medication to produce miosis and trabecular stretching. Commonly used eye drops include epinephrine, echothiophate iodide, timolol, dipivefrin, and betaxolol. Carbonic anhydrase inhibitors such as acetazolamide can also be administered by various routes to reduce IOP by interfering with the production of aqueous humor. All these drugs are systemically absorbed and can, therefore, have anticipated side effects.

It is important to appreciate that maintenance of IOP is determined primarily by the rate of aqueous formation and the rate of aqueous outflow. The most important influence on formation of aqueous humor is the difference in osmotic pressure between aqueous humor and plasma. This concept is illustrated by the equation:

$$IOP = K[(OP_{aq} - OP_{pl}) + CP]$$

where K = coefficient of outflow, OP_{aq} = osmotic pressure of aqueous humor, OP_{pl} = osmotic pressure of plasma, and CP = capillary pressure. The fact that a small change in solute concentration of plasma can dramatically affect the formation of aqueous humor and hence IOP is the rationale for administering hypertonic solutions, such as mannitol, to reduce IOP. Fluctuations in aqueous outflow can also markedly change IOP. The primary factor controlling aqueous humor outflow is the diameter of Fontana's spaces, as illustrated by the equation:

$$A = \frac{r^4 \times (P_{IOP} - P_v)}{8\eta L}$$

where A = volume of aqueous outflow per unit of time, r = radius of Fontana's spaces, P_{IOP} = IOP, P_v = venous pressure, η = viscosity, and L = length of Fontana's spaces. When the pupil dilates, Fontana's spaces narrow, resistance to outflow is increased, and IOP rises. Because mydriasis is undesirable in both closed- and open-angle glaucoma, miotics such as pilocarpine are applied conjunctivally in patients with glaucoma to effect papillary constriction.

The aforementioned equation describing the volume of aqueous outflow per unit of time clearly underscores that outflow is exquisitely sensitive to fluctuations in venous pressure. Because an elevation in venous pressure results in an increased volume of ocular blood as well as decreased aqueous outflow, it is obvious that a considerable increase in IOP occurs with any maneuver that increases venous pressure. Hence, in addition to preoperative instillation of miotics, other anesthetic objectives for the patient with glaucoma include perioperative avoidance of venous congestion and of overhydration. Furthermore, hypotensive episodes are to be avoided because these patients are purportedly vulnerable to retinal vascular thrombosis.

Although glaucoma usually occurs as an isolated disease, it may also be associated with such conditions as Sturge-Weber syndrome, aniridia, mesodermal dysgenesis syndrome, retinopathy of prematurity, Refsum's syndrome, mucopolysaccharidosis, Hurler's syndrome, Stickler's syndrome, Marfan's syndrome, and von Reckinghausen's disease (neurofibromatosis). Additionally, ocular trauma, steroid therapy, sarcoidosis, some forms of arthritis associated with uveitis, and pseudoexfoliation syndrome can also be associated with secondary glaucoma.

Primary closed-angle glaucoma is characterized by a shallow anterior chamber and a narrow iridocorneal angle that impedes the egress of aqueous humor from the eye because the trabecular meshwork is covered by the iris. Relative pupillary block is common in many angle-closure episodes in which iris–lens apposition or synechiae impede the flow of aqueous from the posterior chamber. In the United States, the prevalence of angle-closure glaucoma (ACG) is one tenth as common as open-angle glaucoma. In acute ACG, if the pressure is not reduced promptly, permanent visual loss can ensue as a result of optic nerve damage. It is thought that irreversible optic nerve injury can occur within 24 to 48 hours.

McGoldrick KE. Eye, ear, nose, and throat diseases. In: Fleisher LA, ed. *Anesthesia and uncommon diseases*, 5th ed. Philadelphia: WB Saunders, 2006:4–5.

A.2. What side effects and important anesthetic interactions are associated with eye drops used to treat glaucoma?

Echothiophate is a long-acting anticholinesterase miotic that lowers intraocular pressure (IOP) by decreasing resistance to the outflow of aqueous humor. Useful in the treatment of glaucoma, echothiophate is absorbed into the systemic circulation after instillation in the conjunctival sac. Any of the long-acting anticholinesterases may prolong the action of succinylcholine because, after a month or more of therapy, plasma pseudocholinesterase activity may be less than 5% of normal. It is said, moreover, that normal enzyme activity does not return until 4 to 6 weeks after discontinuation of the drug. Hence, the anesthesiologist should anticipate prolonged apnea if these patients are given a customary dose of succinylcholine. In addition, a delay in metabolism of ester local anesthetics should be expected.

Although topical epinephrine has proved useful in some patients with open-angle glaucoma, the 2% solution has been associated with such systemic effects as nervousness, hypertension, angina pectoris, tachycardia, and other dysrhythmias.

Timolol, a nonselective β-adrenergic blocking drug, has historically been a popular antiglaucoma drug. Because significant conjunctival absorption may occur, timolol should be administered with caution to patients with known obstructive airway disease, severe congestive heart failure, or greater than first-degree heart block. Life-threatening asthmatic crises have been reported after the administration of timolol drops to some patients with chronic, stable asthma. Not unexpectedly, the development of severe sinus bradycardia in a patient with cardiac conduction defects (left anterior hemiblock, first-degree atrioventricular block, and incomplete right bundle-branch block) has been reported after timolol. Moreover, timolol has been implicated in the exacerbation of myasthenia gravis and in the production of postoperative apnea in neonates and young infants. Patients may report feelings of fatigue and/or depression in association with the use of timolol drops.

In contrast to timolol, a newer antiglaucoma drug, betaxolol, a β_1 blocker, is said to be more oculospecific and have minimal systemic effects. However, patients receiving an oral β-blocker and betaxolol should be observed for potential additive effects on known systemic effects of β-blockade. Caution should be exercised in patients receiving catecholamine-depleting drugs. Although betaxolol has produced only minimal effects in patients with obstructive airway disease, caution should be exercised in the treatment of patients with excessive restriction of pulmonary function. Moreover, betaxolol is contraindicated in patients with sinus bradycardia, greater than first-degree heart block, cardiogenic shock, and overt myocardial failure.

McGoldrick KE. Anesthesia and the eye. In: Barash PG, Cullen BF, Stoelting RK, eds. *Clinical anesthesia*, 5th ed. Philadelphia: Lippincott Williams & Wilkins, 2006:980–981.

A.3. Should glaucoma medications be discontinued before elective surgery?

For all the aforementioned reasons, it is important to continue glaucoma medications in the perioperative period. Moreoever, the anesthesiologist must be aware of which medications the patient is taking and the effects of these drugs on anesthetic management.

McGoldrick KE. Anesthesia and the eye. In: Barash PG, Cullen BF, Stoelting RK, eds. *Clinical anesthesia*, 5th ed. Philadelphia: Lippincott Williams & Wilkins, 2006:978.

A.4. Is this patient morbidly obese?

Morbid obesity is defined by a body mass index greater than 35 kg per m². This patient has a body mass index of approximately 30 and would, therefore, be considered obese. See chapter 62, section A.2.

Polk SL. Morbid obesity. In: Roizen MF, Fleisher LA, eds. *Essence of anesthesia practice*, 2nd ed. Philadelphia: WB Saunders, 2002:225.

A.5. What medical conditions may be associated with obesity and morbid obesity?

A plethora of conditions may be associated with obesity and morbid obesity including diabetes, hyperlipidemia, cholelithiasis, gastroesophageal reflux disease, cirrhosis, degenerative joint and disk disease, venous stasis and thrombotic/embolic disease, sleep disorders including obstructive sleep apnea, and emotional disorders. Diseases of the cardiopulmonary system are common and concerning. They include, but are not limited to, systemic hypertension, pulmonary hypertension and cor pulmonale, restrictive lung disease, and right and left ventricular hypertrophy.

Roizen MF, Fleisher LA. Anesthetic implications of concurrent diseases. In: Miller RD, ed. *Miller's anesthesia*, 6th ed. Philadelphia: Elsevier, Churchill Livingstone, 2005:1029–1032.

B. Preoperative Evaluation and Preparation

B.1. What advantages does outpatient surgery offer?

Outpatient surgery typically offers greater convenience to the patient (less time away from home, family, and work), a more pleasant environment with less stress and emotional disturbance, and a reduced risk of infection, particularly for the immunocompromised or the pediatric patient. Additionally, outpatient surgery is more economical and enables more efficient use of operating rooms with greater flexibility in scheduling surgery. Finally, one is not dependent on the availability of hospital beds.

Lichtor JL. Anesthesia for ambulatory surgery. In: Barash PG, Cullen BF, Stoelting RK, eds. *Clinical anesthesia*, 5th ed. Philadelphia: Lippincott Williams & Wilkins, 2006: 1229.

White PF, Freire AR. Ambulatory (outpatient) anesthesia. In: Miller RD, ed. *Miller's anesthesia*, 6th ed. Philadelphia: Elsevier, Churchill Livingstone, 2005:2590.

B.2. What are the goals of the preoperative evaluation of the surgical outpatient?

The objectives of the preoperative evaluation are as follows:

- To perform medical assessments, obtain data, arrange for laboratory tests and consultations, and prescreen for relevant conditions in order to optimize perioperative outcome
- To obtain informed consent
- To provide information and instructions to reduce patient anxiety and improve perioperative management

Organization of the preoperative screening varies among ambulatory surgical facilities throughout the country. The screening process may be organized with an office or facility visit before the day of surgery, by a telephone interview or review of health questionnaire without a visit, or by preoperative screening and visit on the morning of surgery. Each of these systems has its advantages and disadvantages. Nevertheless, the system for preoperative evaluation of ambulatory surgical patients should ensure that screening is performed far enough in advance so that preexisting disease can be evaluated, treatment optimized, and laboratory data recorded before the patient presents for anesthesia. Written instructions should be supplied to the patient in advance describing the preoperative workup, admission, and recovery periods.

Lichtor JL. Anesthesia for ambulatory surgery. In: Barash PG, Cullen BF, Stoelting RK, eds. *Clinical anesthesia*, 5th ed. Philadelphia: Lippincott Williams & Wilkins, 2006: 1229–1231.

White PF, Freire AR. Ambulatory (outpatient) anesthesia. In: Miller RD, ed. *Miller's anesthesia*, 6th ed. Philadelphia: Elsevier, Churchill Livingstone, 2005:2593–2594.

B.3. In order to thoroughly screen for disease, should one put all outpatients through a full battery of laboratory testing?

No. The practice of preoperative "shotgun" laboratory screening for outpatient surgery has received much criticism. In addition to unnecessarily adding several billion dollars annually to the cost of health care, laboratory screening tests in asymptomatic patients have been shown to be of dubious value. History and physical examination are a better means of screening for disease and should serve to reduce expensive, potentially harmful, and inappropriate tests.

Hata TM, Moyers JR. Preoperative evaluation and management. In: Barash PG, Cullen BF, Stoelting RK, eds. *Clinical anesthesia*, 5th ed. Philadelphia: Lippincott Williams & Wilkins, 2006:475–481.

Roizen MF. Preoperative evaluation. In: Miller RD, ed. *Miller's anesthesia*, 6th ed. Philadelphia: Churchill Livingstone, 2005:940–944.

B.4. What preoperative laboratory testing is necessary for the surgical outpatient?

Most outpatient surgical facilities consider the operative procedure and the patient's age, medical condition, medication history, and state and local regulations in determining which preoperative tests are "required." For the healthy ambulatory patient between the ages of 1 and 40 years having a minor surgical procedure, no laboratory testing may be required. Hemoglobin or hematocrit determination is appropriate for surgical procedures associated with blood loss, and for patients at risk for anemia or polycythemia, such as children younger than 1 year or with suspected sickle cell disease, patients with a history of anemia, blood dyscrasia or malignancy, patients with congenital heart disease or chronic disease, menstruating women, and patients older than 60 years old. Additional testing depends on an individual's preexisting condition. For example, serum electrolyte testing would be indicated for a patient with a history of hypertension, diabetes mellitus, renal disease, or for those patients taking diuretics, digoxin, steroids, or angiotension-converting enzyme inhibitors. Likewise, measurement of the partial thromboplastin time (PTT) and the prothrombin time (PT) would be indicated in the presence of a bleeding disorder, anticoagulant use, liver disease, or poor nutritional status. Preoperative urinalysis has not been shown to be useful as a screening test, and is no longer required in a routine anesthetic evaluation.

Stoelting RK, Dierdorf SF, eds. *Anesthesia and co-existing disease*, 4th ed. New York: Churchill Livingstone, 2002:633.

White PF, Freire AR. Ambulatory (outpatient) anesthesia. In: Miller RD, ed. *Miller's anesthesia*, 6th ed. Philadelphia: Elsevier, Churchill Livingstone, 2005:2593–2594.

B.5. Which outpatients should receive a preoperative chest roentgenogram?

Abnormalities in the chest x-ray in asymptomatic patients are rare, and the risks to the patient probably exceed the benefits. A preoperative chest x-ray is indicated only for patients with a history or clinical findings of active pulmonary disease. Extremes of age, smoking, stable chronic obstructive pulmonary disease, stable cardiac disease, or resolved recent upper respiratory infection should not be considered absolute indications for chest x-ray.

American Society of Anesthesiologists Task Force on Preanesthesia Evaluation. Practice advisory for preanesthesia evaluation: a report by the American society of anesthesiologists task force on preanesthesia evaluation. *Anesthesiology* 2002;96:492.

Roizen MF. Preoperative evaluation. In: Miller RD, ed. *Miller's anesthesia*, 6th ed. Philadelphia: Elsevier, Churchill Livingstone, 2005:951.

B.6. In which patients is an electrocardiogram necessary before outpatient anesthesia and surgery?

It has not been established that information obtained from the preoperative electrocardiogram (ECG) affects clinical care. A review of clinical studies on the matter is inconclusive. A retrospective review of adult patients undergoing outpatient surgery, for example, disclosed that the preoperative ECG was not predictive of perioperative risk. Although controversy prevails, current recommendations include the need for a preoperative ECG in men older than 40 years of age, women older than 50 years, and those with systemic cardiovascular disease (e.g., hypertension or peripheral vascular disease). Obviously, those with known cardiac disease, such as patients with a history of myocardial infarction, should have an ECG regardless of their age.

Gold BS, Young ML, Kinman JL, et al. The utility of preoperative electrocardiograms in the ambulatory surgical patient. *Arch Intern Med* 1992;152:301.

Hata TM, Moyers JR. Preoperative evaluation and management. In: Barash PG, Cullen BF, Stoelting RK, eds. *Clinical anesthesia*, 5th ed. Philadelphia: Lippincott Williams & Wilkins, 2006:481.

B.7. Would a patient's age or physical status influence the decision to perform outpatient surgery?

Even patients at the extremes of age (e.g., younger than 6 months and older than 80 years) have been managed successfully at ambulatory centers throughout the country. With the exception of the former preterm infant and newborns in the first few weeks of life, age alone should not be considered a deterrent in the selection of patients for outpatient surgery. Premature infants (gestational age at birth <37 weeks) who undergo general anesthesia during the first months of life are at increased risk for postoperative apnea for up to 12 hours. This risk is greatest for infants younger than 46 weeks postconceptual age, but some investigators have reported apnea in infants as old as 60 weeks postconceptual age. Unfortunately, the postconceptual age at which the former premature infant no longer represents an increased risk for postoperative apnea, and therefore, would be considered an acceptable candidate for an ambulatory surgical procedure is not absolutely known. Therefore, at the present time it is safest to admit to a hospital or to a 24-hour recovery unit all former premature infants less than 46 weeks postconceptual age so that they can be monitored for apnea. If anemia, bronchopulmonary dysplasia, or other neonatal problems are present, this period may need to be extended. Likewise, postoperative apneic episodes have been described in otherwise healthy full-term infants who are anesthetized in the first few weeks of life. For this reason many anesthesiologists are reluctant to proceed with outpatient anesthesia and surgery on a healthy full-term infant of less than 2 to 4 weeks of age.

For the geriatric patient, recent clinical experience has not demonstrated an age-related effect on the duration of recovery or the incidence of postoperative complications after outpatient surgery. However, in determining the acceptability of a geriatric patient for an ambulatory surgical procedure, one must consider the patient's physiologic age and physical status, the surgical procedure, the anesthetic technique, and the quality of care that will be provided at home.

No longer is outpatient surgery restricted to patients of American Society of Anesthesiologists (ASA) physical status I and II. ASA physical status III and IV patients whose diseases are well controlled preoperatively are at no higher risk for postoperative complications, and may be considered acceptable candidates for outpatient surgery.

Gregory GA, ed. *Pediatric anesthesia*, 4th ed. New York, Churchill Livingstone, 2002:773–774.

Lichtor JL. Anesthesia for ambulatory surgery. In: Barash PG, Cullen BF, Stoelting RK, eds. *Clinical anesthesia*, 5th ed. Philadelphia: Lippincott Williams & Wilkins, 2006: 1230–1231.

White PF, Freire AR. Ambulatory (outpatient) anesthesia. In: Miller RD, ed. *Miller's anesthesia*, 6th ed. Philadelphia: Elsevier, Churchill Livingstone, 2005:2593.

B.8. What patients would be considered inappropriate for ambulatory surgery?

An individual may be classified as an inappropriate ambulatory surgery patient for the following reasons:

- The existence of a condition which places an infant at risk
- History of prematurity in an infant less than 44 to 60 weeks postconceptual age
- Apneic episodes, feeding difficulty, or failure to thrive
- Respiratory distress syndrome (RDS) that has required intubation and ventilatory support (may take up to a year for symptoms to resolve)
- Bronchopulmonary dysplasia (BPD) with any degree of significant decrease in pulmonary function or requirement for supplemental oxygen
- Acute concurrent illness
- American Society of Anesthesiologists (ASA) physical status III or IV with poorly controlled disease
- Acute substance abuse
- Morbid obesity with other systemic diseases, such as severe obstructive sleep apnea and ventricular dysfunction
- No available adult at home
- Refusal to have surgical procedure done as an outpatient
- Unwilling to follow instructions

The appropriateness of each patient must be evaluated on an individual basis, taking into account a combination of several factors, such as the patient's circumstances, the nature of the surgical procedure, anesthetic technique, anticipated severity of postoperative pain, and comfort level of the anesthesiologist.

White PF, Freire AR. Ambulatory (outpatient) anesthesia. In: Miller RD, ed. *Miller's anesthesia*, 6th ed. Philadelphia: Elsevier, Churchill Livingstone, 2005:2593.

B.9. **What questions are critically important to ask this patient when obtaining her history?**

It is important to acquire as much information as possible about the patient's eye disease. For example, does she have open- or closed-angle glaucoma? What eye drops is she taking? When she had retinal detachment surgery 3 weeks ago, did the ophthalmic surgeon inject an air or gas bubble to tamponade the retina? If so, which substance was injected and has it been fully resorbed? Additionally, it is important to rule out obstructive sleep apnea in view of the patient's obesity and her complaints of fatigue. Does she snore, have frequent awakenings during the night, and does she fall asleep commonly during the daytime? Obese patients with severe sleep apnea and certain associated conditions (pulmonary hypertension, ventricular dysfunction, etc.) having painful surgery under general anesthesia that may require significant amounts of opioids postoperatively for pain control are typically considered poor candidates for planned outpatient surgery.

American Society of Anesthesiologists Task Force on Perioperative Management. *Practice Guidelines for the Perioperative Management of Patients with Obstructive Sleep Apnea. A Report by the American Society of Anesthesiologists Task Force on Perioperative Management of Patients with Obstructive Sleep Apnea.* Approved by the House of Delegates on October 25, 2005.

McGoldrick KE. Anesthesia and the eye. In: Barash PG, Cullen BF, Stoelting RK, eds. *Clinical anesthesia*, 5th ed. Philadelphia: Lippincott Williams & Wilkins, 2006:977–982, 991.

B.10. How would you premedicate this patient?

Whether the ambulatory surgical patient should receive premedication has been the subject of much interest and debate. Keeping in mind that a prompt recovery is an important consideration in outpatient anesthesia, many authors have recommended that little or no premedication (especially the centrally active depressant premedicants) be given to surgical outpatients so that recovery is not prolonged. Interestingly, most prospective clinical studies have failed to demonstrate a prolonged recovery following premedication with sedative-anxiolytic and analgesic drugs. However, narcotic premedicants have been shown to increase the incidence of postoperative nausea, which could prolong recovery time, and are not recommended unless the patient is in pain preoperatively.

In view of the goals one might want to achieve with outpatient preoperative medication, including anxiety relief, sedation, amnesia, analgesia, vagolysis, prophylaxis against aspiration pneumonia, and prevention of postoperative nausea, premedicant drugs may be safely used if needed by the patient provided the drug and the dosage are carefully chosen. Drugs commonly used as premedicants for outpatients include sedative-hypnotics, opioids, anticholinergics, antacids, gastrokinetics, H_2-receptor antagonists, and antiemetics. Most prospective studies have not found recovery to be prolonged after the use of appropriate doses of sedative premedication (e.g., midazolam 1 to 2 mg intravenous). Indeed, proper use of premedication may actually expedite the discharge process as a result of its ability to reduce postoperative side effects. Clearly, however, lorazepam's very long duration of action makes it unsuitable for use in the ambulatory surgical patient.

Kain ZN, Sevarino F, Pincus S, et al. Attenuation of the preoperative stress response with midazolam: effects on postoperative outcomes. *Anesthesiology* 2000;93:141.

Van Vlymen JM, SaRego MM, White PF. Benzodiazepine premedication: can it improve outcome in patients undergoing breast biopsy procedures? *Anesthesiology* 1999;90:740.

White PF, Freire AR. Ambulatory (outpatient) anesthesia. In: Miller RD, ed. *Miller's anesthesia*, 6th ed. Philadelphia: Elsevier, Churchill Livingstone, 2005:2595–2596.

B.11. Should every outpatient receive prophylaxis against acid aspiration pneumonitis?

Despite early studies demonstrating that a large percentage of outpatients are theoretically at risk for gastric aspiration, the actual incidence of pulmonary aspiration is very low (<1/35,000) in surgical patients with no specific risk factors. The possibility that outpatients have a greater potential for acid aspiration than inpatients had prompted several authors in the past to recommend that some form of aspiration prophylaxis be given to all patients scheduled for outpatient surgery. Unfortunately, this is costly and may result in undesired side effects. Although individual ambulatory surgery centers must determine their own policies, pharmacologic prevention of acid aspiration should not be routine, but rather reserved for outpatients with predisposing factors (e.g., pregnancy, symptomatic hiatal hernia, diabetes mellitus with autonomic neuropathy, morbid obesity, etc).

Lichtor JL. Anesthesia for ambulatory surgery. In: Barash PG, Cullen BF, Stoelting RK, eds. *Clinical anesthesia*, 5th ed. Philadelphia: Lippincott Williams & Wilkins, 2006:1234.

White PF, Freire AR. Ambulatory (outpatient) anesthesia. In: Miller RD, ed. *Miller's anesthesia*, 6th ed. Philadelphia: Elsevier, Churchill Livingstone, 2005:2599–2600.

B.12. Is an overnight fast justified for all outpatients?

Several investigators have questioned the value of the traditional overnight fast for surgical outpatients, particularly pediatric outpatients. Prolonged fasting does not guarantee an empty stomach at the time of induction. It does, however, cause patient discomfort and may produce significant physiologic disturbances in infants and young children. Studies in children and in adults have shown no increase in volume or decrease in pH of gastric fluid when clear liquids were administered as late as 2 hours before induction of anesthesia. Therefore, arbitrary restrictions on the preoperative fast for surgical outpatients without risk factors for pulmonary aspiration, such as "NPO after midnight," appear to be unwarranted. Clear fluids in reasonable amounts (3 mL/kg) may be safely ingested until 2 hours before surgery. Although coffee is not transparent, it is devoid of particulate matter and is accepted as a clear liquid. There is some evidence that briefer periods of preoperative fasting (2 hours) are accompanied by less postoperative nausea and vomiting (PONV), as well as a reduced incidence of dizziness, drowsiness, and thirst. Breast milk should be withheld for at least 4 hours in neonates and infants who are being breastfed. Intake of nonclear liquids, nonhuman milk, and solid food should be discontinued at least 6 hours before the induction of anesthesia.

Gregory GA, ed. *Pediatric anesthesia*, 4th ed. New York: Churchill Livingston, 2002:184–185.

Lichtor JL. Anesthesia for ambulatory surgery. In: Barash PG, Cullen BF, Stoelting RK, eds. *Clinical anesthesia*, 5th ed. Philadelphia: Lippincott Williams & Wilkins, 2006:1231–1232.

White PF, Freire AR. Ambulatory (outpatient) anesthesia. In: Miller RD, ed. *Miller's anesthesia*, 6th ed. Philadelphia: Elsevier, Churchill Livingstone, 2005:2600–2601.

C. Intraoperative Management

C.1. What are the important considerations in choosing an anesthetic technique for outpatient surgery?

- Smooth and rapid onset of action
- Intraoperative amnesia and analgesia

- Hemodynamic stability
- Good operating conditions
- Rapid recovery period without side effects
- Cost-effectiveness

To date, no "ideal" anesthetic drug or technique has been identified for outpatients. No single agent or combination of agents, either inhaled or intravenous, has been clearly demonstrated to reduce recovery time and allow faster discharge of the ambulatory surgical patient. However, with its smooth induction profile and short elimination half-life, propofol may prove to be the induction, if not the maintenance, agent of choice for outpatient anesthesia. The newer halogenated ether compounds, sevoflurane and desflurane, have become increasingly popular in ambulatory anesthesia owing to their rapid onset and quick termination of clinical effects. Currently, desirable anesthetic conditions with an acceptable recovery profile may be produced by a large array of pharmacologically active drugs administered in conjunction with either general, regional, or local anesthesia techniques. It is essential, however, to combine these agents in a rational manner and carefully titrate them to optimal effect.

Lichtor JL. Anesthesia for ambulatory surgery. In: Barash PG, Cullen BF, Stoelting RK, eds. *Clinical anesthesia*, 5th ed. Philadelphia: Lippincott Williams & Wilkins, 2006: 1234–1238.

White PF, Freire AR. Ambulatory (outpatient) anesthesia. In: Miller RD, ed. *Miller's anesthesia*, 6th ed. Philadelphia: Elsevier, Churchill Livingstone, 2005:2601–2613.

C.2. What are the anesthetic implications of recent retinal detachment surgery?

Patients who have had vitreoretinal surgery often have a gas bubble deliberately left within the eye to help tamponade and keep the retina attached as adhesions develop. Filtered room air, sulfur hexafluoride (SF_6), and perfluoropropane (C_3F_8) are the most commonly used gases. By varying the concentration, volume, and type of gas used, bubbles can be produced that will last up to 70 days before being completely absorbed. If nitrous oxide is administered during this time, the bubble will rapidly expand with the attendant risk of retinal and optic nerve ischemia secondary to central retinal artery occlusion. Primate models indicate that irreversible retinal damage occurs after 100 minutes of retinal artery obstruction, suggesting that perhaps some recovery might be expected after briefer anesthetics. However, a narrower window may exist in humans. Therefore, nitrous oxide should be avoided in any patient who has undergone vitreoretinal surgery within the preceding 3 months, unless records are available to confirm that either intraocular gas was not used, or that it has subsequently been completely reabsorbed.

Hart RH, Vote BJ, Borthwick JH, et al. Loss of vision caused by expansion of intraocular perfluoropropane (C_3F_8) gas during nitrous oxide anesthesia. *Am J Ophthalmol* 2002; 134:761–763.

Hayreh SS, Kolder HE. Central retinal artery occlusion and retinal tolerance time. *Ophthalmology* 1980;87:75–78.

Lee EJK. Use of nitrous oxide causing severe visual loss 37 days after retinal surgery. *Br J Anaesth* 2004;93:464–466.

C.3. How would you monitor this patient?

The effects of anesthesia during ambulatory procedures should be monitored using the same standards applicable to inpatient procedures. Standard monitoring in this patient would include a blood pressure cuff, electrocardiogram (ECG), pulse oximeter, precordial or esophageal stethoscope, temperature probe, and measurement of inspired oxygen and end-tidal carbon dioxide. The potential for hypoxia and hypercarbia during laparoscopy requires careful monitoring of oxygen saturation and expired carbon dioxide tension. In addition, intraabdominal pressure must be measured during gas insufflation into the peritoneal cavity. Although standard intraoperative monitoring is appropriate for most outpatients having laparoscopic surgery, American Society of Anesthesiologists (ASA) physical status III or IV patients may benefit from invasive hemodynamic monitoring to carefully and continuously determine the cardiovascular response to pneumoperitoneum and position changes.

Cunningham AJ, Nolan C. Anesthesia for minimally invasive procedures. In: Barash PG, Cullen BF, Stoelting RK, eds. *Clinical anesthesia*, 5th ed. Philadelphia: Lippincott Williams & Wilkins, 2006:1065.

Joris JL. Anesthesia for laparoscopic surgery. In: Miller RD, ed. *Miller's anesthesia*, 6th ed. Philadelphia: Elsevier, Churchill Livingstone, 2005:2297.

C.4. What is the Bispectral Index (BIS) monitor and what information does it convey?

The BIS monitor is a noninvasive monitoring system that is derived from the electroencephalogram (EEG). Using bispectral analysis of the EEG waveform and other features within the EEG, the BIS monitor is used to detect changes in purported depth of anesthesia or hypnosis. A proprietary algorithm translates the complex data generated from the analysis of the EEG over a 30-second period into a single number between 0 (i.e., no brain activity) and 100 (i.e., the patient is fully awake) that is displayed on the BIS monitor. The BIS is one of many brain function monitors that record or process brain electrical activity and convert these signals mathematically into a continuous measure, typically scaled from 0 to 100. It is important to appreciate that intraoperative awareness cannot be measured during the intraoperative phase of general anesthesia, because the recall component of awareness can only be determined postoperatively by obtaining information directly from the patient. Moreover, although clinically important, intraoperative awareness under general anesthesia is a rare occurrence, with a reported incidence of 0.1% to 0.2% in adults.

American Society of Anesthesiologists Task Force on Intraoperative Awareness. *Practice Advisory for Intraoperative Awareness and Brain Function Monitoring. A Report by the American Society of Anesthesiologists Task Force on Intraoperative Awareness*. Approved by the House of Delegates on October 25, 2005

Bergman IJ, Kluger MT, Short TG. Awareness during general anaesthesia: a review of 81 cases from the anaesthetic incident monitoring study. *Anaesthesia* 2002;57:549–556.

Sebel PS, Bowdle TA, Ghoneim MM, et al. The incidence of awareness during anaesthesia: a multicenter United States study. *Anesth Analg* 2004;99:833–839.

C.5. What benefits might be derived from using a Bispectral Index (BIS) monitor?

Information about the patient's hypnotic state obtained from the BIS, in combination with other monitored parameters and clinical signs, may allow better balancing of hypnotic and analgesic administration. Titration of hypnotic agents based on individual requirements arguably is improved, potentially reducing the incidence of relative under- and overdosing. Furthermore, selection of anesthetic interventions (e.g., administration of hypnotics, analgesics, and vasoactive drugs) may be more rational. Reduced drug usage, earlier awakening, and faster recovery have all been associated with using the BIS monitor to help guide anesthesia maintenance. This translates into a higher potential for bypassing the stage one postanesthesia care unit (PACU) and earlier discharge eligibility from the PACU. It is not known yet whether these benefits will ultimately reduce medical costs significantly. Indeed, a recent meta-analysis based on 1,380 subjects from 11 trials disclosed that BIS monitoring reduced anesthetic consumption by 19%, reduced the incidence of nausea/vomiting, and reduced time in the PACU by 4 minutes. However, these benefits did not lead to a significant reduction in time until patient discharge from the ambulatory surgery unit. Additionally, BIS monitoring actually increased the cost per patient by $5.55 owing to the cost of the BIS electrodes.

Johansen JW, Sebel PS. Development and clinical application of electroencephalographic bispectrum monitoring. *Anesthesiology* 2000;93:1336–1344.

Liu S. Effects of bispectral index monitoring on ambulatory anesthesia: a meta-analysis of randomized controlled trials and a cost analysis. *Anesthesiology* 2004;101:311–315.

O'Connor MF, Daves S, Tung A, et al. BIS monitoring to prevent awareness during general anesthesia. *Anesthesiology* 2001;94:520–522.

Pavlin JD, Souter KJ, Hong JY. Effects of bispectral index monitoring on recovery from surgical anesthesia in 1,580 inpatients from an academic medical center. *Anesthesiology* 2005;102:566–573.

C.6. Is Bispectral Index(BIS) monitoring applicable to children?

The BIS was developed and tested on adults. Because the electroencephalogram (EEG) in infants and young children is different from that of an adult and changes as the brain matures, the BIS value may not necessarily apply to the pediatric patient population. Validating the BIS monitor in infants and young children poses significant problems. End points used to confirm BIS in adults, such as assessment of sedation, sleep, or purposeful movement in response to voice commands, cannot be reliably obtained in children. Furthermore, there are serious ethical problems in recruiting healthy children as volunteers in studies of general anesthesia. Nevertheless, recent data from numerous authors comparing BIS values between adults and children at various clinical end points during general anesthesia, such as before anesthesia, during maintenance, at emergence, and with increasing concentrations of volatile anesthetic, suggest that BIS generally performs similarly in adults and children with respect to dose response to anesthetic agents. However, a recent study disclosed that in children, aged 6 months to 12 years, the BIS increased paradoxically as end-tidal sevoflurane concentration increased from 3% to 4%. BIS values showed a wide variation at the same end-tidal sevoflurane concentration, and the age of the patient was considered to be a factor affecting the BIS values. A consensus seems to be forming that BIS monitoring should be used with caution in infants less than 1 year of age. Clearly, further work in this area is needed. Definitive studies correlating level of sedation, awareness, and anesthetic outcome with BIS in children have not yet been published.

Bannister CF, Brosius KF, Sigl JC, et al. The effect of bispectral index monitoring on anesthetic use and recovery in children anesthetized with sevoflurane in nitrous oxide. *Anesth Analg* 2001;92:877–881.

Davidson AJ, Huang GH, Czarnecki C, et al. Awareness during anesthesia in children: a prospective cohort study. *Anesth Analg* 2005;100:653–661.

Davidson AJ, Huang GH, Rebmann CS, et al. Performance of entropy and bispectral index as measures of anaesthesia effect in children of different ages. *Br J Anaesth* 2005;95:674–679.

Kim HS, Oh AY, Kim CS, et al. Correlation of bispectral index with end-tidal sevoflurane concentration and age in infants and children. *Br J Anaesth* 2005;95:363–366.

Watcha MF. Investigations of the bispectral index monitor in pediatric anesthesia: first things first. *Anesth Analg* 2001;92:805–807.

C.7. What are the major limitations of Bispectral Index (BIS) monitoring?

The BIS monitor is not a measure of global anesthetic depth. It is only a measure of the patient's level of sedation and hypnotic state. As such it helps the anesthesiologist assess the potential for patient awareness, but it cannot prevent it. In fact, use of the BIS has not been proved to reduce or eliminate the risk of intraoperative awareness. The BIS will not predict patient movement or hemodynamic response to noxious stimulation, nor will it predict the exact moment when consciousness will return. Sedation produced by both ketamine and nitrous oxide does not produce the expected decrease in BIS. The utility of BIS in patients with neurologic disease has not been adequately studied to validate its use in these patients. Finally, more work is necessary to establish whether BIS is an accurate measure of hypnosis in pediatric patients.

It is important to appreciate that a specific numerical value may not correlate with a specific depth of anesthesia. Moreover, the measured values do not have uniform sensitivity across different anesthetic drugs or types of patients. Artifacts may be introduced by electrocautery, lasers, and warming devices. Clearly, intraoperative monitoring of depth of anesthesia to minimize the risk of awareness should rely on multiple modalities, including clinical observations of purposeful or reflex movement, electrocardiogram (ECG) tracing, blood pressure, heart rate, end-tidal anesthetic analyzer, and capnography.

The consensus of the American Society of Anesthesiologists (ASA) Task Force on Intraoperative Awareness is that brain function monitoring is not routinely indicated for patients undergoing general anesthesia, and that the decision to use a brain function monitor should be made on a case-by-case basis by the individual practitioner for selected patients at increased risk.

Barr G, Jakobsson JG, Öwall A, et al. Nitrous oxide does not alter bispectral index: study with nitrous oxide as sole agent and as adjunct to i.v. anaesthesia. *Br J Anaesth* 1999; 82:827–830.

Chan MTV, Gin T. What does the bispectral EEG index monitor? *Eur J Anaesthesiol* 2000; 17:146–148.

American Society of Anesthesiologists Task Force on Intraoperative Awareness. *Practice Advisory for Intraoperative Awareness and Brain Function Monitoring. A Report by the American Society of Anesthesiologists Task Force on Intraoperative Awareness*. Approved by the House of Delegates on October 25, 2005.

C.8. What does a Bispectral Index (BIS) reading of 56 mean?

The BIS scale is a dimensionless scale from 0 to 100. Typically, BIS values between 40 and 60 correspond with a moderate hypnotic state of general anesthesia, and are associated with a low probability of patient consciousness. Deep sedation with a low probability of explicit recall occurs in the 60–70 BIS range, with higher values up to 85 associated with light to moderate sedation. A BIS number below 40 indicates a deep hypnotic state, with brain isoelectricity increasing as BIS approaches 0. As mentioned previously, however, there are multiple exceptions to these generalities, and the BIS is perhaps best thought of as a trend monitor rather than an "absolute" monitor of hypnotic depth.

Hemmerling TM, Migneault B. Falsely increased bispectral index during endoscopic shoulder surgery attributed to interferences with the endoscopic shaver device. *Anesth Analg* 2002;95:1678–1679.

Johansen JW, Sebel PS. Development and clinical application of electroencephalographic bispectrum monitoring. *Anesthesiology* 2000;93:1337.

C.9. What are the anesthetic options for laparoscopy?

In recent years anesthesiologists have successfully employed local, regional, and general anesthesia for laparoscopy. Local and regional anesthesia offer the potential advantages of faster postoperative recovery and reduced postoperative complications. These techniques also avoid the postoperative discomforts of general anesthesia, such as sore throat, muscle pains, and airway trauma. However, steep Trendelenburg position, pneumoperitoneum, and surgical manipulation often make spontaneous ventilation difficult during local or regional anesthesia. In addition, the potential for postspinal headache may detract from the use of regional anesthesia in the outpatient. The vast majority of laparoscopic procedures continue to be performed under general endotracheal anesthesia. General anesthesia offers the advantages of elimination of patient anxiety, complete amnesia and analgesia, the ability to control ventilation, muscle relaxation, and a motionless operative field.

Cunningham AJ, Nolan C. Anesthesia for minimally invasive procedures. In: Barash PG, Cullen BF, Stoelting RK, eds. *Clinical anesthesia*, 5th ed. Philadelphia: Lippincott Williams & Wilkins, 2006:1065.

Joris JL. Anesthesia for laparoscopic surgery. In: Miller RD, ed. *Miller's anesthesia*, 6th ed. Philadelphia: Elsevier, Churchill Livingstone, 2005:2297–2298.

C.10. What anesthetic agents would you use to induce and maintain general anesthesia in this patient?

A number of anesthetic agents in a variety of combinations can be used successfully to provide general anesthesia in this patient. A reasonable aproach would be to induce anesthesia with propofol or a short-acting barbiturate, such as sodium thiopental, after a preinduction dose of a short-acting benzodiazepine. After intubation, anesthesia is maintained with a volatile anesthetic, such as sevoflurane or desflurane, and an air–oxygen mixture, supplemented with a short-acting narcotic as needed and a muscle relaxant.

Cunningham AJ, Nolan C. Anesthesia for minimally invasive procedures. In: Barash PG, Cullen BF, Stoelting RK, eds. *Clinical anesthesia*, 5th ed. Philadelphia: Lippincott Williams & Wilkins, 2006:1065–1066.

Joris JL. Anesthesia for laparoscopic surgery. In: Miller RD, ed. *Miller's anesthesia*, 6th ed. Philadelphia: Elsevier, Churchill Livingstone, 2005:2297–2298.

C.11. Would you avoid the use of nitrous oxide in this ambulatory patient?

As mentioned in the preceding text, if the patient has an intraocular gas bubble that is not completely resorbed, nitrous oxide is contraindicated for fear of causing devastating visual damage. In the absence of this contraindication, the use of nitrous oxide, albeit somewhat controversial, should be considered. Traditionally, there had been concerns about its ability to diffuse into bowel lumen causing distension and to increase postoperative nausea/vomiting. It has been shown that surgical conditions during laparoscopic procedures lasting 70 to 80 minutes were identical (bowel distension did not increase over time) regardless of whether nitrous oxide was used. In a laboratory study involving porcine subjects, nitrous oxide was shown to diffuse into a carbon dioxide peritoneum and the nitrous oxide fraction exceeded 29%, a level that can support combustion, within 2 hours. Therefore, the clinical risk associated with prolonged laparoscopy remains unclear. Although it had historically been held that nitrous oxide can contribute to postoperative nausea and vomiting (PONV), conclusive evidence is lacking to demonstrate an important effect of nitrous oxide on the incidence of postoperative emesis after laparoscopic cholecystectomy or pelvic laparoscopy. Therefore, any potential benefit from its elimination must be balanced against the potential increased risk of intraoperative awareness.

Cunningham AJ, Nolan C. Anesthesia for minimally invasive procedures. In: Barash PG, Cullen BF, Stoelting RK, eds. *Clinical anesthesia*, 5th ed. Philadelphia: Lippincott Williams & Wilkins, 2006:1065–1066.

Diemunsch PA, Torp KD, Van Dorsselaer T, et al. Nitrous oxide fraction in the carbon dioxide pneumoperitoneum during laparoscopy under general inhaled anesthesia in pigs. *Anesth Analg* 2000;90:951.

Taylor E, Feinstein R, White PF. Anesthesia for laparoscopic cholecystectomy: is nitrous oxide contraindicated? *Anesthesiology* 1992;76:561.

C.12. Discuss the physiologic changes induced by laparoscopy.

Physiologic changes occur as a result of the pneumoperitoneum and the Trendelenburg position that are required during laparoscopy. Carbon dioxide or nitrous oxide can be used to produce the pneumoperitoneum. Insufflation of gas into the peritoneal cavity elevates intraabdominal pressure and impairs venous return. As intraabdominal pressure increases above 20 mmHg, central venous pressure, arterial pressure, pulse pressure, and cardiac output all decrease. Although rare, severe hypotension and cardiac arrest have been reported. The pneumoperitoneum also sequesters blood in the legs, thereby decreasing the circulating blood volume. Vital capacity is significantly reduced as the diaphragm is displaced cephalad by the Trendelenburg position and pneumoperitoneum. Pulmonary compliance is decreased, functional residual capacity is diminished, and aeration of the lower lobes is compromised, predisposing the patient to the development of hypoxia and atelectasis. As the intraperitoneal gas is released and intraabdominal pressure decreases, all cardiovascular and respiratory parameters should return to normal.

Cunningham AJ, Nolan C. Anesthesia for minimally invasive procedures. In: Barash PG, Cullen BF, Stoelting RK, eds. *Clinical anesthesia*, 5th ed. Philadelphia: Lippincott Williams & Wilkins, 2006:1062–1065.

Joris JL. Anesthesia for laparoscopic surgery. In: Miller RD, ed. *Miller's anesthesia*, 6th ed. Philadelphia: Elsevier, Churchill Livingstone, 2005:2286–2294.

C.13. In addition to the physiologic changes described in the preceding text, what other intraoperative complications are associated with laparoscopy?

Absorption of carbon dioxide used for peritoneal insufflation may produce hypercarbia, resulting in hypertension, hypotension, catecholamine stimulation, cardiac arrhythmias, and acidosis. Arrhythmias may also be produced by vasovagal reflexes. Hemorrhage accounts for nearly half of the complications from laparoscopy. A cephalad shift of the mediastinum may cause the endotracheal tube to pass into a bronchus after the Trendelenburg position is assumed. Other complications include gas embolization, tension pneumothorax, pneumomediastinum, perforation and electrical injury of organs, and passive regurgitation and aspiration.

Cunningham AJ, Nolan C. Anesthesia for minimally invasive procedures. In: Barash PG, Cullen BF, Stoelting RK, eds. *Clinical anesthesia*, 5th ed. Philadelphia: Lippincott Williams & Wilkins, 2006:1062–1067.

Joris JL. Anesthesia for laparoscopic surgery. In: Miller RD, ed. *Miller's anesthesia*, 6th ed. Philadelphia: Elsevier, Churchill Livingstone, 2005:2286–2294.

C.14. Why is carbon dioxide the insufflation agent of choice for laparoscopy?

Carbon dioxide is the most commonly used agent for laparoscopy because it is more soluble in blood than air, oxygen, or nitrous oxide. The carbon dioxide–carrying capacity of the blood is high owing to bicarbonate buffering and combination with hemoglobin and plasma proteins. Rapid elimination also increases the margin of safety in the event of intravenous injection of carbon dioxide. All of these properties contribute to the rapid reversal of the clinical signs of carbon dioxide embolism when treated properly. Therefore, the lethal dose of carbon dioxide is approximately five times greater than that of air.

Joris JL. Anesthesia for laparoscopic surgery. In: Miller RD, ed. *Miller's anesthesia*, 6th ed. Philadelphia: Elsevier, Churchill Livingstone, 2005:2289.

C.15. What are some alternatives to carbon dioxide for laparoscopy?

Insufflation of inert gases, such as helium or argon, instead of carbon dioxide avoids the increase in $PaCO_2$ from absorption, thereby avoiding the need for hyperventilation. The ventilatory consequences of the increased intraabdominal pressure persist, however. Although the hemodynamic consequences of pneumoperitoneum from inert gases are similar to those seen with carbon dioxide, the inert gases blunt the increase in arterial pressure but exacerbate the decrease in cardiac output. Unfortunately, the low blood solubility of the inert gases is concerning in the event of gas embolism.

Gasless laparoscopy, using abdominal wall lift from a fan retractor, is another alternative to carbon dioxide. This technique may be attractive for patients with severe cardiac or pulmonary disease because it avoids the respiratory and hemodynamic consequences of increased intraabdominal pressure secondary to insufflation. However, gasless laparoscopy compromises surgical exposure and exacerbates technical difficulty.

Goldberg JM, Maurer WG. A randomized comparison of gasless laparoscopy and CO_2 pneumoperitoneum. *Obstet Gynecol* 1997;90:416.

Joris JL. Anesthesia for laparoscopic surgery. In: Miller RD, ed. *Miller's anesthesia*, 6th ed. Philadelphia: Elsevier, Churchill Livingstone, 2005:2295.

Wolf JS Jr, Carrier S, Stoller ML. Gas embolism: helium is more lethal than carbon dioxide. *J Laparoendosc Surg* 1994;4:173.

D. Postoperative Management

D.1. What are the common causes of nausea and vomiting in outpatients?

Nausea and vomiting are significant problems after ambulatory surgery, causing patient discomfort and delayed recovery and discharge from the ambulatory center. Prolonged vomiting is one of the most frequent causes of unexpected hospital admission from the ambulatory surgical facility. Patients who have a history of motion sickness and a previous experience of postoperative nausea and vomiting (PONV) are more likely to develop postoperative emetic symptoms, as are patients who are obese or pregnant or have diabetes mellitus. PONV are common in children; the incidence decreases with age. Men and women are equally affected until puberty, when the incidence becomes considerably higher in women. Excessive anxiety and noncompliance with fasting can increase gastric volume and predispose patients to PONV. Interestingly, smoking has been shown to decrease the incidence of PONV.

The use of narcotic analgesics, particularly morphine and meperidine, as premedication, as part of the anesthetic technique, or postoperatively to control pain, increases the incidence of PONV after outpatient anesthesia. Methohexital is less likely than either thiopental or etomidate to cause postoperative nausea. Consistently, propofol was shown to have a low incidence of emetic symptoms postoperatively.

Although Apfel's scoring system to predict the likelihood of PONV emphasizes women, nonsmoking status, history of PONV or motion sickness and narcotic administration as the major risk factors, Sinclair also identifies surgical issues. Surgical procedures such as breast augmentation, varicose vein stripping, laparoscopy, dilatation and curettage, strabismus correction, myringotomy and tympanostomy tube placement, and orchiopexy are associated with more PONV, with the incidence escalating with increasing surgical and anesthesia time. Pain, hypotension, and early ambulation are postoperative factors demonstrated to increase nausea and vomiting. Relief of pain often relieves concomitant nausea.

Apfel C, Kranke P, Eberhart LHJ, et al. Comparison of predictive models for postoperative nausea and vomiting. *Br J Anaesth* 2002;88:234–240.

Apfel CC, Laara E, Koivuranta M, et al. A simplified risk score for predicting postoperative nausea and vomiting: conclusions from cross validation between two centers. *Anesthesiology* 1999;91:693.

Sinclair DR, Chung F, Mezei G. Can postoperative nausea and vomiting be predicted? *Anesthesiology* 1999;91:109–118.

White PF, Freire AR. Ambulatory (outpatient) anesthesia. In: Miller RD, ed. *Miller's anesthesia*, 6th ed. Philadelphia: Elsevier, Churchill Livingstone, 2005:2597–2598.

D.2. How would you pharmacologically prevent postoperative nausea and vomiting (PONV) in the susceptible ambulatory patient?

Because of concerns about medication cost and potential side effects, routine prophylactic administration of an antiemetic is not considered appropriate for all ambulatory surgical patients. Instead, antiemetic prophylaxis should be reserved for patients who are considered to be susceptible to developing PONV (see preceding text). A large number of medications have been used to prevent postanesthetic nausea and vomiting in the outpatient, some with only limited success. Unfortunately, the ideal medication for each patient is not known. Serotonin antagonists, such as ondansetron 4 to 8 mg intravenous in adults and 0.1 mg per kg intravenous in children, are highly effective, but the high cost of ondansetron may limit its use. Droperidol has been shown to be effective, inexpensive, and without an increase in postoperative sedation when used in low doses, such as 0.625 to 1.25 mg in adults (or as low as 10 to 20 μg per kg). Recently, however, the U.S. Food and Drug Administration (FDA) issued a so-called black box warning on the use of droperidol for antiemetic prophylaxis owing to purported fears about prolongation of the QTc interval and subsequent potentially dangerous ventricular arrhythmias. Nonetheless, Charbit et al. documented that droperidol and ondansetron induce similar clinically relevant QTc prolongation, and concluded that the safety of 5-hydroxytryptamine type 3 antagonists may not be superior to that of low-dose droperidol.

Prophylactic administration of dexamethasone, 5 to 10 mg intravenous in adults and 0.5 to 1 mg per kg intravenous in children, is effective in the prevention of PONV and appears to offer no evidence of any clinically relevant toxicity. Combining dexamethasone with a serotonin antagonist further decreases the incidence of nausea and vomiting and may prove to be the best prophylactic regimen, although optimal doses of this combination are not currently known. Transdermal scopolamine effectively reduces PONV if given as a premedicant well in advance of the surgery, but the high incidence of anticholinergic side effects and prolonged residual effects on cognitive performance, especially in the elderly, detract from its usefulness in the ambulatory patient.

There is increasing evidence that a multimodal approach may lead to improved outcomes. Double and triple antiemetic combinations, using drugs with different mechanisms of action, are recommended for patients at high risk of PONV. General anesthesia with volatile agents should be avoided, if possible, in high-risk patients. If general anesthesia is necessary, a total intravenous approach with propofol may be advantageous. Moreover, if rescue therapy for PONV is needed within 6 hours of surgery, patients should not receive a repeat dose of the drug that was administered prophylactically. Rather, a rescue drug with a different mechanism of action should be selected.

Apfel CC, Katz MH, Kranke P, et al. Volatile anesthetics may be the main cause of early but not delayed postoperative vomiting: a randomized controlled trial of factorial design. *Br J Anaesth* 2002;88:659–668.

Gan TJ, Meyer T, Apfel C, et al. Consensus guidelines for managing postoperative nausea and vomiting. *Anesth Analg* 2003;97:62–71.

Charbit B, Albaladejo P, Funck-Brentano C, et al. Prolongation of QTc interval after postoperative nausea and vomiting treatment by droperidol or ondansetron. *Anesthesiology* 2005;102:1094–1100.

Scuderi PE, James RL, Harris L, et al. Multimodal antiemetic management prevents early postoperative vomiting after outpatient laparoscopy. *Anesth Analg* 2000;91:1408–1414.

D.3. How is postoperative pain treated?

Pain control is one of the most important factors in determining when a surgical outpatient can be discharged. Pain should be treated rapidly and effectively to minimize postoperative symptoms so that ambulation and discharge are not delayed. The optimal strategy is to use a preemptive, multimodal approach. Begin controlling postoperative pain intraoperatively by supplementing the anesthetic technique with a short-acting narcotic analgesic or a regional block. Intravenous fentanyl is usually the drug of choice for postoperative pain relief. It may be given in small doses of 12.5 μg at 5-minute intervals and titrated to relief of pain. Ketorolac, a nonsteroidal antiinflammatory drug, has become increasingly popular in the management of postoperative pain in the ambulatory patient because of its lack of opioid-related side effects (e.g., sedation, nausea, vomiting, respiratory depression). It is available for oral and parental administration, and its use may decrease a patient's requirement for opioid analgesics. Controversy still surrounds the perioperative use of ketorolac because of the potential for bleeding complications and renal dysfunction. Local and regional anesthetic techniques can be used to provide effective postoperative analgesia, and when used to supplement general anesthesia, facilitate a pleasant emergence, and minimize the need for opioids. Commonly used techniques include local infiltration of the incision site, intraarticular injection, nerve blockade (e.g., dorsal nerve penile block for circumcision, or ilioinguinal and iliohypogastric nerve blocks for inguinal hernia repair), and caudal blocks. When the patient has resumed intake of oral fluids, oral analgesics (e.g., acetaminophen, nonsteroidal antiinflammatory drugs, as well as codeine and other opioid analgesics) may be administered for control of pain after discharge.

Lichtor JL. Anesthesia for ambulatory surgery. In: Barash PG, Cullen BF, Stoelting RK, eds. *Clinical anesthesia*, 5th ed. Philadelphia: Lippincott Williams & Wilkins, 2006:1242.

White PF, Freire AR. Ambulatory (outpatient) anesthesia. In: Miller RD, ed. *Miller's anesthesia*, 6th ed. Philadelphia: Elsevier, Churchill Livingstone, 2005:2614–2616.

D.4. If the patient complained of eye pain postoperatively, how would you manage the situation?

Pain due to corneal abrasion is the most common ocular complication of general anesthesia. Patients with a corneal abrasion usually complain of a foreign-body sensation, pain, tearing, and photophobia. The pain is typically exacerbated by blinking and ocular movement. It is wise to have an ophthalmologic consultation immediately. Treatment typically consists of the prophylactic application of antibiotic ointment and patching the injured eye shut. Although permanent sequelae are possible, healing usually occurs within 24 hours.

If the patient complains of intense pain, he or she should be scrupulously observed for signs of red eye, corneal edema, and a fixed mid-dilated pupil, as well as complaints of blurred vision. These are characteristic signs of acute angle-closure glaucoma (ACG), a serious emergency. Ophthalmologic consultation should be secured immediately to acutely decrease intraocular pressure (IOP) with systemic and topical therapy. Topical pilocarpine 2% is administered to cause miosis and pull the iris taut and away from the trabecular meshwork. A topical β-blocker also should be considered. If a prompt reduction in IOP does not ensue, systemic therapy with an agent such as mannitol should be considered, but its potentially adverse hemodynamic effects should be weighed in a patient with cardiovascular disease. If medical therapy is effective in reducing IOP to a safe level and the angle opens, an iridotomy/iridectomy can be performed immediately, or it can be delayed until the corneal edema resolves and the iris becomes less hyperemic. Failure to act effectively and expeditiously in cases of ACG could result in blindness. The excruciating periorbital pain typically described in these patients is an important aid in differential diagnosis.

Patients with open-angle glaucoma can also experience an acute glaucoma attack after surgery, but the IOP tends to be lower than that seen with ACG. The eye characteristically appears pale, dry, and firm, and the patient generally complains of a dull, periorbital headache. Treatment includes topical miotics and 5 to 7 mg per kg of acetazolamide intravenously. If the patient does not respond to medical therapy, laser trabeculoplasty may be necessary. Should laser treatment be ineffective, conventional filtration surgery, placement of a Molteno valve, or a coablative procedure may be indicated.

McGoldrick KE. Anesthesia and the eye. In: Barash PG, Cullen BF, Stoelting RK, eds. *Clinical anesthesia*, 5th ed. Philadelphia: Lippincott Williams & Wilkins, 2006:991–995.

McGoldrick KE, Kosarussavadi B. Increased intraocular pressure. In: Atlee JL, ed. *Complications in anesthesia*. Philadelphia: WB Saunders, 1999:765–768.

D.5. What criteria would you use to establish that a patient can be safely discharged after ambulatory surgery?

For patients to be discharged from an ambulatory facility, they must satisfy specific criteria that are usually summarized on simplified checklists. Although each ambulatory surgical facility must determine its own set of criteria, generally accepted guidelines for safe discharge home after ambulatory surgery include the following:

- Stable vital signs for at least 1 hour
- No evidence of respiratory depression
- Oriented to person, place, and time
- Able to walk unassisted
- Able to dress unassisted
- Minimal nausea or vomiting
- No active bleeding or oozing
- Pain controllable with oral analgesics
- Responsible adult to escort patient home
- Discharge by both the person who administered anesthesia and the person who performed surgery, or their designees. Written instructions for the postoperative period at home must be supplied to the patient before discharge, as well as a phone number to call in the case of emergency

The requirement for patients to drink and void before discharge is no longer considered mandatory, except in the case of certain patients who had central neuraxial blockade (see subsequent text).

Lichtor JL. Anesthesia for ambulatory surgery. In: Barash PG, Cullen BF, Stoelting RK, eds. *Clinical anesthesia*, 5th ed. Philadelphia: Lippincott Williams & Wilkins, 2006: 1242–1243.

Marshall SI, Chung F. Discharge criteria and complications after ambulatory surgery. *Anesth Analg* 1999;88:514.

White PF, Freire AR. Ambulatory (outpatient) anesthesia. In: Miller RD, ed. *Miller's anesthesia*, 6th ed. Philadelphia: Elsevier, Churchill Livingstone, 2005:2619–2620.

D.6. How would you decide when to discharge a patient after regional anesthesia?

Patients recovering from regional anesthesia must satisfy the discharge criteria listed in the preceding text. In addition, if spinal or epidural anesthesia has been used for outpatients, it is important to ensure recovery from the sympathetic and the motor blocks. Hypotension and syncope on standing may be signs that the sympathetic nervous system is still blocked. An indication that the motor block is no longer functioning is the ability to move the legs and feet freely. A simple test is to have the patient run each heel up and down the opposite leg from the big toe to the knee. A patient's ability to walk to the bathroom and void are excellent recovery tests after epidural or spinal anesthesia, because these abilities reflect recovery of both the motor and the sympathetic functions.

Recently Mulroy et al. have suggested that delaying discharge for voiding after spinal or epidural anesthesia with *short-acting local anesthetics* is unnecessary in *low-risk* patients (e.g., age younger 70 years; no hernia, rectal, or urologic surgery; no history of voiding problems). Nonetheless, appropriate measures must be in place for bladder catheterization if the inability to void persists after discharge home. The use of ultrasonographic monitoring of bladder volume before discharge may reduce the incidence of urinary retention after the patient returns home.

Marshall SI, Chung F. Discharge criteria and complications after ambulatory surgery. *Anesth Analg* 1999;88:511–512.

Mulroy MF, Salinas FV, Larkin KL. Ambulatory surgery patients may be discharged before voiding after short-acting spinal and epidural anesthesia. *Anesthesiology* 2002;97:315.

White PF, Freire AR. Ambulatory (outpatient) anesthesia. In: Miller RD, ed. *Miller's anesthesia*, 6th ed. Philadelphia: Elsevier, Churchill Livingstone, 2005:2620–2621.

D.7. What instructions should be given to an ambulatory surgical patient upon discharge?

Patients should be discharged to the care of a responsible adult. Additionally, they should be instructed that after surgery they should not ingest an alcoholic beverage or depressant medication unknown to their surgeon or anesthesiologist, drive a car, or operate complex machinery for at least 24 hours. In addition, the discharge instructions should provide a list of problems that require immediate notification of the surgeon (e.g., bleeding that does not stop, inability to void, and persistent postoperative nausea and vomiting [PONV]).

Marshall SI, Chung F. Discharge criteria and complications after ambulatory surgery. *Anesth Analg* 1999;88:514.

Lichtor JL. Anesthesia for ambulatory surgery. In: Barash PG, Cullen BF, Stoelting RK, eds. *Clinical anesthesia*, 5th ed. Philadelphia: Lippincott Williams & Wilkins, 2006:1243.

White PF, Freire AR. Ambulatory (outpatient) anesthesia. In: Miller RD, ed. *Miller's anesthesia*, 6th ed. Philadelphia: Elsevier, Churchill Livingstone, 2005:2621.

CHAPTER 61

Magnetic Resonance Imaging

MATTHEW C. GOMILLION • JUNG HEE HAN

A 2-YEAR-OLD BOY

weighing 15 kg is scheduled for a preoperative magnetic resonance imaging (MRI) of his brain for ongoing seizures with possible craniotomy with intraoperative MRI the following week. The technician reports that an attempt to obtain a scan last week was unsuccessful because of patient movement despite adequate sedation by the pediatrician. The child's past medical history is remarkable for partial tonic-clonic seizures since age 1. The child was born full term with no complications at birth, and is otherwise healthy. Medications include carbamazepine and valproic acid, both of which were taken the night prior. NPO (nothing orally) status has been maintained for at least 6 hours.

A. Medical Disease and Differential Diagnosis

1. What is magnetic resonance imaging (MRI), and how does it work?
2. What are some advantages of MRI?
3. What are some disadvantages associated with MRI? What are some safety concerns?
4. What are the contraindications to MRI?
5. What are the biologic effects of clinical MRI?
6. What are the anesthetic considerations for this procedure?
7. What is intraoperative MRI?

B. Preoperative Evaluation and Preparation

1. What type of patients may require sedation or general anesthesia for a magnetic resonance examination?
2. What preoperative laboratory testing would you require for this patient?
3. How would you premedicate this patient?

C. Intraoperative Management

1. What are some of the anesthetic options for this patient?
2. How is an MRI conducted?
3. How would you monitor this patient?
4. What special considerations apply to the monitoring equipment used during MRI?
5. How would you induce and maintain general anesthesia in this patient?
6. How would you maintain the airway during the scan?
7. What is the laryngeal mask airway?
8. What are the advantages of the laryngeal mask airway compared with the face mask?

9. What are the advantages of the laryngeal mask airway compared with the endotracheal tube?

10. What complications are associated with the use of the laryngeal mask airway?

11. What are contraindications to the use of the laryngeal mask airway?

12. What are indications for the use of the laryngeal mask airway?

13. What size laryngeal mask airway is appropriate for this child, and how much air would routinely be required to properly inflate the cuff?

14. How is the laryngeal mask airway prepared?

15. How is the laryngeal mask airway inserted?

16. What additional maneuvers may be attempted if difficulty is encountered when inserting the laryngeal mask airway?

17. Examination of the patient before the table is fed into the MRI scanner reveals wheezing. What most likely is happening, and what do you do?

18. Discuss how the laryngeal mask airway can be used as a conduit for tracheal intubation.

19. Discuss the uses of the laryngeal mask airway in the patient with a difficult airway.

D. Postoperative Management

1. When is the laryngeal mask airway removed?

2. How will you have the patient recover from anesthesia?

A. Medical Disease and Differential Diagnosis

A.1. What is magnetic resonance imaging (MRI), and how does it work?

MRI is a noninvasive diagnostic technique that uses magnetic properties of atomic nuclei to produce high-resolution, multiplanar cross-sectional images of the body. Atoms having an odd number of protons and/or neutrons in their nuclei have an associated electrical charge, and the net rotation of protons or neutrons produces a local magnetic field similar to the electromagnetic field produced by the flow of electrons in a wire loop. Normally, the magnetic fields surrounding these nuclei are randomly oriented. When placed in the powerful static magnetic field of the MRI scanner, the nuclei align themselves longitudinally so they lie parallel to the magnetic field.

Within the MRI, a specific radiofrequency (RF) pulse (a second magnetic field) is directed toward the patient at right angles to the static magnetic field, thereby displacing the orientation of the aligned nuclei from the longitudinal magnetic field. As the RF pulse is removed, the nuclei return to their magnetic alignment positions. This is termed *relaxation*. The energy released as the nuclei relax is detected by the receiver coil of the scanner and used to produce the magnetic resonance image. There are two ways to measure relaxation time. T1 relaxation represents the time to revert to the resting magnetic state and T2 relaxation represents the time to revert to the resting axial spin. The time it takes for relaxation to occur varies for specific body tissues, especially water and fat. This allows for differentiation of body structures, as well as between normal and pathologic tissue. Different atoms respond to different radiofrequencies, with the response being proportional to the strength of the static magnetic field. Hydrogen is the atom most often used for imaging. Resolution of the image requires a strong magnetic field. Most MRI scanners used now have a magnetic field of 0.5 to 3.0 T (the magnetic field of the earth is 5×10^{-5} T). The magnetic field of an MRI takes several days to establish. Therefore, it is constantly applied even in the absence of a patient, and it is deactivated only in an emergency.

Barash PG, Cullen BF, Stoelting RK, eds. *Clinical anesthesia*, 5th ed. Philadelphia: Lippincott Williams & Wilkins, 2006:1337.

Menon DK, Peden CJ, Hall AS. Magnetic resonance for the anaesthetist. Part I. Physical principles, applications, safety aspects. *Anaesthesia* 1992;47:241–242.

Miller RD, ed. *Miller's anesthesia*, 6th ed. Philadelphia: Elsevier, Churchill Livingstone, 2005:2643.

Patteson SK, Chesney JT. Anesthetic management for magnetic resonance imaging: problems and solutions. *Anesth Analg* 1992;74:121–122.

A.2. What are some advantages of magnetic resonance imaging (MRI)?

The advantages of MRI include the lack of ionizing radiation, the capability of using noniodinated intravenous contrast agent, and the production of multiplanar images. MRI also provides excellent resolution of normal tissues (e.g., gray and white matter and soft tissues) without image artifact from bone, and can differentiate between normal and pathologic tissue. MRI may be used to evaluate blood and cerebrospinal fluid flow, contraction and relaxation of organs such as the heart, and provide images of tissues in proximity to bone, because calcium does not interfere with MRI.

Barash PG, Cullen BF, Stoelting RK, eds. *Clinical anesthesia*, 5th ed. Philadelphia: Lippincott Williams & Wilkins, 2006:1337.

Miller RD, ed. *Miller's Anesthesia*, 6th ed. Philadelphia: Elsevier, Churchill Livingstone, 2005:2643.

Rawson JV, Siegel MJ. Techniques and strategies in pediatric body MR imaging. *Magn Reson Imaging Clin N Am* 1996;4:589.

A.3. What are some disadvantages associated with magnetic resonance imaging (MRI)? What are some safety concerns?

The most significant disadvantage is the attraction of ferromagnetic objects to the magnetic field of an MRI. In addition to the risk of dislodgement of implanted metallic objects (i.e., pacemakers, vascular clips, automatic implantable cardioverter-defibrillators, mechanical heart valves, and implanted infusion pumps), a potential exists for injury to patients, personnel, and equipment from propelled ferromagnetic objects brought into the magnetic field. Such objects include gas cylinders, pens, keys, laryngoscopes, scissors, stethoscopes, paper clips, vials, and needles. Therefore, everyone coming near an MRI scanner should be carefully screened for ferromagnetic objects. Owing to the potential for catastrophic events, recommendations for MRI safety have been proposed by the American College of Radiology. Briefly the MRI suite should be separated into four zones: Zone I is the public zone immediately outside the MRI suite, Zone II is the reception area monitored by MRI personnel, Zone III encompasses the control room with access to this area being restricted from the public, Zone IV is the physical MRI scanner room. Adherence to these zones must be maintained especially during emergent situations for the safety of the patient and personnel.

Other disadvantages of the MRI include the potential for malfunction of electronic equipment (such as monitors and infusion pumps), as well as limited access to the patient. The relatively long time necessary to obtain the images (as much as 15 minutes per image, with a total scanning period of 1 to 3 hours), and image degradation from any motion including cardiac contractions, respirations, cerebrospinal fluid (CSF) flow, and bowel peristalsis are additional disadvantages. The small bore of the magnet (i.e., 50 to 60 cm in diameter) makes examination of obese patients impossible and creates a feeling of claustrophobia in some patients.

Barash PG, Cullen BF, Stoelting RK, eds. *Clinical anesthesia*, 5th ed. Philadelphia: Lippincott Williams & Wilkins, 2006:1337.

Kanal E, Borgstede JP, et al. American College of Radiology white paper on MR safety. *Am J Roentgenol* 2002;178:1335–1347.

Menon DK, Peden CJ, Hall AS, et al. Magnetic resonance for the anaesthetist. Part I. Physical principles, applications, safety aspects. *Anaesthesia* 1992;47:248.

Miller RD, ed. *Miller's Anesthesia*, 6th ed. Philadelphia: Elsevier, Churchill Livingstone, 2005:2643–2644.

Patteson SK, Chesney JT. Anesthetic management for magnetic resonance imaging: problems and solutions. *Anesth Analg* 1992;74:122.

A.4. What are the contraindications to magnetic resonance imaging (MRI)?

Patients with implanted biologic devices, such as pacemakers, automatic implantable cardioverter-defibrillators, and pumps, should be excluded from MRI studies because of the possibility of device malfunction, inactivation, or damage in the magnetic field. If exceptions are warranted, they should be performed with the radiologist and cardiologist present and full resuscitation equipment readily accessible in case of an arrthymia or equipment malfunction. Reports indicate that St. Jude implantable cardioverter-defibrillators (ICDs) and Medtronic ICDs when exposed to a constant magnetic field can result in reed switch closure, which can temporarily interfere with tachyarrythmia detection. In Guidant ICDs, response to magnet application can be turned on and off, although constant exposure for more than 30 seconds may deactivate the ICD. This can therefore pose serious risks to the patient should an arrthymia occur. The presence of other implanted metallic materials that might be dislodged by the magnetic field (e.g., vascular clips, wires, and cochlear implants) and interventional radiology devices (e.g., coils, filters, and stents) also preclude MRI examination. Artificial heart valves other than the pre-6000 Starr–Edwards valve do not cause a problem during MRI. Orthodontic braces and dentures and tattoos or cosmetics that contain metallic dyes, although safe, can degrade the image quality significantly.

Chen-Scarabelli CA, Scarabelli TM. Letter regarding article by Roguin et al, "Modern pacemaker and implantable cardioverter/defibrillator systems can be magnetic resonance imaging safe: *in vitro* and *in vivo* assessment of safety and function at 1.5 t".[comment]. *Circulation* 2005;111(23):e390.

Kanal E, Borgstede JP, Barkovich AJ, et al. American College of Radiology white paper on MR safety: 2004 update and revisions. *Am J Roentgenol* 2004;182:1113.

Menon DK, Peden CJ, Hall AS, et al. Magnetic resonance for the anaesthetist. Part I. Physical principles, applications, safety aspects. *Anaesthesia* 1992;47:249.

Miller RD, ed. *Miller's Anesthesia*, 6th ed. Philadelphia: Elsevier, Churchill Livingstone, 2005:2644.

Patteson SK, Chesney JT. Anesthetic management for magnetic resonance imaging: problems and solutions. *Anesth Analg* 1992;74:122.

A.5. What are the biologic effects of clinical magnetic resonance imaging (MRI)?

Though an area of controversy and ongoing investigation, most human data to date suggest that there are no significant deleterious effects to patients or health care professionals from exposure to the static magnetic field of an MRI. However, MRI capabilities were developed relatively recently (the 1960s), and epidemiologic evidence of harmful exposure may not yet be apparent. It seems prudent, therefore, to limit repetitive and readily avoidable exposure to the magnetic field. Also controversial is the use of MRI during pregnancy, as the effects of magnetic fields on the human fetus cannot be easily determined. However, current evidence does not support the suggestion that routine clinical exposure of the pregnant patient to MRI can cause developmental abnormalities in the fetus. Pregnant patients have undergone MRI safely during all stages of pregnancy. Nevertheless, caution is advised. Studies have shown that gadolinium-based contrast agents enter the fetal circulation and are filtered in the fetal kidneys into the amniotic fluid. It is unclear the duration of the substance in the fluid, but it can potentially form free gadolinium ions, which can theoretically pose risks to the developing fetus. The appropriateness of MRI examination and the acuteness of the diagnostic need must be considered. Ultrasonography use is preferred if it can provide equivalent diagnostic information, and consideration should be given to postponing the MRI until late in the pregnancy or until after delivery.

Colletti PM, Sylvestre PB. Magnetic resonance imaging in pregnancy. *Magn Reson Imaging Clin N Am* 1994;2:291.

Kanal E, Borgstede JP, Barkovich AJ, et al. American College of Radiology white paper on MR safety: 2004 update and revisions. *Am J Roentgenol* 2004;182:1113.

McBrien ME, Winder J, Smyth L. Anaesthesia for magnetic resonance imaging: a survey of current practice in the UK and Ireland. *Anaesthesia* 2000;55:741–742.

A.6. What are the anesthetic considerations for this procedure?

The problems that complicate the anesthetic management of any patient outside the operating room environment exist for patients requiring sedation or general anesthesia for magnetic resonance imaging (MRI). The MRI unit is often located some distance from the operating room and anesthesia department, limiting the availability of backup assistance and supplies. As with any remote anesthetizing location, the personnel may not be familiar with the requirements of anesthetized patients, thereby decreasing their ability to provide assistance. Frequently, the MRI suites have been designed without the consideration for anesthetic needs, such as pipeline gases, suction, or an anesthetic exhaust system. Access to a recovery suite for postanesthesia care may not be readily available, thereby necessitating a trip to the main recovery room.

In addition, there are anesthetic challenges unique to the MRI suite. Because of the bulkiness of the unit, the patient is often far removed from the anesthesiologist, and access to the airway is limited. Intravenous lines, anesthesia circuits, oxygen tubings, and monitoring cables must be of sufficient length to reach the patient deep within the scanner. The strong magnetic field necessitates the exclusion of all ferromagnetic objects and equipment. The displays of standard monitoring devices can be distorted or displaced by the magnetic field and the monitors themselves can degrade the MRI image by disturbing the signal/noise ratio of the MRI.

Barash PG, Cullen BF, Stoelting RK, eds. *Clinical anesthesia*, 5th ed. Philadelphia: Lippincott Williams & Wilkins, 2006:1337.

Patteson SK, Chesney JT. Anesthetic management for magnetic resonance imaging: problems and solutions. *Anesth Analg* 1992;74:123.

Rogers MC, Tinker JH, Covino BG, eds. *Principles and practice of anesthesiology*. St. Louis: Mosby, 1993:2345.

A.7. What is intraoperative magnetic resonance imaging (MRI)?

Over the last decade, image-guided surgery systems have been introduced that combine the resources of an operating room with MRI technology and high-performance computing.

Several low-, mid-, and high-field strength interventional magnetic resonance systems have been developed that permit access to the patient by surgeons and provide near–real-time imaging during surgical procedures. Intraoperative MRI furnishes the surgeon with the simultaneous combination of direct vision and beyond-the-surface MRI, allowing for more accurate localization and targeting during surgery. In addition, intraoperative MRI enables the surgeon to detect the full extent of lesions, to devise a surgical approach that is safe with less potential operative morbidity, and to monitor for unseen hemorrhage. Not surprisingly, intraoperative MRI systems are expensive and require the need for MRI-compatible surgical instruments and monitoring equipment. As opposed to MRI, the anesthetic considerations for intraoperative MRI must also include the needs of the ongoing surgical procedure.

Berkenstadt H, et al. Anesthesia for magnetic resonance guided neurosurgery. *J Neurosurg Anesthesiol* 2001;13(2):161.

Hall WA, et al. Intraoperative magnetic resonance imaging. *Top Magn Reson Imaging* 2000;11(3):202–212.

Jolesz FA. Interventional and intraoperative MRI: a general overview of the field. *J Magn Reson Imaging* 1998;8(1):5–6.

B. Preoperative Evaluation and Preparation

B.1. What type of patients may require sedation or general anesthesia for a magnetic resonance examination?

Although magnetic resonance imaging (MRI) is painless, patients must remain still throughout the time required to make each scan (as much as 15 minutes) to obtain images free of movement artifacts. Patients who are unable to cooperate adequately (e.g., infants, young children, and adults who are confused, mentally ill, or intellectually subnormal) usually require an anesthesiologist to help reduce movement during the examination. Small infants may tolerate the procedure well if fed before the examination and swaddled in a blanket. In addition, anesthesiologists frequently care for claustrophobic or anxious adults, and those who require either airway protection (unconscious or critically ill patients) or mechanical ventilation (patients with head injuries or elevated intracranial pressure) to ensure that an adequate examination is obtained safely and efficiently.

Miller RD, ed. *Miller's Anesthesia*, 6th ed. Philadelphia: Elsevier, Churchill Livingstone, 2005:2645.

Peden CJ, Menon DK, Hall AS, et al. Magnetic resonance for the anaesthetist. Part II. Anaesthesia and monitoring in MR units. *Anaesthesia* 1992;47:509.

Rogers MC, Tinker JH, Covino BG, et al. eds. *Principles and practice of anesthesiology*. St. Louis: Mosby, 1993:2345–2346.

B.2. What preoperative laboratory testing would you require for this patient?

For a routine magnetic resonance imaging (MRI) examination in this child, no preoperative laboratory tests would be required as long as anticonvulsant medications have been stable with documented adequate serum levels.

White PF. *Ambulatory anesthesia and surgery*. Philadelphia: WB Saunders, 1997:163–165.

B.3. How would you premedicate this patient?

The goals of premedication for this child would be to provide anxiolysis and facilitate the induction of anesthesia without exacerbating a seizure. At the New York Presbyterian Hospital, ambulatory pediatric patients are not routinely given pharmacologic premedicants; rather, it is our practice to allow a parent to be present at the time of induction, in order to help allay the child's anxiety and ease the induction. If one elects to administer a sedative drug to this child, a logical choice would be oral midazolam (0.5 mg/kg, maximum 10 mg) in a small amount of cherry or strawberry syrup.

Cote CJ, Todres ID, Ryan JF, et al. eds. *A practice of anesthesia for infants and children*, 3rd ed. Philadelphia: WB Saunders, 2001:174.

C. Intraoperative Management

C.1. What are some of the anesthetic options for this patient?

Many different anesthetic techniques have been used for anesthetizing children undergoing magnetic resonance imaging (MRI) or other painless radiologic procedures. These range from simple sedation with orally administered chloral hydrate, or rectally administered barbiturates, to intramuscularly administered meperidine/promethazine/Thorazine, to general anesthesia with ketamine, propofol, or inhaled anesthetics. Because conscious sedation of children is frequently insufficient to prevent patient movement, deeper levels of sedation or general anesthesia are frequently required to successfully anesthetize the pediatric patient for MRI. The ideal anesthetic should allow the anesthesiologist the ability to titrate and maintain stable drug concentrations in order to prevent undesired patient movement during the scan and to provide rapid rates of induction and recovery with a minimal requirement for special MRI-compatible equipment.

Intravenous anesthesia with propofol meets several of the aforementioned criteria and is therefore an excellent technique for MRI. Continuous intravenous infusion of propofol allows for a precise, rapid titration to the desired effect and provides for a rapid recovery. Propofol use eliminates the need for a nonferromagnetic, MRI-compatible anesthesia machine and for a scavenger of waste anesthetic gases, both of which are the major drawbacks of an inhalational technique. Ketamine, although considered a potent bronchodilator with minimal respiratory depression, can increase salivation. This, especially in children, can cause upper airway obstruction, laryngospasm and microaspiration even in the presence of relatively intact upper airway reflexes. In addition, ketamine may elicit undesirable myoclonic movements, increased intracranial pressure, and emergence delirium.

Cote CJ, Todres ID, Ryan JF, et al. eds. *A practice of anesthesia for infants and children*, 3rd ed. Philadelphia: WB Saunders, 2001:576.

Frankville DD, Spear RM, Dyck JB. The dose of propofol required to prevent children from moving during magnetic resonance imaging. *Anesthesiology* 1993;79:953–958.

Martin LD, Pasternak R, Pudimat MA. Total intravenous anesthesia with propofol in pediatric patients outside the operating room. *Anesth Analg* 1992;74:611.

Miller RD, ed. *Miller's Anesthesia*, 6th ed. Philadelphia: Elsevier, Churchill Livingstone, 2005:346–348.

C.2. How is a magnetic resonance imaging (MRI) conducted?

The patient is placed on a long, thin table outside the scanner. After obtaining an adequate level of anesthesia, the patient is positioned. If the head is to be examined, it is often enclosed within a small coil or tube. Next, the table with the patient is fed into the long tube of the magnetic resonance imaging (MRI) magnet. The portion of the body to be examined is usually centered in the magnet approximately 1 m from the end of the tube. During the examination, the delivery of the radiofrequency (RF) pulses produces a loud thumping noise, which can average 95 dB in a 1.5-T scanner. To obtain a high-quality scan, the patient must refrain from moving during the acquisition of an individual cut or from changing position at any time during the entire examination. An individual cut can take several minutes, and the total scanning time may be from 1 to 3 hours.

Menon DK, Peden CJ, Hall AS, et al. Magnetic resonance for the anaesthetist. Part I. Physical principles, applications, safety aspects. *Anaesthesia* 1992;47:246–247.

Peden CJ, Menon DK, Hall AS, et al. Magnetic resonance for the anaesthetist. Part II. Anaesthesia and monitoring in MR units. *Anaesthesia* 1992;47:508.

C.3. How would you monitor this patient?

Reliable and accurate monitoring of an unconscious individual during a magnetic resonance imaging (MRI) is essential because the patient cannot be seen adequately nor easily accessed by the anesthesiologist. During sedation, the American Society of Anesthesiologists (ASA) standard monitors including blood pressure, pulse oximetry, and electrocardiogram (ECG) need to be monitored. During general anesthesia, capnography and temperature should also be monitored. The assessment of ventilation in a spontaneously breathing patient may be difficult especially when the patient is within the magnet and far from view. Monitoring end-tidal carbon dioxide from one limb of the nasal oxygen prongs or through a nasal catheter is frequently successful. Use of a precordial stethoscope may be unsatisfactory due to the length of tubing required and the loud noise of the MRI scanner. Hypothermia can be problematic, especially in the pediatric patient, because of the high airflow through the scanner cavity. The patient should be covered in warm blankets and warm packs wherever possible to minimize heat loss. Temperature monitoring can be accomplished by using nonferromagnetic temperature strips or probes with radiofrequency (RF) filters when feasible. It is currently not mandatory for the anesthesiologist to remain in the scanner room during the examination as long as remote monitoring with direct vision of the patient is possible.

Barash PG, Cullen BF, Stoelting RK, eds. *Clinical anesthesia*, 5th ed. Philadelphia: Lippincott Williams & Wilkins, 2006:1337.

Jorgensen NH, Messiak JM, Gray J, et al. ASA monitoring standards and magnetic resonance imaging. *Anesth Analg* 1994;79:1141–1147.

Miller RD, ed. *Miller's Anesthesia*, 6th ed. Philadelphia: Elsevier, Churchill Livingstone, 2005:2645–2646.

Peden CJ, Menon DK, Hall AS, et al. Magnetic resonance for the anaesthetist. Part II. Anaesthesia and monitoring in MR units. *Anaesthesia* 1992;47:513–516.

C.4. What special considerations apply to the monitoring equipment used during MRI?

Unshielded ferromagnetic materials within monitors and cables can interfere with imaging signals, causing a distortion of MRI results. Similarly, the radiofrequency (RF) signals of the scanner can induce currents in ferromagnetic elements of the monitors, causing a distortion of the monitoring signal, and making the monitor unusable. Fortunately, MRI-compatible monitors and equipment (e.g., ECG electrodes) that use shielding nonferromagnetic components and filters to produce satisfactory functioning without a distortion of signal are readily available. Their use is preferred. In addition, to avoid magnetic pull, monitors should be placed at least 5 to 8 ft from the magnet bore or be permanently mounted.

The ECG may show significant changes within a static magnetic field. In particular the T waves and the late ST segments can mimic the ECG changes associated with conditions such as hyperkalemia and pericarditis. This is due to an induced voltage in blood (a conducting fluid) flowing through the magnetic field. These changes are directly related to field strength, but they do not appear to represent any significant physiologic alteration.

The high RF power used in MRI poses the risk of excessive heat at the monitoring sites and therefore the risk of thermal injury. To minimize the risk of burns from monitoring cables, one should do the following:

- Inspect the insulation on all monitoring wires to ensure that it is intact.
- Place cables and lead wires in straight alignment (do not allow monitoring wires to form loops).
- Remove all leads or wires not in use.
- Separate cables from patient's skin.
- Keep the cable and sensor out of the scanning area (e.g., place a pulse oximeter probe on the toe of a patient whose chest is being examined).
- Avoid excessive power.

Menon DK, Peden CJ, Hall AS, et al. Magnetic resonance for the anaesthetist. Part I. Physical principles, applications, safety aspects. *Anaesthesia* 1992;47:249.

Miller RD, ed. *Miller's Anesthesia*, 6th ed. Philadelphia: Elsevier, Churchill Livingstone, 2005:2645–2646.

Patteson SK, Chesney JT. Anesthetic management for magnetic resonance imaging: problems and solutions. *Anesth Analg* 1992;74:122–123.

Peden CJ, Menon DK, Hall AS, et al. Magnetic resonance for the anaesthetist. Part II. Anaesthesia and monitoring in MR units. *Anaesthesia* 1992;47:513–514.

C.5. How would you induce and maintain general anesthesia in this patient?

With a parent present, induction of anesthesia may be accomplished with an inhalation agent (e.g., sevoflurane) in nitrous oxide and oxygen through face mask in a room adjacent to the MRI scanner or at the greatest possible distance from the magnetic field within the scanner room. After the child has lost consciousness, the parent is escorted back to the waiting room. Then intravenous access is established and all monitors are placed. The anesthetic level is deepened with a loading dose of propofol (e.g., 1 to 2 mg/kg), and the airway is secured. The child is then moved into the scanner room and placed on the MRI table. The patient and monitors are carefully positioned before attempting to advance the table into the magnet bore. Anesthesia is maintained with either a continuous intravenous infusion of propofol or inhalation agent, combined with nitrous oxide in oxygen.

Alternatively, an intravenous catheter may be inserted first and anesthesia induced with intravenous propofol, 3 mg per kg.

Cote CJ, Todres ID, Ryan JF, et al. eds. *A practice of anesthesia for infants and children*, 3rd ed. Philadelphia: WB Saunders, 2001:578.

Frankville DD, Spear RM, Dyck JB. The dose of propofol required to prevent children from moving during magnetic resonance imaging. *Anesthesiology* 1993;79:954.

C.6. How would you maintain the airway during the scan?

Limited access to the patient's airway is one of the greatest challenges for the anesthesiologist during a magnetic resonance imaging (MRI). Because the patient is not visible in the magnet bore and the head is inaccessible, the airways of unconscious or anesthetized pediatric patients should be secured with either an endotracheal tube (ETT) or a laryngeal mask airway (LMA). This avoids the difficulty with airway control that can result in airway obstruction and hypoventilation during anesthesia. Respiration can be spontaneous or controlled depending on personal preference and the needs of the patient. Alternatively, certain patients with good airways can be maintained with nasal cannulae or face mask while keeping them spontaneously breathing. Placing a shoulder roll under the patient with the chin taped up may help prevent future airway obstruction during the scan.

McBrien ME, Winder J, Smyth L. Anaesthesia for magnetic resonance imaging: a survey of current practice in the UK and Ireland. *Anaesthesia* 2000;55:741–742.

Peden CJ, Menon DK, Hall AS, et al. Magnetic resonance for the anaesthetist. Part II. Anaesthesia and monitoring in MR units. *Anaesthesia* 1992;47:511.

C.7. What is the laryngeal mask airway (LMA)?

The LMA is a device introduced by a British anesthesiologist, Dr. Archie Brain. It fills the gap in airway management between use of the face mask and tracheal intubation. Constructed of soft medical-grade silicone rubber, the LMA consists of an elliptical spoon-shaped mask with an inflatable rim fused at a 30-degree angle to an internally ridged tube with a standard 15-mm proximal connector. On the concavity of the laryngeal mask is a fenestrated aperture with three orifices through which the distal end of the tube opens. The cuff of the mask is inflated through a pilot balloon. On the posterior curvature of the tube is a black line running longitudinally to assist in orientating the tube *in situ*. The standard LMA is latex free and contains no ferromagnetic components except a small metal spring in the pilot-tube valve mechanism. It is nondisposable, and can be autoclaved and reused numerous times (as many as 40). In addition disposable LMAs are available which can be safely used as well.

The small amount of metal in the spring valve is not sufficient to be attracted by the magnetic field and dislodge the LMA. However, if the valve lies near the area being scanned, the scan's image can be distorted. There are flexible LMAs reinforced with a stainless steel wire coil, which should not be used during magnetic resonance imaging (MRI).

Barash PG, Cullen BF, Stoelting RK, eds. *Clinical anesthesia*, 5th ed. Philadelphia: Lippincott Williams & Wilkins, 2006:602–605.

Brimacombe JR, Ferson D, Osborn I, et al. Specialized uses of the LMA. *Int Anesthesiol Clin* 1998;36(2):130.

Landsman IS. The laryngeal mask airway. *Int Anesthesiol Clin* 1997;35(3):50–51.

C.8. What are the advantages of the laryngeal mask airway (LMA) compared with the face mask?

When used as an alternative to the face mask, the LMA gives the anesthesiologist more freedom to perform other tasks (e.g., record keeping, monitoring, and drug administration) and decreases the incidence of operator hand fatigue. The LMA allows for more reliable capnography and is capable of maintaining higher hemoglobin oxygen saturations. The contamination of the magnetic resonance imaging (MRI) scanner room environment with inhalational anesthetics is reduced and less manipulation of the airway is required with an LMA. Furthermore, injury to the eyes and facial nerves may be reduced by the avoidance of a face mask.

Boehringer LA, Bennie RE. Laryngeal mask airway and the pediatric patient. *Int Anesthesiol Clin* 1998;36(2):45–60.

Brimacombe JR, Ferson D, Osborn I, et al. The laryngeal mask airway: limitations and controversies. *Int Anesthesiol Clin* 1998;36(2):158.

Landsman IS. The laryngeal mask airway. *Int Anesthesiol Clin* 1997;35(3):50–51.

Miller RD, ed. *Miller's Anesthesia*, 6th ed. Philadelphia: Elsevier, Churchill Livingstone, 2005:2645–2646.

C.9. What are the advantages of the laryngeal mask airway (LMA) compared with the endotracheal tube (ETT)?

Although the LMA does not replace the ETT (especially in longer cases and when protection from aspiration is important), it has some advantages. The ease of LMA placement and provoking less stimulation (i.e., less coughing, gagging, swallowing, breath-holding, bronchospasm, and cardiovascular response) are two advantages over the ETT. Lighter levels of anesthesia can therefore be better tolerated with an LMA than with an ETT. In inexperienced hands, the LMA can be more rapidly and reliably placed than an ETT, suggesting a potential role in resuscitation. Trauma to the vocal cords is limited because the LMA does not pass through this area. In adults, the incidence of sore throat after LMA usage is reduced when compared with the tracheal tube.

Brimacombe JR, Berry AM, White PF, et al. The laryngeal mask airway: limitations and controversies. *Int Anesthesiol Clin* 1998;36(2):158.

Landsman IS. The laryngeal mask airway. *Int Anesthesiol Clin* 1997;35(3):51–52.

C.10. What complications are associated with the use of the laryngeal mask airway (LMA)?

The most serious potential problem of the LMA device is the lack of tracheal protection from aspiration of gastric contents. In patients at low risk of regurgitation, the rate of aspiration during general anesthesia using an LMA is similar to that in all non-LMA general anesthetics (2/10,000 cases). Most authors recommend that it not be used in patients at high risk of regurgitation. Conversely, aspiration of pharyngeal contents has not been shown to be a problem with the LMA, and the use of the device has been reported to be suitable during ear, nose, and throat procedures and dental procedures. Odynophagia occurs in 4% to 12% of patients after LMA use, an incidence that is comparable to the use of a face mask with an oropharyngeal airway. This is still less than that associated with tracheal intubation, which occurs in 30% of the patients. Hoarseness, dysphagia, and several cases of recurrent, hypoglossal and lingual nerve injury have been reported with LMA use. Cuff overinflation, unmonitored increases in cuff pressure secondary to nitrous oxide diffusion, light anesthesia with constriction of pharyngeal musculature, venous engorgement and tissue edema associated with the head-down position, and lidocaine gel lubricant have all been cited as causes of nerve injury. One fatal case has been implicated with the use of an intubating LMA. An unrecognized esophageal tear from an accidental blind esophageal intubation resulted in septic shock and death 9 weeks postintubation. Although this complication was a result of the blind intubation, it nevertheless was associated with an LMA device.

Barash PG, Cullen BF, Stoelting RK, eds. *Clinical anesthesia*, 5th ed. Philadelphia: Lippincott Williams & Wilkins, 2006:605.

Brimacombe JR, Berry AM, White PF. The laryngeal mask airway: limitations and controversies. *Int Anesthesiol Clin* 1998;36(2):159.

Landsman IS. The laryngeal mask airway. *Int Anesthesiol Clin* 1997;35(3):51.

C.11. What are contraindications to the use of the laryngeal mask airway (LMA)?

The following conditions contraindicate the use of the LMA:

- Increased risk of gastric regurgitation
- Limited ability to open the mouth or extend the neck (e.g., severe rheumatoid arthritis and ankylosing spondylitis), making advancement of the LMA into the hypopharynx difficult
- Low pulmonary compliance or high airway resistance
- Airway obstruction at or below the level of the larynx
- Oropharyngeal pathology (e.g., hematoma, abscess, and tissue disruption)
- Single-lung ventilation

Barash PG, Cullen BF, Stoelting RK, eds. *Clinical anesthesia*, 5th ed. Philadelphia: Lippincott Williams & Wilkins, 2006:605.

Landsman IS. The laryngeal mask airway. *Int Anesthesiol Clin* 1997;35(3):52–53.

Pennant JH. The laryngeal mask airway. Its uses in anesthesiology. *Anesthesiology* 1993;79:158–159.

C.12. What are indications for the use of the laryngeal mask airway (LMA)?

The LMA is best suited for use in any patient in whom anesthesia can be safely maintained through a face mask (except in a patient with oropharynx pathology). It has been used routinely in various surgical procedures including minor gynecologic, urologic, orthopedic, bronchoscopic and endoscopic diagnostic procedures. In addition, the device may be useful in surgery around the face in which the trachea is intubated solely due to the physical interference imposed by the face mask. Other types of surgery in which the LMA has been used successfully include dental extraction, adenotonsillectomy, repair of cleft palate, myringotomy and placement of tympanostomy tubes, and eye surgery. Furthermore, use of the LMA in the management of the difficult airway is increasing.

Asai T, Morris S. The laryngeal mask airway: its features, effects and role. *Can J Anaesth* 1994;41:944–945.

Nair I, Bailey PM. Review of uses of the laryngeal mask in ENT anaesthesia. *Anaesthesia* 1995;50:898–899.

C.13. What size laryngeal mask airway (LMA) is appropriate for this child, and how much air would routinely be required to properly inflate the cuff?

In this 15-kg patient, a size 2.0 LMA with a cuff volume of 5 to 10 mL would be appropriate. A guide to selecting the appropriate LMA based on patient weight, as well as the cuff volumes of the different LMAs, is shown in Table 61.1.

Table 61.1 The Selection of Laryngeal Mask Airway Size and Cuff Volume According to Patient's Weight.

LARYNGEAL MASK AIRWAY SIZE	PATIENT WEIGHT (kg)	MAXIMUM CUFF VOLUME (mL)
1	<5	4
1.5	5–10	7
2	10–20	10
2.5	20–30	14
3	30–50	20
4	50–70	30
5	>70	40

Barash PG, Cullen BF, Stoelting RK, eds. *Clinical anesthesia*, 5th ed. Philadelphia: Lippincott Williams & Wilkins, 2006:602.

Boehringer LA, Bennie RE. Laryngeal mask airway and the pediatric patient. *Int Anesthesiol Clin* 1998;36(2):48.

C.14. How is the laryngeal mask airway (LMA) prepared?

Before insertion, the cuff of the LMA should be carefully inspected, tested for leaks, completely deflated, and lubricated. Only water-based gels are used for lubrication and are applied only to the posterior surface of the mask. Care should be taken to avoid lubricating the anterior surface because the lubricant may obstruct the distal aperture or be accidentally aspirated into the larynx. Lubricants containing local anesthetics have been implicated in postoperative numbness, allergic reactions, and nerve damage and are not recommended for use with the LMA.

Barash PG, Cullen BF, Stoelting RK, eds *Clinical anesthesia*, 5th ed. Philadelphia: Lippincott Williams & Wilkins, 2006:602–604.

Brimacombe JR, Berry AM, White PF. The laryngeal mask airway: limitations and controversies. *Int Anesthesiol Clin* 1998;2(36):159.

Ferson DZ. Laryngeal mask airway: preanesthetic evaluation and insertion techniques in adults. *Int Anesthesiol Clin* 1998;2(36):33–34.

Landsman IS. The laryngeal mask airway. *Int Anesthesiol Clin* 1997;35(3):55–56.

C.15. How is the laryngeal mask airway (LMA) inserted?

According to the insertion technique described by the device's inventor, Dr. Brain, the operator places his nondominant hand under the patient's occiput and extends the patient's head at the atlantooccipital joint after induction of general anesthesia. This maneuver tends to open the mouth. The device, which has been lubricated and deflated appropriately, should be held like a pen with the index finger of the dominant hand positioned at the junction of the tube and the mask. It is firmly applied against the hard palate as the LMA is guided over the back of the tongue. Force is applied by the index finger in an upward direction toward the top of the patient's head as the device is directed along the palate and slid into the pharynx and hypopharynx, until the resistance of the upper esophageal sphincter is felt. The LMA is then stabilized with the nondominant hand as the inserting hand is removed from the patient's mouth. The cuff is then inflated with just enough air to form an effective seal. One should be able to observe a rising of the cricoid and thyroid cartilages and the lifting of the tube out of the mouth as the cuff is inflated. The longitudinal black line on the surface of the tube is oriented superiorly and should lie against the upper lip in the midline. Tape is used to secure the LMA in position in a manner similar to that used to secure an endotracheal tube (ETT). A bite block may be inserted between the teeth to prevent biting and occlusion of the LMA barrel.

When correctly positioned, the bowl of the LMA mask lies over the laryngeal inlet with the tip of the LMA cuff resting against the upper esophageal sphincter in the hypopharynx, and the sides of the cuff resting in the pyriform fossae. Although the epiglottis often lies within the bowl of the LMA mask, the device usually creates a satisfactory airway even when the epiglottis assumes an awkward position (e.g., downfolded).

Barash PG, Cullen BF, Stoelting RK, eds. *Clinical anesthesia*, 5th ed. Philadelphia: Lippincott Williams & Wilkins, 2006:602–604.

Ferson DZ. Laryngeal mask airway: preanesthetic evaluation and insertion techniques in adults. *Int Anesthesiol Clin* 1998;2(36):34–35.

C.16. What additional maneuvers may be attempted if difficulty is encountered when inserting the laryngeal mask airway (LMA)?

For the experienced user, the standard insertion technique is successful in most patients (>98%) on the first two attempts. Common reasons for difficult insertion include poor technique, inadequate depth of anesthesia (with resulting cough, retching, and laryngospasm), user inexperience, inability to negotiate the 90-degree turn from the posterior pharynx to the hypopharynx, a large tongue or tonsils, and use of an incorrectly sized LMA. Numerous maneuvers have been described to overcome insertion difficulties, including physically pulling the tongue forward, thrusting the jaw, and using a laryngoscope, a tongue blade, or a Magill forceps to lift the tongue. Inserting the LMA with the mask facing backward and rotating the device 180 degrees after meeting posterior pharyngeal wall resistance has also been advocated. Partially or completely inflating the cuff before insertion has been suggested to ease insertion. Although this maneuver may offer some advantages for an inexperienced user, it has the potential to cause partial airway obstruction if the tip of the LMA travels in front of the arytenoids toward the larynx. Furthermore, it may increase coughing or laryngospasm because of stimulation of protective airway reflexes or result in a high LMA position in the pharynx. In the patient with a high arched palate, approaching the hard palate slightly diagonally from the side with the LMA situated 15 to 20 degrees lateral from the midline may be useful.

Barash PG, Cullen BF, Stoelting RK, eds. *Clinical anesthesia*, 5th ed. Philadelphia: Lippincott Williams & Wilkins, 2006:602–604.

Boehringer LA, Bennie RE. Laryngeal mask airway and the pediatric patient. *Int Anesthesiol Clin* 1998;36(2):50–51.

Brimacombe JR. Problems with the laryngeal mask airway: prevention and management. *Int Anesthesiol Clin* 1998;2(36):141.

Ferson DZ. Laryngeal mask airway: preanesthetic evaluation and insertion techniques in adults. *Int Anesthesiol Clin* 1998;2(36):35–42.

Landsman IS. The laryngeal mask airway. *Int Anesthesiol Clin* 1997;35(3):55–56.

C.17. Examination of the patient before the table is fed into the magnetic resonance imaging (MRI) scanner reveals wheezing. What most likely is happening, and what do you do?

Wheezing in the setting of a laryngeal mask airway (LMA) can be caused by light anesthesia resulting in partial laryngospasm, bronchospasm, or malposition of the device with the tip of the mask encroaching on the glottis. One should deepen the anesthetic in the spontaneously breathing patient or administer muscle relaxant in the mechanically ventilated patient as an initial treatment. If the problem is not relieved, despite an adequate level of anesthesia and/or paralysis, the device should be removed and repositioned.

Brimacombe JR. Problems with the laryngeal mask airway: prevention and management. *Int Anesthesiol Clin* 1998;36(2):141.

C.18. Discuss how the laryngeal mask airway (LMA) can be used as a conduit for tracheal intubation.

The LMA has been used successfully as a conduit for blind tracheal intubation with an endotracheal tube (ETT), intubating tracheal stylet or fiberoptic bronchoscope (FOB)-guided ETT. Blind techniques at intubation through the LMA have the greatest chance of success when the LMA has a perfect central position around the larynx (45% to 60%) versus a noncentral location. The ability to effectively pass an ETT blindly through the LMA into the trachea can be further enhanced with the use of concomitant cricoid pressure. With any blind technique, care must be taken because laryngopharyngeal injury can result.

As opposed to these aforementioned blind techniques, the passage of an FOB through the LMA is approximately 100% successful and often less traumatizing. With an appropriately sized ETT (see later discussion) threaded on the proximal end of the FOB, the scope is passed through the lumen of the LMA and under direct visualization into the trachea. The ETT is then passed over the shaft of the FOB and into the trachea. Unfortunately there are three major disadvantages associated with this technique. First, the ETT needs to be long enough to ensure that the cuff is situated below the vocal cords when the LMA is left *in situ*, especially in patients with long incisor-to-glottis distances. Second, the internal diameter of the LMA limits the size of the ETT that can be used, which can potentially hinder one's ability to provide effective ventilation. Third, the removal of the LMA over the ETT may risk extubation, which may be difficult to replace. Various solutions to these problems have been proposed, including the use of a tube exchanger to replace the LMA and ETT or deflating the LMA cuff to gain another 1.0 to 1.5 cm of depth in which to advance the LMA and ETT together. However, if the ETT that has been passed through the LMA is of adequate size, the LMA should be left in place with its cuff deflated. Table 61.2 lists the LMA size that can accommodate the size of ETT and FOB.

In addition, a specialized LMA designed to provide a superior conduit for blind or fiberoptically guided tracheal intubations was introduced into clinical practice in 1997. The intubating LMA (LMA-Fastrach) permits single-handed insertion from any position without moving the head and neck from a neutral position and without placing the operator's fingers in the patient's mouth. It consists of an anatomically curved, rigid airway tube constructed of stainless steel and covered with a rubberized material that is wide enough to accept an 8-mm cuffed ETT and is short enough to ensure passage of the ETT cuff beyond the level of the vocal cords. A rigid handle is attached to the distal end of the airway tube to facilitate one-handed insertion, removal, and adjustment of the device's position. The mask aperture bars found on the standard LMA are replaced by a hinged epiglottic elevating bar on the LMA-Fastrach. During intubation with the LMA-Fastrach, the epiglottic elevating bar serves to lift the epiglottis as the ETT emerges from the mask aperture, providing the ETT with an unobstructed path through the vocal cords into the

Table 61.2 The Laryngeal Mask Airway Size That Can Accommodate the Size of Endotracheal Tube and Fiberoptic Bronchoscope.

LARYNGEAL MASK AIRWAY SIZE	LARGEST ENDOTRACHEAL TUBE (ID, mm)	FIBEROPTIC BRONCHOSCOPE SIZE (mm)
1	3.5	2.7
2	4.5	3.5
2.5	5.0	4.0
3	6.0 cuffed	5.0
4	6.0 cuffed	5.0
5	7.0 cuffed	6.0

trachea. A special 8-mm, straight, silicone, wire-reinforced ETT is available and should be used for intubation through the LMA-Fastrach, rather than with a standard plastic ETT, to decrease the likelihood of laryngeal trauma.

Campo SL, Denman WT. The laryngeal mask airway: its role in the difficult airway. *Int Anesthesiol Clin* 2000;38(3):34–38.

Ferson DZ, Brimacombe J, Brain AI, et al. The intubating laryngeal mask airway. *Int Anesthesiol Clin* 1998;36(2):185–189.

Landsman IS. The laryngeal mask airway. *Int Anesthesiol Clin* 1997;35(3):52–59.

C.19. Discuss the uses of the laryngeal mask airway (LMA) in the patient with a difficult airway.

In addition to serving as a routine airway during general anesthesia, the LMA has proved to be valuable in supporting airways that are difficult to manage and useful as a conduit for tracheal intubation. Uses of the LMA in the patient with a difficult airway include the following:

- *As a conduit for fiberoptic tracheal intubation in the awake patient.* When the preoperative evaluation indicates that the patient should be tracheally intubated awake, the LMA can be placed in the properly prepared awake patient and used as a conduit for fiberoptic intubation. Insertion of an LMA is a relatively moderate stimulus that may be better tolerated by the awake patient than the very stimulating methods of conventional rigid laryngoscopy and bronchoscopy. Visualization of the laryngeal inlet with a fiberoptic bronchoscope is usually easy through the shaft of a properly positioned LMA. In patients whose airways are potentially difficult but who do not require endotracheal intubation, an LMA can be placed when they are awake and used as the primary means of airway control.

- *As an airway in the anesthetized patient who cannot be tracheally intubated.* The LMA is an alternative to the face mask in the patient under general anesthesia who cannot be tracheally intubated but whose lungs can be ventilated using a mask. An exception to this is the patient in whom cricoid pressure must be continuously applied (e.g., the patient at risk of regurgitation). In this situation, placement of the LMA does not protect the airway from regurgitation and would have little benefit over a conventional mask. As noted in section C.8, the LMA has several advantages over the face mask. An additional advantage of the LMA is that it can be used as a conduit for fiberoptic bronchoscope (FOB) intubation.

- *As a conduit for FOB tracheal intubation in the anesthetized patient who cannot be intubated, but whose lungs can be ventilated.* Refer to section C.18.
- *As an emergency airway in the patient who cannot be ventilated or intubated.* Insertion of the LMA has provided a life-saving emergency airway in this situation and is a reasonable maneuver to try before the tracheal esophageal Combitube or transtracheal jet ventilation, provided that there is no known periglottic pathology. The LMA works well as a routine airway device in most patients, and it is usually easily placed in patients whose airways are Mallampati class 3 or 4 and/or grade III or IV laryngoscopic view. Most anesthesiologists are familiar with the placement of an LMA and can effectively insert one with little trauma.
- *As a conduit for tracheal intubation in the patient who cannot be ventilated or intubated.* If the airway is successfully established with an LMA in this situation, precious time has been obtained to subsequently use the LMA as a conduit for tracheal intubation. If the LMA provides for adequate ventilation, it is likely that the glottic opening lies within the bowl of the LMA, and FOB-guided intubation through the LMA will be successful. If ventilation is poor after LMA insertion, the LMA may not be adequately aligned with the laryngeal inlet or there may be periglottic pathology. In both situations, FOB-guided tracheal intubation may be difficult and may necessitate insertion of a tracheal esophageal Combitube, initiation of transtracheal jet ventilation, or creation of a surgical airway.

Barash PG, Cullen BF, Stoelting RK, eds. *Clinical anesthesia*, 5th ed. Philadelphia: Lippincott Williams & Wilkins, 2006:618–621.

Benumof JL. Laryngeal mask airway and the ASA difficult airway algorithm. *Anesthesiology* 1996;84:694–696.

Campo SL, Denman WT. The laryngeal mask airway: its role in the difficult airway. *Int Anesthesiol Clin* 2000;38(3):29–45.

D. Postoperative Management

D.1. When is the laryngeal mask airway (LMA) removed?

The removal of an LMA during excitation stages of emergence may cause coughing and/or laryngospasm; therefore, it should be removed either when the patient is deeply anesthetized or awake. Suctioning of secretions from the pharynx is usually not necessary before removal of the LMA. If suctioning is to be performed, it is important to ensure that an adequate level of anesthesia is maintained to avoid unnecessary airway stimulation. The cuff of the LMA may be deflated before removal or alternatively it may be left fully inflated to scoop out the secretions collected above the mask as it is withdrawn. As with extubation of the trachea, equipment for managing airway emergencies must be immediately available.

Barash PG, Cullen BF, Stoelting RK, eds. *Clinical anesthesia*, 5th ed. Philadelphia: Lippincott Williams & Wilkins, 2006:605.

D.2. How will you have the patient recover from anesthesia?

Postanesthesia recovery care after a magnetic resonance imaging (MRI) is the same as that required after an anesthetic in the operating room. This can be accomplished in a designated area of the MRI suite provided that adequate facilities and trained personnel are available. For most, such a facility may not be available and the patient will require transport to the main recovery room. To transport the patient quickly and safely, one must ensure that adequate personnel and the proper equipment are organized in advance. It is useful to have the location of recovery and logistics of transport (if necessary) planned before the procedure begins.

Cote CJ, Todres ID, Ryan JF, et al. eds. *A practice of anesthesia for infants and children*, 3rd ed. Philadelphia: WB Saunders, 2001:580.

Miller RD, ed. *Miller's Anesthesia*, 6th ed. Philadelphia: Elsevier, Churchill Livingstone, 2005:2251.

CHAPTER 62

Morbid Obesity and Obstructive Sleep Apnea

JON D. SAMUELS • FUN-SUN F. YAO

A 46-YEAR-OLD WOMAN

was scheduled for elective laparoscopic sleeve gastrectomy. She had a past medical history significant for morbid obesity (MO) (height, 5 ft 4 in.; weight, 176 kg; body mass index [BMI], 66.6 kg/m²), pickwickian habitus, mild rheumatoid arthritis, osteoarthritis, mild asthma, hypertension, adult-onset diabetes mellitus, peptic ulcer disease with severe gastroesophageal reflux, and obstructive sleep apnea. She experienced daytime somnolence, heavy nighttime snoring, and had slept in a seated position for the previous 2 years. She was able to walk around the house with a cane, but was unable to climb any stairs. A preoperative diagnostic polysomnogram (PSG) was performed, and an apnea–hypopnea index of 42 was calculated. Two weeks before surgery, home oxygen therapy with bilevel positive airway pressure settings had been started at the following settings, with symptomatic improvement: FIO_2 of 0.35, respiratory rate 10 breaths per minute, inspired positive airway pressure (IPAP) of +11 cm H_2O, expired positive airway pressure (EPAP) of +4 cm H_2O, spontaneous mode. Cardiology clearance was obtained as a high-risk candidate, after an echocardiogram revealed mild right-sided cardiomegaly and mild pulmonary hypertension. The patient's blood pressure was 155/82 mm Hg, pulse 60 beats per minute, and respirations 20 breaths per minute.

A. Medical Disease and Differential Diagnosis

1. What problems exist with this patient?
2. Define the terms overweight, obesity, morbid obesity (MO), super obesity (SO), normal weight, and ideal body weight (IBW). What is the body mass index (BMI) and how is it measured?
3. What is obstructive sleep apnea syndrome? What are the risk factors for obstructive sleep apnea?
4. How is obstructive sleep apnea diagnosed? What is a sleep study, or polysomnogram (PSG)? How are results obtained from a PSG used to grade the severity of obstructive sleep apnea? What are the criteria for ordering a preoperative screening PSG?
5. What are the different types of obstructive sleep apnea?

6. What is the pickwickian syndrome (PS)? What is the pathogenesis of severe obstructive sleep apnea?

7. What is the association between obesity and obstructive sleep apnea? What is the etiology of pharyngeal pathology in severe obesity?

8. What are the anesthetic implications of obstructive sleep apnea?

9. What kind of metabolic problems would you expect to find in morbidly obese patients?

10. Describe the changes that occur in the following respiratory parameters in morbidly obese patients:

   - *Pulmonary mechanics:* tidal volume (V_T), functional residual capacity (FRC), residual volume (RV), vital capacity (VC), inspiratory reserve volume (IRV), expiratory reserve volume (ERV), and total lung capacity (TLC).
   - Flow volume loops
   - Pressure volume loops
   - Diffusing capacity for carbon monoxide (DLCO)
   - *Compliances:* lung, chest wall, and total
   - *Resistance:* airway, and total respiratory system
   - Closing capacity (CC)
   - Work of breathing

11. What changes occur in Pao_2 and $Paco_2$ in morbidly obese patients?

12. What changes occur in intrapulmonary shunt (Q_S/Q_T) and dead space (V_D/V_T) in morbidly obese patients? Describe the equations.

13. What is the impact of pneumoperitoneum (PNP)on the respiratory and cardiovascular system of the bariatric surgical patient? Are there any other effects?

14. What changes occur in the cardiovascular system of the obese patient? Discuss cardiac output, blood volume, blood pressure, and pulmonary arterial pressure.

15. Are there other disease entities commonly associated with obesity?

16. What anatomic changes that affect the airway are associated with morbid obesity (MO)?

17. What derangements of the gastrointestinal system are associated with MO?

B. Preoperative Evaluation and Preparation

1. How would you evaluate this patient preoperatively?

2. Interpret the following arterial blood gases: pH 7.25; $Paco_2$ 50 mm Hg; Pao_2 58 mm Hg; and HCO_3^- 25 mEq/L on room air.

3. What is the equation for blood pH?

4. What are the normal values for blood pK_a, dCO_2, HCO_3^-, and H_2CO_3?

5. Interpret the following spirometry screening test: vital capacity 2.36 L (expected 3.375 L); forced expiratory volume in 1 second/forced vital capacity 82%; and vital capacity 70% of expected value.

6. How would you premedicate this patient? Why?

7. Describe weight-based dosing.

C. Intraoperative Management

1. How would you monitor this patient?

2. How would you induce anesthesia? Describe the intubation technique.

3. Why is it important to preoxygenate the obese patient? How would you do it? Compare the effectiveness of the four-maximum-breath and 3-minute techniques.

4. How would you maintain general anesthesia? What agents would you choose?

5. Which muscle relaxants would you use?

6. Can regional anesthesia be used intraoperatively and postoperatively to decrease opioid requirements? What are the advantages and disadvantages of regional anesthesia? What are some of the newer techniques available?

7. What is the effect of narcotics on the sphincter of Oddi? Is pharmacologic treatment indicated?

8. During surgery, arterial blood gases showed pH 7.35; PaO_2 57 mm Hg; $PacO_2$ 52 mm Hg; FIO_2 0.6; mechanical ventilator V_T 1 L; and ventilatory rate 15 breaths per minute. The following changes were made to the ventilatory parameters: 10 cm H_2O positive end-expiratory pressure (PEEP) was added, and the V_T was increased to 1.2 L. Twenty minutes later, an arterial blood gas showed pH 7.32; PaO_2 55 mm Hg, $PacO_2$ 55 mm Hg. What is the explanation for these changes?

9. What is apneic oxygenation? Who did the pioneer study?

10. What is diffusion hypoxia? How do you prevent it?

D. Postoperative Management

1. When will you extubate this patient? What are the extubation criteria?

2. What are the major early postoperative complications in the morbidly obese patient? How do health-related risks correlate with obesity? What factors correlated statistically with perioperative mortality?

3. How does position affect respiratory function in the obese patient?

4. How would you prevent postoperative atelectasis?

5. How long would you prescribe supplementary oxygen postoperatively?

6. How would you control postoperative pain?

A. Medical Disease and Differential Diagnosis

A.1. What problems exist with this patient?

Preoperative significant past medical history in this patient consists of morbid obesity, obstructive sleep apnea, possible pickwickian syndrome right ventricular hypertrophy, mild pulmonary hypertension, systemic hypertension, adult-onset diabetes mellitus, osteoarthritis, mild rheumatoid arthritis, and severe gastroesophageal reflux disease. Epidemiologically, this patient is at increased risk of coronary artery disease, cardiac arrhythmias, left- and right-sided congestive heart failure, peripheral vascular disease, venous thrombosis and pulmonary emboli, cerebrovascular disease, biliohepatic disease, hepatic steatosis, hepatic cirrhosis, degenerative joint disease, socioeconomic and psychosocial impairment.

This is a high-risk patient, with increased risk of both perioperative morbidity and mortality. Major anesthetic concerns include risk of difficult airway, difficult mask ventilation, decreased apneic threshold to trace amount of anesthetics, sedatives and narcotics, prolonged anesthesia emergence, postemergence resedation, positional ventilatory collapse, restrictive and obstructive lung disease, ventilation–perfusion mismatch, and worsening of reactive pulmonary hypertension and cor pulmonale. This patient must receive continuation of her preoperative oxygen therapy with continuous positive airway pressure in the immediate recovery period, at the values determined by her sleep study (polysomnogram [PSG]), or greater. Minor anesthetic concerns include difficult monitoring, difficult vascular access, and positioning issues. Additionally, there is a rare risk of postoperative massive pharyngeal collapse, rhabdomyomysis with renal failure, increased risk of infection including pneumonia, positional injuries. Meticulous attention to acute pain management is essential.

Safe perioperative care for this patient requires triage to a specialized facility, additional personnel, surgeons with advanced laparoscopic training, and anesthesiologists with advanced airway skills and optimal equipment.

American Society of Bariatric Surgery. The largest dedicated site to weight reduction surgery. www.asbs.org. 2007.

Bray GA. Pathophysiology of obesity. *Am J Clin Nutr* 1992;55(Suppl):488–494.

Fernandez A, Adolpho Z, Demaria E, et al. Multivariate analysis of risk factors for death following gastric bypass for treatment of morbid obesity. *Ann Surg* 2004;239(5):698–703.

NIH Consensus Development Conference Panel. Gastrointestinal surgery for severe obesity-consensus development conference panel. *Ann Droit Int Med* 1991;115:956–961.

Samuels J. Bariatric anesthesia: a new sub-specialty? *NYSSA Sphere* 2004;56:49–54.

Surgeon general. *Source of demographic trends.* www.surgeongeneral.gov/topics/obesity.

A.2. Define the terms overweight, obesity, morbid obesity (MO), super obesity (SO), normal weight, and ideal body weight (IBW). What is the body mass index (BMI) and how is it measured?

Obesity is a multifactorial chronic disease involving social, cultural, physiologic, psychologic, metabolic, endocrine, genetic, and behavioral components, resulting in excess adipose and tissue mass. The modern basis for the determination of demographics is the BMI, or Quetelet's Index, after the Belgian statistician, Adolphe Quetelet, published in 1842, and is measured in body weight in kilograms divided by the height in meters squared (kg/m^2). The standard for IBW, the sex-specific desirable weight for persons with small, middle, and large frames, is published in the Metropolitan Life insurance tables.

- *Anorexia* is defined as a BMI of less than 17.5 in men or women.
- *Underweight* is defined as a BMI of 17.6 to 19.0 in women, or 17.6 to 20.6 in men.
- *Ideal (normal) weight* is defined as a BMI of 19.1 to 25.8 in women, and 20.7 to 26.4 in men.
- *Marginally overweight* is defined as a BMI of 25.9 to 27.2 in women, and 26.5 to 27.8 in men.
- *Overweight* is defined as a BMI of 27.3 to 32.3 in women, and 27.9 to 31.1 in men.
- *Obese* is defined as a BMI of 32.4 to 34.9 in women, and 31.2 to 34.9 in men. *Severe obesity* is defined as a BMI of 35.0 to 39.9 in both sexes.
- *MO* is defined as a BMI of greater than 40.
- *SO*, a relatively new term, is defined as a BMI greater than 50.

There exist imperial and metric system BMI tables and web-based calculators.

Occasionally, an approximate, non–sex-specific system is used. In this system, a *healthy (normal) weight* is a BMI of 18.6 to 24.9, *overweight* is a BMI of 25 to 29.9, *obesity* is a BMI of 30 to 34.9, *severe obesity* is a BMI of 35 to 39.9, *MO* is a BMI of more than 40.0.

The older definitions of obesity may occasionally suffice. Overweight was formerly defined as a body weight of up to 20% greater than the predicted ideal weight, and obesity of more than 20%. MO was formerly defined as a body weight of 100 lb above the IBW, or alternatively, of twice the IBW. These definitions involved value judgments and inaccuracies, and were later abandoned, in favor of more objective terminology.

Alternative systems for the determination of obesity exist. In the triceps skinfold thickness test, for example, obesity is defined as a value of greater than 23 mm in men or greater than 30 mm in women. In the Broca Index (height in centimeters minus 100 for men and minus 105 for women), the IBW is calculated in kilograms.

- *Men:* ideal body weight (kg) = height (cm) − 100
- *Women:* ideal body weight (kg) = height (cm) − 105

There are different patterns of distribution of obesity. In *peripheral obesity* (e.g., gynoid or gluteal pattern), the individual has a pear shape, and adipose tissue deposition is predominantly in the lower body. In *central obesity* (e.g., android, or cushingoid), and especially upper body obesity, the individual has an apple shape, and adipose tissue deposition occurs predominantly in the upper body. Central obesity has greater associations with perioperative risk and obstructive sleep apnea.

Adams JP, Murphy PG. Obesity in anesthesia and intensive care. *Br J Anaesth* 2000;85: 91–108.

Buckley FP. Anesthetizing the morbidly obese patient. In: *ASA refresher courses in anesthesiology.* American Society of Anesthesiologists, 1990:53–68.

Gidding S, Leibel R, Daniels S, et al. Understanding obesity in youth. A statement for healthcare professionals from the committee on atherosclerosis and hypertension in the young of the council on cardiovascular disease in the young and the nutrition committee, American Heart Association. *Circulation* 1996;94:3383–3387.

Harrison GG. Height weight tables. *Ann Droit Int Med* 1985;103:489–494.

Kasper DL, Braunwald E, Fauci AS, et al. eds. *Harrison's principles of internal medicine,* 16th ed. New York: McGraw Hill, 2005:422–429.

Pai MP, Paloucek FP. The origin of the "ideal body weight" equations. *Annu Rev Pharmacol* 2000;34:1066–1069.

Quetelet LAJ. A treatise on man and the development of his faculties: Edinburgh 1842, reprinted. *Obes Res* 1994;2:72–85.

Scaglione R, Ganguzza A, Corrao S, et al. Central obesity and hypertension: pathophysiologic role of renal haemodynamics and function. *Int J Obes Relat Metab Disord* 1995;19(6):403–409.

www.hallsmd/ideal-weight/met.html. Introduction to the "Metropolitan Life" tables of height and weight. 2007.

www.newimageweightloss.com. Imperial system BMI calculator. 2007.

www.whathealth.com/bmi/chart-metric2.html. Metric system BMI calculator. 2007.

A.3. What is obstructive sleep apnea (OSA)? What are the risk factors for OSA?

OSA is a sleep disorder. Sleep disorders may be grouped into the following types: conditions with excessive daytime somnolence (e.g., OSA), conditions with disorders initiating and maintaining sleep (e.g., insomnia), and circadian rhythm disorders (e.g., jet lag).

In the older terminology, OSA referred to both OSA proper, and to obstructive sleep hypopnea (OSH) syndrome, a milder variant. Currently, it is more precise to refer to obstructive sleep apnea and hypopnea syndrome (OSAHS), when naming the general condition.

OSA is defined as cessation of airflow for more than 10 seconds despite continuing ventilatory effort, five or more times per hour of sleep, associated with a decrease in arterial oxygen saturation (SpO_2) of greater than 4%. *OSH* is defined as a decrease in airflow of more than 50% for more than 10 seconds, 15 or more times per hour of sleep, associated with a decrease in SpO_2 of greater than 4%. Both forms of OSAHS are usually associated with snoring, sleep disruption from increased ventilatory effort–induced arousal, hypersomnolence (daytime sleepiness), altered cardiovascular function, and pathophysiologic alterations, of which hypoxemia and hypercarbia are primary events, and polycythemia, systemic and pulmonary hypertension, various cardiac arrhythmias, myocardial ischemia, right and left ventricular hypertrophy, and eventually failure, are secondary events.

Severe obesity is a strong independent risk factor for OSAHS. Other risk factors include male gender, middle age, evening ingestion of alcohol, and drug-induced sleep. In nonobese individuals, risk factors are craniofacial dysostoses, particularly micrognathia (absolute or relative), cartilaginous abnormalities (e.g., lingual tonsillar hyperplasia), chronic nasal obstruction, and tonsillar hypertrophy.

Benumof JL. Obesity, sleep apnea, the airway, and anesthesia. *ASA refresher courses in anesthesiology*. Park Ridge: American Society of Anesthesiology, 2001; 234.

Benumof JL. Obstructive sleep apnea in the adult obese patient: implications for airway management. *Anesthesiol Clin North America* 2002;20:789–811.

Bestdoctors.com.htm. *An introduction to sleep disorders*. 2007.

Strohl KP, Redline S. Recognition of obstructive sleep apnea. *Am J Respir Crit Care Med* 1996;154:279–286.

A.4. How is obstructive sleep apnea (OSA) diagnosed? What is a sleep study or polysomnogram (PSG)? How are results obtained from a PSG used to grade the severity of obstructive sleep apnea? What are the criteria for ordering a preoperative screening PSG?

OSA may be suspected by history, physical examination, or comorbidities, but definitive diagnosis requires a sleep study. The hallmark of OSA is a history of heavy snoring. Nocturnal apnea, arousal during sleep, and daytime somnolence are commonly reported. Most adults with OSA have upper body obesity, increased neck circumference, micrognathia, and poor Mallampati scores on physical examination. Patient characteristics typically associated with OSA are a higher body mass index (BMI), hypertension, and certain cephalometric measurements. In 90% of cases, the patient has a BMI in excess of 28 kg per m^2. OSA, however, may result from any condition that predisposes to upper airway obstruction. Some examples are pregnancy, upper airway abnormalities (e.g., deviated nasal septum, hypertrophic tonsils, and adenoids), cartilaginous abnormalities (e.g., lingual tonsillar hyperplasia), craniofacial dysostoses, and certain congenital conditions (e.g., Down syndrome, muscular dystrophy). The absence of a typical or compelling presentation, however, does not rule out the possibility of obstructive sleep apnea and hypopnea syndrome (OSAHS). Definitive diagnosis of OSA is made by sleep specialists with a formal sleep study or a *polysomnogram* (PSG). A PSG is an involved study, performed at sleep study centers, that examines nocturnal sleeping patterns by monitoring physiologic parameters. In its most comprehensive form, the following parameters are studied: two to six electroencephalographic (EEG) channels to measure electrical activity of the brain and to document sleep cycles; two electrooculogram (EOG) channels to distinguish rapid eye movement (REM) from non-REM sleep; chin electromyogram (EMG) to monitor arousal and activity of the upper airway (genioglossus and digastric muscles); an airway microphone to monitor airflow from the nose and mouth; elastic belts placed on the chest and abdomen to monitor respiratory effort; an infrared video camera to monitor body position; one channel of electrocardiogram (ECG) to monitor cardiac activity; a pulse oximeter to monitor oxygen saturation; and two-leg EMG channels to monitor leg movements. A PSG may be ordered to definitively diagnose a sleep disorder, as part of medical management, or in the surgical workup of a high-risk population (e.g., preoperative screening of bariatric surgical candidates).

A PSG will diagnose the presence of OSAHS, type (central, peripheral, or mixed), and grade severity. Results are reported in as the total number of apneas and hypopneas per hour of sleep or the *Apnea–Hypopnea Index* (*AHI*). Values of 6 to 20, 21 to 40, and greater than 40 represent mild, moderate, and severe OSA, respectively.

- Mild OSA = AHI of 6 – 20
- Moderate OSA = AHI of 21 – 40
- Severe OSA = AHI of > 40

The total number of arousals hourly is the *Arousal Index* (AI).

- Arousal Index = arousals/hour.

The sum of the AHI and the AI is the Respiratory Disturbance Index (RDI).

- RDI = AHI + AI

American Statistical Association. *Practice guidelines for the preoperative management of patients with obstructive sleep apnea.* Approved by the ASA House of Delegates October 2005.

O'Keefe T, Patterson EJ. Evidence supporting routine polysomnography before bariatric surgery. *Obes Surg* 2004;14(1):23–26.

Shamsuzzaman A, Gersh B, Somers V. Obstructive sleep apnea. *JAMA* 2003; 200(14): 1906–1914.

Strohl KP, Redline S. Recognition of obstructive sleep apnea. *Am J Respir Crit Care Med* 1996;154:279–286.

www.sleep-breathing.bc.ca/sleep.html: An introduction to different types of polysomnograms. 2007.

A.5. What are the different types of obstructive sleep apnea?

Sleep-disordered breathing in children and adults is distinct in pathophysiology, clinical presentation, and therapy.

Childhood obstructive sleep apnea (COSA) consists of a continuum from snoring, to upper airway resistance syndrome, to the fully expressed syndrome. The pathophysiology of COSA is most commonly peripheral in origin, due to nocturnal airway blockage from nasal pathophysiology, hypertrophic tonsils and adenoids, or craniofacial dysostoses. The symptomatology in COSA consists of snoring (usually continuous), rare daytime sleepiness, and frequent behavioral disturbances (e.g., attention deficit/hyperactivity disorder [ADHD]). It is distinguished from adult obstructive sleep apnea (OSA) by the following: snoring is more continuous, there is no sex predilection, and surgery (commonly adenotonsillectomy, rarely uvulopalatopharyngoplasty [UPPP]) is curative. There is no gold standard for the polysomnogram (PSG) diagnosis in children.

Adult OSA or obstructive sleep apnea and hypopnea syndrome (OSAHS) consists of a continuum from asymptomatic, to paraoxysmal snoring, to severe nocturnal airway closure, requiring the patient to sleep in a sitting position, and daytime somnolence. The pathophysiology of OSAHS is central, peripheral, or mixed. Peripheral disease is caused by redundant adipose tissue in the upper airway, in the setting of severe obesity, sometimes with a superimposed craniofacial dysostosis. The symptomatology of OSAHS consists of intermittent snoring, apneic episodes, with daytime somnolence. Obstructive sleep hypopnea (OSH) syndrome, a milder form of OSA, may be clinically indistinguishable. *Obesity–hypoventilation syndrome* (OHS) is severe OSA with chronic daytime hypoventilation, super obesity, and hypercapnia not related to pulmonary disease. *Pickwickian syndrome* (PS) is OHS with cor pulmonale.

American Academy of Pediatrics. Section on pediatric pulmonology, subcommittee on obstructive sleep apnea syndrome. American Academy of Pediatrics: clinical practice guidelines: diagnosis and management of childhood obstructive sleep apnea syndrome. *Pediatrics* 2002;109:704.

Erler T, Paditz E. Obstructive sleep apnea syndrome in children: a state-of-the-art review. *Treat Respir Med* 2004;3:107.

Goldstein NA, Pugazhendhi V, Rao SM, et al. Clinical assessment of pediatric obstructive sleep apnea. *Pediatrics* 2004;114:33.

Rieder AA, Flanary V. The effect of polysomnography on pediatric adenotonsillectomy postoperative management. *Otolaryngol Head Neck Surg* 2005;132:263.

A.6. What is the pickwickian syndrome (PS)? What is the pathogenesis of severe obstructive sleep apnea (OSA)?

The PS was so named by Burwell in 1956, as a reference to Joe, an obese, somnolent boy in the *Posthumous Papers of the Pickwick Club*, written in 1837 by Charles Dickens. In Joe, Dickins had provided the first accurate description of the most severe type of OSA, consisting of a BMI more than 50 kg per m^2, or super obesity (SO), alveolar hypoventilation (hypoxemia and hypercarbia), heavy nighttime snoring with periodic respiration, hypersomnolence (daytime somnolence), secondary polycythmia, right and left ventricular hypertrophy, and right heart failure. This syndrome may occur with or without pulmonary hypertension.

The complete PS, rarely seen, consists of massive obesity, daytime somnolence, alveolar hypoventilation, periodic nighttime respiration, secondary polycythemia, right ventricular hypertrophy, and failure. In these individuals, there are repeated cycles of sleep, arousal, sleep, accompanied by obstructed breathing, with snoring and restlessness. Hypoxemia and hypercarbia result from disruption of a normal sleep pattern; with loss of rapid eye movement (REM) sleep and cardiovascular changes. Loss of REM sleep induces hypersomnolence, personality, behavior, and cognitive changes, and predisposes these individuals to be accident prone. Eventually severe OSA leads to obesity–hypoventilation syndrome, with nocturnal, and later diurnal alterations in the control of breathing, manifested as central apneic events, or apnea without ventilatory efforts. They also develop an alveolar–arterial oxygen gradient by ventilation–perfusion mismatch. The major factor in the pathogenesis of this syndrome is unknown, but may be due to decreased hypoxic and hypercarbic ventilatory drive. Later in the disease process, there is progressive daytime hypoxia and hypercarbia. When cor pulmonale supervenes, the PS is complete.

There are several cardiovascular changes in severe OSA, all related to the episodic airway closure, with hypoxemia and hypercarbia. Hypoxemia and alterations in autonomic tone may induce bradycardia during apneic episodes; in half of these patients long sinus pauses, second-degree heart block, and ventricular ectopy may result. These arrhythmias may lead to nocturnal angina and myocardial infarction in susceptible individuals. Pulmonary hypertension may be caused directly by hypoxic pulmonary vasoconstriction, or indirectly by either increased transmural pulmonary artery pressures from negative thoracic pressure created by a sustained ventilatory effort against the upper airway obstruction, or by increases in pulmonary artery tone from increased sympathetic tone created by episodic hypoxemia. Pulmonary hypertension initially causes right ventricular hypertrophy, resulting in a higher right ventricular end-diastolic pressure (RVEDP), and later culminates in right ventricular failure, or cor pulmonale. The systemic circulation is also affected by episodic increases in sympathetic tone, with systemic hypertension presenting early, and left ventricular hypertrophy, followed by left ventricular failure, presenting much later. Systemic hypertension may also lead to increased stroke rate.

Blankfield RP, Hudgel DW, Tapolyai AA, et al. Bilateral leg edema, obesity, pulmonary hypertension, and obstructive sleep apnea. *Arch Int Neurol* 2000;160:2357–2362.

Bradley TD, Rutherford R, Grossman RF, et al. Role of day-time hypoxemia in the pathogenesis of right heart failure in the obstructive sleep apnea patient. *Am Rev Respir Dis* 1985;181:835–839.

Burwell CB, Robin ED, Whaley RD, et al. Extreme obesity associated with alveolar hypoventilation: a pickwickian syndrome. *Am J Med* 1956;21:811–818.

Guilleminault C, Connelly SJ, Winkle RA. Cardiac arrhythmias and conduction disturbances during sleep in 400 patients with sleep apnea syndrome. *Am J Cardiol* 1983;52: 490–494.

Shafer H, Hasper SE, Koehler U, et al. Pulmonary hemodynamics in obstructive sleep apnea: time course and associated factors. *Eur Respir J* 1998;12:679–684.

Teichtahl H. The obesity-hypoventilation syndrome revisited. *Chest* 2001;120:336–339.

Zwillich CW, Sutton FD, Pierson DJ, et al. Decreased hypoxic ventilatory drive in the obesity-hypoventilation syndrome. *Am J Med* 1975;59(3):343–348.

A.7. What is the association between obesity and obstructive sleep apnea? What is the etiology of pharyngeal pathology in severe obesity?

Obesity and obstructive sleep apnea and hypopnea syndrome (OSAHS) are both common, coexisting, diseases. Obesity has reached epidemic proportions in the industrialized world, and currently poses a greater worldwide health risk than does malnourishment. In the United States alone, obesity is annually responsible for 300,000 premature deaths, and an annual health care cost of $100 billion. Sixty-five percent of the US population, or 127 million adults, are obese. The prevalence of severe obesity, a strong risk factor for OSAHS, is 3.15% in men, and 6.70% in women, according to US population data.

Sixty percent to 90% of patients with OSAHS are obese, and it has been estimated that 9% of women and 24% of men in the United States suffer from the syndrome, a total of 18 million individuals, of which 2% of women and 4% of men are symptomatic. These figures will almost certainly increase, as the demographics shift toward an older and more obese population. Many of these patients are undiagnosed at the time of surgery, representing potential perioperative complications.

There are two reasons why severe obesity *per se* may cause or exacerbate OSAHS. First, there is an inverse relation between obesity and pharyngeal volume. The pharyngeal area decreases in obesity from deposition of adipose tissue into pharyngeal structures: (colon) in particular, the uvula, the tonsils, the tonsillar pillars, the tongue, the aryepiglottic folds, and, most importantly, the lateral pharyngeal walls. The volume of adipose in the lateral pharyngeal walls correlates with the clinical severity of airway obstruction. Increased deposition of pharyngeal adipose increases the likelihood that relaxation of the upper airway muscles will result in collapse of the soft-walled retroglossal space, or the oropharynx, between the uvula and the epiglottis. The shape of the pharynx remodels from an ellipse with the long axis transverse, to an ellipse with the long axis anterior–posterior. The muscles that open the collapsible pharynx on expiration during sleep (e.g., tensor palatini, genioglossus, and hyoid muscles) in response to stretch receptors in the pharynx are located in the anterior pharynx, and do not function well with a remodeled pharynx.

Second, the patency of the collapsible pharynx is determined by the transmural pressure (the difference between the extraluminal and intraluminal pressure) and the compliance of the wall. If the compliance of the wall and intraluminal pressure (inspiratory pressure) are constant, then the remaining important determinant of upper airway patency is extraluminal pressure. In obese patients, extraluminal pressure is increased by superficially located fat masses; that is, the upper airway is compressed externally. Therefore, neck circumference is greater in obese patients with OSAHS compared with obese non-OSAHS patients. The incidence and severity of OSAHS correlates better with neck circumference than does body mass index (BMI).

Benumof JL. Obstructive sleep apnea in the adult obese patient: implications for airway management. *Anesthesiol Clin North America* 2002;20:789–811.

Brodsky JJB, Lemmens JM, Brock-Utne JG, et al. Morbid obesity and tracheal intubation. *Anesth Analg* 2002;94:732–736.

Leiter JC. Upper airway shape. Is it important in the pathogenesis of obstructive sleep apnea? *Am J Respir Crit Care Med* 1996;153:894–898.

Mayer P, Pepin JL, Bettega G, et al. Relationship between body mass index, age and upper airway measurements in snorers and sleep apnea patients. *Eur Respir J* 1996;9:1801–1809.

www.surgeongeneral.gov/topics/obesity. *Official site of the surgeon general. Source of demographic trends*. 2007.

A.8. What are the anesthetic implications of obstructive sleep apnea (OSA)?

Management of anesthesia in patients with severe obstructive sleep apnea and hypopnea syndrome (OSAHS) poses significant risks. These patients are extremely sensitive to minimal doses of central nervous system-depressant drugs, such as anesthetics, sedatives, and analgesics, and may exhibit prolonged sedation, resedation, or apnea, as well as upper airway obstruction or, rarely, massive pharyngeal collapse. For these reasons, premedication with benzodiazepines or narcotics is used sparingly if at all, and sedation is generally reserved for painful or unpleasant situations (e.g., placement of invasive lines) where the patient is under the direct observation of a trained clinician.

Difficult tracheal intubation is expected in 13% to 24% of obese patients with OSAHS. In this particular case, the patient presents for laparoscopic bariatric surgery. Although the "ideal general anesthetic" regimen for these patients is a matter of some discussion, the literature does support the following: a safe induction, a deep maintenance anesthetic with muscle relaxants, and a smooth emergence with rapid offset devoid of active metabolites or trace anesthetic. Anesthetic gases should be insoluble, resistant to metabolic degradation, and without lipid depot compartmentalization, combined with rapid return of airway reflexes. The only weak inhalation anesthetic, nitrous oxide (N_2O), has the advantage of being relatively insoluble, as measured by blood–gas solubility coefficient (0.46), but it causes intestinal inflation, may be emetic, and is not recommended in the presence of pulmonary hypertension, a condition that is more common in morbid obesity. Of the available potent inhalation anesthetics, (desflurane, sevoflurane, and isoflurane), desflurane combines the quickest wake-up, fastest return of airway reflexes, lowest solubility, as measured by the blood–gas solubility coefficient (desflurane, 0.45; sevoflurane, 0.65; and isoflurane, 1.4), and lowest percentage of hepatometabolization (desflurane, 0.02%; isoflurane, 0.2%; sevoflurane, 4% to 5%). Intravenous agents should be either lipophobic (hydrophilic), spontaneously degrade *in vivo*, or be ultrashort acting.

Sedation or awake fiberoptic intubation: ketamine and dexmedetomidine are optimal agents. *Induction of general anesthesia:* all agents have been utilized. *Maintenance agents:* air/oxygen mixtures, desflurane, cisatracurium, and remifentanil. *Last hour of general anesthesia and emergence:* nitrous oxide (except in the presence of pulmonary hypertension), remifentanil, and morphine sulfate.

When feasible, regional anesthesia is useful. Tracheal extubation is considered only when patients are fully awake with intact upper airway reflexes. Episodic arterial hypoxemia may occur early, in the first 24 hours, or late, from the second to the fifth day, postoperatively.

Discharge from the postanesthetic care unit (PACU) may be made in the morbidly obese obstructive sleep apnea, per protocol, after they have been started on continuous positive airway pressure (CPAP) or bilevel positive airway pressure (BIPAP), and have been observed for at least

30 minutes, without stimulation, and found to be free of respiratory arrests. If they have even one respiratory arrest, PACU stay is extended for an additional 3 hours, and consideration is made to transfer the patient to a monitored bed.

Intravenous patient-controlled analgesia (PCA) appears to be well tolerated in the morbidly obese, without deleterious effects on oxygen saturation, respiratory function, blood pressure, or heart rate. Dosing is based on ideal body weight (IBW), without continuous rate. The most common drug used is morphine sulfate, starting at 20 μg per kg every 10 minutes with a 4-hour maximum dose of 80% of the calculated dose. Hydromorphone is an excellent second-line agent. It is important to individualize therapy. There is a paucity of literature on the safety and efficacy of intravenous PCA in the morbidly obese severe OSAHS patient. There are case reports of respiratory complications in this population; postoperative pain management must take into account the exquisite sensitivity of these patients to the ventilatory-depressant effects of opioids.

Babatunde O, Jones S, Jones D, et al. Anesthetic considerations for bariatric surgery. *Anesth Analg* 2002;95:1793–1805.

Benumof Jl. Obstructive sleep apnea in the adult obese patient: implications for airway management. *Anesthesiol Clin North America* 2002;20:789–811.

Choi YK, Brolin YE, Wagner BK, et al. Efficacy and safety of patient-controlled analgesia for morbidly obese patients following gastric bypass surgery. *Obes Surg* 2000;10:154–159.

Eger EI II. Characteristics of anesthetics used for induction and maintenance of general anesthesia. *Am J Health Syst Pharm* 2004;61:S3–S9.

Juvin P, Vadam C, Malak L, et al. Postoperative recovery after desflurane, propofol, or isoflurane anesthesia among morbidly obese patients: a prospective, randomized study. *Anesth Analg* 2000;91:714–719.

McKay RE, Large MJ, Balea MC, et al. Airway reflexes return more rapidly after desflurane than after sevoflurane anesthesia. *Anesth Analg* 2005;100(3):697–700; table of contents.

Strum EM, Szenohradszki J, Kaufman WA, et al. Emergency and recovery characteristics of desflurane versus sevoflurane in morbidly obese adult patients: a prospective, randomized study. *Anesth Analg* 2004;99(6):1848–1853; table of contents.

A.9. What kind of metabolic problems would you expect to find in morbidly obese patients?

In morbid obesity, there is an increase in both low metabolically active tissue (e.g., adipose) and normally active tissue (e.g., muscle). In general, lean body weight (LBW) is equal to ideal body weight (IBW) plus 20% to 40% IBW. IBW is a value, based on population demographics, which could never be realized through weight reduction, in a severely obese individual.

Morbidly obese individuals have an increase in total oxygen consumption and carbon dioxide production due to an increased tissue mass. Increased metabolism demonstrates a linear relation with body weight and body surface area. Basal metabolic rate, however, remains normal in obese individuals.

Kasper DL, Braunwald E, Fauci AS, et al. eds. *Harrison's principles of internal medicine*, 16th ed. New York: McGraw-Hill, 2005:422–429.

White RL, Alexander JK Jr. Body oxygen consumption and pulmonary ventilation in obese subjects. *J Appl Physiol* 1965;20:197–201.

A.10. Describe the changes that occur in the following respiratory parameters in morbidly obese patients:

- *Pulmonary mechanics:* tidal volume (V_T), functional residual capacity (FRC), residual volume (RV), vital capacity (VC), inspiratory reserve volume (IRV), expiratory reserve volume (IRV), and total lung capacity (TLC)
- Flow volume loops
- Pressure volume loops
- Diffusing capacity for carbon monoxide (DLCO)
- *Compliances:* lung, chest wall, and total
- *Resistance:* airway and total respiratory system
- Closing capacity (CC)
- Work of breathing

Morbidly obese patients have reduced lung volumes, increased work of breathing, and alterations in control of breathing and gas exchange. Body fat distribution, as well as body mass index (BMI), determines the effect of obesity on pulmonary function.

Pulmonary mechanics. Pulmonary function tests (PFTs), or lung volumes, are uniformly altered in obesity. VT is normal or increased in the obese, and is decreased in pickwickian obesity. IRV is decreased. ERV is markedly decreased, because the increased weight of the torso decreases the normal expansive tendency of the rib cage and pulmonary parenchyma. RV is normal. FRC or ERV plus RV, is markedly decreased, because of the decrease in ERV. VC or ERV + V_T + IRV, is decreased because of decreased ERV. Total lung capacity (TLC) or RV + ERV + V_T + IRV, is decreased for the same reason as VC. Individuals with central, as opposed to peripheral fat distribution, have greater decreases in the forced vital capacity (FVC), forced expiratory volume (FEV), and TLC. The maximum voluntary ventilation (MVV) may also be reduced.

Diffusing capacity for carbon monoxide. The DLCO is usually normal in individuals with obesity and mildly reduced in those with obesity–hypoventilation syndrome (OHS), because the lung parenchyma is normal, and changes in PFTs are due to abnormal chest wall mechanics and lower lung volumes. DLCO is a useful test to separate intrinsic lung pathology from obesity.

Compliance. There is a decrease in the total respiratory system compliance ($1/C_T = 1/C_L + 1/C_{CW}$), where C_T is the total compliance, C_L is the compliance of the lung, and C_{CW} is the compliance of the chest wall. Total compliance is always decreased because of the weight of the torso and abdominal contents pressing against the diaphragm creating a restrictive component, markedly decreasing the chest wall compliance. Lung compliance is often normal, but is decreased when pulmonary and circulatory comorbidities are present (e.g., pulmonary hypertension).

Resistance. There are increases both in the airway resistance (reduced elastic tension of the lung) and in the total respiratory system resistance (increased elastic tension of chest wall) at lower lung volumes, which leads to reduction in the caliber of the smaller airways. The increase in total resistance is approximately 30% in simple obesity, and 100% in OHS. Resistance increases further in the supine position, possibly due to extrinsic adipose pressure of the supralaryngeal airway, and a decreased FRC.

Closing capacity. FRC is reduced in the morbidly obese patient, and may be below the CC, resulting in small airway closure, ventilation–perfusion mismatch, right-to-left shunting, and possibly hypoxemia, the so-called positional ventilatory collapse. This may be worsened in the supine position, Trendelenberg position, by general anesthesia and muscle relaxants, and improved by the use of lung recruitment strategies (e.g., positive end-expiratory pressure [PEEP]), and reverse Trendelenberg position.

Increased work of breathing. Morbid obesity is associated with a 70% increase in the work of breathing, and a fourfold increase in the oxygen cost of breathing (oxygen consumed by the respiratory muscles per liter of ventilation, used as a surrogate for the energy cost of breathing). This is due to decreased lung compliance, increased respiratory resistance, and threshold inspiratory load from adipose tissue mass. Obese individuals with obstructive sleep apnea syndrome (MO-OSAHS) have elevated pharyngeal and nasopharyngeal resistance, raising the work of breathing 60% above the obese, and 250% above the nonobese.

Alexander JK, Buthrie AE, Sakaguch H, et al. Lung volume changes with extreme obesity. *Clin Res* 1959;7:171.

Campos MA, Wanner A. Lung Physiology. In: *Morbid obesity, peri-operative management*. Cambridge University Press, 2004:45–57.

Collins LC, Hhoberty PD, Walker JF, et al. The effect of body fat distribution on pulmonary function tests. *Chest* 1995;107:1298–1302.

Pelosi P, Croci M, Ravagnan I, et al. Total respiratory system, lung, and chest wall mechanics in sedated, paralyzed morbidly obese patients. *Chest* 1996;109:144–151.

Unterborn J. Pulmonary function testing in obesity, pregnancy, and extremes of body habitus. *Clin Chest Med* 2001;22(4):759–767.

A.11. What changes occur in PaO_2 and $PaCO_2$ in morbidly obese patients?

Hypoxemia is the most common blood gas abnormality in the severely obese patient. The etiology is most commonly due to a low ventilation/perfusion ratio, and less commonly as a result of hypoventilation. Pulmonary perfusion is increased in the obese as a result of increased cardiac output (CO), increased circulating blood volume, and, occasionally, pulmonary hypertension. Alveolar ventilation is decreased in the obese as a result of upper airway closure, and spirometric changes (decreased expiratory reserve volume [ERV], and functional residual capacity [FRC]). In addition, the closing volume is often greater than the expiratory reserve volume, particularly in the supine position, causing airway closure, resulting in right-to-left shunt and hypoxemia.

The second most common blood gas abnormality in the severely obese is a variable change in the carbon dioxide tension ($PaCO_2$), not related to lung disease, and dependent on the alveolar ventilation. There are three patterns of ventilatory derangement described:

- *Alveolar hyperventilation* in response to a hypoxic drive. This occurs in young, active subjects. $PaCO_2$ is approximately 35 mm Hg.
- *Periodic, nocturnal, alveolar hypoventilation* with normal daytime values. This is the hallmark of obstructive sleep apnea and hypopnea syndrome (OSAHS).
- *Daytime, or constant, alveolar hypoventilation*. This occurs in obesity hypoventilation syndrome (OHS), and pickwickian syndrome (PS).

Shamsuzzaman A, Gersh B, Somers V. Obstructive sleep apnea. *JAMA* 2003;200(14):1906–1914.

Stoelting RK, Dierdorf SF. *Anesthesia and co-existing disease*, 4th ed. New York: Churchill Livingstone, 2002:446.

Strolio PJ, Rogers RM. Obstructive apnea. Current concepts. *N Engl J Med* 1996;334:99–104.

A.12. What changes occur in intrapulmonary shunt (Q_S/Q_T) and dead space (V_D/V_T)? Describe the equations.

Q_S/Q_T is normally less than 5%. In the morbidly obese, this is increased, because of the following:

- Lower ventilation/perfusion ratio ($\dot{V}/\dot{Q}$)
- Upper airway closure (e.g., obstructive sleep apnea and hypopnea syndrome [OSAHS])

- Decreased functional residual capacity (FRC), from abdominal compression
- Hypoventilation (e.g., OSAHS)
- Increased pulmonary circulation, from increased cardiac output (CO), increased blood volume, and occasionally pulmonary hypertension

$$\text{Shunt equation} = Q_S/Q_T = (CcO_2 - CaO_2)/(CcO_2 - CvO_2)$$

where CcO_2 is pulmonary capillary oxygen content; CaO_2 is arterial oxygen content; CvO_2 is mixed venous oxygen content.

Dead space is anatomic, alveolar or physiologic. *Anatomic dead space* is the volume of the lung and upper airway that is not involved in gas exchange. Ventilation of this area does not result in gas exchange. The volume of the anatomic dead space in milliliters is approximately equal to the ideal body weight (IBW) in pounds. Fowler's method of measuring anatomic dead space is by analyzing nitrogen concentration after single breath 100% oxygen. *Alveolar dead space* is the area of alveoli with ventilation and no perfusion, which has a ventilation/perfusion ($\dot{V}/\dot{Q}$) equal to infinity, or West Zone 1. *Physiologic dead space*, the sum of anatomic and alveolar dead space, is the total area of lung plus airways not involved in gas exchange. Physiologic dead space is approximately 30% of the V_T. It is decreased in the supine position, and increased with disease states that alter $\dot{V}/\dot{Q}$, and in obesity–hypoventilation syndrome (OHS), because the latter individuals adopt a shallow ventilatory pattern. Physiologic dead space is decreased in the obese, due to increased V_T ventilation and unchanged anatomic dead space. Physiologic dead space, or VD/VT, is measured by the Bohr equation.

$$\text{Bohr equation: } V_D/V_T = (Pa_{CO_2} - PE_{CO_2})/Pa_{CO_2}$$

where PE_{CO_2} is mixed expired CO_2 tension.

Adams JP, Murphy PG. Obesity in anesthesia and critical care. *Br J Anaesth* 2000;85(1): 91–108.

Lumb AB. *Nunn's applied respiratory physiology*, 6th ed. Philadelphia: Butterworth-Heineman, 2005:120–123.

West JB. *Respiratory physiology—the essentials*, 4th ed. Baltimore: Williams & Wilkins, 1990.

A.13. What is the impact of pneumoperitoneum (PNP) on the respiratory and cardiovascular system of the bariatric surgical patient? Are there any other effects?

Currently many surgical procedures, including bariatric surgery, are performed by laparoscopy. The peritoneal cavity is inflated through a trocar with carbon dioxide at a pressure of approximately +15 cm H_2O to displace the abdominal wall, and improve working and visualization conditions for the surgeons. Oxygenation, lung, and chest wall compliance decrease, and peak inspiratory and mean airway pressures increase as a result. These values are further decreased by Trendelenburg position, but may not be improved by reverse Trendelenburg, although this is controversial. Respiratory mechanics are worsened by PNP, due to decreased compliance and increased airway resistance. Increased tidal volume ventilation or ventilatory rate does not improve oxygenation, as long as closing capacity has been exceeded by functional residual capacity (FRC). Large tidal volume ventilation has been associated with volutrauma and low lung water pulmonary edema. Although otherwise healthy morbidly obese patients tolerate these changes relatively well, some patients may require lung recruitment strategies, such as the use of pressure mode ventilation, inspiration/expiration (I:E) of 1:1, and positive end-expiratory pressure (PEEP). Settings should be carefully adjusted to maintain normocarbia, as judged by end-tidal carbon dioxide (ETCO$_2$), and readjusted as conditions change.

PNP effects on the cardiovascular system occur through increases in the systemic vascular resistance (SVR) and the mean arterial pressure (MAP). There is a biphasic pattern: when inflation pressure is below 10 mm Hg, increased venous return, by splanchnic sequestration, raises MAP and cardiac output (CO). When inflation pressure is above 20 mm Hg, the inferior vena cava is compressed, resulting in decreased venous return, decreasing MAP and CO. PNP and reverse Trendelenburg position may decrease femoral venous blood flow, resulting in venous stasis in a patient population already predisposed to venous thromboembolism.

Increased sympathetic output from from PNP may result in decreased urine output by a 30% to 50% decreased glomerular filtration rate (GFR); postoperative renal function is normal. PNP and Trendelenburg position cause cephalad migration of the tracheal tube, and may precipitate endobronchial intubation.

Babatunde O, Jones S, Jones D, et al. Anesthetic considerations for bariatric surgery. *Anesth Analg* 2002;95:1793–1805.

Brodsky JB. Positioning the morbidly obese patient for surgery. In: *Morbid obesity, perioperative management*. Cambridge University Press, 2004:273–286.

Casati A, Comotti L, Tommosino C, et al. Effects of pneumoperitoneum and reverse Trendelenburg position on cardiopulmonary function in morbidly obese patients receiving laparoscopic gastric banding. *Eur J Anaesthesiol* 2000;17:300–305.

Dreyfuss D, Soler P, Basset G, et al. High inflation pressure pulmonary edema: respective effects of high airway pressure, high tidal volume and positive end-expiratory pressure. *Am Rev Respir Dis* 1988;137:1159–1164.

Ezri T, Hazin V, Warters D, et al. The endotracheal tube moves more often in obese patients undergoing laparoscopy compared with open abdominal surgery. *Anesth Analg* 2003;96:278–282.

Harman PK, Kron IL, McLachlan HD, et al. Elevated intraabdominal pressure and renal function. *Ann Surg* 1982;196:594–597.

Kashtan J, Parsons EQ, Holcroft JW. Hemodynamic effects of increased abdominal pressure. *J Surg Res* 1981;30:249–255.

Rosen DM, Chou DC, North L, et al. Femoral venous blood flow during laparoscopic gynecologic surgery. *Surg Laparocs Endosc Percutan Tech* 2000;10:158–162.

Sprung J, Whalley J, Falcone T, et al. The effects of Tidal Volume and Respiratory Rate on Oxygenation and Respiratory Mechanics during Laparoscopy in Morbidly Obese Patients. *Anesth Analg* 2003;97:268–274.

Sprung J, Whalley DG, Falcone T, et al. The impact of morbid obesity, pneumoperitoneum, and posture on respiratory system mechanics and oxygenation during laparoscopy. *Anesth Analg* 2002;94:1345–1350.

A.14. What changes occur in the cardiovascular system of the obese patient? Discuss cardiac output (CO), blood volume, blood pressure, and pulmonary arterial pressure.

Morbid obesity produces changes in cardiac morphology and ventricular function.

As body mass index (BMI) increases, both total and circulating blood volume increase. Although absolute blood volume is expanded, relative blood volume is decreased. Increase in circulating blood volume and decrease in systemic vascular resistance results in augmentation in CO. CO increases by increased stroke volume, and heart rate remains unchanged. CO and stroke volume increase in proportion to oxygen consumption and the degree of obesity, but more closely to the LBW. Left ventricular (LV) wall stress increases according to the law of

Laplace ($P_2 - P_1 = 2T/R$), where P is the change in pressure produced by the increased volume, T is the LV wall stress, and R is the radius. Increase in afterload from hypertension produces eccentric LV hypertrophy, and eventually LV dysfunction. They are therefore sensitive to acute changes in preload and afterload. Morbidly obese patients presenting to the operating room require an electrocardiogram (ECG), chest x-rays, and an echocardiogram. Seventy percent of the echocardiograms in morbidly obese patients contain abnormalities.

Hypertension is more prevalent because of increased CO and increased blood volume. Hypertension is more commonly systolic than diastolic in the obese. Obese patients without comorbidity have normal pulmonary artery filling pressures. Those individuals with obesity–hypoventilation syndrome (OHS) and pickwickian syndrome (PS), however, commonly have pulmonary hypertension, as a result of hypoxic pulmonary vasoconstriction and increased CO. Hypertension and increased CO lead to congestive heart failure in approximately 10% of obese individuals. There are two mechanisms in the pathogenesis of heart failure. In the first, pulmonary and systemic vascular congestion develops as a consequence of chronic volume overload superimposed on diminished diastolic compliance, caused by long-standing ventricular hypertrophy. In the second, chronic volume overload and high CO results in LV hypertrophy. The ventricular wall/cavity ratio decreases, and LV systolic dysfunction results. Echocardiography demonstrates LV hypertrophy in these patients, often in the absence of electrocardiographic evidence. Obesity leads to fatty infiltration of the cardiac conduction system, predisposing to sudden death. Obesity is not a direct predictor of coronary artery disease. As an indirect predictor, obesity is linked to coronary artery disease through hyperlipidemia and systolic hypertension.

Adams JP, Murphy PG. Obesity in anesthesia and intensive care. *Br J Anaesth* 2000;85: 91–108.

Alexander JK, Alpert MA. Hemodynamic alterations with obesity in man. In: Alpert MA, Alexander JK, eds. *The heart and lung in obesity*, Armonk: Futura Publishing, 1998: 45–56.

Alpert MA. Obesity cardiomyopathy: athophysiology and evolution of the clinical syndrome. *Am J Med Sci* 2001;321:225–236.

Alpert MA. Cardiac morphology and ventricular function. In: *Morbid obesity, peri-operative management*. Cambridge University Press, 2004:59–68.

Shenkman Z, Shir Y, Brodsky JB. Perioperative management of the morbidly obese patient. *Br J Anaesth* 1993;70:349.

Stoelting RK, Dierdorf SF. *Anesthesia and co-existing disease*, 4th ed. New York: Churchill Livingstone, 2002:447.

A.15. Are there any other disease entities commonly associated with obesity?

Secondary obesity may be associated with hypothyroidism, Cushing's disease, insulinoma, hypogonadism, and hypothalamic disorders. Although most obese patients are not diabetic, 80% to 90% of nonketotic diabetics are obese. Increased insulin secretion and insulin resistance resulting from peripheral tissue insensitivity are well-characterized features of obesity. Obesity exacerbates the diabetic state. Furthermore, malignancies of breast, prostate, cervix, uterus, colon, and rectum are more common in the obese.

In addition, there is a disproportionate increase in health-related risks from obesity. Above a body mass index (BMI) of 25, the risk of coronary artery disease more than doubles. Above a BMI of 29, there is an increased perioperative risk of pulmonary embolus. Above a BMI of 35, there is more than a 40-fold increase in adult-onset diabetes mellitus, respiratory disease, osteoarthritis, and obstructive sleep apnea/hypopnea syndrome. Perioperative mortality during weight reduction surgery is statistically correlated with BMI, preoperative hypertension, anastomotic leak, and pulmonary embolus.

Bray GA. Pathophysiology of obesity. *Am J Clin Nutr* 1992;55(Suppl):488–494.

Fernandez A, Adolpho Z, Demaria E, et al. Multivariate analysis of risk factors for death following gastric bypass for treatment of morbid obesity. *Ann Surg* 2004;239(5): 698–703.

Kasper DL, Braunwald E, Fauci AS, et al. eds. *Harrison's principles of internal medicine*, 16th ed. New York: McGraw Hill, 2006:422–429.

Stoelting RK, Dierdorf SF. *Anesthesia and co-existing disease*, 4th ed. New York: Churchill Livingstone, 2002:442, 448–449.

A.16. What anatomic changes that affect the airway are associated with morbid obesity (MO)?

Patient-specific anatomic changes in the MO are related to the body mass index (BMI), type of obesity (peripheral vs. central), and presence or absence of obstructive sleep apnea and hypopnea syndrome (OSAHS). Not all morbidly obese patients have airway involvement. The anatomic changes affecting the airway are not always easily diagnosed on routine physical examination. At a given BMI, there is more airway involvement in central obesity compared with peripheral obesity, and the most severe involvement airway involvement occurs in patients with OSAHS.

Significant anatomic alterations in the airway of the morbidly obese include the following:

- Deposit of adipose tissue in the lateral pharyngeal walls, and to a lesser extent in the uvula, the tonsillar pillars, the tongue, and the aryepiglottic folds, causing a decreased in the pharyngeal area.
- Deposit of adipose tissue external to the upper airway (lateral parapharyngeal fat pads, or jowls), extrinsically compressing the airway.
- Presence of hypopharyngeal adipose tissue not evident on external examination that acts as a ball valve, obstructing the upper airway and interfering with the line-of-sight (LOS) at direct laryngoscopy.
- Presense of pretracheal adipose tissue, which pushes the hyoid bone posteriorly into a less favorable position, causing the epiglottis to partially override the glottic entrance, worsening the laryngoscopic view.
- Alteration in shape of the pharynx from an ellipse with the long axis lateral transverse to an ellipse with the long axis anterior–posterior.
- Decreased efficiency of the anterior pharyngeal dilator muscles (tensor palatini [nasopharynx], genioglossus [oropharynx], hyoid muscles [laryngopharynx]), which promotes snoring.

The anatomic changes that occur with MO are important for three reasons. First, these patients may obstruct their airway with light to moderate sedation (peripheral OSAHS). Various surgical procedures have been developed to improve this problem, such as the uvulopalatopharyngoplasty (UPPP). Second, these patients may be difficult to mask ventilate, both because of external adipose tissue, and internal collapse of redundant upper airway adipose. Third, there is a higher incidence of difficult intubation and failed intubation in MO. When coupled with the precipitous desaturation, there is a need to revise the American Society of Anesthesiologists' Difficult Airway Algorithm.

The literature is inconclusive on the relation between obesity and difficult intubation (DI). According to some authorities, obesity is an independent risk factor for DI, due to a disproportionately large tongue base, or a short, thick neck. Other authors found that a higher

BMI is not an indicator of difficult intubation, but that increased neck circumference and poor Mallampati scores (classes 3 and 4) are. MO-OSAHS patients with other risk factors for difficult intubation (e.g., micrognathia) develop worsening of airway closure to an even greater degree than their counterparts.

Benumof L. Obstructive sleep apnea in the adult obese patient: implications for airway management. *Anesthesiol Clin North America* 2002;20:789–811.

Brown DP, Lombard RM, Cadieux RJ, et al. Pharyngeal resistance in normal humans: influence of gender, age and obesity. *J Appl Physiol* 1986;61:890–895.

Collins J, Lemmens HJ, Brodsky J, et al. Laryngoscopy and morbid obesity: a comparison of the "sniff" and "ramped" positions. *Obes Surg* 2004;14:1171–1175.

Horner RL, Mohiaddin RH, Lowell DG, et al. Sites and sizes of the fat deposits around the pharynx in obese patients with obstructive sleep apnea and weight matched controls. *Eur Respir J* 1989;2:613–622.

Leiter JC. Upper airway shape. Is it important in the pathogenesis of obstructive sleep apnea? *Am J Respir Crit Care Med* 1996;153:894–898.

Mayer P, Pepin JL, Bettega G, et al. Relationship between body mass index, age and upper airway measurements in snorers and sleep apnea patients. *Eur Respir J* 1996;9:1801–1809.

Rock DA, Murray WB, Rout CC, et al. Relative risk analysis of factors associated with difficult intubation in obstetric anesthesia. *Anesthesiology* 1992;77(1):67–73.

Rose DK, Cohen MM. The airway problems and predictions in 18,500 patients. *Can J Anaesth* 1994;41(5 Part 1):372–383.

Rose DK, Cohen MM. The incidence of airway problems depends on the definition used. *Can J Anaesth* 1996;43(1):30–34.

A.17. What derangements of the gastrointestinal system are associated with morbid obesity (MO)?

There are several changes in the upper gastrointestinal tract that place severely obese individuals at risk of acid aspiration pneumonitis upon induction and emergence of general anesthesia: prolonged gastric emptying time, decreased gastric pH, increased incidence of hiatal hernia, linear increase in intraabdominal pressure with increasing body weight, and impaired gastroesophageal antireflux mechanism. Ninety percent of fasting morbidly obese patients exceed Mendelson's criteria, a gastric volume of greater than 0.35 mL/kg total body weight, with a pH less than 2.5.

There is a substantially higher incidence of hepatobiliary disease in the morbidly obese, such as cholelithiasis, hepatitis, intra- and extrahepatic cholestasis, hepatic steatosis, and cirrhosis. Seventy-five percent of the morbidly obese have hepatic steatosis. Although there is a 25% incidence of severe hepatic dysfunction in the morbidly obese, there is no clear correlation between liver function tests (LFTs) and hepatic dysfunction, complicating medical and anesthetic management. Pancreatic disease is also more common in this population, specifically gallstone pancreatitis, adult-onset diabetes mellitus, and insulinoma. There is a higher incidence of colorectal malignancies in the morbidly obese.

Adams JP, Murphy PG. Obesity in anesthesia and intensity and intensive care. *Br J Anaesth* 2000;85:91–108.

Babatunde O, Jones S, Jones D, et al. Anesthetic considerations for bariatric surgery. *Anesth Analg* 2002;95:1793–1805.

Mendelson CL. The aspiration of stomach contents into the lungs during obstetric anesthesia. *Am J Obstet Gynecol* 1946;52:191–205.

Ramsey-Stewart G. Hepatic steatosis and morbid obesity. *Obes surg* 1993;3:157–159.

B. Preoperative Evaluation and Preparation

B.1. How would you evaluate this patient preoperatively?

Preoperative evaluation should include a detailed history, review of systems, physical examination, and laboratory tests. Special attention should be paid to circulatory, pulmonary, and hepatic functions. Circulatory evaluation includes signs and symptoms of left or right ventricular failure, history of hypertension, and electrocardiographic abnormalities. Respiratory evaluation includes smoking history, exercise tolerance, history of hypoventilation and somnolence, pulmonary function tests with spirometry and baseline arterial blood gases, and chest x-ray results. Hepatic function tests include serum albumin and globulin, serum aspartate aminotransferase, serum alanine aminotransferase, direct and total bilirubin, alkaline phosphatase, prothrombin time, and cholesterol levels.

A cardiology consultation is needed, with a noninvasive assessment of function by echocardiogram. Patients without an adequate echocardiographic window require radionucleotide ventriculography to assess ventricular function and morphology. It is important to obtain a full assessment by the cardiologist, to determine whether this patient is optimized, and which invasive lines, if any, are appropriate. This patient was found to have mild right ventricular hypertrophy and mild pulmonary artery hypertension. Pertinent negatives were the absence of demonstrated coronary artery disease, and left or right ventricular failure. In this case, it was determined that the patient was optimized, and that an arterial line would be helpful.

Physical examination focuses on the cardiovascular, pulmonary, and the upper airway. The upper airway assessment, in particular, should be thorough. In addition to the routine parameters, atlanto-occipital joint extension, Mallampati classification, temporomandibular joint (TMJ) assessment with interincisor distance, mentohyoid distance, and dentition, the following parameters should be checked: pretracheal adipose thickness, neck circumference, and hypertrophic tonsils and adenoids. Nonreassuring findings related to the latter three variables are a large neck, an abundance of anterior neck soft tissue, and obligate mouth breathing. Neck circumference is an independent predictor of difficult intubation (DI); the odds ratio is 1.13. At 40 cm (15.75 in.), there is a 5% chance of DI; at 60 cm (23.62 in.), this increases to 35%. Pretracheal adipose greater than 1 in. (2.5 cm) at the level of the vocal cords, determined by ultrasonography, may be an even better independent predictor of difficult intubation. Obligate mouth breathing may be a clue that the patient has adenotonsillar hypertrophy, nasal septal blockage, or a craniofacial dysostosis. Factors that render mask ventilation problematic, such as a heavy beard, should be noted.

Prior anesthetic records should be obtained. Patients with a history of heavy snoring should have a formal sleep study or polysomnogram (PSG). Severity of obstructive sleep apnea and hypopnea syndrome (OSAHS), apnea–hypopnea index (AHI), home oxygen therapy with continuous positive airway pressure (CPAP) or bilevel positive airway pressure (BIPAP), response and compliance should be noted.

Brodsky JB, Lemmons JM, Brock-Utne JG, et al. Morbid obesity and tracheal intubation 2002. *Anesthesiology* 2004;94:732–736.

Exri T, Gewurtz G, Sessler D, et al. Prediction of difficult intubation in obese patients by ultrasound quantification of anterior neck soft tissue. *Anaesthesia* 2003;58(11):1111–1114.

Langeron O, Masso E, Huraux C, et al. Prediction of difficult mask ventilation. *Anesthesiology* 2000;92:1229–1236.

Mallampati SR, Gatt SP, Gugino LD, et al. A clinical sign to predict difficult tracheal intubation: a prospective study. *Can Anaesth Soc J* 1985;32:429–434.

B.2. Interpret the following arterial blood gas: pH 7.25; $PaCO_2$ 50 mm Hg; PaO_2 58 mm Hg; and HCO_3^- 25 mEq/L on room air.

This blood gas indicates respiratory acidosis and metabolic acidosis with hypoxemia. HCO_3^- 25 mEq per L is a laboratory error. A pH level of 7.25 is acidosis, which may be respiratory, metabolic, or both. If no metabolic abnormality is present, a PCO_2 of 50 mm Hg should produce a pH level of 7.35 (Table 62.1). The difference in pH ($7.35 - 7.25 = 0.10$) is due to metabolic acidosis. For each 7 mEq per L of acid or base increase, pH changes 0.10 unit in the appropriate direction. A metabolic acidosis of 0.1 unit pH is equivalent to a 7-mEq per L base deficit. The HCO_3^- is expected to be 17 mEq per L ($24 - 7 = 17$), but a change in $PaCO_2$ itself will change the HCO_3^- from chemical equilibrium. Each 10-mm Hg increase in $PaCO_2$ from normal increases the HCO_3^- by 1 mEq in acute CO_2 retention and by 4 mEq in chronic retention. Therefore, expect the HCO_3^- to be $17 + 1 = 18$ mEq in acute CO_2 retention or $17 + 4 = 21$ mEq in chronic CO_2 retention. The blood gas machine provides direct measurement of the pH, $PaCO_2$, and PaO_2

The HCO_3^- is usually derived from an equation or from a nomogram. If a discrepancy is found between the pH, $PaCO_2$, and the HCO_3^-, the technical error is usually in the HCO_3^-. It is important to recheck the blood gases according to clinical conditions. A $PaCO_2$ of 50 mm Hg indicates alveolar hypoventilation due to decreased minute volume or increased dead space. To interpret the PaO_2, the FIO_2 must be known. A PaO_2 less than 200 Hg may indicate ventilatory failure if the FIO_2 is 1.0. Hypoxia in obese patients is usually caused by increased venous admixture from a decreased ventilation/perfusion ratio as a result of low functional residual capacity (FRC) and hypoventilation. Metabolic acidosis with hypoxemia indicates lactic acidosis from anaerobic metabolism.

Dripps RD, Eckenhoff JE, Vandam LD, eds. *Introduction to anesthesia: the principles of safe practice*, 7th ed. Philadelphia: WB Saunders, 1988:267–268.

B.3. What is the equation for blood pH?

The Henderson–Hasselbalch equation is:

$$pH = pK + \log\frac{HCO_3^-}{H_2CO_3}$$

Table 62.1 Predicted pH at Different $PaCO_2$ Levels in the Absence of Metabolic Acid–Base Abnormality.

$PACO_2$	pH (APPROXIMATE)
80	7.20
60	7.30
40	7.40
30	7.50
20	7.60

Each 10-mm Hg decrease in $PaCO_2$ from normal increases the pH 0.1 unit. Each 20-mm Hg increase in $PaCO_2$ from normal decreases the pH 0.1 unit.

The H_2CO_3 concentration is low and cannot be directly measured. Normal blood H_2CO_3 concentration is 0.0017 mmol per L. H_2CO_3 is proportional and not equal to dissolved CO_2. Clinically dissolved CO_2 is used to replace H_2CO_3. Therefore, pK is changed to K_a. Dissolved CO_2 is calculated as αPCO_2; α being the solubility coefficient for carbon dioxide in body fluids, or 0.031 mmol/L/mm Hg PCO_2. For a normal PCO_2 of 40 mm Hg, dissolved CO_2 is calculated to be $40 \times 0.031 = 1.2$ mmol per L. The pK_a is 6.1, but this is variable with temperature and pH. The modified Henderson–Hasselbalch equation is as follows:

$$pH = pK_a + \log \frac{HCO_3^-}{dCO_2} \text{ or } pH = pK_a + \log \frac{HCO_3^-}{0.031 \times PCO_2}$$

Lumb AB. *Nunn's applied respiratory physiology*, 6th ed. Philadelphia: Butterworth-Heinemann, 2005:150–151.

B.4. What are the normal values for blood pK_a, dCO_2, HCO_3^-, and H_2CO_3?

The normal values are pK_a 6.1; dCO_2 1.2 mmol/L; HCO_3^- 24 mEq/L; and H_2CO_3 0.0017 mmol/L.

Lumb AB. *Nunn's applied respiratory physiology*, 6th ed. Philadelphia: Elsevier Butterworth-Heinemann, 2005:149.

B.5. Interpret the following spirometry screening test: vital capacity (VC) 2.36 L (expected 3.375 L);forced expiratory volume in 1 second (FEV₁) per forced vital capacity (FVC) 82%; and vital capacity 70% of expected value.

Preoperative spirometric screening reveals mild restrictive lung disease, with no evidence of obstructive lung disease. *VC* is dependent on sex, age, and height. In restrictive lung disease, the VC is less than 75% of the expected value; a value of 70% is consistent with mild restrictive lung disease. The normal *ratio of FEV₁ to FVC (FEV₁/FVC)* is more than 80%; a value of 82% is normal. In obstructive lung disease, the FEV₁/FVC is less than 75%.

Here are some useful approximations: The expected VC in liters of healthy adult males is approximately equal to the height in meters squared. VC is approximately equal to 65 mL per in. or 25 mL per cm height for men, or 52 mL per in. or 20 mL per cm height for women. The *RV* is approximately equal to 30% of the VC.

Kasper DL, Braunwald E, Fauci AS, et al, eds. *Harrison's principles of internal medicine*, 16th ed. New York: McGraw-Hill, 2005:1448–1449.

Mackem PT. Tests of lung mechanics. *N Eng J Med* 1975;293:339.

B.6. How would you premedicate this patient? Why?

No sedatives or narcotics should be given to an obese, pickwickian patient as premedication. Light sedation may be administered to an otherwise healthy obese patient, if appropriate monitoring and qualified personnel are available to ensure vigilance. Once respiratory depressants have been administered, supplementary oxygen should be administered to prevent hypoxia from respiratory depression. Current practice is not to give sedatives or hypnotics until these patients are on the operating room table, as part of preparation for painful procedures (e.g., arterial line placement), or airway management (e.g., airway topicalization and cranial nerve blocks V, IX, and X). Even then, emphasis should be on minimal respiratory depression. We believe that a well-conducted preoperative visit is more important than is sedation. This patient was not sedated before surgery.

When premedication is used, it should be given orally or intravenously, and not intramuscularly, as it may be inadvertently administered into adipose tissue, leading to unpredictable absorption.

Adams JP, Murphy PG. Obesity in anaesthesia and intensive care. *Br J Anaesth* 2000; 85:91–108.

B.7. Describe weight-based dosing.

Drugs are dosed in the morbidly obese on the basis of their lipophilicity. *Highly lipophilic drugs* have increased volume of distribution (VD) for obese individuals relative to normal-weight individuals. Drug doses are calculated on the basis of the patient's total body weight (TBW). Examples of this group are thiopental, propofol, the benzodiazepines, fentanyl, sufentanil, dexmedetomidine, succinylcholine, atracurium, and cisatracurium. *Weakly lipophilic or lipophobic drugs* have unchanged VD. Drug doses are calculated on the basis of the patient's lean body weight (LBW), which is ideal body weight (IBW) plus 20% to 40% IBW. Examples of this group are alfentanil, ketamine, vecuronium, rocuronium, and morphine sulfate. *Exceptions* are lipophilic drugs with unchanged VD. Drug doses are calculated on the basis of the patient's LBW. An example of this group is remifentanil. In the calculation of weight-based dosing, it is helpful to use Internet calculators. Here is a sample calculation of appropriate dosages in our patient (in bolds are the drugs used).

Demographics: height, 5 ft 4 in. (162.6 cm); weight 387.2 lb (176 kg); body mass index (BMI), 66.6 kg per m^2. *IBW*, assuming a large frame, is 134 to 151 lb (60.9 to 68.6 kg). *LBW*, or 120% to 140% IBW is 174 to 196.6 lb (79.2 to 89.2 kg).

Note: IBW can also be derived from Broca's Index (see section A.2).

- *Highly lipophilic drugs (use TBW)*
  - **Midazolam** 2 to 6 mg background sedation for fiberoptic bronchoscopy (FOB)
  - **Dexmedetomidine** 1 μg/kg over 10 minute, followed by 0.2 to 0.7 μg/kg/hour = 176 μg over 10 minute, 35.2 to 123.2 μg/kg/hour for FOB
  - **Thiopental** 4 to 5 mg/kg × 176 kg = 704 to 880 mg bolus for induction
  - **Propofol** 1 to 2 mg/kg × 176 kg = 176 to 352 mg bolus for induction
  - **Fentanyl** 1 to 2 μg/kg = 176 to 352 μg bolus after intubation
  - **Succinylcholine** 1 to 1.5 mg/kg = 176 to 264 mg for intubation
  - **Cisatracurium** 1.5 to 2 μg/kg/minute = 264 to 352 μg/minute infusion
- *Weekly lipophilic or lipophobic drugs (use LBW = 120% to 140% IBW)*
  - **Ketamine** 10 mg/dose for FOB
  - **Morphine sulfate** 10 to 20 mg in divided doses 1 hour before end of surgery
- *Exceptions (use LBW)*
  - **Remifentanil** 0.2 μg/kg/minute = 17 μg/minute

Babatunde O, Jones S, Jones D, et al. Anesthetic considerations for bariatric surgery. *Anesth Analg* 2002;95:1793–1805.

www.hallsmd/ideal-weight/met.htm. Introduction to the "Metropolitan Life" tables of height and weight. Sex-specific ideal body weight for individuals of small, middle, and large frame. 2007.

www.newimageweightloss.com. Imperial system BMI calculator. 2007.

www.whathealth.com/bmi/chart-metric2.html. Metric system BMI calculator. 2007.

C. Intraoperative Management

C.1. How would you monitor this patient?

In addition to the routine mandated monitors of electrocardiogram, noninvasive blood pressure, pulse oximetry, end-tidal carbon dioxide, and temperature, an arterial line is inserted for frequent assessment of blood gases and for continuous blood pressure tracing. An esophageal stethoscope with thermistor is placed in the axilla to monitor temperature, because any device placed in the esophagus may be inadvertently included in the surgical anastomosis. Hourly urine output is evaluated to assess fluid balance. A peripheral nerve stimulator is used to monitor the effects of muscle relaxants. A processed electroencephalogram, such as the bispectral index(BIS) (Aspect Medical Systems, Inc., Newton, MA), was used to monitor depth of anesthesia.

The advantages of invasive monitoring have to be weighed against the possible complications. Laparoscopic bariatric surgeries have minimal blood loss (typically <100 to 200 mL) and fluid shifts. These are elective cases, and patients are optimized preoperatively. Invasive arterial monitoring is used for the super obese with severe cardiopulmonary disease or poor fit of the noninvasive blood pressure cuff because of the conical shape of the upper arms or unavailability of appropriately sized cuffs. Accurate blood pressure readings may be obtained from the wrist, as it was in this case, or the ankle. Central venous access is typically used when there are difficulties obtaining peripheral access, and was not used here. A pulmonary artery catheter is reserved for patients with documented pulmonary hypertension, cor pulmonale, or left ventricular failure.

Babatunde O, Jones S, Jones D, et al. Anesthetic considerations for bariatric surgery. *Anesth Analg* 2002;95:1793–1805.

Block FE, Schulte GT. Ankle blood pressure measurement, an acceptable alternative to arm measurement. *Int J Clin Monit Comput* 1996;13:167–171.

Emerick DR. An evaluation of non-invasive blood pressure (NIBP) monitoring on the wrist: comparison with upper arm NIBP measurement. *Anaesth Intensive Care* 2002;30:43–47.

Lemons HJ, Brodsky JB. General anesthesia, bariatric surgery, and the BIS monitor. *Obes Surg* 2005;1(15):63.

Pandazi A, Bourlioti A, Kostopanagiotou G.Bispectral index (BIS) monitoring in morbidly obese patients undergoing gastric bypass surgery: experience in 23 patients. *Obes Surg* 2005;15(1):63.

C.2. How would you induce anesthesia? Describe the intubation technique.

This patient should be seen before arriving in the operative suite to ascertain NPO status, and a large bore intravenous access inserted. Nonsedative premedication, such as glycopryollate (0.4 mg), an anticholinergic used to dry the upper airway, and metoclopramide, a prokinetic, is given at this time to increase gastric emptying, because peak effects occur in approximately 45 minutes. The full complement of alternate airway, noninvasive and invasive (e.g., cricothyriodotomy set and surgical tracheotomy set) airway devices should be available.

On arrival in the operating room, the patient is placed on monitors, and given supplemental oxygen. Sedation is administered with very small doses of midazolam (4 mg), dexmedetomidine, a centrally acting α_2 agonist at the usual dosage range (1 μg/kg over 10 minutes, followed by 0.2 to 0.7 μg/kg/hour TBW), and incremental ketamine (10 mg/dose) as needed, titrated to have an awake, sedated cooperative patient. Dexmedetomidine appears to completely override the sympathomimetic effects of the other medications. The decision is made to proceed with fiberoptic intubation, through a nasal route. Topical nasal cocaine (4%, 160 mg) is administered, and the nares are dilated with graduating airways. Additional topicalization is performed with 4% lidocaine on the oropharynx and the anterior surface of the uvula. A nasal fiberoptic intubation is performed, and the vocal cords are sprayed with 4% lidocaine before entering the trachea. A tracheal tube is carefully passed, the position confirmed through auscultation and capnography, and the patient is anesthetized with sevoflurane. After confirmation of acceptable chest wall mechanics, cisatracurium (0.2 mg/kg TBW) is given, and mechanical ventilation is initiated.

Fiberoptic intubation could also have been performed through the oral route, in the event that the anatomic features were unfavorable (small nares). In this case, extensive oropharyngeal topicalization with benzocaine, hypopharyngeal instillation with lidocaine using a mucosal atomization device, and airway blocks (glossopharyngeal, superior laryngeal, and translaryngeal) would provide excellent conditions. Lidocaine ointment placed on the distal surface of an oral airway with a dollop of lidocaine ointment will come into contact with the mucosa adjacent to the superior laryngeal nerves, providing a suitable alternative to a peripheral block, if the external anatomy is unfavorable. The patient is ready for bronchoscopy when they will tolerate an intubating airway (Williams or Ovassapian) without coughing.

If the physical examination and past anesthetic record demonstrated easy orotracheal intubation, a rapid sequence intubation could be contemplated using either thiopental (3 to 5 mg/kg TBW) or propofol (2 mg/kg TBW) with succinylcholine (1 to 1.5 mg/kg TBW), with the patient positioned on a ramp.

If the intubating conditions are suboptimal, a noninvasive alternative airway management device is utilized. Of the various laryngeal mask airways (LMAs), the LMA-fastrach, and the LMA CTrach (LMA North America, San Diego, CA) offer the most versatility, because they allow for conversion of a supraglottic mask into a tracheal tube. The GlideScope (Saturn Biomedical Systems Inc., Burnaby, British Columbia, Canada) may be used on awake or anesthetized patients. Older propriety rigid laryngoscopes (e.g., Bullard Elite Laryngoscopes [Circon ACMI, Racine, WI], UpsherScope Ultra [Mercury Medical, Clearwater, FL] Wu Scope [Achi Corp, Fremont, CA]) have been used effectively on morbidly obese patients. Newer propriety rigid laryngoscopes show initial promise (Bonfils Retromolar Intubating Fiberscope [Karl Storz Endoscopy-America, Inc., Culver City]), and may be helpful in cases with limited mouth opening. A tracheoespohageal Combitube (Tyco, Bermuda) is a useful airway salvage device in the morbidly obese patient. The key to success is extensive operator experience, thorough preparation, a helpful assistant, and willingness to return to a direct laryngoscopy when indicated.

Brown D. *Atlas of regional anesthesia*, 2nd ed. New York: WB Saunders, 1999:197–216.

Della Puppa A, Pittoni G, Frass M. Tracheal esophageal combitube: a useful airway for morbidly obese patients who cannot intubate or ventilate. *Acta Anaesthesiol Scand* 2002;46(7):911–913.

Ferson DZ, Rosenblatt WH, Johansen MJ, et al. Use of the intubating LMA-Fastrach in 254 patients with difficult-to-manage airways. *Anesthesiology* 2001;95:1175–1181.

Foley LJ, Ochroch EA. Bridges to establish an emergency airway and alternate intubating laryngoscopes. *Crit Care Clin* 2000;16:429–444.

Frappier J, Guenoun T, Journois D, et al. Airway management using the intubating laryngeal mask airway for the morbidly obese patient. *Anesth Analg* 2003;96:1510–1515.

Levitan RM, Kush S, Hollander JE. Devices for difficult airway management in academic emergency departments: results of a national survey. *Ann Emerg Med* 1999;33:859–869.

C.3. Why is it important to preoxygenate the obese patient? How would you do it? Compare the effectiveness of the four-maximum-breath and 3-minute techniques.

Thorough preoxygenation is important because intubation may take longer in morbidly obese than nonobese patients; moreover, because obese patients have a small intrapulmonary store of oxygen (low functional residual capacity [FRC]), which is rapidly depleted (high oxygen consumption), they are at particularly high risk of hypoxemia.

Maximal total body preoxygenation, or denitrogenation, requires that the patient breathe 100% oxygen for at least 3 minutes in a well-sealed system, to fill the alveolar, arterial, venous, and tissue spaces, and to obtain a pulse oximeter saturation (SpO_2) of 99% to 100%. This is superior to fast-track preoxygenation, or four-maximum vital capacity breaths. Farmery has created a model to describe the rate of oxyhemoglobin desaturation during apnea. Various preapnea arterial oxygen tensions produce a parallel family of apneic desaturation curves. Not all patients will deoxygenate at the same rate during apnea. In general, the morbidly obese adult desaturates the fastest. The child desaturates next fastest, followed by the moderately ill adult. Only the healthy adult, who desaturates the slowest, recovers from an intubating dose of succinylcholine just as hypoxia ensues.

Drummond et al. have shown that the rate of apneic desaturation after induction of anesthesia is related to the BMI. They suggest that three vital capacity VC breaths of 100% oxygen will allow for 3 minutes of apnea before the onset of hypoxemia. In their study, without preoxygenation, only 1 minute elapsed before significant desaturation occurred. Valentine et al. compared the effectiveness of the four-maximum-breath and 3-minute techniques in elderly patients. They found similar peak oxygen saturation values after preoxygenation with these two techniques. However, a significantly shorter time to all levels of desaturation was associated with the four-maximum-breath method when the patients were kept apneic and exposed to room air. The average times to 90% saturation were $3\frac{1}{2}$ minutes in the four-breath group and $6\frac{1}{2}$ minutes in the 3-minute group. Nakatsuka et al. recommend using pulse oximetry to achieve an SpO_2 of 99% to 100% during induction to ensure maximal oxygen availability and safe duration of apnea (159 ± 60 seconds) in morbidly obese patients. Benumof et al. recommend oxygen insufflation into the pharynx during laryngoscopy through a nasopharyngeal catheter.

Benumof JL. Obstructive sleep apnea in the adult obese patient: implications for airway management. *Anesthesiol Clin North America* 2002;20:789–811.

Benumof JL, Dagg R, Benumof R. Critical hemoglobin desaturation will occur before return to an unparalyzed state following 1 mg/kg intravenous succinylcholine. *Anesthesiology* 1997;87:979–982.

Berthoud MC, Peacock JE, Reilley CS. Effectiveness of preoxygenation in morbidly obese patients. *Br J Anaesth* 1991;67:464–466.

Drummond GB, Park GR. Arterial oxygen saturation before intubation of the trachea: an assessment of oxygenation techniques. *Br J Anaesth* 1984;56:987–992.

Farmery AD, Roe PG. A model to describe the rate of oxyhemoglobin desaturation during apnoea. *Br J Anaesth* 1996;76:284–291.

Gambee AM, Hertzka RE, Fisher DM. Preoxygenation techniques: comparison of three-minutes and four-breaths. *Anesth Analg* 1987;66:468–470.

Jense HG, Dubin SA, Silverstein PL, et al. Effect of obesity on safe duration of apnea in anesthetized humans. *Anesth Analg* 1991;2:89–93.

Nakatsuka M, McVey F. Oxygen desaturation during rapid sequence induction in morbidly obese patients. *Am J Anesthiol* 1996;23:273–276.

Teller LE, Alexander CM, Frumin MJ, et al. Pharyngeal insufflation prevents arterial desaturation during apnea. *Anesthesiology* 1988;69:980–982.

Valentine Sj, Marjot R, Monk CR. Preoxygenation in the elderly: a comparison of the four-maximal-breath and three-minute techniques. *Anesth Analg* 1990;71:516–519.

C.4. How would you maintain general anesthesia? What agents would you choose?

Although the ideal maintenance anesthetic for morbidly obese patients undergoing laparoscopic surgical procedures is a matter of some discussion, there is support in the literature for a technique comprising insoluble anesthetic gases resistant to metabolic degradation and without lipid depot compartmentalization, combined with rapid return of airway reflexes, plus intravenous agents that are either hydrophilic, spontaneously degrade *in vivo*, or are ultrashort acting.

Of the potent inhalation agents, desflurane has several advantages; it is insolubile, has a faster wake-up, a faster return of airway reflexes, and a decreased amount of hepatometabolism. Obesity increases the biotransformation of the inhalation anesthetics, resulting in increased serum toxic products of metabolism. Because of the frequent presence of coexisting liver dysfunction in the morbidly obese (75% have hepatic steatosis, and 25% have severe hepatic dysfunction), and the absence of a clear correlation between liver function tests and hepatic dysfunction, it would seem logical to use the agent with the lowest percentage of hepatometabolism, desflurane (0.02%), compared with isoflurane (0.2%), and sevoflurane (4% to 5%). An agent with a low blood–gas solubility coefficient is better because there will be a smaller body reservoir available for metabolism, and a faster time to steady state at the target organ, the brain. Of the inhaled agents, desflurane has the fastest wake-up, which is followed by sevoflurane, then by isoflurane. Desflurane also has the fastest return of airway reflexes, followed by sevoflurane.

Although nitrous oxide, a weak inhalation anesthetic, has certain advantages, such as a low blood–gas solubility coefficient (0.46), it is not recommended for maintenance use, because it causes intestinal inflation and is emetogenic. Nitrous oxide use is contraindicated with preexisting severe pulmonary hypertension, a condition more common in the severely obese. Short duration use of nitrous oxide, particularly during the surgical closure facilitates offset of relatively lipid soluble agents.

Remifentanil is the intraoperative narcotic of choice because of its rapid onset, consistent profile, and rapid offset. Although it is lipophilic, it has a half-life of 5 minutes, and therefore never enters the lipid compartment. Remifentanil has an equal volume of distribution (VD) calculated as lean body weight (LBW), relative to normal-weight individuals. It is dosed by infusion, starting at 0.2 μg/kg/minute LBW. The lipophilic opioids, fentanyl and sufentanil, that are dosed by total body weight (TBW), and may cause delayed respiratory depression in the high-risk patient, especially obstructive sleep apnea and hypopnea syndrome (OSAHS), are less than ideal.

Babatunde O, Jones S, Jones D, et al. Anesthetic consideration for bariatric surgery. *Anesth Analg* 2002;95:1793–1805.

Cheymol G. Effects of obesity on pharmacokinetics: implications for drug therapy. *Clin Pharmacokinet* 2000;39:215–231.

Egan TD, Huizinga B, Gupta SKZ, et al. Remifentanil pharmacokinetics in obese versus lean patients. *Anesthesiology* 1998;89:562–573.

Eger EI II. Characteristics of anesthetics used for induction and maintenance of general anesthesia. *Am J Health Syst Pharm* 2004;61:S3–S9.

Juvin P, Vadam C, Malak L, et al. Postoperative recovery after desflurane, propofol or isoflurane anesthesia among morbidly obese patients: a prospective, randomized study. *Anesth Analg* 2000;91:714–719.

McKay RE, Large MJ, Balea MC, et al. Airway reflexes return more rapidly after desflurane than after sevoflurane anesthesia. *Anesth Analg* 2005;100(3):697–700.

Minto CF, Schnider TW, Shafer SL. Pharmacokinetics and pharmacodynamics of remifentanil. II Model applications. *Anesthesiology* 1997;86:24–33.

Strum EM, Szenohradszki J, Kaufman WA, et al. Emergence and recovery characteristics of desflurane versus sevoflurane in morbidly obese adult patients: a prospective, randomized study. *Anesth Analg* 2004;99(6):1848–1853; table of contents.

C.5. Which muscle relaxants would you use?

For intubation, a muscle relaxant with rapid sequence induction indication would be used. At the present time, succinylcholine and rocuronium are the available choices. Succinylcholine is used in the vast majority of cases. It is dosed by total body weight (TBW), because the plasma cholinesterase activity increases in proportion to the body mass index (BMI). In the rare patient with contraindications to succinylcholine, rocuronium is an acceptable alternative. It is dosed according to the lean body weight (LBW). When an awake technique is chosen for securing the airway, a nondepolarizing muscle relaxant may be administered, once tracheal intubation has been confirmed.

For maintenance of anesthesia, cisatracurium is the preferred muscle relaxant. It is dosed by TBW. It has a predictable dose–response curve, and no prolongation of recovery due to organ-independent recovery or Hoffman elimination. Dense muscle relaxation is required for laparoscopic bariatric surgical procedures, to facilate ventilation, to maintain adequate space for visualization and manipulation of the surgical instruments, and to permit the introduction of surgical instruments and the removal of excised tissues.

Intraoperative contracture of the abdominal musculature, due to inadequate muscle relaxants, may increase intraabdominal pressure during pneumoperitoneum, driving carbon dioxide out from the inflated abdominal cavity through the trocar sites. The adequacy of intraoperative neuromuscular blockade may therefore be assessed by the anesthesiologist, by following both the train-of-four and the inflation pressures necessary for excellent surgical conditions.

A peripheral nerve stimulator should be used to monitor the extent of relaxation and to avoid underdosing or overdosing of nondepolarizing neuromuscular blocking agents. Extubation should only occur after documentation of full baseline train-of-four ($T_4/T_1 > 0.9$), and return of extubation criteria. Reversal agents should be given in appropriate doses.

Babatunde O, Jones S, Jones D, et al. Anesthetic considerations for bariatric surgery. *Anesth Analg* 2002;95:1793–1805.

Stoelting RK, Dierrorf SF. *Anesthesia and co-existing disease*, 4th ed. New York: Churchill Livingstone, 2002:446.

C.6. Can regional anesthesia be used intraoperatively and postoperatively to decrease opioid requirements? What are the advantages and disadvantages of regional anesthesia? What are some of the newer techniques available?

Several regional anesthetic techniques may be used intraoperatively and postoperatively to decrease opioid requirements. Thoracic epidural anesthesia (TEAA), the best studied of these, has been combined with light general anesthesia, and found by some authors to have a good side effect profile, and to offer advantages over general anesthesia, such as decreased postoperative drowsiness, nausea, and respiratory depression, improved cardiovascular function (decreased left ventricular stroke work index), decreased oxygen consumption, earlier return of lung function, less pulmonary complications, earlier return of gastrointestinal function, and shorter hospitalization times than patient-controlled analgesia (PCA). Regional anesthesia/analgesia remains underutilized (PCA is >90%) in this patient population, because of the following disadvantages: technical difficulties, logistics (slows operating room case flow), increased incidence of epidural failure and catheter dislodgment, decreased epidural space form intraabdominal pressure causing unpredictable spread of local anesthetics, variable block level, and increased incidence of wound infection, possibly from microdehiscence. Both patient-controlled epidural analgesia (PCEA) and PCA offer excellent pain reduction scores without respiratory depression when properly used. It is recommended that epidurals be inserted in the sitting position, using ultrasonic guidance. Laparoscopic cases currently comprise approximately 75% of bariatric surgical volume, reducing the need for postoperative analgesic services.

Other regional anesthesia techniques in the morbidly obese, that have been less studied include continuous spinal anesthesia/analgesia (CSAA), and intrathecal opioids (ITO). CSAA may be used with or without general anesthesia. The advantages are the same as for TEAA, except that technique is technically easier, there is a denser block, motor component, and more predictable and controllable dermatomal spread. With all of these techniques, local anesthetic dose is typically 75% to 80% for the nonobese patient. Local anesthetics (LA) and opioids act synergistically at decreased dosages. Respiratory depression is more common using hydrophilic agents (e.g., morphine) than lipophilic agents (e.g., fentanyl). Respiratory depression induced by morphine follows a longer time course (1 to 18 hours) than with fentanyl (minutes to 2 hours). It is important to identify those individuals with risk factors for neuraxial respiratory depression risk factors: excessive or repeated doses, concommittent sedatives or hypnotics, advanced age, demonstrated lack of opioid tolerance, increased intraabdominal pressure (e.g., pneumoperitoneum), and severe obstructive sleep apnea and hypopnea syndrome (OSAHS) patients, who may be at risk for massive pharyngeal collapse. Our patient was not a candidate for regional anesthesia/analgesia for this reason.

Some of the newer techniques available include multimodal perioperative analgesia (MMPA), nonopioid analgesia (NOA), and dexmedetomidine. MMPA, a combination of preincisional local anesthetics, nonsteroidal antiinflammatory drugs (NSAIDs) and PCA, uses preemptive analgesia. NOA uses a combination of methylprednisolone, ketorolac, clonidine, lidocaine, ketamine infusion, and magnesium sulfate infusion to decrease side effect profile, and speed recovery. Dexmedetomidine, a centrally acting α_2 agonist, may be used intra- and postoperatively to decrease opioid requirements.

For peripheral surgical procedures, the use of peripheral nerve blocks is advocated in the morbidly obese, provided that adequate landmarks exist.

Benumof L. Obstructive sleep apnea in the adult obese patient: implications for airway management. *Anesthesiol Clin North America* 2002;20:789–811.

Chaney MA. Side-effects of intrathecal and epidural opioids. *Can J Anaesth* 1995;42:891–903.

Charghi R, Backman S, Christou N, et al. Patient controlled iv analgesia is an acceptable pain management strategy in morbidly obese patients undergoing gastric bypass surgery. A retrospective comparison with epidural analgesia. *Canadian J Anesth* 2003;50:672–678.

Choi YK, Brolin RE, Wagner BK, et al. Efficacy and safety of patient-controlled analgesia for morbidly obese patients following gastric bypass surgery. *Obes Surg* 2000;10:154–159.

Feld JM, Laurito CE, Berkerman M, et al. Non-opioid analgesia improves pain relief and decreases sedation after gastric bypass surgery. *Can J Anaesth* 2003;50:336–341.

Gelman S, Laws HL, Potzick J, et al. Thoracic epidural vs. balanced anesthesia in morbid obesity: an intraoperative and postoperative study. *Anesth Analg* 1980;59:902–908.

Micheloudis D, Friadakis O, Petrou A, et al. Continuous spinal anesthesia/analgesia for perioperative management of morbidly obese patients undergoing laparotomy for gastroplastic surgery. *Obes Surg* 2000;10:220–229.

Otsu I, Thirlby RC, Allen HW. Patient controlled thoracic epidural analgesia after gastric bypass surgery for morbid obesity. *Reg Anesth Pain Med* 2001;26:A117.

Ramsay M, Jones C, Cancemi M, et al. *Dexmedetomidine improves postoperative pain management in bariatric surgical patients.* ASA Annual Meeting Abstracts 2005.

Rawal N, Sjostrand U, Christoffersson warninge, et al. Comparison of intramuscular and epidural morphine for postoperative analgesia in the grossly obese: influence on postoperative ambulation and pulmonary function. *Anesth Analg* 1984;63:583–592.

Schumann R, Shikora S, Weiss J, et al. A comparison of multimodal perioperative analgesia to epidural pain management after gastric bypass surgery. *Anesth Analg* 2003;96:469–474.

C.7. What is the effect of narcotics on the sphincter of Oddi? Is pharmacologic treatment indicated?

Subcutaneously administered morphine, 10 mg, increases the pressure in the common bile duct more than 10-fold within 15 minutes; this effect can be present for 2 hours or longer. Opioids can cause sphincter of Oddi spasm, which can interfere with intraoperative cholangiography. At equianalgesic doses, fentanyl, and morphine cause larger increases in biliary pressure than meperidine or pentazocine. Butorphanol and nalbuphine probably do not cause sphincter of Oddi spasm. Morphine is not a good analgesic choice for biliary tract surgery. Atropine partially prevents opioid-induced biliary spasm. Glucagon, nalbuphine, nitroglycerine, volatile anesthetics, and opioid antagonists, such as naloxone, effectively prevent or prophylax opioid-induced biliary spasm. Glucagon, 1 or 2 mg intravenously, is the drug of choice, and is also used to decrease upper gastrointestinal tract motility (e.g., for endoscopic procedures). The only common side effects are slight increase in heart rate, and transient hyperglycemia.

Barash PG, Cullen BF, Stoelting RK, eds. *Clinical anesthesia*, 5th ed. Philadelphia: Lippincott Williams & Wilkins, 2006:359.

Radnay PA, Duncalf D, Novakovakovic M, et al. Common bile duct pressure changes after fentanyl, morphine, meperidine, butorphanol, and naloxone. *Anesth Analg* 1984;63:441.

C.8. During surgery, arterial blood gases showed pH 7.35; PaO_2 57 mm Hg; $PaCO_2$ 52 mm Hg; FIO_2 0.6; mechanical ventilator tidal volume 1.0 L; and ventilatory rate 15 breaths per minute. The following changes were made to the ventilatory parameters: 10 cm H_2O positive end-expiratory pressure (PEEP) was added, and the tidal volume was increased to 1.2 L. Twenty minutes later, an arterial blood gas showed pH 7.32; PaO_2 55 mm Hg, $PaCO_2$ 55 mm Hg. What is the explanation for these changes?

Both blood gases are significant for respiratory acidosis and hypoxemia. It is important to look at the surgical field, examine the patient, auscultate the chest, and check the position of the tracheal tube to rule out an endobronchial intubation, kinking of the tube, or mucous plugging. While performing a differential diagnosis, it is advisable to increase the FIO_2, acertain that the level of pneumoperitoneum is less than 20 cm Hg, note the peak airway pressure, hand bag the patient, and consider a bronchial dilator.

In the absence of life-threatening events, there are several pathophysiologic explanations for these blood gases. Usually, PEEP increases PaO_2, and increased tidal volume decreases the $PaCO_2$. Occasionally, PEEP and increased tidal volume may paradoxically decrease PaO_2, and increase the $PaCO_2$, especially in morbidly obese patients. There are several reasons for this. First, high airway pressure can interrupt pulmonary capillary blood flow at the uppermost portions of the lung at peak inspiration. Since these areas already have high ventilation/perfusion, further decreases in perfusion result in an increase in physiologic dead space (V_D/V_T) and increased $Paco_2$. The impeded blood flow will be redistributed to areas of lung that are not affected by the high airway pressure, resulting in an increase in intrapulmonary shunt (Q_S/Q_T) and a decrease in PaO_2. Second, high airway pressures decrease venous return and cardiac output (CO), which may decrease PaO_2 and increase $Paco_2$. Third, high tidal volume and high airway pressures may create low lung water pulmonary edema from volutrauma and barotrauma. Fourth, overdistension of the pleura and turbulent airflow may result from excessive ventilator settings. This may precipitate bronchospasm in susceptible patients, such as asthmatics, especially when associated with light anesthesia. Fifth, at excessive airway pressures, there may be rupture of a preexisting bleb or bulla.

Buckley FP, Robinson NB, Siminowitz DA. Anesthesia in the morbidly obese: a comparison of anesthetic and analgesic regimens for upper abdominal surgery. *Anaesthesia* 1983;38:840–851.

Cunningham AJ, Brull SJ. Laparoscopic cholecystectomy: anesthetic implications. *Anesth Analg* 1993;76:1120–1133.

Dreyfuss D, Soler P, Basset G, et al. High inflation pressure pulmonary edema: respective effects of high airway pressure, high tidal volume and positive end-expiratory pressure. *Am Rev Respir Dis* 1988;137:1159–1164.

In-amani M, Kiduta Y, Nagai H, et al. The increase in pulmonary venous admixture is enhanced in obese patients. *Anesthesiology* 1985;63:A520.

Salem MR, Joseph N, Lim R, et al. Respiratory and hemodynamic response to PEEP in grossly obese patients. *Anesthesiology* 1984;61:A511.

C.9. What is apneic oxygenation? Who did the pioneer study?

Draper and Whitehead conducted the pioneer study on apneic oxygenation in 1944. Apneic oxygenation (formerly known as diffusion respiration) is actually caused by mass movement oxygenation. When the lungs are completely denitrogenized with oxygen and the airway is connected to an oxygen source, continuous oxygenation takes place by mass movement. Normally, every minute, 230 mL of oxygen is removed from the alveoli for metabolism and 200 mL of CO_2 is produced and eliminated from the lungs. When a person is apneic, only 10% of CO_2 accumulates in the alveoli, and 90% of CO_2 stays in the blood as bicarbonate. Consequently, 250 mL of oxygen is removed from the lungs and 20 mL of CO_2 accumulates in the lungs, creating a 230-mL vacuum effect and sucking in oxygen. Carbon dioxide tension continues to rise because no elimination occurs during apnea. The total pressure in the alveoli is constant, so the decrease in PO_2 equals the rise in PCO_2, ranging from 3 to 6 mm Hg per minute. If the patient had been breathing 100% oxygen before respiratory arrest, the starting alveolar PO_2 would be about 650 mm Hg, and therefore, the patient could theoretically maintain PaO_2 above 100 mmHg for about 100 minutes of apnea provided that the airway remained clear and connected to 100% oxygen. However, patients will die of severe respiratory acidosis (pH < 6.80) before hypoxemia occurs. Moreover, as seen in suffocation, gross hypoxia supervenes after about 90 seconds if apnea with airway occlusion follows air breathing at the functional residual capacity. When the airway is patent and the ambient gas is air, gross hypoxia supervenes after about 2 minutes of apnea, as seen during intubation without preoxygenation. However, if the patient is preoxygenated for 3 minutes, gross hypoxia will not occur until 6 minutes of apnea for normal-weight patients and until about 3 minutes of apnea for morbidly obese patients.

Jense HG, Dubin SA, Silverstein PL, et al. Effect of obesity on safe duration of apnea in unanesthetized humans. *Anesth Analg* 1991;2:89–93.

Lumb AB. *Nunn's applied respiratory physiology*, 6th ed. Philadelphia: Elsevier: Butterworth-Heinemann, 2005;160–161.

C.10. What is diffusion hypoxia? How do you prevent it?

Fink and colleagues in 1954 first reported diffusion hypoxia during recovery from nitrous oxide-oxygen anesthesia. A mild degree of hypoxia can develop for more than 10 minutes when nitrous oxide-oxygen anesthesia is concluded and the patient is allowed to breathe room air. The arterial oxygen saturation can fall 5% to 10% and often reaches values less than 90% (PaO_2 <60 mm Hg). This occurs at the times when nitrous oxide is eliminated rapidly through the lungs. Nitrous oxide is 35 times more soluble in blood than nitrogen. Therefore, the amount of nitrous oxide diffused from blood to alveoli is much more than the amount of nitrogen diffused from alveoli to blood. Hence, alveolar oxygen is diluted by nitrous oxide. Diffusion hypoxia can be prevented by the inhalation of high concentrations of oxygen for several minutes before the patient is allowed to breathe room air.

Fink BR. Diffusion anoxia. *Anesthesiology* 1955;16:511–519.

Fink BR, Carpenter SL, Holaday DA, et al. Diffusion anoxia during recovery from nitrous oxide-oxygen anesthesia. *Fed Proc* 1954;13:354.

Sheffer L, Steffenson JL, Birch AA. Nitrous oxide-induced diffusion hypoxia in patients breathing spontaneously. *Anesthesiology* 1972;37:436.

D. Postoperative Management

D.1. When will you extubate this patient? What are the extubation criteria?

In the past, prophylactic ventilatory support throughout the first postoperative night was occasionally utilized for the morbidly obese obstructive sleep apnea and hypopnea syndrome (OSAHS) or obesity hypoventilation syndrome (OHS) patient having an open abdominal weight reduction procedure. Currently, this is rarely the case; due to the huge yearly increases in the number of bariatric surgeries in the United States (16,000 in the early 1990s, to 140,000 in 2004), advanced laparoscopic experience of the surgeons, and advances in the anesthetic care of the morbidly obese, most patients are extubated in the operating room at the conclusion of surgery as soon as the following extubation criteria are met:

- Intact neurologic status, fully awake and alert, with head lift greater than 5 seconds
- Hemodynamic stability
- Normothermia. The core temperature is above 36°C.
- Train-of-four (TOF) reversal documented by peripheral nerve stimulator (T_4/T_1 >0.9). Full reversal of neuromuscular blocking agents.
- Respiratory rate (>10 and <30 breaths/minute)
- Baseline peripheral oxygenation, as judged by pulse oximeter (SpO_2 >95% on FiO_2 of 0.4).
- Rarely, if an arterial line is present, an arterial blood gas may be checked. Acceptable blood–gas results (FiO_2 of 0.4: pH, 7.35 to 7.45; PaO_2, >80 mm Hg; $PaCO_2$, <50 mm Hg).
- Acceptable respiratory mechanics: negative inspiratory force (NIF) (>25 to 30 cm H_2O; vital capacity (VC) >10 mL/kg IBW; tidal volume (V_T) >5 mL/kg ideal body weight [IBW]).
- Acceptable pain control
- No demonstrated or suspected laboratory abnormalities

Extubation criteria should be used systematically in obese patients. In all cases, an attending anesthesiologist with advanced airway skills must be in attendance for extubation. Emergency tracheal reintubation may be necessary. Patients with documented difficult airway should be extubated per protocol. Patients with OSAHS, OHS, and the pickwickian syndrome (PS) have higher incidence of postoperative respiratory dysfunction. They require special attention before and after extubation, and occasionally warrant a monitored bed for observation.

Flores JC. Post-anesthetic care unit management. In: Alvarez A, ed. *Morbid obesity perioperative management*. Cambridge, England, Cambridge University Press, 2004:339–351.

NIH Consensus Development Conference Panel. gastrointestinal surgery for severe obesity—Consensus Development Conference Panel. *Ann Droit Int Med* 1991; 115:956–961.

Samuels J. Bariatric anesthesia: a new sub-specialty? *NYSSA Sphere* 2004;56:49–54.

D.2. What are the major early postoperative complications in the morbidly obese patient? How do helath-related risks correlate with obsesity? What factors correlated statistically with perioperative mortality?

The major early postoperative complications in the morbidly obese are mostly related to the pulmonary and cardiovascular systems. Postanesthetic hypoxemia, respiratory depression, early ventilatory failure with need for reintubation, positional ventilatory collapse, hemodynamic instability, postoperative nausea and vomiting (PONV), and venous thromboembolism are some common examples. Early surgical complications include anastomotic closure with bowel obstruction, anastomotic leak, and wound infection.

At any given weight, the perioperative risk is greater for central obesity than for peripheral obesity, and for patients with preexisting severe comorbidity, especially obstructive sleep apnea and hypopnea syndrome (OSAHS).

The major perioperative risk of death correlates statistically with body mass index (BMI), preexisting hypertension, pulmonary embolus, and anastomotic leak.

Bray GA. Pathophysiology of obesity. *AM J Clin Nutr* 1992;55(Suppl):488–494.

Fernandez A, Adolfo Z, Demaria E, et al. Multivariate analysis of risk factors for death following gastric bypass for treatment of morbid obesity. *Ann Surg* 2004;239(5):698–703.

D.3. How does position affect respiratory function in the obese patient?

In the supine position, intraabdominal contents shift the diaphragm rostrally resulting in diaphragmatic dysfunction, decreased functional residual capacity (FRC), airway closure, increase in venous admixture (Q_S/Q_T), decreased PaO_2, and possibly positional ventilatory collapse. The FRC increases 30% in obese patients by changing from the supine position to the sitting position, both in nonsurgical and postlaparotomy patients. Recovery should take place in a semi-Fowler position (head up at an angle of 30 to 45 degrees) as soon as these patients are hemodynamically stable. Other benefits of a semisitting position are decreased superior vena cava pressure, decreased incidence of positional injuries, which are more common in the morbidly obese. Patients recovered in the semi-Fowler position, who are in need of eventual emergent mask ventilation or tracheal reintubation, present better conditions for the laryngoscopist. There is a higher incidence of tracheal tube misplacement in the morbidly obese; care should be taken when positioning these patients in a semi-Fowler position.

Brodsky JB, Lemmons HJ, Brock-Utne, et al. Anesthetic considerations for bariatric surgery: proper positioning is important for laryngoscopy. *Anesth Analg* 2003;96:1841–1842.

Ezri T, Hazin V, Warters D, et al. The endotracheal tube moves more often in obese patients undergoing laparoscopy compared with open abdominal surgery. *Anesth Analg* 2003;96(1):278–282.

Warner MA, Warner ME, Martin JT. Ulnar neuropathy. Incidence, outcome, and risk factors in sedated or anesthetized patients. *Anesthesiology* 1994;81(6):1332–1340.

D.4. How would you prevent postoperative atelectasis?

In the past, bariatric surgical procedures were often performed open, with an incidence of postoperative atelectasis of 45%. Approximately 75% are now performed laparoscopically, so the incidence would be expected to decline substantially.

Early ambulation, chest physical ambulation with incentive spirometry, and effective coughing are encouraged to improve respiratory function. Prolonged recumbency is avoided whenever because of its adverse effects on the ventilation/perfusion ratio. Careful titration of postoperative analgesics is emphasized to prevent splinting from pain and hypoventilation from excessive sedation.

Babatunde O, Jones S, Jones D, et al. Anesthetic considerations for bariatric surgery. *Anesth Analg* 2002;95:1793–1805.

D.5. How long would you prescribe supplementary oxygen postoperatively?

The incidence of postanesthetic hypoxemia (PaO_2 <60 mm Hg) is increased from a baseline of 25% to 30% in the nonobese to 75% in the obese. For a routine case on an otherwise healthy patient with simple obesity, supplemental oxygen in the postanesthetic care unit (PACU) is probably sufficient. In most morbidly obese patients with comorbidities, oxygen should be prescribed for 24 to 72 hours. The morbidly obese patient with severe obstructive sleep apnea and hypopnea syndrome (OSAHS) on continuous positive airway pressure (CPAP) or bilevel positive airway pressure (BIPAP) will usually have continuation of their therapy overnight, be recovered in a semi-Fowler position (at an angle of 30 to 45 degrees) and should have individualized care, with continuous pulse oximetry, and respiratory monitoring. At The New York-Presbyterian Hospital, most of these patients are discharged to home on the third or fourth postsurgical day.

Downs JB. Prevention of hypoxemia: the simple, logical, but incorrect solution. *J Clin Anesth* 1994;6:180.

Mecca RS, Sharnick S. Nausea and vomiting. In: Brown M, Brown E, ed. *Comprehensive postoperative care*. Baltimore : Williams & Wilkins, 1997:302–318.

D.6. How would you control postoperative pain?

In more than 90% of bariatric surgical procedures, analgesia is provided postoperatively by parenteral narcotics using patient-controlled analgesia (PCA), as it was for our patient. PCA has been shown to be safe and effective in the morbidly obese patient population. It has many advantages: PCA is simple to use, saves nursing time, involves minimal time delay between patient perception of pain and therapy. There is less splinting and pulmonary function tests (PFTs) return early. PCA also facilitates early ambulation and shortens hospital stay. Dosing of morphine, the gold standard, needs to be individualized. Hydromorphone is also frequently used. Dose regimens need to be individualized, according to pain control and side effect profile. There have been some cases of respiratory complications in the MO-OSAHS patient, so extra viligence is needed in this group. PCA dosages for the morbidly obese in the opioid naïve, based on ideal body weight (IBW), are as follows:

- Morphine sulfate 20 μg/kg IBW
- Hydromorphone 4 to 5 μg/kg IBW
- Fentanyl 1 μg/kg.
- Methadone 20 μg/kg IBW

All settings are every 10 minutes, without continuous rate, at 80% of the calculated maximum doses.

Intravenous infusions of opioids may also be administered in a monitored setting. In the past, opioids have been administered intramuscularly. Although this route has been shown to be effective, intramuscular injection is not advisable in the morbidly obese, because of unpredictable pharmacodynamics, arising from inadvert injection into lipid tissue.

There are three regional anesthetic/analgesic options: thoracic epidural anesthesia/patient-controlled epidural analgesia (TEAA/PCEA), intrathecal opioids (IT), and continuous spinal anesthesia/patient-controlled intrathecal analgesia (CSA/PCIA). All of these may be used intraoperatively with or without light general anesthesia (GA). They offer similar side effect profiles and will be described together. *PCEA*, the most commonly used of these, has numerous theoretical advantages. At a lower dose compared with parenteral opioids, there are few side effects and serious complications, effective analgesia, faster recovery, less respiratory complications, decreased total body oxygen consumption, improved cardiac function (decreased left ventricular stroke work index [LVSWI]), and shorter hospitalization times compared with PCA. PCEA dosages in the morbidly obese should be decreased 75% to 80%, due to decreased volume of the epidural space from increased intraabdominal pressure. PCEA is strongly recommended when feasible, yet remains underutilized. Patients should be positioned in a sitting position for epidural catheter insertion, and ultrasonography guidance is recommended. Disadvantages include a higher rate of wound infection, possibly because of microdehiscence from faster return of gastrointestinal function, and the risk of neural injury. There is frequent technical difficulty with catheter insertion, which slows operating room case flow. There is a higher rate of inadequate function, catheter migration and replacement, and variable block height. Side effects include excessive drowsiness, postoperative nausea and vomiting (PONV), pruritis, and urinary retention. Respiratory depression occurs rarely, and is more common with hydrophilic (e.g., preservative-free morphine sulfate [PFMS]) than with hydrophilic agents. With PFMS it may occur from 1 hour until 18 hours. With fentanyl or sufentanil it may occur from minutes until 2 hours. Neuraxial opioid respiratory depression risk factors include advanced age, excessive or repeated doses, lack of opioid tolerance, use of concomitant sedatives or hypnotics, increased intraabdominal pressure (e.g., pneumoperitoneum), and severe OSAHS, which may precipitate massive pharyngeal collapse. *CSA/PCIA* with light GA has been used for gastroplastic surgery. It is technically easier to perform than TEAA/PCEA, and produces a denser block with motor component, which is more predictable and controllable. *IT* opioids, with or without local anesthetics, are technically easier to administer, and offer an excellent alternative for appropriate surgical procedures. Other methods of controlling postoperative pain in bariatric surgery include preemptive analgesia through local anesthetic wound infiltration before and after surgery, pre- and intraoperative nonopioid drug combination (ketorolac, clonidine, lidocaine, ketamine, magnesium sulfate, and methylprednisolone), and perioperative dexmedetomidine.

Charghi R, Backman S, Christou N, et al. Patient controlled iv analgesia is an acceptable pain management strategy in morbidly obese patients undergoing gastric bypass surgery. A retrospective comparison with epidural analgesia. *Can J Anesth* 2003;50:672–678.

Choi YK, Brolin RE, Wagner BK, et al. Efficacy and safety of patient-controlled analgesia for morbidly obese patients following gastric bypass surgery. *Obes Surg* 2000;10:154–159.

Feld JM, Laurito CE, Berkerman M, et al. Non-opioid analgesia improves pain relief and decreases sedation after gastric bypass surgery. *Can J Anaesth* 2003;50:336–341.

Gelman S, Laws HL, Potzick J, et al. Thoracic epidural vs. balanced anesthesia in morbid obesity: an intraoperative and postoperative study. *Anesth Analg* 1980;59:902–908.

Haidbauer AG. Post-operative analgesia. In: Alvarcz A, ed. *Morbid obesity, peri-operative management*. Cambridge, England: Cambridge University Press, 2004:381–396.

Micheloudis D, Friadakis O, Petrou A, et al. Continuous spinal anesthesia/analgesia for perioperative management of morbidly obese patients undergoing laparotomy for gastroplastic surgery. *Obes Surg* 2000;10:220–229.

Otsu I, Thirlby RC, Allen HW. Patient controlled thoracic epidural analgesia after gastric bypass surgery for morbid obesity. *Reg Anesth Pain Med* 2001;26:A117.

Ramsay M, Jones C, Cancemi M, et al. *Dexmedetomidine improves postoperative pain management in bariatric surgical patients*. ASA Annual Meeting Abstracts 2005.

Rawal N, Sjostrand U, Christoffersson warninge, et al. Comparison of intramuscular and epidural morphine for postoperative analgesia in the grossly obese: influence on postoperative ambulation and pulmonary function. *Anesth Analg* 1984;63:583–592.

Schumann R, Shikora S, Weiss J, et al. A comparison of multimodal perioperative analgesia to epidural pain management after gastric bypass surgery. *Anesth Analg* 2003;96:469–474.

Shenkman Z, Shir Y, Brodsky JB. Perioperative management of the obese patient. *Br J Anaesth* 1993;70(3):349–359.

INDEX

Note: Page numbers followed by *f* indicate figures; those followed by *t* indicate tables.

α_2-adrenergic agonist,
for burn patients, 1126
for ischemic heart disease, 380
for myocardial ischemia, 380
α_2 agonist,
for ischemic heart disease, 388–389
α_1-antitrypsin deficiency, lung transplantation for, 89
Abbe flap, 1057–1058
abdominal aortic aneurysm repair,
abdominal aorta's relevance to surgery, 280
anesthesia
for endovascular aortic aneurysm repair, 287
cpidural or intraspinal catheter, placement of, 288, 289t
management of, 283–284
for open repair of the aorta, 287
various techniques used for, 287–288
aortic cross-clamp placement
hemodynamic changes of, *290*, 290–291
infrarenal aneurysm, renal blood flow and, 291
rising pulmonary artery occlusion pressure during, 291
ST-segment depressions, development of, 291
aortic cross-clamp removal
depressed systemic blood pressure and, 293
hemodynamic consequences of, 292, *292*
arterial line
complications of, 285
use of, 285
creatinine clearance, measuring, 279–280
diseases associated with, 273
endovascular repair, risk to kidneys and, 291
extubation parameters, 293
fluid and blood replacement during surgery, 289
monitors used in, 286–287
morbidity and mortality in
causes of, 272–273
elective repair *vs.* emergency repair of, 276

with surgery *vs.* without surgery and, 273
myocardial ischemia
algorithm for patients with, *277*
monitors used for, 286
perioperative myocardial infarction in patients with, 274–275
pulmonary artery catheter, assessing with, 289
postoperative pain
alternatives, 289t, 294–295
controlling, 294
postoperative pulmonary function
anticipated changes in, 293–294
surgical technique's affect on, 294
premedication for, 285
preoperative management
arterial blood gas measurements and, 279
electrocardiogram and, 276–277, 278
laboratory tests for, 276
pulmonary status, evaluating, 278–279
respiratory parameters, maneuvers to maximize, 293–294
small aortic aneurysms, procedure for, 274
spinal cord blood flow, described, 280, *281*
spinal cord ischemia, detecting, *282*, 282–283
surgical approaches to, 283–284
ABO blood group, 833
accelerated atherosclerosis, 830
accidental spinal tap, 921
Accolate (zafirlukast), for asthma, 14
acetylcholine, 4
acetylcholine receptor, 1077, 1078
acetylcholinesterase, 1106
acidemia, 512
acidosis, response to aortic unclamping, 267
activated clotting time, 164–165, 338, 970
activated partial thromboplastin time, 337, 970
acupuncture,
analgesia, mechanisms of, 747–748
for chronic conditions
cancer, 751
headache, 750
nausea and vomiting

acupuncture (*contd.*)
chemotherapy-induced, 749–750
postoperative, 749
neck pain, 750
osteoarthritis, 750–751
complications of, 751–752
defined, 746–747
National Institute of Health Consensus
Conference, conclusions about, 748
practice methods, 747
acupuncture points, 747
acute abdomen,
causes of abdominal pain, gastrointestinal,
and intraperitoneal, 472t
differential diagnosis of, 472
acute chest syndrome, defined, 986
acute left ventricular failure (cardiac asthma), 3
acute lung injury, 55–59, 1198, 1199
defined, 55
pathogenesis of, 56
protective-ventilation strategy in, 57–59, 58
pulmonary compliance, defined, 59
acute myocardial infarction, 142
Acute Pain Service, role of,
in improving postoperative pain management,
744
inadequate, consequences of, 743–744
postoperative outcome, improving, 745
undertreatment, 743
acute renal failure, 1133
in acute respiratory distress syndrome, 55
acute respiratory distress syndrome,
causes of, 55
defined, 55
protective-ventilation strategy in, 57–59, 58
radiographic findings in, 56–57
in trauma patients, 1152–1153
Acute Respiratory Distress Syndrome Network,
58–59
acute symptomatic hyponatremia, 827
acute tubular necrosis, 490, 496, 846
acute vasculitis, in acute respiratory distress
syndrome, 55
adenoidectomy, 1054
adenylate cyclase, 769–770, 770
adjuvant drugs, 690
adrenal cortex, 772
adrenal gland,
anatomy of, normal, 769
embryology of, 769
adrenal medulla, 769

adrenocorticotropic hormone (ACTH;
corticotropin) for myasthenia gravis,
1083
Advanced Trauma Life Support course, 995
aerosol therapy, for asthma, 14
Agency for Health Agency for Health Care Policy
and Research, 709
α-interferon therapy, 1027–1028
air embolism, 150
airflow obstruction, 64
air pollution, asthmatic attacks and, 5
airway fire, managing ("4-E's"), 1033
airway obstruction in childhood,
anesthesia
airway, inability to secure with intubation,
1046–1047
awake intubation, 1047
epiglottitis and
airway, securing, 1045
general used for, in children, 1044–1045
rapid-sequence induction, 1046–1047
frothy secretions from endotracheal tube,
1047–1048
inducing, 1045–1046
medical management of croup and,
1040–1041
nasotracheal or orotracheal tube, 1047
bacterial tracheitis, 1039
croup
anesthetic implications of, 1040–1041
characteristics of, 1048t
defined, 1039
medical management of, 1040–1041
postextubation, 1043
severity of, assessment of, 1039, 1039t
spasmodic, 1039
differential diagnosis of, 1040
epiglottitis
acute, outcomes for child with, 1048
causes of, 1041
clinical manifestations of, 1042
defined, 1041–1042, 1041t
diagnosing, 1042–1043
general anesthesia administered to children
with, 1044–1045
incidence of, 1041
intubation for, 1044
laryngotracheitis, clinical presentation of,
1039
partial, nonacute causes of
extrinsic pathologies, 1044

intrinsic pathologies, 1044
postoperative management
    extubation time, criteria determining, 1048
    intubation
        comfort of patient during, 1048
        duration of, 1047
preoperative evaluation and preparation
    intubation, epiglottitis and, 1044
stridor
    anatomic location of, 1039
    definition of, 1039
airway trauma,
    trauma patient, airway management in
        airway and breathing, evaluating, 995
        circulation, evaluating, 995–996
        diagnostic tests indicated, based on
            mechanism of injury, 996–997
        immediate treatment required before
            diagnostic studies, 997
        impaling object, removal of, 997
        initial assessment of a, 995
        intraoperative management
            of airway, options for, 1000
            anesthetics, maintenance, 1004
            aspiration, minimizing risk of, 1001
            awake fiberoptic intubation
                failure of, other options available, 1003
                risks of, 1003
            awake intubation, anesthetize the airway
                for, 1002
            complications introduced by surgical
                plan, 1004
            cricothyroidotomy, 1003–1004
            exacerbating cervical spine trauma,
                minimizing risk of, 1001
            laryngeal mask airway, 1003
            monitoring, 999
            rapid-sequence induction
                anesthetic agents used for, 1000–1001
                risks of, 1000
            repetitive strain injuries, 1003
            tracheostomy, 1004
            tube thoracostomy, 1000
            Zone III neck injury, surgical approach to,
                1000
        mental status and neurolgic condition,
            evaluating, 996, 996t
        from motorcycle collisions
            other trauma from, 995
            variables mitigating injury from, 994
        postoperative management

alcohol abuse and, affect on, 1005
    extubation
        criteria for, 1005
        techniques used during, 1005
    of pain, 1006
preoperative evaluation and preparation
    airway management, when and where,
        999
    electrocardiogram, necessity of, 998
    intubation before computed tomographic,
        998
    laboratory tests, 997–998
    prophylactic medications, indications for,
        999
    x-rays most important to anesthesiologist,
        998
    zones of the neck, 997
    See trauma patient, airway management in
akinesia, 150
Akineton (biperiden), for Parkinson's disease,
    583
albuterol, for asthma, 14, 19, 26
alcohol withdrawal, signs and symptoms of,
    1127
Alder's sign, defined, 951
aldosterone, 772
algodystrophy, 671
Allen's test, defined, 144
allergens, asthma and, 5
allodynia, 672
allograft rejection, 369
alveolar partial pressure of oxygen,
amantadine, for Parkinson's disease, 583
ambulatory surgery,
    bispectral Index monitor, benefits derived
        from using, 1220–1221
    glaucoma
        anesthetic implications of, 1210–1211
        discontinuing before surgery, 1212
        eye drops used to treat, 1212
    intraoperative management
        anesthesia
            agents, 1223
            for laparoscopy, options, 1223
            technique, for outpatient surgery,
                1218–1219
        bispectral Index monitor
            children and, 1221
            limitations of, major, 1222
            reading of 56, meaning of, 1222
    laparoscopy

ambulatory surgery (*contd.*)
    carbon dioxide, alternatives to, 1225
    carbon dioxide as insufflation agent of
        choice, 1225
    intraoperative complications associated
        with, 1224
    physiologic changes induced by,
        1224–1225
    monitoring, 1219–1220
    nitrous oxide, avoiding, 1223–1224
    retinal detachment surgery, anesthetic
        implications of, 1219
  morbid obesity, 1212
  medical conditions associated with, 1213
  postoperative management
    discharge of patient
      after regional anesthesia, 1229
      criteria for, 1229
      instructions, 1230
    of eye pain, 1228
    of nausea and vomiting in outpatients
      causes of, 1226
      pharmacological treatment of, 1226–1227
    of pain, 1227–1228
  preoperative evaluation and preparation
    chest roentgenogram, 1215
    electrocardiogram, 1215
    goals of, 1213–1214
    history, important questions to ask about,
      1217
    inappropriate candidates for ambulatory
      surgery, 1216
    laboratory testing, 1214
    outpatient surgery
      advantages of, 1213
      patient's age or physical status and,
        1215–1216
    overnight fast, justified, 1218
    premedication, 1217
    prophylaxis against acid aspiration
      pneumonitis, 1218
American College of Obstetricians and
    Gynecologists classification of
    preeclampsia, 905
American Society of Anesthesiologists,
  monitoring, standard guidelines for, 389–390
American Society of Regional Anesthesia and
    Pain Medicine Consensus Conference,
    890
amides, 677
aminocaproic acid, 341

  hemostasis improved by, 348
aminophylline, for asthma, 24–25, 26
amlodipine, for cardiopulmonary bypass, 142
amniotic fluid embolism, 900
anal canal defect (anal atresia), 107
anemia,
  cardiac morbidity and, 830
  in pregnancy, relative, 891
  in progressive renal insufficiency, 824
    blood oxygen-carrying capacity, affect on,
      825
    transfusion and, 825
anesthesia,
  for abdominal aortic aneurysm repair
    for endovascular aortic aneurysm repair,
      287
    epidural or intraspinal catheter, placement
      of, 288, 289t
    management of, 283–284
    for open repair of the aorta, 287
    various techniques used for, 287–288
  for airway obstruction in childhood
    airway, inability to secure with intubation,
      1046–1047
    awake intubation, 1047
    epiglottitis and
      airway, securing, 1045
      general used for, in children, 1044
      rapid-sequence induction, 1046–1047
    frothy secretions from endotracheal tube,
      1047–1048
    inducing, 1045–1046
    medical management of croup and,
      1040–1041
    nasotracheal or orotracheal tube, 1047
  for appendectomy in pregnant patient
    brachial plexus block, 959
    for delivery *vs.* nonobstetric surgery,
      955–956, 956, 957
    epidural, technique and dosage of, 957
    general, technique for, 958
    isoflurane-nitrous oxide-oxygen, 959
    nitrous oxide, controversy surrounding, 959
    options, discussing with patient, 955
    technique of, in pregnant women *vs.*
      nonpregnant women, 955–956,
      956, 957
  for asthma patients
    aminophylline administration, 24–25
    β_y-agonists, administration methods for
      23, *24*

for cyanotic patient not responding to
    aminophylline, 25
halothane mechanisms that produce
    bronchodilation, 20
inhalational *vs.* intravenous techniques, 21
lidocaine for intubation, 19
laryngeal mask airway *vs.* endotracheal
    tube, 17
maintenance of, agents for, 20
methohexital *vs.* thiopental for induction, 18
muscle relaxants that cause histamine
    release, avoiding, 21–22, 22t
propofol, etomidate, ketamine for induction,
    18
rapid sequence induction, precautions, 19
regional *vs.* general, 21
for cardiopulmonary bypass
    desflurane, cardiovascular effects of, 155
    enflurane, cardiovascular effects of, 155
    fentanyl, cardiovascular effects of, 155
    halothane, cardiovascular effects of, 155
    inducing, 153–154
    inhalation *vs.* intravenous agent, 154
    intraoperative management of, 175
    isoflurane, cardiovascular effects of, 155
        dangers of, in patients with coronary
            artery disease, 156
    maintaining, 154
    morphine, cardiovascular effects of, 155
    nitrous oxide, cardiovascular effect of,
        157–158
    sevoflurane, cardiovascular effects of, 155
for carotid endarterectomy
    cerebral blood flow and, effects on, 568–569
    choosing, 566–567
    general, 567
    protective effects of, on cerebral function,
        569–570
    regional, 568
    ventilation, 571
for complex regional pain syndrome, local
    classes of, 677
    epinephrine, addition of, 678
    onset, potency, and duration of, 677, 678t
    systemic toxicity of, 680
        cardiovascular effects, 681
        central nervous system effects, 681
        treatment for, 681
for congenital heart defects
    airway, securing, 1071–1072
    equipemnt, circuit and monitors, 1070–1071

for infant, inducing, 1073
    nitrous oxide, 1073
    severe blood loss and, technique for, 1073
for craniotomy
    CO_2 management, 540
    effects of, on $CMRO_2$, cerebral blood flow,
        and intracranial pressure, 538–539
    goals of, 536–537
    induction, associated risks of, 537
    intracranial hypertension and, 532–533
    intravenous, 539
    monitoring and, effect on, 533
    nitrous oxide, 539
    opiods, 539
    volatile, 538–539, 542–543
for deep brain stimulation
    choosing, 591–592
    electrode implants, anesthetic implications
        for, 590
    implications for, 584–585, 585t
    magnetic resonance imaging unit,
        considerations in, 587–589
    plan for, 586
for diabetes mellitus patients
    insulin and glucose, effects on, 791, 793
    preparing patient for, 790
    techniques, 793
for head injury
    to avoid, 611
    of choice, 611
for heart transplantation
    equipment for, 362
    induction and maintenance of, 363
    left ventricular assist device insertion,
        considerations for, 361
    subsequent noncardiac surgery
        best type for, 368
        implications for, 368
        technique of, 368
for hemophilia
    axillary block, 975
    complications during transfusion,
        immediate steps to take, 976–977
    human immunodeficiency virus, special
        considerations for patients with, 975
for hypertensive patients
    agents for maintenance of, 317–318
    hypokalemia, treating before, 312
    hypomagnesemia and, treating before, 312
    inducing, 315
    postoperative management of, 320–321

anesthesia (*contd.*)
  regional, 320
  for intestinal obstruction
    administration of antacids and/or H$_2$
      blockers, small bowel obstruction
      and, 480–481
    incubation position, 481
    induction, dangers present during, 480
    inspired oxygen, benefits to use high
      concentration of, 483
    muscle relaxants, succinylcholine for
      rapid-sequence induction, 481, 482t
    nasogastric tube and, 482
    nitrous oxide and, 482–483
    Sellick's maneuver, 481
  for ischemic heart disease
    etomidate as an induction agent, 393
    general, inducing, 392–393
    maintenance of, anesthetic agents for,
      393–394
    regional *vs.* general, 392
  for laparoscopic surgery
    agents or adjuvant drugs recommended for,
      863–864
    insufflation and, complications during, 866
    nitrous oxide (N$_2$O), 864, 875–876
    technique, of choice, 862–863
  for laryngeal lesions, laser treatment for
    airway fire, managing ("4-E's"), 1033
    endotracheal tube
      protecting external surface of, 1032
      special, for laser surgery, 1033
    foil-wrapped tubes, disadvantages of, 1033
    intermittent apnea technique, 1037
    setup for, special considerations in,
      1029–1030
    Venturi effect, defined, 1034
    Venturi jet ventilation
      complications of, 1035
      contraindications for the use of, 1035
      defined, 1034
      how anesthesia is maintained during,
        1035
      manual, instituting and conducting,
        1034–1035
  for liver transplantation
    albumin levels and, 493
    combined tecnique, role for, 504
    drugs to avoid, 504
    induction, considerations for, 503
    informed consent, risks included in, 500
    maintenance, agents for, 504
  for lung transplantation
    inducement procedures, 95–96
    volatile, avoided during single-lung
      ventilation, 97
  for neuraxial blocks, pain management and
    agent used for, 652, 653t
    for bilateral block, 653–654
    local, maximum safe dose of, 653, 653t
    local, systemic reaction to, 654
    technique used for, 645
  for pacemaker surgery
    inhalational gases, avoiding certain, 243
    preoperative preparations for, 241
  for preeclampsia, 919
    abnormal fetal heart rate seen with maternal
      hypotension, treatment for, 921
    accidental spinal tap, 921
    choosing, 919
    epidural, bleeding time and platelet count
      evaluation and, 920
    epinephrine and, 921
    ergonovine and, 922
    general, for cesarean delivery, 923
    hypertension, agents to prevent, 923
    level of, 920
    local, 920–921
    postdural puncture headache, 921–922
    prehydration, 919
    spinal, when and how you give, 922–923
    total spinal, 922
  for pregnancy, surgical complications
    airway management, 943–944, *944*
    β-blockade 944
    for emergency cesarean section, 942
    general, 943
    inhalation agents, effect on uterine
      contractility, 945
  for prematurity
    intubation and, 466
    maintaining, 466–467
    requirements of preterm infant *vs.* adult,
      465–466
  for pyloric stenosis
    anatomic characteristics of the airway,
      newborn *vs.* adult, 522–523, 523t
    endotracheal tube size, determining,
      523–524, 523t
    induction–intubation sequence of, 522
    nonrebreathing systems, advantages and the
      disadvantages of, 524

postanesthesia recovery period, complications, 525

preparing patient for, 522

system of, 524

techniques or agents used for, 522

for sickle cell disease, 986–987, 989

comorbidities, effect on, 989–990

general/anesthesia, 987, 989

sickling, precautions to prevent, 990

for subarachnoid hemorrhage

arterial line for induction, necessity of, 625

concerns, during induction, 626–627

hypoxemia and hypercapnia, effects on cerebral blood flow, 628, *629*

induction and maintenance, goals of, 624

rapid-sequence induction and intubation, 627–628

smooth and safe induction and intubation, 627

for tetralogy of Fallot

inducing if intravenous access cannot be established, 416–417

inhalation, effect of, 418

pre–cardiopulmonary bypass goals of, 419

for thoracoabdominal aortic aneurysm repair

evaluation of, 258

inducing, 262–263

see also muscle relaxants

Anesthesia Patient Safety Foundation, 728, 730

aneurysmal rupture, pathophysiology of, 620

see also intracranial aneurysms; subarachnoid hemorrhage

aneurysm clipping,

anesthesia and, emergence from, 634

central venous pressure, monitoring for, 625–626

complications, other neurologic, 638

creatinine phosphokinase MB fractions, elevated, 623–624

fluid management for, 628–629

organ systems manifesting problems in, 638–639

transmural pressure in, decreasing, 630–631

angina pectoris, 142

angiotensin-converting enzyme inhibitors, for hypertension, 307, 307–308

ankle block,

advantages and disadvantages of, 661

landmarks for, 659, *660*, 661

antagonists or blockers, for hypertension, 308

antepartum hemorrhage, 884

anterior longitudinal ligament, 702–703

anteroposterior placement of pacemaker electrodes, 243, 244

antiadrenergic agents, for hypertension, 306

anticholinergic agents, 16

for Parkinson's disease, 583

anticholinergic bronchodilators, for asthma, 14

anticholinesterase, 22, 26

for myasthenia gravis, 1082

anticoagulants,

for cardiopulmonary bypass, 163–164

dosage of, 163–164

heparin and, 163–164

mechanism of, 164

antiemetics, for laparoscopic surgery, 864

antihypertensive drugs,

angiotensin-converting enzyme inhibitors, *307*, 307–308

antagonists or blockers, 308

antiadrenergic agents, 306

brain natriuretic peptides, 308

calcium channel blockers, 307, 307t

chronic angiotensin-converting enzyme inhibition, influence on anesthetic induction, 309

direct vasodilators, 306

discontinuing before surgery, 311

diuretics, 306

influence on hemodynamic responses to induction, laryngoscopy, and intubation, 309

mechanism of action of, 306

pretreat preoperatively with, 313–314

in transurethral resection of the prostate, discontinuing, 801

antiplatelet agents, for ischemic heart disease, 381

antiseizure prophylaxis, for head injury, 614

antithrombotic agents, for ischemic heart disease, 381

antiviral agents, for Parkinson's disease, 583

aorta, cross-clamping of, in cardiopulmonary bypass, 182

aortic aneurysms,

causes of, 253–254

dissecting, classification of, 254, *255*

aortic clamping and unclamping,

in abdominal aortic aneurysm repair

depressed systemic blood pressure and, 293

hemodynamic changes of, *290*, 290–291

hemodynamic consequences of, 292, *292*

aortic clamping and unclamping (*contd.*)
   infrarenal aneurysm, renal blood flow and, 291
   rising pulmonary artery occlusion pressure during, 291
   ST-segment depressions, development of, 291
   in thoracoabdominal aortic aneurysm repair
      pathophysiology of, 266–267
      response to unclamping, 267
aortic dissection, aortic aneurysms and, 253
aortic insufficiency,
   cardiopulmonary bypass, special considerations particular to, 223–224
   etiology of, 199–200
   hemodynamic management goals for, 219, 219t
   pressure/time curves for, 207, *208*
   severity of, using transesophageal echocardiography scales, 215t, 216, 222
   signs and symptoms of, 217, 217t
   see also valvular heart disease
aortic stenosis,
   cardiopulmonary bypass, special considerations particular to, 223
   etiology of, 199
   hemodynamic management goals for, 219, 219t
      combined with mitral regurgiatation, 220
   monitoring patient with, 220
   premedication for, 219
   pressure/time curves for, 206–207, *207*
   severity of, using transesophageal echocardiography scales, 215, 215t
   signs and symptoms of, 217, 217t
   see also valvular heart disease
aortic valve replacement,
apex-anterior placement of pacemaker electrodes, 243, 244
apex-posterior placement, 243, 244
Apgar scoring system,
   defined, 945
   significance of, 945, 945t
apnea, differential diagnosis, 1112
apneic oxygenation, defined, 1278
apneic spells, in prematurity, 455–456
appendectomy for pregnant patient, 949–950
   Alder's sign, defined, 951
   anesthesia
      brachial plexus block, 959
      for delivery *vs.* nonobstetric surgery, 955–956, *956,* 957
      epidural, technique and dosage of, 957
      general, technique for, 958
      isoflurane-nitrous oxide-oxygen, 959
      nitrous oxide, controversy surrounding, 959
      options, discussing with patient, 955
      technique of, in pregnant women *vs.* nonpregnant women, 955–956, *956, 957*
   anesthetic agents
      commonly used, classifications of, 953–954
      teratogenicity of, 952–953
   clinical diagnosis of, 950
   differential diagnosis, 949–950
   gangrenous, incidence of in pregnant *vs.* nonpregnant women, 950–951, *951*
   incidence of, 950
   intraoperative management
      fetal loss
         factors influencing, 958
         incidence of, 958
      for laparoscopic surgery, 960
      medication, supplemental, 958
      uteroplacental perfusion, vasopressor of choice for, 958
   intrauterine fetal asphyxia, preventing, 954
   perforation of the appendix
      incidence of, 952
      trimester most likely to occur in, 952
   postoperative management
      extubation, 960
      monitoring, 960
      precautions, other, 960–961
      preterm delivery following nonobstetric surgery during pregnancy, 961
   preoperative evaluation and preparation
      anesthesia
         for delivery *vs.* nonobstetric surgery, 955
         options, discussing with patient, 955
      premedication, 955
   teratogenicity
      of anesthetic agents, 952–953
      factors influencing, in mammals, 952
   U.S. Food and Drug Administration fetal risk categories for therapeutic agents, 953
   see also pregnancy, surgical complications in
aprotinin, 341–344, *342, 343*
aqueous humor, formation and elimination of, *1009, 1010*
Arndt catheter, 40

Artane (trihexyphenidyl), for Parkinson's
        disease, 583
arterial carbon dioxide (PaCO$_2$),
    in apneic patient, 869–870
    arterial to end-tidal CO$_2$ gradients
            (PaCO$_2$-P$_{ET}$CO$_2$), changes in during
            laparoscopy, 867, 868
    cerebral blood flow and, affect on, 556
    liver transplantation and, 491–492
arterial partial pressure of oxygen,
    age-dependent decrease in, 1180
    evaluating, 12
    during one-lung ventilation, 43
    and PaCO$_2$, 1261
arterial PCO$_2$, intraocular pressure and, affect
        of, 1009
arterial switch operation,
    described, 443
    immediate post cardiopulmonary bypass
            issues following, 446–447
    long-term neurologic outcome after, 449–450
    long-term outcomes after, 448–449
    long-term surgical problems after, 448
    myocardial ischemia, addressing in intensive
            care unit, 447
arterial to end-tidal CO$_2$ gradients
            (PaCO$_2$-PETCO$_2$), changes in during
            laparoscopy, 867, 868
    carbon dioxide (CO$_2$), 867, 868
arteria radicularis magna, 263
aspiration, 50–55
    aspiration pneumonia, 51
    aspiration pneumonitis, 50
        vs. aspiration pneumonia 51
        risk factors for, 50
    bronchial tree irrigation, bicarbonate vs.
            saline solution, 54
    development of, patient characteristics leading
            to, 50
    management strategy, initial, 52
    Mendelson syndrome, 50
        critical pH value causing, 51
        described, 50
        volume of aspirate causing, 51
    prevent during emergency surgery, 54
    prophylactic antibiotics for, 52–53
    steroid therapy for, 53
aspiration pneumonia, 51
aspiration pneumonitis, 50
    vs. aspiration pneumonia 51
    risk factors for, 50

aspirin,
    asthmatic attacks and, 5
    for myocardial ischemia, 381, 383–384
    for perioperative pain management, 732
assist-control ventilation, 62
α-stat regulation, 445
asthma,
    anesthesia
        aminophylline administration, 24–25
        β_y-agonists, administration methods for
                23, 24
        for cyanotic patient not responding to
                aminophylline, 25
        FRC and CC, effects of anesthesia on, 25
        halothane mechanisms that produce
                bronchodilation, 20
        inhalational vs. intravenous techniques, 21
        lidocaine for intubation, 19
        laryngeal mask airway vs. endotracheal
                tube, 17
        maintenance of, agents for, 20
        methohexital vs. thiopental for induction, 18
        muscle relaxants that cause histamine
                release, avoiding, 21–22, 22t
        propofol, etomidate, ketamine for induction,
                18
        rapid sequence induction, precautions, 19
        regional vs. general, 21
    differential diagnosis, compatible symptoms
            of, 3
    etiology of, 4
    intraoperative management
        for asthmatic attack in the operating room,
                17
        atropine, disadvantages of, 16–17
        bronchospasm, differential diagnoses of, 25
        hypoventilation, common causes of, 26
        lidocaine for intubation, 19
        methohexital vs. thiopental, 18
        propofol, etomidate, or ketamine for
                induction, 18
        of weezing attack, 22–23
    ischemic heart disease and, 19
    pathogenesis of, 4, 5
    postoperative management
        endotracheal tube and bronchoconstriction,
                avoiding, 26–27, 27
        extubation, 26
        oxygen administration, in chronic
                obstructive pulmonary disease
                patient, 28

asthma (*contd.*)
  pain control, narcotics for, 27–28
  preoperative evaluation and preparation
    arterial blood gases, interpreting, 12
    cimetidine, effects of, 16
    closing capacity and closing volume, 10, *11*
    closing volume, measuring, 10, *11*
    for chronic obstructive pulmonary disease
        patients, 13
    current/past medications, evaluating, 14
    dead space/tidal volume equation (V_D/V_T),
        12
    distinguish obstructive lung disease from
        restrictive lung disease using
        spirometry, 7, 7t
    flow–volume loops, 8–9, 9, 10
    functional residual capacity
      and closing capacity, effects of age and
          posture on, 10–11
      importance of in oxygenation, 12
      measuring, 12
    hypoxemia, physiologic causes of, 13
    normal lung volumes and lung capacities,
        7–8, *8*
    premedication, 16
    Q_S/Q_T (shunt equation), 12
    steroid preparations, 14–15
      intravenous, onset of action of, 15
    URI, postponing elective surgery due to, 14
    workup for, 6
  prevalence of, 3
  see also Asthmatic attacks; Lung disease
asthmatic attacks, 5–6
  changes in spirometry, lung volumes, lung
      capacities during, 6
  CO_2 retention and, 6
  hypoventilation after, causes of, 26
  hypoxemia and, 6
  postponing surgery due to, 17
  predisposing factors of, 5
  during surgery, most common cause of, 22
  wheezing
    attack during surgery, mangement of, 22–23
    causes of, 25
asymptomatic carotid atherosclerosis study, 551
atelectasis, 31
atenolol, for myocardial ischemia, 378–380
atheromatous aortic disease, 151, 153
atherosclerosis,
  accelerated, 830
  aortic aneurysms and, 253

atracurium, 22, 1019
atrial myxoma, 151
atrial natruretic peptide, 919
atrial septal defect, 107
atrioventricular block,
  first-, second-, and third-degree, diagnosing,
      232
atropine,
  for asthma, 16–17
  for cardiopulmonary bypass, 143
  for intraocular pressure, 1012
    reversal doses of, affect of, 1022
auricular acupuncture, 747
automated percutaneous discectomy, 712
autoregulation, 530
awake craniotomy. See deep brain stimulation,
awake fiberoptic intubation,
  failure of, other options available, 1003
  risks of, 1003
awake intubation, 1002
axillary nerve block,
  commonly missed nerves with, 652
  landmarks of, 648–649
  procedure of, 649
  tourniquet-related pain, managing, 652
Ayre's T-piece, Jackson-Rees modification of, 524
azathioprine, 847

baby lung, 57
back pain, low,
  diagnostic studies, 707–708
  differential diagnosis of, 708
  herniated discs, mechanism of pain from, 704
  history and physical examination, important
      points of, 706, 707t
  incidence and prevalence of, 700
  interventional treatments for, 710–711
  intervertebral disc, anatomy of, 704
  issues of, 699–700
  minimally invasive interventions, advances in,
      712–714
  multiple spine surgeries, causes of, 708
  noninterventional treatments for, 709–710
  persistent, 708–709
  risk factors for, 701–702
  societal cost of, 701
  sources of, in spine, 702–703
  spinal facets, 705
  surgery for
    disc disease, 716, *717–719*
bacteremia, 820

bacterial infection, aortic aneurysms and, 253–254

bacterial tracheitis, 1039

Bacteroides, 52

β-adrenergic antagonists,
asthmatic attacks and, 5
for ischemic heart disease, 378–380

β-adrenergic blockers, for congestive heart failure, 141–142

β_y-agonists, for asthma, 14, 16, 20, 26–27

bain Breathing circuit (Mapleson D system), 524

baker's asthma, 5

β-blockade, 944

benzodiazepines, for cardiopulmonary bypass, 153

benzothiazepines, for cardiopulmonary bypass, 142

benztropine (Cogentin), for Parkinson's disease, 583

bepridil, for cardiopulmonary bypass, 142

Bernard Soulier syndrome, 969

betaxolol HCl (betoptic), 1013

betoptic (betaxolol HCl), 1013

β-globin gene, 981, 982

bicarbonate, for aspiration, 54

bicuspid aortic valve, aortic aneurysms and, 253

Bier method (intravenous regional block), 679

bilateral superior vena cava, 107

bilevel positive airway pressure, 60, 1258

biperiden (Akineton), for Parkinson's disease, 583

bisoprolol, for myocardial ischemia, 378–380

bispectral index monitor, 863
benefits derived from using, 1220–1221
children and, 1221
limitations of, major, 1222
reading of 56, meaning of, 1222

bitolterol, for asthma, 14

Bivona Fome-Cuf, 1033

bladder explosion, 819

bladder irrigation, body temperature and, 804, 804

bladder perforation, 819

Blalock-Taussig shunt, 412, 423–424

bleeding time, 338

blind nasal intubation, 1071

blindness, caused by transurethral resection of the prostate, 817

blood-brain barrier, 541–542

blood compartment, 529

blood donation, preoperative autologous, 162

blood salvage, perioperative, 163

blood urea nitrogen, 239, 836

B-mode, 210, 211

body mass index,
defined, 1252
measuring procedure, 1252–1253

body plethysmography, 12

bolus technique, 12

bowel distension, causes and effects of, 475

bowel obstruction,
location of, small or large bowel, 474
simple and strangulated, differences between, 474
small, fluid shifts during, 475–476, 476t
see also intestinal obstruction

brachial plexus, major branches of, 646, 646

brachial plexus block,
for nonobstetric surgery in pregnant patient, 959
technique of, 646

brain natriuretic peptides, for hypertension, 308

brainstem auditory evoked potential, 530

brainstem auditory evoked response, 533, 537

breech presentation (birth),
cause of, 928
problems associated with, 928
types of, 928

bronchial blockers, 40

bronchial stenosis, 3

bronchial tree irrigation, bicarbonate vs. saline solution, 54

bronchoconstriction, 3, 4, 13, 16, 19, 21, 26

bronchodilation, 23, 24
halothane and, elicited by, 20

bronchodilators, for asthma, 14, 15, 21, 22, 25

bronchogenic carcinomas, 30
manifestations of, less common, 31
staging of, 30
survival rate, 30–31

bronchopulmonary dysplasia, 454–455

bronchoscopes, types of, 34–35

bronchoscopy, 30, 34–35, 38, 40

bronchospasm, 14–28
differential diagnosis of, 25
intraoperative, 3, 4, 23, 25

brush biopsy, 30

Budd-Chiari syndrome, 507

Buerger's disease (thromboangiitis obliterans), 657

Bullard laryngoscope, 1001

burns, 1123

burns (*contd.*)
  carbon monoxide poisoning, 1120
  cardiovascular changes that typify, 1122
  causes of death, most common, 1120
  classifying, 1115, 1115t, *1116*
  combustion, chemical products of, 1120
  Curling ulcers, 1123
  electrical burns, complications associated
      with, 1124
  fluid formula, 1121–1122, 1121t
  hematologic changes occuring in, 1123
  immune system affected by, 1122
  intraoperative management
    anesthetic agents, 1129
      inhalation *vs.* intravenous, 1129
    anesthetic induction, 1128
    arterial line and a pulmonary artery
        catheter, information obtained by,
        1127–1128
    awake intubation, 1128
    body temperature of burn victim, 1129
    hypothermia, 1129
    monitoring, 1127
    muscle relaxants, 1130
      metabolized and eliminated, 1131
      metabolizm and elimination of,
          1131–1132, 1131t
      nondepolarizing, 1131
    succinylcholine
      adverse effects associated with, 1130–1131
      contraindicated in burned patients, 1130
  liver function changes, 1123
    anesthetic implications of, 1123
  major burn, definition of according to
      American Burn Association,
      1117–1118
  major thermal injury
    known mediators released with, 1119, *1119*
    pathophysiologic changes accompanying,
        1118
    prognosis, 1119–1120
  postoperative management
    diffusion hypoxia, 1132
    monitoring during transport, 1132
    oliguria, causes of, 1132–1133
    postanesthetic shivering, 1132
  preoperative evaluation and preparation, 1124
    α_2-adrenergic agonists work
    alcohol withdrawal, signs and symptoms of,
        1127
    blood pressure treatments, 1125–1126
    delirium tremens, 1127
    high P_{CO_2} and low P_{O_2}, causes of, 1126
    mean arterial blood pressure, calculating,
        1124
    oxygen content and oxygen delivery,
        calculating, 1126–1127
    patient concerns, 1124
    tangential excision split-thickness skin graft,
        1125
    tissue hypoxia, causes of, 1127
  resuscitative measure, 1121
  "rule of nines," used on childern, 1117, *1117*
  skin, function of, 1118
  smoke inhalation burn, 1120

C5a complement, 56
calcineurin inhibitors, 847
calcium,
  cardiac electrical activity and, 142
  in pregnancy, 909
calcium channel blockers,
  for cardiopulmonary bypass, 142–143, 143t
  for hypertension, 307, 307t
  for ischemic heart disease, 380–381
  for myocardial ischemia, 380–381
calcium chloride administration, in
        cardiopulmonary bypass, 184
cAMP, 20
cancer,
  lymph node disection for, 852 (*see also*
        laparoscopic surgery)
    pelvic, 851
    prostate, 850–851
cancer pain,
  abdominal pain, differential diagnosis of, 686
  assessment of, 685–686
  causes of, 685
  classifying, 685
  components of, 684
  invasive therapy
    neuraxial neurolysis, 695–696
    neuraxial opioid infusion, 695
    neuroablative procedures, 696
    peripheral nerve blocks, 693–694
      celiac plexus block, complications of,
          694–695
      celiac plexus block, role of, 694
  nonpharmacologic management, 696–698
    distraction and reframing techniques, 698
    hypnosis, role of, 698
    neuromodulation, role of, 697

physical modalities, successfull, 697
psychologic techniques, 698
pancreatic, characteristics of, 685
pharmacologic treatment of
addiction, 690
adjuvant drugs, 690
meperidine, defined, 693
methadone, 688
advantages and disadvantages of, 688
morphine sulfate
classification of, 686–687
synthetic opioids and, difference between, 687
opioids
administration of, 691, 691t
mechanism of action of, 688
meperidine, defined, 693
meperidine and, 688
minimum effective analgesic concentration, 692, *692*
mixed opioid agonist/antagonist *vs.* opioid agonist, 687
patient-controlled analgesia, advantages and complications of, 692
rotation of, 693
side effects of, 689
side effects of, treating, 689
tolerance and physical dependence, defined, 689
tramadol (Ultram), 690
World Health Organization stepladder approach, 686, *687*
psychological factors affecting, 684
radiation therapy, 696
significance of, 683–684
suffering of patients and, 684
cannulation for left heart bypass, 261
capnogram,
common, differential diagnosis of, 1186, *1186,* 1187
normal, appearance of, *1184,* 1184–1185, *1186*
capnography, 1184
capnometer, 1184
carbidopa, for Parkinson's disease, 581–582
carbon dioxide (CO_2), in laparoscopic surgery,
absorption, systemic effects of, 878–879
arterial carbon dioxide ($PaCO_2$)
in apneic patient, 869–870
arterial to end-tidal CO_2 gradients ($PaCO_2$-$PETCO_2$), changes in, 867, 868

diffusion and solubility properties of, significance of, 857–858, 857t
disadvantages of, 856
elevation of, rapid and marked, 869
embolism
vs. air embolism 875–876, 876t
recognizing, 875
treatment of, 876–877
endogenous, 856, 869–870
end-tidal CO_2 tension reflecting CO_2 tension, 868
868, 867, 868
as gas of choice in, 855–856
hypercarbia, effects of
on bowel and gastrointestinal system, 875
on cardiovascular system, 870–871
causes of, 869
on central nervous system, 872–873
on respiratory system, 871–872
rise in, rapid, 869–870
solubility of, in blood, 858
storage of, in body, 856–857
carbonic anhydrase inhibitors, 1011, 1012
carbon monoxide poisoning, 1120
carcinoid syndrome, 31
carcinoid tumors, 3
cardiac allograft vasculopathy, 370
cardiac asthma, 3
cardiac dysrhythmias, in heart transplantation, 365–366
cardiac malformation, 107
cardiac murmurs,
in pyloric stenosis
cause of, 519
evaluate, 520
functional *vs.* organic, differentiating between, 520, 520t
cardiac output, 323–324
cardiac resynchronization therapy device, defined, 236–237
cardiac rhythm management device,
extracorporeal shock wave lithotripsy and, 247–248
magnetic resonance imaging, contraindications for, 249
radiofrequency ablation and, precautions during, 249
type and functionality of, determining, 240, 250

Cardiac Risk Stratification (American Heart
Association/American College of
Cardiology Task), 558
cardiac tamponade,
acute and delayed, difference between,
324–325
coronary blood flow in, 329–330
defined, 324
electrocardiographic abnormalities associated
with, *330*, 330–331
etiology of, 324
intraoperative management
emergency drugs for, 350
hemodynamic effects of intravenous
induction
of etomidate, 351
of fentanyl, 350
of ketamine, 350
of midazolam, 351
of propofol, 351
of thiopental, 350
induction process for cardiac tamponade,
351
monitoring procedures, during transport to
the operating room, 350
myocardial hibernation, 352
myocardial stunning, 352
opening the chest, hemodynamic changes
associated with, 352
resuscitation, management steps required
for, 351–352
low cardiac output postoperatively,
differential diagnosis of, 323–324
pericardial effusion or hematoma, caused by,
151
postcardiopulmonary bypass bleeding,
331–332, *332*
postoperative management
extubation, 353–354
hypertension in the intensive care unit,
managing, 353
preoperative evaluation and preparation
aminocaproic acid, hemostasis improved by,
348
blood component transfusions,
complications associated with,
347–348
coagulation status, evaluating, 345–346
cryoprecipitate, 346
indications for, 347
fresh frozen plasma, 346

indications for, 346–347
hemodynamic findings, interpreting,
344–355
human immunodeficiency virus, risk of
acquiring, 348
low output, treating, 345
platelet concentrate, 347
premedications, 349–350
surgical preparations, 349
and primary pump failure, differentiation
between, 227
roentgenographic and echocardiographic
findings in, 331
ventricular interaction in, 329
cardiac tumors, 151
cardiopulmonary bypass,
Allen's test, defined, 144
anesthesia
desflurane, cardiovascular effects of, 155
enflurane, cardiovascular effects of, 155
fentanyl, cardiovascular effects of, 155
halothane, cardiovascular effects of, 155
inducing, 153–154
inhalation *vs.* intravenous agent, 154
intraoperative management of, 175
isoflurane, cardiovascular effects of, 155
dangers of, in patients with coronary
artery disease, 156
maintaining, 154
morphine, cardiovascular effects of, 155
nitrous oxide, cardiovascular effect of,
157–158
sevoflurane, cardiovascular effects of, 155
anticoagulant given before, choosing, 163–164
dosage of, 163–164
heparin and, 163–164
monitoring, 164
mechanism of, 164
aorta, cross-clamping of, 182
in acute respiratory distress syndrome, 55
arterial blood gases and electrolytes
correcting, according to body temperature,
178, 179t
measuring, blood temperature and, 177–178
arterial switch operation and
immediate post cardiopulmonary bypass
issues following, 446–447
autologous transfusion for, 162–163
β-adrenergic blockers, role of in treating
congestive heart failure 141–142
β-blocker (metropolol)

discontinuing, reasons for, 141
half-life of, defined, 141
intraoperative hypotension, managing, 142
blood conservation for, 162–163
blood sugar level changes, 184–185
calcium chloride administration, 184
cardioplegic solution and, 181–182
coagulation factors, effects of
cardiopulmonary bypass on, 186
coronary artery bypass grafting
indications for, 135
pulmonary artery occlusion pressure
representing left ventricular
end-diastolic volume after, 195
results of, 137
defibrillating internally, 183
digoxin, 141
esmolol, indications and contraindications for,
160–161
fluid balance, estimating, 180
heart rate, adjusting, 184
in heart transplantation, 363–364
hemodilution
advantages and disadvantages of, 167
blood viscosity changes during, 174
pump flow during, adjusting, 173
heparin
neutralizing drugs for, 189
reversing, 187–188
hyperglyccmia, neurologic complications and,
184–185
hypertension
correcting, 159–160
treating, 170–171
hypocapnia and, disadvantages of, 177
hypotension, treating, 160, 170
hypothermia
advantages of, 173
benefits to the brain during low-flow
cardiopulmonary bypass and DHCA,
444–445
blood viscosity changes during, 174
death associated with, main causes of, 175
neuroprotection and, 174
pump flow during, adjusting, 173–174
in infants/children *vs.* adults, for transposition
of the great arteries, 440–441, 440t,
441t
inotropic support, determining need for, 187,
188
intraaortic balloon pump

complications of, 194–195
indications for, 193
principles of, 193–194, *194*
intraoperative transesophageal
two-dimensional echocardiography,
principles and clinical applications of,
150–152, 151, *152*
labetalol, indications and contraindications
for, 160–161
left ventricle, venting of, 165
left ventricular function, evaluating, 138–139,
139
low-flow cardiopulmonary bypass, 444
in lung transplantation, 92, 93, 94, 100
metoprolol, indications and contraindications
for, 160–161
monitoring procedures used in, 143–144, 168
of blood pressure, 169
continuous, for normal pulmonary artery
occlusion pressure, 161
electrocardiogram and
monitoring, using lead V_5, 149
monitoring left ventricle without
precordial leads, 149–150
of heparin, 164
multiple temperature, reason for, 145
of pressure in pulmonary artery
catheterization, 146
muscle relaxants
administered during, 175–176
choosing, 158
reversing, 196
myocardial infarction, preventing, 159
myocardial ischemia
detecting, *148*, 148–149
hemodynamic consequences of, 147–148
intraoperative, preventing, 159
prophylactic nitroglycerin for, 159
myocardial oxygen consumption
calcium channel blockers and, 142–143, 143t
contractility, measuring, 140, *140*
determinants of, 139, 154
determining factors of, 140–141
Myocardial Wall Tension and, estimating,
140
myocardium, preserving, 180–181
nifedipine and, 142–143, 143t
oxygenators
gas flow used, amount of, 177
gas used in, type of, 177
rewarming and cooling patient by, 183

cardiopulmonary bypass (*contd.*)
   types and purposes of, 165–166
   partial bypass, defined, 165
   perfusion during, 176
   plasma hemoglobin, renal threshold for, 182
   platelet factors, effects of cardiopulmonary
      bypass on, 186
   postoperative complications and, 195
   premedication for, 143
   priming solution used in, 166–167
   protamine
      action mechanism of, 189
      complications of using too much, 189–190
      dosage of, 187
      hypotension developing after administration
        of, 190
        treating and preventing, 190–192, 191, 192
   pulmonary artery occlusion pressure
      defined, 146
      increased, correcting, 161
      measurement of, 149
      representing left ventricular end-diastolic
        volume after coronary artery bypass
        grafting, 195
      as sensitive indicator of myocardial
        ischemia, 148–149
   pulmonary artery catheterization
      complications of, 147
        from pulmonary artery catheter, 147
        from venopuncture sites, 147
      placement of, *145*, 145–146
      pressure monitoring and, 146
   pumps used in, 167
      flow of
        adjusting during hemodilution, 173
        adjusting during hypothermia, 173
        amount of, 171
      pulsatile, 167–168
   respirator, weaning patient from, 196
      criteria used for, 197
   results of, 137
   sodium nitroprusside, nicardipine, and
      nitroglycerin intravenous infusion,
      171, 172t
   sternal splitting, procedures during, 161
   ST-segment depression, treating, 158–159
   termination of cardiopulmonary bypass,
      preparing for, 186–187
   tests for, preoperative, 138
   total cardiopulmonary bypass, defined, 165
   triple-vessel coronary artery disease in

   coronary arteries, branches of, 134–135, *135*
      defined, 134
   urine and, pink color of, 182
   valvular heart disease and, 223–224
   valvular regurgitation in, 151
   valvular stenosis in, 151
   venous reservoir, low blood level of, 180
   weaning from cardiopulmonary bypass
      following aortic valve replacement and
        mitral valve replacement, 225
      temperature and, 182–183
cardioversion, in acute respiratory distress
      syndrome, 55
carotid and vertebral artery transluminal
      angioplasty study, 554
carotid artery disease,
   cerebral perfusion in the presence of, 552
   cerebral vasculature and, 552
   natural course of, 550
   prevalence of, 549–550
carotid atherosclerotic disease, surgical
      intervention, 551
carotid endarterectomy, 1204
   diabetes mellitus as a risk factor for, 550–551
   intraoperative management
      anesthesia
        cerebral blood flow and, effects on,
          568–569
        choosing, 566–567
        general, 567
        protective effects of, on cerebral function,
          569–570
        regional, 568
        ventilation, 571
      blood pressure, managing, 571–572
      intravenous fluids, 573
      monitoring, 560–561 (*see also* cerebral blood
        flow)
        of cerebral perfusion, 561, 564–565
        somatosensory evoked potentials, 565
        transcranial Doppler, 565–566
        unprocessed electroencephalogram *vs.*
          processed electroencephalogram,
          561–562, *563*
      reperfusion injury, 573
   postoperative management
      complications, immediate, 575
      of high blood pressure, 574
      neurocognitive dysfunction, 576
      when patient does not wake up, 574
   preoperative evaluation and preparation

blood pressure and, 559
  laboratory data, 559–560
  premedication, 560
  what to look for, 557–558
carotid revascularization, surgical approaches
        to, 553–554
Carotid revascularization using endarterectomy
        or stenting systems, 554
carotid stenosis, presenting symptoms of, 549
carotid stenting, 554
catecholamine,
  for asthma, 19
  pathway for synthesis and breakdown of, 771,
        771
  stimulation of during pheochromocytoma
        surgery, 778
catechol-O-methyltransferase inhibitors, for
        Parkinson's disease, 582–583
causalgia, 671
celiac plexus block, for cancer pain, 694–695
cell savage, role of in obstetric patients, 900–901
central nervous system,
  dysfunction, caused by transurethral resection
        of the prostate, 810
  intraocular pressure and, role of, 1010
central obesity, 1253
central pain, 674
central pontine myelinolysis, 492
central venous pressure, 325, 326
  in kidney transplant, monitoring, 837–838
  in preeclampsia, 915
cerebral autoregulation, 555–556, 556
cerebral blood flow,
  anesthesia and, effects on, 568–569
  critically low, as measured by the
        electroencephalogram, 555
  determinants of, 530, 556
  measuring, intraoperatively, 562, 564
  normal, 554
  $PaCO_2$ and, affect on, 556
  presence of intracranial tumor and, altering
        effects of
cerebral contusion, 599
cerebral hematoma, 599
cerebral perfusion pressure, 535, 608–609
  carotid artery disease and, in the presence of,
        552
  internal carotid stump pressure and, 564–565
  monitoring of, 561
cerebral salt wasting syndrome, 601
cerebral steal syndromes, 531

cerebral vascular accidents, 550
cerebral vasculature,
  anatomy of, 552
  carotid artery disease and, 552
  Circle of Willis and, 552, 553
cerebral vasospasm,
  causes of, 635–636
  defined, 635
  diagnosis of, 636
  pathophysiologic changes seen in, 636
  prevention of, 637
  treatments for, 637
cerebrospinal fluid,
  compartment, 529
  drain, 254
cervical masses, differential diagnosis of,
        1063–1064
  see also congenital heart defects
Charcot joint, 656
Charcot- Marie-Tooth disease, 656
cheiloplasty, 1056
chemical pneumonias, 3
chemonucleolysis, 712
chest roentgenogram, 1215
childhood obstructive sleep apnea, 1255
Child-Turcotte-Pugh score, 490, 490t
cholecystectomy, 17
cholinesterase activity, atypical, 1107
cholinesterase inhibitors, for asthma, 21
chronic airway inflammation, 4
chronic angiotensin-converting enzyme, 309
chronic bronchitis, 3, 31
chronic liver disease,
  fulminant hepatic failure and, 497
  neurologic manifestations of, 497
  problems related to, 489–490
  resulting in referral for liver transplantation,
        causes of, 488–489
  see also liver transplantation
chronic obstructive pulmonary disease, 8
  with asthma
    oxygen administration in recovery room, 28
    special preoperative preparations for, 13
  blood gases compatible with, 12
  carotid endarterectomy and, 559
  cigarette smoking and, 31
  flow–volume loops for, 8
  in lung transplant patients
    manifestations of, expected, 88
    survival rate of, 104
  in thoracic aortic aneurysm pateints, 259

chronic opioid therapy, 733
  chronic opioid-consumtion *vs.* abuse otr
      addiction, 734
  increased postoperative pain and, 733–734
  opioid-tolerant patient
    discharging, 736–737
    perioperative pain management choices for,
      735–736
    surgery and, 734
chronic postsurgical pain syndrome, 743–744
chronic postthoracotomy pain syndrome, 723
chronic renal disease, 824
  hypertension in, 830
cigarette smoking, 31
cimetidine, for asthma, 16
Circle of Willis, 552, 553
circumscribed extrapulmonary extension, 31
cisatracurium,
  for asthma, 19, 21–22
  for open-eye injury, 1019
cleft palate and cleft lip,
  anatomic concept of, 1050, *1051*
  anesthesia
    Abbe flap and, 1057–1058
    complications of, 1057
    crucial problem of, 1058
    management, 1056
    pharyngeal flap and, 1057
  associated conditions, 1052
  cause of, 1050
  closure of, indications and timing of, 1053
  incidence of, 1050
  intraoperative management
    cheiloplasty and palatoplasty, monitors for,
      1056
    complications, 1057
    laryngospasm
      defined, 1058
      diagnosing, 1058
      managing patient with, 1058
    positioning for surgery, 1056–1057
    surgical techniques used to repair, 1057
  pathophysiology of, 1051–1052
  postoperative management
    airway, protecting, 1059
    complications, 1059
    of pain, 1060t
  preoperative evaluation and preparation
    for anesthesia, 1054–1055
    orders, 1055, 1055t
  specialized team care needed for, 1053

velopharyngeal incompetence
  defined, 1054
  diagnosing, 1054
  tonsillectomy and adenoidectomy, relation
    to, 1054
clopidogrel (Plavix), for myocardial ischemia,
    381, 383–384
closing capacity, 11
  age and posture, effects on, 10–11
  anesthesia, effects on, 11
  defining, 10
closing volume, 11
  defining, 10
  measuring, methods of, 12
  normal value of, 10
coagulation, warfarin and, 337
cocaine, as eyedrops, 1013
Cogentin (benztropine), for Parkinson's disease,
    583
Cohen endobronchial blocker, 40
collagen vascular diseases,
  in aortic aneurysm patients, 253
  in valvular heart disease patients, 200
colloid oncotic pressure, 911
Color-coded Doppler flow imaging, 150, 151
combined epidural and general anesthesia, 740
combined high-frequency ventilation, 79
common coagulation cascade, 967–968, 968
complement activation, 56
complex regional pain syndrome,
  anesthesia, local
    classes of, 677
    epinephrine, addition of, 678
    onset, potency, and duration of, 677, 678t
    systemic toxicity of, 680
      cardiovascular effects, 680–681, 681t
      central nervous system effects, 680
      treatment for, 681
  central pain and, differences in, 674
  diagnosing, 670
    criteria for, 671
    intravenous regional block (Bier method)
      and, role in, 679
  differential block, defined, 677
  etiologies of, 673
  Horner syndrome
    defined, 676
    psychogenic in, pain, 676
  incidence of, 671
  nerve injury (type II), 670. 671, 675
  neuralgia and, differences in, 674

noxious stimuli (type I), 670, 671, 675
pathophysiology of development of, 673
pharmacologic management of, 679
social history of patient, relevance to
      development of complex regional
      pain syndrome, 674
spinal cord stimulation and, 679–680
stages of, 672
stellate ganglion, location of, 675
stellate ganglion block
  anatomic landmarks used, 675–676
  clinical signs of, 676
  complications of, 680
  in Horner syndrome patient, 676
  nerve fibers are interrupted in, 676
surgical sympathectomy and, 680
sympathetically independent pain and, 674,
    676, 679
sympathetically maintained pain and,
    673–674, 676, 679
sympathetic nerve supply to the arm,
    described, 675
treatment for, 679
  intravenous regional block and, role in, 679
work up for, 675
computed tomography angiogram,
computed tomography scans,
  for abdominal aortic aneurysm repair
  for aortic aneurysms, 274
  of acute respiratory distress syndrome
    patients, 57
  for head injury, *598*, 604, 607–608
congenital diaphragmatic hernia,
  classification of, 117, *117*
  congenital anomalies associated with, other,
    120
  fetal development of, 118
  hypoxemia and, causes of, 118
  incidence of, 117
  intraoperative management
    anesthesia
      inducing and maintaining, 125–126
      nitrous oxide and, 126
      100% oxygen during, 126
    body temperature, maintaining, 127
    extubation and, 128
    fluid therapy and, 128
    monitoring equipment, 125
    problems, urgent, 127–128
    ventialtion procedures, 127
persistent pulmonary hypertension and, 119

treatment of, 122
postoperative management
  hypoxemia
    causes of, 120, 128
    treatment for, 129
  mortality rate, 128–129
  problems, anticipated, 128
preoperative evaluation and preparation
  arterial blood gas analyses, interpreting,
    120–121
  extracorporeal membrane oxygenation
    advantages of, 123
    establishing, 123
    indications and contraindications to, 124
  nitric oxide, pulmonary and systemic
    circulation and, 122–123
  other measures to take, 125
  oxygenation, improving, 122
  premedication, 125
  repair of
    optimal time to, 124
    urgent, 121
  respiratory status, immediate treatment to
    improve, 121
pulmonary hypoplasia with
  prognosis and, effect on, 118
  severity, assessment of, 119
right-to-left shunting, diagnosing, 120
signs and symptoms, compatible differential
    diagnosis of, 116
congenital heart defects,
anesthesia
  airway, securing, 1071–1072
  equipemnt, circuit and monitors, 1070–1071
  for infant, inducing, 1073
  nitrous oxide, 1073
  severe blood loss and, technique for, 1073
cervical masses, differential diagnosis of,
    1063–1064
cystic hygroma, 1064
ductal patency, maintaining, 1065
hyperoxia test, defined, 1066
interoperative management
  blood loss, monitoring, 1072–1073
  quiet surgical field, accomplishing, 1074
interrupted aortic arch syndrome
  defined, 1064–1065
  pathophysiology of, 1065
postoperative management
  procedures for, 1074
preoperative evaluation and preparation

congenital heart defects (*contd.*)
    for congestive heart failure
        causes of, in infant, 1068–1069
        optimizing properative treatment of, 1069
        signs of, in infant, 1068–1069
        difficult airway in children
        airway, optimizing securing of, 1067
        catagorizing, 1066
        features of, noting on physical exam, 1067
      immobilizing the infant, 1070
      laboratory studies necessary for, 1067–1068
      premedication, 1070
      studies, to evaluate mass, 1066
    prostaglandin infusion, side effects of, 1065
    22q11 deletion syndrome
      associated cardiovascular defects in,
          1062–1063
      defined, 1062
      endocrinologic consequences of, 1063
      immunologic findings in, 1063
congenital heart disease, 151
congenital stenosis, 200
congestive heart failure, 1198
    causes of, in infant, 1068–1069
    increased normal pulmonary artery occlusion
        pressure and, correcting, 161
    optimizing properative treatment of, 1069
    signs of, in infant, 1068–1069
continuous positive airway pressure, 83, 95, 1258
continuous positive pressure ventilation, 77
continuous ultrafiltration, 442
continuous venovenous hemofiltration, 503
continuous wave Doppler, 152, 212, 214, 403,
    457
CO_2 retention, in asthmatic attacks, 6
corneal abrasions, preventing, 1023
coronary arteries, branches of, 134–135, 135
coronary artery bypass grafting,
    in cardiac tamponade, 322
    indications for, 135
    pulmonary artery occlusion pressure
        representing left ventricular
        end-diastolic volume after, 195
    results of, 137
coronary blood flow, aortic
        clamping/unclamping and, 267
cor pulmonale, 31
corticosteroids, 772
    for asthma, 15–16
    for back pain, low, 711
    for myasthenia gravis, 1082

Coumadin therapy, 346, 597, 732
craniotomy,
    awake (*See* deep brain stimulation)
    intraoperative management
      anesthesia
        CO_2 management, 540
        effects of, on $CMRO_2$, cerebral blood flow,
          and intracranial pressure, 538–539
        goals of, 536–537
        induction, associated risks of, 537
        intravenous, 539
        nitrous oxide, 539
        opiods, 539
        volatile, 538–539, 542–543
      deliberate hypotension, achieving, 542–543
      of diuretic therapy, 540–541
      of emergence, 546
      of end-tidal carbon dioxide, dropping of, 545
      of heart rate, dropping, 543–544
      maintenance fluid, 541–542
      monitoring, 537
        for venous air embolism, 544
      for patient who does not wake up, 546
      of serum glucose, 541
      of systemic pressure, dropping of, 545
      for tight brain, 542
      venous air embolism
        monitoring options for, 544
        preventing, 545
    postoperative management
      complications, 547
      monitoring level, 547
    preoperative evaluation and preparation
      anesthesia
        intracranial hypertension and, 532–533
        monitoring and, effect on, 533
      approach to, 532
      intracranial hypertension, preoperative
        management of, 532–533
      positioning and
        determining, 535
        disadvantages associated with, 534
        options for, 533–534
        sitting, 534, 535
      premedication, 536
creatinine clearance, 279–280, 836–837
cricothyroidotomy, 1003–1004
cromolyn, for asthma, 14, 16
cross-clamping of aorta, in cardiopulmonary
        bypass, 182
cross-matching, 834

croup,
  anesthetic implications of, 1040–1041
  characteristics of, 1041t
  defined, 1039
  medical management of, 1040–1041
  postextubation, 525–526, 1043
  severity of, assessment of, 1039, 1039t
  spasmodic, 1039
cryoprecipitate, 346
  components in, 973
  factor VIII activity present in, 973
  indications for, 347, 973
  preparation of, 973
Curling ulcers, 1123
Cushing's syndrome, 31
cyclic adenosine monophosphate, 20
cyclogel (cyclopentolate), 1012
cyclooxygenase 2 inhibitors, 741
cyclopentolate (cyclogel), 1012
cystic fibrosis, lung transplantation for, 89, 90
cystic hygroma, 1064
cystic medial necrosis, 199–200
cytomegalovirus, 101
cytotoxic drugs, for myasthenia gravis, 1082

dantrolene prophylaxis, 1099
dead space/tidal volume equation, 12, 1261–1262
deafferentation pain, 674
declamping shock, 292
deep brain stimulation,
  hemiplegia, differential diagnosis of, 594
  intraoperative management
    airway management, 590
    anesthesia
      choosing, 591–592
      electrode implants, anesthetic
        implications for, 590
      magnetic resonance imaging unit,
        considerations in, 587–589
    blood pressure, control of, 592
    of cough, 593
    fluid administration, 590–591
    monitoring
      of the brain, 591
      invasive, 591
      required, 591
    pain management, 593–594
    prolonged procedure, complications of, 593
    responsivness of patient, 593
  postoperative management
    of comatose patients, 594

hemiplegia, differential diagnosis of, 594
    long-term success rate of procedure, 596
    pain management, 594
    same day discharge, 595
    of second stage of procedure, 595
      electrode insertion and, 595–596
  preoperative evaluation and preparation
    airway management, precautions for, 587
    anesthesia
      implications for, 584–585, 585t
      plan for, 586
    laboratory evaluations, 585–586
    premedication, 586–587
deep hypothermic circulatory arrest, 262
deliberate hypotension, producing in scoliosis,
      1175–1176
delirium tremens, 1127
denervated heart,
  implication of, 369
  pathophysiology of, 365
"De-Qi", 747
dermatomyositis, 981
desflurane,
  for asthma, 20
  cardiovascular effects of, 155
desmopressin D-arginine vasopressin, 966
  for hemostatic management, 340, 974
DHPR genes, 1096
diabetes insipidus, 601
diabetes mellitus,
  anesthesia
    insulin and glucose, effects on, 791, 793
    preparing patient for, 790
    techniques, 793
  autonomic neuropathy, signs and implications
      of, 789–790
  blood glucose control, perioperative, 795
  carotid endarterectomy and, as a risk factor
      for, 550–551
  classifying, 784
  complications of, 784–785
  control of, monitoring, 787
  diabetic ketoacidosis, management of,
      787–788
  etiology of, factors in, 783–784
  forms of, treatment for, 785–786, 785t, 786t
  hyperglycemia, intraoperative, 793–794
  insulin and glucose
    effects of surgery and anesthesia on, 791,
      793
    factors that alter, 787

diabetes mellitus (*contd.*)
managing on day of surgery, 790–791, 792t
nonketotic hyperosmolar coma, defined, 788
perioperative risk in, 795
postoperative control of, 794
complications, expected, 794
premedication, 791
preoperative evaluation of patient, 789
prevalence of, 783
stiff joint syndrome, airway management and, 789
diabetic ketoacidosis, 787–788
diagnostic peritoneal lavage, 1138–1139
diarylaminopropylamine, for cardiopulmonary bypass, 142
dibucaine number, significance of, 1107–1108, 1108t
differential block, defined, 677
diffusion hypoxia, 1132, 1279
DiGeorge syndrome. See 22q11 deletion syndrome,
digitalis, to treat congestive heart failure in prematurity, 457
digits, infections of, 656
digoxin, for cardiopulmonary bypass, 141
dihydropyridines, for cardiopulmonary bypass, 142
diltiazem,
for cardiopulmonary bypass, 142, 143t
for myocardial ischemia, 380–381
dilutional coagulopathy, 512
diphenhydramine, for asthma, 16
diphenylpiperazines, for cardiopulmonary bypass, 142
dipyridamole, for myocardial ischemia, 381
dipyridamole thallium/sestamibi, 831
direct vasodilators, for hypertension, 306
disseminated intravascular coagulation, 512, 607, 818
in peripartum hemorrhage
blood products, use of additional, 895–896
defined, 894–895
emergency release blood, role of, 896
epidural, removing, 902–903
hypotension, concerns with, 903
recombinant factor VII (rFVIIa), role of, 896
distal aortic anastomosis, 262
distal aortic perfusion/left heart bypass, 263–264
distraction techniques, 698
diuretics, for hypertension, 306
dobutamine stress echocardiography, 831

donation after cardiac death, 488
dopamine agonists, for Parkinson's disease, 582
dopaminergic agonists, for hypertension, 306–307
Doppler echocardiography, 150, 152
Color-coded Doppler flow imaging, 150, *151*
color modalities, 208
pressure gradients derived from, 210, 212, *214*
transcranial, carotid endarterectomy and, 565–566
double-lumen tube,
correct positioning of, 38–39, *39*
endotracheal tubes, contraindications to use, 37–38
in lung transplantation, positioning of, 95, 96
right- or left-sided, choosing, 38
Down syndrome, 1052
doxacurium, 22
for cardiopulmonary bypass, 158
droperidol,
for asthma, 16, 21
for laparoscopic surgery, 864
drug overdose, in acute respiratory distress syndrome, 55
D-Tubocurarine, 22
ductus arteriosus, 120
duodenal atresia, 107
dysesthesia, 672
dyskinesia, 150

ε-aminocaproic acid, 974–975
echothiophate iodide (phospholine iodide), 1013
edrophonium (Tensilon), for myasthenia gravis, 1082
Ehlers-Danlos syndrome, aortic aneurysms and, 253
ejection fraction, defined, 202–203
elastance, 59
elastic recoil, pulmonary, 64
electrical burns, 1124
electroacupuncture, 747, 749–750
electrocardiogram,
for abdominal aortic aneurysm repair
for cardiopulmonary bypass
monitoring, using lead V_5, 149
monitoring left ventricle without precordial leads, 149–150
for trauma patient, 998
electrocautery, 245
electroconvulsive therapy, 248
contraindications for, 1202

indications for, 1202
intraoperative management
    airway management, 1207
    anesthetic induction, 1206
    arterial line, need for, 1205
    cerebral hemodynamic effects, 1206
    hemodynamic response, typical, 1204–1205
    hemodynamic stability, attempt to
        maximize, 1205–1206
mechanism of action for, 1202–1203, 1203t
postoperative management
    outpatient therapy, 1208
    postictal agitation, risk factors for, 1207
preoperative evaluation and preparation
    anticoagulation, mangament of, 1203
    cardiac status, assessment of, 1203
    for carotid endarterectomy, 1204
    permanent pacemaker or implantable
        cardiovertor-defibrillator and, 1204
    sleep apnia and, 1204
    for transient ischemic attack, 1204
electroencephalography, 537
electromechanical interference,
    environmental, 250–251
    inappropriate inhibition and, determining, 245
    preventing from electrocautery, 245–246
electromyography, 530, 533
embolic strokes, 550
embolization therapy, preoperative, 531
emotional stress, asthma and, 5
emphysema, 31
    lung transplantation for, 89
end diastolic pressure, 148
endobronchial disease, 3
endocrine adenomatosis, multiple, 773, 773t
endorphins, 688
endothelin 1, 908
endothelium derived relaxing factor, 908
endotracheal spray, 17
endotracheal tube, 17, 37–38
    bronchial blockers and, 40
    for laryngeal lesions, laser treatment for
        protecting external surface of, 1032
    special, for laser surgery, 1033
    for lung transplantation, 96
    for tracheoesophageal fistula repair, 111, 112,
        113
endovascular aortic aneurysm repair,
    anesthesia for, 287
endovascular thoracoabdominal aortic
    aneurysm repair,

anesthetic considerations for, 269
candidates for, 268
complications of, 270
surgical steps for, 269
end-stage liver disease, 489, 490
    electrolyte and acid–base abnormalities in,
        491–492
    hemodynamic changes encountered in, 496
    Na, K, Mg, pH, and $PaCO_2$, discuss, 491–492
    transjugular intrahepatic portosystemic shunt
        procedure and, 493–494
    see also liver transplantation
end-stage renal disease,
    cardiovascular disease in, risk of, 830–831
    causes of, 823
    clinical manifestations of, 823–824
    electrolyte imbalances in, 829
    hematologic issues in, 824
    hyperkalemia, 828
    hypernatremia in, evaluation and treatment
        of, 827
    hyponatremia
        acute symptomatic, 827
        evaluation and treatment of, 826–827, 826t
        hypoosmolar hyponatremia, 826, 826t
        hypovolemic, 826–827
        isoosmolar hyponatremia, 826
    metabolic acidosis, correcting, 829–830
    solute and water disturbances in, 825–826
    transfusion in, 825
end-systolic pressure–volume relation, 202, 203,
    203
end-tidal CO_2 (PETCO2), 417, 545
end-tidal CO_2 (PETCO2), 1184
    arterial to end-tidal CO_2 gradients
        ($PaCO_2$-PETCO2), changes in during
        laparoscopy, 867, 868
enflurane,
    for asthma, 20, 22
    cardiovascular effects of, 155
environment, asthmatic attacks and, 5
eosinophilic pneumonias, 3
epiaortic echocardiography, 151
epidural adhesiolysis, 712
epidural hematomas, 599
epidural neuroplasty, 712
epiduroscopy (or spinal canal endoscopy), 712
epiglottitis,
    acute, outcomes for child with, 1048
    airway, securing, 1045
    causes of, 1041

epiglottitis (*contd.*)
  clinical manifestations of, 1042
  defined, 1041
  diagnosing, 1042–1043
  general anesthesia administered to children
    with, 1044–1045
  general used for, in children, 1044
  incidence of, 1041
  intubation for, 1044
  rapid-sequence induction, 1046
epinephrine, 769–770, 921, 1013
ergonovine, 922
ergot alkaloids, for uterine atony, 898
erythropoietin, preoperative use of, 162
Escherichia, 52
esmolol,
  for cardiopulmonary bypass, 160–161
  for myocardial ischemia, 378–380
esophageal rupture, 110
esters, 677
etomidate,
  for asthma, 18
  for cardiac tamponade, 351
  for cardiopulmonary bypass, 153
  for myocardial ischemia, 393
  for open-eye injury, as an induction agent,
    1020
European Carotid Surgery Trial, 551
exercise, asthmatic attacks and, 5
expanded criteria donor, 832
expiratory reserve volume, 6, 8
extracellular fluid, 826
extracorporeal membrane oxygenation, 76
  for congenital diaphragmatic hernia patients
    advantages of, 123
    establishing, 123
    indications and contraindications to, 124
  for hypoxemia after lung transplantation, 100
  indications/contraindications for, 76
  results of, 76–77
  uses of, 77
extrinsic coagulation cascade, 967–968
extubation,
  of congenital diaphragmatic hernia patients,
    128
  for tracheoesophageal fistula repair, 114
eyedrops, 1012–1013
eye injury. See open-eye injury,

factor IX deficiency, 965
factor VIII,
  administering, bolus *vs.* infusion technique,
    971–972
  advantages and disadvantages of products,
    974, 974t
  bolus injection, failure to respond to, 972
  circulating inhibitors, safety of administering
    to patients with, 977
  coagulation response following infusion, 972
  components of, different, 966
  in cryoprecipitate, 973
  different components of, 966
  fresh frozen plasma and, activity in, 972–973
  inhibitors, transfusions increasing potential
    for development of, 977
  levels of necessary for hemostasis, 969, 969t
  one unit of, 971
  supplements using home infusion, treating
    with, 979
failed back surgery syndrome, 708–709
familial thoracic aortic aneurysm syndrome,
    aortic aneurysms and, 253
fatty acid metabolism, 910
felodipine, for cardiopulmonary bypass, 142
felon, 656
fenoprofen, asthmatic attacks and, 5
fenoterol, for asthma, 14
fentanyl,
  for asthma, 19, 21
  for cardiac tamponade, 350
  for cardiopulmonary bypass, 154
    cardiovascular effects of, 155
  for renal failure, 844
Fetal alcohol syndrome, 1052
fetal heart rate,
  acute fetal distress, causes of, 939
  with beat-to-beat variability, normal, 935
  fetal blood gases, normal values of, 938
  fetal scalp capillary blood pH sampling, false
    signals from, 939
  hypoxia leading to acidosis, assessment of,
    937–938
  monitoring of, 935
  predicting fetal well-being, accuracy of, 937
  transient or periodic decelerations, 935–937,
    936
fetal lie,
  defined, 927
  determining, 927
  transverse lie
    etiology of, 927
    obstetric management for, 928

problems associated with, 928

fetal loss, from nonobstetric surgery for pregnant patient,
  factors influencing, 958
  incidence of, 958
fetal oxygenation, determinants of, 934
fetal scalp capillary blood pH sampling, false signals from, 939
fiberoptic bronchoscopy, for tracheoesophageal fistula repair, 112–113
fiberoptic intubation, 1071–1072
fibrinolysis, 341
fingal infection, aortic aneurysms and, 253–254
flexible FOB bronchoscope, 34–35
flow–volume loops, 8–9, 9, 10
flufenamic acid, asthmatic attacks and, 5
Focused Abdominal Sonography for Trauma, 1138, 1142
Fogarty catheters, 40, 112, 113
Foley catheters, 40, 109
forced expiratory volume, 1159
forced vital capacity, 6, 9, 1159
foreign body aspiration, 3
fraction of inspired oxygen (FIO_2), 12, 22
fresh frozen plasma, 346
  in hemphilia patients
    administration of, indications for, 973
    factor VIII activity present in, 972–973
  indications for, 346–347
  liver transplantation and, 494–495
  in peripartum hemorrhage, 895–896
fulminant hepatic failure, 489
functional residual capacity, 6, 8
  age and posture, effects on, 10–11
  anesthesia, effects on, 6, 8
  measuring, methods of, 12
  oxygenation and, importance of, 12
furosemide, for diuretic therapy in craniotomy, 541

gallamine, 22
gangrenous appendix, 950–951, 951
gastric distension, avoiding in positive pressure ventilation, 109–110, 113
gastroesophageal reflux disease, 1207
Glasgow Coma Scale, 603–604t, 606, 607, 996, 996t
glaucoma,
  in ambulatory surgery
    anesthetic implications of, 1210–1211
    discontinuing before surgery, 1212
    eye drops used to treat, 1212
  defined, 1011
  premedication contraindicated in, 1011
glomerular filtration rate,
  in kidney transplant, 829, 837
  in preeclampsia, 912
glomerular imbalance, 518
glucocorticoids, 772
  replacement therapy, 14–15
glycation, 787
glycine, metabolic byproducts of, 814, 814–815
glycine toxicity, 814
Goldenhar's syndrome, 1052
Goodpasture syndrome, in acute respiratory distress syndrome, 55
G6PD deficiency, 981
graft implantation, hemodynamic alterations during lung transplantation, 99–100
gram-negative sepsis, 485
guanosine monophosphate, 17

Haemophilus influenzae, 51
Haemophilus parainfluenzae, 1039
halothane,
  for asthma, 20, 22
  cardiovascular effects of, 155
  for laparoscopic surgery, 864
hand acupuncture, 747
head injury,
  electrolyte abnormalities and, 602
    sodium and potassium balance, alterations in, 601–602
  female sex hormones, pathophysiology of traumatic brain injury and, 603
  gender, pathophysiology of traumatic brain injury and, 603
  hyperglycemia, effect on neurologic outcome, 601
  intracranial, types of, 599
  intraoperative management
    anesthesia
      to avoid, 611
      of choice, 611
    arterial hypertension, implications of, 609
    of blood pressure, 608
    cerebral perfusion pressure, 608–609
    hypcrventilation and, 608
    hypothermia, 611–612
    intravenous fluid replacement, 609
      of corticosteroids, 609–610
      of hypertonic saline, 610

head injury (*contd.*)
> monitoring
>> during computed tomography and craniotomy, 608
> magnesium, neuroprotective effects of, 602
> mannitol administration, risks and benefits of, 600
> postoperative neurointensive care management
>> antiseizure prophylaxis, role of, 614
>> cerebral oxygenation monitoring, 614
>> hyperthermia, preventing, 614–615, *615*
>> of intracranial pressure, 612
>>> measures, 613
>>> monitoring of, 613
>> ventilation, 612
> preoperative evaluation and preparation
>> airway management, 606
>>> in combative patient, 606
>>> facial fractures/swelling and, 606
>> cervical spine, clearing, 605–606
>> coagulation abnormalities, 607
>> computed tomography scan and, 604–605
>> endotracheal intubation, benefits of early, 606
>> Glasgow Coma Scale and, 603–604t, 606, 607
>> hemostasis, treatment modalities to provide
>> intracranial hematoma expansion, reducing, 607
>> intracranial pressure monitoring
>>> role of, 605
>>> succinylcholine and, effects of, 607
>> of neurologic function, 603–604
> secondary
>> contributing factors of, 600
>> *vs.* primary 600
heart failure,
> New York Heart Association classification of, 218, 375, 449
see also pregnancy, surgical complications of
heart transplantation,
> combined heart/lung transplant, indication for, 360
> important differences in, 360
> diagnoses requiring, 356–357, *357*
> donor heart selection, criteria for, 358
> intraoperative management
>> anesthesia
>>> equipment for, 362
>>> induction and maintenance of, 363

>>> left ventricular assist device insertion, considerations for, 361
>> cardiopulmonary bypass and, 363–364
>> monitors for, 362
>> transesophageal echocardiography, role of, 362–363
> medical and surgical alternatives to, 360
> perioperative donor management, principles of, 358–359
> perioperative evaluation and preparation
>> assessment of patient, 361–362
>> premidication and, 362
> postoperative management
>> cardiac dysrhythmias, common, 365–366
>> complications, early, 364
>> denervated heart, pathophysiology of, 365
>> early graft failure, causes of, 367
>> in intensive care unit, 367
>> nitric oxide, as a selective pulmonary vasodilator, 365
>> posttransplant bleeding
>>> cause of, 366
>>> treating, 366
>> right heart failure
>>> mechanisms of, 364
>>> treating, 364
> posttransplant mortality, risk factors associated with, 359
> recipient selection, indications and contraindications for, 357–358
> subsequent noncardiac surgery
>> allograft rejection, significance of, 369
>> ambulatory surgery and, 371
>> anesthesia
>>> best type for, 368
>>> implications for, 368
>>> technique of, 368
>> cardiac allograft vasculopathy, 370
>> denervated heart, implication of, 369
>> drug interactions, significant implications of, 370
>> infection, significance of, 369–370
>> monitoring, 367
>> muscarinic antagonist with cholinesterase inhibitors, to reverse muscle relaxant, 368
>> posttransplant hypertension, significant implication of, 370–371
>> renal dysfunction, significant implication of, 371
> surgical anastomoses in, sequence of, 359

ventricular assist devices, role of, 360–361

helium dilution, 12

HELLP syndrome, 923–924

hemiplegia, in deep brain stimulation, 594

hemoconcentrators, 442

hemodilution, in cardiopulmonary bypass,
    advantages and disadvantages of, 167
    blood viscosity changes during, 174
    pump flow during, adjusting, 173

hemoglobin C disease, 982

hemoglobinopathies, 981, 982

hemoglobin solutions, 1152

hemophilia,
    A, B, and C, differences between, 965
    clot extending beyond injury site, prevention
        of, 967
    coagulation cascade
        laboratory tests that evaluate, 969, 970t
        procoagulant factors involved in, 967–968,
            968
        specific components measured by each,
            969–970
    endothelial interruption in the blood vessel,
        physiologic events that occur
        following, 967
    intraoperative manaegment
        anethesia
            axillary block, 975
            complications during transfusion,
                immediate steps to take, 976–977
            human immunodeficiency virus, special
                considerations for patients with, 975
            blood loss, transfusing with with packed red
                blood cells or whole blood, 976
            extubation, suctioning endotracheal tube
                and oropharynx before, 978
            human immunodeficiency virus, special
                precations for patients with, 976
            intramuscular injection, safety of, 975
            tourniquet use, 978
    platelet adhesion *vs.* platelet aggregation, 966
    postoperative management
        coagulation status, enhancing, 979
        of pain, 978
    preoperative evaluation and preparation
        coagulation status, steps to correct before
            surgery, 971
        cryoprecipitate
            components in, 973
            factor VIII activity present in, 973
            indications for, 973
            preparation of, 973
        desmopressin D-arginine vasopressin, 966
            for hemostatic management, 340, 974
        ε-aminocaproic acid 974–975
        fresh frozen plasma
            in hemphilia patients
                administration of, indications for 973
                factor VIII activity present in, 972–973
        preoperative factor replacement therapy,
            between hemophilia A or hemophilia
            B, 970–971
        von Willebrand's disease, history and
            pathophysiology associated with,
            965–966
    see also factor VIII

hemoptysis, lung carcinoma and, 30

hemorrhagic strokes, 550

hemostasis,
    cell-based theory of, 968
    desmopressin for, role of, 340, 974
    factor VIII necessary for, levels of, 969, 969t

hemothorax,
    in trauma
        massive, defined, 1137
        signs and symptoms of, 1137
        thoracotomy to treat, indications for, 1137

heparin,
    antagonism mechanism of, by protamine, 336
    for cardiopulmonary bypass, 163–164
        activated coagulation time test, defined,
            164–165
        half-life of, 164
            eliminating, 164
        monitoring, 164
        neutralizing drugs for, 189
        reversing, 187–188
    for tetralogy of Fallot
        in children *vs.* adults, 420
        reversing, 420–421

heparin-induced thrombocytopenia, 334
    low molecular weight heparin and, 335–336,
        338
    therapy for, 335

heparinized saline irrigation-suction device, 866

heparin rebound, 336

hepatitis C, 489

hepatopulmonary syndrome, 495

hepatorenal syndrome, 496

herniated discs, mechanism of pain from, **704**

herniation of the nucleus pulposus, 703

hibernation, 147, 148–149

high-frequency flow interrupters, 79
high-frequency jet ventilation, 78–79
high-frequency oscillatory ventilation, 78, 79
high-frequency positive pressure ventilation and,
    77
  characteristics of, 77
  defined, 77
high-frequency ventilation, 78
  classifications of, 78, *78*
  frequencies used in, 78
  indications/precautions for, 79–80
histamine release, 18, 27
  barbiturate-induced, 18
  from morphine, 27
  from nondepolarizung muscle relaxants,
    21–22, *22*
holmium laser, 821
Horner syndrome,
  defined, 676
  psychogenic in, pain, 676
H_2-receptor antagonists, 16
human immunodeficiency virus,
  cardiac tamponade and, risk of acquiring, 348
  hemophilia, special precations for patients
    with, 976
human leukocyte antigens, 833–834, 847
human papilloma virus, cesarean delivery and,
  1026
humoral events in normal neuromuscular
  transmission, 1106
hydrocortisone acetate, 15
hydrocortisone phosphate, 15
hydronephrosis, 107
hydroxyzine hydrochloride, for asthma, 16
hyperalgesia, 672
hyperammonemia,
  in transurethral resection of the prostate
    prevalence of, 815
    preventative treatment against, 815–816, *816*
    sypmtoms and clinical course of, 815
hypercalcemia, 31
hypercarbia, effects of,
  on bowel and gastrointestinal system, 875
  on cardiovascular system, 870–871
  causes of, 869
  on central nervous system, 872–873
  on respiratory system, 871–872
hypercoagulable state, 911, 912t
hyperesthesia, 672
hyperfibrinolytic state, 511
hyperglycemia,

in cardiopulmonary bypass, neurologic
  complications and, 184–185
in diabetes mellitus, intraoperative, 793–794
in head injury, effect on neurologic outcome,
  601
hyperosmolar hyponatremia and, 826
hyperirritability, 4, 5
hyperkalemia,
  in end-stage renal disease, 828
  in liver transplantation, 508, 512
hyperkalemic cardiac arrest, 1094
hypermagnesemia, 829
hypernatremia, 541
hyperosmolar hyponatremia, 826
hyperoxia, 67
  test, defined, 1066
hypertension,
  anesthesia
    agents for maintenance of, 317–318
    hypokalemia, treating before, 312
    hypomagnesemia and, treating before, 312
    inducing, 315
    postoperative management of, 320–321
    regional, 320
  anesthetic goals for, 314–315
  arterial, in head injury, 608–609
  asymptomatic carotid bruit and, 313
  cardiac tamponade and, postoperative
    management of, 353
  in cardiopulmonary bypass
    correcting, 159–160
    treating, 170–171
  in chronic renal disease, 830
  classification of, general, 299, 299t
  clinical patterns of, 300
  controlled hypotensive technique for, 304–305
  defined, 297
  end-organ damages caused by long-standing,
    302
  essential hypertension, pathophysiology of,
    300
  etiology of, 299
  extubation and emergence, prevent
    hypertension during, 320
  fluid therapy for, 318
  interoperative control of, 319, 319t
  intubation causing hypertension
    drop in blood pressure after, 317
    left ventricular ejection fraction and, 316
    preventative measures, 316
    tachycardia and, 316

isolated systolic hypertension,
  pathophysiology of, 300–301, *301*
in lung transplantation, 89
monitoring, during surgery, 314
perioperative cardiac morbidity and, 303
perioperative cerebral and renal complications
  of, 303–304
in pheochromocytomas, differential diagnosis
  for, 768
portal, in liver transplantation, 493
in post-heart transplantation, 370–371
postponing surgery due to, 311
premedicating patient for surgery, 313
preoperative evaluation, 310
prevalence of, 298
preventing in ischemic heart disease, 396
refractory intracranial, 541
severity of, classifying, 297, 298t
tracheal intubation producing hypertension,
  315–316
in valvular heart disease, diagnosing and
  treating, 225–226
see also antihypertensive drugs; preeclampsia
hyperthermia,
  in head injury, 614–615, *615*
  malignant, 765
  in thyrotoxicosis, differential diagnosis of, 765
hyperthyroidism,
  causes of, 756
  elective surgery and, 763
  signs and symptoms of, 753, 754
hypertrophic obstructive cardiomyopathy,
  increased normal pulmonary artery occlusion
    pressure and, correcting, 161
hypertrophic obstructive cardiomyopathy, 151
hyperventilation, in head injury, 608
hypnosis, 698
hypnotics, for laparoscopic surgery, 864
hypocalcemia, 508, 512
hypocapnia, in cardiopulmonary bypass, 177
hypocarbia, 6
hypoglycemic shock, 794
hypokalemia, 31, 312
hypokinesia, 150
hypomagnesemia, 312, 512, 602
hyponatremia, 31, 492
  in end-stage renal disease
    acute symptomatic, 827
    evaluation and treatment of, 826–827, 826t
    hypoosmolar hyponatremia, 826, 826t
    hypovolemic, 826–827

isoosmolar hyponatremia, 826
  in transurethral resection of the prostate
    effect on the cardiovascular system, 811
    rapid correction of, risks of, 813
    saline administration to correct, 813
hypoosmolar hyponatremia, 826, 826t
hypophosphatemia, 31, 602
hypoplastic left heart syndrome, 441
hypotension,
  in cardiopulmonary bypass, treating, 160, 170
  as complication of endovascular
    thoracoabdominal aortic aneurysm
    repair, 270
  deliberate, 542–543
  in peripartum hemorrhage, 903
  in pheochromocytoma surgery, 780
  in transurethral resection of the prostate,
    causes of, 819
  in valvular heart disease, 227
hypothalamic-pituitary axis, 755
hypothermia,
  in burn patients, 1129
  in cardiopulmonary bypass
    advantages of, 173
    blood viscosity changes during, 174
    death associated with, main causes of, 175
    neuroprotection and, 174
    pump flow during, adjusting, 173–174
  in head injury, 611–612
  in kidney transplant, neuromuscular blockade
    and, 842
  in liver transplantation, 512
  in myocardial ischemia, 398–399
  for spinal cord protection in
    thoracoabdominal aortic aneurysms
    repair, 264
  in tracheoesophageal fistula repair, avoiding,
    111, 113
  in transurethral resection of the prostate, as
    risk factor for myocardial ischemia,
    821
  in trauma
    adverse effects of, 1149
    defined, 1149
    treatment of, 1149
hypoventilation, after asthmatic attack, 26
hypovolemic shock, 64
  crystalloid or colloid therapy to treat, 1141
  dextran or hetastarch (Hespan), 1141
  hypertonic saline, 1142
  pathophysiology of, 1140

hypoxemia, 6
  after lung transplantation, 100
  aortic unclamping and, 267
  in aspiration pneumonitis and acute
      respiratory failure, treatment for,
      66–67
  catagories of, 13
  cigarette smoking and, 31
  in congenital diaphragmatic hernia patients
    causes of, 120, 128
    treatment for, 129
  intraocular pressure and, affect of, 1009–1010
  in liver transplantation, 495
  physiologic causes of, 13
hypoxia and equipment failure,
  arterial-alveolar difference in CO_2, 1187–1188
  capnogram
    common, differential diagnosis of, 1186,
      1186, 1187
    normal, appearance of, *1184*, 1184–1185,
      1186
  capnography, 1184
  capnometer, 1184
  intraoperative management
    for gas leaks, 1196
    monitoring, 1194
      body temperature, 1195
      circulation, 1195
      oxygenation, 1194
      ventilation, 1194–1195
    for respiratory distress, 1195
  postoperative management
    for acute lung injury, 1199
    difference between shunt,
      ventilation/perfusion mismatch, and
      dead space, 1197
    hypoxemia, cause of, 1197
    mechanical ventilation, 1198–1199
    for oxygen administration, 1199–2000
    pulmonary edema, differential diagnosis of,
      1198, 1198t
    tracheal extubation, criteria for, 1196–1197
  preoperative evaluation and preparation
    contemporary anesthesia workstation,
      important safety features of, 1188
    emergency equipment readily available to
      anesthesiologist, 1193
    end-tidal CO_2 (P_{ETCO_2}) concentration, 1184
    gas leakage
      checkin for, 1190
      common sites for, 1189–1190

hemoximeter, 1181
hypoxemia
  defined, 1180
  diagnosing, 1181
hypoxia
  defined, 1180
  mainstream and sidestream gas analyzers,
    1185–1186
  PaO_2, age-dependent decrease in, 1180
  premedication, 1194
  preoperative evaluation and preparation
    equipment checkout, 1191–1193
      breathing system, 1192
      emergency ventilation equipment, 1191
      final position, 1193
      high-pressure system, 1191
      low-pressure systems, 1191–1192
      manual and automatic ventilation
        systems, 1192–1193
      monitors, 1193
      scavenging system, 1192
  pulse oximeter
    defined, 1181
    function of, 1182
    two-wavelength
      accuracy of, 1183
      calibration of, 1182
  SpO_2 readings, effect of dyshemoglobins
    methemoglobin and
    carboxyhemoglobin on, 1183
hypoxic pulmonary vasoconstriction, 42, 97
  anesthetic agents and, effects and implications
    of, 42–43
hysteroscopy, in transurethral resection of the
    prostate, 817

ibuprofen, asthmatic attacks and, 5
ideal body weight, defined, 1252
idiopathic hypertrophic subaortic stenosis, 151
  increased normal pulmonary artery occlusion
    pressure and, correcting, 161
idiopathic pulmonary fibrosis, lung
    transplantation for, 88, 89, 104
ileus, 477
immunoglobulin E (IgE), 4
immunosuppression, in acute respiratory
    distress syndrome, 55
implantable cardioverter-defibrillator,
  atrial pacing only, advantages and
    disadvantages of, 235
  defined, 237–238

indications for, 238
life span of, 237
see also pacemaker surgery
indomethacin, 5, 457
adverse effects of, 457–458
induction options, for tracheoesophageal fistula,
112
infection, aortic aneurysms and, 253–254
inflamation, aortic aneurysms and, 253–254
innervation of the larynx, 758
inspiratory capacity, 8
inspiratory reserve volume, 7
insufflation, 866
intact ventricular septum, 433, 435
intensive care unit ventilator, 23
intercostal arteries, reattachment of, 264
intercostal nerve blocks, 724
interferons, 1027–1028
intermittent positive pressure ventilation, 65
internal carotid stump pressure, and cerebral
perfusion, 564–565
international normalized ratio, 490, 494, 898
interrupted aortic arch syndrome,
defined, 1064–1065
pathophysiology of, 1065
interscalene brachial plexus block,
hemidiaphragmatic paresis after, incidence of,
649
pulmonary function changes occuring after,
650, 650–651
interscalene nerve block,
commonly missed nerves with, 652
dyspnea, 651
landmarks of, 649
procedure of, 649
intervertebral disc, anatomy of, 704
intestinal obstruction,
absorption of bacteria and bacterial products,
systemic effects of, 477
anesthesia
administration of antacids and/or H_2
blockers, small bowel obstruction
and, 480–481
incubation position, 481
induction, dangers present during, 480
inspired oxygen, benefits to use high
concentration of, 483
muscle relaxants, succinylcholine for
rapid-sequence induction, 481, 482t
nasogastric tube and, 482
nitrous oxide and, 482–483

Sellick's maneuver, 481
causes of, 473–474
ileus and, 477
post operative management
gastric contents, aspiration of, 484–485
gram-negative sepsis, 485
principles of, 483
respiratory problems, 484
preoperative evaluation and preparation
abdominal decompression, 478
methods of, 478–479
fluid management
goals of, 479
volume replacement, 479
premedication, 479–480
respiratory implications, 478
tense abdominal wall, implications of, 478
red cell mass, loss of, 477
signs and symptoms of, 474–475
radiologic, 475, 475t
systemic derangements that occur with, 476
see also bowel obstruction
intraaortic balloon pump,
for cardiopulmonary bypass
complications of, 194–195
indications for, 193
principles of, 193–194, *194*
for valvular heart disease
benefits of, for failing heart, 226
contraindications to the use of, 227
cycle of, proper timing of, 227
right heart failure and pulmonary
hypertension, 226
transesophageal echocardiography and,
226–227
intracellular fluid, 825–826
intracerebral hematomas, 599
"intracerebral steal,", 557, 571
intracranial aneurysms,
rupture of
risk factors associated with, 619
steps to be taken in the case of, 634
sizes and locations of, 620
intracranial hematomas, 599
intracranial pressure,
determinants of, 529
fulminant hepatic failure and, 497
in head injury, 612
measures, 613
monitoring
role of, 604–605

intracranial pressure (*contd*.)
  succinylcholine and, effects of, 606
  monitoring of, 613
  mass lesions and, 599
  presence of mass and, altering effects of, 529
intradiscal electrothermal therapy, 713
intraocular pressure,
  arterial P_{CO_2} and, affect of, 1009
  atropine and, reversal doses of, 1022
  carbonic anhydrase inhibitors to decrease,
      1011
  central nervous system, role of, 1010
  coughing and vomiting, affect of, 1009–1010
  deep inspiration, affect of, 1009–1010
  determinants of, 1009
  glaucoma
    defined, 1011
    premedication contraindicated in, 1011
  hypoxemia, affect of, 1009–1010
  inhalation agents affect on, 1020
  intubation and, affect on, 1016
  nondepolarizing muscle relaxants and, affect
      on, 1018
  normal range of, 1009
  osmotic agents and, 1011
  succinylcholine
    affect on, 1016–1017
    induced elevation, nondepolarizing muscle
        relaxants to prevent, 1017
  systemic blood pressure, affect of, 1009
intraoperative hypothermia for aneurysm
      surgery trial, 633
intrapulmonary shunt, 12, 1261–1262
intrauterine fetal asphyxia, preventing, 954
intravenous patient-controlled analgesia, 728,
      729, 730
intravenous regional block (Bier method), 679
intrinsic coagulation cascade, 967–968
intubation options, for tracheoesophageal
      fistula, 112
inverse-ratio ventilation, defined, 72–73
"inverse steal" syndrome, 531, 557, 571
ipratropium bromide, for asthma, 14
irrigation solutions, in transurethral resection of
      the prostate,
  absorption of, 806–807, *807*, *809*, 809–810
    amount of, 807
    effect of, *809*, 809–810
    process of, 806
    on serum sodium level, 811
  characteristics of, 803

distilled water, 803
types of, 803
ischemic heart disease,
  aspirin and, 383–384
  asthma and, 19
  clopidogrel (Plavix) and, 383–384
  coronary artery bare metal stent and, 383–384
  intraoperative management
    anesthesia
      etomidate as an induction agent, 393
      general, inducing, 392–393
      maintenance of, anesthetic agents for,
          393–394
      regional *vs*. general, 392
    extubation, 396
      hypertension and tachycardia, preventing,
          396
    monitoring
      ASA standard guidelines for, 389–390
      electrocardiogram leads used for, 390
      3-mm ST-segment depression, treating,
          394–395
      pulmonary artery catheter for, 390
      transesophageal echocardiography and,
          391
    muscle relaxants for, 394
    perioperative cardiac morbidity, predictors
        for, 389
    prophylactic intravenous nitroglycerin to
        prevent myocardial ischemia, 395
    tight control of the heart rate, significance
        of, 395
  perioperative
    mechanism of, 376–377, *377*
    medical therapy for
    α_2-adrenergic agonist 380
      antiplatelet agents, 381
      antithrombotic agents, 381
    β-adrenergic antagonists 378–380
      calcium channel blockers, 380–381
      nitrovasodilators, 380
      statins, 381
    right bundle branch block/left bundle
        branch block, cardiac complications
        and, 383
  postoperative management
    anemia, adverse cardiac outcome and, 398
    hypothermia associated with postoperative
        myocardial ischemia, 398–399
    pain, controlling, 397

perioperative cardiac morbidity, predictors for, 396–397
perioperative myocardial infarction
   diagnosing, 399–400
   patient management with, 400–401
preoperative evaluation and preparation
   assessment of patient, 384–385
   cardiac risk according to type of surgery, classifying, 386
   coronary revascularization and, 385–386
   medication, discontinuing before surgery, 388
   premedication, 388
   α_2 agonist, role of 388–389
   Q-wave infarction *vs.* non–Q-wave infarction, perioperative reinfarction and, 386–387
   stress test, exercise or pharmacologic, 387
   tests for, 384–385
see also myocardial ischemia
isoflurane,
   for asthma, 20, 22
   coronary artery disease and, 156
isoosmolar hyponatremia, 826
isosorbide dinitrate, for myocardial ischemia, 380
isradipine, for cardiopulmonary bypass, 142

Jehovah's Witness, 1151–1152
Jehovah's Witness, 901–902
Jin Jiao. See acupuncture,
junctional ectopic tachycardia, defined, 424–425

K, liver transplantation and, 491–492
ketamine,
   for asthma, 18, 19, 22–23
   for cardiac tamponade, 350
   for open-eye injury, 1020
Kety-Schmidt method, 562
kidney transplant,
   contraindications to receiving, absolute and relative, 833
   donor kidneys
     preservation of, before transpalnt, 834
   expanded criteria donor, 832
   immunosuppressant agents used in, 831–832
     management of, 832
   intraoperative management
     anesthesia
       agents of choice, 842
       induction, 839–840
       inhalational, effects of, 842–843
       maintaining, 842
       techniques used in, types of, 837
     arterial line used in, 838
     fluid management, 844
     monitoring, central venous pressure, 837–838
     muscle relaxants, nondepolarizing, 840–841, 840t
     neuromuscular blockade, prolongation of, 841
       acid-base imbalance, 842
       drugs, 841
       electrolytes, 841
       temperature, 842
     oliguria, differential diagnosis of, 845–846, 846t
     opioids, pharmacology of, 843–844
     polyclonal and monoclonal antibodies, severe reactions to, 845
     succinylcholine, contraindications for, 840
   matching donors and recipients, 833–834
   new surgical techniques for, 834
   operative procedure of, described, 835
   postoperative management
     acute transplant rejection, diagnosing, 847
     immunosuppressive agents, effects of, 847
   preoperative evaluation and preparation
     blood urea nitrogen, normal values for, 836
     glomerular filtration rate, measurement of, 837
     medications taken by patient before transplant, 836
     renal impairment in living donors, 837
     serum creatinine concentration, normal values for, 836–837
     workup for, 835–836
   see also end-stage renal disease
Klebsiella, 52
Kussmaul's sign, 328–329
kyphoscoliosis, 1092

Lambert–Eaton syndrome, 1079, 1080t
laparoscopic adrenalectomy, 779
laparoscopic surgery,
   advantages and disadvantages of, 853
   autopsies, 855
   cancer, lymph node disection for, 852
     pelvic, 851
     prostate, 850–851
   cholecystectomy, 853–854, 855

laparoscopic surgery (*contd.*)
  contraindications of, 853–854
    general, 854
    gynecologic, 854
    intraoperative management
      anesthesia
        agents or adjuvant drugs recommended
          for, 863–864
        insufflation and, complications during,
          866
        nitrous oxide (N_2O), 864, 875–876
        technique, of choice, 862–863
      arterial line, necessity of, 868
      excubation, 878
      heparinized saline irrigation-suction device,
        purpose of, 866
      of intravenous fluids, 861
      laparotomy, converting to, 867
      laryngeal mask airway, use of, 863
      local *vs.* regional, 865
      monitoring, 860–861
      neuroendocrine changes, 873
      of peritoneal cavity, access to, 866
      pneumothorax or pneumomediastinum,
        causes of, 877–878
      positioning of patient, 862
        hypercarbia and, 870–872
        Trendelenburg position, 862, 872, 879
      renal system and, effects on, 874
      shunting resulting from embolization, 867
  laparoscopy, defined, 852
  lumbar discectomies, 855
  neurosurgical intracranial, 855
  physiology of patient altered during, 852
  postoprerative management
    arterial line, removal of, 880
    carbon dioxide (CO_2) absorption, systemic
      effects of, 878–879
    Foley catheter, removal of, 880
    injuries from instruments, 878
    late complications, 879
    nausea and vomitng, 880
    orders, written, 879
    pneumoperitoneum, complications of, 878
    Trendelenburg position, complications
      caused by, 879
  on pregnant patients, 853–854
  preoperative evaluation and preparation
    history of patient, 858
    informed consent, 859–860
    laboratory tests, 859

  for maximally invasive surgery, 860
  to minimize/prevent complications during
    procedure, 860
  pulmonary complications, factors that
    increase, 859
  thoracoscopic, 855
  in urology, 854
  see also carbon dioxide (CO_2), in laparoscopic
    surgery
laparoscopy, in ambulatory surgery,
  carbon dioxide, alternatives to, 1225
  carbon dioxide as insufflation agent of choice,
    1225
  intraoperative complications associated with,
    1224
  physiologic changes induced by, 1224–1225
laparotomy, 867
Laplace equation, 140
laryngeal lesions, laser treatment for,
  anesthesia
    airway fire, managing ("4-E's"), 1033
    endotracheal tube
      protecting external surface of, 1032
      special, for laser surgery, 1033
    foil-wrapped tubes, disadvantages of, 1033
    intermittent apnea technique, 1037
    setup for, special considerations in,
      1029–1030
    Venturi effect, defined, 1034
    Venturi jet ventilation
      complications of, 1035
      contraindications for the use of, 1035
      defined, 1034
      how anesthesia is maintained during,
        1035
      manual, instituting and conducting,
        1034–1035
  hoarseness, differential diagnosis of, 1028
  human papilloma virus, cesarean delivery and,
    1026
  α-interferon therapy 1027–1028
  intraoperative management
    laryngeal papilloma resection, airway
      management options during, 1036
    laser
      advantages of, 1031
      components of, 1030
      defined, 1030
      disadvantages of, compared to
        microdebriders, 1031–1032
      radiation, characteristcs of, 1031

monitoring, 1036
postoperative management
  complications, common, 1037
preoperative evaluation and preparation, 1029
  laboratory testing, 1029
  preanesthetic history and physical
    examination, key points in, 1028–1029
recurrent respiratory papillomatosis
  cause of, 1026
  presentation of, 1027
  treatment options for, 1027
laryngeal mask airway, 17, 27, 863, 1003, 1015
  advantages of, 1240–1241
    vs. endotracheal tube? 1241
  as conduit for trachea incubation, 1245
  contraindications to use of, 1242
  cuff inflation, 1242, 1242t
  defined, 1240
  difficulty in insertion, additional maneuvers
    for, 1244
  indications for use of, 1242
  insertion of, 1243–1244
  preparing, 1243
  removal of, 1247
  size of, 1242, 1243t, 1246t
  uses of, in patient with a difficult airway,
    1246–1247
  wheezing and, 1245
laryngeal papilloma resection, airway
  management options during, 1036
laryngospasm, 14
  defined, 1058
  diagnosing, 1058
  managing patient with, 1058
laryngotracheal anesthesia, 17
laryngotracheitis, clinical presentation of, 1039
laryngotracheobronchitis, 1039
Laser Flex tube, 1033
laser prostatectomy, 821
Laser Shield II, 1033
lateral decubitus position, 534
lateral positioning, 41
  respiratory effects of, 41–42
left anterior descending branch, 134, 135, *135*
left bundle branch block,
  cardiac complications and, 383
  congestive heart failure and, 236–237
left circumflex branch, 134, 135, *135*
left posterior fascicular hemiblock, diagnosing,
  232
left ventricle,

hypertrophied, 217, 219, 225
imaging, transesophageal echocardiography
  vantage points of, 212, *213*
valvular heart disease and
  changes in loading condition resulting from,
    200–201
  pressure/time curves for, 206, 206, 207
venting, in cardiopulmonary bypass, 165
left ventricular assist device insertion,
  considerations for in heart
  transplantation, 361
left ventricular end-diastolic pressure, 138, 202,
  204, 206, 206, 217, 224, 291
left ventricular end-diastolic volume, 134, 148,
  195, 202, 207, 207, 291, 323–324
left ventricular hypertrophy, 217, 219, 225
leptomeningeal pathways, 572
leukotriene receptor antagonists, for asthma, 14
levodopa ($_L$-dopa), for Parkinson's disease,
  581–582
lidocaine,
  for asthma, 17, 19, 26
  cardiovascular effects of, 678t
lighted stylet intubations, 1001
limb defect (radial aplasia), 107
liposome-encapsulated hemoglobin, 1152
liquid ventilation, 75–76
liver function changes, in burn patients, 1123
  anesthetic implications of, 1123
liver transplantation,
  acute tubular necrosis and, 496
  albumin levels, 493
  chronic liver disease
    fulminant hepatic failure and, 497
    neurologic manifestations of, 497
    problems related to, 489–490
    resulting in referral for liver transplantation,
      causes of, 488–489
  coagulation defects, 494–495
  contraindications to, 498
  early postoperative management
    coagulation disturbances, 511–512
    complications, anticipated, 512–513
    massive transfusion, complications of, 512
    renal function, changes in, 512
    vascular catastrophes, 511
  end-stage liver disease, 489, 490
    electrolyte and acid–base abnormalities in,
      491–492
    hemodynamic changes encountered in, 496
    Na, K, Mg, pH, and $PaCO_2$, discuss, 491–492

liver transplantation (*contd.*)
    transjugular intrahepatic portosystemic shunt procedure and, 493–494
    fulminant hepatic failure, causes of, 489
    graft options, 488
    hepatopulmonary syndrome, 495
    hepatorenal syndrome, 496
    hyponatremia, danger in treating, 492
    hypoxemia and, 495
    intraoperative management
      anesthesia
        albumin levels and, 493
        combined tecnique, role for, 504
        drugs to avoid, 504
        induction, considerations for, 503
        informed consent, risks included in, 500
        maintenance, agents for, 504
      blood vessels that are isolated and ligated, 505
      coagulation disorders, anticipated, 510
      hemodynamic findings, anticipated, 503
      hepatic graft, functioning of, 509–510
      hyperfibrinolytic state, 511
      hyperkalemia, 508
      hypocalcemia, 508
      monitoring, 502
        invasive monitors, placement of, 502
        transesophageal echocardiography, 502–503
      "piggyback" (vena cava preservation) technique, 507–508
      postreperfusion syndrome, 509
      renal replacement therapy, 503
      stages of, 501
        first (preanhepatic phase), 501–502
        second (anhepatic phase), 504–505, 508
        third (postanhepatic phase), 509
      "test clamp" maneuver, 506
      thromboelastography, 510
      vascular anastomoses
        completing, 505–506, *506*
        order of reconstruction of, 506
      venovenous bypass, 506–507, *507*
liver transplantation waiting list, criteria used for determining patient's status on, 490–491, 490t, *491*
orthotopic liver transplant, defined, 488
portal hypertension, sequelae of, 493
preoperative evaluation and preparation
    immunosuppressive agents given perioperatively, 499–500

side efects of, 500t
medications, preoperative, 498
premedication, 501
workup, 498–499
prerenal azotemia and, 496
transjugular intrahepatic portosystemic shunt procedure, 493–494
LMA-ProSeal, 17
lobectomy, life-threatening complications of, 44
lower inflexion point, 58
low molecular weight heparin,
    advantages of, over heparin therapy, 333
    anticoagulant effect of, 333
    heparin-induced thrombocytopenia and, 335–336
    mechanism of action of, 333
    in peripartum hemorrhage, 890
"low pressure" pulmonary edema, 830
lumbar discectomies, 855
lung capacities, 6, 8
    normal, defining, 7–8
lung carcinomas,
    anesthetizing, 34
    broncospes and, 34–35
    diagnoses of, 30–31
    double-lumen endotracheal tubes, contraindications to use, 37–38
    double-lumen tube, choosing right- or left-sided, 38
    5-year survival after primary resection, 30–31
    mediastinoscopy, indications/complications, 35–36
    metabolic manifestations of, 31
    minimal pulmonary function test criteria for, 33t
    monitoring, 34
    mortality rate, 32
    one-lung ventilation, indications for, 36–37
      oxygenation during, improving, 43–44
      pain management, postoperative, 45
        cryoanalgesia, 46
        epidural and intrathecal analgesia, 45–46
        intercostal or paravertebral nerve block, 46
        interpleural regional analgesia, 46
        transcutaneous electrical nerve stimulation, 46
      PaO_2 during, 43
      pulmonary blood flow distribution, during, 43
      shunt flow during, 43

systemic oxygenation during, monitoring of, 41
postoperative complications, predicting, 32–33
premedication, 34
preoperative evaluation, 32
for right middle lobectomy, 36
for thoracotomy, 36
thoracotomy for, 30, 36
lung diseases, obstructive vs. restrictive, 7, 7t
lung transplantation,
    blood products commonly required, 101
    end-stage lung diseases treated with, 88–90, 89, 89t
    history of, 90–91
    intraoperative management
        anesthesia
            inducement procedures, 95–96
            volatile, avoided during single-lung ventilation, 97
        cardiopulmonary bypass, necessity for, 100
        extubation upon conclusion of procedure, 102
        fluid administration, restrictions on, 101
        monitoring procedures, 95
        problems, anticipated
            graft implantation and reperfusion, hemodynamic alterations during, 99–100
            with the lateral position, 98
            pulmonary artery clamping, 99, 99
            with single-lung ventilation, 98
        special equipment for, 95
        ventilation
            endotracheal tube used in, 96
            postoperative, 103
            procedures for, 96–97
            single-lung, affect on cardiopulmonary function, 97
    of one or both lungs, deciding factors in, 91–92
    technical differences in, 92–93
    postoperative management
        alternatives to, surgical, 104
        long-term outcomes, 104
        major complications and, 102
        for recipient requiring general anesthesia for subsequent nonpulmonary surgery, 103–104
        ventilation, 103
    preoperative evaluation and preparation
        desirable, 93
        epidural catheter placement, advantages of, 94
        premedication, 93–94
        vascular access requirements, 94
    selection criteria for recipients, 88, 91
    for single vs. double lung transplants, 91–92
lung volume reduction surgery, 104
lung volumes, 6, 8, 10
    normal, defining, 7–8
lupus erythematosus, 200
"luxury perfusion", 557
lymph nodes, biopsy of palpable, 30

magnesium, for head injury, 602
magnesium sulfate (MgSO4), 779
    toxicity, 917
        mechanism of action of, 918
        therapy, effects of, 918
        treatment of, 917
magnetic resonance imaging,
    advantages of, 1233
    anesthetic considerations, 1235
    in awake craniotomy for deep brain stimulation, 587–589
    clinical, biologic effects of, 1234–1235
    contraindications to, 1234
    defined, 1232
    disadvantages of, 1233
    function of, 1232
    intraoperative, defined, 1235–1236
    intraoperative management
        airway, maintaining, 1240
        anesthetic options 1237
        general anesthesia, inducing and maintaining, 1239
        monitoring, 1238
            equipment, special considerations for, 1238–1239
        procedure for conducting magnetic resonance imaging, 1237–1238
    postoperative management
        laryngeal mask airway removal of, 1247
        postanesthesia recovery, 1247–1248
    preoperative evaluation and preparation
        laboratory testing, 1236
        premedication, 1237
        sedation or general anesthesia, patients requiring, 1236
    safety concerns of, 1233
    see also laryngeal mask airway

major burn, definition of according to American Burn Association, 1117–1118
major thermal injury,
  known mediators released with, 1119, *1119*
  pathophysiologic changes accompanying, 1118
  prognosis, 1119–1120
malignant hyperthermia syndrome, 765
  acute crisis of, laboratory findings during, 1094, 1094t
  clinical features of, 1093
    hyperkalemic cardiac arrest, 1094
    nonspecific, 1093–1094
    specific for malignant hyperthermia, 1093
  clinical features of suseptable patient, 1092–1093, 1093t
  defined, 1092
  genetic disorder resulting in susceptibility to, 1095–1096
  incidence of, 1095
  intraoperative management
    anesthetic techniques and agents, 1100
      agents contraindicated for, 1101
      local, 1101
      succinylcholine, rigidity of jaw muscles after administration of, 1101
    emergency measures for complications, 1102
    monitoring, 1103
  kyphoscoliosis and, 1092
  laboratory tests substantiating susceptibility to, 1097
  mode of inheritance, 1095
  Molecular genetic testing for susceptibility to, 1097–1098
  neuroleptic malignant syndrome and, 1098
  pathophysiology of, 1096–1097
  postoperative management
    advice to patient and family, 1103–1104
    of complications, 1103
    follow-up, 1103
  preoperative evaluation and preparation
    for anesthesia and surgery, 1098–1099
    dantrolene prophylaxis, 1099
    for general anesthesia, 1100
    laboratory tests, 1099
    outpatient surgery, 1099
  suggested resources, 1104
  uneventful sevoflurane anesthesia course, susceptibility and, 1093
malposition, 107

malrotation of the midgut, 107
mannitol,
  for diuretic therapy in craniotomy, 540–541
  for head injury, 600
manual in-line cervical stabilization, 1001
Mapleson D system (Bain Breathing circuit), 524
Marfan syndrome, aortic aneurysms and, 253
masseter muscle rigidity, 1101
mast cell stabilizer, for asthma, 14
maternal mortality,
  anesthesia-related, 883
  causes of, 883
  defined, 883
maximum breathing capacity, 6
maximum midexpiratory flow rate, 6
M3 cholinergic receptors, 4
mean arterial pressure, 168, 169–170, 530, 535
meat wrapper's asthma, 5
mechanical bowel obstruction, 473
mechanical ventilation, 60–66
  adverse effects of, 65
  blood gases, interpreting, 60
  clinical plan for, 60
  criteria for, 60–61
  modes of, basic
    baseline mode, 62
    control mode
      choosing, 62
      pressure-controlled *vs.* volume-controlled modes, 61–62
    cycle mode, 62, *63*
    limit mode, 62
    selecting, 62
    trigger mode, 61
  positive pressure ventilation, hemodynamic effects of, 64–65
  ventilator settings, initial, 64
  see also Ventilatory support
meconium aspiration syndrome,
  defined, 940
  risk of, minimizing, 946
meconium-stained amniotic fluid, significance of, 939
mediastinoscopy, indications/complications, 29, 30, 34, 35–36
mefenamic acid, asthmatic attacks and, 5
Mendelson syndrome,
  critical pH value causing, 51
  described, 50
  volume of aspirate causing, 51
meperidine, 642

for asthma, 21, 28
for cancer pain, 693
psychotropic drugs and, interactions with, 643
for renal failure, 843–844
mesenteric protection, 266
Mestinon (pyridostigmine), for myasthenia
    gravis, 1082
metabolic respone to aortic unclamping, 267
metaiobenzylguanadine, 774
metered-dose inhaler, 17
methadone, 688
advantages and disadvantages of, 688
methohexital, for asthma, 17, 18
methylatropine nitrate, for asthma, 14
methylprednisolone, for asthma, 15
methylxanthines, for asthma, 14
metocurine, 22
metoprolol,
for cardiopulmonary bypass, 160–161
    discontinuing, reasons for, 141
    half-life of, defined, 141
    intraoperative hypotension, managing, 142
discontinuing, reasons for, 141
half-life of, defined, 141
intraoperative hypotension, managing, 142
for myocardial ischemia, 378–380
Mg, liver transplantation and, 491–492
microcirculation, 984
midazolam,
for cardiac tamponade, 351
for cardiopulmonary bypass, 153
middle cerebral artery aneurysm.,
mineralocorticoids, 772
minimum alveolar concentration, 20
mitral regurgitation,
cardiopulmonary bypass, special
    considerations particular to, 224
etiology of, 200
hemodynamic management goals for, 219t,
    220
with aortic stenosis, 220
monitoring patient with, 220
premedication for, 219
pressure/time curves for, 207, *209*
severity of
    impact of AS on, 223
    using transesophageal echocardiography,
      215t, 216, 223
signs and symptoms of, 217, 217t
see also valvular heart disease
mitral stenosis,

cardiopulmonary bypass, special
    considerations particular to, 224
etiology of, 200
hemodynamic management goals for, 219t,
    220
in pregnancy, *933*, 933–934
    ausculatory findings associated with, 932
    echocardiographic findings associated with,
      933, 933–934
    electrocardiogram, indications seen on, 933
    hemodynamic goals of, 942
    physiologic changes, effect of, 934
    physiologic consequences of, 932
    treatment for, 934
pressure/time curves for, 207, *209*
severity of, using transesophageal
    echocardiography scales, 215t, 216
signs and symptoms of, 217, 217t
see also valvular heart disease
mitral valve, 201, 202, 205, 220, 223
mitral valve replacement, 224, 225
mivacurium, 22
M-mode, 210, 211
M2 muscarinic receptor, 4
model for end-stage liver disease, 490, 491
modified Blalock-Taussig shunt, 412, 413
modified ultrafiltration, 442
monoamine oxidase inhibitors,
anesthesia
    implications of, 643, 644t
    precautions in administering, 645
for Parkinson's disease, 582
suregry and, discontinuing before, 644
monoclonal antibodies, 845
montelukast, for asthma, 14
morbid obesity,
airway, anatomic changes affecting,
    1265–1266
anesthetic implications of, 1258–1259
body mass index
    defined, 1252
    measuring procedure, 1252–1253
changes occuring in cardiovascular system,
    1263–1264
defined, 1252
existing problems with, 1251
gastrointestinal system, derangements of, 1266
ideal body weight, defined, 1252
impact of pneumoperitoneum on the
    respiratory and cardiovascular system

morbid obesity (*contd.*)
    of the bariatric surgical patient, 1262–1263
    intraoperative management
      anesthesia, inducing, 1271–1272
      apneic oxygenation, defined, 1278
      complications of, 1277–1278
      diffusion hypoxia, 1279
      four-maximum-breath and 3-minute techniques comparative effectiveness of, 1273
      general anesthesia foe, 1274
      intubation technique, 1271–1272
      monitoring, 1271
      muscle relaxants, 1275
      pioneer study, 1278
      preoxygenating the obese patient, 1273
      regional anesthesia for, 1275–1276
      sphincter of Oddi, effect of narcotics on, 1277
    intrapulmonary shunt (QS/QT) and dead space (VD/VT), cahnges occuring in, 1261–1262
    medical conditions associated with, 1213
    metabolic problems, 1259
    morbid obesity, defined, 1252
    normal weight, defined, 1252
    obesity, defined, 1252
    obstructive sleep apnea
      anesthetic implications of, 1258–1259
      defined, 1253
      diagnosing, 1254
      and obesity, association between, 1257
      risk factors for, 1253–1254
      severe, pathogenesis of, 1256
      types of, 1255
    other disease entities commonly associated with, 1264–1265
    overweight, defined, 1252
    PaO_2 and $PaCO_2$, changes occurring in, 1261
    pickwickian syndrome, defined
    postoperative management
      atelectasis, preventing, 1281
      early postoperative complications, major, 1280
      extubation, 1279–1280
      helath-related risks correlating with obesity, 1280
      mortality, factors correlated statistically with, 1280
      for pain, 1281–1282

      position, affect on respiratory function, 1280
      supplementary oxygen, prescribing, 1281
    preoperative evaluation and preparation
      blood pH, equation for, 1268–1269
      blood values, normal, 1269
      H_2 blockers, side effects of, 1270
      patient evaluation, 1267
      premedication, 1269–1270
      spirometry screening test, interpret, 1269
    respiratory parameters, changes in, 1260–1261
    severe, etiology of pharyngeal pathology in, 1257
    sleep study or polysomnogram, 1254–1255
    super obesity, defined, 1252
morphine,
    for asthma patients, postoperative pain control and, 27–28
    cardiovascular effects of, 155
    classification of, 686
    for renal failure, 843
    synthetic opioids and, difference between, 687
motor evoked potentials, 262, 264–265
    defined and use of, 1169
moxibustion, 746
μ-receptor opioid agonists, 686
multiple aortopulmonary collateral arteries, 405–406, 407
multiple endocrine adenomatosis, 772, 772t
muscarinic antagonist with cholinesterase inhibitors, to reverse muscle relaxant, 368
muscle relaxants,
    for asthma patients
      nondepolarizung, histamine release and, 21–22, *22*
      that cause histamine release, 21–22, 22t
    in cardiopulmonary bypass
      administered during, 175–176
      choosing, 158
      reversing, 196
    in heart transplantation, muscarinic antagonist with cholinesterase inhibitors to reverse, 368
    in ischemic heart disease, 394
    nondepolarizing, affect on intraocular pressure, 1018
    nondepolarizing, in kidney transplant, 840–841, 840t
    for prolonged postoperative apnea
      adequate neuromuscular recovery, defined, 1111–1112

choosing, 1109, 1110t
nondepolarizing, administration of, 1109
reversing, 1111
"train-of-four", 1111–1112
succinylcholine for rapid-sequence induction
for intestinal obstruction, 481, 482t
in valvular heart disease, 222
Mustard and Senning procedures,
described, 443
intraatrial physiologic repairs, transposition of
the great arteries and, 437–438
myasthenia gravis, 31
myasthenia gravis,
cause of, 1076
classifications of
clinical, 1081
in pediatric age-group, 1081
clinical course of, 1076–1077
diagnosing, 1076–1077
differential diagnosis of, 1079
electrical and humoral events that take place
during transmission, 1083
incidence of, 1079–1080
intraoperative management
anesthesia
neuromuscular blocking agents, 1088
options for, 1087
monitoring, 1087
and Lambert–Eaton syndrome, difference
between, 1079, 1080t
postoperative management
for complications, 1090
of pain, 1090
ventilatory support, prolonged, 1089
pregnancy and, effect of myasthenia gravis on,
1084–1085
pregnancy and, effect on course of,
1084–1085
preoperative evaluation and preparation
laboratory data required for, 1086
patient assessment, 1085–1086
premedication, 1086
surgical treatment of, 1084
treatment regimens available for, 1081–1083
mycophenolate mofentil, 847
mydriacyl (tropicamide), 1012
myocardial contractility, 418
myocardial dysfunction,
in liver transplantation, 512
myocardial hibernation, 352
myocardial infarction,

in cardiopulmonary bypass, 159
delaying surgery due to, 378
in transurethral resection of the prostate
perioperative reinfarction, risk of in prior,
800
postponing surgery due to, 800
myocardial ischemia,
in abdominal aortic aneurysm patients
algorithm for patients with, 277
monitors used for, 286
perioperative myocardial infarction in
patients with, 274–275
pulmonary artery catheter, assessing with,
289
in cardiopulmonary bypass, 159
detecting, 148, 148–149
hemodynamic consequences of, 147–148
perioperative and postoperative myocardial
infarction, relation between, 159
perioperative myocardial infarction and,
preventing, 159
prophylactic nitroglycerin for, 159
in transposition of the great arteries, 447
in transurethral resection of the prostate,
hypothermia and, 821
see also ischemic heart disease
myocardial oxygen consumption, in
cardiopulmonary bypass,
calcium channel blockers and, 142–143, 143t
contractility, measuring, 140, 140
determinants of, 139, 154
determining factors of, 140–141
Myocardial Wall Tension and, estimating,
140
myocardial oxygen demand,
clinical measurement of, 376
determinants of, 376
myocardial oxygen supply, determining factors,
376
myocardial stunning, 352
Myocardial Wall Tension, estimating, 140, 140

Na, liver transplantation and, 491–492
Nager syndrome, 1052
naproxen, asthmatic attacks and, 5
narcotics, for asthma, 27–28
nasal intubation with laryngoscope and magill
forceps, 1071–1072
nasogastric tube, 17
National Institute of Health Consensus
Conference, 748–749

National Institutes of Health, 58
near-infrared spectroscopy, 417–418, 441
neck, zones of, 997
needle aspiration biopsy, 30
Nei Guan acupuncture point, 749
neodymium: yttriumaluminum-garnet laser,
    821
neoplasms, 3
neostigmine, 26
neosynephrine, 1012
nephrotic syndrome, 824
nerve blocks of the lower extremities,
    abnormal magnetic resonance angiogram,
        concerns of, 657
    anesthetic options, 658
    ankle block
        advantages and disadvantages of, 661
        landmarks for, 659, *660*, 661
    evaluating patient, 657–658
    local perfusion, assessment of status of,
        657
    monitoring, intraoperatively, 659
    neurologic function, concerns with, 657
    peripheral nerve blocks
        for arthroscopy, *663*, 663–665, *664*
        ultrasound guidance used in, *665–666*,
            665–667
    peripheral regional anesthesia, for incision
        and drainage of an abscess, 661–662,
        662
    postoperative pain management, 667
        neurovascular status, following, 667–668
neuralgia, 674
neuraxial blocks, pain management and,
    advantages and disadvantages of, 647
        perivascular axillary block, 647
        perivascular interscalene block, 647
        perivascular subclavian block, 648
        supraclavicular block, 648
    anesthesia
        agent used for, 652, 653t
        for bilateral block, 653–654
        local, maximum safe dose of, 653, 653t
        local, systemic reaction to, 654
        technique used for, 645
    axillary nerve block
        commonly missed nerves with, 652
        landmarks of, 648–649
        procedure of, 649
        tourniquet-related pain, managing, 652
    brachial plexus block

        technique of, 646
    interscalene brachial plexus block
        hemidiaphragmatic paresis after, incidence
            of, 649
        pulmonary function changes occuring after,
            650, 650–651
    interscalene nerve block
        commonly missed nerves with, 652
        dyspnea, 651
        landmarks of, 649
        procedure of, 649
    meperidine and, 642
        psychotropic drugs and, interactions with,
            643
    monoamine oxidase inhibitors and
        anesthesia
            implications of, 643, 644t
            precautions in administering, 645
        suregry and, discontinuing before, 644
    neurologic dysfunctions, managing, 654
    premedications, 645
    shortness of breath, managing, 654
    tricyclic antidepressants and
        anesthetic implications of, 643, 643t
        suregry and, discontinuing before, 644
neuraxial neurolysis, 695–696
neuraxial opioid infusion, 695
neuroablative procedures, 696
neurogenic pulmonary edema, in acute
        respiratory distress syndrome, 55
neuroleptic malignant syndrome and, 1098
neuromodulation, 697
neuromuscular junction, 1077
neuromuscular blockade, prolongation of,
    in kidney transplant, 841
        acid-base imbalance, 842
        drugs, 841
        electrolytes, 841
        temperature, 842
neuromuscular toxicity, 829
neuroprotective agents, for spinal cord
        protection in thoracoabdominal
        aortic aneurysms repair, 264
neurosurgery,
    intracranial laparoscopic surgery, 855
    intraoperative echocardiography and, 152
New Orleans asthma, 5
New York Heart Association classification of
        heart failure, 375, 449
New York Presbyterian Hospital-Cornell Medical
        Center, 143, 151

nicardipine,
    for myocardial ischemia, 380–381
nifedipine,
    for cardiopulmonary bypass, 142–143, 143t
    for myocardial ischemia, 380–381
nimodipine, for cardiopulmonary bypass, 142
nitric oxide, 80
    for congenital diaphragmatic hernia patients,
        pulmonary and systemic circulation
        and, 122–123
    for congenital heart defects, 1073
    defined, 80
    in heart transplantation, as a selective
        pulmonary vasodilator, 365
    inhaled, for treatment of acute respiratory
        distress syndrome, 80–81
    for lung transplantation, delivery of, 95
    for valvular heart disease, 226
nitrogen washout, 12
nitroglycerin,
    for deliberate hypertension, 542
    for myocardial ischemia, 380
    prophylactic intravenous, to prevent
        myocardial ischemia, 395
    venous air embolism and, 545
nitrous oxide (N_2O),
    avoiding, in ambulatory surgery, 1223–1224
    cardiovascular effect of, 157–158
    in craniotomy, 539
    intestinal obstruction and, 482–483
    in laparoscopic surgery, 864, 875–876
nitrovasodilators, for ischemic heart disease,
    380
N-methyl-D-aspartate antagonist, 602, 611
nonenzymatic glycosylation, 787
nonketotic hyperosmolar coma, 788
nonproductive cough, lung carcinoma and, 30
non-ST-elevation myocardial infarction, 400–401
nonsteroidal anti-inflammatory drugs,
    for asthma, avoiding, 5, 28
    for back pain, low, 710
    for perioperative pain management, 732, 737,
        739, 741
        intravenous, 724
norepinephrine, 769–770
normal sinus rhythm, 322
normal spontaneous vaginal delivery, 1026
normovolemic hemodilution, intraoperative, 162
North American Society of Pacing and
        Electrophysiology and British Pacing
        and Electrophysiology Group,

generic defibrillator code, 238–239, 239t
    pacemaker classification codes, 233, 233t
NorthAmerican Symptomatic Endarterectomy
        Trial, 551, 575
NSAIDs. See Nonsteroidal anti-inflammatory
        drugs,

obese patients, laparoscopic cholecystectomy
        for, 17
obstructive sleep apnea and hypopnea
        syndrome, 1258
obstructive sleep apnea,
    anesthetic implications of, 1258–1259
    defined, 1253
    diagnosing, 1254
    and obesity, association between, 1257
    risk factors for, 1253–1254
    severe, pathogenesis of, 1256
    types of, 1255
oculocardiac reflex,
    afferent and efferent pathways of, 1021
    atropine use, controversy over, 1022
    defined, 1021
    diagnosing and treating, 1021
    incidence of, contributing factors, 1021
    retrobulbar block to prevent, 1022
oliguria, 845–846, 846t
oliguria, causes of, 1132–1133
O_2 metabolites, short-lived, 67
1-desamino-8-D-arginine-vasopressin, 601
open-eye injury,
    aqueous humor, formation and elimination of,
        1009, *1010*
    carbonic anhydrase inhibitors or osmotic
        diuretics for, 1012
    as challenge to anesthesiologist, 1008
    eyedrops, anesthesiologists concern with,
        1012–1013
    intraoperative management
        etomidate as an induction agent, 1020
        intubation, 1015
            awake, 1016
        ketamine and, effect on eye, 1020
        laryngeal mask airway, 1015
        oculocardiac reflex
            afferent and efferent pathways of, 1021
            atropine use, controversy over, 1022
            defined, 1021
            diagnosing and treating, 1021
            incidence of, contributing factors, 1021
            retrobulbar block to prevent, 1022

open-eye injury (*contd.*)
    propofol as an induction agent, 1020
    succinylcholine
        contraindications for, 1016
        elevation in intraocular pressure,
            nondepolarizing muscle relaxants to
            prevent, 1016
        intraocular pressure and, affect on,
            1016–1017
        rapid-sequence induction and intubation
            without using, 1018–1019
    vitreous herniation, risk factors of, 1015
    postoperative management
        corneal abrasions, preventing, 1023
        extubation
            awake *vs.* deep, 1023
            procedures performed before, 1023
        inflamed conjunctiva, reasons for, 1023
        neuromuscular blockade, reversing, 1022
    preoperative evaluation and preparation
        history and physical exam, 1014
        nasogastric tube or emetics to empty the
            stomach, 1014
        open-globe injury as a surgical emergency,
            1014
        premedication, 1015
        retrobulbar block, 1015
        topical anesthesia, 1014
    topically applied ophthalmic medications,
        systemic absorption of, 1012
    see also intraocular pressure
opioids,
    administration of, 691, 691t
    in craniotomy, 539
    mechanism of action of, 688
    meperidine, defined, 693
    meperidine and, 688
    minimum effective analgesic concentration,
        692, *692*
    mixed opioid agonist/antagonist *vs.* opioid
        agonist, 687
    neuraxial opioid infusion, 695
    patient-controlled analgesia, advantages and
        complications of, 692
    rotation of, 693
    side effects of, 689
    side effects of, treating, 689
    tolerance and physical dependence, defined,
        689
opioid therapy. See chronic opioid therapy,
orhepatorenal syndrome, 490

orogastric tube, 106, 109
orthotopic liver transplant, 488
osmotic agents, 1011
osmotic diuretics, 1012
oximetry, mechanism of, 41
oxybarbiturates, 18
oxygenators, used in cardiopulmonary bypass,
    gas flow used, amount of, 177
    gas used in, type of, 177
    rewarmming and cooling patient by, 183
    types and purposes of, 165–166
oxygen delivery, determining factors for, 66
oxygen saturation (SaO2),
oxygen toxicity, 67
    in acute respiratory distress syndrome, 55
    free-radical theory of, 67
    governing factors of, major, 67
    mechanism of, 67

pacemaker classification,
North American Society of Pacing and
        Electrophysiology and British Pacing
        and Electrophysiology Group, 233,
        233t
pacemaker surgery,
    anesthesia
        inhalational gases, avoiding certain, 243
        preoperative preparations for, 241
    bifascicular block, inserting temporary
        pacemaker before general anesthesia,
        232
    cardiac rhythm management device
        extracorporeal shock wave lithotripsy and,
            247–248
        magnetic resonance imaging,
            contraindications for, 249
        radiofrequency ablation and, precautions
            during, 249
        type and functionality of, determining, 240,
            250
    drugs and equipment used during, 243
    electrocautery and, 245
    electroconvulsive therapy, contraindications
        for, 248
    electromechanical interference
        environmental, 250–251
        inappropriate inhibition and, determining,
        245
        preventing from electrocautery, 245–246
    magnets and, effect of, 246
    monitoring

during, 242
in the post–anesthesia care unit, 249
preoperative evaluation, 239
preoperative preparations, 241
reprograming device before surgery, 241–242
transcutaneous external pacer and
defibrillator and, setting up, 243, *244*
ventricular tachycardia during, 247
see also implantable cardioverter-defibrillator;
permanent pacemaker
packed red blood cells, 494, 894, 895–896
PaCO$_2$. See arterial carbon dioxide (PaCO$_2$),
palatoplasty, 1056
palliative shunt, 418
Pancoast's syndrome, 31
pancreatic cancer pain, characteristics of, 685
pancreatitis, in acute respiratory distress
syndrome, 55
pancuronium, 1019
for asthma, 21–22
for cardiopulmonary bypass, 153, 158
PAO$_2$. See Alveolar partial pressure of oxygen
(PAO$_2$),
PaO$_2$. See Arterial partial pressure of oxygen
(PaO$_2$),
parenchymal compartment, 529
park bench (semiprone) position, 534
Parkinson's disease,
clinical symptoms of, 578, *580*, 580t
defined, 578
drug therapy for, 581
anticholinergic agents, 583
antiviral agents, 583
catechol-O-methyltransferase inhibitors,
582–583
dopamine agonists, 582
levodopa/carbidopa, 581–582
monoamine oxidase inhibitors, 582
pathology of, 579, 580t, 581
substantia nigra pars compacta and, 578, *579*
surgical treatment of, criteria for, 583–584 (*see
also* deep brain stimulation)
Unified Parkinson's Disease Rating Scales, 596
paronychia, 656
partial bypass, defined, 165
partial thromboplastin time, 322, 890, 895, 898,
965, 970
patent ductus arteriosus,
prematurity and
diagnosing, 457
incidence and pathophysiology of, 456

treatment for, 457
tracheoesophageal fistula and, 107
patent foramen ovale, 120
patent foramen ovale, 535
PCO$_2$. See arterial PCO$_2$,
Pediatric End-Stage Liver Disease model, 491
pelvic lymph node dissection, 851
pentobarbital, for asthma, 18
percutaneous automated discectomy, 712
percutaneous automated nucleotomy, 712
percutaneous disc decompression,
using 17-gauge Dekompressor probe, 713
using nucleoplasty, 713
percutaneous kyphoplasty, 713–714
percutaneous laser disc decompression, 713
percutaneous manual nucleotomy, 712
percutaneous radiofrequency denervation, 712
percutaneous transluminal coronary
angioplasty,
defined, 136
indications, contraindications, and results of,
136–137
percutaneous vertebroplasty, 713–714
perfluorocarbons, 1152
pericarditis, 830–831
perioperative cardiac morbidity,
predictors for, 389
preoperative predictors for, 373–374
perioperative myocardial infarction,
diagnosing, 399–400
patient management with, 400–401
perioperative pain management,
Acute Pain Sevice, role of
in improving postoperative pain
management, 744
inadequate, consequences of, 743–744
postoperative outcome, improving, 745
undertreatment, 743
for ambulatory surgery
anesthetic technique, postoperative pain
and, 739–740
considerations and advice to the patient, 737
discharge, pain control after, 742
inadequate, consequences of, 738, 738t
nonsteroidal anti-inflammatory drugs, 737
premedication or preoperative analgesic,
role of, 739
surgery technique, influence on pain and,
741–742
analgesic strategy, 724

perioperative pain management (*contd*.)
influence of, on postoperative outcome, 724–725
anesthesia
choice of, 735
technique, choosing, 721–722
chronic opioid therapy, 733
chronic opioid-consumtion *vs.* abuse otr addiction, 734
increased postoperative pain and, 733–734
opioid-tolerant patient
discharging, 736–737
perioperative pain management choices for, 735–736
surgery and, 734
preoperative information, 735
thoracic epidural analgesia, 724, 725
alternatives to, 726, 728
choice of drugs, influencing the efficacy or safety of, 724, 725
doses and concentrations of the anesthetic combinations, 726, 727
efficacy or safety of, choice of drugs that, 725
placement and removal of epidural catheter, 731
for low molecular weight heparin, 731–732
for Oral anticoagulants, 732
for orophylactic unfractionated heparin, 731
for postoperative low molecular weight heparin, 732
for therapeutic intravenous unfractionated heparin, 731
punctures, 726
side effects and complications of, 730
tip of epidural catheter, placement of, 725
for thoracotomy
perioperative reinfarction for noncardiac surgery, incidence of, 377–378
peripartum hemorrhage,
intraoperative management
amniotic fluid embolism, 900
anesthesia
for placenta accreta, 894
for post partum hemorrhage, 897
cell savage, role of in obstetric patients, 900–901
disseminated intravascular coagulation
blood products, use of additional, 895–896
defined, 894–895
emergency release blood, role of, 896
epidural, removing, 902–903
hypotension, concerns with, 903
recombinant factor VII (rFVIIa), role of, 896
Jehovah's Witness, treating, 901–902
postpartum hemorrhage
anesthetic considerations of, 897
defined, 897
resuscitation, laboratory tests ordered during, 898
retained placenta and treatment options, 900
uterine artery balloon placement, role of, 902
uterine artery embolization, role of, 902
uterine atony, treatment options for, 898–899
uterine inversion, treatment options for, 899
postoperative management
epidural, removing, 902–903
hypotension, concerns with, 903
preoperative evaluation and preparation
airway (difficult), due to anatomic changes during pregnancy, 893
anemia of pregnancy, relative, 891
anesthesia
maternal respiratory function changes and, 889
of fetal maturity, 893
laboratory procedures, 890
maternal cardiovascular changes, 889–890
maternal gastrointestinal changes, 892
monitoring, during severe hemorrhage, 892
preoperative medications, 893
supine hypotensive syndrome, 891
transfusion, 891–892, 892t
peripheral nerve blocks, 693–694
for arthroscopy, *663*, 663–665, *664*
celiac plexus block, for cancer pain, 694–695
ultrasound guidance used in, *665–666*, 665–667
peripheral neuritis, 31
peripheral obesity, 1253
peripheral regional anesthesia, for incision and drainage of an abscess, 661–662, 662
perivascular axillary block, 647
perivascular interscalene block, 647
perivascular subclavian block, 648

permanent pacemaker,
  atrial pacing only, advantages and
    disadvantages of, 235
  atrioventricular sequential, indications and
    complications associated with, 235
  biventricular, defined, 236–237
  cardiac resynchronization therapy device,
    defined, 236–237
  energy provided, maximum amount of in
    terms of pulse amplitude and pulse
    width, 236
  functionality of, determining, 240
  heart rate increase, mechanism responsible
    for, 234–235
  indications for, 231
  interrogating, obtaining information from, 241
  leads, acceptable values for in terms of pacing
    thresholds, amplitude of sensed R
    waves, and resistance, 236
  life spans of, 237
  modes of pacing in, 233–234
  types of, identifying, 236
  see also pacemaker surgery
persistent pulmonary hypertension, 90, 92, 119
  treatment of, 122
PETCO2. See end-tidal CO2 (PETCO2),
PFA-100 monitor, 969
pH, liver transplantation and, 491–492
pharyngeal flap, 1057
phenylalkylamines, for cardiopulmonary bypass,
  142
phenylbutazone, asthmatic attacks and, 5
phenylephrine hydrochloride (neosynephrine),
  1012
pheochromocytoma,
  anesthesia, administering, 777–778
  blood loss, 779
  blood pressure management, 778t, 779
  catecholamine stimulation, controlling effects
    of, 778
  clinical features associated with, 772
  defined, 768
  drugs to avoid during surgery, 776–777, 777t
  hypotension, postoperative, 780
  incidence of, 768
  laboratory tests for, 774, 775t
  laparoscopic adrenalectomy, 779
  metaiobenzylguanadine, 774
  monitoring during surgery, 777
  multiple endocrine adenomatosis, 773, 773t
  occurance of, 773, 773t
  postoperative problems, 780
  pregnancy, magnesium sulfate (MgSO4) for
    hypertension and, 779
  sedation for preoperative period, 776
  surgery, pharmacologically preparing for,
    775–776
  tumor, diagnosing and localizing, 774
phosphodiesterase, 25
phospholine iodide (echothiophate iodide), 1013
pH-stat regulation, 446
pial-to-pial collateral pathways, 572
pickwickian syndrome, defined,
Pierre Robin syndrome, 1052
  defined, 1052
  piggyback" (vena cava preservation)
    techniqueD
    507–508
pink Tet, defined, 410
pipecuronium, for cardiopulmonary bypass, 158
placenta accreta,
  diagnosing, 888
  types of, 888
  see also peripartum hemorrhage
placental abruption,
  complications associated with, 886
  diagnosing, 886
  risk factors for development of, 886
placenta previa,
  associated conditions of, 885
  diagnosing, 884
  double setup
    anesthesia for, 885
    defined, 885–886
  management of, 885
  risk factors, 885
  types of, 885
plasmapheresis, intraoperative, 162–163
Plasmapheresis (ACTH; corticotropin) for
  myasthenia gravis, 1083
Plasmodium falciparum, 982
platelet adhesion vs. platelet aggregation, in
  hemophilia, 966
Plavix (clopidogrel),
  for myocardial ischemia, 381, 383–384
Pneumocystis carinii, 102
pneumomediastinum, 877–878
pneumonectomy, life-threatening complications
  of, 45
pneumonia,
  acute respiratory distress syndrome and, 55
  aspiration, 50, 51

pneumonia (*contd.*)
>>> *vs.* aspiration pneumonitis 51
>>> tracheoesophageal fistula and, 110, 114
>> bacterial, lung transplantation and, 102
>> chemical, 3
>> eosinophilic, 3
>> lung resection and, mortality from, 32
>> tracheoesophageal fistula and, 108, 109, 110, 114
pneumoperitoneum, 878
pneumothorax,
>> fatal, 110
>> in laparoscopic surgery, 877–878
polyarteritis, 3
>> aortic aneurysms and, 253–254
polyclonal antibodies, 845
polysomnogram, 1254–1255
porphyria, 981
positive end-expiratory pressure, 12, 68
>> arterial oxygenation and, improvements in, 68
>> asthma and, 12, 23
>> best and optimal, determining, 69, *70*
>> cardiovascular effects of, 69–71
>> criteria for starting, 68
>> double-lumen endotracheal tubes placement and, 38
>> protective-ventilation strategy and, 57–58, *58*
>> weaning from ventilatory support and, 82
positive pressure ventilation,
>> gastric distension occuring with, avoiding, 109–110, 113
>> hemodynamic effects of, 64
postanesthetic shivering, 1132
postcardiopulmonary bypass bleeding, 331–332, 332
postcardiotomy cardiac tamponade, 325, 326
postdural puncture headache, 921–922
posterior cranial fossa pathology, issues specific to, 530
posterior fossa craniotomy. See craniotomy,
posterior longitudinal ligament, 702–703
postextubation "croup,", 525–526
Posthumous Papers of the Pickwick Club, 1256
postictal agitation, 1207
postimplantation syndrome, as complication of endovascular thoracoabdominal aortic aneurysm repair, 270
postlaminectomy syndrome, 708–709
postoperative nausea and vomiting, 1226, 1227
postpartum hemorrhage,
>> anesthetic considerations of, 897

>> defined, 897
>> *see also* peripartum hemorrhage
postrenal acute renal failure (obstruction of urinary outflow), 1133
postrenal olguria, 846
postreperfusion syndrome, 509
posttraumatic seizures, 614
potassium-titanyl-phosphate laser, 821
preeclampsia,
>> American College of Obstetricians and Gynecologists classification of, 905
>> blood pressure predicting occurrence of, 913
>> complications associated with, 914
>> defined, 905–906
>> eclampsia
>>> defined, 906
>>> treatment of, 918
>> intraoperative management
>>> analgesia/anesthesia, 919
>>>> abnormal fetal heart rate seen with maternal hypotension, treatment for, 921
>>>> accidental spinal tap, 921
>>>> choosing, 919
>>>> epidural, bleeding time and platelet count evaluation and, 920
>>>> epinephrine and, 921
>>>> ergonovine and, 922
>>>> general, for cesarean delivery, 923
>>>> hypertension, agents to prevent, 923
>>>> level of, 920
>>>> local, 920–921
>>>> postdural puncture headache, 921–922
>>>> prehydration, 919
>>>> spinal, when and how you give, 922–923
>>>> total spinal, 922
>>> HELLP syndrome, 923–924
>> mortality associated with, 907
>> pathogenesis of, 907
>>> calcium, 910
>>> coagulation factors, 910
>>> endothelial factors, 908, *909*
>>> fatty acid metabolism, 910
>>> genetic factors, 908
>>> immunologic factors, 908
>>> markers of angiogenesis, 910
>>> platelet factors, 909, *910*
>> pathologic alterations of
>>> cardiovascular changes, 911
>>> endochrine changes, 912
>>> hematologic changes, 911, 912t

hemodynamic changes, 911
hepatic changes, 912
neurolgic changes, 912–913
renal changes, 912
respiratory changes, 912
uteroplacental perfusion, 913
postoperative management
   postpartum management, 925
preoperative evaluation and preparation
   immediate delivery, conditions mandating,
     915
   laboratory studies, recommended, 914
   magnesium sulfate toxicity
     mechanism of action of, 918
     therapy, effects of, 918
     treatment of, 917
   monitoring
     of central venous pressure, 915
     importance of, 915
   obstetrical management of, discussing,
     916–917
   seizure prophylaxis, treatment of choice in
     United States, 917
  pulse wave velocity and, 913–914
  risks of developing, 907
  severe, defined, 906
pregnancy, surgical complications in,
  fetal lie
   defined, 927
   determining, 927
   transverse lie
     etiology of, 927
     obstetric management for, 928
     problems associated with, 928
  fetal oxygenation, determinants of, 934
  heart disease
   cardiovascular changes during, 930–931
     electrocardiographic and
      echocardiographic, normal, 931
     in heart sounds, 931
   incidence of, 929
   mitral stenosis, *933*, 933–934
     ausculatory findings associated with, 932
     echocardiographic findings associated
      with, *933*, 933–934
     electrocardiogram, indications seen on,
      933
     physiologic changes, effect of, 934
     physiologic consequences of, 932
     treatment for, 934
   mortality rates, 929

New York Heart Association classification
   of, 930
rheumatic heart disease, cause of, 932
intraoperative management
  anesthesia
   airway management, 943–944, *944*
   β-blockade 944
   for emergency cesarean section, 942
   general, 943
   inhalation agents, effect on uterine
     contractility, 945
  Apgar scoring system
   defined, 945
   significance of, 945, 945t
  meconium aspiration syndrome,
     minimizing risk of, 946
  for mitral stenosis, hemodynamic goals of,
     942
  monitoring
   during cesarean delivery, 941
   invasive, in patient with cardiac disease,
     941–942
meconium aspiration syndrome, defined, 940
meconium-stained amniotic fluid, significance
   of, 939
monitoring
  of fetal heart rate, 935
  of maternal contractions, 935
nonobstertric surgery in pregnant patient
  main concerns associated with, 952
  trauma, as major reason for, 954
position
  defined, 927
  determining, 927
post operative management
  oxygen saturation, decrease in, 946
preoperative evaluation and preparation
  evaluate of pregnant cardiac patient
    noninvasive tests used for, 940
  fetal heart rate
   acute fetal distress, causes of, 939
   with beat-to-beat variability, normal, 935
   fetal blood gases, normal values of, 938
   fetal scalp capillary blood pH sampling,
    false signals from, 939
   hypoxia leading to acidosis, assessment
    of, 937–938
   monitoring of, 935
   predicting fetal well-being, accuracy of,
    937

pregnancy, surgical complications in (*contd.*)
  transient or periodic decelerations,
      935–937, *936*
  premedications, 940–941
  presentation, birth
    breech
      cause of, 928
      problems associated with, 928
      types of, 928
    defined, 927
    determining, 927
  uterine blood flow, determinants of, 935
  see also appendectomy for pregnant patient
prehydration, in preeclampsia, 919
prematurity,
  apneic spells, 455–456
  blood transfusions, 462
  bronchopulmonary dysplasia and, 454–455
  classifying, 453, 453t
  digitalis to treat congestive heart failure, 457
  indomethacin, 457
    adverse effects of, 457–458
  intraoperative management
    anesthesia
      intubation and, 466
      maintaining, 466–467
      requirements of preterm infant *vs.* adult,
          465–466
    blood and fluid therapy, 467–468
    body temperature, maintaining, 465
    dissection of the ductus arteriosus,
        problems during, 468
    Doppler effect, 464
    intubation, endotracheal tube size used in,
        466
    monitoring, 463
      arterial oxygen saturation, 465
    oxygen analyzer, 464
    pulse oximetry, mechanism of, 465
    ventilation, 467
  patent ductus arteriosus and
    diagnosing, 457
    incidence and pathophysiology of, 456
    treatment for, 457
  postoperative management
    extubation, 468
    muscle relaxants, reversing
    persistent cardiac murmur, possible
        diagnosis for, *469,* 469–470
    transporting neonatal intensive care unit,
        minimizing risk in, 469

preoperative evaluation and preparation
  arterial blood gases and pH
    interpreting, 461
    normal values of, 460, 460t
  arterial blood pressure, heart rate, and
      respiratory rate, normal values of,
      461, 461t
  normal levels of white blood cells, red blood
      cells, hemoglobin, glucose,
      electrolytes, calcium, blood urea
      nitrogen, and creatinine, 461–462
  patient evaluation, 460
  premedication, 463
  serum calcium level, 462
  urinalysis, interpreting, 462
problems associated with, common, 453
respiratory distress syndrome and
  pathophysiology of, 454
  survival rates of, 454
retinopathy of prematurity, 458–459
survival rates of, 453–454
temperatures
  natural and critical, 459–460, 459t
  regulating, 460
preoperative, embolization therapy, 531
preoperative evaluation and preparation,
    hemoximeter, 1181
prerenal acute renal failure (hypovolemic), 1133
prerenal azotemia, 496
prerenal oliguria, 845–846, 846t
presentation, birth,
  breech
    cause of, 928
    problems associated with, 928
    types of, 928
  defined, 927
  determining, 927
pressure gradients, measured by transesophageal
    echocardiography, 210, 212, 214
pressure-support ventilation, 71
  advantages of, 71
  defined, 71, *72*
pressure–volume loops,
  defined, 202, *202*
  for valvular lesions, representative, 202–203,
      203, 204, 205
priming solution, used in cardiopulmonary
    bypass, 166–167
Prinzmetal's angina (variant angina), 142
prolonged postoperative apnea,
  acetylcholinesterase, 1106

apnea, differential diagnosis, 1112
atypical cholinesterase activity, incidence of,
  1107
dibucaine number, significance of, 1107–1108,
  1108t
humoral events in normal neuromuscular
  transmission, 1106
muscle relaxants
  adequate neuromuscular recovery, defined,
    1111–1112
  choosing, 1109, 1110t
  nondepolarizing, administration of, 1109
  reversing, 1111
  "train-of-four", 1111–1112
postjunctional receptors blocked before
  transmission is diminished, 1112
pseudocholinesterase
  abnormal, mivacurium used in patients
    with, 1109
  levels, factors that lower, 1108
serum cholinesterase, 1106–1107
succinylcholine
  acetylcholine and, differences in, 1107
  cardiovascular effects of, 1108
  pediatric anesthesia and, 1109
  resemblance to acetylcholine, 1107
prone-position ventilation,
  in craniotomy, 533–534
  oxygenation and, effect on, 74
  rationale for, 73–74
prophylactic antibiotics, for aspirated patient,
  52–53
prophylactic low molecular weight heparin, 731,
  732
propofol,
  for asthma, 18
  for cardiac tamponade, 351
propofol,
  for laparoscopic surgery, 864
prostaglandin infusion, 1065
prostaglandins,
  in asthma, 5
  for uterine atony, 898–899
prostate cancer,
  diagnosing, 850
  incidence of, 850
  treatment choices, 851
protamine,
  for cardiopulmonary bypass
    action mechanism of, 189
    complications of using too much, 189–190

dosage of, 187
    hypotension developing after administration
      of, 190
      treating and preventing, 190–192, 191, 192
  reactions in children, incidence of, 421
prothrombin time/international normalized
  ratio, 732
prothrombin time, 337, 890, 895, 898, 970
proximal aortic anastomosis, 261–262
pseudocholinesterase,
  abnormal, mivacurium used in patients with,
    1109
  levels, factors that lower, 1108
Pseudomonas, 52
pulmonary artery catheter,
  in cardiac tamponade, 325, 351
  in ischemic heart disease, 390
  in myocardial ischemia, assessing with, 289
pulmonary artery occlusion pressure, 325
  cardiopulmonary bypass and, intraoperative
    management before
    defined, 146
    increased, correcting, 161
    measurement of, 149
    monitoring of, continuous, 161
    as sensitive indicator of myocardial
      ischemia, 148–149
  congestive heart failure and, 161
  hypertrophic obstructive cardiomyopathy and,
    161
  idiopathic hypertrophic subaortic stenosis
    and, 161
  representing left ventricular end-diastolic
    volume after coronary artery bypass
    grafting, 195
pulmonary artery catheterization,
  in cardiac tamponade, 325, 344
  in cardiopulmonary bypass
    complications of, 147
      from pulmonary artery catheter, 147
      from venopuncture sites, 147
    placement of catheters in, 145, 145–146
    pressure monitoring and, 146
  in lung transplantation
    clamping, 99, 99
    hypertension, 100
    placement of catheters in, 95
    pressure monitoring and, 98, 100
  with tetralogy of Fallot (TOF/PA), 405–406, 406
    pathophysiology of, 409–410
    surgical procedures for, 414

pulmonary artery catheterization (*contd.*)
  in valvular heart disease, 221
    with pacing capabilities, 221
pulmonary blood flow distribution, during
    one-lung ventilation, 43
pulmonary capillary wedge pressure,
  in burn management, 1124, 1126, 1127–1128,
    1133
  in laparoscopic surgery, 860, 862
pulmonary compliance, defined, 59
pulmonary edema, differential diagnosis of,
    1198, 1198t
pulmonary edema, "low pressure", 830
pulmonary edema in hypoxia, differential
    diagnosis of, 1198, 1198t
pulmonary elastic recoil, 64
pulmonary hypertension, 31. see hypertension,
pulmonary hypoplasia,
  with congenital diaphragmatic hernia
    prognosis and, effect on, 118
    severity, assessment of, 119
pulmonary stenosis,
  with tetralogy of Fallot (TOF/PS), 404–405, *405*
    end-tidal carbon dioxide monitoring in, 417
    palliative surgical procedures available for,
      412
    pathophysiology of, 406–408, *408*
    pre-cardiopulmonary bypass anesthestic
      goals for, 419
    SaO_2 for an infant, 423–424
      following placement of a modified
        Blalock-Taussig shunt, 423–424
    surgical procedures for, 413–414
pulmonary vascular disease, lung
    transplantation for, 89
pulmonary vascular occlusive disease,
  transposition of the great arteries and, 436
pulmonary vascular resistance, 64
  in tetralogy of Fallot interventions to reduce,
    418, 419–420
pulse oximeter,
  defined, 1181
  function of, 1182
  for hypoxia
    defined, 1181
    function of, 1182
    two-wavelength
      accuracy of, 1183
      calibration of, 1182

for pyloric stenosis
  function of, 525
  measurement of oxygen saturation by, 525
two-wavelength
  accuracy of, 1183
  calibration of, 1182
pulsus paradoxus, 328
pyloric stenosis,
  cardiac murmurs
    cause of, 519
    evaluate, 520
    functional *vs.* organic, differentiating
      between, 520, 520t
  diagnosing, 515
  differential diagnosis of, 515
  intraoperative management
    anesthesia
      anatomic characteristics of the airway,
        newborn *vs.* adult, 522–523, 523t
      endotracheal tube size, determining,
        523–524, 523t
      induction–intubation sequence of, 522
      nonrebreathing systems, advantages and
        the disadvantages of, 524
      postanesthesia recovery period,
        complications, 525
      preparing patient for, 522
      system of, 524
      techniques or agents used for, 522
    monitoring, 524
    pulse oximeter
      function of, 525
      measurement of oxygen saturation by, 525
  metabolic alkalosis
    adverse effects of, 516
    correcting, 519
  metabolic problems, 515–516, 516t
    metabolic alkalosis
      adverse effects of, 516
      correcting, 519
  postoperative management
    postanesthesia recovery period,
      complications, 525
    postextubation "croup," 525–526
  preperative evaluation and preparation
    for emergency surgery, 521
    patient evaluation, 519–520
    ventricular septal defect
      risks of surgery and anesthesia, 521

shunt used for, 521
types of, 521
treatment for, 516
diagnostic tests, 517
electrolytes, 517, 518
fluid replacement, 517, 518, 518t, 519t
prevention aspiration, 517
supportive therapy, 517
surgery, 517
pyloromyotomy, 517
pyogenic arthritis, 656
pyridostigmine (Mestinon), for myasthenia
gravis, 1082

"Qi", 747
Q_P/Q_S calculation, 409
QS/QT (shunt equation), 12, 1261–1262
Q-wave infarction vs. non–Q-wave infarction,
perioperative reinfarction and,
386–387, 801

radial aplasia (limb defect), 107
radiation, in acute respiratory distress
syndrome, 55
Ramstedt pyloromyotomy, 517
rapid-sequence induction,
anesthetic agents used for, 1000–1001
risks of, 1000
Rastelli procedures,
described, 444
long-term outcomes after, with left ventricular
outflow tract obstruction, 449
postoperative problems following, immediate,
447
surgical options for repair, transposition of the
great arteries and, 438
rebound alkalemia, 512
recombinant factor VII, 896
recurrent pulmonary emboli, 3
recurrent respiratory papillomatosis,
cause of, 1026
presentation of, 1027
treatment options for, 1027
reduction pneumoplasty, 104
reflex sympathetic dystrophy, 671
reframing techniques, 698
regional cardiac tamponade, 327, 327–328
regional wall motion abnormalities, 147,
148–149, 150

remifentanil, for renal failure, 843–844
renal acute renal failure (acute tubular necrosis),
1133
renal blood flow, 842
renal dysfunction, in heart transplantation, 371
renal dysplasia, 107
renal failure. See kidney transplant,
renal insufficiency,
anemia in, progressive, 824
chronic, 304, 829, 983
renal oliguria, 846, 846t
renal protection, 266
reperfusion injury,
in carotid endarterectomy, 573
in lung transplantation, hemodynamic
alterations, 99–100
repetitive strain injuries, 1003
residual volume, 6, 8
respiratory alkalosis, 6
respiratory distress syndrome and,
pathophysiology of, 454
survival rates of, 454
respiratory tract infections, asthmatic attacks
and, 5, 14
retained placenta, 900
retinal detachment surgery, anesthetic
implications of, 1219
retinopathy of prematurity, 458–459
retrobulbar block, 1015
retrograde cricothyroid wire, 1071
retrolental fibroplasia, 67, 458–459
retropubic prostatectomy, 799
reversible expiratory airflow obstruction, 4
rheumatic fever, 199, 200
rheumatic heart disease, 932
right bundle branch block,
cardiac complications and, 383
with left anterior fascicular hemiblock,
diagnosing, 232
right coronary artery, 134, 135, 135
right heart failure, diagnosing and treating,
225–226
right middle lobectomy, 36
extubation and, 44
right sided arch, 107
right-to-left shunting, diagnosing in congenital
diaphragmatic hernia patients, 120
right ventricle outflow tract,
rigid ventilating bronchoscope, 35

rigid Venturi-effect bronchoscope, 35
ristocetin induced platelet agglutination, 966
"Robin Hood" syndrome, 531, 571
rocuronium,
    for asthma, 21–22
    for open-eye injury, 1019
"rule of nines," used on childern, 1117, 1117
ryanodine receptor, 1096
RYR-1 gene, 1096, 1097

saline solution, for aspiration, 54
SaO_2 for an infant, 423–424
    following placement of a modified
            Blalock-Taussig shunt, 423–424
sarcoplasmic reticulum, 1095, 1096
scalp acupuncture, 747
sciatica. See back pain, low,
scoliosis,
    blood gas abnormality seen in, most common
            arterial, 1162
    cardiovascular system affected by, 1163–1164
    defined, 1156, 1157, 1158
    intraoperative management
        anesthetic technique, optimal, 1171–1172
        deliberate hypotension, producing,
            1175–1176
        estimated blood loss and fluid requirements,
            1172, 1174
        monitoring, 1166–1167
            abnormalities during surgery, actions to
                takes, 1170
            affected by anesthetic agents, 1169
        motor evoked responses, defined and use of,
            1169
        neurologic complications
            monitoring techniques to minimize, 1167
        positioning, complications in, 1172,
            1173–1174
        somatosensory evoked potentials
            abnormalities during surgery, actions to
                takes, 1170
            defined and use of, 1167–1168, *1168*
            reliability of, for predicting spinal injury,
                1168–1169
        transfusion-related acute lung injury, 1174
        transfusion requirements, minimizing,
            1174–1175
        venous air embolism, 1170–1171
            actions to take, 1171

        diagnosing, 1170–1171
            occurance of, 1171
        "wake-up" test, 1170
    and malignant hyperthermia, relation
            between, 1164
    postoperative management
        complications, 1177
        extubation, 1176
        fluid therapy, 1177
        laboratory tests, 1176–1177
        pulmonary status optimizing, 1176
    preoperative evaluation and preparation
        history, important aspects of, 1165
        laboratory testing, 1165–1166
        neurologic assessment, importance of, 1165
        patient preparation, 1166
        physical examination, important aspects of,
            1165
        premedication, 1166
        spinal curve, anethesiologists knowledge of,
            1164–1165
    pulmonary function tests, abnormalities most
            commonly seen in, 1161–1162
    severity of, 1158–1161, 1160, 1161
    types of
        most common, 1156–1157
        other, 1158–1159
    ventilatory drive, abnormalities of, 1163
scopolamine, 1012
seizure prophylaxis, 917
Sellick's maneuver, 481
sensory evoked potential, 530, 533
septicemia, in transurethral resection of the
            prostate, 820
serotonin (5-HT), 909, 910
serum cholinesterase, 1106–1107
serum creatinine concentration, normal values
            for, 836–837
sevoflurane, cardiovascular effects of, 155
sevoflurane, for asthma, 20, 22
Sheehan's syndrome, 903
short-acting local anesthetics, 1229
shunt equation (Q_S/Q_T), 12
shunting,
    defined, 408–409
    resulting from embolization in laparoscopic
            surgery, 867
sickle cell crisis,
    defined, 984

hyperbaric oxygen therapy in treatment of, 992
pathogenesis of, 985, *985*
treatment of, 992
sickle cell disease,
  acute chest syndrome, defined, 986
  anesthesia, 986–987, 989
    comorbidities, effect on, 989–990
    general/anesthesia, 987, 989
    sickling, precautions to prevent, 990
  clinical features of, 982–984
  defined, 981
  diagnosing, 981
  postoperative management
    complications, immediate, 991
    supportive and preventative care, 991
  preoperative evaluation and preparation,
      986–987
    blood transfusion, indications for, 988
    exchange transfusion, 988
  sickle cell crisis
    defined, 984
    hyperbaric oxygen therapy in treatment of,
        992
    pathogenesis of, 985, *985*
    treatment of, 992
  sickle cell trait, defined, 982
  vaso-occlusive crisis, 984
sickle cell trait, defined, 982
sick sinus syndrome, defined, 231
simple bowel obstruction, 474
single-breath nitrogen test, 12
Singulair (montelukast), for asthma, 14
sitting position, 533
sleep apnia, electroconvulsive therapy and, 1204
sleep study or polysomnogram, 1254–1255
smoke inhalation burn, 1120
sodium ions, 810
sodium nitroprusside, nicardipine, and
      nitroglycerin intravenous infusion, for
      cardiopulmonary bypass, 171, 172t
sodium nitroprusside, for deliberate
      hypertension, 542
somatosensory evoked potentials, 264–265,
      533–537, 565
  abnormalities during surgery, actions to takes,
      1170
  defined and use of, 1167–1168, *1168*
  reliability of, for predicting spinal injury,
      1168–1169

Sonic Hedgehog, 106
Sonoclot, 338, 340
spasmodic croup, 1039
specific activity scale of cardiac function, 375
sphincter of Oddi, effect of narcotics on, 1277
spinal cord ischemia,
  in abdominal aortic aneurysm patients, *282,*
      282–283
  endovascular thoracoabdominal aortic
      aneurysm and, 265, 270
    detecting, 265
spinal cord stimulation, 713, 679–680
spinal tap, accidental, 921
spirochete infection, aortic aneurysms and,
      253–254
spirometry, 6, 7
Spitz classification, 108
spontaneous bacterial peritonitis, 489
SpO$_2$ readings, effect of dyshemoglobins
      methemoglobin and
      carboxyhemoglobin on, 1183
sputum cytology, 30
Staphylococcus, 52
statins,
  for ischemic heart disease, 381
stellate ganglion, location of, 675
stellate ganglion block,
  anatomic landmarks used, 675–676
  clinical signs of, 676
  complications of, 680
  in Horner syndrome patient, 676
  nerve fibers are interrupted in, 676
sternal splitting, procedures during, 161
steroids. See Corticosteroids,
steroid therapy, for aspirated patient, 53
Stickler's syndrome, 1052
stiff joint syndrome, 789
strangulated bowel obstruction, 474
Streptococcus pneumoniae, 51
stridor,
  anatomic location of, 1039
  definition of, 1039
stroke volume, defined, 202–203
ST-segment depression, treating, 158–159
ST-segment elevation myocardial infarction,
      400–401
subarachnoid hemorrhage,
  cardiovascular effects of, 621–622
  causes of, 619

subarachnoid hemorrhage (*contd.*)
  diagnosing, 622
  incidence of, 619
  intraoperative management
    anesthesia
      arterial line for induction, necessity of, 625
      concerns, during induction, 626–627
      hypoxemia and hypercapnia, effects on cerebral blood flow, 628, *629*
      induction and maintenance, goals of, 624
      rapid-sequence induction and intubation, 627–628
      smooth and safe induction and intubation, 627
    brain relaxations, achieving, 629–630
    cerebral protection
      intentional mild hypothermia, advantages and disadvantages of, 633
      methods of, 632
    controlled hypotension
      achieving, 631
      drawbacks of, 631
      purpose of, 631
    fluid status, assessment of, 625
    hypothermia
      deep hypothermic circulatory arrest, indications for, 633
      intentional mild, advantages and disadvantages of, for cerebral protection, 633
    monitoring, 626
    surgical exposure, facilitating, 629–630
  pathophysiology of, 620
  postoperative management (*see also* cerebral vasospasm)
    failure to return to preoperative neurologic condition, 635
    complications, other neurologic, 638
    disorientation, 635
    extubation, 634–635
    hemiplegia, 635
  preoperative evaluation and preparation
    coiling of an aneurysm, 623
      anesthesia for, 623
      emergencies occuring during, 623
    interventional neuroradiology suite, concerns in going to, 623
    premedication, 624
  prevalence of, 619
  rebleeding risks, 622
  severity of, assessing, 620–621, 621t
  symptoms and signs of, 620
  see also aneurysm clipping; intracranial aneurysm
subdural hematomas, 599
succinylcholine, 22
  for asthma, 19
  for burn patients
    adverse effects associated with, 1130–1131
    contraindicated in burned patients, 1130
  for cardiopulmonary bypass, 153
  for malignant hyperthermia syndrome
    rigidity of jaw muscles after administration of, 1101
  for open-eye injury
    contraindications for, 1016
    elevation in intraocular pressure, nondepolarizing muscle relaxants to prevent, 1016
    for intraocular pressure
      affect on, 1016–1017
      -induced elevation, nondepolarizing muscle relaxants to prevent, 1017
    intraocular pressure and, affect on, 1016–1017
    rapid-sequence induction and intubation without using, 1018–1019
  prolonged postoperative apnea
    acetylcholine and, differences in, 1107
    cardiovascular effects of, 1108
    pediatric anesthesia and, 1109
    resemblance to acetylcholine, 1107
  for rapid-sequence intubation, 1000
  renal failure patients and, 840
Sudeck's atrophy, 671
superior vena cava syndrome, signs and symptoms of, 759
super obesity, defined, 1252
superoxide dismutase, 67
supine hypotensive syndrome, 891
supine position, 534
suppurative flexor tenosynovitis, 656
supraclavicular block, 648
suprapubic prostatectomy, 799
supraventricular tachyarrhythmias, 142–143
sympathetically independent pain, 674, 676, 679
sympathetically maintained pain, 673–674, 676, 679

sympathomimetics, for asthma, 14, 19
synchronized intermittent mandatory
    ventilation, 62, 84
syndrome of inappropriate antidiuretic hormone
    secretion, 601
systemic glucocorticoids, for asthma, 14
systemic vascular resistance, 418
    in laparoscopic surgery, 862
    in preeclampsia, 911
systolic anterior motion of the mitral valve, 151

tachycardia, preventing in ischemic heart
    disease, 396
Takayasu arteritis, aortic aneurysms and,
    253–254
tangential excision split-thickness skin graft,
    1125
Target of Rapamycin inhibitors, 847
tartrazine, asthmatic attacks and, 5
temperature-uncorrected values, 445
Tensilon (edrophonium), for myasthenia gravis,
    1082
teratogenicity,
    of anesthetic agents, 952–953
    factors influencing, in mammals, 952
terbutaline, for asthma, 14
"test clamp" maneuver, 506
Tetralogy of Fallot, 107
tetralogy of Fallot,
    arterial saturation, determined in single
        ventricle physiology, 410
    definition of, 404
    hypercyanotic spells, 411–412
    intraoperative management
        anesthesia
            inducing if intravenous access cannot be
                established, 416–417
            inhalation, effect of, 418
            pre–cardiopulmonary bypass goals of,
                419
        heparin
            in children vs. adults, 420
            reversing, 420–421
        monitoring
            end-tidal carbon dioxide, 417
            near-infrared spectroscopy, 417–418
        palliative shunt, management issues during
            creation of, 418
        protamine reactions in children, incidence
            of, 421

pulmonary vascular resistance,
    interventions to reduce, 419–420
residual ventricular septal defect following
    separation from cardiopulmonary
    bypass, effect of, 422
transesophageal echocardiography, role of,
    421–422
pink Tet, defined, 410
postoperative management, 423
    junctional ectopic tachycardia, defined,
        424–425
    SaO2 for an infant, 423–424
        following placement of a modified
            Blalock-Taussig shunt, 423–424
    ventilation management following
        placement of transannular patch,
        422–423
preoperative evaluation and preparation
    abnormalities to be considered, 415–416
    history and physical exam, 415
    nothing by mouth guidelines, 416
with pulmonary artery (TOF/PA), 405–406, 406
    pathophysiology of, 409–410
    surgical procedures for, 414
with pulmonary stenosis (TOF/PS), 404–405,
    405
    end-tidal carbon dioxide monitoring in,
        417
    palliative surgical procedures available for,
        412
    pathophysiology of, 406–408, 408
    pre-cardiopulmonary bypass anesthestic
        goals for, 419
    SaO2 for an infant, 423–424
        following placement of a modified
            Blalock-Taussig shunt, 423–424
    surgical procedures for, 413–414
$Q_P : Q_S$, calculation of, 409
shunting, defined, 408–409
thalassemia, 982
theophylline, 16, 42
thermogenesis, 111
thiamylal, 18
thiobarbiturates, 18
thiopental,
    for asthma, 18, 19
    for cardiac tamponade, 350
thoracic aorta, 151
thoracic epidural analgesia, 724, 725
    alternatives to, 726, 728

thoracic epidural analgesia (*contd.*)
   choice of drugs, influencing the efficacy or
         safety of, 724, 725
   doses and concentrations of the anesthetic
         combinations, 726, 727
   efficacy or safety of, choice of drugs that, 725
   placement and removal of epidural catheter,
         731
      for low molecular weight heparin, 731–732
      for Oral anticoagulants, 732
      for orophylactic unfractionated heparin, 731
      for postoperative low molecular weight
            heparin, 732
      for therapeutic intravenous unfractionated
            heparin, 731
   punctures, 726
   side effects and complications of, 730
   tip of epidural catheter, placement of, 725
thoracoabdominal aortic aneurysm,
   classification of, 255, *256*
   history of, 255–256
   medical management of, 256
   surgical intervention, timing of, 256
thoracoabdominal aortic aneurysm repair,
   anesthesia for
         evaluation of, 258
         inducing, 262–263
   anticoagulation used for, 260–270
   aortic clamping and unclamping
         pathophysiology of, 266–267
         response to unclamping, 267
   blood bank support and, 260
   blood transfusion, minimizing
   coexisting diseases of, 259
   complications of, 267–268
   endovascular thoracoabdominal aortic
            aneurysm repair
         anesthetic considerations for, 269
         candidates for, 268
         complications of, 270
         surgical steps for, 269
   mesenteric and renal preservation, strategies
            used for, 266
   monitors used for, hemodynamic, 260
   organ systems threatened during, 263
   rupture, increased risk of, 259
   spinal cord blood supply and, 258–259
   spinal cord ischemia, detecting, 265
   spinal cord protection, strategies used for,
            263–265

surgical approach to, 257, 261–262
   surgical evaluation of, 257
thoracotomy, for lung carcinoma, 29, 30, 31, 34,
         35–36, 36, 46
3-mm ST-segment depression, treating, 394–395
thrombin receptor agonist peptide, 969
thrombin time, 337, 970
thromboangiitis obliterans (Buerger's disease),
         657
thrombocytopenia, 911–912
thromboelastograph, 338, 339, 890, 970
thromboembolic stroke, 550
thromboxane, 18
thyroid function,
   hypothalamic-pituitary axis and, role in, 755
   laboratory assessment of, 760–761, 761t
thyroid gland, enlarged,
   anatomic problems associated with, 759
thyroid hormone,
   cellular effects of, 755
   euthyroid state, medical strategies for
            achieving, 761–762
   organ effects of, 755–756
   synthesis of, 754
   systemic effects of, 756
thyroid-stimulating hormone, 755
thyroid storm,
   cause of, 758
   differential diagnosis of, 765
   occurance of, 766
   thyrotoxicosis and, distinguishing from, 757
thyroid transcription factor-1, 106
thyrotoxicosis,
   adrenergic blockade, benefits of, 762–763
   airway obstruction, possibility of, assessing,
            759–760, *760*
   anesthesia
      endotracheal intubation, necessity of, 764
      extubation, 765
      induction of, 764
      maintaining, 764
   clinical signs and symptoms of, 756–757
   differential diagnosis of, 754
   dyspnea, differential diagnosis of, 765–766
   emergent surgery, preparation for, 763
   hyperthermia, differential diagnosis of, 765
   hyperthyroid patient, elective surgery for, 763
   monitoring, 764
   premedication, 763
   signs and symptoms of, 754

stridor, differential diagnosis of, 765–766
tachycardia, differential diagnosis of, 765
thyroid storm
  cause of, 758
  differential diagnosis of, 765
  occurance of, 766
  thyrotoxicosis and, distinguishing from, 757
thyroid storm and, distinguishing from, 757
thyroxine (T$_4$), 754
ticlopidine,
  for myocardial ischemia, 381
Tidal volume, 7
tight brain, 542, 629–630
Timolol Maleate (timoptic), 1013
timoptic (Timolol Maleate), 1013
tissue hypoxia, causes of, 1127
tissue plasminogen activator, 511
tissue typing, 833–834
TNM system (tumor, node, metastases), 30
Tokyo-Yokohama asthma, 5
Toronto Lung Transplant Group, 92–93
total body oxygen consumption, aortic
    clamping/unclamping and, 266
total intravenous anesthesia, 539, 611, 740
total lung capacity, 6, 8, 11
total parenteral nutrition, 111
tourniquet use, 978
T-piece technique, 83–84
tracheal extubation, criteria for, 1196–1197
tracheobronchial displacement, 31
tracheoesophageal fistula, 105–114
  clinical features of, 106
  diagnosis of, 106
  intraoperative management, 111
    fiberoptic bronchoscopy, role of, 112–113
    of fluid and temperature, 111
    induction and intubation options, 112
    intravenous access and monitoring, appropriate, 111
    problems, discussing, 113
    surgical technique, discussing, 113
  occurance of, during development, 106
  other problems, addressing, 107
  pathophysiology of, 106
  perioperative risk, 108
  postoperative issues, 114
    complications, early and late, 114
    extubatation, when to, 114
    pain control options, 114
  preoperative evaluation and preparation, 109
    laboratory workup, 109
    Neonatal intensive care unit management, described, 110
    patients with severe lung diseases, options for, 109–110
    routine intubation, 110
  types of, Waterson's gross classification of, 107, 108
tracheomalacia, 114
tracheostomy, 1004
Traditional Chinese Medicine, 746–747
tramadol (Ultram), 690
tranexamic acid, 341
transannular patch for tetralogy of Fallot,
    ventilation management following placement of, 422–423
transcranial Doppler ultrasonographic technology, 441
transcutaneous electrical nerve stimulation, 28
transesophageal echocardiography,
  for cardiopulmonary bypass, 144, 149, 150–152
    two-dimensional, 150–152, 151, 152
  for heart transplantation, role of, 362–363
  for ischemic heart disease, 391
  for liver transplantation, 502–503
  for lung transplantation, 95, 99–100
  for valvular heart disease
    basic principles of, 208, 210, *211*
    catheterization criteria for valvular heart disease, 215–216
    images of cardiac tamponade and pump failure, differences in, 227
    intraaortic balloon pump and, 226–227
    left ventrical imaging, vantage points of, 212, *213*
    patient with AS/AI/MR, usual findings in, 222
    pressure gradients measured by, 210, 212, *214*
    severity scales of, 215–216, 215t
    and transthoracic echocardiography, differences in, 210
transfusion-related acute lung injury, 512, 973, 1174
transient ischemic attack, 549, 550, 551
  electroconvulsive therapy and, 1204

transjugular intrahepatic portosystemic shunt, 493–494

transposition of the great arteries,
  cardiac lesions are associated with, 427–428
  clinical subsets of, 432t, 433
  defined, 427–428
  differential diagnosis of, 433, *434*
  intraoperative management
    cardiopulmonary bypass in infants/children
      vs. adults, 440–442, 440t, 441t
    deep hypothermic circulatory arrest, 445
    hypothermia
      benefits to the brain during low-flow
        cardiopulmonary bypass and DHCA,
        445
      defined/classifications for, 444
    induction, 440
    low-flow cardiopulmonary bypass, 445
    modified ultrafiltration, 442–443
    monitoring, 440
    Mustard/Senning surgical procedures,
      described, 443
    Rastelli procedures, described, 444
    α-stat and pH-stat blood gas management,
      difference between 445–446
  natural history of, 428
  oxygen saturation, determining, 429–430, *430*
  pathophysiology of, 428–429
  postoperative management
    arterial switch operation
      long-term neurologic outcome after, 450
      long-term outcomes after, 448–449
      long-term surgical problems after, 448
      myocardial ischemia, addressing in
        intensive care unit, 447
    Rastelli procedure
      long-term outcomes after, with left
        ventricular outflow tract obstruction,
        449–450
      postoperative problems following,
        immediate, 446–447, 448
  preoperative evaluation and preparation
    anesthetic goals before cardiopulmonary
      bypass, 439
    glucose management plan, 439
    information, important, 438–439
  preoperative interventions that stabilize
    intact ventricular septum, 435
    pulmonary vascular occlusive disease, 436
    ventricular septal defect, 435
    ventricular septal defect and left ventricular
      outflow tract obstruction, 435–436
  preoperative issues pertaining to the coronary
    arteries in, 431, *432*
  reverse differential cyanosis and, 430–431
  surgical options for repair, 436–438, *437*
    intraatrial physiologic repairs: Mustard and
      Senning procedures, 438
    Rastelli procedure, 438
transrectal ultrasound, 850
transthoracic echocardiography,
  and transesophageal echocardiography,
    differences in, 210
transurethral resection of the prostate,
  chronic medical conditions, 799
  intraoperative management (*see also* irrigation
    solutions, in transurethral resection
    of the prostate)
    acute hyponatremia, effect on the
      cardiovascular system, 811
    anesthesia
      regional *vs.* general, perioperative
        mortality and, 802
      technique, preferred, 801–802
    bladder explosion, 819
    bladder irrigation, body temperature and,
      804, *804*
    bladder perforation, 819
    blindness caused by, 817
    central nervous system dysfunction, cause
      of, 810
    complications during, 803
    disseminated intravascular coagulopathy,
      triggers of, 818
    excessive bleeding during, causes of, 818
    fluid management, 802
    glycine, metabolic byproducts of, *814*,
      814–815
    glycine toxicity, 814
    hyperammonemia
      prevalence of, 815
      preventative treatment against, 815–816,
        816
      sypmtoms and clinical course of, 815
    hyponatremia
      rapid correction of, risks of, 813
      saline administration to correct, 813
    hypotension, causes of, 819

hysteroscopy and, 817
monitoring, 801
serum sodium level and the incidence of
    neurologic symptoms, 811
sodium ions, physiologic role of, 810
transurethral resection of the prostate
    syndrome
    definition and signs and symptoms of,
        805, *805*
    duration of surgery and the incidence of
        the, 808
    incidence of, factors that increase,
        808
    reducing incidence of, 812
    therapeutic measures, 813
laser prostatectomy and, 821
morbidity and mortality rates in, compared to
    suprapubic or retropubic
    prostatectomy, 799
myocardial infarction
    perioperative reinfarction, risk of in prior,
        800
    postponing surgery due to, 800
postoperative management
    bacteremia, 820
    hypothermia, as risk factor for myocardial
        ischemia, 821
    myocardial infarction, diagnosing, 821
    postoperative shock, bacteria-related cause
        of, 820–821
    septicemia, 820
preoperative evaluation and preparation
    antihypertensives, discontinuing, 801
    of cardiac condition, 800
    coronary angiography, 800
    laboratory tests, 800
    Q-wave infarction and risk of reinfarction,
        vs. non Q-wave infarction, 801
trauma,
    acute respiratory distress syndrome,
        1152–1153
    aortic aneurysms and, 253
    blunt abdominal trauma, most commonly
        injured organs in, 1138
    cardiac, injuries associated with, 1136
    classification of, 1135
    diagnostic peritoneal lavage, 1138–1139
    Focused Abdominal Sonography for Trauma
        examination, 1138

hemorrhage
    classifying, 1140
    initial treatment of, 1141
hemothorax
    massive, defined, 1137
    signs and symptoms of, 1137
    thoracotomy to treat, indications for, 1137
initial assessment and management, 1136
intraoperative management
    anesthesia
        induction of, 1143
        maintaing, agents for, 1144
        for one-lung ventilation was, 1143
    blood given when type and cross-match are
        not completed, 1145–1146
    blood transfusion
        artificial blood substitutes, 1152
        complications associated with, 1146–1147
        guidelines for, 1150–1151
        immune system and, effects of, 1149–1150
        Jehovah's Witness and, 1151–1152
        massive, 1147–1148
    hypothermia
        adverse effects of, 1149
        defined, 1149
        treatment of, 1149
    intraoperative awareness, decressing, 1144
    monitoring, 1143
    muscle relaxants, 1144
    oxygen-hemoglobin dissociation curve,
        quantitating shift of, 1148
    peak airway pressure, increase in,
        1144–1145
    tension pneumothorax
        diagnosising, 1145
        treatment of, 1145
oliguria, 1154
pneumothoraces, categorization of, 1137–1138
preoperative evaluation and preparation
    laboratory tests, 1142
primary survey, objective of, 1136
secondary survey, objective of, 1137
shock
    defined, 1139
    hypovolemic
        crystalloid or colloid therapy to treat,
            1141
        dextran or hetastarch (Hespan), 1141
        hypertonic saline, 1142

trauma (*contd.*)
        pathophysiology of, 1140
     signs and symptoms of, 1139
     types of, 1139
   thoracic, injuries associated with, 1135–1136
Treacher Collins syndrome, 1052
   defined, 1053
treatment dose low molecular weight heparin,
     732
Trendelenburg position, 862, 872, 879
tricyclic antidepressants,
   anesthetic implications of, 643, 643t
   suregry and, discontinuing before, 644
trihexyphenidyl (Artane), for Parkinson's
     disease, 583
triiodothyronine (T$_3$), 754
triple-vessel coronary artery disease,
   coronary arteries, branches of, 134–135, *135*
   defined, 134
tropicamide (mydriacyl), 1012
tssue perfusion distal to the aortic cross clamp,
     aortic clamping/unclamping and, 267
tube thoracostomy, 1000
tubular necrosis, 490
Turner's syndrome, aortic aneurysms and,
     253–254
22q11 deletion syndrome,
   associated cardiovascular defects in,
     1062–1063
   defined, 1062
   endocrinologic consequences of, 1063
   immunologic findings in, 1063

Ultegra (point-of-care monitor), 969
Ultram (tramadol), 690
Unified Parkinson's Disease Rating Scales, 596
United network for organ sharing, 490
upper airway obstruction, 3
upper inflexion point, 58
upper respiratory infection, postponing elective
     surgery due to, 14
uremic cardiomyopathy, 830
ureteral abnormalities, 107
U.S. Food and Drug Administration fetal risk
     categories for therapeutic agents, 953
uterine atony, 898–899
uterine inversion, 899
uterine rupture,
   diagnosing, 887
   risk factors of, 887
   treatment for, 887

VACTERL type anomalies, 106, 107
vagolytic drugs, for laparoscopic surgery, 864
Valsalva's maneuver, 1010
valvular heart disease,
   anesthetic for
     goals of, 219–220
     technique, 221–222
   cardiac tamponade and pump failure,
     distinguishing between, 227
   in cardiopulmonary bypass, 150
     special considerations particular to, 223–224
   echocardiographic and cardiac catheterization
     criteria for, 215–216
   etiologies of, 199–200
   extubation in, 227
   hemodynamic management goals for,
     219–220, 219t
     for aortic stenosis and mitral regurgitation
     combined, 220
   hypotension in, 227
   left ventrical and
     changes in loading condition resulting from,
     200–201
     imaging, transesophageal echocardiography
     vantage points of, 212, *213*
     pressure/time curves for, 206, 206, 207
   monitoring patients with aortic stenosis and
     mitral regurgitation combined, 220
   muscle relaxants used in, 222
   premedication for, 218
   pulmonary artery catheterization and, 221
     with pacing capabilities, 221
   representative pressure–volume loops for,
     202–203, 203, 204, 205
   signs and symptoms of, 216–217, 217t
valvular regurgitation, in cardiopulmonary
     bypass, 151
valvular stenosis, in cardiopulmonary bypass,
     151
Van der Woude's syndrome, 1052
vanillylmandelic acid, 774
variant angina (Prinzmetal's angina), 142
vasa previa,
   defined, 888
   diagnosing, 888
vascular endothelial growth factor, 910

vasoconstrictor thromboxane A_2, 908
vaso-occlusive crisis, 984
vecuronium,
　for asthma, 19, 21–22
　for open-eye injury, 1019
Velocardiofacial (Shprintzen's) syndrome, 1052
velopharyngeal incompetence,
　defined, 1054
　diagnosing, 1054
　tonsillectomy and adenoidectomy, relation to,
　　1054
venous air embolism, 1170–1171
　actions to take, 1171
　in craniotomy
　　monitoring options for, 544
　　preventing, 545
　diagnosing, 1170–1171
　monitoring of, 544
　nitroglycerin and, 545
　occurance of, 1171
venovenous bypass, 506–507, 507
ventilatory support,
　for lung transplantation
　　endotracheal tube used in, 96
　　postoperative, 103
　　procedures for, 96–97
　　single-lung, affect on cardiopulmonary
　　　function, 97
　therapeutic approaches for, 66–86
　　extracorporeal membrane oxygenation, 76
　　　indications/contraindications for, 76
　　　results of, 76–77
　　　uses of, 77
　　high-frequency positive pressure ventilation
　　　and, 77
　　　characteristics of, 77
　　　defined, 77
　　high-frequency ventilation and, 78
　　　classifications of, 78, 78
　　　frequencies used in, 78
　　　indications/precautions for, 79–80
　　hypoxemia, treatment for, 66–67
　　inverse-ratio ventilation, defined, 72–73
　　liquid ventilation and, 75–76
　　nitric oxide, 80
　　　defined, 80
　　　inhaled, role of in the treatment of acute
　　　　respiratory distress syndrome, 80–81
　　oxygen delivery, determining factors for, 66

oxygen toxicity, 67
　governing factors of, major, 67
　mechanism of, 67
positive end-expiratory pressure, 68
　arterial oxygenation and, improvements
　　in, 68
　best and optimal, determining, 69, 70
　cardiovascular effects of, 69–71
　criteria for starting, 68
　weaning from ventilatory support and, 82
pressure-support ventilation, 71
　advantages of, 71
　defined, 71, 72
prone-position ventilation, 73
　oxygenation and, effect on, 74
　rationale for, 73–74
weaning from, 82–86
　by continuous positive airway pressure, 83
　criteria for, 83
　PEEP levels, lowering, 82
　by pressure-support, 84–85, 85
　by synchronized intermittent mandatory
　　ventilation, 84
　by T-piece technique, 83–84
　when to, 83
ventricular assist devices,
　in heart transplantation, role of, 360–361
ventricular septal defect, 107
　left ventricular outflow tract obstruction and,
　　435–436
　in pyloric stenosis
　　risks of surgery and anesthesia, 521
　　shunt used for, 521
　　types of, 521
ventricular tachycardia, during pacemaker
　　surgery, 247
Venturi effect, defined, 1034
Venturi jet ventilation,
　complications of, 1035
　contraindications for the use of, 1035
　defined, 1034
　how anesthesia is maintained during, 1035
　manual, instituting and conducting,
　　1034–1035
verapamil, for ischemic heart disease, 142, 143t,
　　380–381
vertebral anomalies, 107
Veterans Affairs Cooperative Trial, 551
viral infection, aortic aneurysms and, 253–254

visceral aortic anastomoses, 262
Vistaril (hydroxyzine hydrochloride), for
    asthma, 16
vital capacity, 7, 8
vitreous herniation, risk factors of, 1015
volume-controlled mechanical ventilation, 72–73

"wake-up" test, 1170
warfarin, 337
Waterston classification, 107, 108
Westley Croup Score, 1040t
"Why Mothers Die" (report from Great Britain),
    897

woodworker's asthma, 5
World Health Organization stepladder approach
    to cancer pain, 686, 687

X-linked recessive disorder, 965
Xomed Laser Shield, 1033

Yellow Emperor's Classic of Internal Medicine,
    747

zafirlukast (Accolate), for asthma, 14
zones of the neck, 997